MANUAL OF CLINICAL MICROBIOLOGY

Second Edition

MANUAL OF CLINICAL MICROBIOLOGY
Second Edition

EDITED BY

EDWIN H. LENNETTE

Chief, Viral and Rickettsial Disease Laboratory, California Department of Health, Berkeley, Calif.

EARLE H. SPAULDING

Department of Microbiology and Immunology, School of Medicine, Temple University Health Science Center, Philadelphia, Pa.

JOSEPH P. TRUANT

Director of Microbiology-Immunology, Advance Medical and Research Center, Pontiac, Mich.

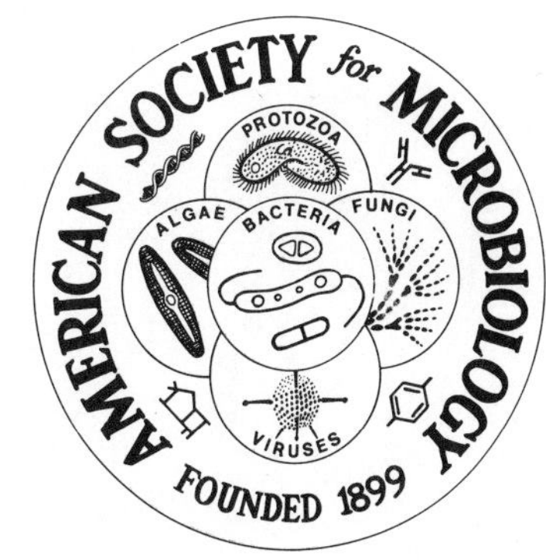

AMERICAN SOCIETY FOR MICROBIOLOGY

Washington, D.C. 1974

Second Printing, 1975

Library of Congress Catalog Card Number 74-81968

ISBN 0-914826-00-X Cloth Binding
ISBN 0-914826-01-8 Plastic Binding

Printed in the United States of America.

AMERICAN SOCIETY FOR MICROBIOLOGY
1913 I St., N.W.
Washington, D.C. 20006

EDITORIAL BOARD

CONTRIBUTORS

Stanley H. Abadie
Professor of Medical Parasitology and Microbiology, Department of Tropical Medicine and Medical Parasitology, Louisiana State University Medical Center, New Orleans, Louisiana

Libero Ajello
Chief, Mycology Division, Center for Disease Control, Atlanta, Georgia

Aaron D. Alexander
Director of Veterinary Medicine, Walter Reed Army Institute of Research, Walter Reed Army Medical Center, Washington, DC

Howard R. Attebery
Research Microbiologist, Research Service, Wadsworth Hospital Center, Veterans Administration; and Research Dentist, Department of Pediatric Dentistry, University of California School of Dentistry (Los Angeles), Los Angeles, California

Robert Austrian
John Herr Musser Professor of Research Medicine, Department of Research Medicine, University of Pennsylvania School of Medicine, Philadelphia, Pennsylvania

Peter K. C. Austwick
Nuffield Research Fellow, Nuffield Institute of Comparative Medicine, The Zoological Society of London, Regent's Park, London, England

Albert Balows
Chief, Bacteriology Division, Center for Disease Control, Atlanta, Georgia

Arthur L. Barry
Lecturer in Infectious and Immunologic Diseases, University of California School of Medicine (Davis); and Director, Microbiology Laboratories, Sacramento Medical Center, University of California (Davis), Sacramento, California

Raymond C. Bartlett
Director, Division of Microbiology, and Assistant Director, Department of Pathology, Hartford Hospital, Hartford, Connecticut

Matilda Benyesh-Melnick
Professor of Virology and Epidemiology, Department of Virology and Epidemiology, Baylor College of Medicine, Houston, Texas

Susan T. Bickham
Microbiologist, Special Bacteriology Unit, Clinical Bacteriology Section, Center for Disease Control, Atlanta, Georgia

Patricia G. Bingham
Public Health Laboratory Technologist, Viral Vaccine Investigations Section, Center for Disease Control, Atlanta, Georgia

Francis L. Black
Associate Professor, Epidemiology and Microbiology, Department of Epidemiology and Public Health, Yale University School of Medicine, New Haven, Connecticut

Philip S. Brachman
Director, Bureau of Epidemiology, Center for Disease Control, Atlanta, Georgia

Marion M. Brooke
Supervisory Microbiologist, Laboratory Training and Consultation Branch, Bureau of Laboratories, Center for Disease Control, Atlanta, Georgia

Thomas R. Cate
Department of Medicine, Duke University Medical Center, Durham, North Carolina

B. Wesley Catlin
Professor of Microbiology, Department of Microbiology, The Medical College of Wisconsin, Milwaukee, Wisconsin

Dan C. Cavanaugh
Chief, Department of Hazardous Microorganisms, Division of Communicable Diseases and Immunology, Walter Reed Army Institute of Research, Walter Reed Army Medical Center, Washington, DC

William B. Cherry
Chief, Analytical Bacteriology Branch, Center for Disease Control, Atlanta, Georgia

Marion T. Coleman
Acting Chief, Respiratory Virology Section, Center for Disease Control, Atlanta, Georgia

B. H. Cooper
Assistant Professor of Microbiology, Temple University Medical School, Philadelphia, Pennsylvania

Clyde G. Culbertson
Lilly Laboratory for Clinical Research, Marion County General Hospital, Indianapolis, Indiana

R. H. Deibel
Professor of Bacteriology, University of Wisconsin, Madison, Wisconsin

Friedrich W. Deinhardt
Professor and Chairman, Department of Microbiology, Rush-Presbyterian-St. Luke's Medical Center, Chicago, Illinois

Walter R. Dowdle
Chief, Virology Branch, Center for Disease Control, Atlanta, Georgia

V. R. Dowell, Jr.
Chief, Enterobacteriology Section, Bacteriology Division, Center for Disease Control, Atlanta, Georgia

Morris Dumoff
Microbiologist, McLaren General Hospital, St. Joseph Hospital, Flint Medical Laboratory, Flint, Michigan

Charles L. Duncan
Associate Professor, Food Research Institute and Department of Bacteriology, University of Wisconsin, Madison, Wisconsin

Henry T. Eiglesbach
US Army Research Institute for Infectious Disease, Frederick, Maryland

George H. G. Eisenberg, Jr.
Plague Section, Department of Hazardous Microorganisms, Division of Communicable Diseases and Immunology, Walter Reed Army Institute of Research, Walter Reed Army Medical Center, Washington, DC

Ana Espinel-Ingroff
Research Technologist, Division of Allergy and Infectious Diseases, Medical College of Virginia, Virginia Commonwealth University, Richmond, Virginia

William H. Ewing
Consulting and Research Microbiologist, Center for Disease Control, Atlanta, Georgia

Richard R. Facklam
Chief, Staphylococcus and Streptococcus Unit, Clinical Bacteriology Section, Bacteriology Branch, Center for Disease Control, Atlanta, Georgia

Silas G. Farmer
Associate Professor of Pathology, Medical College of Wisconsin; Clinical Professor of

Microbiology, Marquette University; and Microbiologist, The Milwaukee County Medical Complex, Milwaukee, Wisconsin

James C. Feeley
Chief, Special Pathogens Unit, Epidemiologic Services Laboratory Section, Bacterial Diseases Branch, Center for Disease Control, Atlanta, Georgia

John C. Feeley
Chief, Bacterial Immunology Section, Bacteriology Branch, Center for Disease Control, Atlanta, Georgia

Mark R. Feldman
Research Associate, Department of Tropical Medicine and Medical Parasitology, Louisiana State University Medical Center, New Orleans, Louisiana

Sydney M. Finegold
Chief, Infectious Disease Section, Wadsworth Hospital Center, Veterans Administration, Professor of Medicine, University of California School of Medicine, Los Angeles, California

Richard K. Forster
Assistant Professor, Department of Ophthalmology, Bascom Palmer Eye Institute, University of Miami School of Medicine, Miami, Florida

E. M. Foster
Professor of Bacteriology and Director, Food Research Institute, University of Wisconsin, Madison, Wisconsin

Vincent A. Fulginiti
Professor and Head, Department of Pediatrics, University of Arizona, Arizona Medical Center, Tuscon, Arizona

Paul Gerber
Chief, Viral Genetics Branch, Bureau of Biologics, Food and Drug Administration, Rockville, Maryland

Gerald L. Gilardi
Microbiologist, Microbiology Division, Department of Laboratories, Hospital for Joint Diseases and Medical Center, New York, New York

J. M. Goepfert
Associate Professor, Food Research Institute, University of Wisconsin, Madison, Wisconsin

Norman L. Goodman
Associate Professor and Director of Mycology Laboratories, Department of Community Medicine, A. B. Chandler Medical Center, University of Kentucky, Lexington, Kentucky

Morris A. Gordon
Director, Laboratories for Mycology, Division of Laboratories and Research, New York State Department of Health, Albany, New York

Donald L. Greer
Assistant Director, ICMR, Tulane University; and Associate Professor, Medical Mycology, Universidad del Valle, Cali, Colombia, South America

Dieter H. M. Gröschel
Associate Professor of Pathology and Microbiology, University of Texas System Cancer Center, M.D. Anderson Hospital and Tumor Institute; and Associate Professor of Medicine and Pathology, University of Texas Medical School, Houston, Texas

Lavelle Hanna
Specialist, Department of Microbiology, University of California, San Francisco, California

William Hausler, Jr.
State Hygienic Laboratory, University of Iowa, Iowa City, Iowa

George J. Hermann
Chief, Enteric Unit, Bacteriology Division, Center for Disease Control, Atlanta, Georgia

Ernest C. Herrmann, Jr.
Associate Professor, Peoria School of Medicine, Peoria, Illinois

F. Blaine Hollinger
Associate Professor of Virology and Epidemiology, Department of Virology and Epidemiology, Baylor College of Medicine, Houston, Texas

Robert H. Huffaker
Chief, Office of Biosafety, Center for Disease Control, Atlanta, Georgia

Rudolph Hugh
Professor of Microbiology, George Washington University School of Medicine, Washington, DC

Henry D. Isenberg
Long Island Jewish-Hillside Medical Center, New Hyde Park, New York

Daniel Ivler
Professor of Pediatrics and Microbiology, University of Southern California School of Medicine; Director, Microbiology Research, Hastings Foundation Infectious Disease Laboratory, Los Angeles County—University of Southern California Medical Center; and Associate Dean, University of Southern California, School of Medicine, Los Angeles, California

Ernest Jawetz
Professor and Chairman, Department of Microbiology, University of California, San Francisco, California

Harald Norlin Johnson
Staff Member, Viral and Rickettsial Disease Laboratory, California Department of Health; and Lecturer, School of Public Health, University of California, Berkeley, California

Wallis L. Jones
Assistant Chief, Bacterial Immunology Section, Center for Disease Control, Atlanta, Georgia

Irving G. Kagan
Chief, Parasitology Branch, Bureau of Laboratories, Center for Disease Control, Atlanta, Georgia

A. G. Karlson
The Mayo Clinic, Rochester, Minnesota

Leo Kaufman
Chief, Fungus Immunology Section, Mycology Branch, Center for Disease Control, Atlanta, Georgia

Douglas S. Kellogg
Chief, Venereal Disease Research Branch, Center for Disease Control, Atlanta, Georgia

Richard T. Kelly
Pathologist, Microbiology Section, Department of Pathology, Baptist Memorial Hospital; and Assistant Professor, Departments of Microbiology and Pathology, University of Tennessee Medical Units, Memphis, Tennessee

George E. Kenny
Department of Pathobiology, University of Washington, School of Public Health, Seattle, Washington

Arden H. Killinger
Associate Professor, Department of Pathology and Hygiene, College of Veterinary Medicine, University of Illinois at Urbana-Champaign, Urbana, Illinois

Franklin P. Koontz
State Hygienic Laboratory, University of Iowa, Iowa City, Iowa

George P. Kubica
Trudeau Institute, Inc., Immunobiological Research Laboratories, Saranac Lake, New York

Howard W. Larsh
Chairman and Research Professor of Microbiology, Associate Director of Laboratories,

University of Oklahoma, Norman, Oklahoma; and Associate Director of Laboratories, Missouri State Chest Hospital, Mount Vernon, Missouri

Edwin H. Lennette
Chief, Biomedical Laboratories, and Chief, Viral and Rickettsial Disease Laboratory, California Department of Health, Berkeley, California

Donald C. Mackel
Deputy Chief, Epidemiologic Services, Laboratory Branch, Bacterial Diseases Division, Bureau of Epidemiology, Center for Disease Control, Atlanta, Georgia

Robert L. Magoffin
Assistant Chief, Viral and Rickettsial Disease Laboratory, California Department of Health, Berkeley, California

George F. Mallison
Assistant Director, Bacterial Diseases Division, Bureau of Epidemiology, Center for Disease Control, Atlanta, Georgia

William J. Martin
Chief, Microbiology Section, Clinical Laboratories, UCLA Hospital and Clinics; and Adjunct Associate Professor of Pathology and Medical Microbiology and Immunology, UCLA School of Medicine, The Center for the Health Sciences, Los Angeles, California

John M. Matsen
Associate Professor of Laboratory Medicine and Pathology, Pediatrics, and Microbiology; and Director, Clinical Microbiology Laboratories, University of Minnesota Hospitals, Minneapolis, Minnesota

Joseph L. Melnick
Professor of Virology and Epidemiology, and Chairman of Department, Department of Virology and Epidemiology, Baylor University, College of Medicine, Houston, Texas

Joseph H. Miller
Professor of Medical Parasitology, Department of Tropical Medicine and Medical Parasitology, Louisiana State University Medical Center, New Orleans, Louisiana

James H. Nakano
Chief, Viral Vaccine Investigations Section, Virology Branch, Bureau of Laboratories, Head, WHO International Reference Center for Smallpox, Center for Disease Control, Atlanta, Georgia

Harry S. Nielsen, Jr.
Director, Allermed Laboratories, Inc., San Diego, California

Lois G. Norman
Research Microbiologist, Parasitology Branch, Center for Disease Control, Atlanta, Georgia

Richard A. Ormsbee
Rocky Mountain Laboratory, Hamilton, Montana

Arvind A. Padhye
Acting Chief, Fungus Reference Section, Center for Disease Control, Atlanta, Georgia

George Paik
Medical Microbiologist, General Hospital Microbiology Laboratory, Los Angeles County—University of Southern California Medical Center, Los Angeles, California

Barbara J. Painter
Long Island Jewish-Hillside Medical Center, New Hyde Park, New York

Donald A. Person
Assistant Professor of Virology and Epidemiology, Assistant Professor of Medicine, Baylor College of Medicine, Texas Medical Center, Houston, Texas

Charles Alan Phillips
Professor of Medicine, Department of Medicine, University of Vermont, Burlington, Vermont

Bertie Pittman
Analytical Bacteriology Branch, Center for Disease Control, Atlanta, Georgia

Bernard Portnoy
Professor, Pediatrics, Community Medicine and Public Health, University of Southern California School of Medicine; and Assistant Medical Director, Los Angeles County—USC Medical Center, Los Angeles, California

William E. Rawls
Professor of Virology and Epidemiology, Department of Virology and Epidemiology, Baylor College of Medicine, Houston, Texas

Gerbert C. Rebell
Research Associate, Department of Ophthalmology, Bascom Palmer Eye Institute, University of Miami School of Medicine, Miami, Florida

Oscar W. Richards
Pacific University, College of Optometry, Forest Grove, Oregon

Morrison Rogosa
Microbiologist, National Institute of Dental Research, Bethesda, Maryland

Leon Rosen
Head, Pacific Research Section, National Institute of Allergy and Infectious Diseases, Honolulu, Hawaii

Jon E. Rosenblatt
Assistant Chief, Infectious Disease Section, Wadsworth VA Hospital Center and Assistant Professor of Medicine, UCLA School of Medicine, Los Angeles, California

Ernest H. Runyon
VA Hospital, Salt Lake City, Utah

Ruth L. Russell
Professor, Microbiology Department, California State University, Long Beach, California; and Consultant Microbiologist, Memorial Hospital Medical Center, Long Beach, California

L. D. Sabath
Associate Professor of Medicine, Harvard Medical School; and Associate Visiting Physician, Boston City Hospital, Boston, Massachusetts

Margaret A. Salvatore
Research Associate in Pediatrics, Community Medicine and Public Health, University of Southern California School of Medicine, Chief Research Analyst, Los Angeles County—USC Medical Center, Los Angeles, California

Julius Schachter
Co-Director, WHO International Reference Centre for Trachoma and Other Chlamydial Infections, 1699-D, HSW, G. W. Hooper Foundation, University of California, San Francisco, California

Jack H. Schieble
Research Specialist, Viral and Rickettsial Disease Laboratory, California Department of Health, Berkeley, California

Nathalie J. Schmidt
Research Specialist, Viral and Rickettsial Disease Laboratory, California Department of Health, Berkeley, California

John D. Schneidau, Jr.
Professor of Medical Mycology, Department of Microbiology and Immunology; and Mycologist, Ochsner Foundation Hospital, Tulane University School of Medicine, New Orleans, Louisiana

Smith Shadomy
Associate Professor of Medicine and Microbiology, Medical College of Virginia, Virginia Commonwealth University, Richmond, Virginia

John C. Sherris
Professor and Chairman, Department of Microbiology, University of Washington, Seattle, Washington

Robert E. Shope
Director, Yale Arbovirus Research Unit, Department of Epidemiology and Public Health, Yale University School of Medicine, New Haven, Connecticut

Grace J. Shramek
Director of Microbiology, St. Francis Hospital, Evanston, Illinois

Margarita Silva-Hutner
Associate Professor and Director, Mycology Laboratory, Columbia University College of Physicians & Surgeons, and Columbia-Presbyterian Medical Center, New York, New York

Louis DS. Smith
Professor of Microbiology, Anaerobe Laboratory, Virginia Polytechnic Institute and State University, Blacksburg, Virginia

Alex C. Sonnenwirth
Director, Division of Microbiology, The Jewish Hospital of St. Louis; and Associate Professor, Departments of Microbiology and Pathology, Washington University School of Medicine, The Jewish Hospital of St. Louis, St. Louis, Missouri

Earle H. Spaulding
Professor of Microbiology and Immunology, School of Medicine, Temple University Health Sciences Center, Philadelphia, Pennsylvania

Marlene Stahl
Chief Technician, Pediatric Virus Laboratory, Department of Pediatrics, University of Arizona, Arizona Medical Center, Tucson, Arizona

Morris T. Suggs
Chief, Biological Products Division, Center for Disease Control, Atlanta, Georgia

Hiroshi Sugiyama
Professor, Food Research Institute, University of Wisconsin, Madison, Wisconsin

Vera L. Sutter
Director, Anaerobic Bacteriology Laboratory, Research Service, Wadsworth Hospital Center, Veterans Administration; and Adjunct Associate Professor, UCLA School of Medicine, Los Angeles, California

J. Clyde Swartzwelder
Professor of Medical Parasitology, and Head, Department of Tropical Medicine and Medical Parasitology, Louisiana State University Medical Center, New Orleans, Louisiana

Harvey W. Tatum
Research Microbiologist, Bacterial Reference Unit, Bacteriology Branch, Center for Disease Control, Atlanta, Georgia

Bernard V. Travis
Emeritus Professor, Department of Entomology, Cornell University, Ithaca, New York

Joseph P. Truant
Director of Microbiology-Immunology, Advance Medical and Research Center, Pontiac, Michigan; Adjunct Professor, Department of Microbiology and Public Health, Michigan State University, Lansing, Michigan; Director of Microbiology, Wayne County Respiratory Disease Control Division, Wayne County, Michigan

Jerome P. Vanderberg
Associate Professor, Department of Preventive Medicine, New York University School of Medicine, New York, New York

Harriette D. Vera
BioQuest Division, Becton, Dickinson and Co., Cockeysville, Maryland

Lionel G. Warren
Associate Professor of Medical Parasitology, Department of Tropical Medicine and Medical Parasitology, Louisiana State University Medical Center, New Orleans, Louisiana

John A. Washington II
Head, Section of Clinical Microbiology, Mayo Clinic; and Associate Professor, Departments of Microbiology and Laboratory Medicine, Mayo Medical School, Rochester, Minnesota

Lawrence G. Wayne
Tuberculosis Research Laboratory, VA Hospital, Long Beach, California

Robert E. Weaver
Chief, Special Bacteriology Unit, Clinical Bacteriology Section, Bacteriology Branch, Center for Disease Control, Atlanta, Georgia

Ronald M. Wood
Chief, Microbial Diseases Laboratory, Division of Laboratories, California Department of Health, Berkeley, California

Viola M. Young
Clinical Branch, National Cancer Institute, Baltimore, Maryland

PREFACE TO SECOND EDITION

This edition represents a continuing effort by the American Society for Microbiology to provide practicing clinical laboratory microbiologists with *a useful manual*. The authors were selected for their extensive, and sometimes unique, knowledge of and experience in their subject areas. The large majority of chapters were peer reviewed, some by coauthors of the same chapter, others by one or more authors of other chapters, and a few by special non-author reviewers.

Since the publication of the first edition in 1970, the acquisition of knowledge, as well as the development of new and improved methods in clinical microbiology, has continued at a constantly accelerating rate. A primary objective of the editors is to keep pace with this process in relevant areas, and they support the policy of the ASM Publications Board which proposes to publish new editions at frequent intervals. Nevertheless, a publication lag is inevitable and unavoidable. Consequently, we welcome the addition of *Cumitechs* as a promising effort to fill this gap.

To a very large extent this edition consists of either extensively revised chapters or entirely new material. A few chapters in the first edition were combined in this one, incorporated into other chapters, or reduced in content to make room for topics of more current importance. Greatly expanded were the following subject areas: collection and transport of specimens, the anaerobic bacteria, control of hospital infections, laboratory tests in chemotherapy, and hepatitis and EB viruses. On the other hand, the section on immunoserological tests was only modestly enlarged because the ASM plans to publish a companion *Manual of Clinical Immunology* in the near future.

We, the co-editors, thank the 125 authors for the generally high quality of their material and for acceptance of the peer review procedure. We are indebted to the other 10 members of the Editorial Board for, as Section Editors, their responsibilities required very heavy commitments of time and effort. It was they, for example, who saw that authors prepared their chapters in accordance with the primary charge ". . . . to provide a working and teaching guide that will be of practical use in the daily routine of the clinical laboratory, and also serve the needs of the student and teacher of clinical microbiology."

A special contribution to the format and content of this edition was made by an ad hoc committee chaired by John C. Sherris; its comprehensive critique of the first edition was the framework for this edition.

Finally, we express our appreciation for the courtesies, patience and cooperation that consistently characterized our treatment by Gisella Pollock, Estella Bradley, and Margaret Miller of Robert A. Day's staff in the ASM Publications Office.

Edwin H. Lennette
Earle H. Spaulding
Joseph P. Truant

3 May 1974

CONTENTS

Section I
GENERAL

Section II
AEROBIC BACTERIA

Section III
SPIROCHETES

Section IV
ANAEROBIC BACTERIA

Section V
LABORATORY TESTS IN CHEMOTHERAPY

Section VI
IMMUNOSEROLOGICAL TESTS

Section VII
FUNGI

Section VIII
PARASITES

Section IX
VIRUSES AND RICKETTSIAE

Section X
INFECTION PREVENTION—QUALITY CONTROL

Section XI
MEDIA, REAGENTS, AND STAINS

Section I

GENERAL

Chapter 1

Introduction

JOSEPH P. TRUANT

PURPOSE AND RATIONALE OF CLINICAL MICROBIOLOGY

Clinical microbiology continues to expand in importance at a very rapid rate throughout the various specialties of medicine. Therefore, the student, the teacher, and others who are interested in clinical microbiology are strongly encouraged to obtain as much academic and practical knowledge as possible in order to keep abreast of current teachings.

The goals of the second edition of the *Manual of Clinical Microbiology* (*MCM*) are that the information provided herein serves as a laboratory manual, reference source, and textbook. Major changes have been made in an attempt to update all the material so that it will conform to current teachings.

In its rapidly expanding role, microbiology has definitely become more complex, thus necessitating frequent revisions in methodologies. The clinical microbiologist not only should attend conferences on specific topics at the local, state, national, or international level in order to keep in step with procedural changes, innovative automation, more rapid techniques, etc., but also should be provided with authoritative reference text books.

This second edition has been expanded from 76 to 96 chapters to allow for more comprehensive treatment of various topics (bacteriology, mycology, parasitology, virology, susceptibility testing, and immunoserology). Considerable effort was expended in rewriting the chapters to update and revise the nomenclature of bacteria.

Additions to the text include many new methods and numerous new tables to permit more rapid evaluation of essential characteristics. The section on bacterial susceptibility testing has been significantly expanded to include more detailed considerations of the clinical relevance and limitations of these procedures.

The primary purpose of the second edition of the *MCM* is to provide information which will give direction and guidance in the isolation and identification of disease-producing organisms and wherever possible to provide data on drug susceptibility. The subsequent reports should assist the physician in making a diagnosis as well as offer guidance in the selection of a therapeutic regimen.

The more than 100 authors and editors have stressed the necessity for the clinical microbiologist and the physician to be acutely aware of the indigenous flora of humans (see chapter 5) so that they can interpret correctly the data obtained by direct smear and culture of clinical specimens. Furthermore, the reader must pay particular attention to the collection of an adequate specimen (see chapter 6) to insure that the clinician will make an adequate evaluation of the microbiological report. Essential prerequisites are to: (i) collect specimens before chemotherapy if possible; (ii) obtain material aseptically from the anatomic site where the pathogen(s) is most likely to be found; (iii) avoid contamination of specimens; (iv) take into consideration the stage of the disease process; (v) inform the laboratory of the clinical considerations to assist the microbiologist in the selection of adequate media and procedures (see chapter 6).

The reader is strongly advised to make frequent reference to section XI, chapters 95 and 96, which provide details on media, reagents, stains, and test procedures. Information on the appropriate methods for dealing with a specific organism or group of pathogens may be found in the chapter dealing with a particular isolate.

Many publications of historical and practical value have appeared relative to the classification of microorganisms. Since clinical microbiologists and physicians need to speak the same language when referring to pathogens, it is necessary to recommend a classificatory key which contains the scientific names of the commonly occurring human pathogens. The key which is referred to most commonly in this country is that which appears in chapter 2. For further details regarding taxonomic information, the reader can refer to the 8th edition of *Bergey's Manual of Determinative Bacteriology* (The Williams & Wilkins Co.).

The nomenclature and classification for the fungi, parasites, and rickettsiae and viruses appear in sections VII, VIII, and IX, respectively. The bacterial classification appears in chapter 2 of this section, but, for a very detailed explanation of bacterial nomenclature and taxonomy, it is imperative to refer to *Bergey's Manual of Determinative Bacteriology* (The Williams & Wilkins Co.).

SAFETY PRECAUTIONS

A large number of disease-producing agents are present, either in clinical specimens or in pure culture, within various areas of a clinical microbiology laboratory (see chapter 94). A summary of the laboratory-acquired infections which have been documented for the period of 1950 to 1965 was published by Pike et al. (4). These authors and others (1–6) discuss the variety of sources for laboratory infections and indicate that in a high proportion of cases the infection was transferred via the aerosol route. Therefore, it is important that microbiology laboratory directors and microbiologists pay particular attention to aseptic procedures and that a safety hood be used whenever one is working with known or suspected highly infectious material. It is not our intent to describe measures or recommend apparatus which will reduce the possibility of laboratory-acquired infections, but the reader is strongly advised to study chapters 91 and 94 and become aware of the guidelines for laboratory safety (2–6).

Since infections may result from the inadequate disposal of contaminated material, it is a good practice to discard all material in a receptacle which has a cover; autoclaving or incineration is necessary. A solution of suitable disinfectant (2–6) may be used for certain contaminated articles. The laboratory supervisor is advised to check frequently the laboratory procedures which are employed for the decontamination of apparatus, equipment, table tops, etc., to reduce the possibilities of laboratory-acquired infections.

It is further recommended that the director of the clinical microbiology laboratory have a definite procedure in effect for the immediate reporting of all laboratory accidents which may lead to the infecting of his personnel (2–6). In this way, the immediate institution of adequate prophylactic measures can be more readily undertaken. In addition, the Center for Disease Control has published two books on infectious agents and laboratory safety: *Classification of Etiologic Agents on the Basis of Hazard* and *Lab Safety at the Center for Disease Control.*

QUALITY CONTROL

The need to control the majority of microbiological tests which are performed in laboratories has been emphasized by many groups and individuals (see chapter 93) throughout the United States during the past decade. The Clinical Laboratories Improvement Act of 1967, in which the Public Health Service updated the regulations for the "licensing of laboratories," in its new section 353 regulates the "maintainence of a quality control program adequate and appropriate for accuracy of the laboratory procedures and services." In October of 1968, a notice of rule published in the Federal Register (33 F.R. 15297–15303) proposed the addition of a new part 74 to the Public Health Regulations of Title 42. Subpart C deals with Quality Control of General (74.20), Microbiology (74.21), and Serology (74.22). Within these three sections, the microbiologist will find that the quality controls must provide for and assure adequate facilities, preventative maintenance of equipment and instruments, labeling of reagents and solutions, availability at all times in the immediate bench area of written procedural descriptions, etc., as well as the availability to all concerned of laboratory records. Recommendations are given for chemical and serological solutions, reagents, media, calibration of the ocular micrometer for size of ova and parasites, and use of positive and negative control antisera, as well as a reference to the new "Manual of Tests for Syphilis 1969" (U.S. Public Health Service Publication No. 411, January 1969).

In addition to the federal regulations briefly discussed above, it should be noted that a large number of cities, states, and countries have proposed their own minimal rules for the performance of microbiological tests. Furthermore, these groups have their own "on the spot" inspections, performance evaluation, and quality control programs. These undertakings have served to improve the quality of microbiological analyses and, as a result, have improved the level of patient care.

Improvement in laboratory testing can come only as a result of desirable changes in test procedures for clinical specimens. The methods described within this manual should serve as a guideline for the individuals who are most concerned with microbiological methods. For example, the reader should pay particular attention to the recommendations discussed in chapters 4–6 and 93–96 of this *Manual*, dealing with quality control recommendations for fluorescent-antibody techniques, processing of specimens, media, reagents, stains, etc. Most laboratories which have quality control programs in use demonstrate considerable improvement in performance as determined by nationwide proficiency surveys.

STERILITY CONTROL

In the preparation of media, reagents, solutions, and stains, it is imperative that "bacteriologically and chemically" clean equipment, glassware, etc. be used because negligence in this regard may result in inhibitory substances being incorporated, especially within media (see chapters 95 and 96). Having assured oneself that traces of detergent, inhibitory metals, etc. are absent, the laboratory worker should concentrate on adequate preparation of the material (i.e., accuracy in weighing, volume of diluent, use of a water or steam bath rather than on a direct flame, etc.) to insure homogeneity of the ingredients. Sterilization may be accomplished by one of the following methods according to the recommendations made in this *Manual* (chapters 93–96) or other references: (i) dry or moist heat, (ii) filtration, (iii) chemical, (iv) radiation, etc. Routine checks on the efficiency of the autoclave by use of filter-paper strips impregnated with spores of vegetative organisms or by other acceptable sterility tests are strongly recommended. Failure to achieve sterilization is demonstrated by the growth of the positive strip which was aseptically transferred to sterile broth and incubated for a 1- to 7-day period. The use of adhesive tape which shows a change in color on autoclaving and the use of dyes in ampoules, etc., are other sterility check procedures which are available for autoclaves.

An uninoculated control (sterility control) which is incubated serves to tell the microbiologist whether or not a particular batch of medium is contaminated. It also gives one a base of reference to read a reaction in the inoculated tube or plate of prepared medium. This inoculum control medium also shows the operator whether the material has undergone any changes (i.e., pH changes, decomposition, etc.) during the incubation period. Thus, the so-called sterility control medium also serves a second important purpose, namely, to show that the observed effect on the test culture represents the action of the organism(s) on the substrate(s).

Any microbiological laboratory that flatly refuses to accept sterility testing of their products, whether they be antisera, media, sterile water or saline used as diluents, supplements, etc., may well encounter false-positive results and contribute to misdiagnosis of disease. The use of known cultures with typical biochemical reactions to evaluate and test the performance not only of the products but also of the technical personnel in the handling of clinical specimens also serves as an additional safeguard.

LITERATURE CITED

1. Benarde, M. (ed.). 1970. Disinfection. Marcel Dekker, Inc., New York.
2. Darlow, H. M. 1969. Safety in the microbiological laboratory, p. 169–204. *In* J. R. Norris and D. W. Ribbons (ed.), Methods in microbiology. Academic Press Inc., New York.
3. Lawrence, C. A., and S. S. Block (ed.). 1971. Disinfection, sterilization and preservation. Lea and Febiger, Philadelphia.
4. Pike, R. M., S. E. Sulkin, and M. L. Schulze. 1965. Continuing importance of laboratory-acquired infections. Amer. J. Pub. Health **55**:190–199.
5. Steere, N. V. (ed.). 1971. Handbook of laboratory safety, 2nd ed. The Chemical Rubber Co., Cleveland.
6. Sulkin, S. E., and R. M. Pike. 1969. Prevention of laboratory infections, p. 66–78. *In* E. H. Lennette and N. J. Schmidt (ed.), Diagnostic procedures for viral and rickettsial infections, 4th ed. American Public Health Association, Inc., New York.

Chapter 2
Classification and Nomenclature of Bacteria

JOSEPH P. TRUANT

Biologists have long been accumstomed to assigning every form of life to one of two kingdoms: (i) the animal kingdom, containing the motile, nonphotosynthetic forms, and (ii) the plant kingdom, consisting of the nonmotile, photosynthetic members. The macroscopic forms of life make the above division rather simple. However, the taxonomic position of microorganisms is not nearly so clear-cut. Some microorganisms possess certain characteristics commonly associated with animals, such as the ability to move or be motile; other microorganisms have chlorophyll and obtain their energy from photosynthesis, as do the green plants; and still others possess characteristics of both animals and plants. Therefore, it has been necessary to make some arbitrary decisions, and the microorganisms have been classified (except the so-called complex microbes known as *Protozoa*) in the plant kingdom. For these and other reasons, the taxonomic position of microorganisms has been the subject of considerable debate and disagreement.

The publication in 1859 of Darwin's *Origin of Species* showed that living organisms did not have to belong to one or the other sharply separated group. The establishment of a third kingdom call *Protista* by Haeckel in 1866 seemed logical. The *Protista*, which are distinguished from animals and plants by their relatively simple organization, became recognized as the third biological kingdom.

A further division of the *Protista* occurred based on the complexity of cellular structure: (i) the higher protists, which include protozoa, fungi, and most algae, have large eucaryotic cells (Gr., "true nucleus") resembling those of plants and animals; (ii) the lower protists, which include all bacteria and the small group of blue-green algae (*Cyanophyceae*), are characterized by smaller, procaryotic cells wherein the nucleus is not organized into individual chromosomes.

The viruses, another group of infectious agents, are not comparable to other microorganisms in cell structure and their mode of replication is fundamentally different. Thus, they cannot fit into the classification discussed above. The classification of the viruses is given in chapter 90A.

It is beyond the scope of this chapter to discuss the arguments and difficulties inherent in attempting to create a universally acceptable and useful system for the classification of bacteria. The most widely used system of classification and nomenclature in the United States is *Bergey's Manual of Determinative Bacteriology*, the first edition of which appeared in 1923 and the seventh edition in 1957. Preparation of the eighth edition has taken much longer than anticipated—namely, 17 years. The bacteria have been placed in 19 parts bearing vernacular and descriptive names as indicated in the classification shown below. For further details, the reader is advised to refer to the eighth edition of *Bergey's Manual of Determinative Bacteriology*, 1974, published by The Williams & Wilkins Co.

Kingdom Procaryotae

Division I. The Cyanobacteria
Division II. The Bacteria

Part 1. Phototrophic Bacteria

Order I. *Rhodospirillales*
- Family I. *Rhodospirillaceae*
  - Genus I. *Rhodospirillum*
  - Genus II. *Rhodopseudomonas*
  - Genus III. *Rhodomicrobium*
- Family II. *Chromatiaceae*
  - Genus I. *Chromatium*
  - Genus II. *Thiocystis*
  - Genus III. *Thiosarcina*
  - Genus IV. *Thiospirillum*
  - Genus V. *Thiocapsa*
  - Genus VI. *Lamprocystis*
  - Genus VII. *Thiodictyon*
  - Genus VIII. *Thiopedia*
  - Genus IX. *Amoebobacter*
  - Genus X. *Ectothiorhodospira*
- Family III. *Chlorobiaceae*
  - Genus I. *Chlorobium*
  - Genus II. *Prosthecochloris*
  - Genus III. *Chloropseudomonas*
  - Genus IV. *Pelodictyon*
  - Genus V. *Clathrochloris*

Part 2. Gliding Bacteria

Order I. *Myxobacterales*
Family I. *Myxococcaceae*
Genus I. *Myxococcus*
Family II. *Archangiaceae*
Genus I. *Archangium*
Family III. *Cystobacteraceae*
Genus I. *Cystobacter*
Genus II. *Melittangium*
Genus III. *Stigmatella*
Family IV. *Polyangiaceae*
Genus I. *Polyangium*
Genus II. *Nannocystis*
Genus III. *Chondromyces*
Order II. *Cytophagales*
Family I. *Cytophagaceae*
Genus I. *Cytophaga*
Genus II. *Flexibacter*
Genus III. *Herpetosiphon*
Genus IV. *Flexithrix*
Genus V. *Saprospira*
Genus VI. *Sporocytophaga*
Family II. *Beggiatoaceae*
Genus I. *Beggiatoa*
Genus II. *Vitreoscilla*
Genus III. *Thioploca*
Family III. *Simonsiellaceae*
Genus I. *Simonsiella*
Genus II. *Alysiella*
Family IV. *Leucotrichaceae*
Genus I. *Leucothrix*
Genus II. *Thiothrix*
Families & Genera of Uncertain Affiliation
Genus *Toxothrix*
Family *Achromatiaceae*
Genus *Achromatium*
Family *Pelonemataceae*
Genus *Pelonema*
Genus *Achroonema*
Genus *Peloploca*
Genus *Desmanthos*

Part 3. Sheathed Bacteria

Genus *Sphaerotilus*
Genus *Leptothrix*
Genus *Streptothrix*
Genus *Lieskeella*
Genus *Phragmidiothrix*
Genus *Crenothrix*
Genus *Clonothrix*

Part 4. Budding and Appendaged Bacteria

Genus *Hyphomicrobium*
Genus *Hyphomonas*
Genus *Pedomicrobium*
Genus *Caulobacter*
Genus *Astilccacaulis*
Genus *Ancalomicrobium*
Genus *Prosthecomicrobium*
Genus *Thiodendron*
Genus *Pasteuria*
Genus *Blastobacter*
Genus *Seliberia*
Genus *Gallionella*
Genus *Nevskia*
Genus *Planctomyces*
Genus *Metallogenium*
Genus *Caulococcus*
Genus *Kusnezovia*

Part 5. Spirochetes

Order I. *Spriochaetales*
Family I. *Spirochaetaceae*
Genus I. *Spirochaeta*
Genus II. *Cristispira*
Genus III. *Treponema*
Genus IV. *Borrelia*
Genus V. *Leptospira*

Part 6. Spiral & Curved Bacteria

Family I. *Spirillaceae*
Genus I. *Spirillum*
Genus II. *Campylobacter*
Genera of Uncertain Affiliation
Genus *Bdellovibrio*
Genus *Microcyclus*
Genus *Pelosigma*
Genus *Brachyarcus*

Part 7. Gram Negative, Aerobic Rods and Cocci

Family I. *Pseudomonadaceae*
Genus I. *Pseudomonas*
Genus II. *Xanthomonas*
Genus III. *Zoogloea*
Genus IV. *Gluconobacter*
Family II. *Azotobacteraceae*
Genus I. *Azotobacter*
Genus II. *Azomonas*
Genus III. *Beijerinckia*
Genus IV. *Derxia*
Family III. *Rhizobiaceae*
Genus I. *Rhizobium*
Genus II. *Agrobacterium*
Family IV. *Methylomonadaceae*
Genus I. *Methylomonas*
Genus II. *Methylococcus*
Family V. *Halobacteriaceae*
Genus I. *Halobacterium*
Genus II. *Halococcus*
Genera of Uncertain Affiliation
Genus *Alcaligenes*
Genus *Acetobacter*
Genus *Brucella*
Genus *Bordetella*
Genus *Francisella*
Genus *Thermus*

Part 8. Gram Negative, Facultatively Anaerobic Rods

Family I. *Enterobacteriaceae*
Genus I. *Escherichia*
Genus II. *Edwardsiella*
Genus III. *Citrobacter*
Genus IV. *Salmonella*

Genus V. *Shigella*
Genus VI. *Klebsiella*
Genus VII. *Enterobacter*
Genus VIII. *Hafnia*
Genus IX. *Serratia*
Genus X. *Proteus*
Genus XI. *Yersinia*
Genus XII. *Erwinia*
Family II. *Vibrionaceae*
Genus I. *Vibrio*
Genus II. *Aeromonas*
Genus III. *Pleisomonas*
Genus IV. *Photobacterium*
Genus V. *Lucibacterium*
Genera of Uncertain Affiliation
Genus *Zymomonas*
Genus *Chromobacterium*
Genus *Flavobacterium*
Genus *Haemophilus* (*H. vaginalis*)
Genus *Pasteurella*
Genus *Actinobacillus*
Genus *Cardiobacterium*
Genus *Streptobacillus*
Genus *Calymmatobacterium*
Parasites of *Paramecium*

Part 9. Gram Negative, Anaerobic Bacteria

Family I. *Bacteroidaceae*
Genus I. *Bacteroides*
Genus II. *Fusobacterium*
Genus III. *Leptotrichia*
Genera of Uncertain Affiliation
Genus *Desulfovibrio*
Genus *Butyrivibrio*
Genus *Succinovibrio*
Genus *Succinomonas*
Genus *Lachnospira*
Genus *Selenomonas*

Part 10. Gram Negative Cocci and Coccobacilli (Aerobes)

Family I. *Neisseriaceae*
Genus I. *Neisseria*
Genus II. *Branhamella*
Genus III. *Moraxella*
Genus IV. *Acinetobacter*
Genera of Uncertain Affiliation
Genus *Paracoccus*
Genus *Lampropedia*

Part 11. Gram Negative Cocci (Anaerobes)

Family I. *Veillonellaceae*
Genus I. *Veillonella*
Genus II. *Acidaminococcus*
Genus III. *Megasphaera*

Part 12. Gram Negative, Chemolithotrophic Bacteria

a. Organisms oxidizing ammonia or nitrate
Family I. *Nitrobacteraceae*
Genus I. *Nitrobacter*
Genus II. *Nitrospina*
Genus III. *Nitrococcus*
Genus IV. *Nitrosomonas*
Genus V. *Nitrosospira*
Genus VI. *Nitrosococcus*
Genus VII. *Nitrosolobus*
b. Organisms metabolizing sulfur
Genus *Thiobacillus*
Genus *Sulfolobus*
Genus *Thiobacterium*
Genus *Macromonas*
Genus *Thiovulum*
Genus *Thiospira*
c. Organisms depositing iron or manganese oxides
Family I. *Siderocapsaceae*
Genus I. *Siderocapsa*
Genus II. *Naumaniella*
Genus III. *Ochrobium*
Genus IV. *Siderococcus*

Part 13. Methane-Producing Bacteria

Family I. *Methanobacteriaceae*
Genus I. *Methanobacterium*
Genus II. *Methanosarcina*
Genus III. *Methanococcus*

Part 14. Gram-Positive Cocci

a. Aerobic and/or facultatively anaerobic
Family I. *Micrococcaceae*
Genus I. *Micrococcus*
Genus II. *Staphylococcus*
Genus III. *Planococcus*
Family II. *Streptococcaceae*
Genus I. *Streptococcus*
Genus II. *Leuconostoc*
Genus III. *Pediococcus*
Genus IV. *Aerococcus*
Genus V. *Gemella*
b. Anaerobic
Family III. *Peptococcaceae*
Genus I. *Peptococcus*
Genus II. *Peptostreptococcus*
Genus III. *Ruminococcus*
Genus IV. *Sarcina*

Part 15. Endospore-Forming Rods and Cocci

Family I. *Bacillaceae*
Genus I. *Bacillus*
Genus II. *Sporolactobacillus*
Genus III. *Clostridium*
Genus IV. *Desulfotomaculum*
Genus V. *Sporosarcina*
Genus of Uncertain Affiliation
Genus *Oscillospira*

Part 16. Gram Positive, Asporogenous Rod-Shaped Bacteria

Family I. *Lactobacillaceae*
Genus I. *Lactobacillus*
Genera of Uncertain Affiliation
Genus *Listeria*
Genus *Erysipelothrix*
Genus *Caryophanon*

Part 17. Actinomycetes and Related Organisms

Coryneform Group of Bacteria
Genus I. *Corynebacterium*
a. Human & Animal Pathogens
b. Plant Pathogenic Corynebacteria
c. Non-pathogenic Corynebacteria
Genus II. *Arthrobacter*
Genera incertae sedis
(*Brevibacterium*)
(*Microbacterium*)
Genus III. *Cellulomonas*
Genus IV. *Kurthia*
Family I. *Propionibacteriaceae*
Genus I. *Proprionibacterium*
Genus II. *Eubacterium*
Order I. *Actinomycetales*
Family I. *Actinomycetaceae*
Genus I. *Actinomyces*
Genus II. *Arachnia*
Genus III. *Bifidobacterium*
Genus IV. *Bacterionema*
Genus V. *Rothia*
Family II. *Mycobacteriaceae*
Genus I. *Mycobacterium*
Family III. *Frankiaceae*
Genus I. *Frankia*
Family IV. *Actinoplanaceae*
Genus I. *Actinoplanes*
Genus II. *Spirillospora*
Genus III. *Streptosporangium*
Genus IV. *Amphosporangium*
Genus V. *Ampullariella*
Genus VI. *Pilimelia*
Genus VII. *Planomonospora*
Genus VIII. *Planobispora*
Genus IX. *Dactylosporangium*
Genus X. *Kitasatoa*
Family V. *Dermatophilaceae*
Genus I. *Dermatophilus*
Genus II. *Geodermatophilus*
Family VI. *Nocardiaceae*
Genus I. *Nocardia*
Genus II. *Pseudonocardia*
Family VII. *Streptomycetaceae*
Genus I. *Streptomyces*
Genus II. *Streptoverticillium*
Genus III. *Sporichthya*
Genus IV. *Microellobosporia*
Family VIII. *Micromonosporaceae*
Genus I. *Micromonospora*
Genus II. *Thermoactinomyces*
Genus III. *Actinobifida*
Genus IV. *Thermomonospora*
Genus V. *Microbispora*
Genus VI. *Micropolyspora*
Addendum to Family

Part 18. The Rickettsias

Order I. *Rickettsiales*
Family I. *Rickettsiaceae*
Tribe I. *Rickettsieae*
Genus I. *Rickettsia*
Genus II. *Rochalimaea*
Genus III. *Coxiella*
Tribe II. *Ehrlichieae*
Genus IV. *Ehrlichia*
Genus V. *Cowdria*
Genus VI. *Neorickettsia*
Tribe III. *Wolbachieae*
Genus VII. *Wolbachia*
Genus VIII. *Symbiotes*
Genus IX. *Blattabacterium*
Genus X. *Rickettsiella*
Family II. *Bartonellaceae*
Genus I. *Bartonella*
Genus II. *Grahamella*
Family III. *Anaplasmataceae*
Genus I. *Anaplasma*
Genus II. *Paranaplasma*
Genus III. *Aegyptionella*
Genus IV. *Haemobartonella*
Genus V. *Eperythrozoon*
Order II. *Chlamydiales*
Family I. *Chalmydiaceae*
Genus I. *Chlamydia*

Part 19. The Mycoplasmas

Class I. *Mollicutes*
Order I. *Mycoplasmatales*
Family I. *Mycoplasmataceae*
Genus I. *Mycoplasma*
Family II. *Acholeplasmataceae*
Genus I. *Acholeplasma*
Genus of Uncertain Affiliation
Genus *Thermoplasma*
Mycoplasma-like Bodies in Plants

In addition, *Bergey's Manual* contains the following:

1. Comprehensive key to the genera.
2. Consolidated list of references.
3. Glossary of terms.
4. Index of scientific names of bacteria.
5. List of culture collections.

Chapter 3
Microscopy

OSCAR W. RICHARDS

KINDS OF MICROSCOPES

Simple microscope

A simple microscope (an ordinary magnifying glass) is a lens thicker at the center than at the edge. Magnifications of 5 to 10× are useful for examining colonies of microorganisms. The greater the magnifying power of a lens, the smaller the field of view is and the closer the lens must be held to the specimen. Lower powers of 2 to 5× magnification are useful for counting and examining bacterial colonies by use of a colony counter (Fig. 1).

The magnification of a simple lens is approximately 10 inches, or 254 mm, divided by the focal length in the same units. The focal length is the distance from the center of the lens to a piece of white paper, when the lens is held at the proper distance to project on the paper an image of a window or light 10 ft (305 cm) or more away. For example, 4 divided into 10 inches equals 2.5× or 254 mm/100 mm equals 2.5×. Distortion and color fringes are seen at the edges of the specimen with a single magnifying glass. Corrected lens systems reduce the aberrations, but the increased cost may be prohibitive for lenses larger than 2.5 cm or so in diameter.

The simple microscope is easy to use. The lens is held close to the eye, and the specimen is brought toward the lens until it is seen clearly in sharp focus. With opaque specimens, some manipulation is necessary to get enough light onto the surface of the specimen for adequate viewing. Lenses with a magnifying power of over 15× are difficult to use for this reason, and when greater magnification is necessary the compound microscope is preferred. Mounting the lens on a stand with an adjustment for focusing is helpful for prolonged dissection or study.

It should be noted that during the 17th century, Leeuwenhoek discovered a number of microorganisms by using simple microscopes with single lenses magnifying 275× or more (8, 46).

Compound, monobjective microscope

Near the beginning of the 17th century, some clever observer discovered that he could use a second magnifying glass to enlarge further the image from the first magnifying glass and invented the compound microscope. Some books attribute this discovery to the Janssens, but examination of the birth records makes this claim very doubtful (43). Continuing this process by using a second microscope, and so on, is not practicable because of loss of light from many lenses and the changes in the sharpness of the image due to the aberrations of the lenses and the nature of light.

Over the centuries, the shape and size of the currently used microscope has changed, although the basic features were available in primitive form during the 17th century. The style of microscope that is popular at the present time is the flattened bar type. (Figure 2 shows the parts of a typical bright-field microscope.) A binocular is better than a monocular instrument because it is more restful to use both eyes. Trinocular models have a third tube for a second observer, a camera, or a projection screen. Illuminating systems are often built into the base of the microscope.

The lens system nearest the specimen, called the objective, magnifies the specimen a definite amount. The second lens system, the eyepiece, further magnifies the image formed by the objective, so that the image seen by the eye has a total magnification equal to the product of the magnifications of the two systems. The individual or initial magnification of the objectives and eyepieces is engraved on each such part. Some microscopes have a third lens system of small magnifying power between the objective and ocular.

The image formed by a compound microscope is inverted; the object is seen upside down and reversed so that the right side is at the left. Movement of a specimen is reversed also, but one soon learns which way to move the specimen slide.

The basic elements of the stand are the stage, the body with nosepiece, prisms to incline the light when a vertical tube is not used, coarse and fine focusing movements, mirror, substage adjustable support for the condenser and auxiliary equipment, objectives and eyepieces.

Present day designs are characterized by interchangeability of parts (within a series of one manufacturer) so that square or round stages, monocular, binocular, or trinocular bodies (vertical or inclined), and accessories may be purchased and used on the same stand. With some makes, the interchanges are readily made; for others, skilled or factory personnel may be needed. A mechanical stage is desirable and essential for counting. When it is necessary to return to a particular part of a slide, a graduated mechanical stage is useful (Fig. 2).

The proposal of the Royal Microscopical Society (40) was one of the first internationally accepted standards and established the diameter of eyepieces and the screw thread for objectives. The size recommended for substage equipment has not been followed. Although it is possible mechanically to interchange oculars and objectives, one should *not* do so because the design of a given manufacturer usually gives best results only when the proper eyepiece of the same make is used with the given objective. Infinity-corrected optics cannot be interchanged with those designed for use with a fixed tube length.

Binocular, biobjective compound microscope

A three-dimensional view of a specimen requires the use of two eyes, seeing the specimen from two slightly different viewpoints (36). The small disparities between the two images are interpreted by the brain as depth or thickness of the specimen. Two separate microscopes, one for each eye, mounted on a common stand make stereoscopy possible in microscopy (Fig. 3). Chérubin de Orleans had one in the latter part of the 17th century. Greenough in 1892 proposed combining a pair of microscopes with lenses to turn the image right side up, and in 1895 Zeiss marketed his design, using prisms rather than lenses to erect the images. Thus, similar biobjective microscopes are commonly called Greenough microscopes. A recent construction uses a common single large objective lens and two separate telescopes, one for each eye (Fig. 4). Changes in magnification utilize different power telescope objectives or field objectives.

Mechanical problems created by placing the objectives close together limit numerical aper-

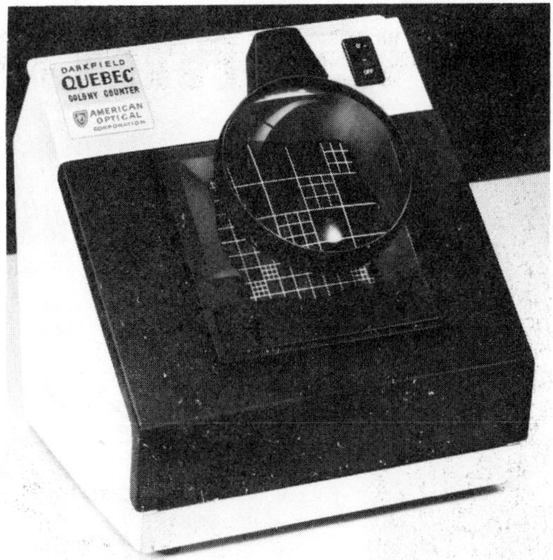

FIG. 1. *Simple microscope, or magnifier, on a colony counter.*

tures to about 0.15, thus limiting the biobjective-type instrument to a useful magnification of about 100 (see below, section on Interpretation of what is seen). When the convergences of the oculars and objectives are similar, the depth and shape of the specimen appear normal. Changing these angles can increase or decrease the apparent depth, and some Greenough microscopes are made to enhance the depth appearance as an aid to dissection under the microscope (36).

Bacteriologists use the binocular, biobjective microscope (stereomicroscope, or Greenough microscope) for counting microcolonies, isolating from a single colony (i.e., L-forms, mycoplasmas, etc.), and dissecting infected material from a specimen when more magnification is needed than is given by a hand lens. The image is right side up, so motions are seen normally. The microscopes can be obtained to fit on the long arm of a stand for examining large areas, with or without an opaque or transparent stage, with a mirror for reflecting light from an external source, or with illumination built in.

The microscope is focused by a rack and pinion motion. The two eyepieces are separated so that each eye looks through the center of the ocular. The main difficulty in using this kind of microscope comes from the fact that each eye is seeing the object from a different direction, making it difficult, or impossible, to light the specimens with a single lamp or one mirror so that it appears equally lighted to each eye. Good lighting uses two separate lamps or a

THE MICROSCOPE

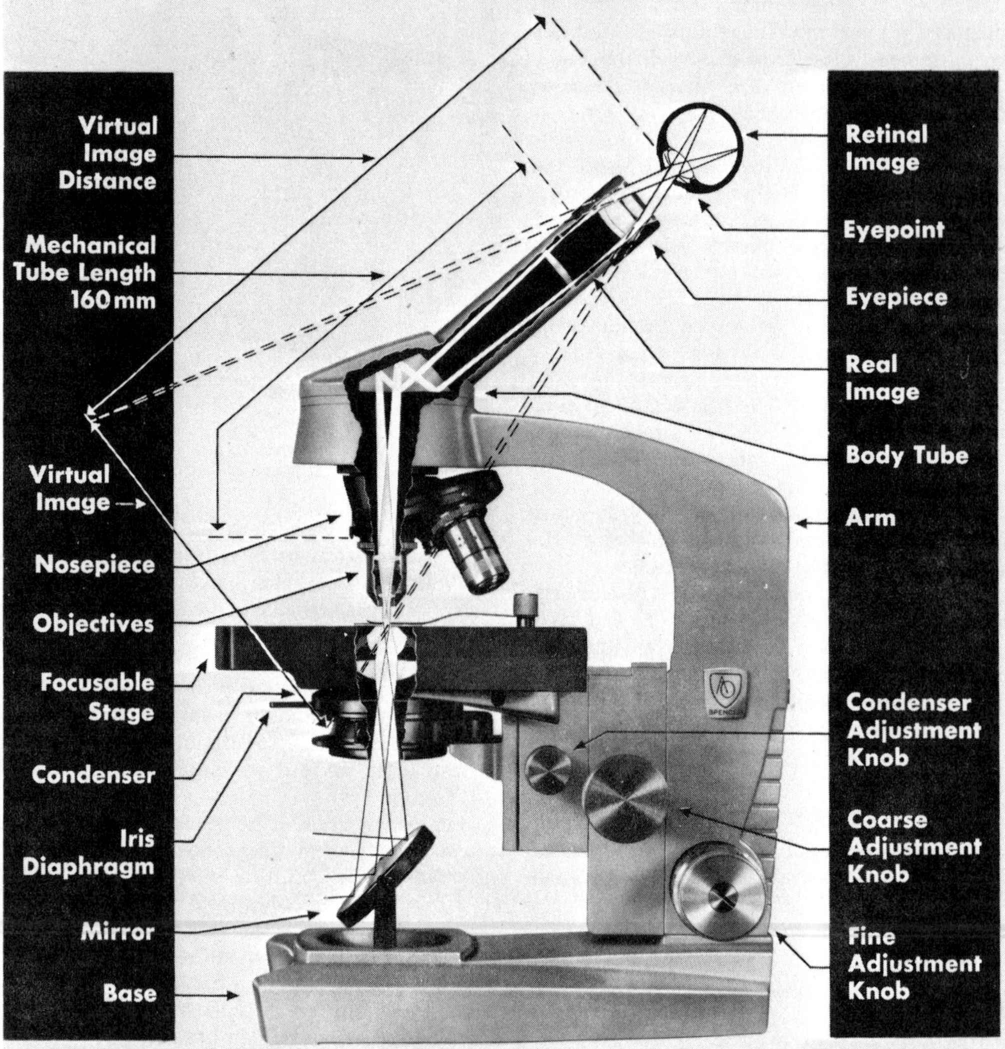

Virtual Image Distance

Mechanical Tube Length 160 mm

Virtual Image

Nosepiece

Objectives

Focusable Stage

Condenser

Iris Diaphragm

Mirror

Base

Retinal Image

Eyepoint

Eyepiece

Real Image

Body Tube

Arm

Condenser Adjustment Knob

Coarse Adjustment Knob

Fine Adjustment Knob

Optical and Mechanical Features of the Microscope.

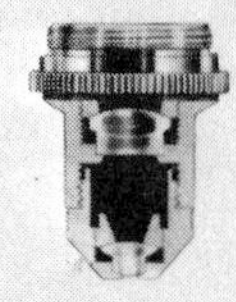

Cross section of low power objective, 10X.

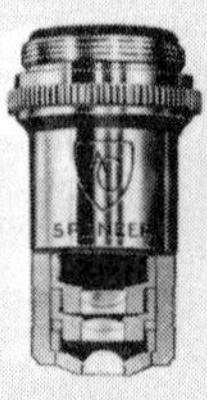

Cross section of "high dry" objective, 43X.

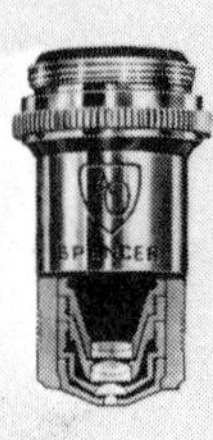

Cross section of oil immersion objective, 97X.

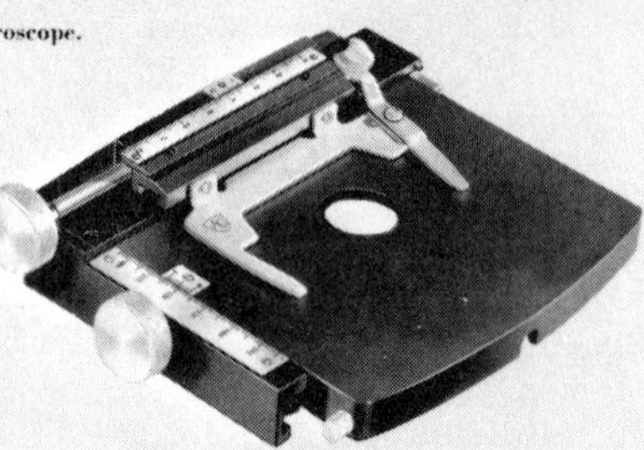

Attachable mechanical stage. Useful for moving slide when complete specimen is to be explored.

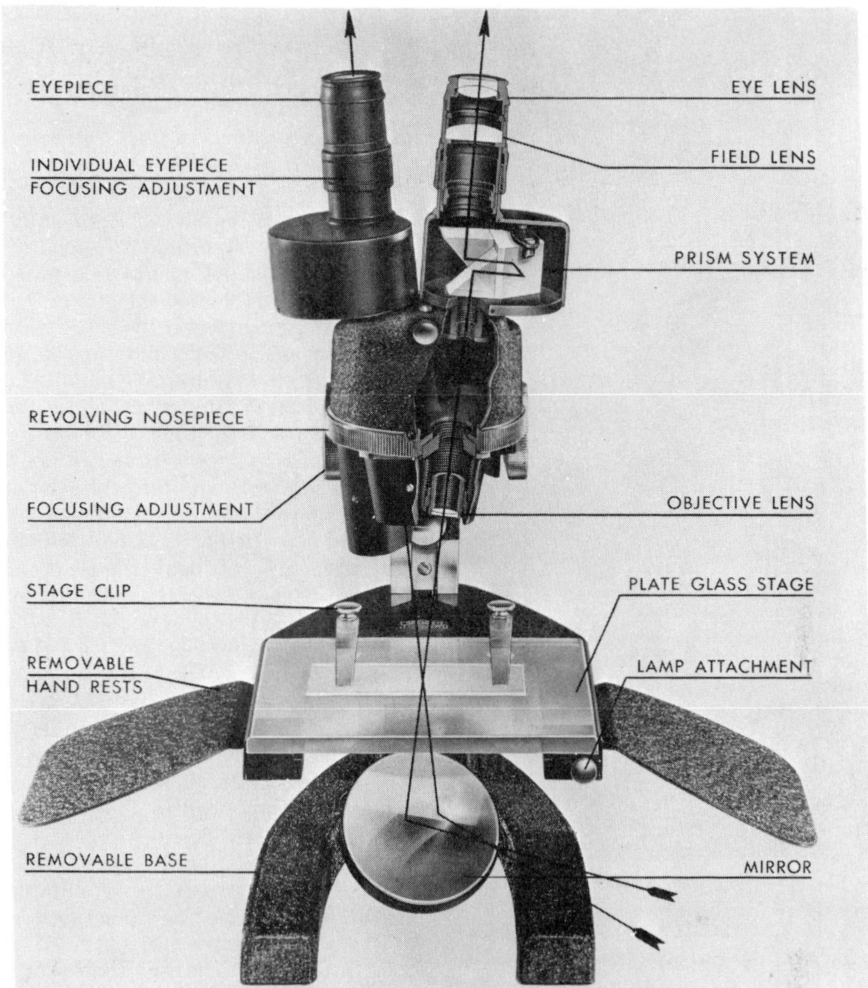

FIG. 3. *Diagram of a binocular, biobjective microscope.*

circular source surrounding the objective. When the light is intense, a piece of white paper placed over the mirror may diffuse the light enough for both eyes. Diffusing the light with a ground glass may also help to equalize the lighting from a single lamp, or a small fluorescent tube may have enough area to light the two views of the specimen.

Most persons see a three-dimensional object very shortly after looking into the stereoscopic microscope, although it does take slightly longer than seeing a single image with one eye. About 5% of people lack stereoscopic vision, and in another 10% it may be weaker than for normal persons. Stereoscopic vision is impossible for those with only one normally functioning eye, although they recognize depth and distance from monocular clues for depth.

Specialized microscopes

The choice of the kind of microscope to use depends on the nature of the specimen and the information required. Often several types of microscopy are needed. Objects which absorb light, or can be made to do so by staining, are readily seen with a bright-field microscope. Very small particles can sometimes be seen better with dark-field. Nearly transparent specimens with optical path details (differences in thickness, in refractive index, or both) are revealed by phase or interference microscopes. With interference microscopes, the optical paths within the specimen can be measured, and when the specimen is relatively homogeneous the mass can be estimated. Specimens which change polarized light can be seen and

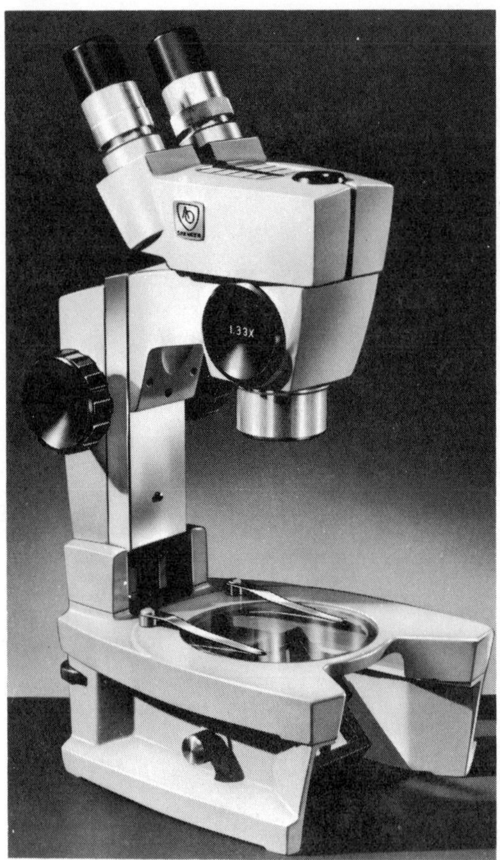

FIG. 4. *Binocular, biobjective microscope with single objective lens.*

often measured with a polarization microscope. Fluorescent chemicals may be absorbed selectively by the specimen, making the detail visible with fluorescence microscopy. Immune reactions can be studied with fluorescence microscopy. Scanning microscopes may measure specimen density for a computer, show it on a television screen, or count particles automatically. Thicker specimens can be photographed with a deep-field microscope. Various industrial contour-projecting, measuring, and surface profile analyzing microscopes are also of use in biomedical fields. Combinations are often useful, e.g., phase and fluorescence.

Specimens which absorb electrons, infrared, ultraviolet, or Roentgen radiation can be studied with special microscopes using electronic translation, television, or photography to record or make the images visible.

OPTICS

So many special optics are available that it is impractical to even list them in a chapter. This general description points to available types. The manufacturers' literature and advanced texts should be consulted for further details (21).

Objectives

The objective is the basic magnifying lens system, and its chief numerical characteristics are engraved on its mount. Magnification is given as times increased linear size (e.g., $10\times$), the ratio of a given length, as of the specimen, to the length of the same part in the magnified image. The kind of objective may be indicated, as Ph for phase, Pol for polarizing, ∞ for infinity correction, etc. The numerical aperture (NA) is an index of its light-gathering power; $NA = n \sin U$, where n is the refractive index of the working space (for air, $n = 1$; immersion oil, $n = 1.52$) and U is one-half of the angle between the maximum rays of light that can enter the objective from a central point in the field of view. The resolving power is a function of the numerical aperture. The greater the numerical aperture is the less the thickness of specimen that can be seen at one time. The brightness of the field of view is proportional to the square of the numerical aperture and inversely proportional to the square of the magnification. These factors are important aids in choosing the proper lens. (See below, section on Interpretation of what is seen.)

White light is composed of different wavelengths, and a single lens cannot focus all to the same point. Longer wavelength red light will focus farther from the lens than shorter wavelength blue light, causing chromatic aberration. Rays of light passing through the lens near its edge focus closer to the lens than those passing through it near its center, which effect is called spherical aberration. Other aberrations are distortion, coma, astigmatism, and curvature of field. By combining lenses of different kinds of glass, or with crystals, the aberration can be corrected, and optimized for the given application.

Achromatic objectives are corrected for one color for spherical aberration and for two colors for chromatic aberration. Apochromats are corrected for three colors and spherically for two colors. Apochromatic objectives are useful for critical microscopy of colored objects either visually or photographically and are made to greater numerical apertures than achromatic objectives. Other objectives are corrected to give flatter fields and minimal distortion, useful in photomicrography. Pathologists, interested in tissue patterns, have stimulated designs for very large flat fields of view, sometimes at a sacrifice of definition at the center of the field. For visual study of small details, it is preferable to have the best possible correction for the center of the field. By giving up the limitation of a fixed tube length, objectives corrected for infinity can have other improved corrections.

The objective and the eyepiece are often designed to work together as a system, and the best imagery can be obtained only when they are used together. Except for some lesser corrected optics, interchanging with those of other design or manufacturers will degrade the performance of the microscope.

Eyepieces, or oculars

Oculars are of two general classes. The negative oculars have the diaphragm between the lenses, which limits how much of the image from the objective can be seen. The Huygenian ocular is a commonly used example because it has a reasonably flat field, but, as it does have distortion at the edge of the field, it is not suitable for measurement.

In the positive-type eyepiece, the diaphragm is below the lenses. There are many kinds of positive eyepieces; some, like the compensating oculars, share in the color aberration correction of the objective and must be used with the corresponding apochromatic objective. Others are designed to provide a flat field for photomicrography, or to give the largest possible reasonably flat field.

Intermediate amplifiers and zoom systems

A third lens system may be added into the body of the microscope between the ocular and the objective. Many microscopes have optics designed for a mechanical tube length of 160 or 170 mm. Adding a binocular body increases the length, and a compensating lens is added to correct for the greater distance. The third lens system can be made adjustable to increase the total magnification, although usually not over three to five times.

Zoom systems change the magnification of the microscope and vary from a movable third lens system to complicated lens systems with means to vary the separation of the lens combinations within the objectives. The zoom system has the advantage of being able to set the magnifications exactly to a given value for a photomicrograph or to avoid fractional values on the micrometer scale when measuring (see below, section on Measuring). Zoom systems may not increase the numerical aperture of the objective and fail to reveal increased detail in the greater (often empty) magnification. When more resolving power is needed, an objective with greater numerical aperture must be used.

When infinity-corrected objectives (∞) are used, the third lens system also is a telescope to bring the image to the focal plane of the eyepiece.

Condensers

A condenser may not be needed for low-power objectives; a concave mirror can be used to concentrate the light onto the specimen. A high-aperture condenser may not light all of the field seen with a low-magnification objective and often has an auxiliary lens that can be swung in front of the condenser for this use, or the top lens of the condenser may be removed and only the lower lens used with 2 to 10× objectives. Use the plane mirror with a condenser.

Objectives with a numerical aperture of 0.5 or greater usually require a condenser to regulate the light to fill both the field and aperture of the lenses. A simple two-lens Abbe condenser is often adequate, but, for best viewing with the better corrected optics, the achromatic, aplanatic corrected condensers should be used.

For the examination of bacteria and small microorganisms, the microscope must give at least 1,000× magnification, with an immersion lens and condenser of at least 1.20 numerical aperture.

USING THE MICROSCOPE

Manipulation

Place a slide with a specimen on the stage, and arrange the stage and the lighting so that the specimen is illuminated. Bring a low-power objective to within a few millimeters of the slide, and focus upward with the coarse adjustment until the detail is seen. Focusing upward will avoid damaging the objective or the slide. Then adjust the light as described below. Turn the nosepiece to the next higher power objective and the specimen should be nearly in focus and nearly centered, so that a partial turn of the fine adjustment will sharply focus the detail. As the magnification is increased, less of the field will remain in view. Before using the oil immersion objective, place a drop of immersion oil on the objective or on the center of the lighted area of the specimen. To obtain full resolution of objectives of higher numerical aperture than 0.92, it is necessary that the microscope condenser be in immersion contact with the slide. This is essential when small objects like bacteria are examined. It is necessary that only immersion liquids recommended by the maker of the instrument be used. Wrong materials can creep into and damage the objective.

Cover glasses should be between 0.17 and 0.19 mm thick (45). Purchasing no. 1½ cover glasses yields the most of correct thickness. High aperture dry objectives give the best image only when used with cover glasses of correct thickness, because spherical aberration is then minimized. United States-made microscopes are usually for 0.18 mm and European for 0.17 mm thick cover glasses.

The detail seen depends on proper illumination. Wrong lighting can produce artifacts that are not in the specimen and result in misinterpretation by the unwary (1). Fortunately, proper lighting of the microscope is easier and quicker than hit-or-miss methods.

Light from a large white cloud is excellent but rarely available; consequently, most microscopy is done with artificial light. Two kinds of illuminators are used: one has a bright surface, such as a table light with a ground or opal diffusing surface, or simple substage lamps; the other kind contains a diaphragm and lenses.

Tungsten light has less blue and more red than average daylight, and a bluish "daylight" filter is often used with tungsten light to give better rendition of colors. The quartz halogen or iodine lamps are tungsten lamps which run hotter for more light and have a longer effective life because of the halogen cycle.

With the first type (bright surface), the lighted surface must be large enough to fill the fully opened diaphragm on the microscope condenser and centered to provide a uniformly lighted field. Remove the ocular and open or close the condenser diaphragm until its edge is just seen within the lighted back lens of the objective. Using a phase telescope, or a built-in Bertrand lens, shows the back lens aperture better than the naked eye. Neutral filters or another ground glass may be put between the lamp surface and the microscope condenser to reduce the intensity where the light is too bright.

The best lighting uses all of the light to form an image of the specimen with no non-image-forming glare light. This is attained with an illuminator with a lens system to focus the light and a diaphragm to limit the area lighted. Some competent microscopists prefer a separate illuminator to the built-in substage lighting systems, because the latter may have to compromise on quality and intensity because of the limited space and the need to avoid heating the microscope.

Light from a reasonably uniform source can be focused by the condenser onto the specimen, but light from a coiled filament lamp used in this way would hide the details in the bright bands of the filament images. Köhler's method avoids this by using the uniformly lighted lens of the illuminator to light the field of view in the microscope.

Focus the lamp filament onto the diaphragm of the microscope condenser by adjusting (focusing) the lamp condenser. If the images of the filament and reflections are not intermeshed, adjust the lamp position within the illuminator to obtain as uniform an area of illumination as possible. Partly closing the lamp iris will make the filament image easier to see. Focus the microscope on the specimen and open or close the lamp iris diaphragm until only the field of view is lighted after focusing the microscope condenser up or down to bring the lamp iris into sharp focus. Then examine the back aperture of the objective (ocular removed, or with a telescopic system), and close the microscope condenser iris diaphragm until about seven-eighths of the aperture is illuminated. An image of the lamp filament will be seen in the back aperture of the objective. This should fill the aperture as uniformly as possible. Note that *no* ground glass is used in the Köhler method.

When a ground glass is put in the illuminating system, much light is lost (30 to 70%), the amount depending on the nature of the ground surface; worse, much of this light is scattered in all directions, making it impossible to avoid some glare from non-image-forming light. A ground glass may be necessary when the light source is too small, or the optics are inadequate, but should be avoided for critical microscopy with systems of numerical aperture 0.6 or greater.

To summarize, the microscope should be adjusted so that field and aperture are as evenly illuminated as possible and the field (lamp iris) and aperture (condenser diaphragm) are opened no more than is necessary to just fill the field of view and the aperture of the back lens of the objective. The light intensity can be reduced by placing neutral filters between the lamp and the microscope condenser. The microscope condenser cannot be used to adjust the brightness without reducing the resolving power of the microscope (see below). Reducing the aperture illumination slightly may increase the crispness of the image, especially when the optics are not fully corrected. Specimens with detail too transparent to be seen with bright field should be examined with phase or other kinds of microscopes.

Microscopes with built-in illuminating systems should have separate controls for the amount of the visual field illuminated and of the aperture. These are used in the same manner described for an external lamp.

Spectacles and care of the eyes

Wearing spectacles while using the microscope is possible and convenient when other nearby tasks are done while observing. Modern oculars, except for the highest magnifications (20 to 30×), have sufficiently high eye points to permit the wearing of spectacles. Individuals with far or near sight correction do not need to wear their spectacles for microscopy as they can focus the microscope to correct for their deficiency, but individuals with a correction for astigmatism should wear their spectacles. Hold the spectacles a few inches from the eye, look at a window or a picture and rotate the spectacle lens. If the object looks normal in shape as the lens is rotated, the lens does not have a correction for astigmatism, but any change of shape of the object indicates a cylindrical lens correction for astigmatism.

A binocular body on the microscope permits the use of both eyes and gives some appearance of depth, although true stereoscopic vision is not obtained ordinarily with this body and a single objective. The binocular bodies usually have inclined eyepiece tubes for greater comfort of the user. The binocular body has two adjustments. One changes the distance between the eyepieces until both eyes see a single field. This interpupillary adjustment permits the observer to place the centers of the lenses in the two eyepieces at exactly the same distance apart as the centers of the observer's eyes. The other adjustment compensates for any difference between the observer's eyes. To make this adjustment, the microscope is focused so as to be sharp to the right eye. Then the right eye is closed and the adjustment on the left eyepiece is turned until the image is equally sharp for the left eye. Both eyes should then see the same image equally well. (Some microscopes may have this adjustment on the right-hand side.)

The amount of light to each eye is less than the amount passed by the monocular body tube, because an equal portion of the light is deflected to each eye and there is some loss of light from absorption and reflections in the prisms and lenses of the binocular body. Antireflection coatings prevent the loss of much of this light. With dense specimens, more intense sources must be used with the binocular than the monocular body.

With proper care, the microscope may be used for hours at a time without undue fatigue. To be comfortable, have the microscope on a table at such a position that you may look into it without stretching or cramping the body. Use both eyes with the binocular body. Alternate the eyes when using a monocular body tube. The eye not used should be kept open to avoid tiring the muscles by trying to hold it tightly shut. At first you will be bothered by seeing with the eye not looking through the microscope, but a very little practice will permit you to keep both eyes open and see with only one. Holding the hand in front of the other eye and gradually taking it away will help one become accustomed to seeing with one eye. Ideally, the room light, or the light at the work table should be nearly as bright, but no brighter, than the observed microscope field. During fluorescence microscopy the room light may need dimming. Sunlight should not be used except for special applications, such as dark-field microscopy.

It is important that the amount of light be adjusted so that there is enough to see the specimen without eyestrain and yet not so much unnecessary light as to cause fatigue from glare. Observers wearing tinted, or absorbing, contact lenses need to increase the lighting of both the microscope and room by the amount of light absorbed in the lenses, for equivalent seeing. Colored contact lenses that alter color appearance should not be worn when color judgment is required. Continual use of the fine adjustment will afford the greatest comfort in observation, as well as indicating the detail in the depth of the specimen.

For best vision with binocular bodies, the distance between the eye pieces should be adjusted carefully until both eyes see the same field. Failure to accomplish this when the eye pieces are centered to the eyes indicates a defect in the microscope, such as misalignment of prisms or paired objectives. Only properly paired oculars should be used with binocular bodies. Eyepieces of different power may have the eye point at different levels, which makes readjustment of the interpupillary distance necessary when the eyepieces are changed.

Interpretation of what is seen

The critical use of a research microscope requires considerable skill and technique, and an understanding of the capabilities and limitations of microscopes. The microscope is an instrument of limited capability. The limitations arise in the nature of the light used to see the specimen, the nature of the transparent materials available for lens manufacture, and the limited sensitivity of the human eye.

Because of the wave nature of light and the fact that the different portions of light waves interfere with one another, the image of a bright point of light is a disk surrounded with alternate dark and bright rings, forming a diffraction pattern and not a point. The image of an opaque edge is a region of graded intensity from light to dark. The image seen is the combination of all of these diffraction patterns, and the micropist must be able to decide to what extent the image reveals the structure of the specimen and is not an artifact.

Magnification alone is not the aim of the finest microscopes. A picture may be faithfully enlarged without showing any increased detail. The enlargement is not helpful unless more detail becomes apparent. Very powerful eyepiece lenses are less useful for visual observation with the microscope. They do not show more detail, and what is seen is less bright because of the increased amplification. The higher powered eyepieces decrease the area of the field seen. Magnification that does not increase the visible detail is called empty magnification. In some photomicrographic, counting, or measurement problems, such magnification may be useful. The least magnification that makes the detail visible to the eye, or slightly more, usually provides the best observation of the brighter, smaller image. The resolving power of the lens is its ability to reveal fine detail, and is measured in terms of the least distance between two lines or points at which they are seen as two rather than as a single blurred object. Resolving power is a function of the wavelength of light used, the lowest refractive index between the condenser and the objective, and the greatest angle between two rays of light that can enter the front lens of the objective. The numerical aperture engraved on the lenses may be used to compute the limit of resolution.

The eye is most sensitive to green light, which has a wavelength of about 0.555 μm (1 μm equals 0.001 mm). The size of the smallest distance between two particles at which they can be seen as two equals the wavelength of light used, divided by the numerical aperture when no condenser is used, or by two times the numerical aperture when the condenser is used to fill completely the back lens of the objective with light. With the low-power 16-mm objective (numerical aperture 0.25), the distance resolved as two points is 1.1 μm with and 2.2 μm without a condenser. The oil immersion objective with a numerical aperture of 1.40 resolves about 0.2 μm with white light. When blue light is used, the resolving power is increased, but it is more difficult to see the specimen. A further increase may be obtained by use of ultraviolet radiation, but it is necessary to use image converters or television, or to record the results photographically, because the eye is not sensitive to this radiation.

The resolving power of the microscope objective indicates which objective should be used to depict any given degree of detail. However, this does not mean that the details can be seen. Before they can be seen by the eye, they must have adequate contrast and be magnified sufficiently to be within the resolving power of the eye. Different observers' eyes are not equally sensitive, but in general the useful magnification should be from 500 to 1,000 times the numerical aperture of the objective.

The working distance of a microscope objective is the distance between the front of the objective and the top of the cover glass when focused on an average preparation. Numerical data for objectives can be obtained from the manufacturer's literature.

The depth of field (i.e., the thickness of the specimen seen in focus at one time) decreases as the numerical aperture and magnification increase. The thickness seen also depends on the accommodation of the observer's eye, which decreases after about age 40. When very thin sections of the specimen are to be examined, sometimes called optical sectioning, lenses of high numerical aperture should be used because of the smaller depth of field. When the general arrangement of the material is to be studied, lenses of longer focal length and less magnification will generally be more satisfactory, despite their lower resolving power, because the image will be brighter and a larger field will be seen. The longer working distance of the lower power objective may also be useful. For example, an 8-mm, numerical aperture 0.50 objective and a 20× eyepiece are useful when searching with fluorescence microscopy, because of the larger field of view and enough resolution for finding the bacteria.

Full and even lighting of the field and aperture are the surest means for good viewing with the least likelihood of finding spurious or false images. Beck (1) published pictures showing some of the weird effects that result from uneven lighting (31). Bad lighting can add or take away flagella on bacteria, and a single coccus can be made to look like a diplococcus or a short chain of streptococci. The commonest misinterpretations arise from oblique lighting. When oblique lighting is used, any specimen with parallel arranged detail should be examined as it is rotated 180° to discover whether the detail is real or caused by the lighting. When the condenser iris is closed too much, it is difficult to know whether odd appearing details are diffraction patterns or actual specimen detail, and small details disappear and are lost because the resolving power diminishes. Problems related to the halos found in phase microscopy are of concern (9, 38).

The image of an edge, being an intensity gradient, makes it difficult to know where the actual edge is. The sharper pictures of living bacteria with phase microscopy made at very short exposures with electronic flash led me to remeasure some bacteria (32). The lack of halos in the images of two-beam interference microscopy pictures has reopened this question (39). Until the mathematics and physics of these problems are solved, accurate measurement is impossible.

Stained preparations require careful interpretation, especially when very small specimens are observed, with regard to color and intensity contrast effects and possible optical illusions. The proper use of color filters can enhance detail of colored objects, both visually and for photography (20, 44). In 8% of men color vision deficiency ranges from slight to the inability to distinguish certain colors. When red Ziehl-Neelsen stained bacteria cannot be seen because of poor color vision, the yellow fluorescent tubercle bacteria with auramine can usually be seen.

Phase detail specimens change a quarter wavelength in path difference as one passes through the sharp focus, and focusing artifacts have been confused with structures. On the other hand, slight defocusing can help one decide whether or not one is looking at a diplococcus (25; see also 5–7, 9, 12, 13, 31, 39).

Care of the microscope

The microscope is a precision instrument made from valuable materials by expert workmen. With reasonable care, it will last a long time, but a single bit of carelessness may damage it.

The microscope should be carried by its arm and, when not in use, placed in its case or properly covered to protect it from dust. When the microscope is brought from a cold to a warm room, it should be allowed to warm up gradually before being used.

The lenses must be kept meticulously clean. Loosen and brush off dust with a camel's hair brush and clean the lens with lens paper. Optical glass is softer than window glass and is easily scratched by any dust on the lens surface or on a cloth used for cleaning. Special lens paper is available, and it is poor economy not to use it.

Dust on the eyepiece lenses is seen as specks which rotate when the eyepiece is turned while looking through it. Dirt on the objective prevents clear vision, and the specimen appears as if it were in a fog. If a wet preparation touches the objective lens, the lens will have to be cleaned before one can see through it clearly.

An eyepiece should always be kept in the tube except when one is examining the back aperture of the objective, to prevent dust from collecting on the objective or on the prisms. If dust does collect, clean it off carefully with a camel's hair brush or blow it off with an aspirator. An all-rubber ear or infants' enema syringe, obtainable at most drug stores, is a useful aspirator. Do not use one with a metal tip which could scratch the glass surfaces.

Blowing the breath on lenses will cover them with minute drops of saliva which are removed from the lens with difficulty. Compressed air from laboratory pipes usually contains traces of moisture or of oil from the compressor and should not be used without a filter on the discharge tube.

If the field does not appear clear, examine the lower surface of the objective with a magnifying glass. Any dirt or damage to the lens is then seen easily.

Objective lenses are carefully adjusted at the factory and should not be taken apart except where they have been made to separate (e.g., the divisible 16-mm objective and the older style immersion objective with funnel stop). The definition depends on all of the component lenses being centered and the right distance from each other. If they must be taken apart, it should be done at the factory where facilities are available for testing the reassembly.

The dry objectives, the condenser, and the eyepieces may be cleaned with distilled water when a liquid is necessary; an immersion objective and condenser top lens may be cleaned with xylene. Only the smallest amount of solvent needed should be used, and the lens should be wiped dry with fresh lens paper immediately after cleaning. Should the immersion oil become gummed on the lens, it should be cleaned off with as little xylene as possible and dried with lens paper. Do not soak the lens with xylene or other solvent, because the mounting of the lenses may be damaged if the solvent gets beyond the seal of the front lens into the objective.

Extreme care should be used in cleaning the surfaces which have antireflection coatings. The best procedure, where these are exposed, is to brush off the dirt gently with a soft camel's hair brush. When this does not clean the surface of prisms, they should be cleaned only by a competent person. Some coated surfaces are more readily damaged than uncoated lenses.

In tropical regions, mold will grow on dirty lens surfaces when the relative humidity and temperature exceed 80% and 26.7 C. When the optical surfaces are kept clean, mold growth can be avoided, or minimized, by keeping the optics in a desiccator, or by keeping the microscope in a warmed, dry cabinet (33).

The surface of the microscope is finished with enamel or metal plating and requires little more care than keeping it free from dirt. These finishes resist most laboratory chemicals, and ordinarily a little mild soap and water is all that is necessary for cleaning.

The slides of the rack and pinion should be cleaned occasionally with a small amount of oil or light grease, unless the manufacturers' instructions advise against this treatment. The fine adjustment does not require oiling. After a time, wear may make the coarse adjustment turn too easily to support the body tube. Various means are provided for restoring the proper tension, such as friction screws, turning one adjustment knob in opposite direction to the other, etc. Adjustments are usually provided to limit the movement of the body tube to the stage, the range of the substage movement, etc. The manufacturers' instructions should always be followed.

Careless handling or dropping may disturb the adjustment of the optical parts of the microscope. If the instrument does not seem to perform properly and there is no dirt on the objective or the eyepiece, it may mean that some of the prisms have become shifted. Do not attempt to adjust any of the prism systems, but rather send the instrument to the factory where tools and tests are available for adjustment and for making certain that the adjustment has been done properly.

Testing microscope lenses is a difficult task, and one which should only be attempted by a skilled microscopist. Instructions for the use of test plates and test objects are given in standard reference books. Adequate comparison requires correct illumination and adjustment of the microscope and considerable experience with lenses of different quality to evaluate the definition and aberrations (23).

ADVANCED METHODS

Oblique lighting

Blocking the light from one side of the microscope condenser or at the emission pupil of the ocular (Ramsden Disc) will give a plastic, pseudo-three-dimensional appearance to some specimens; a variety of attachments have been used for this purpose at one time or another. Specimens with a periodic arrangement will appear differently with a change of the angle of the oblique lighting and the extent of the illuminating aperture. More or fewer lines or dots can be made to appear in such a specimen than are actually present. Great care and experience are needed for the examination of materials with unsymmetrical lighting.

Epi and vertical lighting

Lighting the top of a specimen is difficult when high-power objectives are used unless the light can come from or near the objective. A circular Lieberkühn mirror around the front of the objective was used to reflect light from around the specimen back onto it. Top lighting is essential for opaque specimens and for efficient fluorescence microscopy of other than very thin or transparent materials.

The vertical illuminator (Fig. 5A) has a prism or partially reflecting mirror above the objective lenses to send light through the objective onto the specimen. Light from the specimen passes through the mirror to the eyepiece. Modern partial reflectors can be coated to proportion the light to and from the specimen to favor light toward the eye.

The epi illuminator (Fig. 5B) built around the objective sends the light outside the lenses of the objective to the specimen. Lenses or mirrors can be used to control the direction and concentration of the light.

Special vertical illuminators can provide polarized lighting and lighting for phase and interference microscopy.

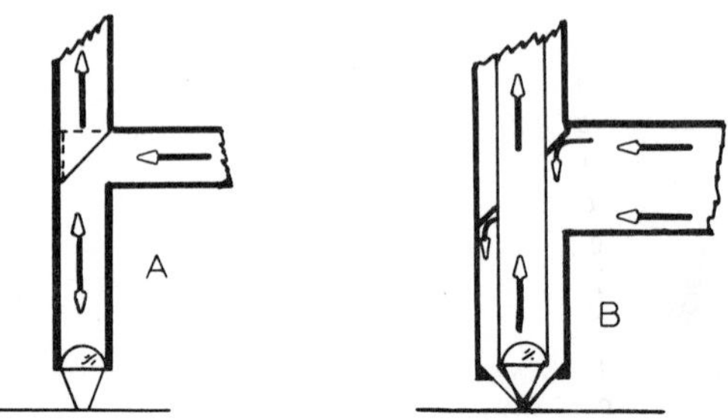

FIG. 5. *(A) Vertical illuminator light path. (B) Epi illuminator light path.*

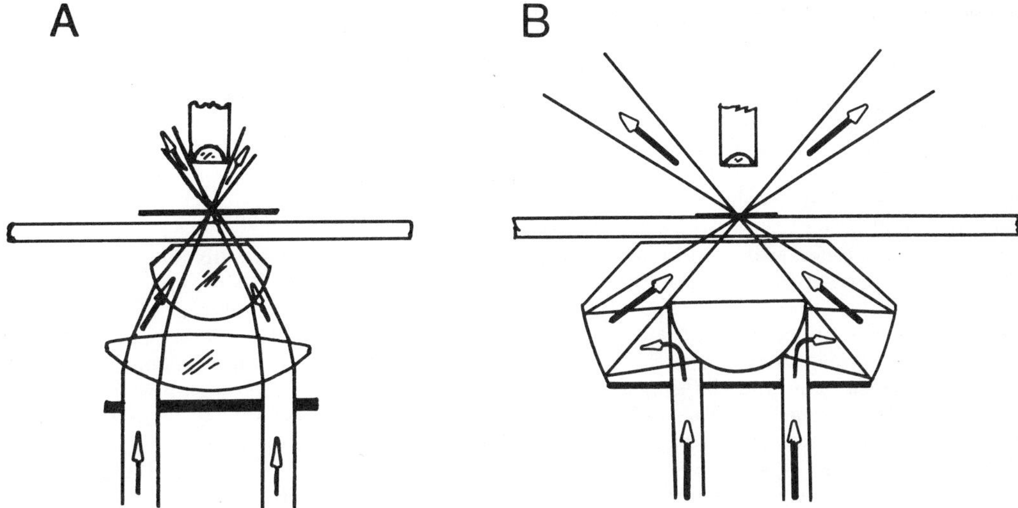

FIG. 6. *Dark-field condenser diagrams. (A) Center stop in a two-lens condenser. (B) Bispheric dark-field condenser.*

Dark-field microscopy

A central stop placed at or near the iris diaphragm of the microscope condenser, of sufficient size to prevent any direct light from reaching the objective, gives a dark field (Fig. 6A). Any specimen, placed at the cross-over point of the light, that scatters or reflects light into the objective will appear bright against the dark background. Dark-field microscopy is useful for nearly transparent specimens with large optical path differences, or for specimens that scatter light. Many biomedical specimens have small optical path difference detail, and dark-field is less useful for them than interference and phase microscopy. Dark field is used for finding syphilis spirochetes in scrapings or exudates from chancres and also when light needs to be concentrated onto the specimen but directed away from the objective, as in fluorescence microscopy, when a crossed-filter system cannot be used (see below). Stained preparations appear self-luminous and may be examined with dark field.

Being bright on dark, the smallest particle revealed depends on the intensity of the light. Intense sunlight shows the smallest particles, but particles smaller than the resolution limit of the objective used are not seen as to size and shape. Estimating the number of particles in a given volume gives some information as to relative size.

Ultramicroscopy (16), with an illuminating beam passing through the specimen at right angles to the direction of viewing, is a special type of dark field used mainly in colloidal chemistry.

Uniform, symmetrical lighting is preferable when structure or shape is to be seen. For the numerical aperture 1.25 Abbe condenser (on the average laboratory microscope), the central stop needs to be about 17 to 19 mm in diameter to block direct light from the objective. Such an arrangement is inefficient as a large amount of light is lost from the stop. Specially designed condensers concentrate more light into smaller volumes at the crossover point. A cardioid reflecting surface is efficient, but expensive to manufacture. Most special dark-field condensers are bispherics using either mirror surfaces or lenses (or both) to concentrate the light onto the specimen (Fig. 6B).

The more light concentrated onto the specimen, the smaller are the details revealed. Intense sources are desirable. Pijper (27) used sunlight for the study of bacterial flagella. A plane mirror must be used when an outside source is being reflected to the microscope condenser, and parallel light should be used (lamp filament focused at a distance of 1.5 meters or more). The specimen must be placed at the light cross-over point by using a slide of the thickness specified for the condenser by the manufacturer. The slides and cover glasses must be very clean and free from dust, scratches, or other surface defects, because such defects scatter so much light that a small bacterium may not be seen in the glare.

Exact centering and focusing of the dark-field condenser is important to concentrate the light.

Some dark-field condensers have an engraved circle, small enough to be seen within the field of the 16-mm objective. The microscope is focused onto the top of condenser, and the bright circle is centered to the field of view, by use of the centering screws on the condenser. When no guide circle is available, one focuses on a specimen and centers the brightness of the specimen and darkens the field to give the best seeing, using the centering screws on the condenser and focusing the condenser to concentrate the light on the specimen. The slide must have immersion oil between it and the condenser. Adjust the system to give the most uniform dark background and the sharpest detail. The better the design of the condenser, the more care is needed for adjustment and the more will be seen.

The field is usually not dark when the numerical aperture of the objective is greater than 0.85, and for objectives of greater numerical aperture it is necessary to reduce the numerical aperture to less than that of the condenser by inserting a funnel stop into the back of the objective, or by closing the iris diaphragm in the objective until the field appears dark. Immersion objectives to be used for dark field should have built-in iris diaphragms.

Violent motion of the specimen as the microscope is focused indicates that the specimen is too thick. Thinner are better than thicker specimens for dark field. Uneven lighting or blotches of colored light are removed by correct centering and focusing of the lamp, condenser, and objective. Hanging-drop preparations in concave slides rarely show well. Cells with flat bottoms should be used. Air in the preparation between the slide and the hanging drop may prevent obtaining a dark-field. A fuzzy picture can result from air bubbles in the immersion oil between the slide and condenser. Thick mounts can be used with special long-focus dark-field condensers. Difficulties of focusing are often due to the cover glass or the specimen being too thick, or occur because the slide is not of the thickness required by the optical design of the condenser.

A variant form uses a polarizing rather than an opaque central stop, and variation from bright field to dark field is achieved by rotating another polarizer in the light beam. The loss of light in the polarizers lessens the advantage of the technique.

Using a colored rather than an opaque central stop colors the background the same as the stop. Placing a colored annulus (preferably of complementary color) around the central stop then reveals the specimen in the color of the annulus, e.g., using a yellow center and blue annulus shows a blue specimen on a yellow background. This is Rheinberg's method of optical staining (30). Usually, not as much is seen with the color stops as with straight dark field, unless advantage can be taken of additional color contrast within the specimen.

Fluorescence microscopy

An early 20th century advance, fluorescence microscopy is useful for examination of minerals, microorganisms, chromosomes, a cell's physiological state, drugs, foods, and industrial materials, and for the rapid diagnosis of otherwise difficult diseases (see chapter 4 also).

Many living tissues absorb ultraviolet radiation, violet light, or blue light and emit green, yellow, or red light. The autofluorescence of microorganisms is usually too weak for useful microscopy. Selective combination with intensely fluorescent chemicals, a process analogous to staining, makes possible fluorescence identification, location, and counting of many microorganisms, as well as differential coloring of the specimen. Such chemicals are called *fluors* (formerly fluorochromes). Conjugating a fluor with an antibody extended fluorescence microscopy to studies of immune reactions and rapid identification of viruses, bacteria, protozoans, and worms causing diseases (chapter 4; references 3, 11, 30, 34, 47, 52).

For fluorescence microscopy, a source of the radiation needed (ultraviolet or other) must be provided, as well as an exciter filter to control the radiation and a barrier filter to limit the light from the specimen to the eye for best contrast and visibility. Silver is not as good a reflector for ultraviolet as aluminum, and the usual glass microscope mirror is replaced with a front-surfaced aluminized mirror. Photography, automated counting, and television observing and recording can also be used. The fluorescence looks bright although the actual amount of light is low and exposures are longer for recording. Some dimming of the room light and efficient, coated optics are helpful. The microscope optics must not themselves fluoresce. Most biological fluorescence microscopy is done with glass optics and does not require short-wavelength ultraviolet or quartz condensers and slides. An external radiation source and attachable filters can convert a laboratory microscope for fluorescence work, although built-in equipment is more convenient.

When the barrier filter transmits none of the exciting energy, (Fig. 7A), the fluorescent specimen is seen against a black background. In this example, the blue-violet exciter filter limits the

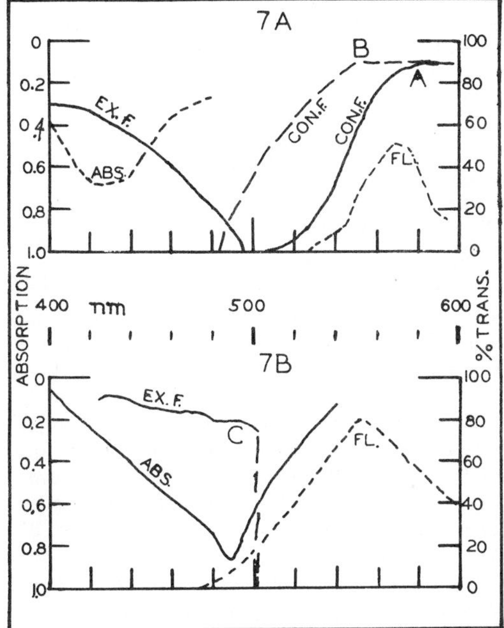

FIG. 7. *(A) Crossed-filter method. A, contrast barrier filter transmission; B, lesser contrast barrier filter; ABS, absorption of auramine O; FL, fluorescence emission auramine O; EX.F., exciter filter transmission. (B) ABS, absorption of, and FL, fluorescence emission of fluoroglobulin; EX.F., exciter filter transmission for fluoroglobulin.*

radiation from the source to wavelengths absorbed by the fluor auramine O. The barrier passes the yellow fluorescence, but blocks any of the exciting blue light. The bright yellow bacteria are easily seen with an 8 mm, numerical aperture 0.5 objective and a 15 or 20× eyepiece (see also chapter 16). This objective has a large field and enough resolving power for rapid searching without the nuisance of immersion techniques. A smear with few bacteria and little debris is difficult to focus, and some microscopists prefer a yellow filter (B) that transmits some of the exciting energy (overlap of the filters), giving a dark, rather than black, background.

The above crossed-filter procedure is most efficient, but not possible when the absorbance (formerly called optical density) and emittance of the fluor overlap (Fig. 7B). A filter limiting the exciting energy to shorter wavelength than the emitted light could give little fluorescence because too little energy would be available at maximal absorbance. A barrier filter of wavelength transmittance to include the absorption peak would give little contrast on a bright field, because of light passing through the preparation between the specimens, or scattered by them.

The earlier solution to this problem was to use a dark-field condenser which spreads the exciting energy at too great an angle to enter the objective of the microscope (Fig. 6). The fluorescence light reaching the objective is seen. Perfect dark field is not always possible, as some exciting energy may be scattered into view by the specimen, other material in the preparation, or defects on the slide. Because of this, a barrier filter is often required for good contrast. The dark-field method does not present as much energy to the specimen as the crossed-filter technique, because of the loss from the center stop (Fig. 6). A combination with phase microscopy is possible by making the center of the phase condenser annulus from ultraviolet (nonvisible) transmitting glass. A similar technique could be applied with the Rheinberg method, although I do not know of its having been used.

Fluorescence is emitted in all directions, but only that passing into the microscope objective is seen. Likewise, the exciting energy can come from all directions, but only that reaching the fluor results in fluorescence. This frees the microscopist from the problems of directional lighting of proper uniformity and aperture required for glare-free, bright-field microscopy, and only requires concentrating the exciting radiation on the specimen. Irradiated from below, little radiation reaches the top of the specimen to excite visible fluorescence where it can be seen unless the specimen is very thin or transparent.

Fluorescence can be brighter when the exciting energy is incident onto the top of the specimen from an epi or vertical illuminator (Fig. 5). The technique is essential for opaque specimens. No loss occurs from absorption within the specimen. The choice between epi and vertical illuminators depends on the efficiency of the illuminator for the given application, and the manufacturers should provide the data necessary for evaluation of the illuminator.

Modern interference filters can be made with sharp cut-off limits for most fluorescence microscopy needs. The use of the filter with a cut-off at 510 nm (Fig. 7B, C) provides most of the energy that can be absorbed by the fluoroglobulin and not too much of the exciting energy to spoil contrast with the background. Fluors with different absorbances will need filters with appropriate cut-offs, to separate the exciting and emitted energy. A barrier filter may be helpful, or not required, depending on the filters and the material viewed. When the excitation and emittance spectra are known, a choice of filters for good seeing can be made, keeping in mind the spectral sensitivity of the human eye, or other observer, to be used. Spectra for commonly used fluors are available (28).

The glass optics of the microscope and the barrier filters do not transmit ultraviolet that damages the human eye (270 to 300 nm). Only when intense shortwave ultraviolet and quartz optics are used is further protection needed. One should not look directly at a high-pressure xenon or mercury arc or at them through a microscope not protected by a barrier filter. When methods are compared, inserting a piece of opal glass into the illuminating beam will remove the excess light for bright-field use. Long-wavelength (340 to 400 nm) ultraviolet entering the eye will cause the lens within the eye to fluoresce, and this fluorescent glare light can spoil seeing by blurring the contrast of the image on the retina. When the barrier filter does not protect the eye from wavelengths shorter than 400 nm, the Wratten 1A, or equivalent, filter should also be used before the eye.

The lowest power of microscope objective with resolving power adequate for the task and the least magnification making the detail seeable is preferable. An example is included under the crossed-filter technique above. When differential color contrast is involved, the choice of filters becomes difficult, with the first choice an exciter filter that does not transmit above 400 nm. Dark field may be adequate. Observation with a spectroscope is helpful. The emitted fluorescence is often polarized, and a suitable analyzer may improve visibility or aid in measurement. Fluorescence can be measured and the amount of materials present can be analyzed. Fluorescence criteria are used in automated microscopy. The 1970 Symposium (3) covers many applications with references. Other useful sources are chapter 4 and references 29, 34, 47, 50, and 52.

Polarization microscopy

Crystal structure, strain and stress, flow of oriented particles, rates of solution, and some changes in structure (e.g., in the mitotic spindle and muscular contraction) are examined and measured from the changes they produce in polarized light passing through them. The polarization microscope adds a polarizer to the condenser, an analyzer in or on the body tube, slots for inserting retardation measuring equipment, and a Bertrand lens to give an enlarged image of the back aperture of the objective. The optics must be strain-free, and a rotating stage is necessary. Strongly curved lenses depolarize light and limit observation to detail resolvable at numerical apertures of about 0.7. By adding a rectifying system, much information has been obtained about fine structure and function of cells (17). Besides it use in analyzing form and stress changes, the polarization microscope is an important aid in the identification of microscopic specimens (17, 41, 50).

Phase microscopy

Phase microscopy is useful to reveal optical path detail due to regions of different refractive index or thickness, when the differences are too small to be seen with bright-field methods. The contrast of the details seen can be changed when different index mounting fluids can be used. Slightly absorbing or faded stained preparations may be seen with B-minus phase contrast. Phase microscopy is useful for the examination of transparent living cells and tissues, glasses, plastics, emulsions, etc. (2, 4, 24, 32, 35, 38).

The phase microscope has an annular stop in the condenser to limit the lighting to a symmetrical hollow cone, which with no specimen comes to a focus within the objective as a bright ring of light. Over this image is placed a diffraction (or phase) plate with retarding or absorbing material over the ring image (conjugate area) or the rest of the area, or part on each. That part covering the image changes the background illumination. When a specimen is in focus, it deviates light, and most of the deviated light does not go through the conjugate area. The diffraction plate can partially absorb and retard the light selectively from the specimen and its background so that the invisible phase differences are changed into visible amplitude differences.

In use, the phase annulus is centered to the condenser of the microscope, and the condenser with annulus is centered to the phase plate seen in the back aperture of the objective (use phase telescope or Bertrand lens). The condenser annulus image and the phase plate must fit so that there is no leakage of the light around the phase plate to spoil the contrast of the phase system. The width and diameter of the phase annulus and the arrangement of the absorbing and retarding materials determine the amount and kind of contrast (bright or dark). A very narrow ring gives harsh contrast that obscures the finer half-tone detail. Variable amplitude and phase microscopy now is possible (37).

Interference microscopy

The image in an interference microscope results from recombining beams of coherent, monochromatic light, some having passed through or been reflected from the specimen, with other comparison beams of light (50). The simplest interference microscope is a multiple-beam system that provides a nearly collimated beam of coherent monochromatic light (24). The specimen is mounted between a metalized surface slide and a cover glass, each having transmissions of about 5%. The light rays inter-reflect repeatedly. Those rays passing through the specimen become out of phase with rays not passing through the specimen and combine into fringes that reveal the optical path differences of the specimen. The mercury green line (546 nm) light is useful for illumination, because it is easily isolated with a filter. When the reference is a plane surface, the surface variations of the specimen are seen as contour lines.

The two-beam interference microscopes divide the coherent light into two beams, either by partially reflecting or by polarizing systems. One beam is used as a reference; the other passes through and is altered by the optical path differences in the specimen. Recombination of the rays forms interference image. Some interference microscopes can be adjusted to present either a fringe (contour system) image or an actual picture of the specimen. White light gives a colored image and monochromatic light gives an intensity image in the color of light used. Measurement of the optical path differences within the specimen is possible when monochromatic light is used, and from the measurement the wet or dry weight of the material may be estimated. The vertical specimen thickness measurement can be more accurate than the lateral resolution (35). The lateral resolution, as with the phase microscope, is the same as with other light microscopes (see above, section on Interpretation of what is seen).

Two kinds of polarized-light interference microscopes are available. In the image-duplicating system, the specimen and reference beams are separated by enough distance to clear a small specimen. The differential, Nomanski, small shearing interference microscope shifts the wavefront only slightly, providing a plastic-appearing or semi-three-dimensional image. The contrast in the image-duplicating system is proportional to the optical path difference, but in the differential interference system the contrast is proportional to the rate of change (partial differential) of the path difference in the direction of the shear, which requires careful interpretation (19, 24, 35, 38, 50).

Electron and scanning electron microscopy

The electron microscope uses electrons instead of light, and the gain in resolving power has greatly increased our knowledge of the finer structure of microorganisms. Electromagnetic or electrostatic fields are used, instead of glass lenses, to focus the electrons through the specimen to form an image on a fluorescent screen or photographic emulsion. The system must work in a vacuum, which usually limits its use to dried specimens. Unless high voltages are used, the specimen must be very thin. Special sectioning methods are required. The transmission electron microscope performs similarly to a light microscope with condensing, primary, and secondary magnification focusing fields. Too transparent materials are "stained" with salts of heavy metals, relatively opaque to electrons. Surface detail can be studied with replicas or by shadowing with thin layers of evaporated metal. Magnifications used vary from five to a thousand times that useful in light microscopy (14, 15, 22, 42).

Electron microscopy includes X-ray microanalysis, field-emission, field-ion, electron reflection, and mirror, as well as transmission microscopes. A beam of electrons onto a specimen is partly transmitted and the rest is reflected, or produces secondary electrons, cathodoluminescence, X-ray excitation, or beam-induced conductivity. These effects are used in different modes of electron microscopy.

The scanning electron microscope moves a small beam of electrons over the surface of the specimen and uses one or more of the above effects to reveal details of the surface examined. The current of primary and secondary emitted electrons from the specimen is used to control the luminance of a fluorescent screen producing an image of the specimen surface. The moving, scanning spot does less damage to the specimen than continuous radiation. The long depth of focus is a real advantage. Resolution is not as yet as good as that obtained with the transmission electron microscope (14, 18, 42, 48).

Electron probe and X-ray microscopy may be used to analyze the chemical elements composing the specimen and to reveal structure. X-ray microscopes have great penetrating power and less resolving power than light and electron microscopes (22, 42).

Automation microscopy

Routine tasks, such as counting, particle sizing, searching to find atypical cells, etc., should not require the personal attention of the microscopist. This and the scarcity of technicians are demanding automation. Coupling a computer to the microscope makes possible counting, identification, area and size distributions (percentage composition), recognition of boundaries, shape, and form, and fluorescence or absorbance measurement without personal attention. Limitations depend on the ability to program the computer and on the sensitivity of the system. One system can place specimens on plastic tape, stain, and examine them, recording preset information, or mark areas where atypical material was found, for later examination by the microscopist. Other systems use standard glass slide preparations. By use of selective absorption of ultraviolet radiation, mixed cell populations are analyzed that are too alike for visual discrimination. Automation microscopy will be useful for counting bacteria in soil and water samples and for scanning smear preparations to sort normal from diseased preparations. Much of the work is experimental, although some commercial equipment is available (10, 51).

USEFUL ACCESSORIES

Location of small specimens

Location of a small specimen can be referenced from the coordinate readings of a graduated stage, but the readings may not be the same as those for the same place on another stage. By marking a dot on the slide label and giving the coordinates for both the dot and the specimen, it is possible to find the specimen with any graduated stage. A simple system is to remove the slide, put a piece of stiff paper or thin cardboard of the same size in place of the slide, and mark the paper in the center of the bright spot from the substage illumination. Either the top or a side should be marked so as to know which side to use in relocating the specimen.

Slides with coordinates printed on them or with numbered spots, e.g., Micro-Visor, Micro-Locator, Field Finder, etc., are available. Another method is to use a stamping or a scribing objective to mark a circle on the cover glass around the area of the specimen to be located. The scribing type is preferable when immersion oil is used, as ink marks may be removed in the cleaning process. These objectives are available from laboratory supply houses.

A simple method is to draw a circle around the lighted area of the slide by use of a small pen and a glass-marking ink. When a permanent mark is not needed, some fountain pen inks can be used to write on a clean cover glass.

A reticle placed on the diaphragm of the ocular is seen in the field of view superimposed on the image of the specimen and can be used to indicate position. Even simpler, a short piece of hair or fine wire cemented onto the eye-piece diaphragm makes a pointer. Demonstration eyepieces or double microscopes permit two people to see the same field.

Counting

Precise counting is best done on a photomicrograph so that each cell is marked as counted. Personal error problems are difficult to avoid. A common counting method is to place the material to be counted in a chamber of known volume, such as hemocytometer, which also has an area scale ruled on the chamber. The particles in a given area are counted, and those on the boundary lines are counted only on two sides, e.g., top and right side. When the sample must be diluted, errors other than enumerating occur and must be evaluated. Counting cells for various volumes are available, and the Sedgwick-Rafter cell is useful for larger volumes when protozoans and sewage samples are examined. The chamber is ungraduated, and the depth of the cell becomes a volume when a Whipple Disc or other suitable reticle is placed in the ocular to establish a definite area in the field of view. Many types of reticles are available for counting and sizing small specimens.

Measuring

The absolute size of a length seen on an ocular micrometer depends on the magnification in use. Consequently, each scale must be calibrated for use for each combination of eyepiece and objective. To calibrate, focus on a stage micrometer and move it until one of the graduations corresponds exactly with one of the divisions of the eyepiece micrometer (Fig. 8). The true distance (x) seen on the stage micrometer, which corresponds to the number of divisions (y) of the eyepiece micrometer, is then read, and dividing this true distance by the number of divisions of the eyepiece micrometer gives the distance each one subtends ($C = x/y$). The number of divisions covered by the specimen multiplied by the calibration constant (C) gives

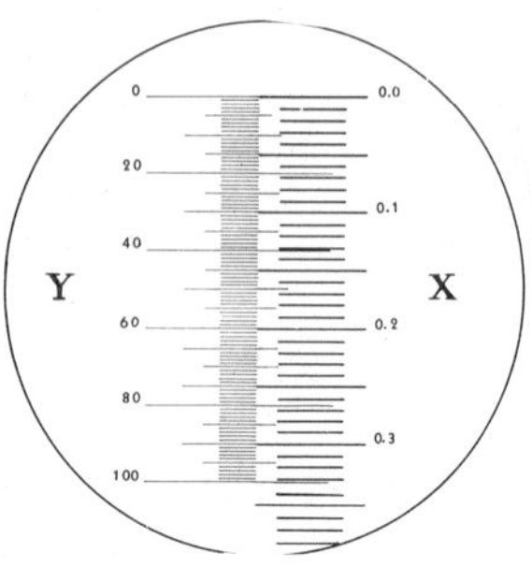

FIG. 8. *Calibration of an ocular micrometer scale.*

the length of the specimen. Once an eyepiece micrometer has been calibrated, it need not be recalibrated when used with the same eyepiece, the same objective, and the same tube length. The calibration can be made an even value when the tube length of the microscope can be changed, because this changes the magnification proportionally. A small change of tube length causes little loss of definition, but any change in tube length from the correct value (160 or 170 mm) increases the spherical aberration and reduces the definition. When small details need not be resolved, a certain amount of distinctness in the image may be sacrificed for convenience in calibrating the eyepiece scale. Microscopes with a zoom system can use the zoom magnification to avoid fractional values, but any further change of the zoom will require recalibration. Filar, or screw, micrometers and other special eyepieces are useful when much work is to be done.

Vertical measurement of a specimen is difficult, and no accurate method is easily available. The fine adjustment is graduated and may be used to measure vertical distance approximately. Focus on the bottom and then on the top of the specimen, and read the difference on the scale. When the measurement is not made in air, the difference must be multiplied by the refractive index of the material measured. The indices of refraction of some common mounting materials are as follows: balsam and damar, 1.52 to 1.54; cedar oil, 1.52; Clarite, 1.54; glycerol, 1.46; Hyrax, 1.73±; Styrax, 1.58±; water, 1.33. Turn the fine adjustment in only one direction during a single measurement. Avoid measuring at the extremes of the fine adjustment. The precision will depend on the model, the wavelength of light used, the accommodation of the observer's eyes, and the depth of field of the objective (35). Unless special precautions are taken, precision may not be much better than ±15%.

Slideways of older microscopes do not have ball bearings, and the movement depends on the condition of the grease (35). When the fine adjustment is to be used for vertical measurement, it should be calibrated at the time of use with an interferometer (1). The use of a dial gauge to read vertical movement of the microscope body tube is no more accurate than is the dial gauge, which also should be calibrated. Every few years, some microscopist puts a long pointer onto the fine adjustment, and, because a larger scale with finer division can be used, he deludes himself into thinking he is measuring better than the capability of the microscope.

Specimens suitable for use with an interference microscope may be measured more precisely than with bright-field microscopes, when the vertical optical path can be related to thickness (homogeneous optically). (See above, section on Interference microscopy.)

Some mechanical stages have millimeter scales and verniers for measuring and to provide location coordinates for later relocation of the specimen. The vernier scale is 9 mm long, divided into 10 parts. Fractions of a millimeter are shown when a scale and a vernier line are coincident; e.g., when the index is slightly beyond a unit millimeter mark and the 6th line of the vernier is exactly in line with a line on the scale, the distance is 0.6 mm more than the value of the unit millimeter mark.

Recording observations

Special drawing eyepieces, or cameras lucida, are used as drawing aids, or the image can be projected onto the drawing paper and traced. Drawing has the advantage that the picture is not cluttered with unnecessary detail and the disadvantage that no other information is available to support or disprove the interpretation made in the drawing.

Present practice makes use of photomicrographs in black and white or color. Some microscopes have built-in cameras; others use small cameras that can be placed over the ocular or trinocular tube. When pictures larger than about 5 cm are made, separate cameras on adjustable stands are more convenient. Apparent time may be increased or decreased with high- and low-speed motion pictures.

The microscopy is of first importance in photomicrography, as the photograph cannot correct a poor image; however, proper filters and longer exposures can provide better contrast in a picture than was seen. Invisible X-ray, ultraviolet, or infrared images may be made visible by photomicrography. The photographic procedures are no different in photomicrography than in other kinds of photography. Exposure is determined by trial and error, or with exposure meters. Many books are available and should be consulted for detailed instruction (20, 23, 26, 44, 49, 50).

When the microscopy is done with the aid of television, records can be made on tape for future use.

LITERATURE CITED

1. Beck, C. 1938. The microscope/theory and practice. R. & J. Beck, London. (For imagery, see p. 78ff; interferometer, p. 194.)
2. Bennett, A. H., H. Osterberg, H. Jupnik, and O. W. Richards. 1951. Phase microscopy. John Wiley & Sons,

Inc., New York. (Out of print. Copies available from University Microfilms, Ann Arbor, Mich.)
3. Beutner, E. H. (ed.). 1971. Defined immunofluorescent staining. Ann. N.Y. Acad. Sci. **177**:1–529.
4. Beyer, H. 1965. Theorie und Praxis des Phasenkontrastverfahrens. Akademische Verlags, Leipzig.
5. Charman, W. N. 1963. Visual factors in size measurement by microscopy. Opt. Acta **10**:130–139.
6. Demptster, W. T. 1944. Principles of illumination and the problems of glare. J. Opt. Soc. Amer. **34**:695–710.
7. Demptster, W. T. 1944. Visual factors in microscopy. J. Opt. Soc. Amer. **34**:711–717.
8. Dobell, C. 1958. Antony van Leeuwenhoek and his little animals. Russell & Russell, New York.
9. Duijn, C. Van. 1957. Visibility and resolution of microscopical detail. Microscope **11**:196–208; 222–230; 254–258; 273–281; 301–309; **12**:16–24, 38–43; 92–101; 131–138; 185–193; 201–211; 269–303.
10. Evans, D. M. D. 1970. Cytology automation. The Williams & Wilkins Co., Baltimore.
11. Francisco, D. E. 1973. Acridine orange epifluorescence technique for counting bacteria in natural waters. Trans. Amer. Microsc. Soc. **92**:416–421.
12. Francon, M. 1961. Progress in microscopy. Harper, New York.
13. Hartridge, H. 1954. The optimal conditions for visual microscopy. J. Quekett Microsc. Club **44**:57–88.
14. Hearle, J. W. S., J. T. Sparrow, and P. M. Cross. 1973. The use of the scanning electron microscope. Pergamon Press, Oxford.
15. Heidenreich, R. D. 1964. Fundamentals of electron transmission microscopy. Interscience Publishers, Inc., New York.
16. Heimstädt, O. 1915. Apparate und Arbeitsmethoden der ultramikroskopie und Dunkelfeld beleuchtung. Handbuch der mikroskop. Technik V. Geschäftsstelle d. "Mikrokosmos" Franckh'sche Verlagshandlung, Stuttgart.
17. Inoué, S., and W. L. Hyde. 1957. Studies on polarization of light at microscope lens surfaces. II. The simultaneous realization of high resolution and high sensitivity with the polarizing microscope. J. Biophys. Biochem. Cytol. **3**:831–838.
18. Johari, O., and I. Corvin (ed.). 1972. Scanning electron microscopy. Illinois Institute of Technology Research Institute, Chicago.
19. Krug, W. J., J. Rienitz, and G. Schulz. 1964. Contributions to interference microscopy. Hilger & Watts, London.
20. Lawson, D. F. 1972. The technique of photomicrography. Macmillan Co., New York.
21. Martin, L. C. 1966. The theory of the microscope. American Elsevier Publishing Co., New York.
22. Mercer, E. H., and M. S. Birbeck. 1972. Electron microscopy. A handbook for biologists. Blackwell Scientific Publications, London.
23. Needham, G. H. 1958. The practical use of the microscope. Charles C. Thomas, Publisher, Springfield, Ill.
24. Osterberg, H. 1955. Phase and interference microscopy, p. 378–437. *In* G. Oster and A. W. Pollister (ed.), Physical techniques in biological research, vol. 1. Academic Press Inc., New York.
25. Osterberg, H., and L. W. Smith. 1961. Defocusing images to increase resolution. Science **134**:1193–1196.
26. Photography through the Microscope. 1970. Eastman Kodak Co., Rochester, N.Y.
27. Pijper, A. 1946. Shape and motility of bacteria. J. Pathol. Bacteriol. **58**:325–342.
28. Porro, T. J. 1963, 1965. Fluorescence and absorption spectra of biological dyes. Stain Technol. **38**:37–48; **40**:173–176.
29. Price, G. R., and S. Schwartz. 1956. Fluorescence microscopy, p. 91–148. *In* G. Oster and A. W. Pollister (ed.), Physical techniques in biological research. Academic Press Inc., New York.
30. Rheinberg, J. 1896. On the addition to the method of microscopic research by a new way of producing colour-contrast between an object and its background, or between definite parts of the object itself. J. Roy. Microsc. Soc. **1896**:373–388; **1899**:142–146.
31. Richards, O. W. 1940. Color and illumination in photomicrography. J. Biol. Photogr. Ass. **9**:77–86.
32. Richards, O. W. 1948. Phase microscopy in bacteriology. Stain Technol. **23**:55–64.
33. Richards, O. W. 1949. Some fungous contaminants of optical instruments. J. Bacteriol. **58**:453–455.
34. Richards, O. W. 1955. Fluorescence microscopy, p. 5/1–5/37. *In* R. C. Mellors (ed.), Analytical cytology. McGraw-Hill Book Co., Inc., New York.
35. Richards, O. W. 1959. Measurement with phase and interference microscopes. Symposium on Microscopy. Amer. Soc. Test. Mater., Spec. Tech. Publ. **257**:6–18.
36. Richards, O. W. 1968. Photography of three dimensions. J. Biol. Photogr. Ass. **36**:155–159.
37. Richards, O. W. 1973. The Polanret variable densiphase microscope. J. Microsc. (London) **98**:67–77.
38. Ross, K. F. A. 1967. Phase contrast and interference microscopy for cell biologists. Edw. Arnold, London.
39. Ross, K. F. A., and G. Galvazi. 1965. The size of bacteria as measured by interference microscopy. J. Roy. Microsc. Sco. **84**:13–25.
40. Royal Microscopical Society Standards. 1936. J. Roy. Microsc. Soc. **56**:377–380.
41. Ruch, F. 1956. Birefringence and dichroism of cells and tissues, p. 149–176. *In* G. Oster and A. W. Pollister (ed.), Physical techniques in biological research. Academic Press Inc., New York.
42. Ruthman, A. 1970. Methods in cell research. Cornell Univ. Press, Ithaca, N.Y.
43. Schierbeek, 1961, found birth records for Zaccharias Jansen, 1588, and Hanns, 1611, which indicates that it is unlikely they invented the microscope in 1590. Doetsch, R. N. 1961. History of the microscope. Science **133**:946–947.
44. Shillaber, C. P. 1944. Photomicrography in theory and practice. John Wiley & Sons, Inc., New York.
45. Standard specifications for cover glasses and glass slides for use in microscopy. 1970. E 211 – 70. American Society for Testing and Materials, Philadelphia.
46. Star, P. van der. 1953. Descriptive catalog of the simple microscopes in the Rijksmuseum voor de Geschiedenis der Naturwetenschappen, Leyden. Commun. No. 87.
47. Strugger, S. 1949. Fluoreszenzmikroskopie und Mikrobiologie. Verlag M. & H. Schaper, Hannover.
48. Thornton, P. R. 1968. Scanning electron microscopy. Chapman & Hall, London.
49. White, G. W. 1966. Introduction to microscopy. Butterworths, London.
50. Wied, G. L. (ed.) 1966. Introduction to quantitative cytochemistry. Academic Press Inc., New York. (Interference, polarization, microspectrophotometry and fluorescence microscopy.)
51. Wied, G. L., and G. F. Bahr. 1970. Automated cell identification and cell sorting. Academic Press Inc., New York.
52. Young, M. R. 1961. Principles and technique of fluorescence microscopy. Quart. J. Microsc. Sci. **102**:419–449.

Chapter 4
Immunofluorescence Techniques

WILLIAM B. CHERRY

INTRODUCTION

This chapter is designed to provide a practical discussion of immunofluorescence (IF) reagents and equipment. Techniques for the preparation and evaluation of fluorescent-antibody (FA) reagents that are discussed include (i) serum production, (ii) fractionation, (iii) labeling and quantitation, (iv) standardization, and (v) preservation. The principles involved in the use of various types of fluorescence optical and lighting equipment are reviewed, and the roles of important components of the system are analyzed. Progress toward automation of IF techniques is cited.

IMMUNOFLUORESCENCE REAGENTS

Many antisera for FA studies are produced in the same way as are those for other serological tests. However, as emphasized elsewhere (5), improvement in the specificity of IF reagents depends both upon the production of purer antigens for use in immunization of animals and upon finding methods for making labeled antibodies monospecific for their respective antigens.

The methods discussed below have been used successfully in the laboratories of the Center for Disease Control (CDC) for several years.

Antiserum production

Many antisera prepared for other serological tests may be suitable for IF work. It is known, however, that some sera give poor IF staining titers although they may exhibit high titers in another type of serological test and vice versa (32). That is, the antibody participating in the IF test may be less active or inactive in other serological tests. Cohen et al. (7) suggested that immunoglobulin G (IgG) antibodies inhibited IgM reactivity in indirect IF tests. They showed that natural antibody to gram-negative bacteria contained IgG as well as IgM class-specific reactivity, a fact which was not evident when bactericidal and agglutination tests were used. IgG antibodies appeared to have greater avidity for gram-negative organisms than did IgM antibodies. Purer antigens and more potent labeled class-specific antibodies are needed for detection of immunoglobulins in indirect IF tests.

Antiserum fractionation

Many methods may be used for separation of antibody protein from serum. Nichol and Deutsch (35) developed ethyl alcohol fractionation procedures which can be applied to the separation of immunoglobulins from a variety of animal sera. Ethyl alcohol precipitation requires careful control of temperature, pH, ionic strength, and alcohol concentration. Several workers have successfully used the methanol fractionation method (9). Others have employed HCl (10), ethodin (2-ethoxy-6,9-diaminoacridine lactate, Winthrop Laboratories, New York, N.Y.; 12, 31), sodium sulfate, DEAE (diethylaminoethyl-cellulose, Schleicher & Schuell Co., Keene, N.H.; 8, 11, 14, 39), Sephadex G-200 and DEAE-Sephadex G-50 (Pharmacia Fine Chemicals, Inc., Piscataway, N.J.; 1, 3, 7, 11, 42), and zonal centrifugation.

The best of the most popular procedures for fractionating serum to obtain antibody are (i) ammonium sulfate precipitation, (ii) ethanol precipitation according to the method of Nichol and Deutsch (35), (iii) column separations on DEAE-cellulose, Sephadex G-200, or DEAE-Sephadex G-50, and (iv) zonal centrifugation. The simplest of these in terms of both equipment and technique is that of salting out the globulins with $(NH_4)_2SO_4$. The antibody may be obtained in rather high yield but is substantially contaminated with alpha and beta globulins and other serum proteins. Density gradient separation in a zonal centrifuge yields highly purified antibody fractions but requires expensive equipment and considerable skill. Globulins of higher purity than those obtained by salt precipitation may be required for more precise determination of fluorescein-to-immunoglobulin ratios because of the high affinity of fluorescein isothiocyanate (FITC) for albumin as contrasted with that of the immunoglobulin (27). Contamination of the product by albumin is decreased as the $(NH_4)_2SO_4$ concentration is reduced below the 50% saturation level of the mixture of salt solution and serum. Some loss of immunoglobulin occurs also so that a balance must be struck depending upon the desired composition of the product. Critical studies to determine the optimal concentration of $(NH_4)_2SO_4$ for precipitating immunoglobulins from the sera of various animal species have not been done until recently (17, 18). The electrophoresis profiles of rabbit serum shown in Fig. 1 illustrate the improved fractionation resulting from serial precipitation with an optimal concentration of $(NH_4)_2SO_4$ (18). Data for 12 animal species whose sera are most frequently used for preparation of diagnostic IF reagents are given in Table 1. From these data and from those given in the literature (17, 18, 21), it is evident that 50% $(NH_4)_2SO_4$ is unsatisfactory for IF reagent preparation from sera of all animal species tested. Follow the guidelines in Table 2 to obtain optimal yield and purity of immunoglobulins from sera of various animal species.

Salting out globulins with $(NH_4)_2SO_4$

1. Prepare a stock-saturated solution of reagent-grade $(NH_4)_2SO_4$ by placing 550 g of the salt in a 1,000-ml volumetric flask and bringing to volume with distilled water. Hold at room temperature for several days and mix frequently. Variations in room temperature between 20 and 30 C, in pH of the $(NH_4)_2SO_4$ between 5.8 and 7.2, and in fractionation of undiluted versus 1:2 or 1:10 dilutions of serum have no important effect on the composition of the serum fractions (18).

2. As needed, prepare fresh working solutions of 60, 70, 80, or 90% (vol/vol) saturated ammo-

TABLE 1. *Concentrations of $(NH_4)_2SO_4$ and number of precipitations for optimal recovery of immunoglobulin from sera of various animal species*

Animal origin of serum	Percent saturation[a] of $(NH_4)_2SO_4$ × no. of precipitations
Rabbit	35 × 3
Sheep	35 × 3
Horse	30 × 2
Goat	30 × 1, 45 × 1
Cattle[b]	30 × 1, 35 × 2
Swine[b]	35 × 3
Chicken[b]	35 × 3
Mouse[b]	35 × 1, 40 × 2
Hamster[b]	35 × 3
Guinea pig[b]	35 × 1, 40 × 2
Monkey[b]	30 × 1, 40 × 2
Chimpanzee[b]	35 × 3

[a] Final concentration in serum-salt mixture.
[b] Data from Hebert (16) with permission of author and publisher.

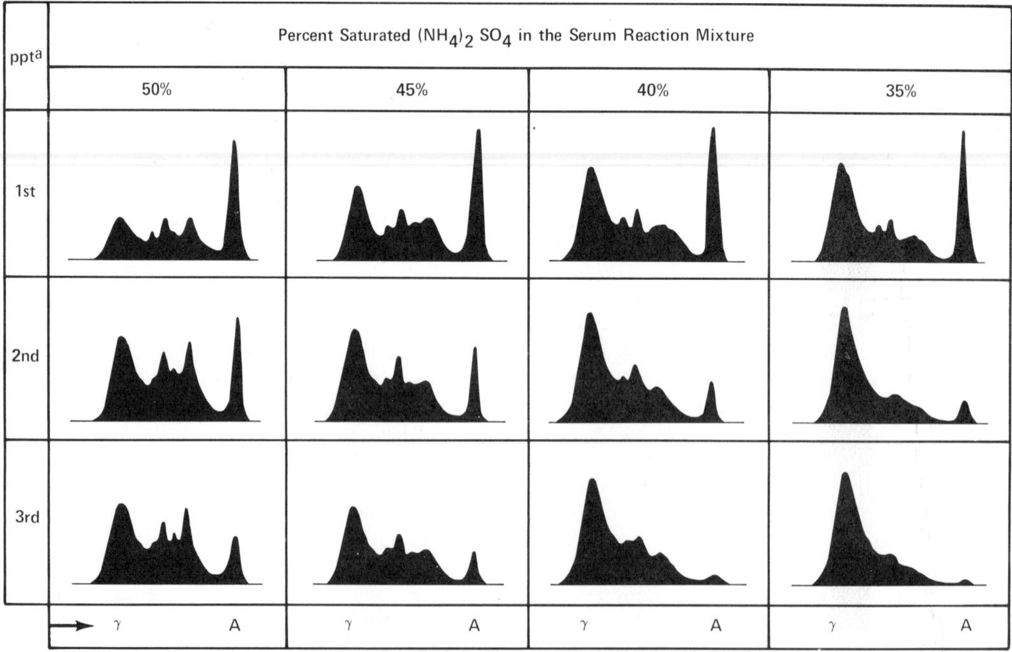

FIG. 1. *Electrophoretic profiles of $(NH_4)_2SO_4$ fractions of rabbit antiserum for E. coli.* [a] *Precipitation.* (*Reproduced from Hebert, Pelham, and Pittman [18] with permission of authors and publisher.*)

TABLE 2. *Recovery of immunoglobulins from antisera after fractionation with* $(NH_4)_2SO_4$

Serum pool[b]	Composition					
	Percent γ[c]	Percent β-α[c]	Percent albumin[c]	Protein (mg/ml)	γ (mg/ml)[d]	Percent γ recovery
Rabbit						
Original	17	25	58	67	11	NA[e]
50% SAS	33	58	9	ND[f]	ND	ND
35% SAS	65	34	1	15	10	91
Sheep						
Original	26	32	42	74	19	NA
50% SAS	44	47	9	ND	ND	ND
35% SAS	68	32	0	24	16	84
Horse						
Original	20	46	34	81	16	NA
50% SAS	23	65	12	ND	ND	ND
30% SAS	74	25	1	14	10	63
Goat						
Original	30	36	34	60	18	NA
50% SAS	48	31	21	ND	ND	ND
30–45% SAS	81	18	1	18	15	83

[a] Data rearranged from references 18 and 21 with permission of authors and publishers.
[b] Optimal concentrations and number of precipitations were: rabbit and sheep, 35%, 3×; horse, 30%, 2×; goat, 30%, 1×, 45%, 1×. SAS, Saturated $(NH_4)_2SO_4$.
[c] Determined by cellulose acetate strip electrophoresis (CASE).
[d] Calculated from total protein and percent γ by CASE.
[e] Not applicable.
[f] Not done: 50% SAS supernatant fluids free from γ.

nium sulfate (SAS) depending upon the animal species from which the serum was obtained.

3. While gently stirring the serum, slowly add a volume of the appropriate $(NH_4)_2SO_4$ concentration equal to the volume of the serum.

4. Allow the mixture to stand at 25 C for a minimum of 4 h or at 4 C for a minimum of 24 h. Pack the precipitated globulin by centrifuging at 4 C for 30 min at a relative centrifugal force of about 1,440 × *g*. Decant and discard the supernatant fluid.

5. While stirring gently, add to the precipitate enough distilled water to result in a globulin solution with a total volume equal to that of the original serum.

6. Reprecipitate the globulin as described in step 3, using a volume of $(NH_4)_2SO_4$ equal to the volume of globulin. Centrifuge immediately as before, discard the supernatant fluid, and resuspend as in step 5. Precipitate the globulin a third time, if necessary for that animal species, and resuspend as in step 5, or to a smaller volume if concentration is desired.

7. Dialyze the globulin at 0 to 5 C against frequent changes of 0.85% NaCl solution (pH 8.0) until sulfate is no longer detected in the saline solution after a period of 16 to 20 h of continuous dialysis. [$(NH_4)_2SO_4$ interferes with the determination of protein by biuret and Kjeldahl techniques and, when present at a concentration of 0.08 M or greater, with the conjugation reaction (24). The time required for removal of the $(NH_4)_2SO_4$ by dialysis is decreased by frequent changes but not appreciably by agitation of the NaCl solution (19).] Presence of sulfate is determined by adding a small amount of saturated $BaCl_2$ solution to an equal volume of the saline. If no cloudiness results, the globulin solution is considered substantially free from sulfate.

DEAE-cellulose. DEAE, an anion-exchange, cellulose absorbent, is useful for obtaining pure gamma globulin fractions from whole serum which has been placed on an appropriate column and subjected to elution with increasing concentrations of buffered NaCl. The disadvantages of the technique are (i) the labor and expense involved in preparing the column and reagents, (ii) the rather high dilution of the antibody obtained, and (iii) the fact that not all DEAE-fractionated antisera appear to be superior to those made from $(NH_4)_2SO_4$-fractionated antiserum (11). The use of DEAE for simultaneous separation of gamma globulin and removal of unreacted fluorescent material from labeled whole serum as described by Riggs et al. (39) is not recommended. The labeling of whole serum, except perhaps as a rapid screening procedure, is not recommended because it does not permit control of the fluorescein to protein (F/P) ratio—an important conjugate characteristic—and wastes FITC.

Sephadex. Sephadex G-200 is a highly cross-linked insoluble dextran polymer which acts as a sieve for separating substances according to the size and shape of their molecules. It is worthy of mention here because of its ability to separate two important classes of globulins—the low- and high-molecular-weight gamma globulins designated 7*S* and 19*S*, respectively. The role of each of these globulins in many common serological reactions has not been established, and even less is known of their participation in FA reactions.

Columns of Sephadex G-200 are relatively easy to prepare and use. Gamma globulin fractions may be prepared by $(NH_4)_2SO_4$ precipitation, labeled with FITC, applied to the column, and eluted with 0.15 M NaCl buffered at pH 7.5 with 0.01 M phosphate (3). Dilution is about threefold. Total protein recovery is good —usually more than 90% of that applied to the column. Elution of the desired material may be followed by its fluorescence when irradiated with a Wood's lamp; the larger molecules pass through the column first.

The disadvantages of gel filtration through G-200 are (i) the length of time required to separate reasonably large amounts of globulin and (ii) the ease of denaturation of the 19*S* fraction.

DEAE-Sephadex. DEAE-Sephadex A-50 (Pharmacia Fine Chemicals, Inc.) has been found to be an excellent matrix for separation of IgG antibodies from other serum components (40). Its activity is primarily a function of the anionic exchange properties of DEAE. A column is prepared for use according to the manufacturer's instruction. The serum is dialyzed against the buffer which has been selected for starting the elution. The serum is then applied to the column and eluted with one of a variety of buffers or salt gradients which are appropriate. The bed material has high capacity so that relatively large amounts (25 to 50 ml) of serum may be fractionated in one operation.

Before DEAE-Sephadex chromatography, it may be desirable to perform a crude fractionation with 50% saturated $(NH_4)_2SO_4$ followed by dialysis against PBS (0.01 M K_2HPO_4 + 0.15 M NaCl, pH 7.6).

Generally DEAE-Sephadex fractionation performed on either conjugates or serum results in the elution of both electrophoretically slow and fast IgG antibody peaks and in better resolution of IgG than is obtained from DEAE-cellulose. The antibody activity within each peak may vary both qualitatively and quantitatively depending upon the antigen used, the method and schedule of immunization, and the technique of fractionation (40).

For processing serum or globulin by any of the above column methods, it is desirable to have a fraction collector monitored by a recorder indicating absorption of the eluate at λ 280 nm. The progress of FITC conjugates through the columns also may be followed by color, by fluorescence under a Wood's lamp, or by absorption at 495 nm.

Labeling of antiglobulins and other serum proteins

The conjugation of protein with FITC is a chemical reaction (Table 3). If the serum contains the desired antibody at a reasonable titer, careful control of production usually results in a specific reagent. Conjugation procedures have been developed which may be used to produce reagents having almost any degree of labeling (F/P) desired (28). The choice of F/P ratio for a conjugate may vary with different antigen-antibody systems and with the use of the conjugate (20, 37). Nonspecific staining (NSS) or nonimmunological staining has been shown to be related directly to the FITC concentration of conjugates (20, 37). Hence, the degree of NSS which can be tolerated is a primary factor in determining the optimal F/P ratio for any antigen-antibody system.

When preparing a conjugate, the most economical means of obtaining the desired F/P ratio is to regulate the initial weight of dye in the reaction mixture and allow the reaction to proceed to completion. An alternate but more expensive method is to increase the weight of dye and interrupt the reaction at a specific time interval (Table 3).

The rate and efficiency of the labeling reaction are greatly influenced by the animal source of the protein, the kind of protein, and the protein concentration (28). Temperature, pH, buffer system, and the buffer concentration at which the reaction is carried out also are important factors. The labeling reaction is most efficient when the conditions are as follows: temperature, 25 C; pH 9.5; 0.05 M Na_2HPO_4.

The procedures outlined here are essentially those of McKinney et al. (28) and were originally designed for use with rabbit gamma globulin obtained by $(NH_4)_2SO_4$ fractionation. They are, however, generally applicable for labeling any protein.

A final but most important factor in the preparation of a conjugate is the purity of the

TABLE 3. *Relationship between labeling conditions and conjugate characteristics of normal rabbit gamma globulin*

No.	Labeling conditions			Conjugate characteristics			
	Protein[a] (g/100 ml)	FITC (μg/mg of protein)	Time (h)	Protein[b] (g/100 ml)	FITC (μg/ml of conjugate)	F/P ratio[c]	NSS[d]
1	0.5	8.3	2.5	0.50	32.5	6.5	7.4
2	0.5	16.6	2.5	0.50	53.5	10.7	11.6
3	0.5	25.0	2.5	0.50	72.5	14.5	22.3
4	1.0	8.3	1.0	1.0	70.0	7.0	16.6
5	1.0	16.6	1.0	1.0	123.0	12.3	33.8
6	1.0	25.0	1.0	1.0	196.0	19.6	44.1
7	1.5	8.3	0.75	1.45	96.0	6.6	18.3
8	1.5	16.6	0.75	1.45	190.0	13.1	35.9
9	1.5	25.0	0.75	1.47	230.0	15.6	40.4
10	2.0	8.3	0.5	2.1	152.0	7.2	23.1
11	2.0	16.6	0.5	2.0	256.0	12.8	39.8
12	2.0	25.0	0.5	2.0	344.0	17.2	53.4

[a] Concentration during the reaction = half the original concentration of 1, 2, 3, or 4 g/100 ml.

[b] Measured values after reconcentration to approximately the labeling condition values.

[c] The labeling efficiency of 100% FITC with rabbit gamma globulin is approximately 60%. The same dye with rabbit albumin would exhibit approximately 98% labeling efficiency. When rabbit gamma globulin is labeled, the final fluorescein to protein (F/P) ratio (e.g., 15) will be about 60% of the dye weight (e.g., 25) in μg/mg of protein, if the reaction is allowed to proceed to completion.

[d] Nonspecific staining.

FITC preparation. Infrared studies revealed a range of approximately 30 to 100% purity in commercially available FITC (29). The purity of the dye used in labeling directly affects the final F/P ratio obtained from a given weight of dye. In addition, conjugates prepared with FITC of low purity exhibit higher levels of NSS than those prepared from pure dyes (20, 37). The labeling procedures and dye weights discussed here are based on the use of pure (100%) FITC preparations. Dyes of less purity may be satisfactory if the weight used is adjusted to account for the impurities and if the impurities do not result in increased NSS. A value of 70% FITC, as determined by the bovine serum albumin test for labeling efficiency, has been adopted as the minimal quality acceptable for certification by the Biological Stain Commission (4). Only dyes of certifiable purity should be used.

To determine the weight of impure dye required to yield a given weight of a pure dye, multiply the desired weight of pure dye by 100 and divide by the percent purity of the dye used. For example, if 25 μg of 100% FITC per mg of protein is required, use 33.34 μg of 75% FITC per mg of protein (25 μg × 100/75 = 33.34 μg).

Conjugation procedure

Direct method. With this method, the total weight of FITC is in contact with the globulin during the entire reaction time. The data in Table 3 may be used as a guide for determining the set of conditions needed to achieve the desired F/P ratio by the direct method of labeling.

Reagents.

1. Na_2HPO_4, 0.2 M, pH 9—28.4 g dissolved and brought to 1 liter with distilled water.
2. Na_2HPO_4, 0.1 M, pH 9—14.2 g dissolved and brought to 1 liter with distilled water.
3. Na_3PO_4, 0.1 M—16.4 g dissolved and brought to 1 liter with distilled water. If $Na_3PO_4 \cdot 12H_2O$ is used, 38.0 g is required.
4. NaCl, 0.85%—8.5 g dissolved and brought to 1 liter with distilled water.
5. Phosphate-buffered saline (PBS), pH 7.6, 0.01 M.

Concentrated (10 ×) stock solution (pH is not 7.6 at this point)

Na_2HPO_4, anhydrous, reagent-grade	12.36 g
$NaH_2PO_4 \cdot H_2O$	1.80 g
NaCl, reagent-grade	85.00 g
Distilled water to a final volume of	1,000 ml

Working solution, PBS, pH 7.6, 0.01 M

Concentrated stock solution	100 ml
Distilled water to a final volume of	1,000 ml

Procedure.

1. Determine the protein concentration of the

globulin to be labeled by using the biuret (15), Kjeldahl (23), or ultraviolet (UV) absorption methods (23).

2. Stabilize the temperature of the globulin and all reagents to 25 C.

3. Calculate the total protein content of the globulin in mg: g of protein per 100 ml × 10 = mg of protein/ml; mg of protein/ml × volume of globulin in ml = total mg of protein

4. Calculate the weight of FITC to be used to achieve the desired F/P ratio. Example: label 12 ml of globulin which contains 1.4 g of protein per 100 ml so that a final F/P ratio of 15 is obtained. Total protein to be labeled = 168 mg (1.4 × 10 × 12). From Table 1, 25 μg of FITC/mg of protein gave an F/P of 15 to 16. Total mg of protein × 25 μg of FITC/mg of protein is the weight of dye needed

168 mg × 25 μg/mg = 4,200 μg = 4.2 mg of FITC.

5. Dissolve the calculated amount of FITC in a volume of 0.1 M Na_2HPO_4, pH 9, equal to half the volume of globulin to be labeled. Using the example in step 4, dissolve 4.2 mg of FITC in 6 ml of buffer. (The FITC solution must be used within 2 h of its preparation since it is unstable.)

6. Place the globulin in a flask large enough to contain more than twice its volume. The initial volume of globulin will be doubled and there must be room for mixing.

7. While gently stirring the globulin, add dropwise a volume of the 0.2 M Na_2HPO_4 equal to one-fourth the volume of the globulin. Using the example in step 4, add 3 ml of the buffer to the 12 ml of globulin.

8. Add, in the same manner, the FITC solution prepared in step 5. The amount of Na_2HPO_4 in this solution added to that used in step 7 results in a 0.05 M concentration of Na_2HPO_4 when the reaction mixture is at its final volume.

9. Immediately measure the pH of the mixture and adjust to 9.5 by dropwise addition of 0.1 M Na_3PO_4. This is necessary because of the reduction of the pH to 8 or below by the addition of the acidic FITC.

10. Add sufficient 0.85% NaCl to bring the final volume to twice the starting volume of globulin, which is 24 ml.

11. Gently mix the final solution, incubate at 25 C, and allow the reaction to proceed without agitation for the required length of time. The speed with which the mixture is brought to a final pH and volume is critical, since the reaction is already in progress. There is no advantage in long periods of labeling because the reaction is essentially complete within a maximum of 4 h under these conditions.

12. Remove by centrifugation even the slightest precipitate which might have formed during conjugation.

13. Remove all unreacted fluorescent material (UFM) from the conjugate by dialyzing for several days, or by passing the conjugate through a Sephadex column. The most economical method is dialysis against pH 7.6 PBS at 0 to 5 C. The important factors in the speed of dialysis are the maintenance of a steep gradient and frequent changes of the dialysate. The removal of UFM is complete when no fluorescence is visible in a sample of the dialysate observed in the dark under a Wood's lamp. Although it is rapid, the Sephadex method results in an approximately threefold dilution of the conjugate.

14. After removing UFM, remove all traces of precipitate by centrifugation.

15. As a preservative, add sodium azide (NaN_3) to a 0.1% concentration or Merthiolate to 1:10,000 and store the conjugates at 0 to 5 C, or freeze in several small portions. Conjugates also may be sterilized by membrane filtration and frozen, or they may be lyophilized. Freezing should be done quickly in a dry ice-alcohol mixture. Afterwards, the conjugates should be stored at −20 C or lower.

Dialysis method (5, 21). Data indicate that conjugates prepared by this method exhibit one-half the level of NSS obtained with those prepared by the direct method when the two are compared at equal FITC concentrations. In the dialysis method, the dissolved FITC slowly diffuses through a dialysis membrane into the globulin mixture and the dye concentration increases with time. For details of labeling by this method consult references 20 and 21.

Titration, sorption, and standardization of conjugates

Conjugates should be titered against the antigens which they are designed to detect, and their ability to stain related antigens should be determined. Usually, twofold dilutions of the conjugate in saline are prepared and used to stain appropriate smears; positive and negative control conjugates and antigens are used. Frequently, a diagnostic dilution can be selected which is specific, and which obviates the need for sorption of the reagent. If sorption is required, it should be performed on the serum or globulin rather than the labeled reagent. Sorption with tissue powders is an empirical method which is sometimes helpful in reducing NSS of tissues. Reagent protein is lost to the extent of

50% or more by tissue powder sorption, and conjugates are often contaminated by residual soluble tissue antigens. Generally, it is more profitable to produce higher-titered conjugates which can be diluted for use. For example, if undiluted conjugates containing 0.5% of antibody protein can be diluted 1:16 or more for use, NSS will be minimal. Important aspects of standardization of IF reagents are discussed in two recent papers (5, 33).

Anti-immunoglobulin reagents for the indirect IF tests should be examined by means of a box or checkerboard titration in which a series of doubling dilutions of both the unlabeled antibody (test serum) and the labeled antiglobulin are tested against each other (2, 16). In these tests the plateau titer is defined as the highest dilution of a positive serum which gives maximal fluorescence with the highest dilution of conjugate. This dilution of the conjugate is referred to as the plateau end point of the conjugate.

The most commonly used diagnostic applications based on indirect IF are probably the fluorescent treponemal antibody, the antinuclear factor, and the *Toxoplasma* tests. Appropriate positive and negative control conjugates constitute a vital part of these tests. In the indirect IF procedure, controls should consist primarily of both homologous and heterologous species antisera known to be either positive or negative for the antigen. The indicator reagent (labeled homologous antiglobulin) control should consist of labeled normal globulin or labeled heterologous antiglobulin.

In addition to performance evaluation, the quality of diagnostic IF reagents can be ascertained by applying physicochemical procedures. The most valuable of these are (i) determination of the F/P ratio, (ii) cellulose acetate strip electrophoresis (CASE), including the fluorescence profile, (iii) immunoelectrophoresis, and (iv) specific antibody globulin. Fluorescein should be determined by the method of McKinney et al. (30) with fluorescein diacetate used as a standard. Protein may be assayed by any of the methods mentioned earlier or by the procedure of Lowry et al. (27). Expressing F/P ratios as the ratio of absorbance at λ 495 nm to that at λ 280 nm cannot be recommended except for screening purposes since the absolute level of FITC as well as the F/P ratio influences NSS and since aromatic compounds having a high absorbance at λ 280 nm are sometimes added to commercial conjugates as preservatives. F/P ratios should be expressed as micrograms of bound FITC per milligram of protein. To obtain this value, divide the protein-bound FITC concentration in μg/ml by the protein concentration in mg/ml. Some workers prefer molar ratios which can be derived from weight ratios by multiplying by the factor 0.411. The latter is derived from the expression

$$\frac{160{,}000}{389 \times 10^3} = 0.411$$

where 160,000 is taken as the average molecular weight of immunoglobulin, 389 as the molecular weight of FITC, and 10^3 converts milligrams to micrograms.

CASE analysis has more value for predicting the performance of a conjugate than any other test, except possibly an independent quantitative assay of specific antibody, which is a much more difficult procedure. Immunoelectrophoresis may yield valuable information about the class specificity of the conjugated antibody and, in conjunction with CASE, indicates the addition to commercial conjugates of other serum proteins as stabilizers or inhibitors.

The relationship of some of the above physicochemical factors to the performance of conjugates has been discussed elsewhere (14, 20, 24, 42, 43, 45).

FLUORESCENT-ANTIBODY MICROSCOPY

Basic principles of fluorescence microscopy are covered in chapter 3, but some important considerations relating to IF must be dealt with here. The essential components of fluorescence lighting and optical equipment for transmitted and incident light fluorescence are shown in Fig. 2 and 3. Lighting sources are usually mercury arc or the newer quartz-iodine-tungsten (halogen) lamps, although xenon lamps also are used for photography, for high intensity excitation at the longer visible wavelengths, and as a stable light source for quantitative IF measurements with incident light. Xenon lamps require DC power supplies which are very expensive. Thus, they will not be discussed further. The HBO-100 mercury arc lamp also is operated from a very expensive DC power supply. Both continuous-wave and pulsed-dye lasers are being introduced for more sophisticated quantitative measurements of fluorescence.

The characteristics of the most useful systems will be discussed as briefly as possible.

Survey of microscopes and illuminators

Those contemplating the purchase of equipment for fluorescence microscopy should realize that this is a new field in which rapid changes are taking place. The choice of equipment is

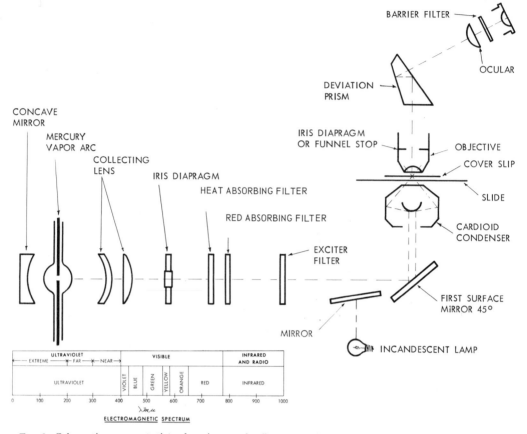

FIG. 2. *Schematic representation of equipment for fluorescence microscopy.*

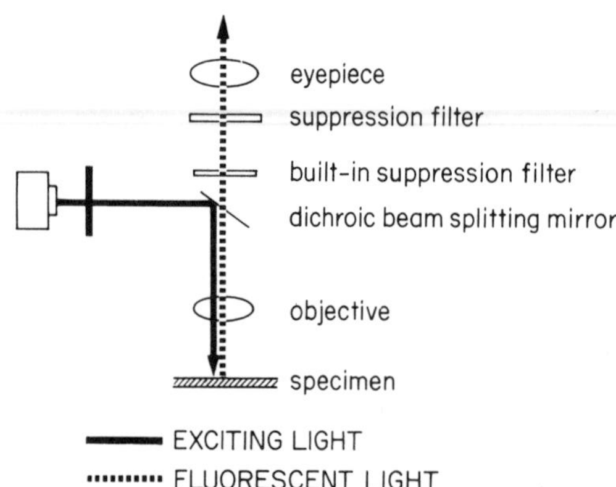

FIG. 3. *Incident-light fluorescence. (Reproduced from Koch [25] with permission of E. Leitz, GMBH, Wetzlar.)*

determined by (i) how it will be used—for research, routine testing, diagnostic work, etc., (ii) the systems to be studied, (iii) personal preference, and (iv) financial considerations. The best arrangement is that which gives the desired result for the biological systems being investigated.

Since the first edition of this *Manual*, two very important developments for IF microscopy have occurred. One was the introduction of the halogen lamp with the interference filter for excitation of fluors whose maximal absorption peaks are at the longer visible wavelengths, e.g., FITC, and rhodamine. These low-wattage (100) lamps are inexpensive and do not require expensive transformers for operation as do mercury or xenon lamps. Because their emission intensity is low in the shorter wavelength portion of the visible spectrum, they could not be used until narrow band-pass interference filters became available which would allow excitation of the fluors at their absorption maximum.

In Fig. 4 is shown a comparison of the relative intensity of various excitation sources. Note that the most commonly used halogen lamp (100 W) has only a fraction of the intensity of the HBO-200 mercury arc lamp at the absorption maximums of FITC (490 nm) and tetramethylrhodamine isothiocyanate (546 nm).

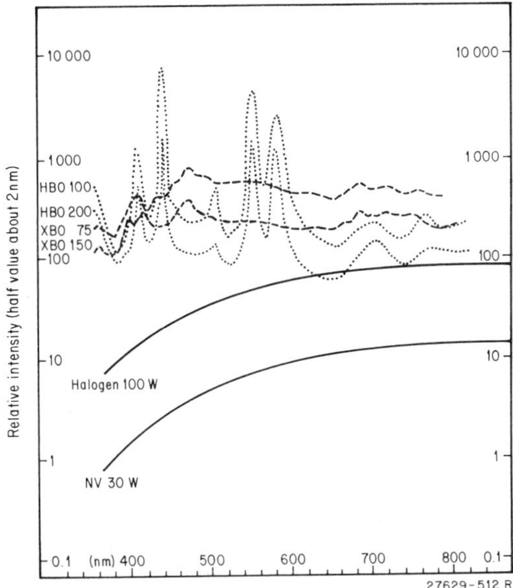

FIG. 4. *Intensity comparison of various light sources suitable for fluorescence microscopy (referred to 6-V 30-W lamp). (Reproduced from Koch [25] with permission of E. Leitz, GMBH, Wetzlar.)*

Nevertheless, experience is proving that halogen lamps are suitable for most routine applications of IF procedures provided that suitable interference filters are used for excitation and that these are matched with appropriate barrier filters.

The second major improvement in IF equipment was the introduction of incident-light or epi-illumination by Ploem (38; see also chapter 3). As shown in Fig. 3, exciting radiation of the desired λ is deflected downward into the objective by a beam-splitting or dichroic mirror (25). The full aperture of the objective is used both for excitation and for transmission of fluorescence to the observer; the light beam is automatically centered because the objective also acts as condenser. For incident lighting, objectives of the largest possible numerical aperture (NA) should be used in order to obtain high intensity. Stimulation of fluorescence in the surface layers of the specimen insures minimal loss of emission intensity by absorption within the specimen itself. The success of incident-light fluorescence depends upon the selection of appropriate dichroic beam-splitting mirrors and suppression filters supplemented by excitation filters selected for their ability to further narrow and separate excitation radiation from fluorescence emission. The crucial selection is performed by the dichroic mirror which, in the case of FITC, deflects, at a 90° angle, the blue light transmitted by the exciting filter while allowing radiation of longer λ to pass through (Fig. 3). Since the yellow-green fluorescence excited by the blue radiation is of longer λ, it is now transmitted upward through the dichroic mirror while blue light reflected from the specimen slide is again reflected by the mirror away from the observer.

The plethora of equipment manufacturers and of illuminating systems makes it impracticable to discuss them individually. The reader should note that the most commonly used excitation sources are the mercury arc and the halogen lamp and that the two basic illumination systems are transmitted-light and incident-light fluorescence. Excitation sources and illumination systems may be combined in many ways, including simultaneous use of incident and transmitted excitation. For example, the latter is well adapted to the demonstration of two different antigens in the same smear when one is labeled with FITC and the other with rhodamine. Since the absorption maxima of the two fluors are quite different, they cannot be excited to maximal fluorescence by a single narrow band-pass filter. In the dual instrument the excitation system most favorable for each fluor may be used; the dichroic mirror serves to transmit both long λ fluorescence emissions.

When the mercury arc lamp is used, many diagnostic applications require auxiliary low-voltage tungsten lamp illumination with a convenient switch-over mechanism. The result is a conventional dark field in which both stained and unstained particles may be observed. This system is helpful in (i) focusing the microscope, (ii) providing information on the nature and number of nonfluorescent objects, and (iii) serving as a control on the preparation and handling of the specimen.

Assuming the availability of both incident- and transmitted-light fluorescence capability in a single system, the following combinations as listed by Koch (25) may be useful for special purposes: (i) conventional transmitted-light dark-field combined with incident-light fluorescence or with transmitted-light dark-field fluorescence, (ii) incident-light fluorescence combined with transmitted-light phase contrast, and (iii) incident-light fluorescence combined with transmitted polarized light. The uses of systems i and ii are essentially those listed in the preceding paragraph. The combination in number iii is useful for simultaneous demonstrations of polarization and fluorescence in birefringent specimens (25).

For research purposes, workers should attempt to purchase fluorescence equipment that has the versatility required for a variety of uses. Expenditures for combined incident- and transmitted-light systems including interchangeable mercury arc and halogen lamp housings will undoubtedly prove to be a good investment. It is unlikely that this equipment will become obsolete for many years. Laser light sources provide much higher excitation intensity than is needed or is desirable except for precise quantitation.

Objectives (see also chapter 3)

There are four major types of objectives that will be of interest to the fluorescence microscopist: (i) achromats, (ii) apochromats, (iii) fluorite, and (iv) plano. All objectives are characterized by certain numerical apertures, magnifications, and working distances.

Achromatic objectives are the least corrected and least expensive lenses. Since they have fewer lenses, there is less light loss by reflection. Fluorite objectives lie between the achromats and the apochromats; they are corrected both chromatically and spherically for two colors. At least one lens of the fluorite objectives consists of calcium fluorite, which exhibits autofluorescence. However, difficulties arising from autofluorescence are minimal when the objective is used with a dark-field condenser. Apochromats consist of seven or more lenses, some of which are fluorite. Their focusing is more critical, reflected light losses are greater, and they are more expensive than the above objectives. However, if maximal resolution and brightness are required, these highly corrected objectives with their larger apertures may be used.

In fluorescence microscopy, there are certain factors which encourage the use of the less expensive achromatic objectives. Most microscopists use the cardioid or bispheric dark-field condenser for illumination because the contrast is better than it is with a bright-field condenser. In addition, the fluorescence spectrum is frequently almost monochromatic, and, in the case of fluorescein, it is emitted in the green band, a region in which the retina is maximally sensitive.

Plano objectives are designed primarily for photomicroscopy where flatness of the field is of great importance. The improved performance is gained at the price of higher sensitivity to the thickness of the slide and cover glass, and substantially increased costs.

Very recently, some very good water immersion objectives have become available. One series consists of the following lenses (25):

W 25/0.60
W 50/1.00
W 100/1.20

They obviate the messiness of oil and are particularly recommended for incident-light fluorescence.

Eyepieces

See chapter 3 for a detailed discussion of oculars and an interpretation of the microscopic images.

Condensers

Dark-field condensers are used almost exclusively for IF work because (i) it is difficult to achieve the desired contrast with bright-field condensers and because (ii) objectives containing fluorite lenses can be used successfully with a dark-field condenser.

The two major types of dark-field condensers are (i) refracting and (ii) reflecting. The basic difference is the NA achievable with each. The former may be used with objectives whose NA does not exceed 0.85, i.e., low- and medium-power lenses. The latter are required for higher-power objectives and are used for most IF work. Either the bispheric or cardioid type of doubly reflecting condenser is preferred. Both types of condensers produce a hollow cone of light having a range of NA from about 1.20 to about 1.40. The maximal NA of the oil immersion objectives which can be used successfully with such condensers is approximately 0.05 less than the NA of the condenser. If this relationship is not maintained, light enters directly into the objective and destroys the dark-field effect. Control is achieved preferably by an iris diaphragm which permits variable adjustment of the NA of the objective. It should be remembered that light from these high NA condensers cannot fill the field of low-power objectives, e.g., 10×. All condensers must be oiled to the undersurface of the slide on which the preparation is mounted. For dark-field fluorescence microscopy, the importance of maintaining a homogeneous optical system from condenser to oil immersion objective cannot be overemphasized.

Slides

According to Needham (34), all light-field and dark-field condensers will focus through slides of an average thickness of 1.1 mm, and he suggested that these be adopted for all high-power microscopy. Assuming good quality and uniformity of the glass, slide thickness is not too critical. However, it must be realized that serious problems arise when the slide is either so thick that the focal point of the condenser is within the glass itself or so thin that oil contact cannot be maintained either between the condenser and slide or between the objective and cover slip. For some years, we have used successfully, with a variety of fluorescence microscopes, special slides whose thickness specification is 1.1 to 1.2 mm and on which are etched two circles, each 14 mm in diameter (Trident Fluoro Slides #V58958, A. S. Aloe Co., St. Louis, Mo.). Cel-Line Associates (P.O. Box 213, Minotola, N.J.) markets standard slides printed with various numbers and sizes of wells, and the company will custom prepare special slides of any design. If used with acetone, specifications should call for an acetone-resistant coating. Slides with any desired number of wells outlined by a Teflon-like compound (Fluoro-Glide, Chemplast, Inc.) can be prepared very cheaply in the laboratory (12). These multi-well slides expedite the performance and decrease the cost of routine IF testing.

The American Optical Co.'s dark-field condenser is designed for use with slides of 1.15- to 1.25-mm thickness on which no. 1 (0.13 to 0.17 mm) cover glasses are mounted. Both slides and cover glasses should be made of clear nonfluorescent glass and should be cleaned thoroughly before use.

Cover glasses

The thickness of the cover glasses used for IF microscopy is critical (see chapter 3.) Commercial cover slips are rather uniform in refractive index (n) but vary widely in thickness; the latter condition is frequently responsible for the hazy, bleached appearance of the image (Technical Information Bulletin, vol. 1, no. 4, 1961, E. Leitz, Inc., New York, N.Y.). The allowable deviation in thickness beyond which image quality is impaired decreases rapidly with an increase in NA of the objective. For example, with a dry objective at an NA of 0.95, a deviation of 0.003 mm in cover slip thickness will cause a noticeable decrease in image quality. Oil immersion objectives are less sensitive to cover slip thickness than high dry lenses. If the refractive index of the mounting medium differs from that of the cover glass, it may have considerable influence upon the image quality. The microscopist should strive to achieve as homogeneous a dispersive system as possible.

Binocular versus monocular

The choice of binocular versus monocular heads for microscopes used in IF studies is purely a matter of utility. The binocular head is more comfortable. With lower power objectives and larger specimens, it may be used to advantage. Enough light can be obtained with certain fluorescence equipment to permit binocular viewing of bacteria by oil immersion.

Immersion oil

For fluorescence microscopy, it is imperative that a nonfluorescent oil such as Cargille's type A very low fluorescence, nondrying immersion oil for microscopy be used (Fisher Scientific Co., Pittsburgh, Pa.). It has an n of 1.515 at 25 C. Excess oil or oil of high viscosity on either the condenser or the cover slip should be avoided, and all oil should be removed from the former when the day's work is finished. Care must be taken to keep the oil clean and clear.

Mounting fluid

Buffered glycerol saline (nine parts of glycerol to one part [vol/vol] of buffered saline, pH 9.0) has been used extensively as a semipermanent mounting medium. Cover slips may be sealed with clear fingernail polish, and some preparations may be preserved at 4 C for periods of several weeks or months. However, results are not consistent from one antigen or one specimen to another.

In the CDC laboratory, polyvinyl alcohol mounting media consisting of either 10 or 15% Elvanol (Elvanol Grade 51-05, E. I. DuPont de Nemours and Co., Electrochemicals Dept.) or 5% Gelvatol (Gelvatol 3-60, Shawiningan Resins Corp., Springfield, Mass.) mounting media permitted storage of smears of pure cultures of *Escherichia coli* and *Shigella sonnei*. The *E. coli* could be stored for 13 months and the *S. sonnei* for 5 months at 25, 4, and −40 C without detectable loss of specific fluorescence (43). However, fecal smears containing either *E. coli* or *S. sonnei* were unsatisfactory after 3 months of storage at any temperature. With all mounting media, the cover glass should be pressed down firmly so that its thickness will not be increased by the mountant and result in hazy images.

Mounting media may be adjusted to any pH compatible with the fluorescence of the fluorochrome used, but for FITC it should not be lower than 7.0 because fluorescence decreases rapidly below this pH. It has been recommended that FITC preparations be mounted in glycerol saline buffered to a pH of 9.0 to increase the intensity of fluorescence (36). The apparent specific titer of a conjugate is increased by this procedure, but nonspecific staining is increased concomitantly. Also the pH decreases with time because of oxidation of the glycerol and absorption of CO_2 by the mounting fluid. A pH of 8.0 is easier to maintain. In any event, fresh mountant should be prepared at least once a month, or more often if any color or turbidity appears. The pH should be taken with a meter and the fluid should be adjusted to the desired level.

Filters (see also chapter 3)

Selection of an appropriate combination of exciter (primary) and barrier or suppression (secondary) filters is essential for successful IF work. Complexity has resulted from the introduction of interference filters and dichroic mirrors. The nature of the preparation being observed, the kind of information desired, and the personal preferences of the observer also are important factors in filter selection. In general, the barrier filter is chosen to absorb most, if not all, of the exciting radiation passed by the exciting filter (Fig. 5). This arrangement maximizes the darkness of the background and enhances contrast. On the other hand, some workers use a barrier filter which allows some of the exciting radiation to pass. Thus, the filter serves as an optical blue counterstain against which the yellow-green fluorescence of FITC is observed; the demonstration of rabies antigen in tissue sections or imprints is an excellent example of the use of this technique. Some IF experts also prefer near UV (365 nm) excitation because the various colors produced by autofluorescence of tissue components aid in the histological localization of the specific fluorescence.

Until the introduction of interference filters, which made possible the use of weaker light sources, mercury arc lamps were used almost exclusively for excitation. When these lamps are used with glass filters, the fluorescence of FITC-stained specimens usually is excited with light in the λ band 350 to 450 nm, although fluorescein absorbs maximally at 490 nm (Fig. 6). Conversely, the intensity spectrum of the mercury vapor arc is relatively low at 490 nm (Fig. 4).

Interference filters combined with appropriate dichroic mirrors and suppression filters make it possible to utilize halogen lamps for excitation by either transmitted- or incident-light microscopy.

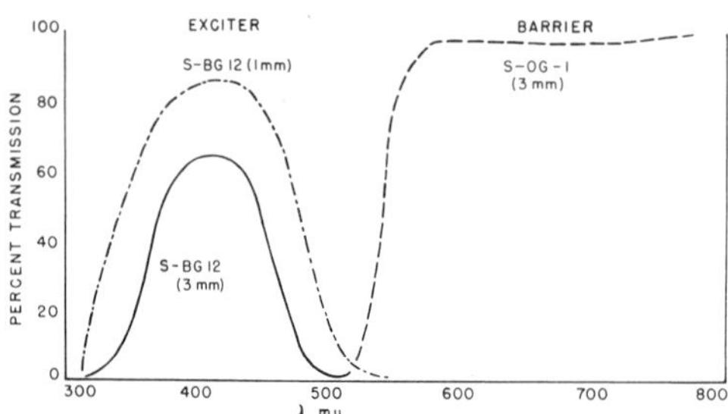

FIG. 5. *Principle of complementary filters.*

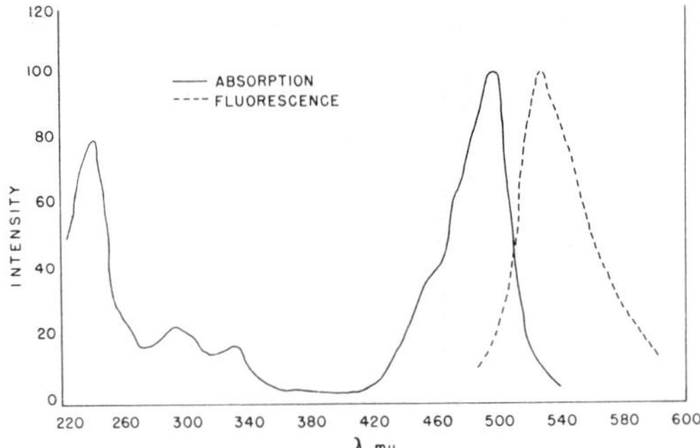

FIG. 6. *Absorption and fluorescence of fluorescein in alkaline solution.*

Some of the most popular and useful combinations of filters for IF work are given in Table 4. No attempt is made to include filter designations used by all manufacturers or to suggest combinations for specific applications. Table 4 includes both glass and gelatin filters which have been in use for transmitted-light fluorescence for many years and also the newer narrow band-pass interference filters used for both transmitted- and incident-light excitation. Dichroic (beam splitting) mirrors required for incident-light fluorescence are not included in the table. Filters should be identified by the designations used by their makers rather than by those of the distributor. The user can then consult the appropriate specifications catalogues. Each filter should be accompanied by a transmittance versus wavelength curve plotted on two-cycle semilog paper. These graphs should be plotted to the same scale and size so that the user can make a rapid and direct comparison of filters from different sources.

Most filters used in IF work are manufactured by Schott and Gen., Mainz, West Germany (Schott Optical Glass, Inc., Duryea, Pa., U.S. factory), by Balzers in Liechtenstein (Optonetics, Inc., Manhasset, N.Y., U.S. distributor). by Barr and Stroud, Ltd., Glasgow, Scotland, or by Corning Glass Works, Corning, N.Y. Gelatin filters are made by Eastman Kodak Co., Rochester, N.Y.

In Table 4 data are given only for the HBO-200 and tungsten-halogen sources. Slight modifications in type or thickness of filters may be necessary if xenon or other wattage mercury vapor lamps are used for excitation. Filter thicknesses are given for most of the glasses since thickness strongly influences light transmission at a given λ, especially if the maximal transmission is rather low. This is because the transmittance of a filter decreases exponentially

TABLE 4. *Some useful filter combinations for immunofluorescence work*[a]

Light source	Type, thickness, and designation of filter systems for FITC and TRITC							
	Heat-absorbing	Thickness (mm)	Red-absorbing	Thickness (mm)	Primary	Thickness- (mm)	Secondary	Thickness (mm)
					FITC			
HBO-200	KG[b] 1; BG[b] 22; AO[c] 713 or AO 308	2–4	BG 38 or BG 14	2–3	BG 12; AO 702 or AO 2064; or S 400/Leitz	3	OG[b] 1; AO 1124 or AO-OG 515; OG 4; Zeiss/50 or 53; K 510 or K 530; Leitz/Blau Abs 3384[d] or W12[e]	1–2 3
	KG 1 or BG 22	2–4	BG 38 or BG 14	2–3	BG25	3	OG 1 or OG 4 3384 or W12	1–2 3
	KG 1 or BG 22	2–4	BG 38 or BG 14	2–3	UG[b] 1; 5840[d]; AO 693 or AO 2066; FL 405/Zeiss; or S 360 (Leitz)	2	W2A (EK2A); AO 1106; Zeiss/41, 44, or 47; Leitz/UV Abs, Euphos, or UV 2; GG[b] 9; AO 1123	1–2
	KG 1 or BG 22	2–4	BG 38 or BG 14	2–3	BG 3 + UG 5, or S 370 (Leitz) AL[f] 405	2	Zeiss/47 K 460 K490	1–2
	KG 1	2–4	BG 38	2–4	KP[f] 490 or 2× KP 490[g] KP 500[g] + K 480[h]		K 510 (OG 4) or K 530 (OG 1) K 510 or K 530 or Zeiss/53	1–2
Tungsten-halogen 12 V 100 W	B1/K2		BG38	2–4	KP 490 or KP 500		K 510; K 530; AL 525	1–2
					TRITC			
HBO-200 or tungsten-halogen	KG 1	2	BG 38	2–4	BG 36 (2 mm) + AL 546 (S[f] 546 Leitz); AO-IF 530; FL[f] 546/Zeiss		K 580; K 590; K 610 AO-OG 570; 58/Zeiss	1–2

[a] All filters may be used with both transmitted and incident lighting. Dichroic mirrors required for incident-light fluorescence and frequently used for transmitted-light fluorescence are not included in the table. The TK series of beam splitters is made by Leitz. FITC, fluorescein isothiocyanate; TRITC, tetramethylrhodamine isothiocyanate.

[b] KG, BG, OG, UG, S, and GG = Schott filters.

[d] 3384 and 5840 = Corning filters.

[e] W and EK2A = Kodak Wratten Gelatin filters.

[f] KP, AL, FL and S 546 = interference filters. The KP series is made by Balzers.

[g] 2× KP 490 = two separate KP 490 filters; KP 500 = two combined KP 490 filters.

[h] K 480 = edge filter to eliminate autofluorescence of λ below 480 nm. All K-series filters are distributed by Leitz. A similar series of edge filters designated LP is listed by Zeiss.

as its thickness increases arithmetically. This may be expressed as

$$\log T_2 = \frac{d_2}{d_1} \log T_1$$

where d_1 and d_2 are filter thickness and T_1 and T_2 are transmittance of the filters. Decreasing filter thickness increases light transmission, but it also broadens the transmission band which may result in loss of filter complementarity.

Photomicroscopy

The photography of fluorescent microscopic specimens is important to the laboratory worker because of its value in training and in the illustration of published reports. It is unfortunate that the reproduction of color photographs is so expensive, since they are far superior to black and white images for illustrative purposes. Color slides are used almost exclusively for projection because they are inexpensive and can reproduce faithfully the visual impression of the microscope field. If black and white prints are desired, they can be prepared from color transparencies.

For fluorescence photomicroscopy with a dark-field condenser, 35-mm film is most practical. Some workers attach a camera back (without lens) directly to the ocular. The spherical aberration produced causes a significant decrease in image clarity, especially with high dry objectives. A lens system which focuses the eye lens image onto the film plane should not be omitted.

The simplest way to obtain an exposure calibration is to perform a series of trial exposures. Bring into focus a specimen to be photographed. Place an ordinary pocket exposure meter over the aperture which directs light into the condenser, and measure and record the intensity. Expose the film. Repeat the process five or more times, doubling the exposure time at each step. Develop the film, select the best photograph, and note the exposure time. Subsequently, if the same optical arrangement and film are used, the most favorable exposure times should be near those determined by the trial series.

Using the same geometry as before, periodically measure the intensity of the light source. If the original intensity is divided by that fraction remaining after some period of time, the quotient is the relative increase in exposure time required to normalize photographic results. For example, if the meter indicates three-fourths the light intensity used for the trial exposure, the exposure time should be multiplied by 1.0/0.75 = 1.3. The photographer should be aware that reciprocity failure may occur, especially with slow color film at long exposures.

In our laboratories, good photographic results have been obtained by using the Leitz Micro-Ibso photographic attachment for a 35-mm camera back. The unit houses a lens to focus and flatten the image in the film plane, a cable-operated shutter with time and bulb settings, a lateral observation and focusing telescopic lens for viewing the image on a glass screen, and a prism which can be moved in or out of position by means of a cable. The best viewing telescopes contain a totally reflecting prism and a clear glass screen; both modifications are required to produce images bright enough for sharp focusing. In practice, the film holder and attachment unit incorporating the microscope ocular is placed into the barrel of the microscope. Usually, the primary and secondary filters which are used for visual observation also are used for photomicroscopy (Table 4). However, some experimentation with other combinations of filters is highly desirable because the colors recorded on film seldom parallel their visual interpretation. When the image is in focus through the telescopic viewer, the prism is moved from the light path and the film is exposed. Good fluorescent images have been obtained even at film plane magnifications of 400 or more (1,200 × at microscope ocular). Anscochrome D/200 (ASA-200) film made by General Aniline and Film Corp. gives excellent results; exposure times generally range from 30 s to 3 min. Eastman Ektachrome film (ASA-200) may give very satisfactory results with incident-light excitation systems (KP-490 and K-510 filters); however, special processing of the film to approximate ASA-400 may be required. Either daylight or indoor-type film may be used; the former is preferred because its color temperature response more nearly matches the fluorescence emission of FITC. Little is to be gained by exposures longer than 3 min because of the rapidity with which the fluorescence fades. Kodak Tri X black and white film has been used at exposure times varying from a few seconds to 1 min. The photographic area should be free from vibration. It should be remembered that the field of the 10× objective cannot be filled with light by dark-field illumination.

The objective of color photomicroscopy is to obtain on film all of the pertinent information available by visual observation of the microscope field.

Quantitation

The quantitation of fluorescence in routine

diagnostic work usually is based on visual observation of the brightness or relative contrast of the specifically stained antigen. This furnishes a rough but satisfactory estimate when used in conjunction with positive and negative controls. For mercury arc lamps, excitation intensity can be adjusted, within limits, by means of an inexpensive voltage regulator placed between the power pack and the power source. For the HBO-200 mercury arc lamp, care should be taken not to increase the voltage times amperage (VA) across the lamp above 230.

IF microscopy has developed to the point where quantitation by precise photometric measurements of fluorescence is being seriously investigated. Commercial equipment is available for measuring the fluorescence of single cells, even those as small as bacteria. Usually the results have been expressed in units relative to an arbitrarily selected fluorescence standard such as a preserved stained preparation, a uranyl glass slide, or a known volume of fluorescein enclosed in a microcapillary. More recently, combined immunological-fluorescence standards have been devised. These consist of known amounts of purified antigen or antibody covalently bound to cellulose or agarose beads. When, for example, antigen-treated beads are exposed to FITC-labeled antibody and the fluorescence activity is measured, the results can be related to a given weight of antigen or a number of international units. In this way a valid basis for comparison of the potency of conjugates is established. The above techniques have been reviewed (5, 22).

Recently, Taylor and Heimer (41) succeeded in developing a system for expressing the fluorescence of single cells of *E. coli* in international physical units of candelas per square meter.

Automation

Although several papers dealing with the automation of IF procedures have appeared, I am not aware of anyone routinely using a system including both specimen processing and automatic recording of fluorescence. The Seromatic system (Aerojet Medical and Biological Systems, El Monte, Calif.) encompasses a mechanical slide processor, but the fluorescence is read visually (26). The same company has an electronic readout system under evaluation at the present time. A major problem is finding a way to differentiate specific from unwanted fluorescence without increasing the cost of equipment until it is prohibitive.

ACKNOWLEDGMENTS

I am indebted to personnel of the Analytical Bacteriology Section of the CDC for having provided some of the data used in the preparation of this chapter. I would especially like to thank Ann Hebert, Bertie Pittman, and Roger McKinney for revisions of the serum fractionation and labeling procedures and for their constructive criticism.

LITERATURE CITED

1. Bergquist, N. R., and W. G. E. E. Schilling. 1970. Preparation of antihuman immunoglobulin for indirect fluorescent tracing of auto-antibodies, p. 171. *In* E. J. Holborow (ed.), Standardization in immunofluorescence. Blackwell Scientific Publications, Oxford, England.
2. Beutner, E. H., M. R. Sepulveda, and E. V. Barnett. 1968. Quantitative studies of immunofluorescent staining. Bull. W.H.O. **39:**587–606.
3. Brooks, J. B., V. J. Lewis, and B. Pittman. 1965. Separation of fluorescent antibody conjugates into 7S and 19S globulin components by gel filtration. Proc. Soc. Exp. Biol. Med. **119:**748–751.
4. Cherry, W. B., R. M. McKinney, V. M. Emmel, J. T. Spillane, G. A. Hebert, and B. Pittman. 1969. Evaluation of commercial fluorescein isothiocyanates used in fluorescent antibody studies. Stain Technol. **44:**179–186.
5. Cherry, W. B., and C. B. Reimer. 1973. Diagnostic immunofluorescence. Bull. W.H.O. **48:**737–746.
6. Clark, H. F., and C. C. Shepard. 1963. A dialysis technique for preparing fluorescent antibody. Virology **20:**642–644.
7. Cohen, I. R., L. C. Norins, and A. J. Julian. 1967. Competition between, and effectiveness of, IgG and IgM antibodies in indirect fluorescent antibody and other tests. J. Immunol. **98:**143–149.
8. Curtain, C. C. 1961. The chromatographic purification of fluorescein-antibody. J. Histochem. Cytochem. **9:**484–486.
9. Dubert, J. M., P. Slizewicz, P. Rebeyrotte, and M. Macheboeuf. 1953. Nouvelle methode de separation des proteines seriques par le methanol. Ann. Inst. Pasteur (Paris) **84:**370–375.
10. Fife, E. H., and L. H. Muschel. 1959. Fluorescent antibody technique for serodiagnosis of *Trypanosoma cruzi* infection. Proc. Soc. Exp. Biol. Med. **101:**540–543.
11. Flodin, P., and J. Killander. 1962. Fractionation of human-serum proteins by gel filtration. Biochim. Biophys. Acta **63:**402–410.
12. Frommhagen, L. H., and M. J. Martins. 1963. A comparison of fluorescein-labeled γ-globulins purified by Rivanol and DEAE chromatography. J. Immunol. **90:**116–120.
13. Goldman, M. 1968. Fluorescent antibody methods. Academic Press Inc., New York.
14. Goldstein, G., I. S. Slizys, and M. W. Chase. 1961. Studies of fluorescent antibody staining. I. Nonspecific fluorescence with fluorescein-coupled sheep anti-rabbit globulins. J. Exp. Med. **114:**89–110.
15. Gornall, A. G., D. J. Bardawill, and M. M. David. 1949. Determination of serum proteins by means of the Biuret reaction. J. Biol. Chem. **117:**751–766.
16. Hardy, P. H., and E. E. Nell. 1971. Characteristics of fluorescein-labelled anti-globulin preparations that may affect the fluorescent treponemal antibody-absorption test. Amer. J. Clin. Pathol. **56:**181–186.
17. Hebert, G. A. 1974. Ammonium sulfate fractionation of sera: mouse, hamster, guinea pig, monkey, chimpanzee, swine, chicken, and cattle. Appl. Microbiol. **27:**389–393.
18. Hebert, G. A., P. L. Pelham, and B. Pittman. 1973.

Determination of the optimal ammonium sulfate concentration for the fractionation of rabbit, sheep, horse, and goat antisera. Appl. Microbiol. **25:**26–36.

19. Hebert, G. A., and B. Pittman. 1965. Factors affecting removal of $(NH_4)_2SO_4$ from salt fractionated serum globulins employing a spectrophotometric procedure for determination of sulfate. Health Lab. Sci. **2:**48–53.
20. Hebert, G. A., B. Pittman, and W. B. Cherry. 1967. Factors affecting the degree of nonspecific staining given by fluorescein isothiocyanate labeled globulins. J. Immunol. **98:**1204–1212.
21. Hebert, G. A., B. Pittman, R. M. McKinney, and W. B. Cherry. 1972. The preparation and physicochemical characterization of fluorescent antibody reagents. Center for Disease Control, Atlanta, Ga.
22. Jongsma, P. M., W. Hijmans, and J. S. Ploem. 1971. Quantitative immunofluorescence. Histochemie **25:**329–343.
23. Kabat, E. A., and M. M. Mayer. 1961. Experimental immunochemistry, 2nd ed. Charles C Thomas, Publisher, Springfield, Ill.
24. Kaufman, L., and W. B. Cherry. 1961. Technical factors affecting the preparation of fluorescent antibody reagents. J. Immunol. **87:**72–79.
25. Koch, K. F. 1972. Fluorescence microscopy. Instruments, methods, applications. Ernst Leitz GMBH, Wetzlar.
26. Lewis, J. S., W. P. Duncan, and G. W. Stout. 1970. Automated fluorescent treponemal antibody test: instrument and evaluation. Appl. Microbiol. **19:**898–901.
27. Lowry, O. H., N. J. Rosebrough, A. L. Farr, and R. J. Randall. 1951. Protein measurement with the Folin phenol reagent. J. Biol. Chem. **193:**265–275.
28. McKinney, R. M., J. T. Spillane, and G. W. Pearce, 1964. Factors affecting the rate of reaction of fluorescein isothiocyanate with serum proteins. J. Immunol. **93:**232–242.
29. McKinney, R. M., J. T. Spillane, and G. W. Pearce. 1964. Determination of purity of fluorescein isothiocyanates. Anal. Biochem. **7:**74–86.
30. McKinney, R. M., J. T. Spillane, and G. W. Pearce. 1964c. Fluorescein diacetate as a reference color standard in fluorescent antibody studies. Anal. Biochem. **9:**474–476.
31. Mostratos, A., and T. S. L. Beswick. 1969. Comparison of some simple methods of preparing γ-globulin and antiglobulin sera for use in the indirect immunofluorescence technique. J. Pathol. **98:**17–24.
32. Nadel, M. K., and T. R. Carski. 1964. Investigation into factors influencing staining intensities of rabies immunofluorescent conjugates. Health Lab. Sci. **1:**60–64.
33. Nairn, R. C. 1968. Standardization in immunofluorescence. Clin. Exp. Immunol. **3:**465–476.
34. Needham, G. H. 1958. The practical use of the microscope. Charles C Thomas, Publsiher, Springfield, Ill.
35. Nichol, J. C., and H. F. Deutsch. 1948. Biophysical studies of blood plasma proteins. VII. Separation of γ-globulin from the sera of various animals. J. Amer. Chem. Soc. **70:**80–83.
36. Pital, A., and S. L. Janowitz. 1963. Enhancement of staining intensity in the fluorescent-antibody reaction. J. Bacteriol. **86:**888–889.
37. Pittman, B., G. A. Hebert, W. B. Cherry, and G. C. Taylor. 1967. The quantitation of nonspecific staining as a guide for improvement of fluorescent antibody conjugates. J. Immunol. **98:**1196–1203.
38. Ploem, J. S. 1967. The use of a vertical illuminator with interchangeable dichroic mirrors for fluorescence microscope with incident light. Z. Wiss. Mikrosk. **68:**129–142.
39. Riggs, J. L., P. C. Loh, and W. C. Eveland. 1960. A simple fractionation method for preparation of fluorescein-labeled gamma globulin. Proc. Soc. Biol. Med. **105:**655–658.
40. Sela, M., D. Givol, and E. Mozes. 1963. Resolution of rabbit γ-globulin into two fractions by chromatography on diethylaminoethyl-sepahdex. Biochim. Biophys. Acta **78:**649–657.
41. Taylor, C. E. D., and G. V. Heimer. 1974. Measuring immunofluorescence emission in terms of standard international physical units. J. Biol. Standard. **2:**11–20.
42. The, T. H., and T. E. W. Feltkamp. 1970. Conjugation of fluorescein isothiocyanate to antibodies. I. Experiments on the conditions of conjugation. Immunology **18:**865–874.
43. The, T. H., and T. E. W. Feltkamp. 1970. Conjugation of fluorescein isothiocyanate to antibodies. II. A reproducible method. Immunology **18:**875–881.
44. Thomason, B. M., and G. S. Cowart. 1967. Evaluation of polyvinyl alcohols as semipermanent mountants for fluorescent-antibody studies. J. Bacteriol. **93:**768–769.
45. Wood, B. T., S. H. Thompson, and G. Goldstein. 1965. Fluorescent antibody staining. III. Preparation of fluorescein-isothiocyanate labelled antibodies. J. Immunol. **95:**225–229.

Chapter 5
Indigenous and Pathogenic Microorganisms of Man

HENRY D. ISENBERG AND BARBARA G. PAINTER

CHANGING CONCEPTS OF INFECTIOUS DISEASE

Traditionally, the clinical microbiologist has been charged with the responsibility of identifying microorganisms in a clinical specimen as accurately and as quickly as possible. There is also a tacit, almost universal agreement between clinicians and microbiologists that the microorganisms of interest are the so-called pathogens. This attitude suggests that a very small number of microorganisms are endowed with the capacity to incite infectious disease processes without regard to their number, their portal of entry, or the presence of other microorganisms. Most significantly, this view neglects the determinative role of the host and of the environment in the clinically overt manifestations of infectious disease, placing the onus for the disease squarely on the microorganism.

Dubos (2) and Burnet (1) have expanded the appraisal by Theobald Smith (10) of the numerous host and parasite interactions which culminate in clinically overt infectious disease. The studies of these investigators make it quite evident that the general health of the host, his previous contact with particular microorganisms, his past clinical history, and a variety of toxic, traumatic, or iatrogenic insults, not of microbial origin, are significant determinants of infectious disease. Implied in the appreciation of this work is the understanding that members of the so-called indigenous microflora can, given the opportunity by an unrelated lowering of the host's resistance, become involved in infectious disease. (In deference to editorial policy, the authors have omitted certain terms which appear to be gaining some degree of acceptance. They have indicated a personal preference for the term "protista" to designate all microorganisms and the term "amphibiont" to designate the large group of microorganisms found in and on humans which often are harmless while still being capable of inciting disease [ed.].)

The dilemma of the clinical microbiologist is deciding which of the several microorganisms isolated from a clinical specimen are involved in the disease. There are very few microorganisms to which the term "pathogenic" can be applied invariably, if "pathogenic" is defined to mean causing infectious disease at all times (8). Yet, the clinical microbiologist is expected by an increasing number of clinicians to decide the causal relationship between a microorganism and a patient's disease even though most of the organisms from clinical material are at best "sometimes" pathogenic. All that can be presented here is a very limited discussion and outline of some of the factors which affect the categorizing of microorganisms as "harmless," "potentially hazardous," or "actively involved in a lesion."

Clinical microbiologists will have to contend with an additional albeit artificial complication in the near future. Recent previews of the forthcoming eighth edition of *Bergey's Manual* indicate that the diagnostic designations of bacteria, helpful to the clinician as well as the laboratorian in distinguishing between closely related microorganisms, have been ignored to a considerable degree by the editors and authors of this authoritative work. We believe that clinical microbiologists cannot abandon a system of classification useful and generally accepted. As but one example, the order which the painstaking investigations of Ewing and his colleagues at the Center for Disease Control has brought to the confusion hitherto known as the family *Enterobacteriaceae* cannot be ignored for a system which will not allow the ease of recognition and confirmation. The clinical microbiologist has responsibilities to the clinician and most significantly to the patient. This obligation should never be subjected to the vagaries of taxonomic disagreements.

Microorganisms, i.e., bacteria, yeasts, fungi, protozoa, and viruses, are not only ubiquitous in man's environment; they also abound in enormous numbers on and in his body while he is in the best of health. Thus, from the time of birth people live in a microbial biosphere composed of innumerable individuals representing types, variants, strains, species, genera, families, orders, etc. The composition of this microbial environment is by no means static. Numerous additions and deletions both qualitative and quantitative are taking place constantly. Many populated and sterile areas are found in and on the human body as well as sparsely populated areas or regions harboring transient microbiota. These temporary habitats of microorganisms include the larynx, trachea, bronchi, accessory nasal sinuses, esophagus, stomach and upper portions of the small intestines, the upper urinary tract including the posterior urethra, and the corresponding distal areas of the male and female genital organs. The persistent finding of numerous microorganisms in these temporarily inhabited areas or in blood provides, according to Rosebury (8), as reliable a marker as can be found for the imaginary line that divides health from disease. Conclusions concerning the significance of a laboratory isolation from areas usually without microorganisms must be based on properly obtained specimens which were properly handled and transported, which were examined promptly, and which yielded an obviously large number of microorganisms unusual in this locale or recovered occasionally in small numbers.

One other aspect of microbiology cannot be ignored. Not all of the microorganisms present in many specimens can be cultivated. Some are isolated when clinical suspicion is communicated immediately to the microbiologist. The conscientious, well-trained clinical microbiologist is constantly aware of the existence of microorganisms that have not as yet been cultivated or are very difficult to cultivate. He insists on viewing stained preparations from clinical material, especially when specimens are obtained directly from pathological lesions and from suspect areas usually populated by a mixed microflora.

A description of the indigenous and pathogenic microorganisms in various body areas is hampered further by several other important considerations. The specimen submitted for microbiological analysis must be obtained from the suspect lesion and not from an adjacent, healthy area. The site of sampling must be properly prepared. Furthermore, there is little if any information concerning the so-called normal host or the variations in microflora from one geographical locale to another. Very frequently, the socioeconomic background, diet, climate, and other equally significant factors may modify the definition and the suitability of a normal host and impose harmless changes in his microbiota.

Obviously, no hard and fast rule can be presented which divides the microorganisms of people into clear-cut categories of harmless, commensal organisms and pathogenic species. Instead, and at best, the most commonly encountered microbial species are listed in the various tables of this chapter, along with the anatomical locale in which they are encountered most usually and the infectious diseases in which they become involved (3). The list of organisms lacks several which could have been included without stretching the definition of "sometimes pathogenic microorganisms." Also omitted are those microorganisms which are usually restricted to domestic or wild animals, as well as ordinary inhabitants of soil and plants. As an example, the omnipresent bacilli cannot be designated as invariably harmless. *Bacillus subtilis* may cause severe eye disease, especially iridocyclitis and panophthalmitis. In debilitated patients, this same organism has been involved as the causative agent of meningitis and bacteremia. Occasionally, *B. subtilis* has complicated the healing of surgical wounds. Some other bacilli, which elaborate toxins in profusion, may give rise to food poisoning (11).

BODY AREAS

Microbiologists have listed, since the inception of this discipline, the indigenous or autochthonous and the pathogenic microorganisms of the various body areas. They have isolated them from lesions, although many times the causal relationship between the microbe recovered and the presenting disease was tenuous, at best. Despite the dearth of basic information and the very cautious presentation of such publications, these listings have been accepted as authoritative. Organisms not mentioned as either indigenous or pathogenic are treated with an extreme degree of suspicion or, worse, ignored entirely. This practice still prevails despite considerable improvement in cultural technology and a changed approach toward the basic tenets of infectious disease. Therefore, it must be stated categorically that the following compilations are not exhaustive; the omission or inclusion of a microbial species in any category does not imply that it cannot be isolated from a particular or any other body area nor that it cannot incite disease, complicate underlying disease, or colonize anatomical abnormalities of congenital, traumatic, or iatrogenic origin. Of course, it is understood that all microbiological practices and scientific cautions, which comprise this volume, have been applied diligently to such extraordinary microbes.

The areas to be described are divided into two major categories: those which usually bear microorganisms and those which are usually sterile or only occasionally harbor a few protista, but which may become heavily colonized if diseased. The microorganisms will be classified as indigenous and pathogenic in various degrees.

RESPIRATORY TRACT

Areas which usually harbor microorganisms (Table 1)

Mouth. The mouth will be considered as composed of the buccal cavity, teeth, tongue, gingivae, palates, and saliva. The following organisms are commonly found in this region. Micrococci, including *Staphylococcus epidermidis*, *Staphylococcus aureus*, various pigmented micrococci, and anaerobic varieties are especially numerous in the saliva and on tooth surfaces, but they are not usually encountered in gingival crevices of healthy individuals. *S. aureus* and the anaerobic varieties are rare in the predentulous mouth. The viridans streptococci, including both the *mitis* and *salivarius* groups, are ubiquitously distributed on all surfaces of the mouth. Enterococci are usually present. *Streptococcus pyogenes* is present in a certain small percentage (5 to 10%) of normal mouths, usually in those individuals who yield this organism in throat cultures. This finding of group A streptococci in healthy individuals is restricted to adults and their saliva or tooth surfaces. Peptostreptococci are commonly

TABLE 1. *Respiratory tract*

Organism[a]	Anatomic locale	Infectious disease process
Acinetobacter spp.	Nasopharynx	Meningitis, bacteremia, pneumonia
Actinomyces spp.	Mouth, tonsils	Actinomycosis, salivary calculi
Bacteroides spp.	Mouth, tonsils	Lung abscesses, lung gangrene
Borrelia refringens	Mouth	? Vincent's angina
Candida albicans and other yeasts	Mouth, throat	Thrush, pneumonitis
Corynebacterium spp.	Mouth, nose	Subacute bacterial endocarditis, lung abscesses
Dialister pneumosintes	Throat	Chronic disease of meninges and other organs (rare)
Entamoeba gingivalis	Mouth	Not determined unequivocally
Enterobacteriaceae	Mouth, throat	Pneumonia, lung abscesses
Enterococcus	Mouth, tonsils, nose	Bacteremia, meningitis, pneumonia, endocarditis
Fusobacterium spp.	Mouth, tonsils	? Vincent's angina, lung abscesses, complication of human bite
Haemophilus spp.	Mouth, nasopharynx, throat	Laryngotracheobronchitis, meningitis, conjunctivitis, pneumonitis, bacteremia
Lactobacillus spp.	Mouth, saliva	Bacterial endocarditis (very rare), lung abscess (one report)
Leptotrichia buccalis	Mouth, tooth surface	Not determined unequivocally
Micrococcus spp.	Mouth, tonsils	Not determined unequivocally
Moraxella spp.	Nasopharynx, nose	Conjunctivitis
Mycoplasma spp.	Mouth	Primary atypical pneumonia by one species
Neisseria spp.	Mouth, nasopharynx, nose	Meningitis (by one species; very rare by others)
Peptostreptococcus spp.	Mouth, tonsils	Lung gangrene, abscesses
Staphylococcus aureus	Mouth, nasopharynx, tonsils, nose	Pneumonia, otitis, parotitis, abscess
S. epidermidis	Mouth, nasopharynx, tonsils, nose	Subacute bacterial endocarditis
Streptococcus pneumoniae	Mouth, nose, tonsils, throat	Pneumonia, conjunctivitis, meningitis, otitis media
Treponema denticum	Mouth	Not determined unequivocally
Trichomonas tenax	Mouth	Not determined unequivocally
Veillonella spp.	Mouth, tonsils	Bacterial endocarditis
Vibrio sputorum	Mouth	Not determined unequivocally
Viridans streptococci	Mouth, throat	Subacute bacterial endocarditis

[a] Several species of the genera listed may be found; not all of these species are involved in disease processes.

found. *Streptococcus pneumoniae* may be present in the predentulous mouth and has been recovered from saliva and tooth surfaces of as many as 25% of healthy adults. Pigmented *Neisseria* spp., *Veillonella* spp., and aerobic corynebacteria are very common in saliva and in gingival crevices. *Actinomyces bifidus* and *A. israelii* can be isolated from the gingiva. The lactobacilli are commonly in saliva, whereas the leptotrichia are more frequently encountered on tooth surfaces. The family *Enterobacteriaceae* is well represented, with *Escherichia coli* and the *Klebsiella-Enterobacter* group the most common representatives, especially in saliva and on teeth. The hemophiline rods, especially *Haemophilus influenzae* and *H. parainfluenzae*, are very often recovered from or demonstrated in normal mouths, as are representatives of *Bacteroides* and *Fusobacterium*, *Vibrio sputorum*, and a variety of spirochetes, especially *Treponema denticum* and *Borrelia refringens*. Several mycoplasmata have been isolated from the saliva of healthy individuals, and *Candida albicans* and occasionally other *Candida* spp. apparently exist in the oral cavity without disease production. The protozoa *Entamoeba gingivalis* and *Trichomonas tenax* are found in the gingival crevices of some healthy adults.

This very large array of microorganisms found in healthy mouths makes it almost impossible not to find a goodly number represented whenever pathology is present. Undoubtedly, some appear in lesions accidentally. Findings from gum lesions, root canals, caries, etc. reflect this state. Debilitated patients or those on prolonged chemotherapy often present with lesions of the tongue from which fungi are isolated; others with nutritional deficiencies or possibly hygienic neglect present with membranous lesions involving the entire oral cavity. Numerous bacteria can be demonstrated in this disease picture, often identified as Vincent's angina. Only very few of these have been cultured. The causal relationship between the microbes and the disease is not at all clear.

Throat, including the nasopharynx, oropharynx, and tonsils. Micrococci are among the organisms usually found. *S. epidermidis* may be found in the nasopharynx and on the tonsillar area of children older than infants. *S. aureus* is frequently present in the nasopharynx, the oropharynx, and the tonsils. The tonsils may harbor anaerobic micrococci. Viridans streptococci are almost always present in the throat. Various hemolytic streptococci, among them *S. pyogenes*, can be found in the nasopharynx and especially in the tonsillar region of normal, healthy individuals, but in small numbers. Enterococci, the group D streptococci, may be present on tonsils. The anaerobic streptococci are occasionally isolated from tonsils. *S. pneumoniae* and the neisseriae which tolerate 20 to 25 C are present in the healthy throat, accompanied in the nasopharynx, at times, by *N. meningitidis*, usually without the slightest evidence of a disease process or contact with individuals ill with meningococcemia or meningococcal meningitis. *Veillonella* spp., corynebacteria, and *A. israelii* are present especially on the tonsils. *E. coli*, *Klebsiella-Enterobacter* group, and the various species of *Proteus* all can be found with greater or lesser frequency in the various regions of the throat. A large number of healthy throats harbor *H. influenzae* or *H. parainfluenzae*, and the tonsils especially contain various *Bacteroides* spp., *Fusobacterium* spp., the salivary vibrio, and spirochetes. In addition, culture or special preparations of healthy throat specimens indicate the presence of *Dialister pneumosintes*, tiny gram-negative rods capable of passing most bacterial filters, mycoplasmata, *C. albicans*, and other *Candida* spp., as well as the same protozoa described for the mouth.

Infectious disease of the throat can be caused by an appreciable number of microorganisms. Undoubtedly, a considerable number of lesions may be initiated by different viruses only to be followed quickly by bacteria and fungi. Large numbers of pathogenic microbes in the throat may, in addition, reflect infectious disease of the lower respiratory tract, and their detection in the throat, especially in the absence of sputum, can constitute helpful guidance for the clinician. Immunization against at least two of the most dreaded pathogenic bacteria, *Corynebacterium diphtheriae* and *Bordetella pertussis*, has lessened the incidence of the associated diseases in those geographical areas where such protection is available. The rapid means of transportation and ready interchange with representatives from endemic areas are sufficient reasons to keep the clinical microbiology laboratory prepared to evaluate the suspicions of alert physicians. In many geographical areas, *S. pyogenes* remains the major pathogenic bacterium involved in throat disease. The importance of ready detection and rapid recognition of this organism in a pathological process in the throat cannot be stressed too often, since treatment can frequently prevent the sequelae of streptococcal sore throat—rheumatic fever and acute glomerulonephritis. *S. pneumoniae* may not contribute at all to pathological processes in the throat. However, large numbers of pneumococci in the nasopharynx, oropharynx, or the tonsils are very suggestive of pathology in the lower respiratory tract. Their presence in this locale may also denote sinusitis and, by the persistence of large numbers, otitis media. Although the hemophilic bacteria are frequently present in the human throat, *H. influenzae* serogroup B has been involved in a variety of diseases, among them those confined to this anatomical area. Especially serious are supraglottal edema and laryngotracheal bronchitis, both diseases of children with grave prognoses. *S. aureus* may be involved in a variety of disease processes in the throat. Its presence is probably the most difficult to interpret. Certainly, isolation of this bacterium in large numbers from a carefully cultured lesion obviates such doubts. As a rule, the number of coagulase-positive staphylococci in this region is small. The opportunistic nature of the organism and the proximity of the throat to its natural habitat allow rapid seeding of any pathological process with these bacteria. They may, thus, complicate secondarily any disease process, and their presence in mixed cultures cannot be interpreted as reflecting contamination only. Should there be infectious disease due to staphylococci in any other part of the body, it is very likely that an inordinately large number of representatives will be recovered from the throat. *Mycoplasma pneumoniae*, *Klebsiella pneumoniae*, and *Pseudomonas aeruginosa* isolated in large numbers from throat cultures most often reflect pathology of the lower respiratory tract; this is true especially of the gram-negative rods which tend to complicate the noninfectious diseases of the lung in debilitated patients. As with the pneumococcus, *P. aeruginosa* may cause sinusitis. This organism has gained notoriety recently as the most prevalent agent contaminating inhalation equipment and being seeded in large numbers by these pressure machines into the lower respiratory tract (6). Thrush, already described for the mouth, may also involve the throat. Candidal lesions may be found in the throat accompanying a variety of drug regimens, as well as in patients with debilitating and neoplastic diseases and in neonatal infants. The throat and especially the tonsils may be the site for primary lesions of syphilis. Recent reports (5) suggest that *N. gonorrhoeae* may also be detected and may occasionally give rise to a local disease in this area.

Nose. The indigenous microflora of the nasal passages and the nares is more limited than that of the adjacent anatomic regions. The nares are the usual habitat of the staphylococci. *S. epidermidis* and *S. aureus* are recovered with great frequency from this site. Although both organisms may not be present at all times in any one individual, their recovery from the nares is to be expected. On rare occasions, viridans streptococci can be isolated from the nasal passages. In children, and especially in infants, enterococci and other bacteria reflecting the fecal microbiota are not uncommon. The noses of healthy, unexposed individuals have also yielded occasionally *S. pyogenes* and *S. pneumoniae*. The so-called nonpathogenic neisseriae are transients in this location as well. Healthy contacts of patients with meningococcal disease may harbor *N. meningitidis*. Additional residents of the nose are the various aerobic corynebacteria and occasionally *Moraxella lacunata*.

Actual disease of the nasal passages must be differentiated carefully from disease of adjacent areas, including the skin, nasopharynx, oropharynx, tonsils, and sinuses. It is not uncommon to recover microorganisms in great numbers which reflect the diseased state of these neighboring areas or even more distant areas. Such isolations are of significance and represent, to a large degree, the rationale for this frequently performed microbiological analysis. However, the nasal passages themselves do become involved. Regardless of the primary causative agents, viral or chemical, staphylococci, especially *S. aureus*, will complicate as a secondary invader any disease process in this area. Independent staphylococcal disease in the form of boils, furunculosis, etc., may be present as well. In premature and newborn infants, lesions due to hemolytic *E. coli*, *P. aeruginosa*, and *C. albicans* may be encountered, but these usually represent more generalized disease, as is augured by the isolation of *Acinetobacter lwoffi* (*Mima polymorpha*), *Moraxella duplex* (*Mima polymorpha* var. *oxidans*), *A. anitratus* (*Herellea* sp.), and various flavobacteria. Ozaena, a disease characterized by atrophy of the nasal mucosa (11), is caused by gram-negative rods. An infective granuloma, rhinoscleroma, most often does involve the nose, although the pharynx and the remaining upper respiratory tract may be involved as well. Certain distinct klebsiellae, of the species *K. rhinoscleromatis*, are regarded by most investigators of this disease, which is uncommon in the United States, as the etiological agent. Mild rhinitis due to *N. meningitidis* has been reported.

Usually sterile areas

The larynx, trachea, bronchi, bronchioles, alveoli, and the accessory nasal sinuses are usually sterile. Contamination by occasional microorganisms is usual, but the various defense mechanisms of these organs remove such offenders quickly and efficiently. The usual specimen submitted to the clinical microbiological laboratory for establishing infectious disease of the respiratory tract is the sputum specimen. Bronchial washings, thoracentesis fluid, transtracheal aspirates and aspirates from tracheostomies or lung lesions are gaining in frequency of submission for microbiological analysis. Sputum and some aspirates may be contaminated by the microbiota of the throat, nose, and mouth. Rapid, efficient processing is imperative to prevent these contaminating protista from obscuring etiological agents. The most commonly encountered bacteria in the sputum are *S. aureus*, *H. influenzae*, representatives of the family *Enterobacteriaceae*, *P. aeruginosa*, and *C. albicans*. These organisms may be involved in the disease, they may be contaminants, or they may reflect superinfection following therapy. It must also be remembered (7) that in any infective lesion of the lungs the demonstration of the causative organisms in sputum can hardly be expected unless escape of exudate into the bronchus has occurred.

It is perhaps most suitable to list the various diagnoses of chest disease and those etiological agents most frequently recovered. Acute infectious bronchitis, most frequently seen during winter in children and the aged, and associated with viruses of the adenovirus-influenza groups, may be caused or complicated by *S. pneumoniae*, *S. pyogenes* and related serogroups, *S. aureus*, and *H. influenzae* (*Bordetella pertussis* when whooping cough is present). Chronic bronchitis, of unknown etiology and associated frequently with pulmonary emphysema, is assuming increasing importance. Sputum from such patients displays a variety of microorganisms, not necessarily the same species on repeat examinations. The presence of bacteria associated with pathology of the respiratory tract, such as pneumococci or group A streptococci, *H. influenzae*, and staphylococci, may be significant. *P. aeruginosa*, flavobacteria, and other environmental microorganisms which contaminate inhalation equipment may also be important. The laboratory work-up for chronic bronchitis should invariably include cultures for mycobacteria, actinomycetes, and those fungi involved in pneumonic disease. Acute mediastinitis is usually the result of perforation of the esophagus in conjunction with instrumentation, obstruction, external wounds, downward propagation of deep cellulitis of the neck, forceful vomiting, and occasionally the extension of infectious disease of the lungs, pleural cavity, or pericardium. The bacteria usually found are those common to the mouth and pharynx which are drained into the area. The bacteria which contribute most frequently to the disease picture are the peptostreptococci, *Bacteroides* spp., fusobacteria, and occasionally clostridia. Pneumonia may be caused by *S. pneumoniae*, *S. pyogenes*, *H. influenzae*, *S. aureus*, *Klebsiella pneumoniae*, *Francisella tularensis*, *C. albicans*, *E. coli* (usually the hemolytic serogroups), *P. aeruginosa*, *Proteus* spp., and *P. hemolytica*. Pulmonary abscesses may result from staphylococcal or Friedlander pneumonias or the aspiration of particulate matter. The organisms most commonly cultured from such lesions are *Bacteroides* spp., *Fusobacterium* spp., peptostreptococci, enterococci, staphylococci, clostridia, klebsiellae, escherichiae, and pseudomonads. The examination of such abscesses should always include a search for acid-fast organisms, aerobic and anaerobic actinomycetes, and the fungi associated with pulmonary lesions. Empyema is usually a secondary disease, i.e., an extension of the primary disease. Some special attention must be accorded certain clinical variants of empyema, especially empyema of infants usually caused by *S. aureus*, empyema due to *Entamoeba histolytica*, and empyema due to *Actinomyces* spp. or *Nocardia* spp.

GASTROINTESTINAL TRACT

Areas which usually harbor microorganisms (Table 2)

The part of the gastrointestinal tract which invariably harbors microorganisms is the large intestine, although some fecal organisms have been recovered in aspirates of the lower ileum of normal individuals (8). Once past the ileocecal valve, the contents of the large intestine reflect the microbiota of feces. It is surprising that information concerning the fecal microflora is so meager (8). It seems almost superfluous to list the organisms which can be encountered; many of them are ignored in the search for "enteric pathogens," i.e., salmonellae and shigellae, which certainly do not represent the only microbes endowed with the potential of disease production. Rosebury (8) lists the following microorganisms as indigenous: *S. epidermidis*, *S. aureus*, viridans streptococci, enterococci, occasionally *S. pyogenes* and related serogroups, peptostreptococci, lactobacilli (especially in infants), corynebacteria, some mycobacteria, clostridia, actinomycetes, the various members of the family *Enterobacteriaceae*, *P. aeruginosa*, *Alcaligenes faecalis*, occasionally

TABLE 2. *Gastrointestinal tract*

Organism[a]	Anatomic locale	Infectious disease process
Achromobacter spp.	Large intestine, lower ileum	Post-operative and post-traumatic wound infectious complications
Aeromonas spp.	Large intestine, lower ileum	Diarrhea (rare), septicemia (rare), osteomyelitis, postoperative complications
Alcaligenes faecalis	Large intestine, lower ileum	Gastroenteritis (rare), bacteremia
Bacteroides spp.	Large intestine, lower ileum	Peritonitis, abscesses, cholecystitis
Candida albicans and other yeasts	Large intestine, lower ileum	Pseudomembranous enterocolitis
Clostridium spp.	Large intestine, lower ileum	Food poisoning, choledochitis, cholecystitis
Corynebacterium spp.	Large intestine, lower ileum	Not known
Enterobacteriaceae	Large intestine, lower ileum	Abscesses,[a] peritonitis, bacteremia, diarrhea, enteric fevers, typhoid fever, postoperative and post-traumatic complications, meningitis, endocarditis
Enterococcus	Large intestine, lower ileum	Peritonitis, cholecystitis, postoperative complications
Flavobacterium spp.	Large intestine, lower ileum	Meningitis, bacteremia
Fusobacterium spp.	Large intestine, lower ileum	Abscesses, bacteremia
Lactobacillus spp.	Large intestine, lower ileum	Not known
Mycobacteria spp.	Large intestine, lower ileum	Not by indigenous bacteria
Mycoplasma spp.	Large intestine, lower ileum	Not determined unequivocally
Peptostreptococcus	Large intestine, lower ileum	Cholecystitis, abscess
Pseudomonas aeruginosa	Large intestine, lower ileum	Gastroenteritis, meningitis, bacteremia, postoperative complications
Staphylococcus aureus	Large intestine, lower ileum	Pancreatic abscesses, enteritis, pseudomembranous enterocolitis, food poisoning
Viridans streptococci	Large intestine, lower ileum	Not known
Vibrio spp.	Large intestine, lower ileum	Not by indigenous bacteria

[a] Several species of the genera listed may be found; not all of these species are involved in disease processes.

the various *Achromobacter* spp., and flavobacteria, *Bacteroides* spp., *Fusobacterium* spp., mycoplasmata, *C. albicans*, various other yeasts, and a large variety of protozoa such as *Entamoeba coli, Endolimax nana, Dientameba fragilis, Iodameba butschlii, Trichomonas hominis, Giardia lamblia*, and *Chilomastix mesnili*. Of course, not all microbial groups are present in each and every individual at all times. Undoubtedly, many other genera can be found with frequency. Geographical distribution, dietary habits, and sanitary habits will also be active in the selection of a resident microflora. It is unfortunate that the paucity of information does not permit even a short statement concerning the role of the intestinal microbiota in the economy of the host and as a first line of defense against colonization by microorganisms less adapted to the human environment. A similar state of ignorance shrouds the host-parasite relationship between this large microbial aggregate and people, and no really authoritative treatment has been accorded the fecal microflora as potential etiological agents of infectious disease in other areas of the body.

The most readily recognized diseases of the gastrointestinal tract, usually initiated in the colon or ileum but often involving other parts of the tract or other organs, are salmonellosis and shigellosis. All of the various members of the genus *Salmonella*, as well as the arizonae, are capable of evoking the various clinical symptoms of salmonellosis and its complications. The various shigellae can cause the syndrome recognized as bacillary dysentery. *Vibrio cholerae* and the attendant disease are encountered increasingly in some parts of the world. In the newborn period, enteropathogenic *E. coli* may cause fatal epidemics of diarrhea. *S. aureus, Proteus mirabilis*, and occasionally *C. albicans* may be involved in pseudomembranous enterocolitis. Staphylococcal food poisoning must also be considered as affecting the gastrointestinal tract, as does food poisoning due to clostridial toxins in addition to botulism. In these cases, as distinct from the pseudomembranous enterocolitis, the toxins, rather than the microorganisms, cause the symptomatology and the bacteria need not be demonstrable in feces or vomitus. Acute diarrhea may at times be associated with *P. aeruginosa, Proteus* spp., or *C. albicans*. *Entamoeba histolytica* is the etiological agent of amoebic dysentery and its complications. Large numbers of *Giardia lamblia* may reflect a subacute infectious colitis due to this organism in susceptible individuals. Balantidiasis, quite rare in the United States, can occasionally be suspected when biopsies of the rectal mucosa reveal the ciliate *Balantidium coli*. Localized pathology of the large intestine may involve *Aeromonas* spp. or *Yersinia enterocolitica*, the latter not only causing occasional gastroenteritis but also appendicitis. Hemolytic serotypes as well as enterotoxigenic varieties of *E. coli* have been isolated from intestinal disease processes. In addition, *Vibrio parahaemolyticus* may be involved in food poisoning episodes after the ingestion of seafood.

Usually sterile areas

The esophagus and the stomach are contaminated with bacteria whenever food is ingested. The microbial population does not survive in these two sections of the gastrointestinal tract. Similarly, most of the small intestine, with the exception previously mentioned, the liver, and the gall bladder are usually free from microbial contamination. This also applies to the peritoneum. Microorganisms in these areas usually are secondary to underlying diseases such as carcinoma or reach various sites because the large intestine has been punctured or ruptured. Peritonitis, regardless of its initial cause, can be caused by any of the fecal organisms listed. They may occur as part of the bacteremia, but usually mixed aerobic and anaerobic, gram-positive and gram-negative microorganisms participate. Peritonitis may give rise to intra-abdominal abscesses, especially pelvic, paracolic, intermesenteric, subphrenic, and retroperitoneal. All may show the mixed microbial population or single causative agents, *S. aureus*, *Bacteroides* spp., enterococci, *P. aeruginosa*, and hemolytic *E. coli*. In an appreciable number of cholecystitis cases, bacteria have been isolated. These were possibly involved as secondary opportunists. *E. coli*, enterococci, peptostreptococci, and clostridia are the most frequently encountered, but many other common and uncommon representatives of the fecal microflora in health and disease may be found. Bacterial cholangitis usually is secondary to intra- or extrahepatic obstruction in the area of the bile duct. Cholangitis caused by salmonellae, staphylococci, and streptococci may be accompanied by septicemia due to these bacteria (7). Again, the organisms usually recovered reflect the microbiota of the intestinal tract. Amoebic abscesses of the liver obviously constitute complication of the primary dysentery. Pyogenic hepatic abscesses in the antibiotic era yield *E. coli* most frequently. Pancreatic abscess formation is a secondary complication of pancreatitis. The microorganisms most frequently found are *S. aureus* and *E. coli*. Clostridial diseases are uncommon but not rare (6). They include acute gaseous cholecystitis due to *Clostridium perfringens*, but other clostridia, *E. coli*, and aerobic and anaerobic streptococci have been associated with this entity. Invasion of the bile ducts from the intestinal tract results in clostridial choledochitis, from which *C. perfringens* has been isolated exclusively. Enteritis necroticans is caused by heat-resistant *C. perfringens* type F. Clostridial cellulitis of the abdominal wall is a complication of perforation of intestinal neoplasm with local peritonitis or of colon or biliary tract surgery.

GENITOURINARY TRACT

Areas which usually harbor microorganisms (Table 3)

External genitalia. Rosebury (8) has listed the following organisms as those present on the surface of genitalia: *S. epidermidis*, viridans streptococci, enterococci, peptostreptococci, corynebacteria, mycobacteria, various members of *Enterobacteriaceae*, *Bacteroides* spp., *Fusobacterium* spp., mycoplasmata, *C. albicans*, and other yeasts.

The external genitalia are subject to the same infectious disease as other skin areas. The special lesions of the external genitalia are venereal in nature and include the lesions of syphilis, chancroid or soft chancre, and granuloma inguinale, which is widespread in the tropics and is caused by an agent variously thought to be a *Klebsiella* variant or a separate pathogenic organism *Donovania granulomatis* (11).

Anterior urethra. An appreciable number and variety of microorganisms can usually be recovered from this region in normal healthy individuals of both sexes: coagulase-negative and occasionally coagulase-positive staphylococci, enterococci, various nonpathogenic neisseriae, aerobic corynebacteria, rarely certain mycobacteria, the various enteric gram-negative rods, *A. lwoffi* (*Mima*), *Haemophilus vaginalis*, mycoplasmata, and *Candida* spp. including *C. albicans*. *Trichomonas vaginalis* may on occasion gain access to this part of the urethra without overt disease.

It is difficult to delineate exactly where the anterior portion of the urethra ends, especially when disease is present. In the male, it is indicated to consider disease involving the en-

TABLE 3. *Genitourinary tract*

Organism	Anatomic locale	Infectious disease process
Acinetobacter spp.	Anterior urethra, vagina	Urethritis, disease of newborn, complication of instrumentation and surgery, complications of burns
Bacteroides spp.	External genitalia	Complication of surgical procedures especially in females
Candida albicans and other yeasts	External genitalia, anterior urethra, vagina	Candidiasis
Clostridium spp.	Vagina	Complication of surgical procedures, criminal abortion
Corynebacterium spp.	External genitalia, anterior urethra, vagina	Not determined unequivocally
Enterobacteriaceae	External genitalia, anterior urethra, vagina	Pyelonephritis, cystitis, bacteriuria
Enterococcus	External genitalia, anterior urethra, vagina	Pyelonephritis, cystitis, bacteriuria
Fusobacterium spp.	External genitalia, vagina	Not determined unequivocally
Haemophilus vaginalis[a]	Anterior urethra, vagina	Vaginitis
Lactobacillus spp.	Vagina	None
Mycobacterium spp.	External genitalia, anterior urethra, vagina	Not by indigenous organisms
Mycoplasma spp.	External genitalia, anterior urethra, vagina	Nonspecific urethritis
Neisseria spp.	External genitalia, anterior urethra, vagina	Not by indigenous organisms
Peptostreptococcus spp.	External genitalia, vagina	Puerperal fever
Staphylococcus aureus	External genitalia, rare anterior urethra, vagina	Urethritis, furunculosis
S. epidermidis	External genitalia, rare anterior urethra, vagina	None
Trichomonas vaginalis	Anterior urethra, vagina	Vaginitis
Viridans streptococci	External genitalia, rare anterior urethra, vagina	None

[a] This bacterium is identified by some as *Corynebacterium vaginalis*.

tire urethra. Urethritis may be caused specifically by the gonococcus, or nonspecifically by a variety of bacteria which include the staphylococci, the fecal gram-negative rods, and *Listeria*. In the female, contamination by vaginal-labial disease of the anterior portion of the urethra is also unavoidable. It is perhaps appropriate to maintain that *Neisseria gonorrhoeae* can be recovered from the anterior urethra of the female at times when its detection in the vagina has failed.

Vagina. The usual microflora of this organ from the menarche to the menopause is dominated by lactobacilli, designated as Doderlein bacillus and actually *L. acidophilus*. Premenstrual girls shortly after birth and postmenopausal women harbor the skin microbiota in this region. Despite the control over the vaginal environment exerted by the lactobacilli, many other microorganisms can be cultured from vaginal samples of healthy women. Thus, *S. aureus* and *S. epidermidis*, viridans streptococci, enterococci, peptostreptococci, group B streptococci, the low temperature-tolerant neisseriae, corynebacteria, some actinomycetes, members of the family *Enterobacteriaceae*, the acinetobacters corresponding to *Mima*, *H. vaginalis*, occasionally clostridia and other anaerobic rods, mycoplasmata, *C. albicans*, other yeasts, and *Trichomonas vaginalis* may be isolated.

The major infectious diseases of the female pudenda are the venereal diseases syphilis and gonorrhea as well as candidiasis, trichomoniasis, and nonspecific vaginitis caused by a variety of organisms which may very well act as opportunistic secondary invaders reflecting disturbances in the microbiological balance as a complication of diseases elsewhere and their treatment. *Haemophilus vaginalis* infection ranks high among the so-called nonspecific vaginitides, but fecal and skin organisms including staphylococci, enterococci, *Listeria*, etc. may contribute to clinically overt disease (11). *Vibrio fetus* and related unclassified organisms have been isolated from the vaginas of women who have aborted repeatedly. The vaginal microflora, especially the anaerobic members, contribute to the complications of criminal abortions. Postpartum sepsis and salpingitis, frequently caused by the enteric gram-negative rods, and to a lesser degree by clostridia and staphylococci, probably reflect the microbiota of the vagina. Similarly, colonization and infectious disease of the newborn reflect the protistal population of the vagina.

Usually sterile areas

As a rule, the remaining structures of the genitourinary tract are without permanent microbiota. Infectious disease of the kidneys is still not completely understood, with two major theories advanced to explain the seeding of this organ by infectious particles. There are many predisposing factors for pyelonephritis, especially host factors and underlying diseases, which appear mandatory for establishment of infectious disease. The major bacterial offenders are the gram-negative enteric rods, especially *E. coli*, *Proteus* spp., *P. aeruginosa*, and the *Klebsiella-Enterobacter* group; enterococci are not uncommon and can be demonstrated in adequate numbers repeatedly in untreated acute pyelonephritis. *Mycobacterium tuberculosis* can infect the kidney and can be demonstrated in urine. The prostate in the male may become a secondary seat of gonorrheal disease. However, other microorganisms including staphylococci, enterococci, listeriae, *E. coli*, mycoplasmata, pseudomonads, and achromobacters may lodge in this organ, especially in middle-aged and older individuals.

SKIN, EAR, AND EYE

Areas which usually harbor microorganisms (Table 4)

It seems superfluous to remark that the outermost border of the body is constantly populated with microorganisms which reflect the contacts of the individual, his habits, his profession, etc. Still, the organisms which are universally present on the skin number far fewer than one would expect (Table 4). They are the staphylococci, among which *S. epidermidis* by far outdistances *S. aureus*, occasionally *S. pyogenes*, aerobic corynebacteria, *Propionibacterium acnes*, mycobacteria, and a variety of usually harmless yeasts. No doubt certain areas, especially those adjoining the various body openings, reflect the microbiota of these adjacent sites.

The most common, at least the most obvious, skin diseases are caused by the staphylococci; *S. aureus* is involved most frequently in boils and furuncles, and *S. epidermidis* is found in pimples and acne, often accompanied by *P. acnes*. Pustulosis, especially of the newborn, also has *S. aureus* as the etiological agent. The most common agents of impetigo are *S. aureus* and *S. pyogenes*. Coagulase-positive staphylococci are also involved in superficial folliculitis and sycosis barbae. Although streptococci and other oral bacteria may also be found, *S. aureus* is the major etiological agent of acute suppurative parotitis. Actinomycosis, as the name implies, is usually caused by *Actinomyces* spp., and represents a chronic suppurative or granulomatous disease, culminating in abscesses. Deep cellulitis of the neck is most frequently caused by streptococci, both aerobic and anaerobic, as well as staphylococci. *S. aureus* is also responsible for hydradenitis suppurativa, a disease more common in women and usually involving the axillae, and it is the most frequent disease-producing agent in acute mastitis and breast abscess. Paronychia most often involve staphylococci and streptococci, and less commonly *C. albicans*. These former organisms are also most frequently recovered from tenosynovitis. Clostridia are usually responsible for anaerobic cellulitis mixtures of bacteria for crepitant cellulitis and *S. pyogenes* for necrotizing fascitis or hemolytic streptococcal gangrene. Erysipelas is a superficial form of streptococcal cellulitis. Erysipeloid, an acute, cutaneous, bluish-red inflammation of the hands and wrists, which is usually confined to certain vocations, is caused by *Erysipelothrix insidiosa*. The eruptions of secondary syphilis may be most obvious on the skin. The various skin disorders caused by the dermatophyte fungi are well known, and the skin infections due to *C. albicans* have already been mentioned.

The external auditory canal usually reflects the microbiota of skin. Perhaps *S. pneumoniae* and the gram-negative rods including *P. aeruginosa* have been recovered with greater frequency from this site than from other skin areas. The middle and inner ear are usually sterile. Diseases of the outer ear reflect the disorders of skin. The other parts of the auditory organ may be involved during generalized disease or may be affected only locally by *S. aureus*, *S. pneumoniae*, *S. pyogenes*, *P. aeruginosa*, *H. influenzae*, and occasionally other microorganisms.

The healthy conjunctiva of the eye may harbor a number of skin organisms. Among those most frequently recovered from the healthy eye are the staphylococci; viridans streptococci, *S. pyogenes*, the pneumococcus,

TABLE 4. *Skin, ear, and eye*

Organism	Anatomic locale	Infectious disease process
Candida albicans and other yeasts	Skin	Paronychia (rare)
Corynebacterium spp.	Skin, ear, eye	Bacterial endocarditis, complication of cardiac surgery
Micrococcus spp.	Skin	Not determined unequivocally
Neisseria spp.	Eye, skin	Not known for indigenously occurring representatives
Peptostreptococcus	Skin	Not known
Propionibacterium acnes	Skin	Pimples, acne, bacterial endocarditis
Staphylococcus aureus	Skin, ear, eye (rarely)	Boils, furuncles, impetigo, pustulosis, mastitis
S. epidermidis	Skin, ear, eye	Pimples, acne, endocarditis, complication of cardiac surgery, thrombophlebitis
Viridans streptococci	Skin, eye	None

neisseriae, and corynebacteria are recovered rarely. The fecal gram-negative rods have been isolated even less frequently from this site, but *H. influenzae* has an incidence second only to the coagulase-negative staphylococci. Some eyes have also yielded *C. albicans* and other yeasts. Eye disease has, of course, been caused by *S. aureus* and *P. aeruginosa* (very often iatrogenically), and occasionally by *S.* pneumoniae. More often, infectious diseases peculiar to the eye have yielded *M. lacunata*, *H. influenzae*, *H. aegyptius*, and *Noguchia granulosis*, m addition to *B. subtilis.*

BLOOD, CEREBROSPINAL FLUID, EXUDATES, AND TRANSUDATES

The blood and spinal fluid of healthy individuals are usually sterile. However, during an appreciable number of infectious diseases or during infectious complications of a primary disease, microorganisms may be recovered from blood. They may be present only transiently or persistently. Positive blood cultures reflect a variety of conditions and diseases and encompass a large array of microorganisms. Positive blood cultures may result from traumatic and surgical wounds, as well as from burns, injury to bones and joints, brain abscesses, furunculosis, cellulitis, meningitis, pneumonia, lung abscesses, empyema, mucoviscidosis, mycotic aneurysm, cardiac anomalies, peritonitis, intestinal or biliary obstruction, cholangitis, carcinoma, urinary obstruction, nephropathies, postpartum endometritis, and septic abortion. Immunosuppressive, cytotoxic, or X-ray therapy and conditions such as arteriosclerosis, chronic debility, diabetic acidosis, hematological diseases, hepatic insufficiency, and malignancies of all sorts may lead to positive blood culture findings. No hard and fast rule concerning the types of microorganisms of significance can be stated. Certainly, staphylococci have been recovered repeatedly, not only *S. aureus* but also *S. epidermidis*. The latter can be involved in bacterial endocarditis and has complicated cardiac catheterization and prostheses procedures. The gram-negative rods, especially *E. coli*, *Klebsiella-Enterobacter* organisms, *P. aeruginosa*, and the various *Proteus* spp. have been recovered following trauma or after surgery of contaminated body areas, or as nosocomially acquired microorganisms complicating protracted hospitalization of patients with a great variety of diseases. The recovery of salmonellae from the blood of individuals with systemic salmonellosis is not uncommon. Other so-called fevers of unknown origin may yield bruceliae, pasteurellae, pneumococci, *N. meningitidis*, *L. monocytogenes*, etc. Bacterial endocarditis patients may harbor *S. mitis*, coagulase-negative staphylococci, enterococci, corynebacteria, *Bacteroides* spp., *Candida albicans*, etc. The rare recovery of environmental or so-called commensal microbes from the blood of patients with bacterial endocarditis need not be surprising. Fungi have been found in blood cultures from patients with lung abscesses, mycotic aneurysms, and hematological disorders. Clostridia have been recovered in the blood of accident victims and from patients with cholangitis and postpartum complications. In the newborn with bacteremia or septicemia during the first week of life, the organisms most often responsible are *S. aureus* and *E. coli*, and with some frequency *Streptococcus agalactiae.*

Positive cultures obtained from cerebrospinal fluids also reflect a variety of conditions. Besides meningitis, trauma, infectious complications of surgery, cranial and spinal epidural abscesses, subdural abscess, septic thrombophlebitis of the venous sinuses, and brain abscesses contribute to positive findings. There are systemic infectious diseases which may afflict the meninges, including severe pneumococcal pneumonia, salmonellosis, *H. influenzae* pneumonia and bacteremia, tuberculosis, listeriosis, *A. lwoffi* (*Mima*) septicemia of the newborn, generalized candidiasis, and advanced sepsis with every type of gram-negative rod, especially *E. coli* and *P. aeruginosa*. Meningitis is caused primarily by *H. influenzae* group B in children and by the meningococcus and pneumococcus in a majority of adults; the aged are most frequently involved with the latter organism. Of course, *S. aureus*, *E. coli*, *P. aeruginosa*, *Salmonella* spp., and *L. monocytogenes* are recovered not uncommonly. *Flavobacterium meningosepticum* has been isolated occasionally. Traumatic or surgical injury may be complicated by any one of the microorganisms, but the staphylococci and gram-negative rods predominate, along with enterococci. In intracranial abscesses, anaerobic microorganisms are most common. These included peptostreptococci, *Bacteroides* spp., *Actinomyces* spp., *C. acnes*, and less frequently *Veillonella* spp. Cranial epidural abscesses have yielded staphylococci, streptococci, pneumococci, and occasionally some gram-negative rods. Spinal epidural abscesses have involved *S. aureus* and *P. aeruginosa*. Other gram-positive cocci have been isolated as well as *Salmonella* spp. which, while infecting vertebrae, caused epidural abscesses (7). Subdural abscess is a comparatively rare complication of *H. influenzae* meningitis in children. *Cryptococcus neoformans*, *M. tuberculosis*, and leptospiral disease of the meninges must also be considered.

Transudates and exudates accompany a large variety of clinical conditions. They may be sterile or contain varied microflora. Any and all microorganisms involving the afflicted organs may be recovered. The organisms found reflect the anatomical site of the disease nidus or adjacent areas. The usual organisms outlined in the foregoing sections may of course be encountered. This includes the anaerobic microorganisms, fungi, and *M. tuberculosis*.

WOUNDS AND BURNS

The microbiota of wounds reflects their anatomical site, the mode of infliction, i.e., traumatic or surgical, the environment in which they were inflicted, and the degree of microbial contamination of adjacent areas which were perforated in the process. These considerations supplement rather than substitute for the general considerations which maintain an adequate host-parasite equilibrium. Traumatic wounds are most usually complicated by aerobic indigenous microorganisms, especially *S. aureus*, group A streptococci, enterococci, *P. aeruginosa*, *E. coli*, *Proteus* spp., flavobacteria, and *Acinetobacter* spp. Among the anaerobic bacteria associated with traumatic wounds, the histotoxic and neurotoxic clostridia are most prominent, leading, under proper conditions, to gas gangrene or tetanus. The most common clostridia of gas gangrene are *C. perfringens* type A, *C. septicum*, and *C. novyii*, but these organisms may be harmless contaminants of wounds. The diagnosis of gas gangrene is strictly a clinical one; isolation of clostridia may alert a clinician but does not constitute the diagnosis of clostridial cellulitis or clostridial myonecrosis. *C. tetani* should not present a problem in a community of properly immunized individuals. Criminally inflicted stab wounds, often intentionally contaminated with feces, require not only expert surgical but also exquisite microbiological attention.

Infections complicating surgery may be of two kinds. The so-called wound infection usually denotes a complication of a clean surgical procedure, a procedure performed under the best available aseptic conditions on tissues usually sterile and not found grossly contaminated during surgery. These wounds may yield *S. aureus*, enterococci, or gram-negative rods, and today rarely microorganisms such as *S. pyogenes*, corynebacteria, pneumococci, *B. subtilis*, etc. When the surgeon performed all or part of his procedures in a contaminated area, resulting infectious disease complications are expected in a certain percentage, often reflecting the state of health of the patient. The microorganisms mirror the microbiota of the particular anatomical site, but all too frequently certain minority members of microflora attain a majority in the usually sterile tissue insulted surgically and gravely complicate the recovery of the patient. Among the bacteria involved in this complication are *E. coli* (especially the hemolytic serotypes), *P. aeruginosa*, *Proteus* spp. and the *Klebsiella-Enterobacter-Serratia* group, flavobacteria, and *Acinetobacter* spp. (*Herellea*).

Microbial contamination of severe burns can be a life-threatening complication. The organism most commonly encountered and most difficult to eradicate is *P. aeruginosa*, often in conjunction with flavobacteria and other gram-negative rods and staphylococci which abound in the institutional environment or on the uninvolved skin of the patient. Early microbiological analysis of burns usually shows a large number of a great variety of microorganisms, many of which are eventually supplemented by the bacteria cited above.

SURGICAL SPECIMENS

The microbiology of surgical specimens depends on the anatomical site and the underlying disease, the care exercised at the time of excision and during subsequent handling, and the available information which will help to narrow the number of etiological agents. The usual pyogenic organisms may be recovered, often as single components. Systemic fungi, nocardiae, actinomycetes, and various mycobacteria including, of course, *M. tuberculosis*, as well as mixtures of anaerobic bacteria, have been found. In addition to bacteria such as *S. aureus*, primarily infected bone has yielded peptostreptococci, *Salmonella* spp. (especially in children with sickle cell disease), gonococci, *Veillonella* spp., representatives of the fecal gram-negative rods, and rarely actinomycetes and blastomycetes. Foreign bodies including prostheses, old sutures, and indwelling catheters have been sources of many species or organisms, among them *P. aeruginosa*, salmonellae, escherichiae, and staphylococci.

AUTOPSY SPECIMENS

Autopsy specimens can yield invaluable information when the examination is performed promptly and aseptically and when cultures are plated immediately and accompanied by smears. Routinely, the kidney, spleen, liver, and lung are negative unless distinct lesions are cultured or an appreciable portion of the organ is diseased. If an excess of 6 h has elapsed between death and the examination, heart blood cultures and the tissues will reflect postmortem or perimortem invasion by organisms from the large bowel. An experienced and interested prosector will culture the areas of tissues possibly involved in an infectious disease process. A large variety of suspected and totally unexpected microorganisms can be recovered and demonstrated subsequently in tissue sections. The microorganisms range from the usual bacteria to lesions populated by brucellae, nocardiae, penicillia, aspergilli, pneumococci, group A streptococci, phycomycetes, clostridia, salmonellae, and shigellae, to name but a few.

MICROBIAL NUMBERS AND CLINICAL DISEASE

The preceding considerations underline the lack of understanding, in quantitative terms, of the many factors which contribute to overt symptoms of infectious disease in any particular person. Certainly, the notion that disease production in any host resides solely in the pathogenic and virulent properties of the microbial particle cannot be accepted any longer. Obviously, the numerous specific and nonspecific defense mechanisms of a particular host, the general health of this individual, and the stresses and insults to which he has been subjected recently have considerable influence if not the determinant role in the initiation and progression of an infectious disease process. Undoubtedly, the quality and quantity of the microbiota in this individual's intimate biosphere at any given moment play significant roles in the process. These roles are as multifarious as the genera and species of microorganisms which constitute the microbial ecosystem of the person. The understanding of microbial ecological relationships between the constituents of this large pool of protista is lacking, especially with regard to the host's health. We know very little about the selectivity exercised by the tissues and organs of the host in the establishment of a local, autochthonous microbiota. There are but a few indications that age, physical environment, and nutrition may affect the minimal infectious dose of some microorganisms with more pronounced pathogenic proclivities. As with other areas of human biology, it is the abnormal condition which permits an intimation of understanding. If infectious disease is viewed as the disturbance of the equilibrium between two very complex systems, the host and his microbiota at a specific moment, then the information derived from the study of the compromised patient and nosocomially significant organisms may be useful in the comprehension of the many factors operative in the maintenance of the host-parasite equilibrium. Microorganisms of nosocomial significance are widely distributed in nature but are involved in disease complications in medical facilities only. They may be minority members of an individual's microbiota or they may be residents of the hospital where they are concentrated as a result of antibiotic-associated selective pressures (4). Patients, compromised in their capacity to resist microorganisms for various medical and surgical reasons, most often find themselves under an umbrella of antimicrobial therapy.

Since their humoral and cellular defense mechanisms may be suppressed pharmacologically, antibiotic-resistant endogenous or institutional protista establish themselves quite readily as a majority in usually contaminated anatomic sites or even in tissues considered sterile. The original number of such protista may be very small, certainly much less than required with healthy individuals if the environmental surveillance and epidemiological studies can be applied as indicators of the distribution of such nosocomial microorganisms. The impaired patient mechanisms and probably the disturbed microbial ecology resulting from antibiotic therapy allow these hospital organisms to reach critical levels with attendant overt clinical disease. It is not completely clear whether these microorganisms must reach a certain critical number or whether the access of just a few suffices as long as host impairment and lack of competition of normal microbiota persist. These observations emphasize that pathogenicity and virulence cannot be applied to a microbial genus or species without reference to the host and the host's environment or special circumstance. While it is obvious that much must be learned before a clear understanding of infectious disease is established (9), it is equally clear that the concern and responsibility of the clinical microbiologist must transcend the narrow borders of microbial diagnosis or recognition and encompass aspects of the patient's history and condition, his treatment, his present and past environment, and his community. This more encompassing view is required to allow proper distinction of significant microorganisms isolated from pathological specimens. Without such information, the unclear lines of separation between the indigenous and pathogenic microbiota of people will be confused still more, depriving the clinician of information and the capability to intercede effectively against microorganisms for the benefit of his patients.

LITERATURE CITED

1. Burnet, F. M. 1962. Natural history of infectious disease, 3rd ed. Cambridge Univ. Press, Cambridge.
2. Dubos, R. J. 1958. The evolution and the ecology of microbial diseases, p. 14–27. *In* R. J. Dubos (ed.), Bacterial and mycotic infections of man, 3rd ed. J. B. Lippincott Co., Philadelphia.
3. Isenberg, H. D., and J. I. Berkman. 1966. Recent practices in diagnostic bacteriology, p. 237–317. *In* M. Stefanini (ed.), Progress in clinical pathology, vol. 1. Grune and Stratton, New York.
4. Isenberg, H. D., and J. I. Berkman. 1971. The role of drug-resistant and drug-selected bacteria in nosocomial disease. Ann. N.Y. Acad. Sci. **182**:52–58.
5. Fiumara, N. J., H. M. Wise, Jr., and M. Many. 1967. Gonorrheal pharyngitis. N. Engl. J. Med. **276**:1248–1250.
6. McNamara, M. J., M. C. Hill, A. Balows, and E. B. Tucker. 1967. A study of the bacteriological patterns of hospital infections. Ann. Intern. Med. **66**:480–488.
7. Pulaski, E. J. 1954. Common bacterial infections. W. B. Saunders Co., Philadelphia.
8. Rosebury, T. 1961. Microorganisms indigenous to man. McGraw-Hill Book Co., Inc., New York.
9. Smith, H. 1972. The little-known determinants of microbial pathogenicity, p. 1–24. *In* H. Smith and J. H. Pearce (ed.), Microbial pathogenicity in man and animals. Cambridge Univ. Press, Cambridge.
10. Smith, T. 1934. Parasitism and disease. Princeton Univ. Press, Princeton.
11. Wilson, G. S., and A. A. Miles. 1964. Topley and Wilson's principles of bacteriology and immunology, 5th ed. The Williams & Wilkins Co., Baltimore.

Chapter 6

Collection, Handling, and Processing of Specimens

HENRY D. ISENBERG, JOHN A. WASHINGTON II, ALBERT BALOWS, AND ALEX C. SONNENWIRTH

A. INTRODUCTION

A major concern of clinical microbiologists has been with the rapid identification of significant microorganisms isolated from clinical specimens. The scientific literature contains many publications directed at genus and/or species identification in the fastest possible time, yet the subject of this chapter has been almost totally ignored, despite the fact that it constitutes the foundation for all subsequent work. It is not possible to present in the space available an all-encompassing guide to the procurement, proper management, and primary inoculation procedures of clinical specimens (see Table 1). Our interest is to present a working outline that is admittedly not all inclusive, but which is an approach which knowledgeable clinical microbiologists insist on pursuing in the handling of clinical specimens in their laboratories. There are many variations on the approach presented here, and many situations will arise not covered by this chapter.

It is necessary to establish certain quasi-philosophical ground rules for clinical microbiology. The purpose of the clinical microbiology laboratory in the medical facility is to rapidly and accurately provide the clinician with information concerning the presence or absence of a microbial agent, specifically or potentially involved in an infectious disease process in a patient. This information should be speedily supplemented with an antibiotic profile (16, 34). It is more significant for a physician to know that a gram-negative rod susceptible to various antimicrobial agents is present than to wait several days or weeks for a properly identified microorganism. Clinical microbiologists must admit that when they identify a microorganism, they base their identification on a number of salient characteristics. Clinical microbiologists are *not* taxonomists in the strict sense; they do not weigh each microbial character on an equal scale and, after having collected an appreciable number, determine the identity of the organism according to Adansonian precepts. It is, therefore, not surprising to find that a variety of identification schemes are used by clinical microbiologists which do not necessarily reflect the classification schemes of taxonomists or even follow *Bergey's Manual of Determinative Bacteriology*. It is necessary that the staff of the clinical microbiology laboratory be aware of the numerous synonyms which may be attached to the organism they identify by the "accepted" genus and species designation to bridge any communication gap that may occur with the medical staff.

B. COLLECTION OF SPECIMENS

Anatomic and surgical pathology

The microbiologic examination of tissues obtained at the time of surgery or autopsy is of considerable importance because the specimen may represent the entire pathologic process. Surgical specimens are obtained at considerable expense and some risk to the patient. Further surgery to obtain more material may be contraindicated or refused; additional autopsy specimens often are not available because the remains may have already been embalmed and buried. The microbiologist must be prepared to do whatever is necessary to establish the diagnosis frequently with assistance from the pathologist. Many of the necessary procedures have been described in detail (28, 36, 37) and form the basis of the discussion which follows.

Selecting the proper specimen and collecting an adequate sample for examination are essential. When the lesion is large or when there are several lesions, multiple specimens from different sites must be collected. Samples from an abscess should include pus along with a portion of the wall of the abscess. The use of a cotton swab to collect a small amount of pus from an abscess cavity is tantamount to malpractice! It must be remembered that abscesses of the brain, lung, pleural space, peritoneal cavity, liver, pelvis, and wounds commonly contain anaerobes or a mixed flora and that an adequate sample of infected material should be collected and transported to the laboratory in an anaerobic container. When granules are observed in the pus, they should suggest infection with actinomycetes.

Gross surgical specimens submitted for histopathologic examination are ideal for microbiological study since portions of the specimen may be carefully selected for analysis prior to placing the tissue in fixative. A close rapport between microbiologist and pathologist is invaluable. Histologic examination reveals whether or not the lesion is malignant and, if it is inflammatory, whether it is granulomatous or suppurative. If the lesion is malignant, it may not be necessary to perform cultures. If it is inflammatory, the type of reaction seen may indicate what type of cultures are necessary; however, it is well to bear in mind that the histopathology of infections due to mycobacteria, fungi, and brucellae is quite variable and not mutually exclusive. Histopathologic diagnosis of an infection depends on the visualization of a sufficient number of organisms in characteristic form. Tissue stains for acid-fast bacilli provide positive results in only 30 to 40% of those specimens with positive cultures, whereas special stains for fungi may not show the organisms recovered in cultures, or they may show structures resembling the organisms but lacking definitive characteristics (36). Cultures, therefore, are absolutely necessary to establish or to confirm the diagnosis of an infectious process.

A gross surgical specimen may be bisected aseptically by the surgeon. One-half is submitted to surgical pathology and the other half is placed in a sterile, wide-mouthed, screw-capped jar and sent to the microbiology laboratory. The tissue is finely minced with sterile scissors and ground aseptically in a mortar with a pestle with 60-mesh aluminum oxide (alundum). A 20% suspension of the ground material is made in broth and placed into a sterile dropper bottle to be used for inoculating culture media and for storage. Because preparing and examining special histologic stains may take several days and because further microbiologic studies may be indicated thereby, it is advisable to store any residual emulsion at 5 C for a week or two before discarding it. It is recommended that as much material as possible be examined microbiologically by the massive inoculation of multiple plates or tubes containing the appropriate media.

It is generally thought that cultures of embalmed tissue are useless; however, Weed and Bagenstoss were able to isolate tubercule bacilli, *Histoplasma capsulatum*, *Nocardia asteroides*, and various species of bacteria from tissues that had been embalmed for 24 to 48 h (38). Embalming certainly will diminish the probability of recovering an organism; however, in certain cases cultures of tissues embalmed for as long as 48 h may be worthwhile, provided nothing else is available and the area selected for cultures is centrally located.

The value of postmortem microbiology remains controversial. In some institutions the heart blood is routinely cultured; in others, cultures are limited to cases and organs in which infectious disease is suspected. In recent years, attempts have been made to determine whether or not clinical or autopsy evidence of infection is an appropriate mechanism for selecting cases to culture, whether sampling should be limited to tissues or organs suspected of being infected, and whether the microbiologist should attempt to correlate postmortem culture results with those obtained antemortem (12, 17, 40). In general, the results of these studies have demonstrated that man possesses an indigenous tissue flora, that there does not appear to be postmortem transmigration of organisms, that the frequency of positive cultures is poorly related to clinical or autopsy evidence of infectious disease, that there is a substantial lack of correlation between ante- and postmortem culture results, that cultures performed on a single postmortem tissue only are rarely of value, and that in some cases postmortem cultures of multiple tissues may be of value in identifying the etiologic agent of the infection, especially if these represent cases with well-recognized clinical entities caused by a single organism or cases with an overwhelming infection. The value of postmortem cultures is, therefore, limited except in selected cases.

When postmortem cultures are indicated, the prosector should obtain at least a 6-cm-cubed portion of tissue, with one serosal or capsular surface intact. The tissue should then be placed in a sterile, sealed, plastic container and sent to the laboratory for immediate processing or storage at 5 C. Subsequent procedures are based on those described by Dolan (11). In the laboratory, the capsular or serosal surface is throughly seared with a soldering iron and incised with a sterile instrument. A 1-cm-cubed portion of tissue is removed aseptically from the core of the tissue block; it is used to prepare impression smears and is then ground, as described above, to provide a 10 to 20% emulsion to be used as inoculum for cultures. When a small specimen is received, it may be immersed in boiling water for 3 to 5 s to decontaminate its surface. Any residual portion of surgical or anatomical specimens should be retained in the refrigerator by the microbiologist until it is reasonably well established that there is no longer any need to retain the tissue.

The routine described by Isenberg and Berkman for postmortem examination (16) has also been found useful by a number of pathologists and entails qualitatively surveying lungs, liver, spleen, and kidney, as well as obtaining heart blood. Smears and cultures are made of the material aseptically obtained at the time of autopsy. Comparison between the findings from the direct smear and especially the inoculated blood plates usually indicates correlation. One of the major points which must be stressed is the need to obtain microbiological cultures from areas grossly appearing infected or involved in an infectious process. The past history of the patient and his treatment and the agonal events must also be considered so that cultures for organisms which do not grow readily on the media used routinely can be obtained.

Blood cultures

The prompt and accurate isolation of the etiologic agents of septicemia remains one of the most important functions performed by the clinical microbiology laboratory. The indications for obtaining blood cultures are a sudden relative increase in the patient's pulse rate and temperature, a change in sensorium, and the onset of chills, prostration, and hypotension. Other indications include a prolonged, mild, and intermittent fever in association with a heart murmur. Whereas in endocarditis or endarteritis, uncontrolled infections, typhoid fever, and brucellosis the bacteremia is continuous, it is usually intermittent in other cases of bacteremia. Timing in the collection of cultures in endocarditis, for example, is, therefore, not critical; however, in other cases, timing of collection presents a problem because the bacteremia is usually intermittent and precedes the onset of fever or chills by as much as an hour.

In patients with suspected bacterial endocarditis, three blood cultures have been shown to be sufficient to isolate the etiologic agent in nearly all instances. These should be collected separately at no less than hourly intervals within a 24-h period of time. In intermittent bacteremias, three separate blood cultures within 24 to 48 h are usually sufficient to isolate the etiologic agent. In such instances, the time interval between cultures is frequently determined by clinical circumstances and the urgency to initiate antimicrobial therapy. In patients who have received antimicrobics prior to blood collection, a total of four to six separate blood cultures may be necessary to isolate the etiologic agent.

Because of the microflora normally resident in the skin and the misinformation which may result from contamination of blood cultures, it is essential that their collection be performed aseptically, first by cleansing the skin with 70 to 95% alcohol and, secondly, by applying 2% iodine in concentric fashion to the venipuncture site. Because of the lower incidence of skin hypersensitivity to iodophors, they may be used in lieu of iodine. "Instant" antisepsis never occurs, and the iodine or iodophor should remain intact on the skin for at least one minute. The intended venipuncture site should not then be touched unless the fingers used for palpation are similarly disinfected. After the venipuncture, any residual iodine should be removed with an alcohol sponge or pad.

It is recommended that 10 to 20 ml of blood be collected for each culture. Culture of a lesser volume may be responsible for lower recovery rates because of the low order of magnitude of most bacteremias. In infants and children, collection of 1 to 5 ml appears to be satisfactory. In most instances the blood is inoculated directly into culture media at the patient's bedside, either with a syringe and needle or a transfer set. Alternatively, the blood may be transported to the laboratory in a sterile, evacuated tube containing sodium polyanetholsulfonate (SPS) and then inoculated into culture media.

It is essential to inoculate blood into culture media on a 10% vol/vol basis in order to counteract the normal bactericidal activities of chemical and cellular mediators of immunity. Any residual bactericidal effects following this dilution of blood in the culture media have been shown to be abolished by the presence of 0.05 and 0.025% SPS which is a polyanionic anticoagulant which is also anticomplementary and antiphagocytic.

Any general-purpose, commercially available, nutrient broth medium may be used for the culture of blood. Soybean casein digests, such as tryptic (Difco) or Trypticase (BBL) soy broth, Columbia broth, and brain heart infusion broth have been found to be satisfactory. Strict reliance on fluid thioglycolate, Thiol (Difco), or supplemented, prereduced anaerobically sterilized media is not recommended because of lower isolation rates of aerobic or facultatively anaerobic bacteria in these media. Commercially available liquid media are generally bottled under vacuum with CO_2 and contain 0.025% SPS. As such, they are satisfactory for cultivation of anaerobes from blood (see Chapter 43 for more details about anaerobic blood cultures). Bottles containing 50 or 100 ml of media should be employed. Liquid media made hyperosmotic, generally by the addition of sucrose, should still be considered to be experimental, but have, in general, not been found to increase the detection rates nor to decrease the time interval for detection of bacteremia.

If only one blood culture bottle is used, it should not be vented; however, it is desirable to use two bottles, one which should not be vented and the other of which may be vented. Venting should be performed by inserting aseptically a sterile, cotton-plugged needle through the bottle's rubber stopper and then withdrawing it after the vacuum within the bottle has been released. If the venting unit is left in place, the bottle should be incubated in an atmosphere containing 10% CO_2.

Cultures are incubated at 35 C and are inspected later on the same day of their collection and daily thereafter for at least 7 days for evidence of turbidity, hemolysis, gaseousness, or discrete colonies. Clinically significant bacteria are recovered in at least 95% of instances within this period of time; however, longer periods of incubation may be necessary in seriously ill patients who are receiving antimicrobics and who have not responded to initial antimicrobial therapy or in patients with endocarditis or endarteritis due to fastidious microorganisms. Recovery of such bacteria beyond the first 7 days of incubation may provide the opportunity for administration of more specific and effective antimicrobics.

Gram-stained smears and aerobic and anaerobic subcultures of obvious or suspected positive cultures should be prepared immediately, and the results of the microscopic examination of the smear, if positive, should be reported by phone and in writing to the patient's physician as quickly as possible. Subcultures for direct susceptibility testing may be performed; however, these results should be considered to be tentative and should be confirmed by retesting the isolate with standardized methodology.

Routine ("blind") subcultures of grossly negative cultures should be performed within the first 24 h after blood collection and after 4 or 5 days of incubation. Subcultures are inoculated onto quadrants of chocolate blood agar plates which are incubated in 10% CO_2 for 48 h. Subcultures are necessary to ensure the recovery of *Pseudomonas aeruginosa*, *Haemophilus*, meningococci and gonococci, and yeasts, particularly when blood culture bottles are not vented. In some instances a routine Gram-stained smear within 24 h after blood collection has been found to be helpful.

The recovery of diphtheroids (aerobic and anaerobic), *Bacillus*, and *Staphylococcus epidermidis* nearly always signifies contamination, unless they are present in multiple cultures. Nonhemolytic streptococci, excluding group D streptococci, and alpha hemolytic streptococci in single cultures are of uncertain significance. *Bacteroidaceae*, *Enterobacteriaceae*, *P. aeruginosa*, *Haemophilus*, *Staphylococcus aureus*, pneumococci, and yeasts are nearly always clinically significant.

Pour plates are not generally recommended because quantitation of bacteremia is rarely of clinical significance and because isolation rates of bacteria in pour plates are usually lower than those encountered in liquid media. The routine addition of penicillinase to blood culture media does not appear to be justified, except in selected cases which are receiving high doses of a penicillin or cephalosporin at the time of blood collection. In such instances, it is essential to prepare concurrent cultures of the penicillinase solution, contamination of which has been associated with outbreaks of "pseudosepticemia."

The isolation of brucellae may be performed by inoculation of the blood into Castañeda's double medium or into soybean casein digest broth which must be subcultured at least twice weekly for 4 weeks. In either case, prolonged capneic incubation is required.

Leptospiremia is usually present only during the first week of illness. One to three drops of freshly drawn blood are inoculated into each of several tubes containing 5 ml of a suitable semisolid medium, such as Fletcher's, which are incubated in the dark at 30 C for 28 days. A portion of each culture is examined weekly by dark-field or fluorescence microscopy.

Although it has been recommeded by some that detection of fungemia should be accomplished by inoculation of blood, on a 10% vol/vol basis, into a soybean casein digest broth or into brain heart infusion broth with subcultures to fungal isolation agar media at 48-h intervals, it appears that fungal isolation rates are improved by inoculation of the blood into a Castañeda double medium, preparation of pour plates, or direct inoculation of fungal isolation agar media.

For more details regarding blood cultures readers may consult the *Cumitech* (in press, America Society for Microbiology, Washington, D.C.) devoted to blood cultures.

Ear

The bacteriological findings from persons with acute otitis media have been sufficiently consistent in many reported studies that there would seem to be little justification in performing tympanocentesis, except in therapeutic failures or in neonates in whom the bacterial etiology differs from that found in older children. Since the correlation between nasopharyngeal cultures and middle ear cultures is poor, cultures of the nasopharynx may provide misleading results. Most studies show that *Streptococcus pneumoniae*, *Haemophilus influenzae*, and *Streptococcus pyogenes* are the most common etiologic agents of acute otitis media; however, in neonates, *Escherichia coli*, *Klebsiella pneumoniae*, and *Staphylococcus aureus* represent the most frequent isolates (7), and in therapeutic failures *S. aureus* and *Pseudomonas aeruginosa* are predominant (1, 7).

Eye

In patients with conjunctivitis and, especially, with keratitis, there are special problems in specimen collection and processing. Swabs are generally inadequate for establishing the presence of microorganisms because of the small sample size. An additional problem is the antimicrobial activity of topical anesthetics (26). Microbes responsible for keratoconjunctivitis include bacteria, actinomycetes, fungi, and viruses. It is, therefore, recommended that swabs for cultures be taken before topical anesthetics are applied and that corneal scrapings be taken after they are applied. Ideally, a laboratory technologist should assist the opthalmologist in collecting the specimen and preparing the cultures.

Examination of Gram- and Giemsa-stained smears of the corneal scrapings may provide preliminary clues as to the nature of the disease. If necessary, stains for acid-fast bacteria or a potassium hydroxide wet mount can be made. Because of the limited amount of material available, it is recommended that the scrapings be spot-inoculated directly on to each one of the following media: chocolate-blood-agar, brain heart infusion-agar with 5% sheep's blood, inhibitory mold agar, and Lowenstein-Jensen agar. Swab cultures may be inoculated on to one half of each agar plate and the scrapings on the other half.

Feces

Proper collection and preservation of feces is a frequently neglected but important requirement for the isolation of microorganisms contributing to intestinal disease. Unless the specimen can be taken immediately to the laboratory and properly handled there, a number of significant microorganisms will not survive the changes in pH which occur with a drop in temperature. This is especially true of most shigellae and an appreciable number of the salmonellae. When the above-mentioned delays are unavoidable, it should be a standard rule that all stool specimens be submitted in a stool preservative, such as 0.033 M phosphate buffer mixed with equal volumes of glycerol. An indicator may be added which will assure an approximate pH of 7. Stool specimens are then introduced into a screw-capped glass container with stool preservative immediately after they have been passed. A 0.3- to 2-g quantity is quite sufficient. If sterile swabs are used in obtaining the specimen, they should be passed beyond the anal sphincter, carefully rotated, and withdrawn. The swabs may be added to a screw-capped tube containing preservative and transported to the laboratory for culture. The indicator added to the specimen provides visual proof that the pH drop has not been inordinate. Difficulties are occasionally encountered when patients have diarrhea and are unable to use a bedpan. Under those circumstances, paper toweling may be deposited into the toilet bowl and the diarrheal stool obtained above the water level. Toilet paper which has been impregnated with bismuth salts in the manufacturing process should not be used, since a number of organisms found in feces are inhibited or killed by these salts.

If the patient is hospitalized, personnel obtaining the specimen should be instructed explicitly to choose portions of the stool that display either mucus or blood. These areas usually harbor a large number of the organisms that are involved in the disease process.

It cannot be stated too often that the very vast majority of bacteria found in feces are anaerobic gram-negative rods. They are usually ignored in the attempt to diagnose infectious intestinal disorders. This is not to imply that such organisms may not be involved in disease processes of the intestinal tract. However, to date such a causal relationship has not been established, with the exception of foodborne *Clostridium perfringens* intoxication. It is important to remember that the biochemical activities of the anaerobic microbiota contribute to the detriment of the *Enterobacteriaceae*. Therefore, the facultative anaerobic enteric bacteria require the type of buffering provided by a stool preservative.

There are times when surveys for carriers as well as institutional outbreaks indicate a need to use rectal swabs to obtain specimens. Under these circumstances, the stool preservative should not be used; the swab should immediately be placed, instead, into a medium such as GN broth, especially if the responsible organism has already been identified and contacts or carriers are being sought. Enrichments such as tetrathionate broth or Selenite F may be used, particularly if salmonellae are involved.

As with most other specimens, a single stool specimen with little or no accompanying information is inadequate. The laboratory can be much more helpful to the clinician if a brief history is provided. If necessary, the physician of record should be called for this information so the clinical microbiologist can be particularly attentive to culturing the stool on media most likely to yield the responsible bacteria, fungi, or parasites. Without such information, procedures cannot be modified to accommodate as complete a microbiological analysis as is required. Of equal concern is the increased cost and time lost in searching for impossible organisms.

A single negative stool culture can not be regarded as being sufficient for laboratory confirmation of noninvolvement of infectious bacteria. Although the number three is not inviolate, repeated cultures are indicated if the clinical picture suggests the involvement of bacteria and the first two cultures are unrewarding in spite of the symptoms. Similarly, after the diagnosis has been made, microbiological surveillance of the convalescent individual and of contacts that may have become carriers should be conducted at regular intervals until at least three negative specimens have been obtained consistently.

When the history or early examination suggests the possibility that anaerobes or staphylococci, *Vibrio cholerae*, or *V. parahaemolyticus* may be involved, special media should be used for direct inoculation of the stool. When gastrointestinal tuberculosis is suspected, the clinical microbiology laboratory should follow the suggestions in Chapter 16. Specimens collected for the demonstration of parasites and ova will be discussed in the section on parasitology. Gram-stained smears for the demonstration of bacteria have not been used frequently in recent times. In the past, this examination was popular for determining the ratio of gram-negative to gram-positive bacteria. It is not possible to determine the type of microorganisms present simply by observing the morphology and staining characteristics of bacteria in a stool specimen. The usefulness of such a method should be restricted to cases such as pseudomembranous colitis, staphylococcal enterocolitis, or monilial disease where the overwhelming number of gram-positive cocci or yeast-like cells would easily be demonstrated in a properly made Gram stain of a portion of the stool specimen or rectal swab.

Fluids, body

Cerebrospinal fluid. Examination of cerebrospinal fluid (CSF) from patients suspected of having meningitis represents one of the major emergency procedures faced by personnel in the clinical microbiology laboratory. The reasons for this urgency are that bacterial meningitis is a rapidly fatal disease if untreated or inadequately treated and that appropriate antimicrobial therapy often requires prompt identification of the etiologic agent. Lumbar puncture and examination of the CSF should be undertaken whenever the physician suspects meningitis or wants to rule it out. It must be remembered that the typical signs of meningeal irritation in the adult, such as fever, headache, vomiting, nuchal rigidity, hypereflexia, etc., are usually absent in infants and neonates in whom the clinical manifestations of meningitis are vague and nonspecific. An unexplained febrile illness in an irritable infant who is doing poorly should lead one to suspect meningitis. Meningitides due to myocbacteria, fungi, leptospira, and protozoa are generally insidious in onset. The diagnosis of viral meningoencephalitis is frequently one established by exclusion and one that may be established by virus cultures of sources other than spinal fluid or by serologic means.

Lumbar puncture must be performed under conditions of strict asepsis, since contamination of the specimen can occur readily and confuse the identification of the etiologic agent. The skin should be disinfected with povidone-iodine. Specimens should be collected in sterile containers which can be sealed with a screw cap in order to preclude leakage and loss or contamination of the contents. Cotton-plugged or rubber-stoppered tubes should not be used, and snap-top containers should be checked to ensure that a tight seal does occur and that some contents are not aerosolized on opening. The absence of microorganisms in CSF specimen containers should not only be confirmed by culture but also presumptively by Gram stain (22). Prompt transport of the specimen to the laboratory is mandatory, since fastidious organisms, such as *Haemophilus influenzae* and *Neisseria meningitidis*, may not survive storage or variations in temperature. For these reasons, some advocate that smears be prepared and cultures inoculated at the patient's bedside when the CSF is obtained. Though such a practice may be ideal, it is seldom practical. The clinical microbiologist, therefore, should (i) examine the lumbar puncture tray routinely used in the hospital to ensure that the CSF containers are of satisfactory quality (not all commercially available trays have airtight specimen containers), (ii) attempt to establish a standardized skin preparation, and (iii) develop the systems whereby the specimen can be transported promptly to the laboratory. An adequate sample of CSF ("as much as possible") should be available for microbiologic examination, particularly when a diagnosis of tuberculous or fungal meningitis is considered, since the numbers of microorganisms present are often small. If only one specimen container is filled, it should be submitted to the microbiology laboratory first so that it can be opened aseptically and samples for chemical and cytological studies can be removed at the time cultures are inoculated. The microbiology laboratory should process the fluid immediately by preparing Gram-stained smears and inoculating the appropriate media.

Since there are usually only small numbers of microorganisms present in infected CSF, some procedure for the concentration of any organisms present should generally be performed. The simplest of these procedures is to centrifuge the specimen at 2,500 rpm for 15 min, and then to remove the supernatant fluid for chemical or serologic studies and use the sediment for both smear and culture purposes. This centrifugation is adequate for those fluids in which there is an increase in inflammatory cells; however, its limitations are that in very early cases of bacterial meningitis and in fungal meningitis the cell count may be normal despite a positive culture. Furthermore, a force of $10,000 \times g$ for 10 min is required to sediment *H. influenzae*, which means that with most standard clinical laboratory centrifuges, which develop a maximum of $1,000 \times g$, 60 min may be necessary (30). For these reasons, prolonged ($\geq$30 min) examination of the Gram-stained smear under oil immersion may be necessary. The same sampling problem occurs when attempts are made to culture the specimen from a nonexistent sediment. In instances in which there is no cellular response or a poor one, it is recommended that the specimen be concentrated instead by filtration through a 0.45-μm membrane filter which is directly placed on an appropriate culture medium. Sterile, disposable, 13- and 25-mm filter units (Swinnex, Millipore Corp.) are satisfactory and convenient for this purpose.

A variety of immunological procedures have been developed for the rapid diagnosis of bacterial meningitis; however, they are not widely used because of the specialized reagents and equipment required. Fluorescent microscopy, capsular swelling, counter immunoelectrophoresis and latex particle agglutination are the principal techniques used. In most laboratories, however, the Gram-stained smear remains the most reliable and convenient rapid diagnostic tool.

The host's inflammatory and noninflammatory responses may be helpful in the differential diagnosis of meningitis. Whereas the leukocytic response in the CSF in acute bacterial meningitis is usually polymorphonuclear, that in tuberculous, fungal, leptospiral, or protozoal meningitis is usually lymphocytic and less intense. Although polymorphonuclear leukocytes may be predominant in the CSF early in the course of aseptic meningitis, there is usually a clear shift to mononuclear cells within 8 h (13). The CSF glucose is usually depressed in acute bacterial and tuberculous meningitis and normal in the other meningitides; CSF protein is usually elevated. Cytological and chemical changes in the CSF may occur in patients with brain abscess; however, smears and cultures of the CSF are generally negative in these cases unless the abscess ruptures into the subarachnoid space or the ventricles.

One final point in partially treated cases of bacterial meningitis deserves emphasis, and that is that cellular and chemical tests and the recovery rates of bacteria in cultures may be altered (9, 10). Furthermore, a tendency has been noted for gram-positive organisms to appear to be gram-negative in such cases (9), so that findings in a Gram-stained smear must be interpreted cautiously.

When fungal meningitis is suspected, a drop of the CSF sediment should be mixed with a drop of India ink (Pelikan, Gunther, and Wagner, Hanover, Germany) or nigrosin (Harleco, Div. of Hartman-Leddon Co., Philadelphia, Pa.) solution on a clean glass slide, covered with a cover slip, and examined with a decreased intensity of light. Nigrosin is preferable to India ink because it is free of discernible particulate matter. The presence of encapsulated, budding yeast-like cells in the wet preparation is virtually diagnostic of cryptococcal meningitis; however, special care must be exercised in differentiating nonencapsulated yeasts from red or white blood cells, air bubbles, or even talc. In some cases of cryptococcal meningitis, there is little or no cellular response or depression of the sugar value in the CSF.

Cryptococcal meningitis is frequently associated with disseminated infection, and it is not uncommon to recover *C. neoformans* from sources other than CSF (urine, blood, sputum, bone marrow, etc.). In patients from whom *C. neoformans* has been recovered initially from such other sources, serious consideration must be given to lumbar puncture and examination of the CSF, since symptoms referable to the central nervous system may be absent. In cases with suspected cryptococcal meningitis, performance of the latex-cryptococcal antigen test (LCAT) with CSF and serum may be helpful.

The development of meningoencephalitis of obscure etiology in patients with a recent history of swimming in brackish water before the onset of symptoms should lead to the prompt examination of the CSF for motile amoebas (12a).

Fluids other than CSF. As with the lumbar puncture, the percutaneous aspiration of pleural, pericardial, peritoneal, and synovial fluids must be performed aseptically to avoid contamination of the specimen and to prevent the accidental introduction of microorganisms into these anatomical spaces. The specimen should immediately be injected into a sterile tube or bottle. Since infection of these spaces may be due to anaerobes, it is recommended that fluid or pus be collected with a sterile syringe and needle, that any air bubbles present in the syringe be expelled, and that the material then be injected into an anaerobic transport tube or vial containing CO_2. Again, as much material as is feasible and practical to collect should be submitted to the laboratory. A small amount of sterile heparin may be added to the fluid to prevent coagulation, since clots may trap microorganisms. Coagulated material should be emulsified and cultured along with a portion of its surrounding fluid.

Gram-stained smears of the centrifuged sediment of clear or slightly cloudy fluids should be examined carefully; however, frankly purulent material should be smeared directly and examined after it has been stained for the presence of bacteria.

Respiratory tract

Cultures of the respiratory tract must be interpreted cautiously because of the microflora normally present in the nose, oral cavity, and pharynx and because of the frequency of nosocomial acquisition of potentially pathogenic microorganisms by seriously ill patients. Since potential pathogens such as *Staphylococcus aureus*, *Haemophilus influenzae*, *Streptococcus pneumoniae*, *Pseudomonas aeruginosa*, *Enterobacteriaceae*, and yeasts may be present in the oropharynx, their isolation from cultures of the respiratory secretions does not represent a priori evidence of their etiological role in respiratory infections.

Nasopharyngeal cultures should be performed to detect carrier states of *Neisseria meningitidis*, *Corynebacterium diphtheriae*, and *Streptococcus pyogenes*. In addition, such cultures aid in the diagnosis of whooping cough, croup, and pneumonia in infants and children unable to expectorate sputum for examination. Nasopharyngeal specimens should be obtained with a dacron, cotton, or calcium alginate swab on a flexible wire which is gently passed through the nose into the nasopharynx, rotated, removed, and placed into a suitable transport medium or inoculated directly into the appropriate medium for isolation. Since coughing may force organisms from the lower respiratory tract into the nasopharynx, there may be some virtue in stimulating coughing in an infant or child by attempting to obtain a throat culture before the nasopharyngeal specimen is obtained for culture. Examination of a Gram-stained smear of material obtained by nasopharyngeal swab may be helpful in providing a preliminary indication of the etiology of a pulmonary infection if there is a predominance of one type of organism.

Although nasopharyngeal cultures are sometimes recommended in comatose patients unable to expectorate a sputum sample, the frequency of aspiration and subsequent anaerobic pleuropulmonary infection in these patients and the misleading results provided by oropharyngeal contamination make percutaneous transtracheal aspiration mandatory (5).

H. influenzae type B may cause a form of croup known as acute epiglottitis. The distinctive appearance of the epiglottis and the rapidly progressive and fulminating course which may lead to death within 24 h demand prompt initiation of therapy. Nasopharyngeal and blood specimens should be cultured for *H. influenzae*. Since it is important to rule out diphtheria, specimens from the larynx should also be cultured for *C. diphtheriae*.

It should be kept in mind that orolaryngeal involvement is not uncommon in both acute and chronic disseminated forms of histoplasmosis and blastomycosis (6), in tuberculosis, and in leishmaniasis. Cultures for these agents and biopsy with histological demonstration of the organisms are necessary to establish the correct diagnosis. It is imperative that the clinician communicate his clinical suspicions to the microbiologist immediately. Otherwise valuable time and specimens may be lost.

Throat cultures are most frequently obtained for the diagnosis of streptococcal pharyngitis and, less commonly, for the diagnosis of pertussis, diphtheria, and pharyngitis due to gonococci or viruses. There is no need to identify other microorganisms in routinely submitted throat cultures, since there is little or no evidence to document their role in producing pharyngitis. Exudative pharyngitis, enlarged cervical nodes, headache, nausea, vomiting, and abdominal pain are commonly associated with streptococcal pharyngitis, whereas cough, rhinorrhea, and hoarseness are commonly associated with viral pharyngitis (14). There are, however, many viral infections which are confused clinically with streptococcal pharyngitis. Acute tonsillopharyngitis with vesicles or shallow ulcers on the anterior fauces, palate, and buccal mucosa is usually due to herpes simplex or to coxsackie A virus. A history of an incomplete immunization series or no immunization during childhood should alert the clinician to the possibility of infection with *Bordetella pertussis* or *Corynebacterium diphtheriae*, particularly when coupled with the characteristic signs and symptoms of these diseases. Gonococcal pharyngeal infection should be suspected in patients with gonococcal infections at other sites, especially among those practicing fellatio (39).

Requisitions for culture or specimens from the upper respiratory tract should specify the suspected etiological agent so that laboratory personnel may take appropriate steps to ensure its isolation. The culture should be obtained, under direct visualization with a dacron, cotton, or calcium alginate swab, by vigorously swabbing both tonsillar areas, the posterior pharynx, and any areas of inflammation, ulceration, exudation, or capsule formation. The tongue should be depressed with a tongue blade or spoon to minimize contamination of the swab with oral secretions which may dilute, overgrow, or inhibit the growth of pharyngeal flora.

Bacterial culturing of sputum is fraught with error, and clearcut results are seldom obtained. Specimens are frequently collected haphazardly by paramedical personnel who are not aware of the necessity for a fresh, clean specimen resulting from a deep cough and who fail to transport the specimen to the laboratory promptly. Expectorated sputum is frequently contaminated with oropharyngeal flora, and it is difficult to determine which of the many different potential pathogens isolated is responsible for pulmonary infection. Rarely, a potential pathogen is isolated in pure culture and may be presumed to represent the etiological agent. To quote E. Barrett-Connor (3), who found no pneumococci in 45% of the sputum and nasopharyngeal cultures examined from patients with pneumococcal bacteremia, "The routine sputum culture for the diagnosis of acute bacterial pneumonia may be a sacred cow. Not only can the results lead to serious mismanagement of the patient, but also sputum cultures represent one of the largest workloads and expenses for the hospital bacteriology laboratory." Correlation between results of cultures of transtracheal aspirates and results of qualitative and quantitative cultures of the sputum has been poor (15). There is, therefore, no completely satisfactory method for isolating bacterial pathogens from expectorated sputum at the present time. Under no circumstances is anaerobic bacterial culturing of sputum performed.

Lower respiratory secretions collected by nasotracheal aspiration with a catheter may also become contaminated with upper respiratory flora. Bronchial washings or brushings may be collected with minimal risk of contamination through the lumen of a bronchoscope which can be directed towards the site of a lesion or drainage. A third method, which bypasses oropharyngeal contamination completely, is percutaneous transtracheal aspiration, a relatively harmless procedure that can be performed rapidly with local anesthesia (5). This procedure is recommended for seriously ill or comatose patients who have pneumonia and cannot raise sputum. Serious complications are rare when experienced personnel perform this procedure (35); nonetheless, patients must be followed carefully. In preparation for transtracheal aspiration, the patient is placed in the supine position with a pillow under the shoulders in order to hyperextend the neck. The skin is disinfected with povidone-iodine. An intradermal wheal is raised over the inferior edge of the thyroid cartilage with lidocaine or xylocaine. A commercially available intravenous catheter (12 inches [ca. 30.5 cm] in length) set with a 14-gauge needle (Bardic) is inserted through the skin and cricothyroid membrane into the trachea, and the catheter is directed caudad. The needle is withdrawn and the catheter is left in place. A 30- or 50-ml syringe is attached to the catheter, and suction is applied. If no material is aspirated in this manner, 2 to 4 ml of sterile saline free from bacteriostatic agents may be injected rapidly through the catheter and aspirated for culture. Since the saline itself may be bactericidal, any specimen so collected should be cultured promptly; if this is not feasible, a balanced salt solution, such as lactated Ringer's, should be used instead (25). At the conclusion of the procedure, the catheter is withdrawn, and pressure is applied over the puncture site for several minutes. It is recommended that a Gram-stained smear of the material collected by transtracheal aspiration be examined and that aerobic and anaerobic bacterial cultures be performed with all possible speed. In some instances, culturing for mycobacteria and fungi may also be indicated. The above procedure should be performed by a qualified physician.

Culture of early morning freshly expectorated sputum, or of expectorated sputum induced by a heated aqueous aerosol of 10% glycerin and 15% sodium chloride, followed in about 1 h by a gastric washing (8) is useful for recovery of mycobacteria and fungi. Gastric washings obtained after induced coughing may have more mycobacteria (8). A series of such collections may be desirable. Ideally, the specimens should be cultured on the day they are collected. Pooled specimens are sometimes collected for culture; however, to prevent overgrowth of contaminants, it is necessary to refrigerate each specimen until the pool is processed. Twenty-four-hour sputum collections are unnecessary, in fact, undesirable.

In some instances, the etiology of pulmonary infections may be diagnosed by percutaneous transthoracic needle biopsy of the lung, thoracentesis, needle aspiration of an abscess or empyema cavity, or open lung biopsy. When open biopsy is performed, multiple specimens should be obtained from different sites if the lesion is large or multiple lesions are present. In addition, a portion of an abscess wall should be removed, as well as a sample of the pus within (37). Histological examination serves two purposes: to determine whether the lesion is inflammatory and, if so, to provide clues as to the nature of the infectious agent. These clues may, in turn, lead to further histological studies with special stains and to additional special cultures. Open lung biopsy may be necessary to establish the diagnosis of infection due to *Pneumocystis carinii*, and it may be helpful in either establishing or confirming infections due to mycobacteria, fungi, and viruses. In experienced hands, the diagnosis of pneumocytosis may be made by staining appropriately material obtained by bronchial or by transbronchial biopsy.

Urine

Urinary tract infections encompass diseases that affect areas ranging from the kidney to the urethra, with the urethra and bladder most commonly affected. Infections are classified as uncomplicated (medical) when there are no anatomical or neurological abnormalities present and as complicated (surgical) when residual inflammatory changes, obstructive uropathy, calculi, or neurological lesions are present (19). Infections usually arise via the urethra by the ascending route and, less commonly, hematogenously. In most hospitals, urinary tract infections represent the most common form of nosocomial infection.

Females of child-bearing age seen for the first time with symptoms of uncomplicated urinary tract infection are nearly always infected with *Escherichia coli*. These strains are usually susceptible to antimicrobics, including sulfonamides, which are active against gram-negative bacilli. Because a high degree of correlation exists between urinary sterilization and in vitro susceptibilities (32), some argue that it is unnecessary to obtain cultures on these patients. However, the prevailing viewpoint is that it is essential to obtain urine cultures during therapy. According to Stamey, "Better medicine is practiced, at less expense to the patient, if a culture is repeated 48 to 78 hours after starting therapy than if a useless antimicrobial agent is continued for ten days in the face of ineffective therapy" (33). Urine cultures obtained during therapy should be sterile, and the patient's symptomatic response is a poor indicator of successful therapy. Pyuria is not a totally reliable index of the presence of disease because it may be absent during the process or may occur in disorders other than in bacterial infection, such as extreme dehydration, trauma secondary to instrumentation or calculi, chemical inflammation, renal tuberculosis, acute glomerulonephritis, and nonbacterial gastroenteritis and respiratory infections (24).

The reliability of a culture of a single, cleanly voided specimen from a female is about 80% and is virtually 100% in the adult male if he is circumcized or has carefully retracted the foreskin and cleansed the glans. In females, the reliability of a clean-voided specimen increases to 90% and to nearly 100% if two and three specimens, respectively, are obtained and contain the same organism. Obviously, in symptomatic patients one specimen only is usually collected before therapy is initiated; however, in asymptomatic patients two or three specimens should be collected to document the presence of bacteriuria.

Guidelines for the diagnosis of urinary tract infections and minimal diagnostic criteria have been presented in detail by Kunin (19). In most females, the clean-voided midstream method of specimen collection is satisfactory, provided the patient is capable of cleansing herself and collecting her own specimen, or the nursing personnel, in the case of the bedridden patient, clearly understand printed or stated instructions (19). All too frequently, instructions are given casually. The result is a grossly contaminated specimen. In addition, the task of obtaining a specimen from the bedridden patient is frequently assigned to the most inexperienced hospital aide or orderly. Hospitals should be encouraged to establish urine collection teams or select individuals who are trained in the proper methods of urine collection and transport.

Urine collection for culture by urethral catheterization is seldom indicated, except in those cases in which catheterization must otherwise be done for diagnostic or therapeutic reasons. There is a small risk of infection after urethral catheterization which varies according to the type of patient catheterized. Because of normal urethral colonization with bacteria, it may be difficult to determine whether organisms isolated from a catheterized urine sample are of urinary or urethral origin.

Contamination of the urine by urethral or introital microflora may be obviated by suprapubic aspiration. This is a rapid, safe, and simple technique when performed by a qualified physician. Suprapubic aspiration is indicated in patients with clinical evidence of urinary tract infection but in whom bacterial counts in clean-voided specimens are low and, therefore, indeterminate, in neonates, in young infants, and in patients in whom catheterization may be contraindicated. The patient should have a full bladder at the time the procedure is performed. After the skin has been properly disinfected, a 19- or 20-gauge needle attached to a syringe is passed through the skin in the midline at a point approximately one-third the distance from the symphysis pubis to the umbilicus. Urine is aspirated into the syringe.

In patients with chronic indwelling urethral catheters attached to closed drainage, urine is collected for culture by disinfecting with a suitable agent the wall of the catheter at its juncture with the drainage tube and puncturing it with a 21-gauge needle attached to a syringe into which the urine is aspirated. It is possible to puncture such a catheter repeatedly without leakage occurring from the puncture sites. The connection between the catheter and the drainage tube should *not* be broken for specimen collection, nor should material for culture be taken from the drainage bag.

During the course of cystoscopy, ureteral catheterization, or retrograde pyelography, urine may be collected for culture. In the case of an obstructed ureter, bladder urine may be sterile whereas the urine proximal to the obstruction may be infected; hence, the urologist will often collect several specimens and request that each be handled separately.

Transport and storage of urine specimens are important adjuncts to the reliability of culture results. A sterile, screw-capped container or tube should be used. Urine is an excellent culture medium, and a small or insignificant number of bacteria can multiply rapidly to a significant number unless certain precautions are taken. If the urine cannot be cultured within an hour after its collection, it can be refrigerated with satisfactory results for at least 24 h and, according to one report (21), for as long as 5 to 10 days. The wisdom of prolonged refrigeration has recently been questioned and should be done only if absolutely necessary.

Significant bacteriuria occurs when there are 100,000 colonies or more per ml in a clean-voided, midstream specimen obtained from asymptomatic patients. Lower counts in a catheterized specimen require reculturing for confirmation of the results. Any count in a suprapubic aspirate is significant, although recovery of skin contaminants, such as diphtheroids and staphylococci, may not be significant and may require repetition of the procedure to confirm or rule out their presence in the urine. Clean-voided, midstream specimens containing between 1,000 and 100,000 colonies of a single microbial species per ml represent possible or probable infections and should be repeated, whereas those with less than 1,000 colonies per ml represent contamination. It must be recognized, however, that bacteriuria may be low on a diurnal basis when the patient is well hydrated, if the urine pH is below 5.0 or its specific gravity is less than 1.003, in the presence of an antimicrobic, with complete ureteral obstruction, and in chronic pyelonephritis (24). The role of cell wall-defective variants in urinary tract infections has not been established clearly. Anaerobic bacteriuria, although not uncommon in cleanly voided, midstream specimens, has been only rarely confirmed by suprapubic aspiration (29), which represents the only reliable means by which to establish this diagnosis.

Chemical and other newer screening tests notwithstanding, significant bacteriuria may be established with 80 to 90% accuracy by microscopic examination of a Gram-stained smear of a well-mixed, unspun urine or of a wet preparation of unstained urinary sediment. Finding bacteria by either method signifies bacteriuria of 100,000 or more colonies per ml.

Candiduria is abnormal; its quantitation is of little importance and may even be misleading if standards currently applicable to bacteriuria are applied (27). What is important is its relationship to the clinical picture, and it may serve not only as a warning of generalized candidiasis but also as an indication of the presence of an underlying disease. *Candida* and *Torulopsis* are frequently grown on conventional bacteriological media; however, their recovery is improved, particularly when present in small numbers mixed with bacteria, on fungal agar media containing antibiotics, e.g., inhibitory mold agar. A microscope examination of a wet preparation of urinary sediment may serve easily and inexpensively to demonstrate the presence of yeasts and pseudohyphal elements.

Pyuria without bacteriuria indicates the possibility of renal tuberculosis. There may be gross or microscopic hematuria, and secondary bladder involvement may produce symptoms of cystitis. Three consecutive clean-voided, early morning specimens should be collected for cultures. Twenty-four-hour urine collections are undesirable because of the frequent overgrowth of bacteria other than mycobacteria.

Finally, a urinary calculus should be split so that cultures can be made of its interior, as well as of its surface, since it is not uncommon to isolate bacteria from within the stone which are not present on its surface (23).

Venereal disease

Concern with gonorrhea has dominated the field of venereal disease. At this time, the only diagnostic test is the microbiological demonstration of viable gonococci in the various exudates and lesions which are present in persons with this disease. In the male, the microscopic observation of gonococci in a Gram-stained smear of a urethral discharge remains unproblematic. There is excellent correlation between the presumptive diagnosis of uncomplicated gonorrhea in the male based on the microscopic examination of a Gram-stained smear of urethral exudate and the confirmation of the diagnosis by culturing and identifying the organisms by standard techniques. However, it must be kept in mind that some individuals do not arrive at a clinic or consult their physician in the early stages of the disease. On such occasions, a Gram smear obtained from such a urethral discharge may still contain numerous pus cells but little or no evidence of microorganisms. In this circumstance, it is advisable that the urethral exudate of the male be cultured as well as smears obtained. Direct inoculation of Thayer-Martin (TM) medium or modified TM medium (20) is advisable in situations where an inoculated plate can be immediately transported to the laboratory. If the history and symptoms suggest exposure, but only a small urethral discharge can be obtained, prostatic massage should be performed by the clinician, the secretions cultured appropriately, and a smear examined. If it is known or suspected that homosexuality exists, oropharyngeal and rectal cultures are indicated. TM agar or modified TM agar plates are indicated. Recent reports of cryptic carriage of gonococci in the distal urethra of clinically asymptomatic men exposed to infected women makes the culturing of this site with bacteriologic loops inserted into the urethra for a short distance a significant test.

Obtaining an adequate specimen in female patients may present greater problems. The presence of a cervical discharge is helpful in the diagnosis. However, the Gram-stained smear obtained from such a discharge cannot be relied upon to establish the absence or presence of the gonococcus, and cultures should be made without exception. A cervical culture and, where possible, an anal culture have been recommended. If pelvic examination suggests that the vaginal glands or the urethra are involved, swabs from these areas should also be cultured for the gonococcus on TM medium. Should transport to the laboratory be delayed, modified TM may be employed.

Skin lesions, especially in the female, have been observed with increasing frequency. Very often they appear at the same time as pudendal involvement. Cultures of scrapings from the base of such lesions have been successful but are positive in a comparatively low percentage of the cases. Careful uprooting of the skin lesion with a sterile needle should be employed for obtaining specimens from these sites.

When a diagnosis of gonococcal arthritis is suspected, properly obtained specimens should be cultured on a blood-agar plate and a noninhibitory plate of chocolate-agar. Caution must be exercised before needling such joints, with particular emphasis on adequate skin preparation. It is advisable that smears be made from the aspirated material and that it be cultured also for organisms other than the gonococcus. The use of hypertonic media for the detection of cell wall-deficient variants is advisable. Finally, when gonococcemia is suspected, the blood culture bottles should be subcultured minimally at 1-, 2-, and 4-day intervals on noninhibitory chocolate-agar.

Either TM medium or modified TM is advocated for cultures of the exudate in ophthalmia neonatorum. Endocervical cultures of the mother should also be obtained immediately.

The immediate inoculation and proper incubation of the culture medium should be stressed by the clinical microbiology laboratory. It is comparatively easy to indoctrinate clinic and hospital personnel in the proper fashion of carrying out this procedure. Illustrative materials, available from the Center for Disease Control, are most helpful in presenting the proper procedures. The microscopic observation of bacteria on smears prepared carelessly is often obscured by the thickness of the material allowed to dry on a slide. Ward and clinic personnel should be reminded continuously that thinner smears are more helpful, instructed how to prepare slides in a proper fashion, and shown the difference between thick and thin smears for the purposes of recognizing gonococci.

It is also necessary to instruct and inform physicians, nurses, and attendants that the gonococcus can remain viable for some periods of time in certain body fluids and that precautions to protect themselves and laboratory personnel handling the material are required. Containers contaminated on the outside, swabs not properly transported in enclosures, and smears dripping with discharge should not be handled in the laboratory without all individuals using every precaution to prevent personal contamination.

Dark-field demonstration of *Treponema pallidum* from primary and secondary lesions of syphilis is the only direct microbiological examination that may be requested of a clinical laboratory. This is a useless procedure if performed on material obtained and transported to the laboratory. Patients with such lesions must be examined within the vicinity of a dark-field microscope. Proper preparation of these lesions, the preparation of the slide, and the recognition of the treponemae are not within the scope of this chapter. However, it should be evident that, because of the infrequency with which this examination is performed in the routine clinical microbiology laboratory, only very experienced personnel should be assigned the task of identifying *T. pallidum* in the dark-field preparations made from lesions. It may even be advisable to send patients to a laboratory where the test is performed routinely. The misdiagnosis of syphilis can be a traumatic and damaging experience to the patient and must be avoided at all costs.

Chancroid is rarely reported. A presumptive identification of *Haemophilus ducreyi* may be made on a smear obtained from the soft center of the lesion produced by the organism. However, inexperienced laboratory personnel should not attempt to make a final diagnosis of this agent but insist on corroboration by experienced microbiologists, usually found at governmental or central laboratories.

Wounds

Material from a previously undrained wound abscess, if properly collected and transported to the laboratory, should contain the etiological agent(s) of disease in most instances. An opened wound, ulcer, or sinus tract, however, frequently becomes contaminated with skin, mucosal, or airborne microorganisms. In general, the use of a swab to collect material from these sites is of limited value, since the amount of material supplied for examination is not only very small but also likely to represent an inadequate sample. Moreover, nothing is more worthless than a dry swab from a dry lesion. In chronic, localized lesions the number of organisms present may be small. A sterile needle and syringe should be used to collect a generous quantity of liquid material. Since anaerobes are commonly recovered from certain wounds, such material should be sent to the laboratory immediately or preferably injected into an anaerobic tube or vial for transport. Since sinus tracts usually originate in bone or in lymph nodes, the orifice of the tract should be cleansed thoroughly with a suitable antiseptic, then curettings of the tract's lining should be taken as close to its base as possible. Ulcerative lesions of the skin and mucosa should be biopsied or, if they are small, excised for histopathological and microbiological studies. Irrigation, intravenous, or intraarterial catheters should be carefully removed after their entry site in the skin is disinfected; the tips should be cut off aseptically and submitted in a sterile container to the laboratory for culture.

Repeated cultures of open draining wounds or of large areas of devitalized tissue will frequently yield a profusion of microorganisms. Their significance is uncertain, their numbers and variety will tax the laboratory, and their presence is unlikely to be affected by rational systemic antimicrobial therapy. Repetitive antimicrobial susceptibility testing of isolates from such cultures not only wastes the laboratory's time and the patient's money, but may also provide misleading results, inasmuch as attempts at therapy may simply favor superinfection by resistant microorganisms.

Although acute infections are generally recognizable clinically and their etiology is usually established by conventional bacteriological procedures, the recognition and establishment of the etiology of chronic localized infections are not so readily accomplished. Whereas staphylococci, streptococci, *Enterobacteriaceae*, and *Pseudomonadaceae* predominate in the former type of infection, actinomycetes, brucellae, mycobacteria, and fungi must be considered in the differential diagnosis of the latter. As we have already emphasized, biopsy and histopathological examination are valuable adjuncts in the diagnosis of the latter type of infection. The importance of microscopic study of the tissue is emphasized further by the occasional resemblance between neoplasms and infectious processes.

Burn wounds represent a somewhat unique problem because they are initially contaminated with staphylococci, streptococci, and clostridia and subsequently with such opportunists as *Pseudomonas* species, *Klebsielleae*, *Providencia*, *Candida albicans*, phycomycetes, and viruses. The burn eschar is a nonviable, devascularized structure which provides a milieu favorable for microbial growth. Cultures of biopsies of black, degenerated, or unhealthy areas of the burn or of drainage from burn wounds may be helpful in establishing the etiology of local or invasive infections. Gram-stained smears of any drainage may be helpful in providing an early clue as to the nature of the infectious process. Such patients must be monitored with blood cultures at frequent intervals.

C. TRANSPORT OF SPECIMENS TO THE LABORATORY

Inefficiency in transporting specimens to the laboratory after they have been obtained from the patient is a major problem. It becomes a convenient excuse that laboratory workers use for not finding organisms suspected to be present by the clinician. When a specimen is lost, it also becomes a convenient excuse for the clinician who has left the specimen with allegedly responsible personnel who, in turn, have instructed others to transport it to the laboratory. Although this activity is not directly under the jurisdiction of a clinical microbiology laboratory, every effort must be made to control its operation. The best possible way to obtain acceptable results is to insist that transportation time be as short as possible. Some laboratories refuse to accept specimens if they have been in transport too long. Certain specimens should be transported in a medium or vehicle which preserves the organisms in the specimen and helps to maintain the ratio of one organism to the other in the specimen. This is especially important for those specimens in which a normal microbiota may be admixed with bacteria or other microorganisms foreign to the location. It becomes even more necessary to use a transport medium if significant microorganisms are present in very low numbers. In hospitals, the various responsible administrators or supervisors should keep appropriate personnel aware that prompt and proper transport of specimens from the patients' floors to the laboratory is important. Many laboratories have established a policy of refusing to process specimens that have been handled improperly.

Microbiological specimens may be transported to the laboratory by various means. A variety of media may be used directly for this purpose. A nonproliferating, buffer type of transport medium such as that of Stuart, Toshach and Patfula may be employed; however, the charcoal transport medium is preferred by some. Ordinary nutrient broth or anaerobic broth may be used when swabs or aspirates are involved. In other instances, microbiologists insist that, for example, throat cultures for streptococci be inoculated just as the swab is obtained onto blood-agar plates and that the inoculations be made near the periphery over an area of approximately 2 cm in diameter. The swab used for obtaining the specimen is then broken into a fluid transport medium and submitted in conjunction with the blood-agar plate. Modified TM medium (20) is recommended for gonococcal specimens when transport to a laboratory is to be done. For the isolation of *Bordetella pertussis*, direct inoculation of Bordet-Gengou agar is advocated. Many laboratories do not accept stool specimens for culture unless they are transported in various buffered preservatives. Preparation of these transport media is described in various manuals (see chapter 95). One of the best and up-to-date references which should be consulted when problems arise concerning transport of specimens is Public Health Publication number 976, revised September 1973, entitled *Collection, Handling and Shipment of Microbiological Specimens*. The major points advocated in this manual may be summarized as follows. (i) Aspirated specimens, such as fluids, etc., should be collected with a sterile needle and syringe instead of with swabs which permit rapid drying and subsequent loss of viability of the bacteria. (ii) Microorganisms survive better if 0.5% agar is added to media such as thioglycolate, chopped meat, etc. (iii) Smears for staining should be prepared at once. This is especially true when the material is from pathological lesions which have not been aspirated with a syringe and needle and from which a large quantity of material cannot be obtained. It is important for adequate and proper smears to be prepared at the bedside by clinicians who fully understand the significance of this procedure and are aware that thick smears are of very little help. Thin smears can be prepared from material that seems thick and tenacious by firmly pressing two slides together over the areas containing the applied specimen. This method is recommended for urethral discharges, wound exudates, aspirated material from abscesses, etc. By simply sliding the slides apart, thin areas of smear are made which are useful as a guide for the clinical microbiologist in the selection of media for primary culturing.

Special treatment is required for specimens when the etiological agent is thought to be anaerobic. The material is aspirated with a needle and syringe. It may be practical to remove the needle, cap the syringe with its original seal, and bring the specimen directly to the laboratory. No more than 10 min ought to be allowed for the transport of such specimens. The laboratory must be alerted that a specimen for anaerobic cultures is on the way. If prereduced media are available, they must be inoculated as soon as the specimen is obtained. It is the responsibility of the microbiology laboratory to insure that personnel using this approach fully understand the method of inoculation. Swabs for anaerobic culture are usually less satisfactory than aspirates, even when transported in an anaerobe tube.

Transport of urine specimens to the laboratory presents some problems. The urine must be obtained properly and transported and processed as soon as possible. No more than an hour should elapse between the time the specimen is obtained and incubation. If this time schedule cannot be followed, the urine specimen must be refrigerated immediately. If transport to the laboratory takes more than a few minutes, the urine specimen should be placed in an insulated bag containing scotch ice. Upon delivery to the laboratory, the urine specimen should be cultured immediately; if not, it should be refrigerated again. In any event, it is not advisable to refrigerate urine for longer than 18 to 25 h before culture under routine circumstances (see Inoculation of Media and Colony Isolation Methodology).

All laboratory personnel must be aware that material submitted for culture which is not in a supported environment must be handled immediately, especially spinal fluids, urines, pus, or any material not transported in a preservative. All smears should be fixed and stained immediately. In addition, laboratory personnel doing the primary culturing of specimens should acquaint themselves with the clinical diagnosis and any other pertinent laboratory findings, especially with select specimens such as blood, spinal fluids, wounds, burns, etc. Thus, hematological and chemical data, immunochemical findings on levels of immunoglobulins, complement, etc., may be helpful frequently in interpreting the findings of the laboratory and planning for the isolation of certain specific microorganisms.

D. RECORDING OF LABORATORY SPECIMENS

The person collecting the specimen is responsible for ensuring that the patient's name, registration, and location are correctly (and legibly!) written or imprinted on the culture request form and that this information corresponds with that written or imprinted on a label affixed to the specimen container. The type or source of the sample and the physician's choice of tests to be performed must be specified on the request form. Errors in specimen identification may have disastrous consequences and must be avoided. Correct identification of the specimen, however, continues in the laboratory where the number of different types of cultures, subcultures, and other appropriate tests and procedures may proliferate and, ultimately, are compiled into one or more reports. Multiple specimens from the same patient may be collected for diagnostic purposes or for following the progress of therapy; for these specimens, sample source, timing, and type of test performed must be clearly recorded.

In most laboratories, a system of accession numbers has been developed to expedite record keeping. There are undoubtedly many variations of the system at all levels of sophistication, depending on whether human or machine systems are employed. Since off- or on-line computer systems are relatively uncommon in clinical microbiology laboratories today, most accessioning systems are human and, therefore, subject to an incidence of random errors from 1/100 operations to 1/1,000 operations (18).

One approach to accessioning is the use of sequentially numbered self-adherent labels produced with sufficient replicates so that one can be affixed to each copy of the culture request form, the specimen container, work card(s), each of the primary plates or tubes of media inoculated, and the average number of plates or tubes of media used in subcultures. Further categorization according to the type of specimen and the year it was received can be achieved by color coding the labels and using a numbered prefix to indicate the year of accession, followed by one or two letters to designate the type of specimen received. A list of accessions by laboratory and by specimen type is helpful in documenting whether or not the specimen was received and can be used for rapid location and tracking of work in progress. Such a listing may also be used to tabulate the monthly and annual workloads received by the laboratory. These figures enable the laboratory director to anticipate his requirements for technical assistance and space (4).

In addition to the specimen records discussed above, the date and time the specimen was collected and received should be recorded on the request forms. If the specimen was received in an unsatisfactory condition, this fact should be noted in the accession list, on the request forms, and in an incidence record. Compliance with these standards is not only required by laboratory inspection and accreditation agencies but also provides data which are useful in the delivery of proper patient care.

Most laboratories use some type of work card on which a record of the work in progress is noted and updated as each step is completed. If the work card format is systematized, an individual who is unfamiliar with a particular culture can answer inquiries about it before the final report is ready. Inspection of the work card to determine the appropriateness of the tests performed and the accuracy of their interpretation is an important responsibility of the laboratory director when the final report is prepared.

Final reports need to be retained in the laboratory at least until the results are recorded in the patient's history. Retention beyond this point is not practical unless it fulfills a specific purpose, be it epidemiological or investigational, since record storage is expensive; retention of records is especially unnecessary if the data are also a part of other permanent records. Microbiological results provide the data base for a hospital's epidemiology program and should be organized in a manner facilitating analysis of infection rates by medical or surgical services and hospital location. This will enhance detection of hospital endemics or epidemics. Antimicrobial susceptibility data should be tabulated by organism and by antimicrobic on a yearly basis to detect trends in susceptibility and provide clinicians with the information needed for selecting initial therapy for serious infections.

Many variations of this procedure are extant. The essential features of the approach described must be part of all record-keeping efforts. It should be stressed that the record must reflect, in addition, the various steps which comprised the analytical process to ensure accuracy and detection of aberrant reactions while enabling other laboratorians to follow the decision-making process at a later date. All quality controls exercised in the interest of the particular specimens must be recorded. Although it may not be an absolute requirement that each specimen record reflect this concern, the various controls exercised must be logged to provide the reassurance of proper materials, reagents, media, etc.

E. PREPARATION OF SPECIMENS FOR PRIMARY CULTURING

A variety of considerations must be entertained by the technical personnel when any specimen is delivered to a laboratory: the source of the specimen, the transport medium or status of the specimen, the accompanying smear or the nature of the specimen from which a smear is to be made, the established routine in the particular laboratory for a given specimen, the established routine for the laboratory in general. All of these matters must be brought into play for the technical personnel to determine the steps to be taken in preparing specimens for primary culture.

Section B (Collection of Specimens) lists a variety of anatomical sources from which laboratory specimens may be obtained. It seems reasonable that in any laboratory all of the specimens should be cultured on a certain series of microbiological media. Which media will be used in any given laboratory can largely be left to the experience of the director or supervisor of the clinical microbiology laboratory. The consideration of possible anaerobic microorganisms in a particular specimen must be accompanied by use of prereduced media or other media capable of supporting growth of anaerobic bacteria. Another important factor is the antibiotic history of the patient from whom the specimen was obtained. The physician submitting the specimen should provide the microbiologist with his working diagnosis, so that the latter may then consider the addition of special media which might help in isolating those microorganisms consistent with the clinical impression. If the specimen contains large or inhibitory amounts of the antimicrobial agent administered, it may be necessary to dilute the specimen.

If the organisms suspected of being present are not frequently encountered in the particular laboratory, a representative of such microorganisms should be cultured in duplicate media to insure that proper support and conditions for their proliferation are provided and to permit comparison of cultural characteristics when the unknown organism has grown. The use of such control cultures has been advocated by some for years (16). It is a helpful measure which frequently aids in a speedier recognition of organisms encountered only rarely.

As mentioned earlier, certain specimens require dilution. This is especially true of urine specimens submitted for quantitative microbiological analysis. There are many ways of ascertaining the number of bacteria per milliliter of urine. Whichever the method chosen, it must be of proven efficacy and accuracy when performed in the laboratory. The most common approach is the use of a calibrated loop that delivers a specified volume of urine to an agar plate which is then streaked. Another approach is diluting the specimen through several tubes until a 1:1,000 dilution has been obtained. A small portion, usually 0.1 ml, is then delivered to the plates used for assessing the number of bacteria, and this small volume is then spread across the plates either with a glass spreader, a bacteriological loop or needle, or with the pipette itself. Finally, the dilution method by shake-agar technique is used occasionally. Various dilutions of the urine specimen are added to melted, measured volumes of agar. After addition, the agar is mixed and the mixture delivered into a petri dish where it is allowed to harden.

When a piece of tissue is submitted for microbiological analysis, it should be cut into small pieces or, if available, a tissue grinder should be used for maceration (see section B, Collection of Specimens). If the material submitted is very viscous, it may be treated with sterile *N*-acetyl cysteine or an equal volume of 1.5% amyl acetate, both of which have been shown not to inhibit microorganisms. This treatment is very helpful with certain body fluids and sputum.

Before primary culturing is begun, all media and equipment must be well organized on a clean bench top. A sequence of the steps to be performed should be established so that the inoculating procedure can be executed smoothly. Proper entries in workbooks, on worksheets, or on patient records should be made to indicate that each particular step has been executed. Adequate safeguards should be within easy reach; a disinfectant solution must always be on hand. The proper placement of a Bunsen burner, a microincinerator, loop carriers, or sterile swabs, if they are to be used, is a prerequisite for efficient working. Whenever possible, safety cabinets should be used. These are mandatory if aerosolization may occur during the processing of the specimen.

F. INOCULATION OF MEDIA AND COLONY ISOLATION METHODOLOGY

Many methods of inoculating various media are available to the laboratory. The bacteriological inoculating loop is used most often, particularly when a homogenous specimen is available. When broth cultures are being transferred to agar media, sterile cotton or synthetic fiber swabs, Pasteur pipettes, calibrated pipettes, syringes and needles are used for distributing certain specimens to various or several solid and liquid media. In general, it is unwise to utilize these various transfer devices for spreading the culture across the entire agar plate. Most laboratories, therefore, plant a portion of specimens to an area near the periphery of the plate(s). After having distributed the specimen to all the various substrates upon which it is to be cultured, one proceeds to distribute the specimen across the agar in a fashion that permits an ongoing dilution of the specimen. This is best accomplished with a bacteriological loop. The specimen is spread back and forth over the surface of perhaps one-quarter to one-third of the plate, with the bacteriological loop held loosely between the thumb and index finger. The weight of the bacteriological loop is allowed to exert its own pressure. There is no need to exert additional pressure with the hand. After the first quadrant has been inoculated, the plate is turned 90° and the first few cross-streaks touch the original inoculum. After that, the laboratory worker continues to inoculate the surface of the agar, avoiding the first inoculated quadrant. When another quarter of the plate is covered, it is once more turned 90° and the process is repeated. Many individuals prefer to complete the process by turning an additional 90° at the end and permitting, therefore, a small area to be inoculated after the fourth turn has been made. This is to ensure the presence of isolated colonies.

The microbiologist must keep in mind the purpose of the medium being inoculated. For example, highly selective media require a heavier inoculum, and one drop of the specimen may be inadequate to yield growth of the microorganism in question. Therefore, for those media, it may be appropriate to utilize a swab which is used to inoculate the first quadrant of the plate.

Table 1. *Recommended media and Gram-stain requirements for various specimens*[a]

Specimen	Media										
	Supplemented thioglycolate[c]	BA	EMB or McC	PEA	CBA	TM[d]	HE, XLD, GNB	Actinomyces	Anaerobic	Mueller-Hinton broth	Gram stain
Autopsy tissue	X	X	X	X							
Bowel drainage by mechanical means (Gomco, sump, etc.)	X	X	X	X			X (not gastric)				X
Ear, nose, parotid, antrum, mouth, bronchial, sinus (head)	X	X	X	X	X			Mouth, nose tissue only	Tissue only		
Eye	X	X	X	X	X				BA only		X
Fluids: dialysis, chest, abdominal, pericardial, peritoneal	X	X	X	X					X		X
Fluids: spinal, scalp flap, subgaleal, ventricular	X	If not filtered			X				BA only	X	X
Prostate	X	X	X	X	X	If swab					(from males only)
Stools and rectal swabs		X	X	X			X				
Surgical tissue from lung, lymph nodes, spleen,	X	X	X	X	Lung only			X	X		X
Suprapubic aspirate	1 ml of urine	X	X								
Throat, sputum, tonsil, nasopharynx, tracheal		X	X		X						
Throat swab for *Neisseria meningitidis*					X	X					
Transtracheal aspirate, synovial and joint fluids	X	X	X	X	X				X		X
Urethra, vagina, cervix, prostate for *Neisseria gonorrhoeae* ("GC") only[c]					X	X					X
Urine		X	X								

Vagina, lochia, cervix, urethra, pelvic area, perineum	X	X	X	X	X	If MT-M not received[c]			Pelvic and perineum		Pelvic and perineum
Vaginal swabs for *Haemorphilus vaginalis*	X	X			X						
Wounds, abscesses, ulcers, exudates, tissues, etc.	X	X	X	X	Brain		Perianal neck and rectal tissue abs. only		X		X

[a] Adapted from J. A. Washington II, *Laboratory Procedures in Clinical Microbiology*, Little, Brown Co., Boston, in press.

[b] Abbreviations: BA, blood-agar; EMB, eosin methylene blue-agar; PEA, phenylethyl alcohol-blood-agar; CBA, supplemented chocolate-blood-agar; TM, Thayer-Martin agar; HE, Hektoen enteric agar; XLD, xylose-lysine-deoxycholate agar; GNB, gram-negative broth (Hajna); McC, MacConkey agar; MT-M, modified Thayer-Martin medium.

[c] Thioglycollate-135C (BBL) supplemented with either 0.5 to 1.0 ml of rabbit serum (Thio-135C with 1.0 ml of serum, used for all anaerobic cultures) or 1.0 ml of ascitic fluid.

[d] Cultures for *Neisseria gonorrhoeae* may be inoculated directly into modified Thayer-Martin before being submitted to the laboratory.

[e] Supplemented thioglycolate, blood-agar, kanamycin-vancomycin-blood-agar, and PEA.

Resorting to a bacteriological loop thereafter is helpful in obtaining isolated colonies. Familiarity with the composition and purpose of each medium plus experience is the ultimate way to master this aspect.

If the purpose of the procedure is to obtain an evenly distributed inoculum of a diluted specimen, a bent glass rod may be used. This rod is designed in such a way as to make approximately a 45° angle. The side used for inoculation usually covers the radius of a standard petri dish. This sterile glass applicator is then placed over the inoculum, and the plate carrying the agar is rotated until an even layer of liquid is above the agar. Care must be exercised that the inoculating volume is proper (usually 0.5 to 1.0 ml).

The special requirements for inoculating specimens for anaerobic cultivation will be discussed in Chapter 38. Animal inoculations are performed with decreasing frequency in the average clinical microbiology laboratory. It would be useful to consult standard texts describing this procedure should the need arise. As a word of caution, individuals not experienced in performing animal inoculations should send the specimens to central or reference laboratories which are equipped to provide this service. It is also important that animal facilities and animal care meet prescribed regulations.

Occasionally there is a need to use the pour plate technique. Pour plates are used infrequently in the quantitation of urinary microorganisms, but the method is often used to quantitate the microorganisms in environmental cultures. For this type of inoculation, sterile pipettes are required. If dilutions are to be made, tubes containing measured amounts of sterile diluent are needed. A Bunsen burner is usually required. The other types of inoculations can all be accomplished with microincinerators, a device safer and easier to use when pathological material is involved.

If the specimen for primary inoculation is of very tenacious or friable material and is to be cultured for fungi, such as skin scraping, nail scraping, hairs, etc., it may be necessary to use a small sterile scalpel to cut the specimen into smaller pieces on the surface of an agar medium. This will permit the pathological specimen to be submerged into the agar and further inoculated in the plate by using the scalpel to make additional cuts in the medium.

The inoculation methods described are to be used only for the inoculation of primary isolation media. Other methods are appropriate for transferring laboratory-grown microorganisms; these are not covered here.

G. MEDIA FOR PRIMARY ISOLATION

At the risk of redundancy, it must be stated once more that the purpose of using a number of different solid and broth media is twofold. It permits the isolation of many of the various microbial agents in a specimen. At the same time, a number of media select specific members of the microbial population by suppressing other microorganisms present in the specimen.

Table 1 represents the recommended media and Gram stain requirements for primary bacteriological cultures as used at the Mayo Clinic, Rochester, Minn. It is reproduced here to serve as a guide to the selection of media as practiced in one of the outstanding institutions in the United States. It is obvious that for each medium chosen others may be substituted. It is equally obvious that the choice of media may be expanded considerably. This recommendation encompasses the requirements for the isolation of microorganisms usually looked for in these specimens and is in no way all encompassing. Additional media must be chosen when information concerning specific microorganisms is available from the clinician. This guide is similar to others that have been published by various media manufacturers such as BioQuest and Difco or advocated in such texts as Bailey and Scott (2), Sonnenwirth (31), Isenberg and Berkman (16), etc.

Detailed discussion of the many media for primary isolation could not be included. It must be remembered that the choice of which medium to use for a specific purpose represents perhaps best the mystique of clinical microbiology, a mystique compounded by habit, preferences of favorite teachers, personal experience, and occasionally solid data. It is also determined to a degree by the availability of commercially available, prepackaged agar plates and broth.

H. INCUBATION OF INOCULATED MEDIA

After inoculation on proper substrates, cultures should be incubated at an optimal temperature as quickly as possible. Delay in bringing certain organisms to the desired temperature may hamper their ability to grow in the desired period of time. Turbidity or other manifestations in broth will be impaired. Overgrowth by undesirable microorganisms will be encouraged especially in liquid media. The question of proper temperature has preoccupied clinical microbiologists for some time. Although it is theoretically desirable to come close to body temperature for many of the organisms involved in disease production, there are a number of microorganisms which cannot tolerate the optimal temperature for man. Therefore, most incubators in clinical laboratories are set at 35 C, which permits the growth of virtually all organisms capable of existing at 37 C. A single incubator set at 35 C is obviously inadequate for many of the temperature requirements of a large clinical laboratory. Provision for changes of incubation temperature should be available and can be provided even in the smallest laboratory by the judicious use of temperature blocks, water baths, or small incubators. If only one major incubator is available, it is recommended that the temperature be set at 35 C. A drawer or a closed cabinet can be used in laboratories that do not have multiple incubators for room temperature incubation. A water bath may be adjusted to a temperature beyond that of the main incubator, such as 42, 56, or 60 C.

It is desirable that most cultures be inspected after 15 to 18 h of incubation, the so-called "overnight" incubation. Not only are most cultures readable after this time, it is important to the clinician and his patient that a preliminary report be issued within the first 24 h. Even a negative report on certain cultures, especially those of body fluids, has significance to the clinician. However, many of the bacteria in clinical specimens require additional incubation for visible growth. Good clinical microbiologists inspect all cultures that were negative during the first 18- to 24-h period routinely on a daily basis for a period ranging from 1 to 2 weeks. In fact, recovery of bacteria after 4 to 5 days is not a frequent occurrence. However, this observation is offset by the isolation of bacteria after a 1- to 2-week incubation period, especially from blood cultures. Although the percentage of such delayed isolations is of low frequency, it nevertheless constitutes isolation of significant organisms of consequence to the diagnosis and the treatment of the patient. Only broth media containing portions of the clinical specimen are so treated. Incubation of agar media in excess of 3 days is unnecessary unless specific information for slow-growing microorganisms or a suspicion of prolonged lag phase exists. Should the clinical information suggest that bacterial L-forms, the so-called cell wall-defective variants are suspected in the specimen submitted, hypertonic conditions should be established in the media used for primary and subculture purposes. This may be accomplished even after ordinary media have been inoculated by the addition to fluid media of suitable hypertonic solutions.

Adequate moisture is a further requirement of all the incubation chambers. Even the most primitive incubator should be supplied with such a source. Many of the new incubators have water reservoirs attached or are equipped to regulate the evaporation of water into the incubator. Pans of water may be placed on the lowest shelf of an incubator not adequately equipped for this purpose. When automatic regulation of moisture is present, a relative humidity of 70 to 80% should be provided. Provision and control of atmospheric conditions are other important aspects for proper incubation for primary isolation. Many bacteria prefer a carbon dioxide atmosphere for growth. A capnophilic environment may be provided in special incubators equipped with a CO_2 gas tank which regulates adequate carbon dioxide content in the atmosphere. Burning a candle in a tightly closed jar, the candle extinction method, is still considered quite adequate in providing the increased CO_2 required by all such bacteria. Another method to provide an increased CO_2 environment is to tip a 1% HCl solution into a beaker containing $NaHCO_3$ previously placed in a wide-mouth jar with a secure-fitting lid. The special atmospheric requirements of mycobacteria and anaerobic microorganisms are described in Chapters 16 and 38.

All incubators must be equipped with a thermometer. Whereas many of the newer models have mechanical recording devices, those incubators which do not should at least be monitored by a high- and low-indicator thermometer a device which will record the lowest and highest temperature achieved between inspections. Daily checking and recording of the temperature are necessary. Similarly, the sanitary care of walk-in incubators is of the highest order. Accidental spills, collections of old overlooked specimens, dust and other soil must be avoided by meticulous attention to a cleaning schedule. Even the smaller table-top or closet-type incubators should be inspected periodically to insure proper sanitary conditions. All personnel with access to the incubator must be aware that accidental spillage of the specimen, culture media, etc., represents a serious hazard and must be quickly disinfected and cleaned up.

I. EXAMINATION OF CULTURES FOR PRESUMPTIVE RECOGNITION AND IDENTIFICATION OF ISOLATES

One of the most decisive steps in clinical microbiology is the preliminary inspection of growth on primary isolation media after the first period of incubation. Once growth has been recognized or its identity suggested by the various manifestations in and on isolation media, an accepted set of standardized procedures should be followed to initiate presumptive and definitive identification. The recognition that a potentially significant microorganism is present in a clinical specimen must result from consideration of the source of the specimen; namely, is it from a body area in which microorganisms are rarely, if ever, found in the normal state or does the organism come from an anatomic site which has a normal microbial flora? It is important that not only the appearance of certain organisms on generally supportive media is allowed to bear on the decision, but also the numbers and kind of bacteria which manifest themselves on various selective media used for the cultivation of the original specimen.

The experienced microbiologist or his technical staff requires a glance at a series of selective and general media used to gain an appreciation of the organisms present. However, no one should misunderstand or underestimate the importance of this first approach to acquaint oneself with the organisms present as being sufficient for further action. It is imperative that this first scanning be followed by close inspection of each primary isolation medium employed. More often than not such agar plates should be inspected with the aid of a hand lens, an illuminated magnifying lens, if available, or best of all, a stereoscopic microscope. Much of the morphology of bacteria, fungi, and yeasts on primary isolation media is a self-taught pattern recognition system which combines the aspects of colonial morphology on one medium with the appearance of the same organism on the various other selective media used. Even the absence of detectable colonial growth on one medium is important to the identity. It is customary for laboratorians in the clinical microbiology laboratory to utilize magnification to search out and to inspect β-hemolytic streptococcal and possibly pneumococcal colonies. However, an inspection of all plates with some magnification helps to acquaint workers in the clinical microbiology laboratory with subtle differences in colonial morphology on a variety of media. Colony inspection with magnification should be encouraged in all laboratories. Even the laboratory which does not receive large numbers of clinical specimens can afford to train neophytes in clinical microbiology by providing them with known cultures which can be studied on the various media used in that laboratory. Learning to describe the morphological characteristics of each significant bacterium on each medium will enhance one's ability to recognize these organisms in mixtures that are common from contaminated body areas and also enable a prompt preliminary decision when the bacteria appear in cultures of blood and other body fluids.

The characterization of colonial morphology follows well-established guidelines. There are many authoritative texts which will acquaint clinical microbiologists with the easiest manner of describing the appearance of a colony. Many methods are useful in recording these particular differences. Some prefer to sketch the appearance of the colony in their notebooks. Others utilize the terms used to describe the appearance. It is also helpful to establish comparable size differences of the colonies. Although "eyeballing" and guessing the size of a colony lacks all quantitative aspects, it is helpful to note these impressions. Recording the findings of colonial morphology aids in the final recognition of organisms if such data are recorded immediately and permanently, rather than attempting to reconstruct the reasons for further studies long after the original impressions of the primary colonies have become blurred in the minds of the worker.

The properties of surface colonies on solid

TABLE 2. *Growth on primary plate cultures*[a]

Blood-agar (aerobic) after overnight incubation			
Colonies 1 mm or more in diameter		Colonies less than 1 mm in diameter	
Gram-positive cocci:	Staphylococci	Gram-positive cocci in pairs or chains (short):	
	Micrococci	1. Growth on MacConkey medium	Enterococci
	(Streptococci)		(*Streptococcus* group D)
Gram-negative cocci:	*Neisseria*		Streptococci of groups, B, C, G
Gram-positive rods:	*Corynebacterium*		
	Bacillus		
Gram-negative rods:		2. No growth on MacConkey medium[c]	Group A (beta-hemolytic) streptococci
1. Growth on MacConkey agar	*Enterobacteriaceae*		*S. pneumoniae*
	Yersinia		Viridans (α) streptococci
	Aeromonas	Gram-positive cocci in clumps:	Staphylococci
	Vibrio		Micrococci
	Flavobacterium	Gram-negative cocci:	*Neisseria*
	Acinetobacter	Gram-positive rods:	*Corynebacterium*
	Pseudomonas		*Lactobacillus*
	(*Actinobacillus*, *Pasteurella*)[b]		*Nocardia*
2. No growth on MacConkey agar[c]	(*P. multocida*, few other *Pasteurella* sp.)		*Erysipelothrix*
			Listeria
	Haemophilus	Gram-negative rods:	*Haemophilus*
			Brucella[b]
			Pasteurella[b]
			Bordetella[b]
Blood-agar (anaerobic, with 2 to 4% CO_2) after overnight incubation (no equivalent growth on aerobic culture)			
Colonies about 1 mm or spreading		Gram-positive rods:	*Bifidobacterium*
Gram-positive rods:	*Clostridium*		*Corynebacterium*
Colonies minute[d]			*Actinomyces*
Gram-positive cocci:	Anaerobic streptococci		*Eubacterium*
	Anaerobic micrococci	Gram-negative rods:	*Bacteroides*[e]
Gram-negative cocci:	*Veillonella*		*Fusobacterium*

[a] Revised from: A. C. Sonnenwirth, 1970. Collection and culture of specimens and guides for bacterial identification, p. 1122–1169. *In* S. Frankel, S. Reitman, and A. C. Sonnenwirth (ed.), Gradwohl's clinical laboratory methods and diagnosis, 7th ed. C. V. Mosby Co., St. Louis.

[b] These organisms often require special media and conditions for primary isolation; occasionally they will grow on the media shown above. *Brucella abortus* does not grow on primary isolation without CO_2; *F. tularensis* usually does not grow on ordinary media; *P. multocida* does not grow on MacConkey agar.

[c] No growth on MacConkey agar; sensitive to bile salts.

[d] Many of these small colonies fail to appear for several days. Some may prove to be microaerophilic, not true anaerobes.

[e] Occasionally 1 mm or larger.

media can be described very simply as summarized in many of the standard texts of microbiology. It is important to note whether the shape of a colony is circular, irregular, radiate, or rhizoid. The size of the colony should be expressed in millimeters. Those who use calipers or millimeter rules for the measurement of zones of inhibition in antibiotic susceptibility tests have learned to make such measurements quickly and accurately. The elevation of the colony must be described either by sketching or by words such as raised, low convex, convex or dome shaped, umbonate, umbilicate, and with or without beveled margins. Wilson and Miles (41) add to this description the structure of the colony which they describe as amorphous, fine medium or coarsely granular, filamentous and/or curved. The surface may be described as smooth, contoured, beaten-copper, rough, fine medium or coarsely granular, ringed, papillate, dull, or glistening. The word matt has been used to describe the appearance of colonies somewhere between the dull and glistening state. The edge of the colony may be described as being entire, undulate, lobate, crenated, erose, fimbriate, curved, or effuse. The pigmentation of a colony should be detected by reflected or transmitted light. Pigment may be described as fluorescent, iridescent, and opalescent, as well as by color description. It should also be noted whether these pigments are carotenoid or water insoluble, i.e., confined to the colony itself or diffused into the surrounding medium. Another variable is the opacity of the colony. Opacity may be classified as transparent, translucent, or opaque. The consistency of the colony becomes apparent to the experienced microbiologist; therefore, descriptions such as butyrous, viscid, friable, and membranous may help in characterizing the colonial morphology as well as serving as a guide to the handling of a colony should it be necessary to subculture it. The manner in which a colony behaves when it is picked for making a Gram stain may serve as a distinctive characteristic with a particular medium. This is referred to as emulsifiability and is either easy or difficult; it may be noted that the colony forms a homogeneous or granular suspension and remains membranous when rubbed in a drop of water with an inoculating needle. These notations are helpful, especially when training individuals to describe the appearance of colonies and continue to aid in the recognition of organisms by their colonial morphology. Certain organisms will produce characteristic odors on various media. The ability to distinguish some bacteria by the odor produced can be of great help. However, odor detection is to be done with care and caution and is not totally reliable.

Growth in fluid media helps in the presumptive identification of microorganisms. Fluid media may be evaluated by first noting the degree of growth present. It is reported as none, scant, moderate, or abundant. Another variable is the degree of turbidity. This may be recorded as absent and, if present, as slight, moderate or dense. Another useful descriptive observation is whether the turbidity is uniform, granular, or flocculent. Variation in these properties will occur in different fluid media. It is not possible to compare the appearance of an organism in thioglycolate broth with its appearance in brain-heart infusion broth. The presence or absence of precipitates in broth media is also important. The degree of precipitate, slight, moderate, or abundant, should be noted. The precipitates may also be described as powdery, granular, flocculent, membranous, or viscid. In some instances, slight shaking will resuspend the precipitates formed, whereas no effect may be noted with others. The formation of a pellicle on the surface of the broth is still another characteristic that should be observed. If a pellicle is present, it may have a ring of growth around the inner surfaces of the tube. The pellicle may be thick, thin, smooth, granular, or rough. This manifestation may also be destroyed by shaking or remain intact.

Growth on selective media may constitute a clue to the identification of certain microorganisms. Tables 2, 3, and 4 present summaries of some of the bacteria which may be recognized presumptively at this stage. It must be emphasized that it is not the purpose of these tables to serve as other than a guide to assist the microbiologist in deciding whether it is necessary to identify a particular organism further. This decision is influenced by the source of the specimen, the microorganism recovered, and the history of the patient. As an illustration, consider the recovery of *Escherichia coli* from a stool specimen of a 30-year-old male. If all the colonial morphology patterns indicate that this organism is *E. coli* and that it is not being confused with other members of the *Enterobacteriaceae*, especially not *Shigella*, or that such an identification error is of no consequence in this specimen, then no further work needs to be done. This is true especially if the history of the patient does not indicate any gastrointestinal symptoms. The same organism isolated from the same individual from a urine specimen would require additional tests to identify the organism.

The clinical microbiologist must decide

TABLE 3. *Growth characteristics of frequently isolated bacteria on some commonly used agars*[a]

Organism	Growth on agar						
	EMB	MacConkey	HE	SS	BS	XLD	SEA
Arizona	Translucent, colorless	Uncolored, transparent; red (LF)	Similar to *Salmonella*	Black centered, clear periphery	Black; green brown (LF)	Black-centered red colonies	Inhibited
Citrobacter	Translucent colonies, greenish metallic sheen (LF)	Uncolored transparent; red (LF)	Usually inhibited when present, colonies are small and bluish-green	Similar to *Arizona*	Black; green-brown	Opaque, yellow	Inhibited
Enterobacter *Serratia*	Metallic sheen, similar to *E. coli* but somewhat larger	Red-pink	Green centers with yellow to brown periphery	White or cream colored, opaque, mucoid	Raised mucoid colonies, silvery sheen	Opaque; yellow	Inhibited
Escherichia coli (rapid lactose fermenters)	Dark center; greenish metallic sheen	Red or pink, may be surrounded by a zone of precipitated bile	Moderately inhibited; orange to salmon-pink	Red to pink; colorless with a pink center	Mostly inhibited; black-brown greenish surface; no metallic sheen	Opaque; yellow	Inhibited
Klebsiella	Larger than *E. coli*, mucoid, brownish, tend to coalesce, often convex	Pink, mucoid	Yellow centers, periphery orange	Red to pink; colorless with a pink center	Mostly inhibited	Opaque; yellow	Inhibited
Proteus	Translucent, colorless	Uncolored, transparent	Most strains are inhibited; dark centered, greenish (H_2S producers), similar to *Salmonella*	Black centered, clear periphery	Green; black (H_2S producers), mostly inhibited	Opaque, yellow (*P. mirabilis*, *P. vulgaris*), red (*P. rettgerii*, *P. morganii*)	Small grey colonies (few)
Pseudomonas	Translucent, colorless; amber	Uncolored, transparent	Most strains are inhibited; colonies are small, flat and green to brown	Mostly inhibited, transparent, colorless colonies	Inhibited	Sometimes red colonies	Inhibited
Salmonella	Translucent amber colonies; colorless	Uncolored, transparent	Blue to blue-green; most colonies have black centers, (H_2S producers)	Opaque; transparent; uncolored; black centered, clear periphery	*S. typhi* black with sheen or dotted black or greenish-gray; other *Salmonella* are black or green	Black-centered red (H_2S producers); red color (no H_2S)	Inhibited
Shigella	Translucent, amber colonies; colorless	Uncolored, transparent	Blue to blue-green, periphery of colonies lighter than center portion	Opaque, transparent	Mostly, inhibited; *S. flexneri* and *S. sonnei* are brown, raised and craterlike	Red	Inhibited

	SEA	110	Mannitol, Salt	MS	Choc. agar	Thayer Martin	
Enterococci	Translucent to whitish colonies surrounded by dark-brown to black zones	Mostly inhibited	Mostly inhibited	Blue-black, shiny center, clear periphery	White to gray		
Listeria	Pin-point colonies with reddish to black-brown zones	Inhibited	Inhibited	Inhibited	Gray		
Neisseria sp.					Opaque, grayish white	Mostly inhibited	
N. gonorrhoeae					Opaque, grayish white	Gray	
N. meningitidis					Opaque, grayish white	Gray	
Staphylococcus	Small, white-gray colonies	White; orange to yellow	Colonies with yellow zones (mannitol fermenters); colonies with red or purple zones (mannitol not fermented)	Mostly inhibited	White to gray	White to gray, mostly inhibited	
Streptococci	Tiny colonies	Mostly inhibited	Mostly inhibited	Small blue colonies		White to gray	
Beta-hemolytic	Tiny colonies						
Alpha-hemolytic							
Nonhemolytic							
S. salivarius				Blue gum drop colonies			
S. mitis				Small blue colonies			

[a] Abbreviations: EMB, eosin methylene blue-agar; HE, Hektoen enteric agar; SS, *Salmonella-Shigella* agar; BS, bismuth sulfite agar; XLD, xylse-lysine-desoxycholate-agar; SEA, selective enterococcus agar; 110, *Staphylococcus* 110 agar; MS, Milis-Salivarius agar; Choc. agar, chocolate-agar; LF, lactose fermenter.

TABLE 4. *A simplified guide to the presumptive recognition of common groups of bacteria*[a]

I. Aerobic cultures
  A. Gram-positive cocci
    1. Catalase positive
      a. Arranged in clusters, large colonies: *Staphylococcus* (chapter 7)
      b. In pairs, fours, or small clusters; utilize dextrose oxidatively or not at all: *Micrococcus* (chapter 7)
    2. Catalase negative
      a. Short and long chains and even pairs; fermentative (anaerobic) utilization of sugars: *Streptococcus* (chapter 8) Note: beta-hemolytic streptococci may belong to pyogenes or enterococcus group; alpha-hemolytic streptococci may belong to viridans or enterococcus group; nonhemolytic streptococci (gamma) may be viridans or enterococcus group
        (1) Pyogenes group: usually, but not always, beta-hemolysis; do not grow at 45 C; do not survive 30 min at 60 C; serological groups A, B, C, F, G, H, K, L, M, O; Lancefield grouping or fluorescent-antibody technique; most group A strains susceptible to bacitracin
        (2) Viridans group: alpha-hemolysis or none; not soluble in bile; not inhibited by Optochin; usually grow at 45 C (*Aerococcus*)
        (3) Enterococcus group: some beta-hemolytic, others alpha- or gamma-; bile-esculin agar positive; grow at 45 C and survive 30 min at 60 C; grow on MacConkey agar
      b. Usually lancet-shaped, pairs, single or short chains, bile-soluble, inhibited by Optochin, alpha-hemolysis, no growth at 45 C, virulent for mouse: pneumococci (*Streptococcus pneumoniae;* chapter 9)
  B. Gram-negative cocci: mostly in pairs
    1. *Neisseria* (all oxidase positive)
      a. No growth at 22 C or on nutrient agar; growth on Thayer-Martin agar (35 C)
        (1) Requires enriched medium; acid from dextrose and maltose: agglutination by antimeningococcal serum: *N. meningitidis* (chapter 10)
        (2) Requires enriched medium; acid from dextrose only: *N. gonorrhoeae* (chapter 11)
      b. Growth at 22 C and on nutrient agar
        (1) Yellow pigment, no acid from dextrose, maltose, sucrose, or lactose: *N. flavescens*
        (2) Grow well on ordinary media; acid from dextrose and maltose: pharyngeal group
    2. Rule out *Acinetobacter* (chapter 24), *B. anitratum* (chapter 24), (*Mima-Herellea*) (see C.1.e)
  C. Gram-negative rods
    1. Grow well on ordinary media, including MacConkey agar[b]
      a. **Fermentative,**[c] **oxidase negative,**[d] nitrate reduced to nitrite
        (1) Lactose usually fermented,[e] phenylalanine deaminase not produced
          (a) Voges-Proskauer (V-P), citrate, urease, and H_2S negative, indole and methyl red positive: *Escherichia* (chapter 18)
          (b) V-P and citrate positive, grow in KCN, indole negative, urease positive or delayed, motile: *Enterobacter;* nonmotile: *Klebsiella* (chapter 18)
          (c) H_2S and citrate positive, lysine decarboxylase not produced, V-P, urease, and indole negative, grows in KCN: *Citrobacter* (chapter 18)
          (d) Lysine decarboxylase and H_2S produced, malonate positive, no growth in KCN, lactose prompt or delayed; *Arizona* (chapter 18)
        (2) Lactose usually not fermented,[e] phenylalanine deaminase not produced
          (a) H_2S, citrate, and lysine decarboxylase positive, indole, V-P, urease, and KCN negative: *Salmonella* (chapter 18); exceptions—no gas, little H_2S: *S. typhi* and others (use specific antisera); β-galactosidase and malonate positive: *Arizona* (chapter 18)
          (b) H_2S citrate, V-P, and urease negative, nonmotile, usually no gas: *Shigella* (or nonmotile *Escherichia*); some *Shigella* sp. ferment lactose slowly (chapter 18)
          (c) V-P and citrate positive, urease delayed positive, motile, pigment often formed, especially at room temperature: *Serratia* (chapter 18)
          (d) H_2S, indole, lysine, and methyl red positive, urease, V-P, citrate, and KCN negative, most sugars (except glucose and maltose) not fermented: *Edwardsiella* (chapter 18)
        (3) Phenylalanine deaminase produced
          (a) Urease positive: *Proteus* (chapter 18)
            (i) H_2S positive, indole positive: *P. vulgaris*
            (ii) H_2S positive, indole negative: *P. mirabilis*
            (iii) H_2S negative, indole and ornithine positive: *P. morganii*
            (iv) H_2S negative, indole positive, ornithine negative: *P. rettgeri*
          (b) Urease negative: *Providencia* (chapter 18)
      b. **Fermentative, oxidase negative,** motile at 20 to 25 C but not 35 C; urease positive, phenylalanine negative: *Yersinia pseudotuberculosis, Y. enterocolitica* (chapter 19)
      c. **Fermentative, oxidase positive**
        (1) Catalase positive, nitrate reduced, usually motile, arginine dehydrolase produced: *Aeromonas* (chapter 20)

TABLE 4—*continued*

(2) Cells spiral or comma shaped, motile, fermentative, lysine and ornithine decarboxylase produced: *Vibrio* (chapter 21)
(3) No growth on MacConkey (see *Pasteurella* [chapter 22] *multocida, urea,* etc.): *Cardiobacterium* (chapter 24)
(4) Grows on MacConkey: *Pasteurella haemolytica* (chapter 22)

d. **Oxidative utilization of sugars** (O-F medium, no fermentation)[c]
(1) Oxidase positive, no gas, motile, grow on MacConkey, *Salmonella-Shigella* (SS), and cetrimide agar, many have soluble pigments (green or yellow): *Pseudomonas* spp. (chapter 23)
(2) Oxidase positive (or variable), growth variable on MacConkey agar, oxidative or no utilization of sugars, yellow pigment, no reduction of nitrate: *Flavobacterium* (chapter 24)
(3) Oxidase negative, grow on MacConkey agar, nitrate reduction variable, malonate negative; nonmotile, no reduction of nitrate, no decarboxylases: *Acinetobacter*
(4) No growth on MacConkey agar, oxidase negative: *Pseudomonas mallei* (chapter 23)

e. **Carbohydrates not attacked** (no oxidation or fermentation, O-F medium)
(1) Oxidase positive, grows on MacConkey and cetrimide agar, nitrate reduced to nitrite, no decarboxylases, motile: *Alcaligenes*
(2) Oxidase positive, nonmotile, usually no growth on MacConkey agar (exceptions), citrate and urease negative: *Moraxella*
(3) Oxidase negative, grows on MacConkey agar: *Acinetobacter* (chapter 24), *Pseudomonas maltophilia* (chapter 23), *Bordetella parapertussis* (chapter 27)
(4) Oxidase positive, grows on MacConkey, microaerophilic, slow growth: *Vibrio fetus* (Chapter 21)

2. Some grow on ordinary media, others need enriched media; **fermentative,** no gas produced; usually no growth on MacConkey, sucrose fermented, nonmotile, oxidase usually positive: *P. multocida,* other *Pasteurella* sp. (chapter 22)
3. Slow growth, pleomorphic cells, nonmotile, **fermentative,** no gas, often polar staining, oxidase and catalase variable, slow coagulation of milk, no decarboxylases: *Actinobacillus* (chapter 29); grow on MacConkey, oxidase positive: *A. lignieresi. A. equuli;* no growth on MacConkey, oxidase negative: *A. actinomycetemcomitans* (chapter 29); **oxidative,** no growth on MacConkey, oxidase negative: *P. mallei*
4. **Some requirement of special media** (no growth on MacConkey) and conditions, no capsule, nonmotile: *Brucella* (members of this group have to be differentiated by CO_2 requirement, H_2S production, dye inhibition test, and agglutination tests; (chapter 25)
5. **No growth or poor growth without special factors in media,** capsule variable, nonmotile
   a. Require factors X and/or V: *Haemophilus;* characteristic satellitism along *Staphylococcus* streak or other colonies, no growth on plain agar, encapsulated strains (mainly from cerebrospinal fluid identified by type-specific antisera: *H. influenzae;* grows on plain agar along a *Staphylococcus* streak or other colonies providing factor V: *H. parainfluenzae, H. ducreyi* (cultivation rarely done for diagnostic purposes), *H. aphrophilus* (chapter 26)
   b. Do not require factors X and/or V, growth improved by addition of serum or ascitic fluid, sugars not attacked, oxidase positive: *Moraxella;* no growth on blood-agar, characteristic pitting on Loeffler serum slant, typical diplobacillus: *M. lacunata* (from angular conjunctivitis): *M. nonliquefaciens* [see C.1.e.(2); chapter 24]
6. **Primary isolation best on complex media with blood, oxidase positive,** shows characteristic colonies on Bordet-Gengou agar, agglutination by specific antiserum: *Bordetella pertussis* (rough variant of *B. pertussis* grows on ordinary media; *B. parapertussis* and *B. bronchiseptica* grow on MacConkey agar (chapter 27)
7. **No growth on ordinary media,** requires special media (cystine-glucose-blood agar): *Francisella tularensis* (chapter 28)
8. **Grow best on enriched media,** crescent-shaped or spiral cells (long screws or portions of a turn): *Spirillum* (chapter 31)

D. Gram-positive rods
1. **Catalase positive, no spores formed,** no growth on MacConkey agar
   a. Nonmotile, arranged in Chinese figures, stain unevenly with bands and granules: *Corynebacterium;* toxin production, fermentative: *C. diphtheriae* and *C. ulcerans;* other corynebacteria and "diphtheroids" differentiated by biochemical and toxigenicity tests, some fermentative, others do not attack sugars at all (chapter 12)
   b. Motile (at 20 C but usually not at 37 C), short, "diphtheroid"-like rods, often narrow zone of beta-hemolysis: *Listeria monocytogenes* (chapter 13)
   c. Motile, do not attack sugars, indole and nitrate reduction negative, long rods, some form filaments and coccoid bodies in broth: *Kurthia* (chapter 2)

TABLE 4—*continued*

2. **Catalase negative, no spores formed**
   a. Nonmotile, frequently form long filaments, usually no growth in litmus milk, fermentative (dextrose, lactose). H_2S in butt of TSI agar, nonbranching: *Erysipelothrix* (chapter 14)
   b. Form chains, grow better on tomato juice agar, H_2S negative in butt of TSI agar: *Lactobacillus*
3. **Acid fast,** no branching, no spores
   a. Nonmotile, no branching, no hyphae: *Mycobacterium* (chapter 16)
      (1) Special media required, slow growth: *M. tuberculosis* (distinguish by biochemical and cultural characteristics); "atypical" mycobacteria, groups I, II, III (see various species)
      (2) Rapid growth: group IV; "saprophytes"
4. **Nonmotile, some branching,** some acid fast; hyphae, but no true conidia produced, oxidative: *Nocardia* (chapter 17)
5. **Catalase positive, spores formed,** many motile
   a. One species medically important, characteristic colonies, nonmotile, usually nonhemolytic: *B. anthracis* (chapter 15)

II. Anaerobic cultures
   A. Gram-positive cocci
      1. Occurring mainly in clusters but also in pairs: anaerobic *Staphylococcus* (*Peptococcus;* chapter 40)
      2. Mainly in pairs and chains: anaerobic *Streptococcus* (*Peptostreptococcus;* chapter 40)
   B. Gram-negative cocci—in irregular masses, very small cocci: *Veillonella* (chapter 40)
   C. Gram-negative rods
      1. Usually nonmotile of varying sizes and shapes, non-sporeforming, often foul smelling, cells greater than 0.6 μm, do not produce butyric acid: *Bacteroides* (chapter 41)
      2. Some with pointed ends, effuse colonies; many very pleomorphic, produce butyric acid: *Fusobacterium* (chapter 42)
      3. Motile, polar flagella: *Campylobacter, Butyrivibrio, Succinimonas*
      4. Spiral forms: *Treponema, Borrelia* (chapters 35, 36)
   D. Sporeformers (majority gram-positive, certain species may appear gram-negative)
      1. Catalase negative, anaerobic or aerotolerant, motile or nonmotile: *Clostridium* (some, e.g., *C. perfringens* rarely produce spores except in special media; chapter 39)
   E. Gram-positive rods
      1. Vegetative mycelium produced, which fragments: true branching, non-acid-fast, catalase negative; slow-growing, dry crumbly colonies on solid media; in fluid medium granules adherent to walls of tube; unstained preparation of crushed granule shows typical clubs; succinic acid produced: *Actinomyces* (chapter 17)
      2. No catalase or indole produced, no butyric acid: *Bifidobacterium* (chapter 42)
      3. Catalase and indole positive, nitrate reduced, gas from glucose, produce propionic acid: *Propionibacterium* (chapter 42)
      4. Nonmotile, nonbranching, do not ferment lactose, produce butyric acid, catalase negative: *Eubacterium* (chapter 42)

[a] Revised from: A. C. Sonnenwirth. 1970. Collection and culture of specimens and guides for bacterial identification, p. 1122–1169. *In* S. Frankel, S. Reitman, and A. C. Sonnenwirth (ed.), Gradwohl's clinical laboratory methods and diagnosis, 7th ed. C. V. Mosby Co., St. Louis.

[b] Some do not grow on MacConkey agar; exceptions listed.

[c] Oxidation-fermentation (O-F) medium; fermentation observable in triple sugar iron (TSI) medium and in ordinary fermentation media ("sugars").

[d] Cytochrome (indophenol) oxidase test.

[e] Lactose is valuable in the case of prompt fermenters (on differential plates overnight or in 24 to 48 h in fermentation media): some strains of the groups listed show delayed or no fermentation of lactose. See *Enterobacteriaceae* (chapter 18).

which of the organisms isolated on primary culture must be identified. There are no easy guidelines that can be advanced which would cover all eventualities. If, after careful inspection, the organisms represent the normal microbiota of the part of the body from which the specimen was obtained, further identification of these organisms by additional testing is superfluous. If the specimen was obtained from an anatomical site which is normally sterile, the laboratory must proceed to establish the identification of genus and species but not at the expense of presumptively reporting the initial impressions.

This need for presumptive identification is in response to the major responsibility of the clinical microbiology laboratory. As mentioned at the onset, it is the function of the clinical microbiology laboratory to report as accurately and as quickly as possible the presence of a significant microorganism in a clinical specimen and to provide the clinician with a guide to antibiotic therapy. This aim can be met by the judicious application of the principles outlined in this chapter and by the early and quick use of diagnostic tests available for the recognition of certain microorganisms. An example is the isolation and recognition of *Staphylococcus* from a specimen. A coagulase test would quickly confirm that this organism is *S. aureus* without requiring additional testing. This does not rule out the possible future need to perform phage typing for epidemiological purposes. Similarly, the recognition of either *Salmonella* or *Shigella* in a stool specimen may require the use of grouping antisera to confirm the identity of the organism. The species or serotype designation must be obtained, and the biochemical tests to confirm the identification of the organism must be carried out. However, the certainty and authority with which one can report the presence of such an organism in a specimen are enhanced largely by the ability to perform rapid tests leading to strong presumptive identification.

The special circumstances of the patient frequently requires the testing of a microorganism further than would appear necessary at first. An example is the serotyping of *E. coli* in the stools of neonates and infants up to the age of 2. Also, the persistent isolation of an organism from a usually sterile body area ought to lead to identification tests, even if under ordinary circumstances such an organism would be described as "nonpathogenic." Early presumptive reporting is imperative. It is the practice in many laboratories to render a verbal report to the clinician. This is followed by a written report reiterating its preliminary nature. Laboratories (and clinicians) must also be aware that occasionally the preliminary report may prove to be incorrect. One should never hesitate to retract the initial report and indicate the correctness of the final report. This is done with explanations if required. Clinical microbiologists must not hesitate to alert the physician and the institution's infection committee when they have presumptive evidence of organisms that are potentially dangerous to the institution and the community at large.

The classical purpose of primary isolation is the separation of microorganisms into groups which can be identified according to the principles of sound microbiology. Primary isolation constitutes the starting point for the detective work which leads to the diagnosis, if not the identification, of microorganisms in a manner expounded by the experts to guide the reader to the level of genus and species recognition. The dynamic state of the intimate human biosphere makes it imperative that the clinical microbiologist remain aware of the changes which bring new populations into this environment and that the role of these newcomers in disease production or complication is recognized with dispatch. This responsibility can only be met by the judicious use of the chapters which follow.

LITERATURE CITED

1. Bass, J. W., T. M. Cashman, A. L. Frostad, et al. 1973. Antimicrobials in the treatment of acute otitis media. Amer. J. Dis. Child. **125:**397–402.
2. Bailey, W. R., and E. G. Scott. 1966. Diagnostic microbiology. C. V. Mosby Co., St. Louis.
3. Barrett-Connor, E. 1971. The nonvalue of sputum culture in the diagnosis of pneumococcal pneumonia. Amer. Rev. Resp. Dis. **103:**845–848.
4. Bartlett, R. C., G. O. Carrington, and C. Mielert. 1968. Quality control in clinical microbiology (revised). Commission on Continuing Education, Council on Microbiology, ASCP, Chicago.
5. Bartlett, J. G., J. E. Rosenblatt, and S. M. Finegold. 1973. Percutaneous transtracheal aspiration in the diagnosis of anaerobic pulmonary infection. Ann. Int. Med. **79:**535–540.
6. Bennett, D. E. 1967. Histoplasmosis of the oral cavity and larynx: a clinicopathologic study. Arch. Int. Med. **120:**417–427.
7. Bland, R. D. 1972. Otitis media in the first six weeks of life: diagnosis, bacteriology, and management. Pediatrics **49:**187–197.
8. Carr, D. T., A. G. Karlson, and G. G. Stillwell. 1967. A comparison of cultures of induced sputum and gastric washings in the diagnosis of tuberculosis. Mayo Clin. Proc. **42:**23–25.
9. Converse, G. M., J. M. Gwaltney, D. A. Strassburg, and J. Q. Hendley. 1973. Alteration of CSF findings by partial treatment of bacterial meningitis. Clin. Res. **21:**120.
10. Dalton, H. P., and M. J. Allison. 1968. Modification of laboratory results by partial treatment of bacterial meningitis. Amer. J. Clin. Pathol. **49:**410–413.
11. Dolan, C. T. 1972. Postmortem microbiology, p. 207–216. *In* J. Ludwig (ed.), Current methods of autopsy practice. W. B. Saunders, Philadelphia.
12. Dolan, C. T., A. L. Brown, and R. E. Ritts Jr. 1971. Microbiological examination of postmortem tissues. Arch. Pathol. **92:**206–211.

12a. Duma, R. J., H. W. Ferrell, C. Nelson, and M. Jones. 1969. Primary amebic meningoencephalitis. N. Engl. J. Med. **24:**1315–1323.

13. Feigin, R. D., and P. G. Shackelford. 1973. Value of repeat lumbar puncture in the differential diagnosis of meningitis. N. Engl. J. Med. **289:**571–574.
14. Hable, K. A., J. A. Washington II, and E. C. Hermann Jr. 1971. Bacterial and viral throat flora: comparison of findings in children with acute upper respiratory tract disease and in healthy controls during winter. Clin. Pediat. **10:**199–203.
15. Hahn, H. H., and H. N. Beaty. 1970. Transtracheal aspiration in the evaluation of patients with pneumonia. Ann. Int. Med. **72:**183–187.
16. Isenberg, H. D., and J. I. Berkman. 1966. Recent practices in diagnostic bacteriology, p. 237–317. *In* M. Stefanini (ed.), Progress in clinical pathology, vol. 1. Grune and Stratton, New York.
17. Koneman, E. W., T. M. Minckler, D. B. Shires, and D. S.

de Jongh. 1971. Postmortem bacteriology. II. Selection of cases for culture. Amer. J. Clin. Pathol. **55**:17–23.

18. Krieg, A. J., T. J. Johnson, C. McDonald, and E. Cottore. 1971. Clinical laboratory computerization. University Park Press, Baltimore.
19. Kunin, C. M. 1972. Detection, prevention and management of urinary tract infections: a manual for the physician, nurse and allied health worker. Lea and Febiger, Philadelphia.
20. Martin, J. E., J. H. Armstrong, and P. B. Smith. 1974. New system for cultivation of *Neisseria gonorrhoeae*. Appl. Microbiol. **27**:802–805.
21. Mou, T. W., and H. A. Feldman. 1961. The enumeration and presentation of bacteria in urine. Amer. J. Clin. Pathol. **35**:572–575.
22. Musher, D. M., and R. F. Schell. 1973. False-positive Gram stains of cerebrospinal fluid (Letters). Ann. Intern. Med. **79**:603–604.
23. Nemoy, N. J., and T. A. Stamey. 1971. Surgical, bacteriological, and biochemical management of "infection" stones. J. Amer. Med. Ass. **215**:1470–1476.
24. Pryles, C. V., and B. Lustik. 1971. Laboratory diagnosis of urinary tract infection. Pediat. Clin. N. Amer. **18**:233–244.
25. Rein, M. F., and G. L. Mandell. 1973. Bacterial killing by bacteriostatic saline solutions—potential for diagnostic error. N. Engl. J. Med. **289**:794–795.
26. Schmidt, R. M., and H. S. Rosenkranz. 1970. Antimicrobial activity of local anesthetics: lidocaine and procaine. J. Infect. Dis. **121**:597–607.
27. Schonebeck, J. 1972. Studies on Candida infection of the urinary tract and on the antimycotic drug 5-fluorocytosine. Scand. J. Urol. Nephrol. Suppl. **11**:1–48.
28. Segal, E. L., G. E. Starr, and L. A. Weed. 1959. Study of surgically excised pulmonary granulomas. J. Amer. Med. Ass. **170**:515–522.
29. Segura, J. W., P. P. Kelalis, W. J. Martin, and L. H. Smith. 1972. Anaerobic bacteria in the urinary tract. Mayo Clin. Proc. **47**:30–33.
30. Smith, A. L. 1973. Diagnosis of bacterial meningitis. Pediatrics **42**:589–592.
31. Sonnenwirth, A. C. 1970. Collection and culture of specimens and guides for bacterial identification, p. 1122–1169. *In* S. Frankel, S. Reitman, and A. C. Sonnenwirth (ed.), Gradwohl's clinical laboratory methods and diagnosis, 7th ed. C. V. Mosby Co., St. Louis.
32. Stamey, T. A., D. E. Govan, and J. M. Palmer. 1965. The localization and treatment of urinary tract infections: the role of bactericidal urine levels as opposed to serum levels. Medicine **44**:1–35.
33. Stamey, T. A., and A. Pfan. 1970. Urinary infections: a selective review and some observations. Calif. Med. **113**:16–35.
34. Steel, K. J. 1962. The practice of bacterial identification. Symp. Soc. Gen. Microbiol. **12**:405–432.
35. Unger, K. M., and K. M. Moser. 1973. Fatal complication of transtracheal aspiration: a report of two cases. Arch. Int. Med. **132**:437–439.
36. Weed, L. A. 1954. Microbiologic methods in surgical pathology. Mayo Clin. Proc. **29**:393–399.
37. Weed, L. A. 1958. Technics for the isolation of fungi from tissues obtained at operation and necropsy. Amer. J. Clin. Pathol. **29**:496–502.
38. Weed, L. A., and A. H. Bagenstoss. 1951. The isolation of pathogens from tissues of embalmed human bodies. Amer. J. Clin. Pathol. **23**:1114–1120.
39. Wiesner, P. J., E. Tronca, P. Bovin, et al. 1973. Clinical spectrum of pharyngeal gonococcal infection. N. Engl. J. Med. **268**:181–185.
40. Wilson, W. R., C. T. Dolan, J. A. Washington II, A. L. Brown, and R. E. Ritts, Jr. 1972. Clinical significance of postmortem cultures. Arch. Path. **94**:244–249.
41. Wilson, G. S., and A. A. Miles (ed.). 1964. Topley & Wilson's principles of bacteriology and immunity, 5th ed. Williams and Wilkins Co., Baltimore.
42. Winn, W. R., et al. 1966. Rapid diagnosis of bacteremia with quantitative differential membrane filtration culture. J. Amer. Med. Ass. **197**:539–548.

Section II

AEROBIC BACTERIA

Chapter 7

Staphylococcus

DANIEL IVLER

CHARACTERIZATION

Member of the family *Micrococcaceae*. Two species: *Staphylococcus aureus* and *Staphylococcus epidermidis*. Frequently found on normal human skin and mucous membranes. *S. aureus* usually associated with disease; *S. epidermidis* rarely pathogenic. Anaerobic gram-positive cocci of the genus *Peptococcus* becoming increasingly important in human disease (see chapter 40). Responsible for abscesses, pustules, and furuncles; less frequently, for septicemia, endocarditis, meningitis, enterocolitis, osteomyelitis, and pneumonitis. Some strains elaborate an exotoxin capable of producing food poisoning. Infect both humans and animals. Isolated from clinical specimens, carriers, food, and environment.

Spherical forms; usually occur in irregular characteristically "grapelike" clusters, but may appear singly, in pairs, in short chains, or in tetrads; 0.5 to 1 μm in diameter. Gram-positive. Nonmotile. Usually noncapsulated. No spores.

Growth. Aerobic and facultatively anaerobic. Some strains dependent on increased carbon dioxide tension. Grow on ordinary unenriched media and in the presence of a high salt concentration (7.5 to 10% sodium chloride). May produce pigmentation varying from white, orange, or yellow to gold. May be beta-hemolytic on blood-agar. Optimal temperature, 37 C; temperature range, 10 to 45 C.

Biochemical characteristics. Catalase positive. Acid from glucose under aerobic and anaerobic conditions. Usually acid from mannitol: *S. aureus*. No acid from mannitol: *S. epidermidis*. Phosphatase and coagulase produced and nitrate reduced to nitrites by *S. aureus*. No coagulase produced by *S. epidermidis*. Nitrate reduction by *S. epidermidis* is delayed, and phosphatase production is unusual.

Animal pathogenicity. *S. aureus* strains may be pathogenic to mice on intravenous or intraperitoneal injection with gastric mucin adjuvant. Also may be pathogenic to rabbits on intravenous and intradermal injection.

CLINICAL SIGNIFICANCE

S. aureus causes most superficial suppurative infections. Serious infections, always a problem in hospitalized patients, have much greater clinical importance since the advent of antibiotics. The majority of life-threatening infections now arise within hospitals. Twenty to sixty percent of humans carry the organism in the anterior nares. Hospital personnel and patients have significantly higher carrier rates than the general populations, and these organisms are generally resistant to penicillin and to other antibiotics. Direct person to person contact is the most important means of transmission.

The anaerobic gram-positive cocci, *Peptococcus*, are being found more often as agents of disease. These agents, although capable of producing disease by themselves, are more often found in association with other genera, e.g., *Streptococcus* and *Peptostreptococcus* (see chapter 40).

COLLECTION, TRANSPORT, AND STORAGE OF SPECIMENS

The staphylococci are relatively resistant to adverse environmental conditions. No special precautions are necessary for preservation of clinical specimens for culture. As with all specimens for culture, it is desirable to culture as soon after collection as possible. Should any delay be expected, the specimen should be refrigerated. The wide distribution of these organisms warrants particular care in the collection of certain specimens, particularly when the nature of the infection is such that material for culture must be obtained by aspiration. It is essential that particular precautions be taken in sterilizing the skin. Although the organisms have a rather complex nutritional requirement, no special cultural conditions are required, and they will develop well on ordinary media such as nutrient or Trypticase soy agar. Sheep blood-agar is preferred for primary isolation from biological specimens.

DIRECT MICROSCOPE EXAMINATION

The morphological arrangement of the individual cells forming irregular clusters enables one to identify the staphylococci presumptively on the basis of a proper Gram stain of the biological specimen. This is particularly true with cerebrospinal fluid, tracheal aspirates, peritoneal fluid, pus, and biopsy specimens. However, this characteristic morphological appearance is not fixed, and definitive identification of *S. aureus* and *S. epidermidis* cannot be made without culture of the specimen, a coagulase test, and, when warranted, mannitol fermentation. Failure of growth under ordinary conditions from a positive smear may indicate the presence of CO_2-requiring strains or an anaerobic micrococcus (genus *Peptococcus*).

ISOLATION AND CULTIVATION

Specimens suspected of containing staphylococci should be streaked on blood-agar and inoculated into thioglycolate broth (see chapter 95 for media composition). Human blood should not be used for the preparation of blood-agar because nonspecific inhibitors or antibodies present in human blood may inhibit or alter the appearance of staphylococcal colonies on this medium.

Pus, purulent fluids, sputum, and urine

Streak specimens directly on a blood-agar plate and inoculate a tube of thioglycolate broth. Incubate at 37 C. Specimens from patients receiving penicillin may be treated with penicillinase (see chapter 6) to inactivate the drug prior to inoculation of the medium.

Feces and heavily contaminated specimens

In addition to blood-agar, phenylethyl alcohol-agar or mannitol-salt-agar (see chapter 95) should be inoculated. These selective media will suppress bacteria of many other genera.

Blood cultures

Add 3 to 5 ml of venous blood to 50 ml of a medium such as tryptose-phosphate broth, Trypticase soy broth, brain heart infusion broth, etc., and incubate at 37 C. It is important to remember that, for patients receiving penicillin, penicillinase should be added to the blood culture bottle at the time of specimen inoculation. See the procedures for blood cultures described in chapter 6.

IDENTIFICATION

Identification of staphylococci and the separation of the two species in the genus are based upon colonial and microscopic morphology, catalase production, coagulase production, and mannitol and glucose fermentation.

Colonial appearance

On blood-agar, abundant growth occurs in 18 to 24 h. Colonies will generally be 1 to 3 mm in diameter; they are usually opaque, circular, smooth, and raised, with a butyrous consistency. Colonies conforming to this description should be Gram-stained and observed for typical morphology.

On primary isolation, *S. aureus* may produce a golden-yellow pigment (a lipochrome soluble in alcohol and ether). In many instances, however, the colony may be white or colorless. Although the presence of porcelain-white or colorless colonies has been used as a criterion to identify *S. epidermidis*, the production of pigment *is not* a valid means of separating the two species. White or colorless colonies of *S. aureus* are not infrequently found on primary isolation from clinical material, and pigmented colonies of *S. epidermidis* have been observed.

Pathogenic varieties of staphylococci may elaborate soluble hemolysins which produce a zone of beta-hemolysis surrounding the colony on blood-agar. Although hemolytic activity is usually suggestive of *S. aureus*, some *S. epidermidis* strains are also beta-hemolytic, particularly in primary isolation. As with pigment production, the elaboration of hemolysins is a variable characteristic of the staphylococci, and hemolytic activity should not be, by itself, used to separate the two species.

Except for a somewhat smaller colony size on other media, the characteristics described for the appearance of *S. aureus* and *S. epidermidis* on blood-agar will apply when these organisms are cultured on media other than blood-agar, e.g., nutrient or Trypticase soy agar.

Mannitol-agar with a high salt concentration is a selective medium for staphylococci and may be used to differentiate *S. aureus* from *S. epidermidis* on the basis of mannitol fermentation. *S. aureus* strains capable of fermenting mannitol usually do so within 24 h, and colonies belonging to this species will therefore be surrounded by a yellow zone indicating acid production. Delayed fermentation of mannitol may occur with some strains, so negative plates should be held an additional 24 to 48 h before a final reading is made. Most strains of *S. epidermidis* fail to ferment mannitol, and consequently no change of the indicator in the medium will occur.

The anaerobic gram-positive peptococci grown on blood-agar are convex, gray to white, with a shiny appearance and entire edges. Hemolysis of the alpha or beta type may occur.

Catalase production

Procedures for detection of catalase are described in chapter 96. Staphylococci and micrococci are catalase-positive; pneumococci and streptococci do not possess this enzyme. Peptococci may or may not produce catalase, and this test for the differentiation of *Peptococcus* from *Peptostreptococcus* is open to question. When the colony testing method for catalase is performed, extreme care must be exercised if a colony is taken from a blood-agar plate. The enzyme catalase is present in red blood cells, and the carryover of blood cells along with the colony can give rise to a false-positive reaction.

Coagulase test

Although staphylococci produce many extracellular products, only one is generally accepted as a marker of pathogenic strains: the production of the enzyme coagulase, which clots rabbit and human plasma. Coagulase production is also one of the major criteria employed to differentiate *S. aureus* from *S. epidermidis*. Approximately 97% of staphylococci associated with pathological processes in humans are capable of elaborating this enzyme and are thus classified as *S. aureus*. All strains of *S. aureus* are, by definition, coagulase-positive. (*Editor's note*. Coagulase-negative strains of *S. aureus* which meet the other criteria for this species have been described in the literature.)

The coagulase test can be performed as a slide test for the measurement of bound coagulase (clumping factor) or as a tube test for the measurement of free coagulase. Because some difficulty has been encountered in the performance and reading of the slide test, because of necessity of using *fresh human* plasma rather than commercially available dehydrated rabbit plasma, and because of the necessity of confirming negative slide tests by the tube method, the slide test is not recommended for the routine diagnostic laboratory and will not be described here. Its primary use is for screening large numbers of staphylococci, and the methodology for conducting this test is well-described in other publications (1). It is understood, however, that lyophilized rabbit plasma is used in some laboratories for slide and tube coagulase tests.

To perform the tube test, add to 0.5 ml of undiluted or 1:4 diluted rabbit plasma one loopful of the growth of a gram-positive coccus from an 18- to 24-h-old agar culture, 0.1 ml of a broth culture, or a single colony from a blood-agar plate. Cultures of a known coagulase-positive organism, a coagulase-negative organism, and, if possible, a weak coagulase producer must be set up as controls with each test. Incubate in a water bath (37 C), and examine for clotting at intervals of 30 min for 4 h. If no clot is observed at the end of this period, examine tubes again at 6 and 24 h.

A positive coagulase test is represented by any degree of clotting—from a loose clot suspended in plasma to a solid clot that is immovable when the tube is inverted. The majority of coagulase-positive strains will produce a firm clot within the first 4 h; many, within 1 h. False-positive tests may occur with mixed cultures or with pure cultures of some gram-negative rods, e.g., *Pseudomonas*, but the mechanism of clotting is different.

Carbohydrate fermentations

Determining the ability of isolates to produce acid from various carbohydrates is not usually necessary for the identification of staphylococci. *S. aureus* and *S. epidermidis* can be, and usually are, differentiated by the coagulase test alone. On rare occasions, however, freshly isolated strains of *S. aureus* may be coagulase-negative on primary isolation but become positive after several transfers. As an additional procedure to identify these strains in a short period of time, the mannitol fermentation test is employed.

An 18- to 24-h slant culture or a typical colony from a blood-agar plate is used to inoculate a tube of phenol red-mannitol broth. Mannitol acid fermentation is indicated by a change of the phenol red from red to yellow. *S. aureus* will usually ferment mannitol within 24 to 48 h. *S. epidermidis* is mannitol-negative. Alternatively, a mannitol-salt-agar plate can be streaked with the isolate. Colonies of *S. aureus*, but not *S. epidermidis*, will be surrounded by a yellow zone indicating fermentation of mannitol. The possible variations in coagulase and mannitol reactions of the two species are indicated in Table 1.

TABLE 1. *Possible coagulase and mannitol reactions of Staphylococcus aureus and S. epidermidis*

Species	Coagulase production	Acid from mannitol
S. aureus	+	+
	+	−
	Delayed	+
S. epidermidis	−	−
	−	+

Serological examination

Serological procedures for the identification of staphylococci and for the classification of isolates into specific serological types have been developed. The procedures employed are extremely complicated, and consequently such studies are restricted to a few research laboratories engaged in a full-time study of the antigenic composition of these organisms. At the present time, therefore, serological identification of isolates is not a practical procedure for use in the diagnostic laboratory. In addition, because of the ubiquitous distribution of these organisms and the frequency of exposure of humans, many normal human sera will agglutinate staphylococci in vitro to various degrees. Consequently, agglutination tests per se have no special diagnostic significance.

Animal inoculation

Virulence testing of isolates by inoculation of laboratory animals correlates extremely well with the coagulase test and therefore is not needed for the identification of *S. aureus*.

Bacteriophage typing

Staphylococci, particularly *S. aureus*, can be identified and classified into groups on the basis of their susceptibility to various bacteriophages (3; Table 2). The production of enterotoxin is confined primarily to phage groups III and IV. Bacteriophages 52, 52A, 80 (group I), and 81 (not allotted) predominate in the hospital environment and among hospital personnel. Phage type 71 appears to be specifically related to vesicular skin lesions (impetigo), and many *S. aureus* strains resistant to antibiotics fall into phage group III. Comparison of patterns of lysis produced by a battery of phages enables determination of relationships among strains of bacteria as well as their source. Phage typing is thus of great value in epidemiological investigations, but, because of the rather involved procedure necessary, it is not recommended for use by the diagnostic laboratory for the routine identification of a clinical isolate. The study of phage typing is not complete since many strains are isolated which cannot be typed.

SUSCEPTIBILITY TO ANTIMICROBIAL AGENTS

Before the introduction of antibiotics, the mortality from staphylococcal septicemia was over 80%. After the introduction of penicillin, the mortality fell to 28% between 1942 and 1944, but it has risen to over 50% since the appearance of staphylococci resistant to penicillin and other antibiotics. Table 3 lists the current national pattern of staphylococcal susceptibility to a variety of antimicrobial agents. Susceptibility testing methodology is described in chapter 46.

Resistance of staphylococci to penicillin is now found in 60 to 90% of staphylococci isolated from hospitalized patients in the western world. This resistance is due to the elaboration of the enzymes β-lactamase and/or amidase (penicillinases), which inactivate the antibiotic. Resist-

TABLE 3. *Antibiotic susceptibility of staphylococci*

Antibiotic	Percent susceptible	
	S. aureus	*S. epidermidis*
Ampicillin	22	41
Bacitracin	92	78
Cephalothin	99	97
Chloramphenicol	98	94
Cloxacillin	96	84
Dicloxacillin	99	81
Erythromycin	93	80
Gentamicin	99	98
Kanamycin	96	85
Lincomycin	95	86
Methicillin	92	82
Nafcillin	93	88
Neomycin	94	89
Oxacillin	94	84
Penicillin G	21	37
Streptomycin	89	79
Tetracycline	84	52
Vancomycin	99	96

TABLE 2. *Lytic groups of Staphylococcus typing phages which are included in the internationally agreed set of basic typing phages*

Lytic group	Phages in group								
I	29	52	52A	79	80				
II	3A	3B	3C	55	71				
III	6	7	42E	47	53	54	75	77	83A
IV	42D								
Not allotted			81	187					

ance to other antimicrobials may also occur by a variety of mechanisms on a genetic basis.

The incidence of resistance to a specific antimicrobial has correlated closely with the frequency of its administration.

DISCUSSION

The criteria employed for the identification of staphylococci are colonial appearance on blood-agar, Gram reaction and microscopic morphology, catalase and coagulase production, and, when warranted, mannitol fermentation. Although many other biochemical tests can be performed, e.g., gelatin liquefaction, acetyl methyl carbinol production, carbohydrate fermentations, reaction in litmus milk, etc., they are not necessary for identification purposes.

Procedures have been proposed for the measurement of extracellular products, other than coagulase, elaborated by the pathogenic *S. aureus*. Toxins, lipases, fibrinolysin, phosphatase, deoxyribonuclease, etc., all correlate in varying degrees with coagulase production and have no advantage over the coagulase test for the identification of this organism.

For those laboratories dealing primarily with food and dairy products, a procedure for the separation of the genera *Staphylococcus* and *Micrococcus* may be of value. The recommended method has been published (2).

LITERATURE CITED

1. American Public Health Association. 1963. Diagnostic procedures and reagents. American Public Health Association, Inc., New York.
2. Subcommittee on Taxonomy of Staphylococci and Micrococci. 1965. Recommendations. Int. Bull. Bacteriol. Nomencl. Taxon. **15**:109–110.
3. Wentworth, B. B. 1963. Bacteriophage typing of the staphylococci. Bacteriol. Rev. **27**:253–272.

Chapter 8

Streptococci

RICHARD R. FACKLAM

CHARACTERIZATION

Streptococci are gram-positive cocci; cells are spherical, oval, or occasionally elongated into rods and occur in pairs or as short or long chains. Growth on agar surface is scanty; enriched infusion medium (brain heart infusion, Trypticase soy, heart infusion agar, etc.) is required. Streptococci are fastidious with respect to their nutritional requirements. A number of B vitamins and amino acids are required for growth.

Streptococci are facultative with respect to oxygen. Many strains grow better anaerobically than aerobically. Carbohydrate fermentation is homofermentative with dextrorotatory lactic acid as the major end product. Lactic acid is not the major end product among anaerobic streptococci, i.e., peptococci and peptostreptococci (41).

Streptococci do not produce catalase or reduce nitrate. These physiological characteristics, in addition to cellular arrangement, serve to differentiate the streptococci from the staphylococci. One species of streptococci has been reported as having the capacity to decompose hydrogen peroxide (3). However, this release of O_2 from H_2O_2 is very weak, and these strains have not been documented as having a role in any human pathological condition (12). One species of staphylococci, *Staphylococcus salivarius*, fails to decompose hydrogen peroxide; however, *S. salivarius* reduces nitrate and is similar to other staphylococci in cellular and cultural morphology (20).

Streptococci are oxidase-negative. This property, together with the Gram strain characteristics and cellular morphology, differentiates streptococci from *Neisseria*. *Neisseria* is also catalase-positive.

Most streptococcal species contain specific polysaccharide antigens. These *group*-specific antigens are useful in differentiating and classifying streptococci.

Not all streptococci found in pathological conditions have group-specific antigens, and other methods of identifying these strains are necessary. The hemolytic action of streptococci on animal red blood cells varies (see below, section on Hemolysis, for definitions). The different types of hemolytic action are an aid in identification of species. There is a wide range of physiological characteristics among streptococci, and many overlap; therefore, they are of little value in identifying the species. Microbiologists can take advantage of useful physiological characteristics to help identify the pathogenic streptococci (13–15).

A combination of antigenic, hemolytic, and physiological characteristics must be determined to identify the pathogenic streptococci.

CLINICAL SIGNIFICANCE

Members of the genus *Streptococcus* form the dominant bacterial flora of the mouth and pharynx of humans and other animals. Some species of streptococci are normally found in the intestines. The principal streptococcal species producing communicable disease in humans, Lancefield's group A streptococci or *S. pyogenes*, is primarily a resident of the pharynx. Apart from respiratory tract diseases (pharyngitis, rhinitis, tonsillitis, pneumonia, and scarlet fever), group A streptococci are found in pyoderma lesions, in wound infections, and in the blood of patients with erysipilas, puerperal fever, cellulitis, and septicemia. The severity of some streptococcal infections has been recently described by Quintiliani and Engh (37). Nonsuppurative disease such as acute rheumatic fever and acute glomerulonephritis may follow streptococcal pharyngitis. Nephritis may follow streptococcal impetigo, but acute rheumatic fever does not. Neonatal meningitis and sepsis, omphalitis, and vaginitis can be caused by group A streptococci (19) and group B streptococci (*S. agalactiae*) (10, 22). Bacterial endocarditis, urinary tract infection, and wound infections are common diseases caused by group B streptococci. Group B streptococci are also implicated in a variety of other diseases, including upper respiratory tract infections (52). Group D streptococci are found in the urine of patients with urinary tract infection and in the blood of patients with bacterial endocarditis (6,

34). Blazevic et al. (2) reported that alpha-hemolytic streptococci (which were probably all enterococci) were identified from 10% of their urinary tract infection patients over a 10-year period. The antibiotic susceptibility of enterococci (members of the group D) is markedly different from that of other streptococci; therefore, the identification of enterococci is important. Knowledge of the infecting organism in patients with urinary tract infection and bacterial endocarditis helps the physician prescribe the best antibiotic therapy. The viridans streptococci (alpha-hemolytic streptococci without defined specific polysaccharide antigen) are still the leading cause of bacterial endocarditis (24), and the identification of these organisms can save patients undue discomfort and the expense of enterococcal antibiotic therapy. Many other species of streptococci, including the beta-hemolytic group C, G, and F and alpha-hemolytic group H, K, and O streptococci, can cause disease in humans. Duma et al. (8) have summarized their clinical and bacteriological findings with streptococcal bacteremia. Their findings are typical of the distribution of streptococcal species found in bacteremias. Reinarz and Sanford (40) and Feingold et al. (16) also discuss infections caused by non-group A or D streptococci. These papers should be studied for the clinical significance of non-group A streptococci isolations from human diseases.

Streptococci cause a wider variety of clinical manifestations than any other genus of bacteria. The group A streptococcus remains the bacterium most commonly isolated from human infections. One hundred thousand Americans develop post-streptococcal heart disease each year, and some 16,000 die from such complications. We need not point out the importance of reliable laboratory procedures and tests for the identification of streptococci.

COLLECTION, TRANSPORT, AND STORAGE OF SPECIMENS

Methods of collection

Throat. The technique of swabbing the throat is as important in isolating streptococci as is cultivation of the specimen obtained. The two most common pitfalls which result in inadequate specimens are (i) swabbing the tongue or uvula tissues rather than the pharynx and (ii) inadequate exposure of the pharynx. The pharynx must be adequately exposed and illuminated. Rub the tonsils and pharynx with a cotton- or dacron-tipped applicator (swab) while avoiding the tongue and uvula tissues. Any exudate should be touched with the swab.

Nose. Nasal cultures should be taken with a sterile cotton-tipped flexible wire. The swab may be moistened with sterile water or saline before it is introduced into the patient's nose. The tip of the nose is raised with one hand, and the swab is introduced gently along the floor of the nasal cavity, under the middle turbinate, until the pharyngeal wall is reached. Force should not be used; if any obstruction is encountered, the nasopharyngeal culture cannot be taken on that side.

Skin. Skin lesions are best cultured by removing the crusts of the cap of the pustule or vesicle. The sterile swab should be firmly rubbed into the lesion. This may cause some discomfort to the patient, but it is important to ensure maximal recovery of streptococci. Wound cultures should be treated in the same manner. If the lesions or wounds are dry, a moistened swab should be used.

Blood, cerebrospinal fluid, urine, and other body fluids. The methods used for collecting and processing these specimens are described in chapter 6.

Transport

Swabs may be cultured on blood-agar plates or in infusion broth immediately after collection. Plates and broths should be incubated as soon as possible after inoculation. Freshly inoculated media should never be refrigerated since streptococci will not survive under such conditions. Swabs may be transported to the laboratory in simple, sterile, dry envelopes such as pill envelopes (3). Survival of streptococci by this method is satisfactory for short periods of time (1 to 3 h). An efficient and reliable method of transport is the silica gel transport method described by Redys et al. (39). Streptococci will survive for weeks in silica gel packets (47).

Storage

Streptococci survive for several months on tightly capped blood-agar slants stored at 4 C. Streptococci do not survive well in broth cultures; some strains die after only 3 or 4 days. Streptococci survive lyophilization and sand desiccation for more than 20 years, with over 95% viability (17).

DIRECT EXAMINATION

Direct examination of throat, nose, and skin cultures is of no value in identifying pathogenic streptococci. Nonpathogenic streptococci are normal inhabitants of these areas and do not differ from the pathogenic streptococci in their staining characteristics or cellular morphology.

Gram-stained smears of blood, cerebrospinal fluid (CSF), and other body fluids will be of some help in identifying the pathogen as a streptococcus.

CULTURE AND ISOLATION

Recommendations for primary culture

Ideally, swabs should be placed in an enriched broth and a pour-streak plate should be made. Sheep blood in an infusion agar base that is free from fermentable carbohydrates and has a final pH of 7.3 to 7.4 is preferred. Rabbit or horse blood may be substituted in the base, but the user should be aware of the subtle variations in hemolytic activity that can result (48, 50).

Pour-streak plate:

1. Place throat swab in 1 ml of broth and incubate at 37 C for 2 h. Specimens received in the laboratory within 2 to 4 h after they are taken may be cultured wth 0 to 2 h of incubation in broth. Specimens which have been in transit for 4 to 8 h should have a minimum of 2 h of incubation in broth, whereas those in transit over 8 h should have 4 to 5 h of incubation in broth.
2. Remove the swab from the 1 ml of broth, drain against inside of tube, and place in a sterile tube.
3. Melt a 15- to 20-ml tube of blood-agar base and hold in a water bath at 50 C.
4. Add 0.8 to 1.0 ml of sterile defibrinated blood to melted and cooled agar.
5. From the broth with the swab washings transfer a drained loop to the blood-agar tube.
6. Mix thoroughly, flame lip, and pour into sterile petri dish.
7. When the agar is hard, rotate the swab over a small section of the surface. Using an inoculating loop, spread the inoculum over *half* of the plate, streaking for isolation. Stab into agar after each cross-hatch series.

Overnight broth swabs:

1. From an overnight broth culture, mix the tube contents to get an even suspension of organism.
2. Transfer one loopful of broth culture to 15 ml of sterile saline and mix well. (If growth is light, it may be necessary to use two to three loops.)
3. Follow procedure for steps 3 through 7 above, except in step 5 use a loopful of the saline dilution, not a drained loop.

Other cultural methods

Swabs may be cultured on blood-agar plates immediately after collection. The swabs should be rolled firmly over one-sixth of the plate. A sterile wire loop is used to streak the remainder of the plate. The agar should be stabbed several times with the wire loop. There is no need to resterilize the wire loop at any stage of the streaking or stabbing of the plate. The American Heart Association (AHA) has prepared an excellent statement describing this method of culturing beta-hemolytic streptococci (51).

Body fluid cultures

Body fluids such as CSF, blood, etc., may be processed by either the pour-streak plate or the streak plate method. Use a loopful of the body fluid as the inoculum. All streak plates should be incubated anaerobically in the presence of 10% CO_2. Pour plates, however, exclude some of the air from the subsurface colonies and these plates can be incubated aerobically with satisfactory results. Streak plates should also be incubated under conditions of increased CO_2 tension for enhancement of growth. The conditions achieved in candle jar incubation permit the detection of hemolytic activity by streptococci on streaked blood plates if the hemolytic activity is read from the growth in the stabbed areas of the plate as described by AHA (51). All media should be incubated at 35 to 37 C unless otherwise stated.

IDENTIFICATION

Recognition of the colonies

Typically, after 18 to 24 h of incubation on blood-agar the colonies of *S. pyogenes* are about 0.5 mm in diameter, transparent to opaque, and domed; they have a smooth or semi-matt surface and an entire edge. They are surrounded by a well-defined zone of complete hemolysis, usually two to four times the diameter of the colony; however, considerable variations occur. Appearance of the colonies depends markedly on the medium used, and not all colonial characteristics are manifested on a single medium. Subsurface colonies also vary. Some colonies are lancet-shaped, whereas others are oval or round. The appearance of beta-hemolytic group B, C, or G streptococcal colonies does not differ enough from the variations in group A colonial morphology to be of any value in identification (surface or subsurface). Group D streptococcal colonies are somewhat larger than group A colonies on the surface of blood-agar. They are usually opaque, and some strains are glossy-white, resembling staphylococcal colonies on blood-agar. Group D streptococci may exhibit beta, alpha, or no hemolytic action on red blood cells, either surface or subsurface. The beta zones produced by hemolytic action of group D streptococci are usually larger than the beta zones produced by other streptococci. Group F streptococci generally form "minute colonies." These pinpoint colonies will have large zones of hemolysis surrounding the tiny colony. This characteristic has little diagnostic value, however, since some strains of group G and even some strains of group A also form minute colonies.

Some strains of group B streptococci form dull brick-red pigmented colonies after anaerobic incubation. Again, this characteristic is of little value for identification, since not all strains of group B streptococci form this pigment. The most important cultural characteristic for recognition of streptococci is the hemolytic action on the red blood cells in the medium.

Hemolysis

The hemolytic action of streptococci on red blood cells was described and defined by Brown in 1919 (4). Taranta and Moody (48) have recently photographed streptococci representative of Brown's definitions. These definitions are as follows:

Alpha (α)—an indistinct zone of partial destruction of red blood cells about the colony, often accompanied by a greenish to brownish discoloration of medium.

Beta (β)—a clear, colorless zone around the streptococcus colonies, in which the red blood cells have undergone complete discoloration.

Gamma (γ)—no apparent hemolytic activity or discoloration produced by the colony.

Alpha Prime (α') or *Wide Zone Alpha* (WZα)—a small halo or envelope of intact or partially lysed red blood cells lying adjacent to the bacterial colony, with a zone of complete hemolysis extending further out into the medium. When examined macroscopically, α' hemolysis can be confused with β hemolysis.

These observations by Brown were based on microscope examination of subsurface colonies in blood-agar pour plates. Through the years, these definitions have been applied to the characterization of colonies arising on the surface of streaked blood plates. This extended application has not been achieved smoothly because of the character of the hemolysins responsible for beta hemolysis and because of the misinterpretation of alpha prime as beta hemolysis.

In 1932 and subsequently, Todd described two distinct hemolysins responsible for beta-hemolytic activity. He differentiated these hemolysins on the basis of antigenicity and susceptibility to inactivation by oxidation. He designated the antigenic, oxygen-labile hemolysin as streptolysin O and the nonantigenic oxygen-stable hemolysin as streptolysin S. He found that oxygen-sensitive streptolysin O could be reactivated in the presence of reducing agents. Furthermore, streptolysin S was not produced in serum-free broth, and its production was inhibited in media rich in fermentable carbohydrate. When these restrictive properties are kept in mind, it becomes obvious that aerobic incubation of streaked blood plates neutralizes the hemolytic activity of streptolysin O and restricts the characterization of the beta-hemolytic streptococcus to streptolysin S activity, which may vary greatly from strain to strain. By using streaked blood plates incubated in the presence of atmospheric oxygen, the investigator unknowingly imposes limitations upon the hemolytic expression of the organism which could cause the beta-hemolytic characteristics to be overlooked. Cultures which possess these hemolytic traits are called "poor surface hemolyzers."

Much has been written in the literature about the influence of blood obtained from a variety of animal species on the hemolytic expression of streptococci. The inference that the type of hemolysis changes dramatically from alpha to beta or beta to gamma, depending on the species of blood incorporated into the medium, is frightening in its implications. Although there is some basis for these disquieting revelations, presently available information indicates that variations in hemolytic activity are restricted to the enterococci. Updyke (50) reported the following:

> "In a study at the CDC (Center for Disease Control) 100 group A strains and 45–50 each of group B, C, and G strains grew equally well and gave identical hemolytic reactions in pour plates prepared from sheep, rabbit, horse, and human blood bank blood. The only differences in hemolytic activity occurred among the enterococci: 99% of 90 group D strains were alpha hemolytic in sheep blood agar and beta hemolytic in rabbit, horse, and human blood agar . . . . "

Thus, the change in beta hemolysis in blood from different animals is usually manifested (except for the enterococci) as a variation in size of the hemolytic zone and the sharpness of the edge of the zone; slight change in the opacity of the medium in the hemolyzed zone is *not* due to incomplete hemolysis. The variations in alpha hemolysis are much more pronounced and, for this reason, misinterpretation of alpha hemolysis accounts for much of the confusion in the literature. Differences in alpha hemolysis in a variety of blood media may range from delicate variations in intensity of greening, on one hand, to the demonstration of alpha prime hemolysis on the other. On cursory examination, alpha prime hemolysis may be confused with beta hemolysis, and they can be differentiated with certainty only by microscope examination of subsurface colonies in pour plates. The frequency of the occurrence of alpha prime hemolysis is unknown.

In recent years, investigators have recommended that sheep blood be incorporated in blood-agar plates for the isolation of beta-hemolytic streptococci. Sheep blood does not support the growth of most strains of *Haemophilus*; of particular importance, it does not support beta-hemolytic *H. haemolyticus*, which tends to confuse the isolation of beta-hemolytic streptococci. Conversely, some investigators feel that failure of sheep blood to support growth of *Haemophilus* is a distinct disadvantage to the use of this blood. They argue that inability to isolate *Haemophilus* on sheep blood necessitates the use of a second blood medium to augment the sheep blood plate. However, using rabbit or horse blood as an alternative to sheep blood requires that particular care be exercised in selecting beta-hemolytic colonies for characterization and that *all colonies be Gram-stained.*

In selecting a medium for use as a blood-agar base, choose an infusion medium that is free from fermentable carbohydrate and has a final pH of 7.3 to 7.4 before addition of the blood. The presence of dextrose in the basal medium for blood plates results in the inhibition of hemolysis by beta-hemolytic streptococci. The deleterious effect of dextrose upon hemolytic activity may be partially explained by the fact that streptolysin S is inactivated by the acid produced during fermentation. Brown stated that, whereas small amounts of dextrose were beneficial to demonstration of alpha hemolysis, actively fermenting gamma-hemolytic strains produced discoloration of the blood medium which confused the differentiation of the types of hemolysis.

Specific recommendations. For plating the specimen, use media and growth conditions which favor the demonstration of streptococcal characteristics. Inoculate the specimen into a carbohydrate-free infusion medium, pH 7.3 to 7.4, containing 4 to 5% defibrinated sheep blood. Ideally, the specimen should be plated in a pour plate to allow for microscope examination of subsurface colonies. The suspect colony should be examined under low-power magnification (total magnification, 100×) with a conventional microscope. It is imperative that the edge of the colony be in sharp focus during the determination of hemolytic activity. A portion of the surface of the hardened pour plate can be streaked in the usual manner to permit ease of isolation of the obvious beta colonies. If streak plates remain the method of choice, at the very least stab the streaked plate with the inoculating loop to get subsurface growth and to permit detection of both O and S streptolysin.

Group identification

Fluorescent-antibody (FA) technique. The primary swab can be tested for group A streptococci by the following method (33, 35).

Preparing and fixing the smear:

1. Place swabs in 1 ml of broth and incubate for 2 to 5 h at 37 C.
2. Remove the swab from broth and place in a sterile tube.
3. Centrifuge broth for 5 min at approximately 2,000 rpm.
4. Pour off broth into disinfectant solution and wipe lip with disinfectant-soaked cotton; resuspend cells in 1 ml of sterile buffered saline, pH 7.5, and recentrifuge.
5. Pour off buffered saline into disinfectant solution. Wipe lip with disinfectant-soaked cotton while tube is in inverted position to remove all visible diluent.
6. Place tube in rack for 2 to 3 min and let residual buffered saline collect in bottom of tube. (Usually no additional diluent will be necessary).
7. Mix cells thoroughly in diluent.
8. With a Pasteur capillary pipette, transfer sediment to area within circles on an FA slide. An attempt should be made to transfer most of the sediment to the smears.
9. Let smear dry in air. If atmosphere is humid, smears may be dried in an incubator at 37 C.
10. Cover each smear with 95% ethanol. Keep wet for 1 min; then let ethanol evaporate. After smears are thoroughly dry, they may be stained, or they may be frozen and stored and then stained at a later date if *absolutely no thawing* occurs in the interim.

Staining the smears: Apply procedure to thoroughly dried, fixed smears. Include a known positive control slide in each test run.

1. Cover smear nearest etched end of slide

with small drop of control conjugate (normal rabbit globulin labeled with fluorescein-isothiocyanate and treated to remove nonspecific staining). Cover the other smear with group A antistreptococcus conjugate (group A antistreptococcus globulin labeled with fluorescein-isothiocyanate and treated to remove nonspecific staining). Spread each conjugate over entire smear with an applicator stick held in a horizontal position. After the desirable sensitivity and specificity of a particular vial of group A antistreptococcus conjugate has been established with groups A, C, and G *Streptococcus* and *Staphylococcus aureus* control cultures, it is permissible to omit staining with the normal rabbit globulin control conjugate routinely.

2. Let stand for 30 min at room temperature in a moist chamber. Half of a 15-cm petri dish fitted with moist filter paper makes a suitable chamber.

3. Shake excess conjugate onto disinfectant-soaked paper towel.

4. Dip slides momentarily into buffered saline, pH 7.5, in a staining dish.

5. Transfer to a second vessel of buffered saline and let stand for 10 min.

6. Dip momentarily into distilled water and air-dry.

7. Add a drop of buffered glycerol saline mounting fluid and a cover slip. Avoid formation of bubbles in mounting fluid. Apply one drop of nail polish (or similar adhesive) to each cover slip corner.

Storing and examining the smear: Stained and mounted smears may be refrigerated (not frozen) and examined anytime within 24 to 48 h without significant loss of brilliance of fluorescence. Smears may be stored in a refrigerator for longer periods to be used later for reference purposes, although there may be a gradual loss of staining intensity. Slides to be stored in a refrigerator overnight or longer should be sealed completely with nail polish.

Recommended filter system: BG12 exciter, OG1 barrier.

Estimation of fluorescence—intensity of stained cells:

4+ = Maximal fluorescence, brilliant yellow-green clear-cut cell outline; sharply defined nonstaining center of cell.

3+ = Less brilliant yellow-green fluorescence; clear-cut cell outline; sharply defined nonstaining center of cell.

2+ = Less brilliant, but definite fluorescence; less clear-cut cell outline; nonstaining center area fuzzy.

1+ = Definite fluorescence, but very subdued; peripheral and center staining at same intensity.

A satisfactory working dilution of the test reagent is one which stains all of the group A strains at 3+ or 4+ fluorescence intensity and the other strains at not more than 1+ or 2+.

A satisfactory control conjugate should not stain group A streptococci. Occasionally *S. aureus*, group C, and group G streptococci, and rare group A streptococci stain at low levels.

In reporting the FA results, the laboratorian must report only his findings. If the hemolysis is not known before the FA results, his report should be "group A streptococci by FA," or "not group A streptococci by FA." If the hemolysis is known, then a report of "beta streptococci group A by FA," "beta streptococci not group A by FA," or "no beta streptococci isolated" can be made.

Bacitracin grouping for group A streptococci. Commercial disks are available that will differentiate between beta-hemolytic group A streptococci and other beta-hemolytic streptococci. The users of bacitracin disks should be aware of several important factors.

1. Be sure to purchase *differential, not sensitivity* disks. Disks sold and used for bacitracin susceptibility testing have too high a concentration of bacitracin to differentiate accurately between group A and non-group A streptococci. Commercial differential bacitracin disks contain approximately 0.04 units of bacitracin per disk, whereas sensitivity disks contain 10 units per disk.

2. A heavy inoculum of a pure culture is advisable. According to one report, when the differential disk was placed on primary plates that had been inoculated with throat swabs, only 70% of the group A streptococci were correctly identified (36). The test has been designed for use with pure cultures, not mixed cultures (25, 29).

3. The test is designed for differentiating beta-hemolytic streptococci. Hemolysis must be determined correctly before this differential test can be reliable. Many alpha-hemolytic streptococci, including pneumococci, are sensitive to the bacitracin differential disk (29).

4. There have been reports of variation in lots of commercial disks; therefore, each new lot of disks obtained should be tested with known strains of group A and non-group A streptococci. Biweekly tests with control strains should be performed to assure the continued reliability of the disks.

5. The following criteria should be used to read the tests. Any zone of inhibition, regardless

of diameter, is positive. No zone of inhibition (growth right up to the edge of the disk) means that the culture is resistant. Reports of zone size requirements are in the literature (9, 36), and the technical bulletin of one manufacturer implies that a zone of a certain size is necessary for presumptive identification of group A streptococci. The originator of the test (29) did not specify that zones should be a certain size. No experimental data are available to show that measurement of zone diameters is necessary for the differentiation of group A from non-group A streptococci. We prefer false-positive rather than false-negative results. By requiring zones of 10 mm or more for presumptive identification of group A streptococci, at least one group of investigators (9) increased the error in results of the test by 10% (false negatives). The users of differential disks should realize that growth of some strains of beta-hemolytic streptococci other than group A is inhibited by the bacitracin disk. Therefore, findings should be reported as follows: (i) "presumptive beta-hemolytic group A by bacitracin," or (ii) "beta-hemolytic streptococci, not group A by bacitracin."

There are reports of excellent agreement between the results of the FA and the bacitracin tests for identifying group A streptococci (31, 44). Also, there are reports of the failure of the bacitracin test to correlate with the FA procedure (11). We believe that with correct determination of hemolysis, proper testing of differential disks, proper reading of the resulting inhibition or lack of inhibition, and the use of proper (heavy) inoculum, a 95% accuracy can be achieved for presumptive identification of group A streptococci.

Extraction of the group antigen and serological grouping. The most definite identification of streptococci can be made by demonstrating the group-specific carbohydrate antigen that can be extracted from the isolated streptococci. There are four methods for extracting the group carbohydrate (CH) antigen: the hot-acid method of Lancefield (46), the hot-formamide method of Fuller (18), the autoclave method of Rantz and Randall (38), and the enzyme method of Maxted (28). A second enzyme method (Pronase B extraction) has been proposed (9) but is of questionable value, unless highly potent antisera are used. In a short study conducted in our laboratory, the Lancefield, Fuller, and Rantz methods extracted all of the 21 group A, 26 group B, 22 group C, 30 group D, 7 group F, and 24 group G strains equally well. No cross-reactions were observed, and all reactions occurred within 10 min. The Pronase extraction procedure extracted all of the group A strains, but failed to extract 13 of 26 group B, 8 of 20 group C, 12 of 12 group D, 5 of 5 group F, and 2 of 11 group G strains. All antisera used were prepared by the Biological Reagents Section of the CDC. Although the Maxted enzyme extraction procedure does not extract group D antigens, it can be used to extract group A through G (except D) beta-hemolytic streptococci.

The four extraction procedures are given below. However, if M-typing of group A streptococci or subtyping of group B streptococci is desired, only the Lancefield method will extract all type antigens. In addition, Todd-Hewitt broth should be used if typing results are sought. Typing antisera are evaluated and standardized with Lancefield extracts of streptococci grown in Todd-Hewitt broth. Interested readers are referred to Moody et al. (32) and Wilkinson et al. (53) for information on procedures for *typing* group A and group B streptococci, respectively.

Lancefield's hot acid extraction method:

1. Inoculate the organism into 30 ml of suitable infusion broth and incubate overnight (18 to 20 h) at 35 to 37 C.
2. Pack the cells by centrifugation.
3. Discard the supernatant fluid; save the sedimented cells.
4. Add one drop of 0.04% *meta*-cresol purple and about 0.3 ml of 0.2 N HCl to the sedimented cells. Mix well and transfer to a Kahn tube. If the suspension is not a definite pink color (pH 2.0 to 2.4), add another drop or so of the 0.2 N HCl. The 0.2 N HCl is made up in 0.85% NaCl.
5. Place in boiling water bath for 10 min, shaking several times.
6. Remove from water bath and pack the cells by centrifugation.
7. Decant supernatant fluid into a clean Kahn tube and discard sediment.
8. Neutralize the extract by adding 0.2 N NaOH (in distilled water) drop by drop until it is slightly purple (pH 7.4 to 7.8). A deep purple indicates that the pH is too high. Adjust back to light purple with 0.2 N HCl because a pH that is too high may cause nonspecific cross-reactions. Whenever possible, this additional dilution resulting from back-titration should be avoided.
9. The extract should be clarified by centrifugation and the supernatant fluid decanted into a small screw-cap vial. Store at 4 C. To preserve the extract, prepare a 1:100 Merthiolate solution in 1.4% sodium borate and then dilute

up to 1:500. One drop of 1:500 solution is added to the extract.

10. React with grouping antisera.

Fuller's formamide extraction method:

1. Inoculate 5 ml of suitable infusion broth and incubate overnight (18 to 20 h) at 35 to 37 C.

2. Centrifuge at 2,000 rpm; discard supernatant fluid and *keep* precipitate.

3. Add 0.1 ml of formamide to cells; mix by shaking.

4. Place in oil bath (150 C) for 15 min. Cool.

5. Add 0.25 ml of acid alcohol mix. This mix is 95 parts of anhydrous (100%) alcohol with 5 parts of 2 N HCl (one part concentrated acid with four parts water).

6. Centrifuge in a clinical centrifuge. Transfer supernatant fluid to a Kahn tube. Keep supernatant fluid.

7. Add 0.5 ml of acetone. Shake.

8. Centrifuge in a clinical centrifuge. Discard supernatant fluid. *Keep pellet* (precipitate).

9. Add 1 ml of saline and 1 drop of phenol red indicator to precipitate. Shake. Neutralize with trace of sodium carbonate. (If after shaking a part does not dissolve, centrifuge and neutralize supernatant fluid).

10. React with grouping antisera.

Rantz, Randall's autoclave extraction method:

1. Inoculate a 30-ml suitable infusion broth; incubate overnight (18 to 20 h) at 35 to 37 C.

2. Pack cells by centrifugation.

3. Discard the supernatant fluid; save the cells.

4. Add 0.5 ml of 0.85% NaCl solution.

5. Shake the tube to suspend the cells.

6. Autoclave the tube for 15 min at 15 psi (120 C).

7. Transfer to a Kahn tube.

8. Centrifuge to sediment the cellular debris.

9. Decant the supernatant fluid into a clean sterile container.

10. React with grouping sera.

Maxted's enzyme extraction method:

1. Pipette 0.25 ml of enzyme solution (*Streptomyces albus* enzyme; available commercially) into a small test tube (12 by 75 mm or smaller).

2. Suspend in this solution a loopful of growth from a 16- to 24-h blood-agar plate culture of beta-hemolytic streptococci.

3. Place in a water bath at 45 C until solution is clear (about 1.5 h).

4. Cool to room temperature and centrifuge for 10 min at 2,000 rpm.

5. Perform precipitin grouping as with acid-heat extracts.

Precipitin grouping of beta-hemolytic streptococci:

1. Dip capillary (vaccine capillary tubes, Kimble borosilicate glass, both ends open and lightly fire-polished) into serum (in screw-cap vial) until a column about 1 cm long has been drawn in by capillary action. (To maintain sterility of the sera, sterilize the capillaries and keep them sterile at the lower end until after the serum is taken up.)

2. Wipe off capillary with facial tissue, taking care to hold tube so air does not enter the end.

3. Dip capillary into extract until an amount equal to the serum column is drawn up. If an air bubble separates serum and extract, discard capillary and repeat.

4. Wipe capillary carefully. Fingerprints, serum, or extracts on the outside of the capillary may simulate or obscure a positive reaction.

5. Plunge the lower end of the capillary into the plasticine until a small plug fills the opening.

6. *Invert* capillary and insert gently into the plasticine-filled groove of the rack.

7. After 10 min, examine with a bright light against a dark background. A white cloud or ring at the center of the column represents a positive result. A strong reaction appears in 5 to 10 min; a weaker reaction develops more slowly. Since after 30 min the reaction may fade or a false positive may appear, it is important to examine the capillary tubes at frequent intervals between 10 and 30 min.

Since serological grouping is considered the definitive means of identifying streptococci, the report can state "Lancefield group A streptococcus" or whatever the group reaction that was observed. Group A streptococci are *S. pyogenes*, group B streptococci are *S. agalactiae*, group G and F streptococci do not have species names. There are several species of group C and D streptococci. The report should include the hemolytic reaction observed. Occasional beta-hemolytic streptococci occur that do not react with grouping antisera A, B, C, D, F, or G. When this happens, other characteristics of the strain should be determined to identify the strain. The majority of beta-hemolytic strains that fail to react with CDC grouping antisera resemble group F streptococci morphologically and physiologically. Beta-hemolytic streptococci that are group A variant or group L are found only rarely in humans. Beta streptococci belonging to groups E, M, P, and U are not found in humans. Extracts of some alpha-hemolytic streptococci react with group H, K, or O antisera; however, the antisera are not standardized. Reference centers are not in agreement as to what strains should be used as vaccine strains for production of these antisera. Therefore, many discrepancies have resulted between grouping results obtained in different laboratories. Some alpha-hemolytic or nonhemolytic streptococci that react with grouping antisera may be found. Nonhemolytic varieties of group A and group B streptococci have been reported (21, 54). The frequency of occurrence of these isolations from human infections is unknown, but they are thought to be rare. Not all group reactions observed can be read as positive identification of a species. Extracts of *Streptococcus* MG react with group F antisera, yet the species is not considered a group F streptococcus. Other alpha-hemolytic streptococci react with grouping sera of various streptococcal groups but are not true members of that group. The grouping antisera A through G are produced with vaccines of beta-hemolytic strains. With the exception of group D, the antisera are tested with specific strains only. It is obvious that we do not know whether these sera will react with alpha-hemolytic strains of streptococci. The grouping sera (A, B, C, F, and G) should be used routinely only to test extracts of beta-hemolytic streptococci. Under special circumstances, the sera can be used in the gel diffusion technique to test extracts of alpha-hemolytic streptococci for group antigens. A positive control with a known beta-hemolytic streptococcus is necessary to show that the reaction is valid.

Group N streptococci are nonpathogenic streptococci and are found in dairy products. Group R, S, and T streptococci are alpha-hemolytic streptococci, which are found rarely, if at all, in humans.

We suggest that a clinical laboratory dealing with human infections need purchase only groups A, B, C, D, F, and G antisera for the reasons stated above. If the laboratory should desire to divide group C streptococci further, the physiological reactions described by Swift (45) can be used. I have previously described the procedures for group D streptococcal speciation of human isolates (12).

Physiological differential characteristics. Group A, C, and G streptococci cannot be reliably differentiated by physiological characteristics. Bacitracin can be used to recognize group A, but groups C and G cannot be differentiated by physiological reactions.

Group B streptococci can be recognized by either the hippurate hydrolysis test (1) or the CAMP test (5). We have had considerable experience with the hippurate hydrolysis test and have found it to be a satisfactory presumptive test for identifying group B streptococci.

All group B streptococci hydrolyze hippurate and, hence, yield a positive test. A few group D streptococci are also positive. Other beta-hemolytic streptococci (groups A, C, G, and F) do not hydrolyze hippurate. Some alpha-hemolytic streptococci (*S. uberis* and *S. acidominimus*) hydrolyze hippurate. These strains should not interfere with the identification of the beta-hemolytic group B streptococci because of their hemolytic reaction, and they are found rarely, if at all, in human infections. *S. uberis* is found in bovine infections; therefore, investigators studying diseases of animals other than humans will need to rely on other characteristics to identify the isolated species. The few group D strains that hydrolyze hippurate are also bile-esculin (BE)-positive; thus, strains with positive BE and hippurate reactions are presumptive group D streptococci (or enterococci if the NaCl test is positive). The BE-negative, hippurate-positive, beta-hemolytic streptococci should be reported as "presumptive group B streptococci by hippurate hydrolysis."

Nonhemolytic group B streptococci of human origin have been reported (54). These strains hydrolyze hippurate; thus, they could be identified as non-beta-hemolytic "presumptive group B streptococci by hippurate hydrolysis." Unusual strains that hydrolyze hippurate, such as non- or alpha-hemolytic streptococci, should be sent to your state health department for confirmation and definitive identification.

Group D streptococci can be identified by the BE reaction (13, 14). Care must be taken to select the proper BE medium since there are major differences in commercial products (13).

BE medium will differentiate between group D streptococci and non-group D streptococci (13, 14). All group D streptococci (this group includes all enterococci) will blacken the BE slant, usually within 48 h (13). Most non-group D streptococci do not blacken the medium. We correctly reported 100% of the group D streptococci and only 3% of alpha-hemolytic non-group D streptococci (viridans; 14). Not all group D streptococci are enterococci (penicillin-resistant); *S. bovis* and *S. equinus* are group D species but not enterococci. *S. bovis* (BE-positive) is found in a significant number of group D infections and is penicillin-susceptible; therefore, further tests are needed for adequate differentiation of the enterococci from non-enterococci (12). A streptococcus that gives a positive BE reaction should be reported as a "presumptive group D streptococcus by bile-esculin hydrolysis." BE does not differentiate enterococci from non-enterococci; thus, a positive BE reaction should not be reported as presumptive identification of enterococci.

The enterococci can be identified by determining the salt tolerance of BE-positive streptococci (13). Enterococci (*S. faecalis* and its varieties, *zymogenes* and *liquefaciens*, *S. faecium*, and *S. durans*) will usually give heavy growth and an indicator change within 24 h; however, some enterococcal strains take 48 h to change the indicator, and some will grow with no accompanying indicator change even after 72 h. About 80% of group B streptococci will also grow in this medium; some change the indicator. Beta groups A, C, G, and F usually do not grow in the medium. The alpha-hemolytic, nongroupable streptococci (viridans) such as *S. mitis*, *S. sanguis*, *S. salivarius*, *S. mutans*, and *Streptococcus* MG do not grow in 6.5% NaCl medium, nor do the group D species *S. bovis* and *S. equinus*.

A positive BE test and growth in 6.5% NaCl broth confirm the presence of enterococci. Even if serological reactions are determined, growth in 6.5% NaCl broth should be used to confirm that the group D streptococcus is an enterococcus. Salt-tolerant beta-hemolytic strains other than group B and D streptococci occur very rarely. Salt-tolerant group A streptococci (bacitracin-positive) occur occasionally. Strains that give positive salt-tolerant tests, and that are not presumptive group B (hydrolyze hippurate) or presumptive group D (BE-positive) streptococci, should be tested for purity by streaking the growth from the salt-tolerance test medium onto a blood-agar plate and comparing the morphology with that of the original strain. If the morphology differs, a Gram stain and a catalase test should be performed.

Presumptive identification of the pathogenic streptococci can be achieved with satisfactory results when the following determinations are made (Table 1).

1. An accurate determination of hemolysis. This is an absolute necessity for all laboratories concerned with proper identification of streptococci.
2. Susceptibility to bacitracin differential disks.
3. Hydrolysis of hippurate.
4. Blackening of BE medium.
5. Tolerance to 6.5% NaCl broth.

Beta-hemolytic streptococci that are susceptible to bacitracin, fail to hydrolyze hippurate, and fail to blacken BE medium are presumptive group A streptococci. Beta-hemolytic streptococci that hydrolyze hippurate and fail to blacken BE medium are presumptive group B streptococci. Beta-hemolytic, bacitracin-susceptible streptococci that hydrolyze hippurate are also presumptive group B streptococci. Beta-hemolytic streptococci that are resistant to bacitracin, fail to hydrolyze hippurate or blacken BE medium, and are not 6.5% NaCl tolerant are beta-hemolytic streptococci not group A, B, or D. Group C, G, and F streptococci fall into this presumptive classification. An occasional salt-tolerant strain will occur among these streptococci. BE-positive streptococci are group D streptococci; BE medium-positive and 6.5% NaCl-tolerant streptococci are enterococci. The enterococci can be beta-, alpha-, or nonhemolytic. Approximately 8% of the enterococci hydrolyze hippurate, but group B streptococci fail to blacken BE medium. Thus, streptococci that are BE medium-positive, salt-tolerant, and hippurate-positive are enterococci. BE-positive streptococci that fail to tolerate 6.5% NaCl are group D streptococci but not enterococci. Like nearly all group D streptococci, these non-enterococcal group D

TABLE 1. *Presumptive identification of streptococci*

Group identification	Hemolysis	Bacitracin susceptibility	Hippurate hydrolysis	Bile-esculin hydrolysis	Tolerance to 6.5% NaCl
Group A	Beta	+	−	−	−
Group B	Beta	−[a]	+	−	V[b]
Non-group A, B, or D	Beta	−[a]	−	−	−[a]
Group D enterococcus	Beta, alpha, or none	−	V	+	+
Group D not an enterococcus	Alpha or none	−	−	+	−
Viridans non-group D	Alpha or none	V	−[a]	−	−

[a] An occasional exception occurs.
[b] V, variable.

streptococci are resistant to bacitracin; they are nonhemolytic and fail to hydrolyze hippurate. They are found frequently in human infections (12). Alpha-hemolytic streptococci that fail to blacken BE medium, fail to hydrolyze hippurate, and are not tolerant to 6.5% NaCl broth are viridans streptococci. About 8 to 12% of the viridans streptococci are susceptible to bacitracin; these figures indicate the importance of the correct determination of hemolysis for presumptive identification.

Bacitracin-susceptible group C and G streptococci would be erroneously identified as group A streptococci with these presumptive tests. However, we have shown that 99.4% group A, 99.7% group B, 81.6% beta-hemolytic streptococci not A, B, or D, 99.7% of the enterococcal group D, 97.8% of the non-enterococcal group D, and 94.7% of the viridans streptococci can be presumptively identified with the above-mentioned tests (15).

SUSCEPTIBILITY TO ANTIMICROBIAL AGENTS

Group A streptococci are universally susceptible to penicillin; therefore, susceptibility of group A streptococci to antimicrobial agents need not be determined unless the physician is considering an antimicrobial agent other than penicillin for therapy. The only acceptable reason for considering an alternative drug is patient sensitivity to penicillin (26). Erythromycin or lincomycin, but not tetracycline, should be substituted in these cases (6). Resistance to erythromycin and lincomycin has been documented (42), but the frequency with which it occurs is unknown. Sanders (42) suggested that antimicrobial susceptibilities should be determined on all group A streptococci if the patient is not receiving penicillin therapy. It is advisable to determine antimicrobial susceptibilities of all streptococci isolated from patients with systemic infection and penicillin allergy. Apparently susceptibility testing is not necessary on streptococci isolated from the throat or skin unless a treatment failure is documented.

Although there is very little data on antimicrobial susceptibility of beta-hemolytic non-group A or D streptococci, it appears that beta-hemolytic streptococci of groups B, C, and G are slightly less susceptible to erythromycin and penicillin, and those of group B are the least susceptible to penicillin (23). Recently, Matsen et al. (27) reported that all the throat and skin streptococci that they tested were susceptible to penicillin, erythromycin, and four cephalosporins. They included strains of group A, B, C, and G streptococci in the study. Weinstein (52) recommended penicillin G as the drug of choice for all streptococcal infections except enterococcal infections. The enterococci are penicillin-resistant and require combined antibiotic therapy (52). Techniques for demonstrating antibiotic synergism can be obtained from Moellering et al. (30) or Standiford et al. (43). Toala et al. (49) and Wilkowske et al. (55) reported on similarities and differences in the susceptibility of the group D streptococcal species to various antibiotics; the major point they made was that the enterococcal species are resistant to penicillin but the non-enterococcal species (*S. bovis*) are susceptible to this drug. Our own studies with 30 strains of *S. bovis* isolated from bacterial endocarditis patients indicate that all *S. bovis* strains are susceptible to penicillin. The susceptibility of this species was more similar to that of the viridans streptococci than to that of the enterococci. Antibiograms should be determined in all alpha-hemolytic and nonhemolytic streptococci isolated from systemic infections.

EVALUATION

The laboratorian must convey information that will best help the physician to manage his patient. In the case of throat cultures, the report should include: (i) the identity of the organism isolated, either presumptive or otherwise, and (ii) the relative number of organisms present.

A convenient method for estimating the number of organisms present on the culture plate is as follows (7): 1+ = 10 colonies or less; 2+ = 10 to 50 colonies; 3+ = more than 50 colonies; 4+ = predominant or pure culture.

Laboratory results of skin cultures should be reported in the same manner as results of throat cultures (7). Physicians are interested primarily in beta-hemolytic group A streptococci from throat and skin swabs.

Reports of results with blood, CSF, and other body fluids should include the identity of the organism if possible. Reports on urine samples must include the number of organisms per milliliter.

Feingold et al. (16) presented an evaluation of both clinical and laboratory findings in an attempt to assess the importance of the various serological groups of streptococci isolated from extra-respiratory sources. They found that the clinical picture as well as the laboratory findings were important in assessing the importance of streptococci isolated from blood and urine specimens. Readers are urged to study Feingold's criteria and to communicate with the attending physician about laboratory findings. The laboratorian's responsibility does not end with a simple report of his findings; he is obliged to have knowledge of the clinical significance of the bacteria he identifies. In this way, he can at least tell the physician what other scientists believe and relate his findings to theirs. The streptococci offer the physician and the laboratorians a challenge. The tests and procedures offered here should enable the laboratorian to meet the challenge.

LITERATURE CITED

1. Ayers, S. H., and P. Rupp. 1922. Differentiation of hemolytic streptococci from human and bovine sources by the hydrolysis of sodium hippurate. J. Infect. Dis. **30:**388-399.
2. Blazevic, D. J., J. E. Stemper, and J. M. Matsen. 1972. Organisms encountered in urine cultures over a 10-year period. Appl. Microbiol. **23:**421-422.
3. Breese, B. 1965. The use of cotton-tipped swabs as a simple method of transporting cultures of beta-hemolytic streptococci. Pediatrics **36:**599-603.
4. Brown, J. H. 1919. The use of blood agar for the study of streptococci. Rockefeller Inst. Med. Res., Monograph no. 9.
5. Christie, R., N. E. Atkins, and E. Munch-Petersen. 1944. A note on a lytic phenomenon shown by group B streptococci. Aust. J. Exp. Biol. Med. Sci. **23:**193-197.
6. Denny, F., et al. 1970. Prevention of rheumatic fever. A statement prepared by the Rheumatic Fever Committee of the Council on Rheumatic Fever and Congenital Heart Disease of the American Heart Association.
7. Dillon, H. G., and B. A. Dudding. 1970. Streptococcal infections, p. 1-15. *In* Brennemann's practice of pediatrics, vol. 2. Harper and Row Publishing, Inc., Hagerstown, Md.
8. Duma, R. J., A. N. Weinberg, T. F. Medrek, and L. J. Kunz. 1969. Streptococcal infections. A bacteriological and clinical study of streptococcal bacteremia. Medicine **48:**87-127.
9. Ederer, G. M., M. M. Herrmann, R. Bruce, J. M. Matsen, and S. S. Chapman. 1972. Rapid extraction method with Pronase B for grouping beta-hemolytic streptococci. Appl. Microbiol. **23:**285-288.
10. Eickhoff, T. C., J. O. Klein, A. K. Daly, D. Ingall, and M. Finland. 1964. Neonatal sepsis and other infections due to group B beta-hemolytic streptococci. N. Engl. J. Med. **271:**1221-1228.
11. Estela, L. A. and H. E. Shuey. 1963. Comparison of fluorescent antibody, precipitin, and bacitracin disk methods in the identification of group A streptococci. Amer. J. Clin. Pathol. **40:**591-597.
12. Facklam, R. R. 1972. Recognition of group D streptococcal species of human origin by biochemical and physiological tests. Appl. Microbiol. **23:**1131-1139.
13. Facklam, R. R. 1973. Comparison of several laboratory media for presumptive identification of enterococci and group D streptococci. Appl. Microbiol. **26:**138-145.
14. Facklam, R. R., and M. D. Moody. 1970. Presumptive identification of group D streptococci: the bile-esculin test. Appl. Microbiol. **20:**245-250.
15. Facklam, R. R., J. F. Padula, L. G. Thacker, E. C. Wortham, and B. J. Sconyers. 1974. Presumptive identification of Group A, B, and D streptococci. Appl. Microbiol. **27:**107-113.
16. Feingold, D. S., M. L. Stagg, and L. J. Kunz. 1966. Extrarespiratory streptococcal infections. Importance of the various serologic groups. N. Engl. J. Med. **275:**356-361.
17. Frobisher, M., E. I. Parsons, S. E. Pai, and S. Hakim. 1947. A simplified method for the preservation of bacteria by desiccation in vacuo. J. Lab. Clin. Med. **32:**1008-1015.
18. Fuller, A. T. 1938. The formamide method for the extraction of polysaccharides from hemolytic streptococci. Brit. J. Exp. Pathol. **19:**130-139.
19. Geil, C. C., W. K. Castle, and E. A. Mortimer. 1970. Group A streptococcal infections in newborn nurseries. Pediatrics **46:**849-854.
20. Gordon, D. F., Jr. 1967. Reisolation of *Staphylococcus salivarius* from the human oral cavity. J. Bacteriol. **94:**1281-1286.
21. James, L., and M. McFarland. 1971. An epidemic of pharyngitis due to a nonhemolytic group A streptococcus at Lowry Air Force Base. N. Engl. J. Med. **284:**750-752.
22. Jelinkova, J., M. Neubauer, and J. Duben. 1970. Group B streptococci in human pathology. Zentralbl. Bakteriol. Parasitenk. Infektionskr. Hyg. Abt. I Orig. **214:**450-457.
23. Jones, W. F., H. Feldman, and M. Finland. 1957. Susceptibility of hemolytic streptococci other than those of group D to eleven antibiotics in vitro. Amer. J. Clin. Pathol. **27:**159-169.
24. Lerner, P. I., and L. Weinstein. 1966. Infective endocarditis in the antibiotic era. N. Engl. J. Med. **274:**199-206.
25. Levinson, M. L., and P. F. Frank. 1955. Differentiation of group A from other beta hemolytic streptococci with bacitracin. J. Bacteriol. **69:**284-287.
26. Markowitz, M., and A. Taranta. 1971. Problems and pitfalls in the management of streptococcal infections. Excerpta Medica (Special Issue), p. 3-11.
27. Matsen, J. M., D. J. Blazevic, and S. S. Champan. 1970. In vitro susceptibility patterns of beta-hemolytic streptococci. Antimicrob. Ag. Chemother. 1969, p. 485-488.
28. Maxted, W. R. 1948. Preparation of streptococcal extracts for Lancefield grouping. Lancet (14 August 1948), p. 255-256.
29. Maxted, W. R. 1953. The use of bacitracin for identifying group A hemolytic streptococci. J. Clin. Pathol. **6:**224-226.
30. Moellering, R. C., Jr., C. Wennersten, T. Medrek, and A. N. Weinberg. 1971. Prevalence of high-level resistance to aminoglycosides in clinical isolates of enterococci. Antimicrob. Ag. Chemother. 1970, p. 335-340.
31. Moffett, H. L., H. G. Cramblett, and J. P. Black. 1964. Group A streptococcal infections in a children's home. I. Evaluation of practical bacteriologic methods. Pediatrics **33:**5-10.
32. Moody, M. D., J. F. Padula, D. Lizana, and C. T. Hall. 1965. Epidemiologic characterization of group A streptococci by T-agglutination and M-precipitin tests in the public health laboratory. Health Lab. Sci. **2:**149-162.
33. Moody, M. D., A. C. Siegel, B. Pittman, and C. C. Winter. 1963. Fluorescent-antibody identification of group A streptococci from throat swabs. Amer. J. Pub. Health **53:**1083-1092.
34. Mundt, J. O., and W. F. Graham. 1968. *Streptococcus faecium* var. *casseliflavus*, nov. var. J. Bacteriol. **95:**2005-2009.
35. Peeples, W. J., D. W. Spielman, and M. D. Moody. 1961. Field application of fluorescent antibody technique for identification of group A streptococcus. Pub. Health Rep. **76:**651-654.
36. Petran, E. I. 1964. Comparison of the fluorescent antibody and the bacitracin disk method for the identification of group A streptococci. Amer. J. Clin. Pathol. **41:**224-226.

37. Quintiliani, R., and G. A. Engh. 1971. Overwhelming sepsis associated with group A beta hemolytic streptococci. J. Bone Joint Surg. **53:**1391-1399.
38. Rantz, L. A., and E. Randall. 1955. Use of autoclaved extracts of haemolytic streptococci for serological grouping. Stanford Med. Bull. **13:**290-291.
39. Redys, J. J., E. W. Hibbard, and E. K. Borman. 1968. Improved dry-swab transportation for streptococcal specimens. Pub. Health Rep. **82:**143-149.
40. Reinarz, J. A., and J. P. Sanford. 1965. Human infection caused by non group A or D streptococci. Medicine **44:**81-96.
41. Rogosa, M. 1971. Peptococcaceae, a new family to include the gram-positive, anaerobic cocci of the genera Peptococcus, Peptostreptococcus, and Ruminococcus. Int. J. Syst. Bacteriol. **21:**234-237.
42. Sanders, E., M. T. Foster, and D. Scott. 1968. Group A beta-hemolytic streptococci resistant to erythromycin and lincomycin. N. Engl. J. Med. **278:**538-540.
43. Standiford, H. D., J. B. deMaine, and W. M. M. Kirby. 1970. Antibiotic synergism of enterococci. Arch. Intern. Med. **126:**255-259.
44. Streamer, C. W., P. M. Williams, W. L. L. Wang, R. S. Johnson, C. D. McGuire, I. J. Abelow, and R. J. Glaser. 1962. Identification of group A streptococci. Amer. J. Dis. Child. **104:**157-160.
45. Swift, H. F. 1948. The streptococci, p. 237-294. *In* R. Dubos (ed.), Bacterial and mycotic infections in man. J. B. Lippincott Co., Philadelphia.
46. Swift, H. F., A. T. Wilson, and R. C. Lancefield. 1943. Typing group A hemolytic streptococci by M-precipitin reactions in capillary pipettes. J. Exp. Med. **78:**127-133.
47. Taplin, D., and L. Lansdell. 1973. Value of desiccated swabs for streptococcal epidemiology in the field. Appl. Microbiol. **25:**135-138.
48. Taranta, A., and M. D. Moody. 1971. Diagnosis of streptococcal pharyngitis and rheumatic fever. Pediat. Clin. N. Amer. **18:**125-143.
49. Toala, P., A. McDonald, C. Wilcox, and M. Finland. 1970. Comparison of antibiotic susceptibility of group D streptococcus strains isolated at Boston City Hospital in 1953-54 and 1968-69. Antimicrob. Ag. Chemother. 1969, p. 479-484.
50. Updyke, E. L. 1957. Laboratory problems in the diagnosis of streptococcal infections. Pub. Health Lab. **15:**78-80.
51. Wannamaker, L. W. 1965. A method for culturing beta hemolytic streptococci from the throat. *In* Statement prepared for the American Heart Association.
52. Weinstein, L. 1970. Chemotherapy and microbial diseases, p. 1176-1180. *In* L. S. Goodman and A. Gelman (ed.), The pharmacological basis of therapeutics, 4th ed. The MacMilliam Co., London.
53. Wilkinson, H. W., R. R. Facklam, and E. C. Wortham. 1973. Distribution by serological type of group B streptococci isolated from a variety of clinical material over a five-year period (with special reference to neonatal sepsis and meningitis). Infect. Immunity **8:**228-235.
54. Wilkinson, H. W., L. G. Thacker, and R. R. Facklam. 1973. Non-hemolytic group B streptococci of human, bovine, and ichthyic origin. Infect. Immunity **7:**496-498.
55. Wilkowske, C. J., R. R. Facklam, J. A. Washington II, and J. E. Geraci. 1971. Antibiotic synergism: enhanced susceptibility of group D streptococci to certain antibiotic combinations. Antimicrob. Ag. Chemother. 1970, p. 195-200.

Chapter 9

Streptococcus pneumoniae (Pneumococcus)

ROBERT AUSTRIAN

CHARACTERIZATION

Streptococcus pneumoniae (pneumococcus) is a gram-positive, capsulated, nonmotile, facultatively aerobic coccus which occurs singly, in pairs, or in short chains in its natural habitat, the upper respiratory tract of humans and of other mammals. Typical forms are paired (as the former American generic name implies), and the cocci are often lanceolate, with the somewhat pointed ends occurring at the distal ends of each pair. Eighty-four serotypes are now known, type specificity being based upon the composition of the highly polymerized capsular polysaccharides of the organism.

GENERAL DESCRIPTION

Although pneumococcus was classified formerly in the genus *Diplococcus* by American taxonomists, it is more properly designated *Streptococcus pneumoniae*, which nomenclature has been adopted in the eighth edition of *Bergey's Manual of Determinative Bacteriology*. In culture media, the organism frequently grows in short chains, and genetic variants growing in long chains can be selected in the laboratory (1). Its close relationship to other alpha-hemolytic streptococci inhabiting the respiratory tract can be demonstrated by comparative study of deoxyribonucleates of the organisms in question (10) and by the genetic transfer of drug resistance and of capsular polysaccharide from streptococci to pneumococcus by means of transformation reactions (17). It is of historical interest that Sternberg, a co-discoverer of the pneumococcus, preferred the name *Streptococcus pneumoniae* for this organism (15).

A common inhabitant of the upper respiratory tract, the pneumococcus can be isolated from the pharynx of 30 to 70% of normal humans at different seasons of the year. From this site, it can invade the sinuses or middle ear, and, if unchecked by the natural defensive mechanism of the host, it can extend to give rise to mastoiditis and to meningitis. It may also cause purulent conjunctivitis. In addition, the pneumococcus can invade the lower respiratory tract, giving rise to pneumonia, of which it is the most common bacterial cause. Failure of normal cellular and humoral mechanisms to check the spread of the organism within the pulmonary parenchyma or at the secondary line of defense in the mediastinal lymph nodes is followed by passage of pneumococci into the thoracic duct and thence into the systemic circulation, giving rise to bacteremia. Infection may then spread to the endocardium, pericardium, meninges, peritoneum, or joint cavities. The pleural cavity may be involved by direct extension from the lung. Pneumococci may be isolated occasionally from the vagina, and it has been hypothesized that they may gain access to the peritoneal cavity through the female genital tract to cause peritonitis. Swallowed organisms have been recovered from the stools of patients with pneumonia.

From the foregoing resume, it is evident that pneumococci may be sought in specimens of throat and nasopharyngeal swabbings, sputum, blood, pus, and body fluids (cerebrospinal fluid, pleural fluid, etc.). The pneumococcus is a delicate organism and does not withstand drying at room temperature or residence in sterile physiological salt solution. For these reasons, swabs to be cultured for pneumococcus should be placed in tubes containing a sterile nutrient medium which will support growth of the organism during transport to the laboratory. Sputum should be collected in a sterile container, glass or plastic, and held at refrigerator temperature (4 C) until cultured. Collection of sputum is properly the responsibility of the physician, and it should be expectorated in his presence to insure its origin from the lungs. If the container is left at the bedside, the sample obtained is all too frequently saliva. Sputum may be difficult to obtain from infants with pneumonia, and material for culture from such patients must often be obtained from the nasopharynx.

Pneumococcus has complex nutritional requirements and, although chemically defined media have been devised for its growth (14), they are impractical for routine work. For this purpose, one of a variety of media which are derived from meat extracts or tryptic digests of soy bean is usually employed. For routine laboratory work, Trypticase soy broth and Trypticase soy agar have proved satisfactory. Although pneumococcus grows aerobically, it lacks cytochromes and is closely related biochemically to the anerobes. It can utilize oxygen through a flavoprotein enzyme system, and the end product of its oxygen metabolism is hydrogen peroxide, which it cannot degrade. Because hydrogen peroxide is toxic to the pneumococcus, the organism cannot survive long in cultures from which catalase is lacking. It is usual practice, therefore, to add defibrinated blood (rabbit, sheep, horse, or human) to media in or on which pneumococci are to be grown. If human blood is used, it is essential to know that it does not contain antibiotics. Pneumococci survive poorly in media containing added glucose; the glucose is metabolized to lactic acid, and the low pH resulting therefrom is inimical to the organism. About 5 to 10% of pneumococci require a higher than atmospheric concentration of carbon dioxide to grow on the surface of solid media at the time of primary isolation (2), and such cultures should be incubated in a CO_2 incubator or a candle jar. CO_2-requiring strains of pneumococci will grow in liquid media, however, in the absence of increased atmospheric concentrations of carbon dioxide.

Strains of pneumococci isolated from humans are capsulated. Noncapsulated mutants of pneumococcus may arise spontaneously in cultures of capsulated strains maintained in the laboratory, however, and their recovery may be facilitated by the addition of homologous anticapsular antibody to cultures of capsulated forms. The capsule of the pneumococcus protects the organism partially from phagocytosis and is essential to its virulence. The capsular polysaccharides of the pneumococcus, however, are nontoxic to humans. Noncapsulated variants of pneumococcus are phagocytized readily in the absence of antibody and lack virulence for humans and laboratory animals.

Cultures of pneumococci will remain viable for 6 to 8 weeks at 4 C if grown for 18 to 24 h in tubes containing 5 to 7 ml of fresh beef heart infusion broth with Neopeptone to which 0.3 ml of defibrinated rabbit blood has been added. Pneumococci may also be lyophilized for preservation.

Reference strains of pneumococcal capsular types 1 to 34 and of noncapsulated pneumococci may be obtained from the American Type Culture Collection.

DIRECT EXAMINATION

Pneumococci present in the secretions or exudates of untreated subjects or in young cultures may be decolorized by acetone-alcohol ized by acetone-alcohol. Material from patients treated with antimicrobial drugs and from older cultures may be decolorized by acetone-alcohol and appear gram-negative. By means of the Gram stain alone, it is impossible to distinguish pneumococcus from some strains of alpha-hemolytic or nonhemolytic streptococci on morphological grounds, and it is important to avoid this potential source of error in the interpretation of stained preparations. Pneumococci are stained readily by methylene blue. The capsule of the organism can be demonstrated by a variety of staining techniques (16) and by the use of wet mounts made with India ink. These techniques are employed rarely, however, the capsule of pneumococcus being demonstrated more readily by use of the quellung or capsular precipitin technique.

In typical cases of lobar pneumonia, the sputum has a characteristic rusty color; however, this color is not invariably present. For best results in examining sputum, it should be homogenized with 1 to 2 ml of sterile broth by refluxing gently with a 2- or 5-ml sterile syringe without a needle attached, care being taken to avoid spattering of the infectious material. Smears of sputum so treated should be placed on a glass slide, air-dried, fixed by passage several times through the flame of a Bunsen burner, and stained by the Gram technique. In the sputum from most patients with pneumococcal pneumonia, except from those with low white blood cell counts, considerable numbers of polymorphonuclear leukocytes will be present, in addition to the gram-positive lanceolate pneumococci which are found singly, in pairs, and in short chains. Exudates from patients with pneumococcal infection can be applied to slides directly without preliminary treatment, and the smears so prepared are treated in a fashion similar to those of sputum.

The most simple, rapid, and accurate method for the identification of pneumococci by direct examination is the quellung or capsular precipitin reaction. This technique is described below in the section on Serological Identification.

CULTURAL IDENTIFICATION

As noted earlier, the nutritional requirements of pneumococci are complex. The organism can be grown on solid media or in liquid media without difficulty, however, if the proper nutrilites and environmental conditions are provided. Growth on solid media such as brain heart infusion agar or Trypticase soy agar enriched with 5% blood is essential if the organism is to be isolated from other bacteria present in specimens such as sputum. A loopful of sputum homogenized in the manner described in the preceding section should be streaked on the surface of a nutrient blood-agar plate and incubated at 37 C for 18 h in a candle jar or CO_2 incubator. Colonies of pneumococci have a fairly typical appearance on such plates. The colony is round with entire edges, mucoid in appearance, about 1 mm in diameter (Fig. 1), and surrounded by a zone of alpha-hemolysis. On similar media incubated anaerobically, pneumococcal colonies are surrounded by a zone of beta-hemolysis. Young colonies are domed or hemispherical, but, as the culture ages, autolysis results in sinking of the central portion of the colony to give rise to a flattened surface, likened to the head of a nail, or to a central depression surrounded by an elevated rim, described by some as resembling a checker. Colonies of pneumococcus types 3 and 37 are often two or three times the size of those of other types and have a more watery appearance (Fig. 2). Because of their small size, pneumococcal colonies are recognized best when magnified. For this purpose, a colony or dissecting microscope should be used, and the surface of the plate should be examined with oblique reflected light at a magnification of 40 to 50 times. Despite their widespread use, hand lenses providing a magnification of 10 times are not satisfactory for recognizing pneumococcal colonies. The colony microscope is of great value also in isolating cells from single colonies on the surface of solid media.

Liquid media for the cultivation of pneumococci may be made from the same nutrient bases employed for solid media without the addition of agar. The organism grows satisfactorily also in thioglycolate media. The addition of 5% defibrinated blood (rabbit, sheep, horse, or human) as a readily available source of catalase will permit longer survival of the culture. In most media, glucose is the limiting growth factor, and the addition of glucose to a final concentration of 1% will permit a 10-fold increase in the bacterial population. To achieve this end, however, it is necessary to neutralize periodically the lactic acid formed from the metabolism of glucose by use of an alkalizing agent such as sodium hydroxide, sodium bicarbonate, or calcium carbonate. Pneumococci grow best at pH 7.6 and survive poorly outside the pH range of 7 to 7.8. The hydrogen ion concentration of pneumococcal cultures can be determined from a sample removed and tested in a pH meter or can be approximated more simply by the addition of a 0.5% alcoholic solution of phenol red to a final concentration of 0.0005%. Pneumococcus grows diffusely in liquid media and does not form a pellicle. In old cultures, the organisms may settle to the bottom of the container, giving rise to some sediment.

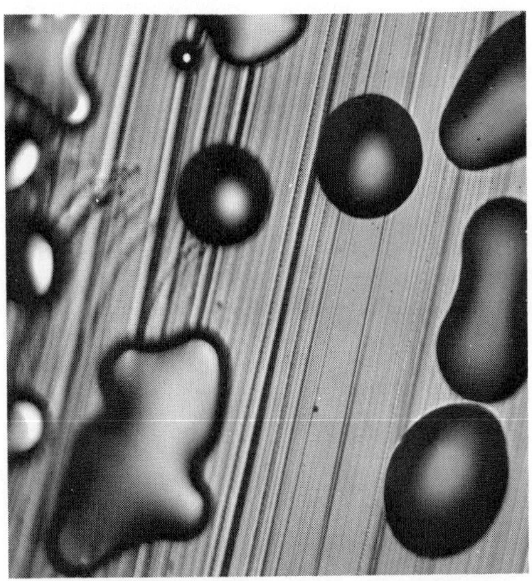

Fig. 2. *Colonies of pneumococcus type III. Note the watery appearance of the colonies and their large size. ×21. (Reprinted with permission of the Journal of Experimental Medicine.)*

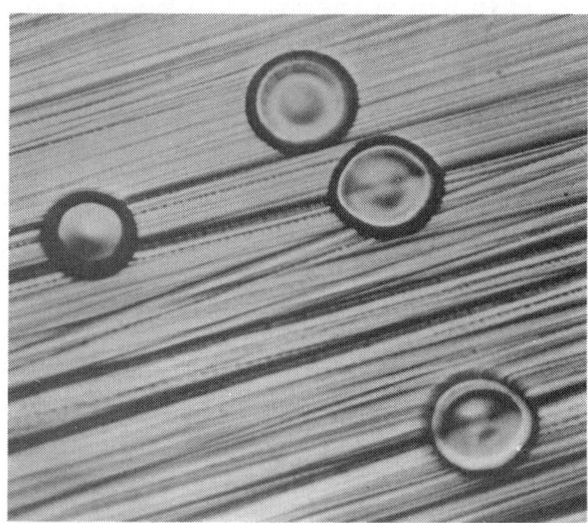

Fig. 1. *Colonies of pneumococcus type II on the surface of a blood-agar plate. Note the checker-like appearance of the three colonies on the left which have undergone partial autolysis. Unautolyzed colony is shown on the right. ×21. (Reprinted with permission of the Journal of Experimental Medicine.)*

The blood of any patient suspected of having a pneumococcal infection should be cultured. The ratio of the amount of blood to the medium into which it is inoculated should approximate 1:10, 5 to 15 ml of blood should be used. The culture should be examined after 24 and 48 h of incubation with the aid of strong transmitted illumination; if turbid, a subculture should be made by streaking a blood-agar plate, and a smear of the culture stained by the Gram technique should be examined. If organisms resembling pneumococci are seen in the smear, they may be typed directly from the culture fluid. Viable pneumococci are rarely recovered from the blood of patients treated with antimicrobial drugs, and parenterally administered penicillin will generally render the blood sterile within 1 h of its administration. The addition of penicillinase to blood cultures from treated patients has not proved to be very useful, in my experience.

Body fluids should be cultured by streaking the surface of a blood-agar plate and by inoculating a suitable liquid medium with 0.5 to 1 ml of the specimen. The cultures should be handled in a fashion similar to that employed for blood cultures.

Although serological methods provide the most suitable means for the identification of pneumococci, there are several additional tests for the presumptive identification of this organism. Most pneumococci strains ferment inulin. The test is not specific, however, as this carbohydrate is also fermented by some strains of streptococci, such as *S. salivarius*. The test is carried out in a liquid medium such as Hiss serum water (7) or in a semisolid medium such as that described in reference 3.

A second test for the presumptive identification of pneumococci is the so-called bile solubility test. Surface-active agents such as bile, bile salts, and sodium dodecyl sulfate alter pneumococcal structure in such a fashion as to lead to the dissolution of the cell as a result of activation of its autolytic enzymes. The test should be carried out with live cells at neutral pH and in the absence of significant concentrations of protein which exert an inhibitory effect on cell lysis. Most pneumococci lyse rapidly, though rare strains are known which are relatively resistant to autolysis. In addition, occasional strains of alpha-hemolytic and nonhemolytic streptococci may show a tendency to dissolution in the presence of bile salts. For these reasons, bile solubility can be regarded as a highly useful but not rigorous test for the identification of pneumococci.

Most strains of pneumococcus are sensitive to ethylhydrocupreine hydrochloride (optochin), whereas most strains of alpha-hemolytic streptococci are not. This difference in sensitivity to optochin of pneumococci and alpha-hemolytic streptococci forms the basis of another test employed widely to distinguish organisms in these two groups (4). The test can be carried out in a variety of ways, but perhaps most conveniently by employing the filter-paper disk technique in the manner used for testing bacterial susceptibility to antimicrobial drugs. Only pure cultures of the organism to be examined should be used to provide the bacterial lawn on the surface of the blood-agar plate. To this, a dry 6-mm disk of filter paper impregnated with 5 μg of optochin (0.02 ml of a 1:4,000 solution) should be applied. The plate should be incubated aerobically rather than in an atmosphere containing an increased concentration of CO_2 (13), as the inhibitory zone about the disk is reduced in size when pneumococci are incubated under the latter conditions. A zone of growth inhibition 18 mm or more in diameter is indicative of sensitivity. The test should not be employed to identify pneumococci in mixed cultures, such as sputum.

ANIMAL INOCULATION

The white mouse is exquisitely sensitive to infection with many pneumococcal types when inoculated by the intraperitoneal route. One colony-forming unit of some types will result in fatal infection. The virulence of other types is seemingly enhanced by mucinous material in sputum. In addition, the inoculum employed exceeds by 500- to 1,000-fold that which can be used to streak a blood-agar plate. These considerations make the white mouse an unusually useful tool for the isolation of pneumococcus from the mixed bacterial populations normally found in sputum. Because the white mouse will usually eliminate other bacteria present in sputum prior to being killed by the pneumococcus, it is often possible to isolate the latter in pure culture from the blood of an animal infected by the intraperitoneal route.

The test is performed in the following fashion. A 1-ml amount of sputum emulsified as described above is injected into the peritoneal cavity of a white mouse through a 21- or 22-gauge needle. When pneumococci are present in the inoculum, the mouse will usually sicken and die within 96 h. About 5% of mice injected with material containing pneumococci will survive for a longer period, however, and it is desirable to sacrifice all survivors at the end of 4 days (12). Longer than average survival may occur after infection with a variety of pneumococcal types. Pneumococcus type 6 is noteworthy in being responsible for about 15% of such protracted infections. Although many texts state that pneumococcus type 14 is unusual by virtue of its limited virulence for mice, it is not unique in this regard, this property being shared by a number of other types (11).

Animals dying of infection or sacrificed should be autopsied with sterile precautions. After washing the animal with 70% ethyl alcohol, the skin of the thorax and abdomen is dissected from the body wall. Next, the thorax is opened, the tip of the heart is cut off with sterile scissors, and the drop of blood obtained is streaked with a loop on a blood-agar plate. A second drop should be inoculated into a tube of blood broth medium.

After the heart blood has been cultured, a small opening is made in the peritoneum, and 1 ml of sterile broth or saline is introduced with a sterile pipette. The fluid is refluxed gently with the pipette, and 0.2 to 0.5 ml is withdrawn and placed in a sterile test tube. The fluid generally has a cloudy or ground-glass appearance. A loopful of the fluid should be streaked on a blood-agar plate. A second loopful should be smeared on a slide which is stained by the Gram technique. If organisms resembling pneumococci are present, the pneumococcus may then be typed directly from smears made with the remainder of the fluid. The fluid should be diluted, if necessary, prior to making preparations for typing, to yield a density of 50 to 100 organisms per oil immersion field.

Mice should be autopsied promptly after death, as postmortem growth of intestinal bacteria will result in contamination of the peritoneal cavity. If autopsy is to be delayed, the animal should be stored at 0 to 4 C.

SEROLOGICAL IDENTIFICATION

The simplest, most rapid, and most accurate way to identify pneumococci present in biological specimens or in cultures is by means of the serological test known as the quellung reaction. Discovered by Neufeld, the optical phenomenon which occurs when pneumococci are brought into contact with homologous anticapsular serum is often referred to as the "capsular swelling" reaction. This descriptive term is probably a misnomer, and the phenomenon might be described more accurately as the capsular precipitin reaction. When the precipitate formed by the union of a capsular polysaccharide with its homologous capsular antibody is viewed microscopically, it has refractile properties which differ from that of the aqueous menstruum in which the reaction has occurred. When the reaction takes place at the surface of a pneumococcus, the organism is seen to be surrounded by a sharply demarcated halo which has the refractile properties sometimes described as resembling ground glass (Fig. 3). To make the bacterial cell more readily visible, it is stained by mixing an equal volume of 1% aqueous methylene blue with the anticapsular serum, both of which are applied to the preparation prior to microscope examination. The test has the added value that it can be used to identify nonviable intact organisms early in the course of antimicrobial therapy.

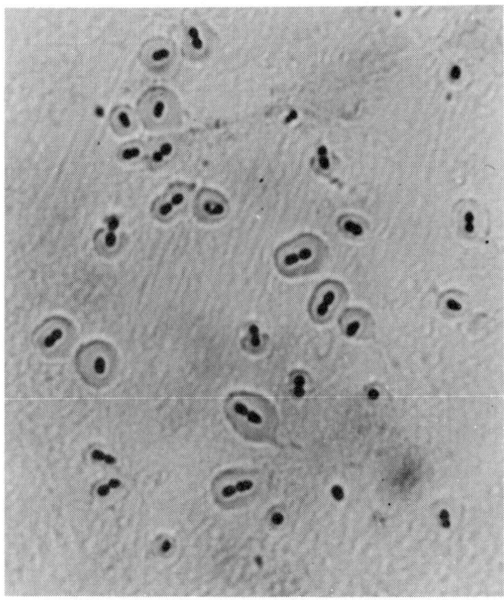

FIG. 3. *Capsular precipitin or Neufeld's quellung reaction of capsulated pneumococci in contact with homologous anticapsular serum. ×1,100. The halo surrounding the organisms is clearly visible. (Reprinted with permission of the Journal of Experimental Medicine.)*

To carry out the quellung or capsular precipitin test, the following details should be followed. A loopful of emulsified sputum, body fluid, mouse peritoneal washings, or liquid culture is spread over an area 0.5 to 1 cm in diameter on a slide and allowed to dry at room temperature. In similar fashion, the cells from a single colony of pneumococcus may be emulsified in a drop of sterile physiological salt solution or of nutrient broth on a slide and allowed to dry. A loopful of 1% aqueous methylene blue is placed on a cover slip, and a loopful of typing serum is then applied to the dried spot on the slide. The residual antiserum on the loop is next mixed with the drop of methylene blue on the cover slip and then applied to the antiserum on the slide which is spread over the area of the dried preparation. The cover slip is inverted over the wet preparation and blotted lightly; a drop of immersion oil is then applied to the cover slip. The preparation is examined under the oil immersion lens of a microscope.

For best results, it is essential to employ

oblique illumination; a microscope with a fixed substage lamp will be unsatisfactory for this purpose. The light source should be reflected by a concave substage mirror through the condenser so that only the lower left third of the microscopic field is brightly illuminated when viewed through a low-power (10 ×) objective. The other factor of importance is the density of pneumococci in the preparation. It should be limited to 50 to 100 bacteria per oil immersion field. A greater number of pneumococci may result in a prozone phenomenon when homologous anticapsular serum is applied, with inhibition of the quellung or capsular precipitin reaction by the excess antigen in the preparation. This phenomenon is most likely to occur with pneumococci of types 3 and 37.

Because of the large number of individual pneumococcal types, typing is expedited by combining antisera of three or more types into pools. The quellung reaction is carried out with successive pools until a positive reaction is encountered. The antisera to the individual types comprising the pool are then tested until a type-specific reaction can be identified. Because more than one type of pneumococcus may be present in sputum, it is important to observe whether or not all organisms morphologically resembling pneumococci react with a given serum. If not, testing with the remaining pools of antiserum should be carried out.

In the United States, pools of antisera reacting with the first 33 capsular types are available commercially, but those for individual types are not. Similar pools and unitypic sera for the first 33 individual capsular types are produced by the laboratories of the Center for Disease Control, Atlanta, Ga., and are available to Public Health Laboratories and to those engaged in government-sponsored research. Antisera reacting with all 84 pneumococcal capsular serotypes may be purchased from the Statens Seruminstitut, Copenhagen, Denmark. Because the nomenclature of pneumococcal types differs somewhat in the American and Danish systems of classification, a suitable reference should be consulted for reconciliation of these differences (8), and reports should indicate which system is employed in designating specific types. The Statens Seruminstitut provides also a highly concentrated polyvalent antiserum, "omniserum" (9), which reacts with all 84 pneumococcal capsular types and which is a most useful reagent for prompt recognition of pneumococci regardless of capsular type. It has especial value in the prompt and accurate identification of pneumococci in body fluids. Although capsulated strains of alpha-hemolytic and nonhemolytic streptococci from the human respiratory tract which cross-react with pneumococci are known, the reactions observed are usually very small and unlikely to cause confusion.

INTERPRETATION AND REPORTING

The clinical significance of pneumococcus varies with the source from which it has been isolated. Because many normal persons carry pneumococci in their upper respiratory tract, the role played by a pneumococcus isolated from this part of the body or from material passing through it, such as sputum, cannot be assessed by the laboratory in many instances in the absence of additional information. On the other hand, the recovery of one of the recognized highly pathogenic types (types 1, 2, 3, 4, 7, 8, 12, and 14) from typical rusty sputum containing large numbers of polymorphonuclear leukocytes is usually indicative of a pneumonic process resulting from pneumococcal infection. Confirmation of the diagnosis of pneumococcal infection can be obtained in some cases as the illness evolves by demonstrating a rise in the titer of antibodies to the capsular type recovered from sputum or the presence of capsular polysaccharide in blood or in urine. Pneumococci isolated from cultures of blood or body fluids or from cultures of the lower respiratory tract obtained by transtracheal or lung puncture are highly significant and indicate the presence of infection caused by this organism.

Antibiotic agents such as penicillin exert a marked and rapid inhibitory effect on the growth of pneumococci, and, if the organism is to be isolated, specimens must be obtained prior to the initiation of antimicrobial therapy. Although most strains of pneumococci isolated from humans are susceptible to 0.02 to 0.05 μg of penicillin/ml, capsulated strains resistant to concentrations as high as 0.5 μg/ml have been recovered infrequently from human respiratory secretions (6), and capsulated mutants resistant to higher concentrations (10 μg/ml) have been selected in the laboratory (5). Strains of pneumococci resistant to tetracyclines, macrolides (erythromycin), lincomycin, sulfonamides, or streptomycin have been recovered from humans and may be cultivated from patients receiving a drug to which the organism is resistant. Pneumococci are not susceptible to gentamicin.

Intact nonviable pneumococci can be identified in sputum and body fluids by the capsular precipitin test, and the quellung reaction should be employed in the study of such specimens from treated patients if organisms resembling pneumococci are demonstrable in Gram-stained preparations. Cultures of blood obtained from treated patients are rarely positive, and the addition of penicillinase when appropriate is of doubtful utility. Staining of blood to demonstrate pneumococci is also of little value, for the organism rarely reaches densities permitting its direct visual recognition except in the occasional untreated terminal patient.

LITERATURE CITED

1. Austrian, R. 1953. Morphologic variation in pneumococcus. I. An analysis of the bases for morphologic variation in pneumococcus and description of a hitherto undefined morphologic variant. J. Exp. Med. **98:**21–34.
2. Austrian, R., and P. Collins. 1966. Importance of carbon dioxide in the isolation of pneumococci. J. Bacteriol. **92:**1281–1284.
3. Austrian, R., and M. S. Colowick. 1953. Modification of the fermentative activities of pneumococcus through transformation reactions. Bull. Johns Hopkins Hosp. **92:**375–384.
4. Bowers, E. F., and L. R. Jeffries. 1955. Optochin in the identification of *Str. pneumoniae*. J. Clin. Pathol. **8:**58–60.
5. Gunnison, J. B., M. A. Fraher, E. A. Pelcher, and E. Jawetz. 1968. Penicillin-resistant variants of pneumococcus. Appl. Mcrobiol. **16:**311–314.
6. Hansman, D., H. Glasgow, J. Sturt, L. Devitt, and R. Douglas. 1971. Increased resistance to penicillin of pneumococci isolated from man. N. Engl. J. Med. **284:**175–177.
7. Hiss, P. H., Jr., J. H. Borden, and C. B. Kropp. 1905. A comparative study of pneumococci and allied organisms. J. Exp. Med. **7:**547–591.
8. Lund, E. 1960. Laboratory diagnosis of *Pneumococcus*. Bull. World Health Organ. **23:**5–13.
9. Lund, E., and P. Rasmussen. 1966. Omni-serum. Acta Pathol. Microbiol. Scand. **68:**458–460.
10. Marmur, J., S. Falkow, and M. Mandel. 1963. New approaches to bacterial taxonomy. Annu. Rev. Microbiol. **17:**329–372.
11. Mørch, E. 1943. Serologic studies on the pneumococci, p. 160–162. Humphrey Milford, Oxford Univ. Press, London.
12. Mørch, E. 1947. Mechanism of pneumococcus infection in mice. Acta Pathol. Microbiol. Scand. **24:**169–180.
13. Ragsdale, A. R., and J. P. Sanford. 1971. Interfering effect of incubation in carbon dioxide on the identification of pneumococci by optochin discs. Appl. Microbiol. **22:**854–855.
14. Sicard, A. M. 1964. A new synthetic medium for Diplococcus pneumoniae and its use for the study of reciprocal transformations of the *amiA* locus. Genetics **50:**31–44.
15. Sternberg, G. M. 1897. The etiology of croupous pneumonia. Nat. Med. Rev. **7:**175–177.
16. White, B. 1938. The biology of pneumococcus, p. 33–35. The Commonwealth Fund, New York.
17. Yurchak, A., and R. Austrian. 1966. Serologic and genetic relationships between pneumococci and other respiratory streptococci. Trans. Ass. Amer. Physicians **79:**368–375.

Chapter 10

Neisseria meningitidis (Meningococcus)

B. WESLEY CATLIN

CHARACTERIZATION

Gram-negative cocci typically arranged in pairs with adjacent sides flattened. Nonmotile, no spores; capsules are not conspicuous.

Growth. Aerobic. Primary cultures may require or benefit by incubation in an atmosphere of air with 2 to 8% carbon dioxide. Preferred medium: blood (or "chocolate")-agar or Mueller-Hinton agar. Colonies on blood-agar incubated at 37 C for 20 h are greater than 1 mm in diameter, and are smooth, nonpigmented, and nonhemolytic. Autolyzes readily. Typical strains do not grow on sodium chloride-free nutrient agar. Narrow temperature range: optimum about 36 to 37 C; no growth at 22 C. Optimal pH 7.2 to 7.4.

Biochemical characteristics. Oxidase-positive. Catalase-positive. Acid, no gas, from glucose and maltose; no acid from sucrose or fructose.

Serological identification. Four accepted serogroups (A, B, C, D) and five provisional groups (X, Y, Z, 29E, 135) are determined by agglutination with group-specific antisera. Most meningococcal disease is produced by groups A, B, C, and Y.

CLINICAL SIGNIFICANCE

Neisseria meningitidis is a primary cause of septicemia and meningitis. It may be isolated from blood and spinal fluid, from the nasopharynx, and less commonly from other sites. It is an obligate parasite which has been recognized only in humans. Although a primary pathogen and one of the commonest causes of meningitis, *N. meningitidis* may be isolated from nasopharyngeal or throat cultures of healthy humans. The incidence of the carrier state varies with the season and the nature of the population being studied, but it is always appreciable (30). The relationship between the carrier state and meningococcal disease remains obscure. However, after a mild rhinopharyngitis, an acute or chronic meningococcemia may develop. Meningitis ensues in some cases, but not in all. A blood-borne infection may lead to the development of a petechial rash, septic arthritis, endocarditis, or other conditions associated with dissemination to different sites.

When a gram-negative diplococcus is isolated, a pure culture must be examined for typical biochemical and serological reactions. Even though a strain is found in specimens of cerebrospinal fluid or blood, it may be a member of a species other than *N. meningitidis*. Meningitis or bacteremia may be caused occasionally by *N. gonorrhoeae* (12), by *N. catarrhalis* (15, 24, 46, 47), or by various chromogenic *Neisseria* species which are usually not pathogenic (8, 40, 46). Furthermore, occasional cases of meningitis are caused by various gram-negative coccobacilli which bear a morphological resemblance to neisseriae and which may be oxidase-positive (e.g., *Moraxella osloensis*; see chapter 24). Another possible source of error is introduced by an exclusive reliance on serological identification procedures. For example, antigenic relationships exist between *Escherichia coli* and *N. meningitidis* group B (29) or group C (45).

The use of antibiotic-containing selective media for nasopharyngeal cultures has simplified the problem of detecting meningococcal carriers (52, 54). Vancomycin and ristocetin, when used at appropriate concentrations, inhibit growth of many gram-positive cocci without suppressing neisseriae. The addition of polymyxin B or colistimethate to a medium which contains either vancomycin or ristocetin (Thayer-Martin selective medium [53]) suppresses most of the normal bacterial flora, including some species of *Neisseria*, without significantly affecting *N. meningitidis*. In addition to meningococci, strains of gonococci and *N. lactamica* may be present in throat cultures and are recovered on Thayer-Martin medium (12, 37).

DIRECT MICROSCOPE EXAMINATION

Specimens of cerebrospinal fluid are prepared for examination as described in chapter 6. A film on a microscope slide is air-dried, fixed in absolute methanol for 10 min to preserve the morphology of the leukocytes, and stained by the Gram method. Although the bacteria may be too few in number to be observed during a 10-min search, they are usually seen. Their location may be extracellular or intracellular, i.e., found within the cytoplasm of polymorphonuclear neutrophiles as a result of phagocytosis.

Meningococci, in common with other strains of *Neisseria*, are gram-negative cocci which are typically arranged in pairs with their abutting sides flattened. Each coccus averages 0.8 by 0.6 μm in diameter; however, considerable variation in size and staining quality is observed with cells that are beginning to undergo autolysis.

Cellular division occurs in two planes, the second plane of division being at a right angle to the first. Thus, there is a transient formation of tetrads by diplococci that are actively multiplying (Fig. 1). Tetrads are best observed in a wet mount or an impression preparation of bacteria from a 3 to 6-h blood-agar culture; they are less evident in older cultures. Knowledge of the mode of division is an aid in differentiating strains of *Neisseria* from very short rod forms which divide in a single plane and, therefore, may form short chains as well as pairs.

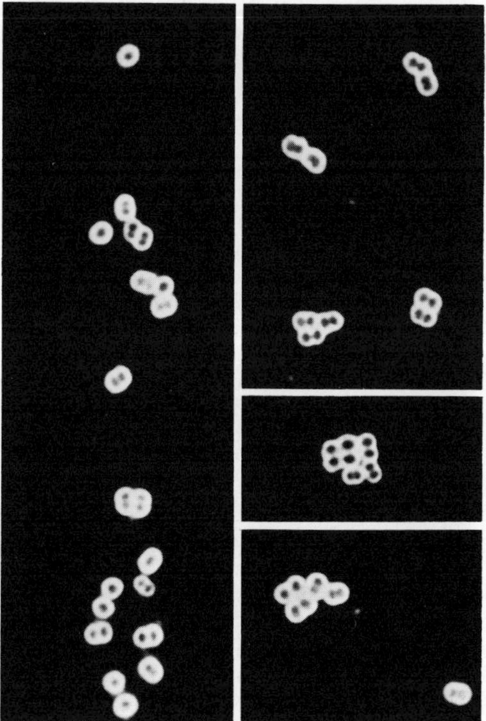

FIG. 1. *Neisseria meningitidis group C. Impression preparation of cocci cultivated on blood-agar for 3 h, stained with group C antibody conjugated to fluorescein isothiocyanate, and photographed with ultraviolet light and dark-field condenser.* ×*2,500.*

The characteristic antigens of meningococci of serogroups A and C, but not B, are organized in the form of capsules (7). The capsular swelling, or quellung, reaction can be observed when the capsulated bacteria are mixed with homologous group-specific antiserum. The meningococci in cerebrospinal fluid or in pure cultures (on blood-agar incubated at 37 C for 4 to 6 h) can be examined by use of the quellung test method described in chapter 9. A sharply delimited, swollen capsule which surrounds and partly obscures a pair of blue-stained bacteria is characteristic of a positive reaction.

PRIMARY ISOLATION AND EXAMINATION OF CULTURES

Specimens from which *N. meningitidis* may be isolated include spinal fluid, blood, material from petechial skin lesions, fluid aspirated from joints, pus, and nasopharyngeal or throat swabs. Rarely, *N. meningitidis* may be cultured from the urogenital tract (12). Thayer-Martin selective medium (53) is used only for culture of material which is expected to contain a mixed flora. The mixture of antibiotics can be obtained from BBL and is added to previously sterilized, melted "chocolate"-agar or, preferably, to a transparent medium, such as Mueller-Hinton agar. The final concentrations of antibiotics are as follows: vancomycin, 3 μg/ml; colistin, 7.5 μg/ml; and nystatin, 12.5 units/ml. This medium is inoculated heavily.

Specimens of patient's blood or spinal fluid, preferably drawn prior to initiation of chemotherapy, are processed as described in chapter 6. A commercially available blood culture bottle containing 100 ml of tryptic soy broth with CO_2 under vacuum is an appropriate medium. Also, several drops of the specimen can be spread over the surface of blood- or "chocolate"-agar media.

An automated method has been developed for detecting the presence of bacteria in broth cultures of specimens of blood or spinal fluid (18, 19). Bacterial growth is measured by the conversion of carbon-14-labeled glucose to $^{14}CO_2$.

Viability of *N. meningitidis* is readily lost as a result of drying, chilling, exposure to unfavorable pH, lysis by tissue enzymes or autolytic meningococcal enzymes, or the antimeningococcal activity of other bacteria. Therefore, cultures should be made with a minimum of delay. If stored in a refrigerator, media should be allowed to warm to 25 C before use. The surface of agar plates should be practically free from moisture, but not wrinkled, a state that indicates a degree of dryness likely to inhibit or delay growth of *N. meningitidis*.

Agar media should be incubated at 36 to 37 C in an atmosphere of air with increased contents of carbon dioxide (2 to 8%) and moisture. It is convenient to place them in a wide-mouth jar containing moistened filter paper and a short length of smokeless candle, which is lighted just before applying an airtight cover; 2 to 3% CO_2 is generated as the flame burns to extinction. A method for generating CO_2 by interaction of $NaHCO_3$ and H_2SO_4 is described by Reyn (48). Commercial CO_2 incubators are satisfactory if the necessary degree of humidity (50 to 70%) is maintained. Many strains of *N. meningitidis* do not require added CO_2; much of the apparent beneficial effect is due to the higher moisture content of the air in a small container compared to that of a large incubator.

Growth of *N. meningitidis* should be evident after incubation of plate cultures for 18 to 20 h. Negative plates are reincubated. Careful examination of primary cultures is of critical importance, as the final bacteriological diagnosis depends on the original judgment regarding selection of colonies to be subcultured. Moreover, the bacteriologist should be alert to the possibility of simultaneous mixed bacterial meningitis involving *N. meningitidis* together with some other organism, such as *Haemophilus influenzae*, *Diplococcus pneumoniae*, or *Escherichia coli* (34).

N. meningitidis colonies are round, smooth, glistening, and practically nonpigmented, although some group B strains become yellowish with age. On a transparent medium, such as Mueller-Hinton agar, young colonies are translucent and often iridescent. Their size depends on the culture medium, the degree of crowding, and age; well-isolated colonies may be 1 mm or more in diameter within 18 h. When touched with a needle, they have a butyrous consistency, and a homogeneous suspension of the bacteria is easily made in saline solution. Upon further incubation, the colonies become viscid or rubbery, as a result of liberation of nucleoprotein from the autolyzing cells. Such older cultures exhibit atypical cellular morphology and reduced viability. Therefore, examination of primary cultures should not be delayed. Several colonies composed of oxidase-positive gram-negative diplococci should be picked and separately subcultured by streaking sections of a blood-agar plate.

The oxidase reaction can best be shown by the method of Kovacs (as elaborated by Steel [51]). A portion of a colony is removed with a sterile platinum loop (iron-containing wire gives a false-positive reaction) and rubbed on filter paper impregnated with a fresh 1% solution of tetramethyl-*p*-phenylenediamine dihydrochloride. The moist paper where the bacteria were deposited turns dark purple within 10 s for a positive reaction. A delayed reaction (color development in 10 to 60 s) is not typical of *Neisseria*, but may be encountered if the bacteria are too old or are taken from an acid environment (medium containing a utilizable carbohydrate); the test should be repeated with an 18-h culture on blood-agar. An alternate oxidase test is described in chapter 95.

DIFFERENTIAL TESTS OF PURE CULTURES

Representatives of the genus *Neisseria* are gram-negative cocci which are oxidase-positive and catalase-positive. *Neisseria* are aerobic; *N. meningitidis* and *N. gonorrhoeae* do not grow on "chocolate"-agar that is incubated in a strictly anaerobic atmosphere at 37 C for 2 days. Growth of *Clostridium tetani* in the same atmosphere provides a positive control for this test. Significant reactions which differentiate *N. meningitidis* from other species encountered in clinical material are given in Table 1. All of these species are parasites of humans; therefore, they are adapted to growth in a nutritionally rich environment at 37 C. *N. meningitidis*, *N. gonorrhoeae*, and most strains of *N. lactamica* do not initiate growth at 22 C, whereas strains of other species commonly (but not invariably) form colonies on a rich medium during incubation at 22 C for 7 days. Likewise, many of these less fastidious bacteria grow on nutrient agar that contains only beef extract, peptone, agar, and distilled water. In contrast, only 11 of 822 nasopharyngeal isolates of *N. meningitidis* were able to grow on salt-free nutrient agar incubated at 37 C in 8% CO_2 for 24 h (43). Addition of 0.8% NaCl to the nutrient agar enabled 74% of the meningococci to grow (43). Diluted inocula should be used for all tests of growth to avoid spurious reactions due to feeding or protection by large numbers of bacteria. For control purposes, corresponding tests should be made of known strains of *N. meningitidis* and *N. subflava*.

Tests of the metabolism of carbohydrates by *Neisseria* are complicated by certain characteristics of these aerobic bacteria. A soft-agar basal medium, such as cystine Trypticase agar, affords better growth than most fluid media. However, some workers prefer to use Mueller-Hinton broth (1). (Sterile solutions of each carbohydrate should be added aseptically to

TABLE 1. *Differentiation of Neisseria species associated with humans*

Species	Capsulation	Colonies: Yellow pigmentation	Colonies: Appearance and consistency	Production of acid from: Glucose	Maltose	Sucrose	Lactose	Fructose	Synthesis of polysaccharide from sucrose	Reduction of: NO_3	NO_2
N. gonorrhoeae	0	0	Smooth, granular or butyrous	+	0	0	0	0	0[a]	0	0
N. meningitidis	D[b]	0	Smooth, transparent, butyrous	+	+	0	0	0	0[a]	0	D
N. lactamica	0	+	Smooth, transparent, butyrous	+	+	0	+	0	0	0	+
N. sicca	D	D	Wrinkled, dry, adherent	+	+	+	0	+	+	0	+
N. subflava	D	+	Smooth, transparent or opaque, often adherent	+	+	D[c]	0	D[c]	D	0	+
N. mucosa	+	D	Mucoid, often adherent	+	+	+	0	+	+	+	+
N. flavescens	0	+	Smooth, opaque	0	0	0	0	0	+	0	+
N. catarrhalis[d]	D	0	Smooth, opaque, often granular	0	0	0	0	0	0	+	+

[a] Often no growth on medium with 5% sucrose; negative with 1 to 2% sucrose.
[b] D, some strains positive, some negative.
[c] Strains formerly designated *N. perflava* are positive.
[d] Reclassified as *Branhamella catarrhalis*.

give a final concentration of 1% in the previously autoclaved basal medium.) Strains which metabolize glucose (dextrose) do so primarily by an oxidative pathway rather than by fermentation (2, 38); consequently, the production of acid may be rather slight. During growth of neisseriae, other enzymes degrade peptone and produce alkaline products which tend to neutralize the acid and may cause reversion to an alkaline pH. Therefore, the reaction should be observed after incubation of the inoculated medium for 16 to 20 h. Tubes which show growth without acid should be reincubated and examined daily for up to 5 days. An uninoculated control tube of medium containing each carbohydrate should be incubated for the same length of time to reveal acid which may possibly develop spontaneously (e.g., in fructose medium).

Occasional strains of *Neisseria* produce atypical reactions in growth medium containing carbohydrate (1, 12, 31). Use of a nongrowth synthetic medium, such as a nitrogen-free solution of salts with 1% carbohydrate (23), may detect instances in which apparent failure to produce acid was actually due to excess production of alkali from a nitrogenous source. (See chapter 95 for composition of Elrod and Braun solution.) Tubes of this solution with each carbohydrate, together with a control tube of the carbohydrate-free basal solution, should be inoculated with about 10^{10} bacteria taken from a 16- to 20-h culture on blood-agar. A large bacteriological loop (4-mm internal diameter) held at an angle and moved slowly through confluent colonial growth will readily pick up a solid ball of bacteria. The cells should be suspended in the fluid to make a final density much greater than that of a broth culture. Tubes are incubated in a water bath at 35 C for up to 24 h; however, the preformed enzymes often produce detectable acid in less than 6 h. Using this same idea, other workers have recently recommended a sustaining fluid which has an increased buffering capacity and an indicator (phenol red) with a higher pH range (39).

Some strains of *N. meningitidis* and *N. gonorrhoeae* which give an equivocal acid reaction in 1% glucose do give clear positive reactions in Elrod and Braun solution that contains 10% glucose (Catlin, unpublished data). All isolates of *Neisseria* examined in my laboratory which are recorded as negative in 1% glucose are retested in 10% glucose.

Another valuable differential test (not yet sufficiently appreciated) is based on detection of an iodine-reacting polysaccharide which is synthesized from sucrose by amylosucrase produced by some *Neisseria* strains (3, 4, 32). A culture streaked on 5% sucrose agar is incubated aerobically at 35 to 37 C for at least 48 h. The growth is then treated with 1 to 2 drops of a solution containing 0.2% iodine and 0.4% potassium iodide (Burke's modification of Gram's iodine solution, freshly diluted 1:5 with water).

A positive test shows a rapid darkening of the colonies (a dark reddish-blue or blue-black color which fades, but which can be restored by reapplication of iodine solution). A corresponding culture on sucrose-free medium, tested with iodine for comparison, will not turn blue (a negative reaction). This test differentiates *N. meningitidis*, *N. gonorrhoeae*, and *N. lactamica*, which do not produce the polysaccharide, from many other neisseriae which do synthesize the polymer. It is of practical importance to recognize that some strains of *Neisseria* polymerize sucrose, although they do not cleave it to acid products. By this means, some nasopharyngeal isolates, which on other grounds might be reported as ungroupable *N. meningitidis*, are identified as members of *N. subflava*.

The enzyme (β-galactosidase) of *N. lactamica* that hydrolyzes lactose also cleaves the chromogenic substrate *o*-nitrophenyl-β-D-galactopyranoside (ONPG; 16, 37). A dense bacterial suspension is made in 0.5 ml of a solution containing 5 mM ONPG (dissolved in phosphate-buffered saline, pH 6.7). Development of a yellow color, often within a few minutes, indicates hydrolysis; a negative test remains colorless after 1 day at 22 to 25 C. *N. meningitidis* and *N. gonorrhoeae* are invariably negative.

Tests of reduction of nitrates or nitrites are an aid in identifying some species (4, 56). The substrate (KNO_3 or KNO_2), at a final concentration of 0.1% (or less if it impairs growth), is added to Mueller-Hinton broth (BBL) or heart infusion broth. Sterile serum may be added to the broths to improve growth of fastidious strains. Nitrate broth is tubed in 10-ml volumes, and nitrite broth in 15-ml volumes, with an inverted Durham tube for collection of nitrogen gas. Inoculated media are incubated at 37 C for up to 5 days and are tested periodically by use of sulfanilic acid and α-naphthylamine (chapter 96). Verify an apparently negative nitrate reduction reaction by adding powdered zinc to confirm the presence of NO_3.

The ability of meningococci to form colonies on Dubos oleic acid agar medium has been used to differentiate them from gonococci, which do not grow (21).

Chemically defined agar media have been developed which support normal growth of recent isolates of *N. meningitidis*, *N. gonorrhoeae*, and *N. lactamica*. Each species has a distinctive nutritional profile which serves to differentiate and identify it (12). On a series of defined media lacking different groups of compounds, the meningococci are relatively homogeneous in their growth responses and are more competent biosynthetically than strains of the other species. Gonococci exhibit a diversity of nutritional requirements, but all strains examined (more than 400 clinical isolates) require cystine (or cysteine) to form colonies on the defined medium (12; unpublished data).

The technique of gas-liquid chromatography provides a rapid and accurate means of determining the composition of bacteria and identifying metabolic products. Analyses of the fatty acid composition of extracts of whole cultures of *Neisseria* (9, 41, 44), and also of the hydroxy acids present in spent culture media (10), have been reported.

ANTIGENIC GROUPS

Differences in the composition of surface antigens of *N. meningitidis* cells are detected by serological tests. The currently accepted classification subdivides the species into four groups, which are usually determined by agglutination tests (7). Groups A, B, and C account for most cases of meningitis. Group D strains are now isolated only very rarely (7, 55). Many of the isolates from meningococcal carriers fall within groups A, B, and C, but a fraction of the strains fail to agglutinate in antisera prepared separately against antigens of the four groups (20, 25, 35, 49, 50, 55). Collections of such ungroupable meningococci have been examined recently by a number of investigators using newer methods. Additional serogroups have been identified (Table 2), which in time must be consolidated into a new, internationally acceptable, serological classification.

Underlying the various superficial group-specific antigens are somatic antigens common to bacteria of the various groups, which may account for some cross-reactions (i.e., agglutination in antiserum of more than one group or species). RAS-10 is a designation for some meningococci which agglutinate in a number of grouping sera (20). Cross-reactions create practical problems for laboratory diagnosis. Some strains of other *Neisseria* species, such as *N. gonorrhoeae* and *N.* (*Branhamella*) *catarrhalis*, may agglutinate in meningococcal grouping sera (12, 48). Furthermore, antigenic similarities have been found in unrelated bacteria (45). Thus, a strain of *E. coli* isolated from the spinal fluid of an infant was agglutinated by group B antiserum and therefore was identified initially as *N. meningitidis* group B (29).

The suspension of cells which serves as the

TABLE 2. *Serological groups of meningococci: occurrence and relations between various designations*

Common usage 1940–1950 (7)	International Committee, 1950 (7)	Slaterus (49, 50)	Evans et al. (25)	Other studies (20, 35, 55)	Frequency of disease production[a]
I	A	A	A	A	Varies[b]
II	B	B	B	B	Common
II alpha	C	C	C	C	Common
IV	D	D	D	D	Very rare
		X		E (35)	Rare
		Y	Bo	F (35), E (55)	Occasional
		Z		G (35)	Rare
		Z′	29E		Rare
			135		Rare

[a] The nasopharynx of carriers harbors strains of all groups, except D which is currently very rarely identified.
[b] Common during classic epidemics, infrequent during interepidemic periods.

antigen for agglutination tests must be prepared from cultures of actively growing bacteria, as the surface structures of older cultures tend to deteriorate (7). Blood-agar cultures incubated at 36 C in CO_2 for 5 to 6 h are preferred. A smooth suspension of bacteria is made in a saline solution (0.85% [wt/vol] NaCl) containing Formalin (0.5% [vol/vol]). The antigen for the slide test must be of sufficient density to permit the antigen-antibody reaction to proceed to completion within 1 min. In a strong positive reaction, all bacteria are agglutinated, and the fluid between the clusters is clear. A weaker reaction shows incomplete clearing of the fluid because only a fraction of the cells are aggregated. As some strains are autoagglutinable in normal serum plus saline, a serum control must be run with each antigen.

High-titer meningococcal antiserum is difficult to prepare and is not readily available (54). Different lots of antiserum are not equally satisfactory. Some instances of cross-reactions apparently are due to the presence of antibody to RAS-10 meningococci in sera (20). Antisera for some meningococcal groups are available from Burroughs-Wellcome Co. (Research Triangle Park, N.C.) and from Difco. Antiserum is often obtained as a lyophilized preparation. For agglutination tests, this should be reconstituted with the appropriate volume of a sterile solution of 50% glycerol in distilled water. Fewer instances of cross-agglutinations are obtained with antisera reconstituted with 50% glycerol than with distilled water alone (35).

Group B and group C meningococcal isolates can be further subdivided into types for epidemiological investigations (27, 28). This is done by a bactericidal assay in which a known low number of bacteria are incubated for 30 min in the presence of antibody and complement, and then the number of viable colony-forming units is determined by plating on agar. A different system of typing also has been developed based on the sensitivity of meningococci to bacteriocins that are produced by some strains of meningococci (17).

IMMUNOSEROLOGICAL DIAGNOSIS

Immunofluorescence microscopy provides a rapid and relatively sensitive method for detecting *N. meningitidis* in smears of cerebrospinal fluid sediments (5). Figure 1 shows the appearance of a pure culture of group C meningococci which have undergone a reaction with fluorescein-tagged group C antibody. The capsules are swollen and fluoresce brightly in the ultraviolet light. In the hands of trained personnel, the method may be particularly valuable for detecting bacteria which have been rendered nonviable as a result of prior chemotherapy. However, cross-reactions are encountered with immunofluorescence, as well as with other serological procedures (29, 35, 42). A polyvalent meningococcal antiserum conjugated to fluorescein isothiocyanate is available from Sylvana Co. (Millburn, N.J.) and from Difco.

Countercurrent immunoelectrophoresis is another rapid diagnostic method for the identification of meningococcal infection in blood, spinal fluid, and synovial fluid (22, 26). The presence of soluble meningococcal antigen in the specimen is detected by its precipitation reaction with group-specific *N. meningitidis* antiserum.

NEISSERIA SPECIES

Table 1 includes most of the *Neisseria* species that are likely to be isolated from human clinical material. However, it does not include a rod-shaped organism named *Neisseria elongata* (6) whose status as a member of the genus has not yet been adequately evaluated. Also, a number of *Neisseria* species that have been isolated thus far only from domestic or laboratory animals are omitted (4).

Current applications of sophisticated biochemical methods and new genetic approaches are providing fresh insights into the relationships among various neisseriae. This inevitably affects their classification. The forthcoming edition (8th) of *Bergey's Manual of Determinative Bacteriology* combines the former species *N. subflava*, *N. flava*, and *N. perflava* into one species, *N. subflava*. In practice, these species have been difficult to differentiate on the basis of pigmentation and production of acid from fructose and sucrose. Thus, an organism isolated from a fatal case of meningitis was identified as *N. flava* by three laboratories and as *N. perflava* by a fourth (46). Furthermore, *N. subflava* and the two former species are all part of the normal pharyngeal flora, all have been recorded as rare causes of meningitis, and all are closely related as determined by genetic transformation and by nucleic acid homologies (13, 33).

An oxidase-negative species has been transferred to a new genus, *Gemella haemolysans* (2). The former *N. catarrhalis* also has been transferred to a new genus, *Branhamella* (11), as recommended by others (33) because it differs substantially from *Neisseria* species (13, 14, 41). These changes are reflected in Table 1, and two new species are added which have been described since the 7th edition of *Bergey's Manual* (1957). *N. lactamicus* (36), more correctly named *N. lactamica*, is encountered frequently in throat or nasopharyngeal cultures (36, 37) and rarely in specimens of spinal fluid or secretions from the urogenital tract (12, 36, 37). *N. mucosa* is found occasionally in the nasopharynx and (rarely) in spinal fluid. Although it has a number of similarities to *N. sicca* and *N. subflava*, *N. mucosa* differs from them antigenically (57).

REFERENCE STRAINS

Standard strains are needed as controls to accompany serological and biochemical tests. Cultures may retain their viability for a few days at 36 C (if drying is prevented), but they tend to undergo genetic variation and become atypical. Storage of *Neisseria* cultures in a refrigerator is unsatisfactory, but the bacteria may be preserved in a low-temperature (below −40 C) freezer or dry ice chest (48). A large mass of bacteria is removed from an 18-h culture on blood-agar and placed in a 1-ml volume of broth containing 10% glycerol or 10% serum, and is immediately fast-frozen. The freezing and subsequent thawing may destroy large numbers of neisseriae, but the strain can usually be recovered if promptly streaked on blood-agar and incubated. Strains also may be preserved by freeze-drying.

LITERATURE CITED

1. Beno, D. W., L. F. Devine, and G. L. Larson. 1968. Identification of *Neisseria meningitidis* carbohydrate fermentation patterns in Mueller-Hinton broth. J. Bacteriol. **96**:563.
2. Berger, U. 1960. Über den Kohlenhydrat-stoffwechsel von *Neisseria* und *Gemella*. Zentralbl. Bakteriol. Parasitenk. Infektionskr. Hyg. Abt. I Orig. **180**:147–149.
3. Berger, U. 1961. Polysaccharidbildung durch saprophytische Neisserien. Zentralbl. Bakteriol. Parasitenk. Infektionskr. Hyg. Abt. I Orig. **181**:345–349.
4. Berger, U. 1963. Die anspruchslosen Neisserien. Ergeb. Mikrobiol. Immunitaetsforsch. Exp. Ther. **36**:97–167.
5. Biegeleisen, J. Z. Jr., M. S. Mitchell, B. B. Marcus, D. L. Rhoden, and R. W. Blumberg. 1965. Immunofluorescence techniques for demonstrating bacterial pathogens associated with cerebrospinal meningitis. I. Clinical evaluation of conjugates on smears prepared directly from cerebrospinal fluid sediment. J. Lab. Clin. Med. **65**:976–989.
6. Bøvre, K., and E. Holten. 1970. *Neisseria elongata* sp. nov., a rod-shaped member of the genus *Neisseria*. Re-evaluation of cell shape as a criterion in classification. J. Gen. Microbiol. **60**:67–75.
7. Branham, S. E. 1953. Serological relationships among meningococci. Bacteriol. Rev. **17**:175–188.
8. Breslin, A. B. X., J. C. Biggs, and G. V. Hall. 1967. Bacterial endocarditis due to *Neisseria perflava* in a patient hypersensitive to penicillin. Australas. Ann. Med. **16**:245–249.
9. Brooks, J. B., D. S. Kellogg, L. Thacker, and E. M. Turner. 1971. Analysis by gas chromatography of fatty acids found in whole cultural extracts of *Neisseria* species. Can. J. Microbiol. **17**:531–543.
10. Brooks, J. B., D. S. Kellogg, L. Thacker, and E. M. Turner. 1972. Analysis by gas chromatography of hydroxy acids produced by several species of *Neisseria*. Can. J. Microbiol. **18**:157–168.
11. Catlin, B. W. 1970. Transfer of the organism named *Neisseria catarrhalis* to *Branhamella* gen. nov. Int. J. Syst. Bacteriol. **20**:155–159.
12. Catlin, B. W. 1973. Nutritional profiles of *Neisseria gonorrhoeae*, *Neisseria meningitidis*, and *Neisseria lactamica* in chemically defined media and the use of growth requirements for gonococcal typing. J. Infect. Dis. **128**:300–320.
13. Catlin, B. W., and L. S. Cunningham. 1961. Transforming activities and base contents of deoxyribonucleate preparations from various neisseriae. J. Gen. Microbiol. **26**:303–312.
14. Catlin, B. W., and L. S. Cunningham. 1964. Genetic transformation of *Neisseria catarrhalis* by deoxyribonucleate preparations having different average base compositions. J. Gen. Microbiol. **37**:341–352.
15. Cocchi, P., and A. Ulivelli. 1968. Meningitis caused by *Neisseria catarrhalis*. Acta Paediat. Scand. **57**:451–453.
16. Corbett, W. P., and B. W. Catlin. 1968. Galactosidase activity of lactose-positive *Neisseria*. J. Bacteriol. **95**:52–57.
17. Counts, G. W., L. Seeley, and H. N. Beaty. 1971. Identification of an epidemic strain of *Neisseria*

meningitidis by bacteriocin typing. J. Infect. Dis. **124:**26-32.
18. DeBlanc, H. J. Jr., F. DeLand, and H. N. Wagner, Jr. 1971. Automated radiometric detection of bacteria in 2,967 blood cultures. Appl. Microbiol. **22:**846-849.
19. DeLand, F., and H. N. Wagner, Jr. 1970. Automated radiometric detection of bacterial growth in blood cultures. J. Lab. Clin. Med. **75:**529-534.
20. Devine, L. F., and C. R. Hagerman. 1970. Relationship of serogroups of *Neisseria meningitidis*. I. Microagglutination, gel diffusion, and slide agglutination studies of meningococcal antisera before and after absorption with RAS-10 strain of meningococci. Infect. Immunity **1:**226-231.
21. Diena, B. B., R. Wallace, C. P. Kenny, and L. Greenberg. 1970. Dubos oleic acid agar medium in the differentiation of meningococci and gonococci. Appl. Microbiol. **19:**1025.
22. Edwards, E. A. 1971. Immunologic investigations of meningococcal disease. I. Group-specific *Neisseria meningitidis* antigens present in the serum of patients with fulminant meningococcemia. J. Immunol. **106:**314-317.
23. Elrod, R. P., and A. C. Braun. 1942. Pseudomonas aeruginosa; its role as a plant pathogen. J. Bacteriol. **44:**633-644.
24. Elston, H. R., H. J. Quigley, Jr., and D. M. Fitch. 1970. Meningitis due to *Neisseria catarrhalis*. Nebr. State Med. J. **55:**369-371.
25. Evans, J. R., M. S. Artenstein, and D. H. Hunter. 1968. Prevalence of meningococcal serogroups and description of three new groups. Amer. J. Epidemiol. **87:**643-646.
26. Feldman, S. A., and T. DuClos. 1973. Diagnosis of meningococcal arthritis by immunoelectrophoresis of synovial fluid. Appl. Microbiol. **25:**1006-1007.
27. Frasch, C. E., and S. S. Chapman. 1972. Classification of *Neisseria meningitidis* group B into distinct serotypes. I. Serological typing by a microbactericidal method. Infect. Immunity **5:**98-102.
28. Gold, R., J. L. Winklehake, R. S. Mars, and M. S. Artenstein. 1971. Identification of an epidemic strain of group C *Neisseria meningitidis* by bactericidal serotyping. J. Infect. Dis. **124:**593-597.
29. Grados, O., and W. H. Ewing. 1970. Antigenic relationship between *Escherichia coli* and *Neisseria meningitidis*. J. Infect. Dis. **122:**100-103.
30. Greenfield, S., P. R. Sheehe, and H. A. Feldman. 1971. Meningococcal carriage in a population of "normal" families. J. Infect. Dis. **123:**67-73.
31. Hajek, J. P., M. J. Pelczar Jr., and J. E. Faber, Jr. 1950. Variations in the fermentative capacity of neisseriae. Amer. J. Clin. Pathol. **20:**630-636.
32. Hehre, E. J., and D. M. Hamilton. 1948. The conversion of sucrose to a polysaccharide of the starch-glycogen class by Neisseria from the pharynx. J. Bacteriol. **55:**197-208.
33. Henriksen, S. D., and K. Bøvre. 1968. The taxonomy of the genera *Moraxella* and *Neisseria*. J. Gen. Microbiol. **51:**387-392.
34. Herweg, J. C., J. N. Middelkamp, and A. F. Hartmann, Sr. 1963. Simultaneous mixed bacterial meningitis in children. J. Pediat. **63:**76-83.
35. Hollis, D. G., G. L. Wiggins, and J. H. Schubert. 1968. Serological studies of ungroupable *Neisseria meningitidis*. J. Bacteriol. **95:**1-4.
36. Hollis, D. G., G. L. Wiggins, and R. E. Weaver. 1969. *Neisseria lactamicus* sp. n., a lactose-fermenting species resembling *Neisseria meningitidis*. Appl. Microbiol. **17:**71-77.
37. Hollis, D. G., G. L. Wiggins, R. E. Weaver, and J. H. Schubert. 1970. Current status of lactose-fermenting *Neisseria*. Ann. N.Y. Acad. Sci. **174:**444-449.
38. Hugh, R., and E. Leifson. 1953. The taxonomic significance of fermentative versus oxidative metabolism of carbohydrates by various Gram negative bacteria. J. Bacteriol. **66:**24-26.
39. Kellogg, D. S., Jr., and E. M. Turner. 1973. Rapid fermentation confirmation of *Neisseria gonorrhoeae*. Appl. Microbiol. **25:**550-552.
40. Lewin, R. A., and W. T. Hughes. 1966. *Neisseria subflava* as a cause of meningitis and septicemia in children. J. Amer. Med. Ass. **195:**821-823.
41. Lewis, V. J., R. E. Weaver, and D. G. Hollis. 1968. Fatty acid composition of *Neisseria* species as determined by gas chromatography. J. Bacteriol. **96:**1-5.
42. Mitchell, M. S., D. L. Rhoden, and B. B. Marcus. 1966. Immunofluorescence techniques for demonstrating bacterial pathogens associated with cerebrospinal meningitis. III. Identification of meningococci from the nasopharynx of asymptomatic carriers. Amer. J. Epidemiol. **83:**74-85.
43. Mitzel, J. R., J. A. Hunter, and W. E. Beam, Jr. 1972. Influence of sodium chloride on growth of *Neisseria meningitidis*. Appl. Microbiol. **24:**155-156.
44. Moss, C. W., D. S. Kellogg, Jr., D. C. Farshy, M. A. Lambert, and J. D. Thayer. 1970. Cellular fatty acids of pathogenic *Neisseria*. J. Bacteriol. **104:**63-68.
45. Myerowitz, R. L., R. Schneerson, J. B. Robbins, and M. Turck. 1972. Urinary-tract *Escherichia coli* with cross-reactive antigens to encapsulated pyogenic bacteria. Lancet **2:**250-253.
46. Noguchi, T. T., R. Nachum, and C. A. Lawrence. 1963. Acute purulent meningitis caused by chromogenic Neisseria. Med. Arts Sci. **17:**11-18.
47. Pfister, L. E., M. V. Gallagher, T. G. Potterfield, and D. W. Brown. 1965. *Neisseria catarrhalis* bacteremia with meningitis. J. Amer. Med. Ass. **193:**399-401.
48. Reyn, A. 1965. Laboratory diagnosis of gonococcal infections. Bull. World Health Organ. **32:**449-469.
49. Slaterus, K. W. 1961. Serological typing of meningococci by means of micro-precipitation. Antonie Van Leeuwenhoek J. Microbiol. Serol. **27:**305-315.
50. Slaterus, K. W., A. C. Ruys, and I. G. Sieberg. 1963. Types of meningococci isolated from carriers and patients in a non-epidemic period in the Netherlands. Antonie van Leeuwenhoek J. Microbiol. Serol. **29:**265-271.
51. Steel, K. J. 1961. The oxidase reaction as a taxonomic tool. J. Gen. Microbiol. **25:**297-306.
52. Thayer, J. D., P. F. Frank, and J. E. Martin, Jr. 1965. Thayer-Martin selective medium for the cultivation of *Neisseria meningitidis* from the nasopharynx. Amer. J. Pub. Health **55:**923-927.
53. Thayer, J. D., and J. E. Martin, Jr. 1966. Improved medium selective for cultivation of *N. gonorrhoeae* and *N. meningitidis*. Pub. Health Rep. **81:**559-562.
54. Van Peenen, P. F. D., L. E. Suiter, A. D. Mandel, and M. S. Mitchell. 1965. Field evaluation of Thayer-Martin medium for identification of meningococcus carriers. Amer. J. Epidemiol. **82:**329-333.
55. Vedros, N. A., J. Ng, and G. Culver. 1968. A new serological group (E) of *Neisseria meningitidis*. J. Bacteriol. **95:**1300-1304.
56. Véron, M., P. Thibault, and L. Second. 1959. *Neisseria mucosa* (*Diplococcus mucosus* Lingelsheim). I. Description bactériologique et étude du pouvoir pathogène. Ann. Inst. Pasteur (Paris) **97:**497-510.
57. Véron, M., P. Thibault, and L. Second. 1961. *Neisseria mucosa* (*Diplococcus mucosus* Lingelsheim). II. Etude antigènique et classification. Ann. Inst. Pasteur (Paris) **100:**166-179.

Chapter 11

Neisseria gonorrhoeae (Gonococcus)

DOUGLAS S. KELLOGG, JR.

CHARACTERIZATION

Neisseria gonorrhoeae, the gonococcus, is the cause of gonorrhea, a venereally transmitted disease whose only natural host is the human.

Occur in pairs of diplococci that have flattened or curved adjacent sides ("coffee beans"); no detectable capsules in vitro; nonmotile, gram-negative, and nonsporulating. In exudates, size varies from 0.6 to 1.0 μm; large cells 1.2 to 1.5 μm are found from in vitro growth. Four colony types: T_1 and T_2, virulent types from exudates; T_3 and T_4, avirulent (6, 8).

Growth optimal aerobically under increased CO_2 tension on protein hydrolysate media enriched with bovine red cells and growth supplements such as Thayer-Martin (TM) selective medium (20) or Transgrow (12). Growth favored by moist medium surfaces; colonies are nonpigmented; does not grow on nutrient agar, eosin-methylene blue agar, or MacConkey medium.

Biochemical characterization. Catalase, oxidase, and deoxyribonuclease positive; glucose only fermented with acid (no gas). Some strains require accessory factors for proper fermentation (22). Rapid confirmation of presumptive positive growth can be accomplished by using a specific fluorescent-antibody (FA) reagent which has been sorbed with *N. meningitidis* serogroup B cells (15).

CLINICAL SIGNIFICANCE

N. gonorrhoeae, the gonococcus, one of the two pathogenic species of the genus *Neisseria*, is the cause of gonorrhea, a venereally transmitted disease whose only natural host is the human. Infection in the male usually causes an anterior urethritis accompanied by a purulent discharge; however, asymptomatic gonorrhea may exceed a 10% incidence in males who are contacts of known infected females. In the female, who is usually asymptomatic and presents few signs of the disease, the cervix is the most frequently infected site. In both males and females, other sites that may become infected primarily or secondarily are the conjunctiva, rectum, and nasopharynx. The infection may spread to other sites of the genitourinary system in both sexes and in certain cases may also involve the joints, blood, or skin. The disease is transmitted by sexual intercourse, except for gonorrheal ophthalmia of the newborn and vulvovaginitis in children, and is rarely if ever transmitted by intermediary objects. Humans are the only natural host of the gonococcus, although the disease can be reproduced in chimpanzees and is venereally transmissible from male to female (4). Smaller laboratory animals such as rabbits, guinea pigs, hamsters, rats, and mice can be experimentally infected through the inoculation of subcutaneous chambers (2, 3).

COLLECTION OF SPECIMENS

Females

Diagnosis of infection in females is made by obtaining a specimen principally from the cervix and secondarily from the rectum, urethra, or nasopharynx with a sterile cotton-tipped applicator. Careful specimen acquisition is necessary to ensure the maximal sensitivity of the culture procedure, since there may be a very small number of gonococci at the site sampled (18).

Urethritis. Digitally strip a small amount of exudate from the urethra and Skenes ducts; inoculate the exudate onto selective medium, and prepare a smear for Gram staining.

Bartholonitis. Use a platinum loop or swab to collect exudate from a palpable gland, and inoculate onto selective medium.

Cervicitis. Using a bivalve vaginal speculum to expose the cervix, take a specimen on a swab and inoculate selective media. The speculum may be moistened with warm water, but do not use any other lubricant.

Vaginitis. Obtain specimen from the posterior fornix, and streak selective media.

Vulvovaginitis. Care should be taken to obtain the specimen from well within the vagina; an ear-type speculum may be necessary to obtain a satisfactory specimen.

Males

In males a diagnosis of gonorrhea is usually based on history, characteristic clinical signs, and symptoms. The diagnosis is usually confirmed by the finding of gram-negative "coffee bean" shaped diplococci within the pus cells of the urethral discharge.

Urethritis. Collect a small amount of urethral pus on a swab. When there is no discharge at the time of examination or the male is asymptomatic, it will be necessary to obtain a specimen from within the urethral canal for culture. Urethral canal specimens are acquired by inserting into the canal, approximately 2.5 cm, either a 2-mm platinum-iridium loop, commercially produced without spurs, or a sterile small-head cotton-tipped applicator moistened with either saline or water. Avoid contact with the exterior aspect of the urethral meatus.

Nongonococcal urethritis. A clinical picture and exudate characterized as nongonococcal urethritis is encountered with increasing frequency. Differential diagnosis for this condition requires a negative finding for gonococcal cultures on selective media. Since the etiological agent or agents for this condition have not been established, place specimens upon blood and chocolatized (heated) blood-agars to determine the presence of streptococci, staphylococci, candida, chlamydia, mycoplasma, and other agents. In addition, examine a wet preparation microscopically for *Trichomonas vaginalis*.

Prostatitis. Prostatic fluid may be inoculated directly onto TM medium; if a sufficiently large specimen is obtained, centrifuge the specimen and culture the sediment.

Males or females

Presumed positive findings from the following sites must be confirmed by sugar fermentations or FA staining since meningococci and other potentially confusing microorganisms may be isolated from these sites.

Proctitis. The rectum is frequently infected in females, and in 5 to 10% of the cases it is the only site infected (18). In males rectal infections are found in homosexuals almost exclusively. A sterile swab is used to obtain a specimen from the crypts just inside the rectal ring; care should be taken not to contact feces in the rectum itself. Inoculate the specimen upon TM medium which has trimethoprim added to it to suppress the spreading growth characteristic of *Pseudomonas* and *Proteus* species (12).

Arthritis. Obtain synovial fluid by aspiration, and dilute with sterile Trypticase soy broth; mix well, and centrifuge at high speed. Inoculate selective medium and prepare smears for Gram and FA staining (23). Antibiotic therapy or certain characteristics of the patient's condition may reduce the effectiveness of culture; however, FA staining will specifically detect either living or dead gonococci.

Ophthalmia. Collect pus from the conjunctiva with a sterile swab and inoculate selective media. Also prepare slides for both Gram and FA staining.

Gonococcemia. Obtain blood by the usual method, and inoculate 5 ml into a biphasic medium of 20 ml of Trypticase soy broth with added glucose (0.5%) over an agar base (GC Medium Base). Incubate the specimen in such a manner that the blood and broth are in a shallow layer to allow for maximal aeration. Place loosely capped bottles in a candle jar or other CO_2-generating system at 35 to 36 C for a period of at least 10 days. (Examine bottles daily for turbidity, and subculture to chocolate agar with supplement at 2, 7, and 10 days.)

Pharyngitis. Swab areas of inflammation in the tonsils and posterior pharynx, and inoculate selective media.

Cutaneous lesions. These are the various erythematous, papular, urticarial, and hemorrhagic lesions that occur with arthritis and/or fever with a certain predominance on the extremities and periarticular regions. Although these lesions can be cultured, positive cultures are rarely obtained and the aspirated material is most profitably examined by FA staining of smears (5, 23).

Transport

Ideally, specimens from suspected gonococcal lesions or infection sites should be inoculated upon selective media when collected and placed under increased CO_2 at 35 to 37 C. However, many clinics and physicians' offices do not have local laboratory support, and the specimens must be transported under adverse circumstances or over considerable distances which may require as long as 4 days.

An approach to the ideal was set forth by Stuart, Toshach, and Patsula (19) and Amies and Douglas (1). Their methods called for placing the specimen swab in a favorably buffered and reduced nonnutrient semisolid agar gel for transport. When planting of the specimen was delayed no longer than 12 h, 95% of the positive cultures were recovered. When planting was delayed for periods greater than 12 h, the efficiency of the method decreased rapidly.

Recently a transport-growth system (Transgrow) has been developed for the transport of gonococcal specimens to a processing laboratory (12). The bottle medium is inoculated with the specimen swab, the cap is firmly tightened, and the bottle is incubated overnight. After specimens treated in this manner had been in the mail 48 to 96 h, the recovery was 99%. The commercially produced Transgrow system has a storage life of 3 months and is quite reliable since the early problems with reproducibility have been solved. Although typical colonial morphology is not useful for making a presumptive diagnosis because the optical character of the bottle distorts the image, there does not seem to be an appreciable loss of sensitivity or specificity for the system. Coloration or other obvious nongonococcal characteristics are still useful in eliminating other bacteria which are able to grow on this medium.

Stock

Gonococcal strains that are to be used later for checking the quality of media and the efficacy of staining reagents, and for further examinations, can best be stored by lyophilization or freezing. Although lyophilization results in specimens that can be readily stored, the equipment is expensive and not widely available. The freezing procedure is simple and available to any laboratory with freezer facilities. Supplement Trypticase soy or a similar protein hydrolysate broth with 20% glycerol and sterilize. Use a plate of 20- to 24-h gonococcal growth to make a turbid suspension in 2 ml of glycerol broth which can be stored as a unit or split into 0.1-ml quantities for freezing at either −20 or −40 C. Survival is longest at −40 C but is satisfactory for at least 2 weeks at −20 C.

DIRECT EXAMINATION

Except in the diagnosis of male urethritis, Gram-stained smear preparations for microscope examination are highly unproductive. For specimens from cervical, vaginal, and rectal sites, better results are obtained by culturing on selective media. A smear preparation can be valuable as an index of suspicion when many gram-negative diplococci are seen. An occasional gram-negative diplococcus in specimens from such sites would probably be a false-positive observation since saprophytic *Neisseria* species and other morphologically confusing organisms do occur at these sites.

A negative finding should not be given since the sensitivity of the smears is very low because of the small amount of sample examined and the nonspecific character of the stain. It is well to remember that overly decolorized staphylococci, streptococci, and diphtheroids, or old cells that have lost their ability to stain gram-positive, occur in the normal flora of the urogenital tract and on other mucous membranes and may lead to an incorrect microscopic diagnosis of gonorrhea. Certain coliform bacteria and gram-negative diplobacilli also may closely resemble gonococci. The morphology of *Mima polymorpha* var. *suboxydans* (presently designated as *Moraxella*-like) is also quite similar to that of gonococci, especially in exudates and when cultured on enriched media. These microscopically confusing bacteria are of little importance when specimens are cultured on TM selective medium since their growth is not subcultured on this medium. The practice of some clinics of staining smears with methylene blue or Seller's stains multiplies the difficulties of microscopic identification and is not recommended as a diagnostic laboratory procedure.

Synovial fluid and smears from conjunctival pus may be examined by either Gram or FA staining, and smears from cutaneous lesions may be profitably examined by FA staining.

CULTURE AND ISOLATION

Inoculation of media

Figure 1 depicts the method of inoculating the TM medium by rolling the swab over the medium surface and streak diluting with a bacteriological loop. Care should be taken to ensure that all of the swab tip encounters the medium during the roll inoculation. Streak dilution is usually performed in the laboratory although it may be done by the clinic nurse or assistant. If the streak diluting is to be done several hours after swab inoculation, it may be desirable to roll inoculate the entire surface of the medium. In either event, the plate should be immediately placed in an elevated CO_2 atmos-

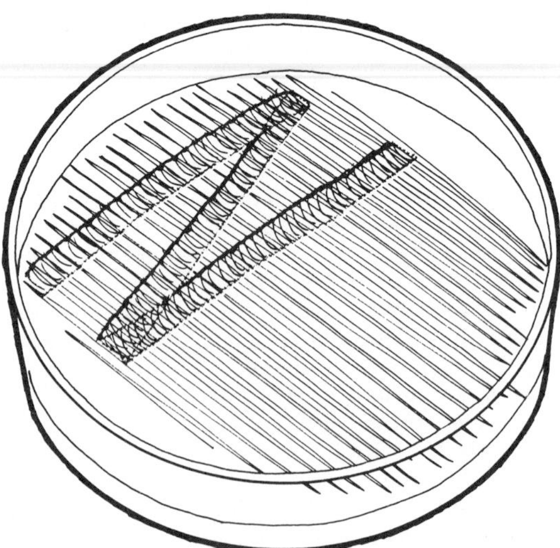

FIG. 1. *Method for inoculating plate medium with specimens from patients. (Note the close streaking across the swabbed area.)*

phere (such as a candle extinction jar) and within 4 to 8 h incubated at 35 to 37 C.

Inoculation of Transgrow (Fig. 2) is accomplished by rolling the swab back and forth over the medium surface, starting at the base of the bottle and withdrawing the swab across the medium toward the bottle opening. It will facilitate inoculation of the medium if the swab is used to soak up any free moisture at the bottom of the bottle before roll inoculating. The cap should be replaced and tightened. The Transgrow system was designed for use when there is no local laboratory support and when the specimen must be transported for 1 to 4 days through the mails or by courier service to a laboratory. Optimal recovery of *N. gonorrhoeae* from the Transgrow specimens requires overnight incubation at 35 to 36 C before shipment. Under circumstances where neither TM nor Transgrow is available, the swab should be placed in 0.5 ml of Trypticase soy or other protein hydrolysate broth and kept at 4 C until appropriate media can be inoculated.

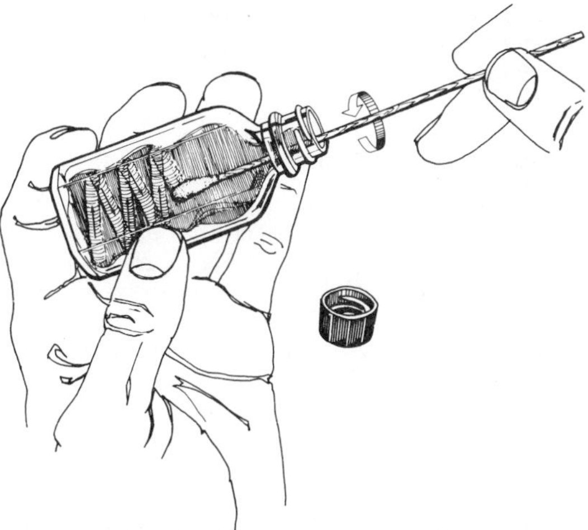

FIG. 2. *Method for inoculating Transgrow bottles with specimens from patients.*

Incubation of media

Invert and place inoculated plates in an air-tight container such as a large pickle jar or suitable tin canister as soon as possible after inoculation. Light a smokeless candle fixed to a glass microscope slide and place it in the jar with the plates. Effervescent tablets which release CO_2 when exposed to moisture can also be used as a CO_2 source. The 3% CO_2 developed by the candle method is adequate to stimulate growth; CO_2 levels up to 20% do not inhibit growth. Incubator temperatures should be 35 to 36 C. When available and when the volume of specimens warrants, a CO_2 incubator, with control of CO_2, humidity, and temperature, will provide adequate conditions.

Examination of cultures

Inspect the cultures for "typical" colonies of gonococci after 20 to 24 h. Return negative plates to the incubator for further incubation. When VCN (vancomycin-colistimethate-nystatin) antibiotic supplement is used, growth may be apparent after 20 h of incubation; on approximately 40% of those plates that ultimately become positive, growth may not be apparent until after 40 to 48 h. Cultures have been described that required 3 days for expression of colonial growth. Before discarding negative plates, flood them with oxidase reagent to detect microcolonies.

On chocolate agar or TM media, colonies of gonococci are usually opaque, grayish-white, raised, finely granular, glistening, and convex. Almost all strains will be mucoid after 48 h of incubation. The colony size may vary from 1 to 4 mm in diameter. Only first-hand experience in observing colonies of gonococci will make the meaning of "typical colonies" apparent to the worker.

Neisseria species and certain other bacteria and yeasts possess an oxidizing enzyme which, in the presence of air, acts on certain aromatic amines to produce colored compounds. The color changes produced by the indicator in contact with the colony are readily observed. The oxidase reagent is a 1.0% solution of dimethyl-*p*-phenylenediamine hydrochloride in distilled water and is prepared fresh each day. The solution cay be kept for 1 week stored at 4 C in a glass-stoppered bottle and protected from light. The tetramethyl form is preferred by some workers. Since the oxidase reagent is toxic and allergenic for some individuals, care should be exercised to protect the skin from direct contact. The dimethyl compound is oxidized slowly by the gonococcal colony; it is pink at first, but within 60 s changes to a bright red and finally to a purplish-black. The oxidase test may be performed also by picking colonial growth onto filter paper impregnated with the oxidase reagent. Contact with the reagent for 5 to 10 s is lethal for gonococci. However, gonococci killed by the reagent may still be specifically identified as *N. gonorrhoeae* by FA staining. The oxidase test is *not* confirmatory for gonococci. However, a positive oxidase reaction by colonies of gram-negative diplococci cultured on TM medium constitutes a *presumptively positive* test for *N. gonorrhoeae*. More than 95% of the *presumptively positive* cultures from urogenital specimens are confirmed as *N. gonorrhoeae* by either sugar fermentations or FA staining with a specific reagent (15).

Purification and confirmation

Difficult, time-consuming procedures formerly used to purify the culture and establish identification as *N. gonorrhoeae* are no longer necessary when the selective medium is used. Confirmation of a culture as *N. gonorrhoeae* is accomplished by either fermentation patterns or FA staining. (It would be more accurate to use the term carbohydrate degradation since the gonococcus is principally aerobic in its growth character, even though *Bergey's Manual* lists it as a facultative anaerobe.)

Inoculation of growth fermentation media should not be done by picking a colony from selective media, since the antibiotics in the media are bacteriostatic. It is necessary first to transfer a typical gonococcal colony to a chocolate agar plate and use the resulting growth for a carbohydrate utilization pattern. This is done by picking two or three typical colonies with a bacteriological loop and emulsifying them in a tube containing 0.2 ml of Trypticase soy broth. As a precautionary measure, apply a loop of oxidase reagent to the site from which the colonies were removed to check the oxidase reactivity. Inoculate a drop of the emulsified growth onto a TM plate and streak over the entire medium surface. Incubate the purification plate in the usual manner for 24 h. Select typical gonococcal colonies for oxidase testing and Gram staining. If the reactions are proper, a very turbid suspension is made in 0.5 ml of physiological saline. Use a 1.0-ml plastic pipette to inoculate 0.05 ml of cell suspension onto the surface of the fermentation tube media. Push the suspension to one-third of the depth of the medium. An effective fermentation medium is cystine-tryptophan-peptone agar (BBL CTA medium; Difco Cystine tryptic agar) to which appropriate filter-sterilized carbohydrates are added. Tighten tube caps, and incubate the tubes at 36 C in an environment without CO_2. Check all tubes showing fermentative activities (phenol red changes from red to yellow) for growth and for purity of the growth by Gram stain.

An alternate fermentation procedure is available in which growth from either the primary isolation plate or a purification plate is used to inoculate a lightly buffered salts-indicator system with a heavy inoculum of cells (9). Growth does not take place, but carbohydrate fermentation occurs in 1 to 4 h at 36 C. Obvious contaminants on plate media should be avoided, but otherwise inhibited organisms do not interfere with the fermentation patterns. The procedure was designed to confirm the identity of *presumptively positive* growth.

With either of these fermentation procedures, the quality of the carbohydrates is very important because, if the maltose contains fermentable materials, false-positive fermentation patterns will result.

Unsatisfactory primary cultures may be encountered when plates are overgrown by *Proteus* "spreaders." In this event, report the culture as "unsatisfactory" and request another specimen. The addition of trimethoprim lactate (5 μg/ml) to either the TM or Transgrow media will inhibit the spreading growth of both *Proteus* and *Pseudomonas*.

Rapid confirmation may also be obtained by using FA procedures (7, 15). High-titer antigonococcal conjugates are sorbed twice with group B meningococci (1.0 ml of packed cells to 10.0 ml of conjugate incubated at 60 C for 2 h) to eliminate cross-reactions with meningococci and stain only the gonococci. Such conjugates are also sorbed with staphylococci or blocked with staphylococcal antiserum. Presently, only one commercial conjugate has demonstrated requisite specificity for confirmation. Every lot of conjugate should be tested for reactivity with known gonococcal cells and for specificity with meningococcal and staphylococcal cells before and during use.

Serology

At present, there are no serological tests which are diagnostically useful for gonorrhea. In recent years, several tests have been developed or revised which may offer limited diagnostic assistance for this disease. They are the precipitin (17), microflocculation (16), microhemagglutination (11), flocculation (10), indirect fluorescent-antibody (13, 21), and complement fixation (14) procedures. There are several other tests under development but, even though preliminary results are encouraging, they have not been published as of this date. Current information on the published procedures indicates that with each of them there are problems in distinguishing between infected and uninfected persons. In gonorrhea, detectable antibody appears approximately 7 to 10 days after initiation of infection and may be detectable for weeks to months after adequate treatment. In a patient from a low gonorrhea incidence group, a reaction may be indicative of an infection. However, in a population having a high incidence of gonorrhea, the false-positive reactor rate varies between 5 and 15% because of repeated episodes of gonorrhea. Generally speaking, currently available serological tests detect antibodies in 80 to 85% of the sera from culturally positive patients.

LITERATURE CITED

1. Amies, C. R., and J. I. Douglas. 1965. Some defects in bacteriological transport media. Can. J. Pub. Health **56:**27.
2. Arko, R. J. 1972. *Neisseria gonorrhoeae:* experimental infection of laboratory animals. Science **177:**1200–1201.
3. Arko, R. J. 1973. Implantation and use of a subcutaneous chamber in laboratory animals. Lab. Animal Sci. **23:**105–106.
4. Brown, W. J., C. T. Lucas, and U/S. G. Kuhn. 1972. Gonorrhea in the chimpanzee. Brit. J. Vener. Dis. **48**(3)**:**177–178.
5. Danielsson, D., and G. Michaelsson. 1966. The gonococcal dermititis syndrome. Acta Dermato-Venereol. **46:**257–261.
6. Kellogg, D. S., Jr., I. R. Cohen, L. C. Norins, A. L. Schroeter, and G. Reising. 1968. *Neisseria gonorrhoeae.* II. Colonial variation and pathogenicity during 35 months in vitro. J. Bacteriol. **96:**596–605.
7. Kellogg, D. S., Jr., and W. E. Deacon. 1964. A new rapid immunofluorescent staining technique for identification of *Treponema pallidum* and *Neisseria gonorrhoeae.* Proc. Soc. Exp. Biol. Med. **115:**963–965.
8. Kellogg, D. S., Jr., W. L. Peacock, Jr., W. E. Deacon, L. Brown, and C. I. Pirkle. 1963. *Neisseria gonorrhoeae.* I. Virulence genetically linked to clonal variation. J. Bacteriol. **85:**1274–1279.
9. Kellogg, D. S., Jr., and E. M. Turner. 1973. Rapid fermentation confirmation of *Neisseria gonorrhoeae.* Appl. Microbiol. **25:**550–552.
10. Lee, L., and J. D. Schmale. 1970. Identification of a gonococcal antigen important in the human immune response. Infect. Immunity **1:**207–208.
11. Logan, L. C., P. M. Cox, and L. C. Norins. 1970. Reactivity of two gonococcal antigens in an automated microhemagglutination procedure. Appl. Microbiol. **20:**907–909.
12. Martin, J. E., Jr., and A. Lester. 1971. Transgrow, a medium for transport and growth of *Neisseria gonorrhoeae* and *Neisseria meningitidis.*
13. O'Reilly, R. J., B. G. Welch, and D. S. Kellogg, Jr. 1973. An indirect fluorescent-antibody technique for study of uncomplicated gonorrhea. II. Selection and characterization of the stain of *Neisseria gonorrhoeae* used as antigen. J. Infect. Dis. **127:**77–83.
14. Peacock, W. L., Jr. An automated complement fixation procedure for detecting antibody to *N. gonorrhoeae.* HSMHA Health Rep. **86:**706–710.
15. Peacock, W. L., Jr., B. G. Welch, J. E. Martin, Jr., and J. D. Thayer. 1968. Fluorescent antibody technique for identification of presumptively positive gonococcal cultures. Pub. Health Rep. **83:**337–339.
16. Reising, G. 1971. Microflocculation assay for gonococcal antibody. Appl. Microbiol. **21:**852–853.
17. Reising, G., and D. S. Kellogg, Jr. 1965. Detection of gonococcal antibody. Proc. Soc. Exp. Biol. Med. **120:**660–663.
18. Schmale, J. D., J. E. Martin, Jr., and G. Domescik. 1969. Observation on the culture diagnosis of gonorrhea in women. J. Amer. Med. Ass. **210:**312–314.
19. Stuart, R. D., S. R. Toshach, and T. M. Patsula. 1954. The problem of transport specimens for culture of gonococci. Can. J. Pub. Health **45:**73–83.
20. Thayer, J. D., and J. E. Martin. 1966. Improved medium selective for cultivation of *N. gonorrhoeae* and *N. meningitidis.* Pub. Health Rep. **81:**559–562.
21. Welch, B. G., and R. J. O'Reilly. 1973. An indirect fluorescent-antibody technique for study of uncomplicated gonorrhea. I. Methodology. J. Infect. Dis. **127:**69–76.
22. White, L. A., and D. S. Kellogg, Jr. 1965. An improved fermentation medium for *Neisseria gonorrhoeae* and other neisseria. Health Lab. Sci. **2:**238–241.
23. White, L. A., and D. S. Kellogg, Jr. 1965. *Neisseria gonorrhoeae* identification in direct smears by a fluorescent antibody-counter stain method. Appl. Microbiol. **13:**171–174.

Chapter 12

Corynebacterium

GEORGE J. HERMANN AND S. T. BICKHAM

CHARACTERIZATION

Corynebacterium diphtheriae

Member of the *Corynebacteriaceae*.

Morphology. Pleomorphic, gram-positive bacilli. Cells vary considerably in size and shape; some curved, may stain unevenly; frequently contain metachromatic granules that appear as polar bodies; cells arrange themselves in pairs and angles producing L, V, and "Chinese character" formations. No capsules; no spores and not acid-fast.

Growth. Aerobic. Grows well on ordinary media. Human isolates grow best at 35 to 37 C. Potassium tellurite medium used for isolation. Loeffler (coagulated serum) or Pai (coagulated egg) media used for microscopic morphology. Colonies on cystine-tellurite media are grayish black or gunmetal gray; brownish zone or halo on Tinsdale medium. Three colony types.

Biochemical characterization. Nonmotile. Acid (no gas) from glucose and maltose; starch and glycogen fermented only by gravis strain. Trehalose not fermented. Nitrate usually reduced to nitrite; gelatin, urea, and indole negative.

Toxigenicity tests. In vivo (rabbit or guinea pig) or in vitro.

Clinical significance. Toxigenic strains cause diphtheria in humans. Isolated from throat (tonsils, posterior pharynx), nasopharynx, and nose. Rarely causes primary cutaneous diphtheria in North America. Secondary infections by *C. diphtheriae* may occur in wounds or other skin lesions such as abrasions, burns, insect bites, and rashes.

Corynebacterium haemolyticum

Morphology. Similar to *C. diphtheriae*.

Growth. Grows poorly on tellurite medium. Resembles hemolytic streptococci on blood-agar plate; hemolysis better on plates containing rabbit or human blood than on those containing sheep blood. Growth in broth is poor without added serum enrichment.

Biochemical characterization. Glucose, lactose, and maltose fermented; sucrose usually fermented. Mannitol and xylose not fermented. Catalase, indole, and urease negative; gelatin not liquefied.

Clinical significance. Have been reported from cases of acute pharyngitis and cutaneous infections. Organism may morphologically resemble *C. diphtheriae* but can be readily differentiated by cultural and biochemical characterization. It does not produce diphtheria toxin.

Corynebacterium ulcerans

Morphology. Pleomorphism more marked than described for *C. diphtheriae* above. Coccal forms with diphtheria-like rods and short rods may all be found in same field; fewer metachromatic granules than *C. diphteriae*.

Growth. Similar to *C. diphtheriae* described above on tellurite medium; growth more luxuriant on Loeffler or Pai medium.

Biochemical characterization. Nitrate not reduced to nitrite; urea hydrolyzed; gelatin slowly liquefied. Trehalose fermented in 1 week.

Toxigenicity tests. Some strains produce diphtheria toxin in addition to a toxic factor that is not an exotoxin. Use same tests as with *C. diphtheriae* to demonstrate the diphtheria exotoxin.

CORYNEBACTERIUM DIPHTHERIAE

Collection of specimens

The clinical laboratory usually receives the specimen on a swab or on a medium, such as Loeffler medium, upon which a swab of the patient's throat has been inoculated. *C. diphtheriae* commonly spreads into the nasal passages, and a nasopharyngeal specimen should be requested for culture in addition to the throat swab. In the case of the convalescent patient and the asymptomatic carrier, the latter specimen may be positive when the former is negative, as pointed out by Russell (14) and by Lyman and Youngstrom (10). The throat swab should be rubbed vigorously over any membrane, white spots, or inflamed areas in the throat. The nasal swab should be inserted into the nasopharynx and not confined to the anterior nares.

Primary cutaneous diphtheria occurs rarely in North America. Secondary infection by *C. diphtheriae* may occur in wounds or other skin lesions, such as abrasions, burns, insect bites, and rashes. Cultures from cutaneous lesions may be obtained directly by using a dry cotton swab which is inoculated onto Loeffler or Pai medium. There is an apparent association between respiratory tract infection and skin infection, although skin infection may occur in the absence of respiratory tract infection (1).

Laboratories that must refer the specimen for bacteriological examination may ship the swabs in tubes or packets containing silica gel, as recommended by Sinclair et al. (15).

Microscope examination

In frank cases of diphtheria, the organism is present in large numbers in the lesion and membrane. The swab should be cultured onto a slant of Loeffler or Pai medium, and the growth is used to prepare smears for staining with Loeffler alkaline methylene blue. After overnight incubation, the cells vary considerably in size and shape, and some of the rods are distinctly curved. They stain unevenly and frequently contain granules that appear as polar bodies. The cells arrange themselves in pairs and at angles, producing L- and V-shaped formations that produce the "Chinese character" effect when groups of these formations lie adjacent to each other.

The results of microscope examination of the stained smear can only constitute a presumptive identification. Other *Corynebacterium* species, certain actinomycetes, and pleomorphic streptococci, which may be present, can morphologically resemble *C. diphtheriae* in stained smears made from Loeffler or Pai medium. Confirmation requires that *C. diphtheriae* be isolated in pure culture and identified by means of cultural, biochemical, and toxigenicity tests.

Culture and isolation

A procedure for processing the specimen received from a suspect case of diphtheria is outlined in Fig. 1. As shown, a swab of the throat membrane should be used to make a smear to be stained for the fusospirochetal symbionts of Vincent's angina. When extended to the tonsils, this ulceromembranous stomatitis can simulate the clinical appearance of diphtheria.

To obtain a pure culture, the swab from the overnight Loeffler or Pai medium slant should be inoculated to a plate of blood-agar and a plating medium containing potassium tellurite. Although the swab may be used to inoculate the plating media directly, growth may not result if only small numbers of bacteria are present on the swab because of the inhibitory effect of tellurite on the organism.

The colonies of *C. diphtheriae* are not readily distinguished from those of certain other bacterial flora on blood-agar. However, the blood plate is recommended because occasional strains of *C. diphtheriae* are very sensitive to potassium tellurite and may not grow on tellurite media. In addition, the blood plate will

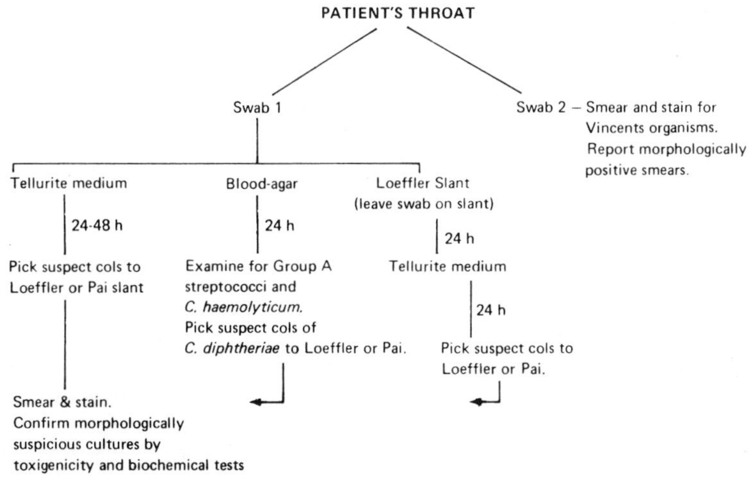

FIG. 1. *Processing specimens for laboratory confirmation of diphtheria.*

reveal the presence of group A beta-hemolytic streptococci that may be responsible for the throat lesions. The group A streptococcus infection may occur simultaneously with diphtheria, and its presence would not be detected on a medium containing potassium tellurite in the concentration used for the isolation of *C. diphtheriae*.

Many media incorporating the salts of tellurite have been formulated for the isolation of *C. diphtheriae*. At the Center for Disease Control (CDC), cystine-tellurite (CT) medium described by Frobisher (5) and a modification of Tinsdale's medium (12) have been used extensively for isolating *C. diphtheriae* from mixed cultures. The CT medium is less difficult to prepare and can be stored for a longer period than the latter medium. Furthermore, in our experience the CT plate has yielded positive cultures when a commercial preparation of Tinsdale's medium failed to support growth of *C. diphtheriae*. For these reasons, CT medium is preferred if only one tellurite medium can be used for isolation.

The colony of *C. diphtheriae* on CT medium is grayish black, sometimes described as gunmetal gray. One of the cultural biotypes of *C. diphtheriae* called *intermedius* produces a small flat colony, whereas the cultural biotypes called *gravis* and *mitis* are larger (2 to 3 mm), with a raised or convex surface. On modified Tinsdale's medium, the black colonies of *C. diphtheriae* are surrounded by a brownish zone or halo, which is an aid to their recognition when growing on this medium. Unfortunately, on both of the above media colonies are not well developed after overnight incubation, and colony characteristics are more clearly defined after a second night of incubation. However, if stabs are made in the Tinsdale's medium during the streaking process, the brownish zone often appears in the stab area after overnight incubation when *C. diphtheriae* is present.

Suspicious colonies should be picked carefully with a straight wire and inoculated to a Loeffler or Pai medium slant. After overnight incubation, a smear can be made from the slant growth and stained with methylene blue. The morphological characteristics described previously should be evident if the colony selected was that of *C. diphtheriae*. Pure culture growth from a slant showing morphological evidence of *C. diphtheriae* may be used for subsequent biochemical and toxigenicity tests.

Toxigenicity tests

Detection of diphtheria toxin, sometimes called the diphtheria virulence test, may be accomplished by an in vivo or in vitro method. The in vivo method, with the guinea pig, is recommended for laboratories that seldom isolate *C. diphtheriae*. The in vitro test is less laborious and the results are obtained faster. However, the method must be carefully controlled because of variability in the animal serum, in the peptone constituent in the base medium, and in the purity of the antitoxin (3). Recently, a commercial medium (Difco) for the in vitro test, in which a serum substitute (8) is used, has been found to be satisfactory in our laboratory.

In vivo test. Inoculate, from the pure culture on Loeffler or Pai medium, a tube of infusion broth without dextrose (for example, heart infusion broth) which has been adjusted to pH 7.8 to 8.0. Allow this to incubate at 37 C for about 48 h. The tube should contain at least 10 ml of broth because the test requires 8 ml of the broth culture. Fill a syringe fitted with a 22-gauge needle with 8 ml of the 48-h broth culture. This is the inoculum for the test.

Use two guinea pigs weighing about 300 to 400 g each. Shave or clip an area about 3 cm in diameter on the abdomen of each animal. Clean the shaven area with a pledget soaked in alcohol. Inject one animal intraperitoneally with 250 units of diphtheria antitoxin. This is the protected or control animal. Wait 2 h, and then inject each animal subcutaneously with 4 ml from the syringe containing the broth culture. The second unprotected guinea pig is the test animal. If the culture is that of a toxigenic strain of *C. diphtheriae*, the unprotected guinea pig will die within 24 to 96 h. The animal protected by antitoxin will exhibit no ill effects from the injection. If both animals show no ill effects, the organism under test may be a nontoxigenic strain of *C. diphtheriae*. If both animals show ill effects, the organism is not *C. diphtheriae*.

In vitro test. A modification of the Elek method (3) is used at the CDC and in many state health laboratories in this country. For this method, a tube of melted basal medium is cooled to about 48 C and poured into a plate that contains 2 ml of sterile rabbit serum and 1 ml of 0.3% potassium tellurite. The medium is thoroughly mixed and allowed to almost harden. Then, to the serum-medium mixture is added a strip of sterile filter paper (1.5 by 7 cm) that has been immersed in a tube containing diphtheria antitoxin which has been diluted to contain 100 units of antitoxin per ml. The strip is allowed to drain against the side of the tube before it is placed, with sterile forceps, on the serum medium surface, where it is gently pressed into place in the center portion of the plate. After the strip has been placed, the plate is put in an incubator to dry. If the top is slightly tilted, this usually requires about 1 h. The plate should be inoculated within 2 h after drying.

The culture being tested may be inoculated from the growth on a slant of Loeffler or Pai medium or from suspicious colonies growing on the tellurite isolation plate. Each culture to be tested is streaked with a loop in a single line on each side perpendicular to the strip. Each culture should be spaced about 1 cm from the preceding culture. Four test cultures and a known positive and negative control can be tested on a single plate without crowding. The positive control culture is usually a stock strain of *C. diphtheriae* intermedius biotype.

Toxigenic strains will show a positive reaction within 24 to 48 h after incubation. A positive reaction is evidenced by white lines of precipitated toxin-antitoxin mixture that appear about 2 to 5 mm from the impregnated filter-paper strip. The white lines begin at and extend out from the line of bacterial growth at an angle of approximately 45°. The lines are usually quite visible to the naked eye and can easily be read by transmitted light against a dark background. A negative test should not be reported if there is no positive reaction with the known toxigenic control culture. *C. diphtheriae* strains that are negative in vitro should be tested by an animal method.

Biochemical tests

A positive toxigenicity test constitutes proof of the identity of the organism as *C. diphtheriae* in virtually all cases, since the only other organism that produces a toxin specifically neutralized and precipitated by diphtheria antitoxin is C. ulcerans. This organism is quite rare, as evidenced by the relatively few cultures received at the CDC or reported in the literature. It will be described later.

Biochemical tests are helpful in differentiating *C. diphtheriae* from other corynebacteria which are often present in nose and throat cultures. The biochemical tests also support other criteria, such as morphology and colony characteristics, in identifying nontoxigenic strains of *C. diphtheriae*. The role of nontoxigenic strains in the epidemiology of diphtheria is not known. However, these strains are capable of converting to the toxigenic state, as Freeman (4), Parsons (13), and Groman (6) have shown.

C. diphtheriae ferments glucose and maltose, producing acid only. Lactose, mannitol, trehalose, and xylose are not fermented. Sucrose is rarely fermented by strains found in the United States or Europe. Only the *gravis* biotype ferments starch or glycogen. Nitrate is usually reduced to nitrite; however, some *mitis* strains of the "belfanti variety" uniformly fail to reduce nitrate (2). Indole is not formed, urea is not hydrolyzed, and gelatin is not liquefied. Table 1 lists some of the biochemical reactions of *C. diphtheriae* and a few other corynebacteria.

In addition to the morphological and cultural characteristics, one can often utilize the biochemical results to support a decision as to whether or not an isolate is *C. diphtheriae*. For example, the ability to hydrolyze urea of an isolate that morphologically somewhat resembles *C. diphtheriae* should rule it out from further consideration. On the other hand, a strain that has the morphological, cultural, and biochemical characteristics of *C. diphtheriae* should be reported as a nontoxigenic strain if the toxigenicity test is negative. When there is doubt, the culture should be sent to a reference laboratory for identification.

CORYNEBACTERIUM HAEMOLYTICUM

C. haemolyticum is occasionally mistaken for *C. diphtheriae* because it is isolated from patients with acute pharyngitis and from cutaneous lesions (11). When a smear made from Loeffler medium is stained, the morphology of the organism is suggestive of *C. diphtheriae*. However, this organism grows poorly on isolation media containing tellurite and is likely to be isolated only from a blood-agar plate upon which the colonies resemble those of hemolytic streptococci. Unlike the hemolysis of most streptococci, that of *C. haemolyticum* is poorer on agar media containing sheep blood than on media containing human or rabbit blood (7).

TABLE 1. *Biochemical differentiation of some Corynebacterium species*

Test	*C. diphtheriae*	*C. ulcerans*	*C. haemolyticum*	*C. hoffmanii*	*C. xerosis*
Glucose	+	+	+[a]	−	+
Maltose	+	+	+	−	+
Sucrose	−	−	+ or −	−	+
Starch	− or +[b]	+	−	−	−
Trehalose	−	+	−	−	−
Nitrate	+ or −[c]	−	−	+ or −	+
Urease	−	+	−	+	−
Catalase	+	+	−	+	+

[a] Fermentation of carbohydrates is slow and irregular unless sterile serum is added to the base medium.

[b] Only the *gravis* biotype of *C. diphtheriae* produces acid from starch.

[c] Some strains of the *mitis* biotype fail to reduce nitrate.

C. haemolyticum grows poorly in most broth media unless a small amount of sterile serum is added to the broth. At the CDC, fermentation tests are done in infusion broth (3 ml) to which a drop of sterile rabbit serum is added. Under these conditions, the organism ferments glucose, lactose, and maltose within 24 to 48 h. Sucrose is fermented by most but not all strains. Mannitol and xylose are not fermented. The tests for catalase, indole, and urease are negative. This organism fails to liquefy gelatin or digest the casein of milk; these characteristics differentiate it from *C. pyogenes*, which it closely resembles.

The poor growth on tellurite media, failure to produce catalase, and fermentation of lactose readily differentiate *C. haemolyticum* from *C. diphtheriae*. If a diagnosis of diphtheria is considered on morphological grounds, the bacteriologist should have no trouble in dismissing this organism from further consideration, once cultural and biochemical results are examined.

CORYNEBACTERIUM ULCERANS

C. ulcerans would be found in the same type of specimen that yields *C. diphtheriae*. It grows well on tellurite isolation media and its colonies resemble those of *C. diphtheriae*. However, it grows much more luxuriantly on Loeffler or Pai medium than does *C. diphtheriae* (9). Morphologically, it does not resemble *C. diphtheriae* in that the pleomorphism exhibited is more pronounced. A stained smear from Loeffler medium will often reveal an almost coccal form with diphtheria-like rods, short rods, and cocoid elements all being found in the same field. Metachromatic granules may be present, but they are few in comparison with those found in a smear made from a culture of *C. diphtheriae*.

The biochemical reactions of *C. ulcerans* differ from those produced by *C. diphtheriae*, notably in that this organism does not reduce nitrate to nitrite, hydrolyzes urea, and slowly liquefies gelatin. It also is capable of fermenting trehalose within 1 week, whereas *C. diphtheriae* does not ferment this carbohydrate.

Some strains of *C. ulcerans* produce diphtheria toxin in addition to a toxic factor that is not an exotoxin. The latter toxic factor is not present in sterile filtrates of a broth culture as is the diphtheria toxin. This nonfilterable toxic factor is not neutralized by diphtheria antitoxin and is present in broth cultures of strains that fail to produce diphtheria antitoxin.

LITERATURE CITED

1. Belsey, M. A., M. Sinclair, M. R. Roder, and D. R. LeBlanc. 1969. *Corynebacterium diphtheriae* skin infections in Alabama and Louisiana. A factor in the epidemiology of diphtheria. N. Engl. J. Med. **280:**135–141.
2. Bezjak, V. 1954. Differentiation of *Corynebacterium diphtheriae* of the mitis type found in diphtheria and ozaena. Antonie van Leeuwenhoek J. Microbiol. Serol. **20:**269–271.
3. Bickham, S. T., and W. L. Jones. 1972. Problems in the use of the *in vitro* toxigenicity test for *Corynebacterium diphtheriae*. Amer. J. Clin. Pathol. **57:**244–246.
4. Freeman, V. J. 1951. Studies on the virulence of bacteriophage-infected strains of Corynebacterium diphtheriae. J. Bacteriol. **61:**675–688.
5. Frobisher, M. 1937. Cystine-tellurite agar for *C. diphtheriae*. J. Infect. Dis. **60:**99–105.
6. Groman, N. B. 1956. Conversion in *Corynebacterium diphtheriae* with phages originating from nontoxigenic strains. Virology **2:**843–844.
7. Hermann, G. J. 1961. The laboratory recognition of *Corynebacterium haemolyticum*. Amer. J. Med. Technol. **27:**61–66.
8. Hermann, G. J., M. S. Moore, and E. I. Parsons. 1958. A substitute for serum in the diphtheria *in vitro* toxigenicity test. Amer. J. Clin. Pathol. **29:**181–183.
9. Hermann, G. J., and E. I. Parsons. 1957. Recognition of *C. diphtheriae*-like corynebacteria (*Corynebacterium ulcerans*) in the laboratory. Pub. Health Lab. **15:**34–37.
10. Lyman, E., and J. Youngstrom. 1956. Diphtheria cases and contacts: is it necessary to take cultures from both nose and throat? Nebr. State Med. J. **41:**361–362.
11. McLean, P. D., A. A. Liebow, and A. A. Rosenburg. 1946. A haemolytic corynebacterium resembling *Corynebacterium ovis* and *Corynebacterium pyogenes* in man. J. Infect. Dis. **79:**69–90.
12. Moore, M., and E. I. Parsons. 1958. A study of a modified Tinsdale's medium for the primary isolation of *Corynebacterium diphtheriae*. J. Infect. Dis. **102:**88–93.
13. Parsons, E. I. 1955. Induction of toxigenicity in nontoxigenic strains of *C. diphtheriae* with bacteriophages derived from nontoxigenic strains. Proc. Soc. Exp. Biol. Med. **90:**91–93.
14. Russell, W. T. 1943. The epidemiology of diphtheria during the last forty years. Med. Res. Counc. (Gt. Brit.) Rep. No. 247.
15. Sinclair, M. C., S. Bickham, and J. H. Schubert. 1972. Silica gel as a transport medium for *Corynebacterium diphtheriae*. S. Med. J. **65:**1383–1384.

Chapter 13

Listeria monocytogenes

ARDEN H. KILLINGER

CHARACTERIZATION

Member of the *Corynebacteriaceae*.

Diphtheroid-like bacilli; usually occur in pairs and may resemble diplococci; 1.0 to 2.0 by 0.5 μm. Gram-positive. Motile (tumbling motility in cultures grown at 18 to 20 C). Nonencapsulated. No spores.

Growth. Aerobic; facultatively anaerobic. Grows on ordinary media; most, but not all, strains produce a narrow zone of hemolysis on blood-agar; may require refrigeration at 4 C of tissue suspensions, fluids, swabs, etc., for periods of a few days to 3 months before initial culture is successful. Optimal temperature, 30 to 37 C; temperature range, 3 to 45 C. Umbrella-type growth 3 to 5 mm below surface after stab of motility medium incubated at 20 to 25 C. Characteristic blue-green colony on clear solid media when viewed by oblique light.

Biochemical characteristics. Catalase positive. Voges-Proskauer positive. Methyl red usually positive; may depend on peptone used. Litmus milk acidified slowly, eventually decolorized but not coagulated. Arginine hydrolyzed to ammonia. Nitrate not reduced. Indole not produced. Gelatin and coagulated serum not liquefied. Starch and urea not hydrolyzed. Esculin hydrolyzed. H_2S production irregular.

Carbohydrate fermentation. Acid but no gas in 24 h at 37 C from glucose, levulose, trehalose, and salicin. Acid but no gas in 3 to 10 days sometimes produced in arabinose, galactose, lactose, maltose, rhamnose, sucrose, dextrin, sorbitol, glycerol, and melezitose. No fermentation in adonitol, dulcitol, inositol, inulin, and mannitol.

Serological identification. Serological confirmation possible for most cultures with slide or tube agglutination tests with type 1 or type 4 antisera. Serotypes determined on basis of somatic (O) and flagellar (H) antigens (3).

Animal pathogenicity. Purulent conjunctivitis 24 to 36 h after instilling culture into conjunctival sac of rabbits or guinea pigs (Anton reaction). Monocytosis (up to 40%) develops in rabbits 3 to 5 days after intravenous injection of culture. Lethal for mice after intraperitoneal injection; enhanced by gastric mucin (10).

CLINICAL SIGNIFICANCE

Listeriosis is a disease of humans, domesticated animals, and wildlife species. Purulent meningitis, meningoencephalitis, and septicemia are the clinical conditions from which *Listeria monocytogenes* is most frequently isolated in humans. About half of the cases are perinatal infections, illustrated by the mother who develops mild "flu-like" symptoms, possibly with low grade fever and diarrhea, during the last trimester of pregnancy. She may abort subsequently or have a stillborn child, or the child may develop meningitis soon after birth. Listeric meningitis or septicemia sometimes is a secondary complication in debilitated patients with neoplastic disease, alcoholism, or diabetes.

In clinical cases of meningitis in humans, *L. monocytogenes* can be isolated most easily from cerebrospinal fluid and in some cases from the blood early in the infection. The organism may be recovered from spinal fluid or blood for several weeks after clinical recovery. Initial isolation of *L. monocytogenes*, however, may be difficult, particularly from materials containing mixed microbial populations, such as specimens from the uterus, cervix, vagina, meconium, feces, nasopharynx, or tissues. Often, for reasons unknown, storage of broth suspensions of these specimens at 4 C for periods up to 3 months is required before initial isolation is possible. An awareness of the peculiarities of the bacterium and an ability to differentiate *L. monocytogenes* from diphtheroids are essential to bacteriological diagnosis of listeric infections.

SPECIMENS

The standard procedures described in chapter 6 are satisfactory for the collection and processing of cerebrospinal fluid, including biochemical tests for glucose and protein, for total and differential leukocyte counts, and blood for the primary culture of *L. monocytogenes* from cases of meningitis, meningoencephalitis, and bacteremia.

Swab specimens are collected from the female reproductive tract and from abscesses.

Necropsy tissue specimens, placenta, and feces are triturated with sterile 60-mesh alundum or sand in a mortar and pestle and diluted with tryptose broth to a 10% suspension. Allow tissue and alundum to settle; decant supernatant material to a sterile screw-cap vial.

Special "cold enrichment" at 4 C of L. monocytogenes suspect specimens

Suspect specimens, particularly those containing mixed bacterial flora, should be routinely stored at 4 C for at least 4 weeks and possibly up to 6 months. Subculture weekly for 4 weeks and monthly thereafter. For storage of specimens at 4 C for "cold enrichment," inoculate 5 ml of blood into 50 ml of fluid blood culture medium. Transfer swabs to screw-cap tubes containing 5 ml of tryptose broth. Store 10% tissue or fecal suspensions in screw-cap tubes.

DIRECT EXAMINATION

Cerebrospinal fluid

Centrifuge the tube of spinal fluid submitted for bacteriological examination at 1,500 × *g* for 15 min. Remove the supernatant fluid except for about 0.4 ml which is used to resuspend the sediment.

Gram stain. Smear a loopful of sediment on a slide, gently fix with heat, and Gram stain. Examine for gram-positive coccobacilli or diplobacilli, which may be intracellular or extracellular. The organisms may stain unevenly and may resemble *Haemophilus influenzae*.

Fluorescent-antibody staining. Prepare smears of cerebrospinal fluid sediment, air-dry, fix for 1 min by immersion in 95% ethyl alcohol, and stain with fluorescent antibody (FA). *Listeria* type 1, type 4, and polyvalent FA, as well as counterstain, control materials, and directions for conducting the FA tests, are available (Difco). Additional information on FA procedures is given in chapter 4. Interpretation of FA results may be difficult. Intensive efforts to culture *L. monocytogenes* should be made from specimens positive to the FA procedure.

Meconium

Microscope examination of Gram-stained smears of meconium is very useful in the early diagnosis of neonatal listeriosis and should be done whenever possible. The presence of easily detectable small gram-positive coccobacilli in meconium prompts suspicions that they are *L. monocytogenes*. Examine hanging-drop preparations for motility of such organisms. If positive, report the findings to the physician, who may wish to attempt antibiotic prophylaxis against the development of listeric meningitis or septicemia in the child.

Consider FA staining of suspect meconium.

Even though *L. monocytogenes* cells may be present in large numbers in Gram stains of smears of meconium, it may be difficult to isolate them in culture without long periods of "cold enrichment" at 4 C.

Swabs from the reproductive tract of the mother after infectious abortion or stillbirth or postnatal infection of the neonate

Prepare smears and stain by the Gram method. *L. monocytogenes* may be present in large numbers in some cases. Information gained from the smear examination is useful in planning cultural procedures.

CULTURE AND ISOLATION

Laboratory workers are divided in their preference of solid media for isolating *L. monocytogenes*. Some persons prefer sheep blood-agar and look for characteristic narrow zones of beta-hemolysis around the colonies; others prefer clear tryptose-agar and look for colonies of characteristic blue-green color which can be seen with oblique light transmission through the colony at an angle of 45°. A microscope lamp, with filters removed, is tilted at a 45° angle toward a flat mirror placed in front of the microscope. Light is reflected obliquely through the colonies on the surface of clear medium. The petri dish cover is removed, and colonies are examined at 10 to 15× magnification.

Cerebrospinal fluid

Inoculate sediment from centrifuged cerebrospinal fluid. (i) Transfer a drop to a sheep blood-agar plate, streak, and incubate at 35 C in a candle jar or a 10% CO_2 atmosphere. (ii) Transfer a drop to a tryptose-agar plate; incubate at 35 C. (iii) Transfer a drop (or remainder of the sediment) to 5 ml of tryptose broth; store at 4 C, and subculture to blood- or tryptose-agar plates weekly for at least 4 weeks if no isolations occur on earlier subcultures.

Blood

Inoculate 5 ml of blood into 50 ml of fluid blood culture medium in blood culture bottles containing 10% CO_2 or in flasks which will be incubated in an atmosphere of 10% CO_2. Useful fluid blood culture media are Trypticase soy broth, tryptic soy broth, thiol broth, and brain and heart broth. Incubate at 35 C. Subculture to a blood-agar or tryptose-agar plate when growth appears or on the 2nd, 4th, 7th, and 12th days.

Inoculate 5 ml of blood into 50 ml of fluid blood culture medium. Store at 4 C. Subculture weekly for 4 weeks on blood- or tryptose-agar plates.

Subculture from swab, tissue, and fecal suspensions after cold enrichment in tryptose broth at 4 C

Subculture 0.2 ml of the cold-enriched tryptose broth suspension to 5 ml of KCNS-tryptose broth (3.75% potassium thiocyanate, reagent grade, is added to tryptose phosphate broth [Difco] before sterilization [5]) at weekly intervals for the first month and monthly for 4 to 6 months if no isolations occur on earlier subcultures. Incubate at room temperature (22 to 25 C) for 48 h. Transfer a loopful from just below the surface of the KCNS-tryptose broth and streak a blood-agar, tryptose-agar, or McBride Listeria agar plate. Incubate for 24 to 48 h at 35 C.

Primary isolation in mice

Inoculate 16- to 20-g mice intraperitoneally with 0.2 ml of tryptose broth suspect suspension of tissue or swab extract. From mice that die, culture pooled liver and spleen suspensions on blood- or tryptose-agar plates. Sacrifice all living mice on the seventh postinoculation day. Culture pooled liver and spleen suspensions on blood- or tryptose-agar plates. Reculture after storage at 4 C.

Alternate procedures for handling specimens containing mixed bacterial flora (1–4, 8)

McBride Listeria medium (9). After cold enrichment in tryptose broth, subculture the broth directly to plates of McBride Listeria medium.

Polymyxin B (10). Hold tissue suspensions and swabs at 4 C for cold enrichment in tryptose broth containing 25 units or 3.12 μg of polymyxin B sulfate per ml. Subculture from the polymyxin B-tryptose broth culture directly to tryptose-agar plates containing 25 units of polymyxin per ml.

IDENTIFICATION

Examination of plates

Examine blood-agar plates for round translucent, slightly raised bluish-gray colonies with fine-textured surface that varies from 0.3 to 1.5 mm in diameter and has a narrow zone of beta-hemolysis.

Examine clear agar plates with a binocular scanning microscope (10 to 15× magnification) with obliquely transmitted light. *L. monocytogenes* colonies are distinctively blue-green.

Differential tests for suspect colonies

Gram stain. *L. monocytogenes* grows on solid media as small gram-positive, diphtheroid-like rods, usually diplobacilli with rounded ends. The dimensions are 1.0 to 2 by 0.5 μm. Frequently, in a microscopic field there are a few long rods measuring 5 to 7 μm or chains composed of three to five cells. Smears reveal typical palisade formation (Chinese lettering).

Motility test on semisolid agar. Inoculate two tubes of semisolid motility medium by stabbing with a straight needle. Incubate one tube at room temperature (20 to 25 C) and the other at 35 C for 2 to 5 days. Motility is determined by the spread of the growth from the line of the stab and the development of an "umbrella" 3 to 5 mm below the surface. Motility is minimal at 35 C.

Catalase and fermentation pattern

L. monocytogenes produces catalase.

For routine determination of the fermentation pattern, suspend a loopful of bacterial growth from an agar slant in 2 ml of broth. Add a drop of the suspension to tubes of Phenol Red Broth (Difco) or CTA medium (BBL) containing 1% glucose, lactose, maltose, sucrose, trehalose, salicin, mannitol, or dulcitol. Incubate at 35 C. Record the results after 24 h and after 4 days. *L. monocytogenes* produces acid from glucose, trehalose, and salicin in 24 h; acid is produced irregularly or slowly from lactose, maltose, and sucrose. Acid is not produced from mannitol or dulcitol. Determination of additional fermentation activity and biochemical tests may be valuable in specific research on the organism.

SEROLOGICAL METHODS

Rapid slide test for presumptive identification

Carefully wash bacterial growth from the agar slant and suspend it in 2 ml of 0.85% NaCl buffered to pH 7.2 with 0.067 M potassium phosphate mixtures. Place the tube of bacterial suspension in a boiling-water bath for 1 h. Identify the resulting O antigen with *Listeria* O antiserum, type 1, type 4, or polyvalent, by mixing 1 drop of antigen with 1 drop of 1:20 antiserum in a slide agglutination test. Antiserum, control antigens, and detailed directions for the rapid slide and tube agglutination tests are available commercially (Difco). A binocular scanning microscope is useful in reading the test.

Complete serological identification

Complete serological identification of strains of *L. monocytogenes* is based on both somatic (O) and flagellar (H) antigens (3). Cultures presumptively identified as *L. monocytogenes* should be submitted for complete serological identification through the state health department to: General Bacteriology Unit, Bacteriology Section, Center for Disease Control, Atlanta, Ga. 30333. As a part of the serological typing service, the Center for Disease Control supplies a Listeriosis Case Investigational Report form to gain epidemiological information about patients from whom *L. monocytogenes* has been isolated.

ANIMAL INOCULATION

Identification of cultures

Anton test. Instill a drop of 24-h broth culture in the conjunctival sac of a young rabbit or guinea pig; the opposite conjunctival sac will serve as the uninoculated control. Observe the animal for 5 days. Marked purulent conjunctivitis develops within 24 to 36 h after instillation of *L. monocytogenes*.

Monocyte production by rabbits. Inoculate the marginal ear vein of a young rabbit with 0.5 ml of a suspension of culture in distilled water standardized to tube 1 of the McFarland nephelometer (3×10^8 organisms per ml). Marked monocytosis, up to 40%, will develop within 3 to 5 days if the culture is *L. monocytogenes*.

Pathogenicity of L. monocytogenes cultures for mice

Inject 0.2 ml of a 24-h tryptose broth culture intraperitoneally in 16- to 20-g mice. *L. monocytogenes* cultures usually kill mice within 5 days. The organism may produce necrotic foci of the liver and may be recovered from the liver and spleen.

IMMUNOSEROLOGICAL DIAGNOSIS

The results of serological tests are too difficult to interpret to be of much assistance in the diagnosis of listeriosis (3, 6, 7, 9).

DIFFERENTIATION

An awareness that *L. monocytogenes* may cause acute meningitis and septicemia is essential in training laboratory staff. Periodic use of a known culture of *L. monocytogenes* is helpful in becoming familiar with the morphology of the organism, its characteristic beta-hemolysis of colonies on sheep blood-agar, the blue-green colonies that can be seen on clear tryptose-agar when viewed by oblique light, and the characteristic microaerophilic "umbrella" growth in semisolid motility medium incubated at room temperature (20 to 25 C). Differentiation of *L. monocytogenes* from other diphtheroids is often necessary.

L. monocytogenes is a small diphtheroid. The gram-positive organisms form coccobacilli in pairs with characteristic palisade arrangement in stained smears from agar cultures. Morphology and staining are more uniform than with many other diphtheroids. If decolorized excessively during Gram staining of spinal fluid sediment, the organisms may stain unevenly and resemble *H. influenzae*.

With experience, colonies of *L. monocytogenes* on blood-agar and on tryptose-agar can be differentiated from those of diphtheroids. Many diphtheroid organisms produce pigmented colonies. Motility at 20 C and the characteristic type of microaerophilic growth 3 to 5 mm below the surface of motility media are important differential characteristics. Very few diphtheroids are motile, and most grow on the surface of motility media rather than in the microaerophilic zone below the surface. Fermentation of salicin differentiates *L. monocytogenes* from most diphtheroids.

In practice, if colonies on blood-agar are typical and Gram stain morphology is suggestive of *L. monocytogenes*, colonies are picked to agar slants and incubated for 24 h. The growth from these agar slants is washed off, the suspension is heated, and the organism is presumptively identified serologically by a slide or tube agglutination test with *Listeria* antisera. Additional biochemical tests are done.

EVALUATION

Since early and intensive administration of antibiotics is necessary in the management of listeric infections, the results of preliminary and presumptive laboratory findings should be promptly submitted to the clinician; in the meantime, intensive efforts to isolate the organism should be continued. If bacteriological diagnosis is possible in retrospect, it may assist

Chapter 15

Bacillus anthracis

JAMES C. FEELEY AND PHILIP S. BRACHMAN

CHARACTERIZATION

Bacillus anthracis causes anthrax in humans and animals. Taxonomically it belongs to the family *Bacillaceae*, of which most other members are soil saprophytes and insect pathogens. It is rod-shaped, 1.0 to 1.3 by 3.0 to 10.0 μm, and gram-positive, and grows best aerobically but can grow anaerobically. It is nonmotile and nonhemolytic, and produces central or paracentral spores without significant swelling of the rods. Growth is supported best by ordinary media at 35 to 37 C, with a temperature range of 22 to 42 C. On special media in a CO_2 atmosphere, pathogenic strains produce mucoid colonies, as contrasted to rough colonies when grown ordinarily. Mice, guinea pigs, and rabbits are killed when injected with small numbers of bacteria.

SAFETY REGULATIONS

Although most of the historical background of anthrax has led to an exaggerated fear of working with the agent, any competent laboratory practicing good bacteriological safety techniques should be able to isolate and identify *B. anthracis* (including animal injection) safely. The most important precaution is avoiding the production of aerosols, which may occur with certain laboratory manipulations.

Any work with spore suspensions or processing of contaminated soil or animal hair must be done only in a safety cabinet and must be performed by immunized individuals. For persons working in these special situations, a vaccine is available from the Center for Disease Control (CDC). After use, work surfaces must be decontaminated with either 5% hypochlorite or 5% phenol (carbolic acid).

All glassware, autopsy equipment, needles, and syringes used must be considered contaminated. Before cleaning, they must be placed in an iodine solution (2,500 ppm with 0.4% sodium nitrate to prevent corrosion) and autoclaved.

Inoculation of animals should be performed with great care. Individuals should wear lab coats, masks, and surgical gloves. Safety apparel worn should be decontaminated before it is reused or discarded.

Inoculated animals should be housed in a separate room or in an isolated part of the general animal quarters, and warning signs should be posted. All carcasses must be autoclaved and incinerated. Cages (including bedding with excreta) must be autoclaved before cleaning, and the quarters must be decontaminated after use.

In the event of a laboratory accident, with possible deposition of viable organisms beneath the skin, cleanse the affected area of skin and administer penicillin or broad-spectrum antibiotics in the usual therapeutic doses.

COLLECTION OF SPECIMENS

Appropriate specimens are extremely important if a clinical diagnosis of anthrax is to be confirmed by the laboratory. The type of clinical specimens collected depends on the recognition of the form of illness. Human illness may be in the form of a cutaneous lesion, pulmonary disease, or gastrointestinal involvement. The most common has been cutaneous (95%). Secondary meningitis may develop in all forms. It must be noted that the probability of having an actual case of anthrax in the United States is very low. Fewer than five cases have occurred annually since 1970, and these were primarily industrially acquired (80%); the remainder were agriculturally related. These figures emphasize that extreme care must be exercised in the identification. Most often the isolate will be recognized as a soil saprophyte. However, the seriousness of the disease and the public health significance demand that the isolate be considered suspect *B. anthracis* and thoroughly examined before being dismissed.

Cutaneous anthrax

Two sterile swabs should be soaked in the clear serous fluid of the vesicle or ring of vesicles that develops 3 to 7 days after exposure and appears initially as a pruritic pimple. Smears should be made, air-dried, and gently heat-fixed from one of the swabs for both Gram and fluorescent-antibody staining. The second swab should be used for culture immediately or transported to the laboratory in a dry sterile tube.

For lesions with developed eschars, moisten two sterile swabs in sterile broth (squeeze excess fluid from swabs by pressing and rotating the swabs against the inside walls of the sterile container), and then rotate the moistened swabs beneath the edge of the black eschar without causing its detachment from the skin. Make smears and cultures as described for vesicular fluid. Cultures will usually be negative within 24 h after initiation of antibiotic therapy.

Inhalation anthrax

Obtain sputum, prepare smears, and inoculate culture media. Perform blood cultures.

Gastrointestinal anthrax

Collect fecal and food specimens (if available) and culture. Also do a blood culture.

Note that blood should be cultured whenever the patient shows systemic symptoms and when the bacteria are present in sufficient numbers to be observed in smears. Furthermore, if there is meningeal involvement, spinal fluid should be collected, and both smears and cultures should be made. In any event, acute and convalescent serum specimens (5 ml) should be obtained.

MICROSCOPE EXAMINATION

One of the air-dried, heat-fixed smears from the patient must be Gram stained. The second should be reserved for fluorescent-antibody staining. Additional stains such as spore and capsule should be performed with culture isolates.

Gram stain

The rods are typically large, square-ended, gram-positive, 1.0 to 1.3 by 3.0 to 10 μm, and occur singly or in chains of two or three bacilli. Capsules will be present but not observable. Spores will not develop if the smears are prepared immediately on collection and fixed. Note that occasionally round-ended bacilli will be detected. Long parallel chains of rods will be seen in smears of colonies.

Fluorescent-antibody stain (3, 4)

The fluorescent-antibody technique may prove extremely important, especially when cultures are collected after initiation of antibiotic therapy. Smears may be sent to the CDC. Note that, although this test is only persumptive, it can provide ancillary evidence for the clinical diagnosis. If isolates are to be examined by this technique, they must be grown on sodium bicarbonate media under a CO_2 atmosphere to allow capsules to develop.

CULTURAL EXAMINATION

Primary inoculation

Inoculate specimen on 5% blood-agar plates prepared from defibrinated or citrated sheep, rabbit, or human blood which is free from antibiotics. It should be noted that a variety of selective media have been described (6–8).

Although these media may be used effectively in such applications as air monitoring, they may partially or totally inhibit some strains of *B. anthracis*. Consequently, nonselective media are usually preferable. Incubate plates aerobically for 18 h at 35 C.

Colonial morphology

Examine under a fluorescent lamp by tilting the plate back and forth so that the light will be reflected from the colonies at various angles. The colonies are nonhemolytic, 4 to 5 mm in diameter, and off-white, with a ground-glass appearance. They are usually flat with an irregular margin and may have many comma-shaped outgrowths (Fig. 1). When the margin of the colony is pushed inward and gently lifted with an inoculating needle, the disturbed part of the colony stands up like beaten egg whites, a characteristic termed "tenacity" (Fig. 2).

FURTHER CHARACTERIZATION

Motility

Either perform a hanging-drop test or inoculate a motility medium and incubate for 4 days at 37 C. *B. anthracis* is nonmotile.

Capsule production

Inoculate sodium bicarbonate agar (see chapter 95) with the test organism and incubate under 5% CO_2. If CO_2 gas is not available, use a candle jar; colonies will be less mucoid. Some strains may not encapsulate (5). Virulent strains of *B. anthracis* are the only organisms that produce rough colonies when grown aerobically and mucoid colonies when grown on sodium bicarbonate medium under a CO_2 atmosphere. If the plates are re-incubated aerobically after mucoid colonies have formed, rough outgrowths from the margins will appear, showing reversion to the rough form.

Gamma phage (1)

Prepare a lawn of the test organism by inoculating 0.1 ml of an 18- to 24-h broth culture or a swab soaked in the broth culture onto an agar plate with a dry surface. Cross-spread this inoculum at right angles. Add one drop of

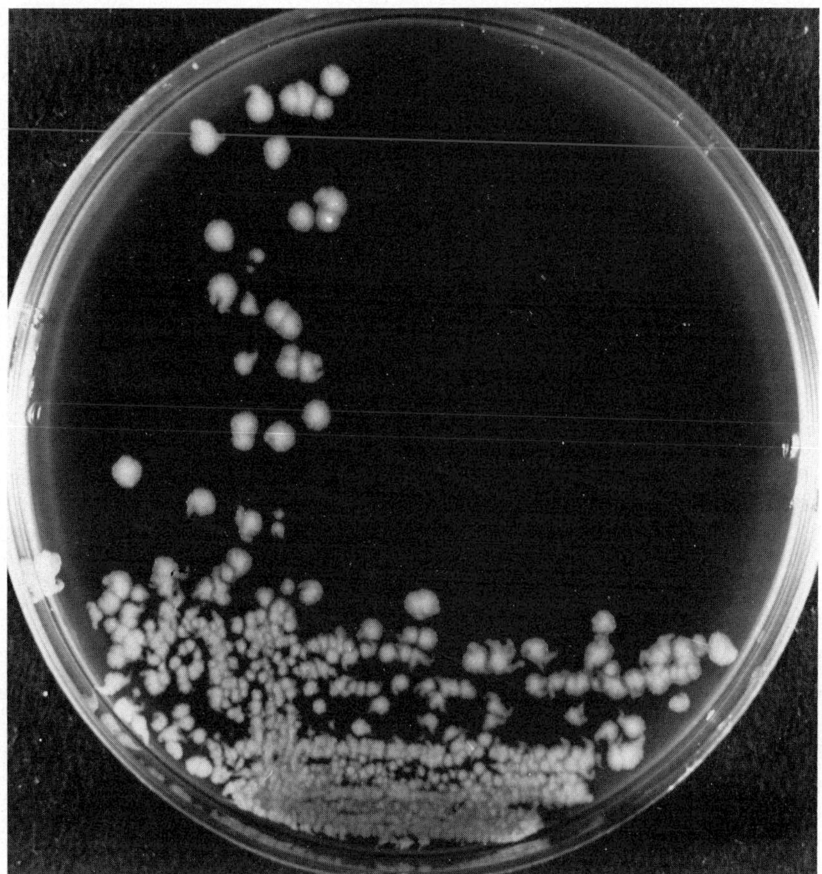

FIG. 1. *Colonies of Bacillus anthracis on blood-agar for 24 h at 37 C (no magnification).*

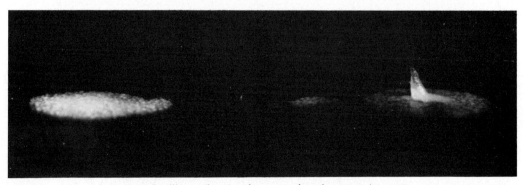

FIG. 2. *Bacillus anthracis colony teased to show tenacity. ×10.*

undiluted phage suspension (CDC can supply gamma phage only to state laboratories) and one drop of sterile heart infusion broth to different parts of the area prepared for testing. Let the phage and broth inocula dry; invert the plates and incubate them for 18 h at 37 C.

If time is critical, a colony from initial isolation can be used to prepare a test lawn. Inoculate the colony on a plate and reduce the inoculum by streaking one-quarter of the test plate with a loop. Prepare an area 5 cm by 5 cm by cross-streaking at right angles. This test is suggested as an additional test and should not replace the overnight broth culture method for phage testing.

Preliminary readings can usually be made in 4 to 6 h, but all plates should be incubated for 18 h. A positive reaction consists of an area devoid of growth where the phage was dropped, surrounded by a mat of luxuriant growth. A few resistant colonies may be seen in the phage-inoculated area. Known cultures of *B. anthracis* and *B. cereus* should be run concomitantly as controls.

Animal pathogenicity

Inoculate each of 10 mice (2 to 3 weeks old) subcutaneously with 0.2 ml of a saline suspension of the test organism. Rabbits and guinea pigs may also be used. Prepare the inoculum by scraping some growth from an agar plate (18 to 24 h) with a loop having a diameter of approximately 4 mm. Carefully emulsify into a test tube containing 10 ml of sterile saline by holding the tube at a 45° angle and rubbing some of the growth into the area of the meniscus so that the upper 0.5 ml of saline is slightly turbid. Mix the tube contents. The resulting suspension should not show any turbidity and will have approximately 10^5 to 10^6 organisms per ml. Broth cultures must not be used because nonspecific deaths might occur.

Death resulting from anthrax infection usually occurs in 2 to 5 days but may be as late as 10 days. Confirm all deaths by culturing the liver, spleen, or heart blood.

Biochemical tests

Additional tests may be helpful for characterization. Inoculate the following fermentation media with the suspect *B. anthracis*: arabinose, glucose, maltose, mannitol, salicin, sucrose, and xylose (see chapters 95 and 96). Also inoculate Voges-Proskauer, litmus milk, semi-solid agar containing 0.0004% methylene blue, egg yolk-agar, and gelatin tube media. Incubate these media at 37 C aerobically for 18 to 24 h; the Voges-Proskauer medium requires an additional 24 h of incubation (see chapters 95 and 96).

Results of the biochemical and other tests on *B. anthracis* are listed in Table 1 and compared with the reactions of *B. cereus*, the organism most easily mistaken for *B. anthracis*. Refer to *Bergey's Manual of Determinative Bacteriology* to identify other members of the family *Bacillaceae*.

Although salicin is usually negative, a few *B. anthracis* strains may produce slight acidity. No opaque zone of lecithinase activity on egg yolk-agar should be seen around *B. anthracis* colonies in 24 h; further incubation usually results in lecithinase activity. Gelatin tubes show liquefaction after prolonged incubation.

TABLE 1. *Characteristics of Bacillus anthracis and B. cereus*

Characteristic	*B. anthracis*	*B. cereus*
Blood-agar colony	Rough, flat, usually many comma-shaped outgrowths	Rough, flat, no or few comma-shaped outgrowths
Hemolysis	None or very weak	Usually beta-hemolytic
Tenacity	Positive	Negative
Bicarbonate medium (CO_2)	White, round, raised glistening, mucoid	Flat, dull
Fluorescent-antibody test	Positive	Negative
Gamma phage	Susceptible	Resistant
Animal pathogenicity	Positive	Negative
Litmus milk	Not reduced or slowly reduced and peptonized	Usually reduced in 2 to 3 days
Methylene blue	Not reduced or slightly reduced in 24 h	Usually reduced in 24 h
Motility	Negative	Usually positive
Voges-Proskauer test	Positive	Positive
Gelatin liquefaction (7 days)	Negative or partial	Usually complete
Fermentation tests:		
Glucose	Acid, no gas	Acid, no gas
Maltose	Acid, no gas	Acid, no gas
Sucrose	Acid, no gas, or negative	Acid, no gas, or negative
Arabinose	Negative	Negative
Mannitol	Negative	Negative
Xylose	Negative	Negative
Salicin	Usually negative or late	Usually positive in 24 h

SEROLOGICAL EXAMINATION

Biotype determination

Currently there is no method for differentiating *B. anthracis* into serological types. However, there is indication that biotypes exist.

Antibody detection

An indirect hemagglutination test for detection of antibodies to *B. anthracis* is performed at the CDC on an investigational basis (2). Paired serum specimens should be submitted from persons with suspect cases of anthrax.

Antigen detection

The Ascoli test has been used to detect *B. anthracis* antigens in animal products. However, the necessary hyperimmune serum is not commercially available in the United States.

LITERATURE CITED

1. Brown, E. R., and W. B. Cherry. 1955. Specific identification of *Bacillus anthracis* by means of a variant bacteriophage. J. Infect. Dis. **96**:34–39.
2. Buchanan, T. M., J. C. Feeley, P. S. Hayes, and P. S. Brachman. 1971. Anthrax indirect microhemagglutination test. J. Immunol. **107**:1631–1636.
3. Cherry, W. B., and E. M. Freeman. 1959. Staining bacterial smears with fluorescent antibody. V. The rapid identification of *Bacillus anthracis* in culture and in human and murine tissues. Zentralbl. Bakteriol. Parasitenk. Infektionskr. Hyg. Abt. I Orig. **175**:582–597.
4. Cherry, W. B., M. Goldman, T. R. Carski, and M. D. Moody. 1961. Fluorescent antibody techniques. U.S. Public Health Service Publication No. 729.
5. Chu, H. P. 1952. Variation of *Bacillus anthracis* with special reference to the noncapsulated avirulent variant. J. Hyg. **50**:433–444.
6. Knisely, R. F. 1966. Selective medium for *Bacillus anthracis*. J. Bacteriol. **92**:784–786.
7. Morris, E. J. 1955. A selective medium for *Bacillus anthracis*. J. Gen. Microbiol. **13**:456–460.
8. Pearce, T. W., and E. O. Powell. 1951. A selective medium for *Bacillus anthracis*. J. Gen. Microbiol. **5**:387–390.

Chapter 16
Mycobacterium

ERNEST H. RUNYON, A. G. KARLSON, GEORGE P. KUBICA, AND LAWRENCE G. WAYNE

INTRODUCTION

The contribution of the clinical laboratory to the diagnosis of mycobacterial disease may be conveniently considered in three phases, the detection and isolation of mycobacteria, the identification of the mycobacteria isolated, and the determination of drug susceptibilities of these organisms. These procedures are quite time-consuming and require facilities and reagents not routinely used in the study of bacteria in other genera. A laboratory report suggesting mycobacterial disease has serious consequences for the patient, which may affect his life for many months, or even years. There is a general trend for tuberculosis to be treated in the general hospital or on an outpatient basis, rather than in the specialized setting of a tuberculosis sanatorium, as in the past. With the decline in incidence of tuberculosis, and this decentralization of treatment, it may be expected that the volume of tuberculosis bacteriology will be distributed rather evenly among many laboratories in a community, with few laboratories receiving large numbers of such specimens. Therefore, the clinical bacteriologist should become well acquainted with the procedures described here, and then decide whether the number of specimens he receives for mycobacterial examination is large enough to warrant maintaining the expertise and special materials necessary for optimal performance. In some cases, he may decide he receives too few specimens to permit him to maintain full proficiency and that it may be more practical to delegate one or more phases of this work to another laboratory (either private or public) which does handle a large volume of such work.

SOME GENERAL CHARACTERISTICS OF MYCOBACTERIAL PATHOGENS

The mycobacteria are acid-fast, alcohol-fast, aerobic or microaerophilic, nonsporeforming, nonmotile bacilli. Their lipid content is high. Growth is slow. The most rapidly growing species require 2 to 3 days on simple media at a temperature of 20 to 40 C, and most pathogens require 2 to 6 weeks on complex media at restricted temperatures. *Mycobacterium leprae* fails to grow in vitro. *M. ulcerans* and *M. marinum* require a temperature lower than 37 C; *M. xenopi* and *M. avium* are favored by temperatures above 37 C. Colonies may be rough, the bacilli compacted in dense coils (e.g., *M. tuberculosis*); they may be smooth and transparent, the bacilli being in no discernible pattern (e.g., *M. intracellulare*); or they may be intermediate in roughness (e.g., *M. kansasii*). Colonies of some species (*M. xenopi* and some rapid growers) form fragile branching filamentous extensions in a radial pattern on the surface of the medium; other extensions may penetrate the medium or even project into the air. Pigmentation may be photochromogenic (light required for formation of pigment), scotochromogenic (pigment formed in dark or light), lacking, or sporadic, according to the species.

About a dozen species are pathogens, producing slowly developing, destructive granulomas that may necrose with ulceration or cavitation, or heal with possible disfiguration. Disease may be confined to cooler superficial parts of the body or may invade internal organs. Tuberculosis of the lungs may disseminate to other parts of the body via the blood stream, lymphatics, or the intestinal tract. Pathogenicity for experimental animals varies with the mycobacterial species. Animals may be useful for both primary isolation and identification, although, with the more gentle digestion techniques and multiple in vitro tests currently available, cultural methods alone are generally considered to be adequate. Identification of mycobacterial diseases by test of patients' sera has not become a clinical laboratory procedure. For some species, bacillary agglutination tests with hyperimmune animal sera are useful for culture identification. Several species are only occasionally or very rarely pathogenic for humans, occurring in clinical specimens usually as saprophytes. Mycobacteria occur in soil, in water and food, and in several kinds of animals.

"Atypical"

The designation "atypical" is much used for mycobacteria other than *M. tuberculosis* or *M.*

bovis which occur in clinical specimens. Since these bacteria in reality are *not atypical*, but rather are characteristic of their particular species, it is better to avoid this designation. Often the word "mycobacterial" is preferable, or one may refer to "mycobacteria other than tubercle bacilli" or "mycobacteria of Group I–IV" (or of whatever group is indicated).

Groups (Runyon)

The groups are of mycobacteria exclusive of *M. tuberculosis* or *M. bovis* occurring in clinical specimens; they are not species, rather each group is comprised of several species. Group I consists of photochromogenic species of slow growers. Members of Group II are the scotochromogenic slow growers. Group III contains the nonphotochromogenic and often, at least initially, nonchromogenic slow growers. Group IV consists of rapid growers, defined as maturing in less than 1 week at 25 C (room temperature) or at 37 C. Thus, although Group I is generally and correctly said to consist of the species *M. kansasii* and *M. marinum*, very rarely a strain of *M. kansasii* is encountered which qualifies for Group II or III. *M. intracellulare* and *M. avium* are the major pathogens of Group III, but variants of both of these species may be yellow (i.e., be Group II scotochromogens). If species names are available, reference to groups is superfluous and undesirable.

Species

The species of acid-fast pathogens that may be encountered and should be distinguished in clinical laboratories are listed in Table 1. Besides the most important species, *M. tuberculosis*, the other tubercle bacillus, *M. bovis*, must still be recognized as a threat to humans. Although *M. bovis* in the United States is now very rare as a cause of human disease, it still occurs sporadically in cattle and other animals. Recent investigations have indicated that some previously named species are complexes of probably three or more related species. However, since taxonomic status and distinctive clinical importance of these newly named species are not established, it may be adequate to identify only as far as to the complex. A proposed new species, *M. africanum*, possesses variable properties intermediate between *M. tuberculosis* and *M. bovis*. It is currently known only as a pathogen of humans in certain parts of Africa, but its occurrence elsewhere is anticipated. Little information is available concerning *M. szulgai*; however, all strains so far identified have been thought to be causes of disease. *M. simiae* was originally found in monkeys, but very similar strains have been isolated from humans in Cuba; the latter strains were given the species name *M. habana*. Species listed as being commonly nonpathogens (Table 1) may very rarely be identified as pathogens in some especially susceptible patient. These species include the tap water scotochromogens (*M. gordonae*), the nonpigmented *M. gastri*, *M. terrae*, and *M. triviale*, and others. In this category also are strains of the species *rhodochrous* which has often been listed, though incorrectly, in the genus *Mycobacterium*.

Equipment and supplies

Sources of equipment and supplies required in mycobacterial laboratories are well detailed in brochures and manuals available from the Center for Disease Control, Atlanta, Ga. (22, 47).

SAFETY PRECAUTIONS IN THE MYCOBACTERIAL LABORATORY

Intelligent observance of a few rules and precautions makes the hazard of work in a well-equipped mycobacterial laboratory small. Minimizing the dispersal of mycobacteria into the air and avoidance of inhalation of airborne bacilli are of utmost importance. Any contact with tubercle bacilli is, of course, to be avoided. Maintenance of optimal health is a primary precaution. The pathogenic potential of mycobacteria demands unwavering respect.

Special precautions

Avoid production of infectious aerosols or dust; avoid inhalation of contaminated air. The following preventive devices or measures should be intelligently applied.

Safety transfer hoods. Negative pressure safety transfer hoods should be spacious, should impose a glass barrier between face and source of infection, and should provide for all the operations dealing with tuberculosis, with the possible exception of centrifugation (see below). *Mycobacterial examinations should not be permitted in a laboratory lacking an adequate safety hood.* (See brochure, *Biological Safety Cabinet*, Center for Disease Control, Atlanta, Ga., 1966.) Ideally, the hood should be in a room which is kept scrupulously clean; the surfaces should be swabbed with phenolic germicide and irradiated with ultraviolet light at appropriate times, and air movement should be restricted to that provided by the hood exhaust, with air entry into the chamber only through an appropriate filter except when the door is open for passage. Exhaust from hoods should be

TABLE 1. *Distinctive properties of mycobacteria encountered in clinical specimens*[a]

Runyon group	Complex name[b]	Species name	Incorrect or illegal synonym(s)	Clinical significance[c]	Growth rate[d] 45 C	37 C	31 C	24 C	Colony type: Usual colony morphology[e]	See Fig. no.	Pigmentation[f]	Niacin	Susceptibility to isoniazid (1 μg/ml)	Susceptibility to T2H (10 μg/ml)	Nitrate reduction	Semiquantitative catalase (>45 mm)	68 C catalase	Tween hydrolysis, 5 days	Tellurite reduction, 3 days	Tolerance to 5% NaCl	Iron uptake	Aryl sulfatase, 3 day	MacConkey agar	Urease	Agglutination tests available
		M. leprae		1																					
		M. ulcerans	*buruli*	1	–	–	S	–	R		N	–	–	–	–		+	–		–					
	TB	*M. tuberculosis*		1	–	S	S	–	R	2	N	+	+	–	+	–	–	–		–				+	
	TB	*M. bovis*		1	–	S		–	Rt		N	–	+	+	–	–	–	–		–				+	
I		*M. marinum*	*balnei, platypoecilus*	2		∓	M	M	S/SR		P		+		–	–	+	+		–					+
I		*M. kansasii*	*luciflavum*	2		S	S	S	SR/R	3C	P		+		+	+	+	+		–				+	+
I		*M. simiae*	*habana?*	3–2	–	S			S		P	+	–		–	+	+	–		–					
II	scrofulaceum	*M. scrofulaceum*	*marianum, paraffinicum*	3–2		S	S	S	S		S		–		–	+	+	–		–	–			+	+
II		*M. szulgai*		1		S	S	S	S or R		S/P		±		+			∓		–		±			+
II		*M. gordonae*	*aquae*	4		S		S	S		S		–		–	+	+	+		–	–			–	±
III		*M. xenopi*	*littorale*	3	S	S			Sf	3D	S[g]		+		–	–	+	–		–	–			–	
III	avium	*M. avium*		2	–/+	S		∓	St	4	N	–	–	–	–	–	+	–	+	–	–			–	+
III	avium	*M. intracellulare*	*brunense*, Battey bacillus	2	–/+	S		+	St	4	N	–	–	–	–	–	+	–	+	–	–			–	+
III		*M. gastri*		4		S		S	S		N	–	+	–	–	–	–	+	–	–	–			+	
III	terrae	*M. nonchromogenicum*		4		S		S	SR		N	–	–	–	+	+	+	+	–	–	–			–	
III	terrae	*M. novum*		4		S		S	SR		N	–	–	–	+	+	+	+	–	–	–			–	
III	terrae	*M. terrae*		4		S		S	SR		N	–	–	–	+	+	+	+	–	–	–			–	
III	terrae	*M. triviale*		4		S		S	R		N	–	–	–	+	+	+	+	–	+	–				
IV	fortuitum	*M. fortuitum*	*ranae, minettigiae*	4–3	–	R		R	Sf/Rf	3E	N		–		+	+	+	±	V	+	+	+	+	+	+
IV	fortuitum	*M. chelonei*	*borstelense*	4–3	–	R		R	S/R	3A, B	N	V	–		–	+	+	–	V	–	–	+	+	+	+
IV	fortuitum	*M. chelonei* subsp. *abcessus*	*runyonii, abscessus*	3–2	–	R		R	S/R		N		–		–	+	+	–	V	+	–	+	+	+	+
IV		*M. diernhoferi*		4		R		R	S		N				+	+	+	+		–	+	–	–		
IV		*M. flavescens*		4		M		M	S		S				+	+	+	+	–	+	–	–	–	+	
IV		*M. phlei*	*moelleri*	4	R	R		R	R		S				+	+	+	+	+	+	+	–	–		
IV		*M. smegmatis*		4	R	R		R	R/S		N				+	+	+	+	+	+	+	–	–		
IV		*M. vaccae*		4		R		R	S		S				+	+	+	+	+	V	+	–	–		

[a] Plus and minus signs indicate presence or absence of feature; blank spaces indicate either that information currently is not available or that the property is unimportant.
[b] For most clinical laboratories, designation to "complex" is usually sufficient.
[c] Potential clinical significance: 1, only as pathogens; 2, usually as pathogens; 3, commonly as nonpathogens; 4, usually as nonpathogens.
[d] S, slow; M, moderate; R, rapid.
[e] R, rough; S, smooth; SR, intermediate in roughness; t, thin or transparent; f, filamentous extensions.
[f] P, photochromogenic; S, scotochromogenic; N, nonphotochromogenic. NB; *M. szulgai* is scotochromogenic at 37 C, photochromogenic at 25 C.
[g] Young cultures may be nonchromogenic or possess only pale pigment which may intensify with age.

monitored by flow meters. Filter change, as needed, must be done with due precaution. It should be recognized that *working in a hood with the exhaust turned off may cause an air flow into the face of the operator, constituting a greater hazard than working in an open laboratory.*

Proper ventilation. Proper ventilation requires filtration of air exhausted from laboratories as well as from hoods. Centrifuges and shaking machines, if not in safety hoods, should be in specially ventilated enclosures. Air movement in rooms should be gentle, not such as to maintain dust dispersal.

Aerosol-proof containers. For material subjected to shaking or centrifugation, use containers sealed with rubber-, plastic-, or Teflon-lined screw caps.

Effective masks. Effective masks are available (Bordic, Deseret Filtermask, C. R. Bard, Inc., Murray Hill, N.J.; Aseptex Surgical Mask, #1800, 3-M Co., St. Paul, Minn.), but too infrequently used. Properly fitting masks of a kind which has been demonstrated to minimize passage of airborne bacteria are highly recommended (32). They continue to be effective for many hours and are not appreciably affected by moisture from the breath. Avoid touching the masks with contaminated hands.

Ultraviolet irradiation. Ultraviolet irradiation is a useful adjunct to surface decontamination procedures and is helpful for control of airborne contaminants in restricted areas. Keep ultraviolet tubes clean and *test output of germicidal wavelengths each month* by use of a meter.

Atomizer or fogging machine. Some type of atomizer should be used for fogging phenolic germicide in the area of accidental or unavoidable dispersal of infectious material.

Sand-alcohol bottle. A 250- to 500-ml Erlenmeyer screw-top flask filled with washed sea sand and 95% ethyl alcohol may be used to "wipe" off inoculating wires, loops, and spades before flaming; an alternative is the glass-enclosed incinerator attached to some Bunsen burners. Use of disposable cotton swabs, applicator sticks, Pasteur pipettes, or paper straws for transferring inoculum eliminates the necessity of flaming an inoculating wire. Prior to sterilization of applicator sticks, their ends may be sliced to make effective "spades" for colony transfer.

Splash-proof discard containers. Do not pour contaminated fluids down the drain. Rather, discard them into autoclavable, covered containers (preferably of stainless-steel construction).

Manual-operating pipettes. Put nothing into the mouth in the mycobacterial laboratory. A number of safety pipettors are available commercially which obviate the need for mouth pipetting. With a little practice they are extremely accurate.

Phenolic germicide-soaked towels. These towels should be frequently used. Cheesecloth or paper toweling soaked in 3% Lysol or 5% phenol should be spread over the immediate work area to minimize spattering and to decontaminate spills.

Avoid skin, mouth, or other contact with contaminated surfaces. Procedures for minimizing direct contact with contaminated material are widely recognized, and at times needlessly extreme. To have tubercle bacilli briefly in contact with healthy skin is no calamity. Any person leaving a mycobacterial laboratory should routinely wash his hands thoroughly. While hands are still wet, flood them with 70% isopropyl alcohol and allow to air-dry. Gowns, caps, and gloves which have been worn while dealing with contaminated material must be removed before entering clean areas.

Provide handy dispensers of effective germicides at every work area. Use freely. The faucets and a germicide dispenser at the hand-washing sink should have pedal controls.

Not all so-called germicides are effective against tubercle bacilli. Avoid any that have not been demonstrated to be effective against tubercle bacilli. Quaternary ammonium disinfectants do *not* kill tubercle bacilli. Suitable (41) disinfectants are as follows:

(i) Isopropyl or ethyl alcohol, 70%. Residual action: none. (Only these or some dilute phenolics should be used on the skin.)

(ii) Phenolic-soap mixtures employing *o*-phenylphenol or other phenol derivatives with contact periods of 10 to 30 min are adequate. Residual action: 2 to 3 days. Various proprietary products are available (Amphyl: Lehn and Fink, Toledo, Ohio; Osyl: National Laboratories, Toledo, Ohio; Staphene and Vesphene: Vestal Laboratories, St. Louis, Mo.).

(iii) Sodium hypochlorite, 1:200 to 1:1,000. Contact should be for 10 to 30 min. Residual action: none. Clorox or other household product may be used.

(iv) Formaldehyde, 3 to 8%; alkaline glutaraldehyde, 2%.

(v) Phenol, 5%.

Maintain good health. A program of periodic skin sensitivity testing as long as the reaction is negative, and X-raying of those who are tuberculin-positive, is important. If skin test converts from negative to definitely positive, prophylactic isoniazid administration is commonly recommended. Seek medical advice.

COLLECTION OF SPECIMENS

The greatest single problem in culturing clinical specimens for mycobacteria is the presence of large numbers and kinds of other microorganisms. This problem is partially solved by procurement of the freshest possible specimens and by refrigeration of any which cannot be processed promptly. The microbiologist should be prepared to exert strong influence to correct any deviation from proper procedure in procuring optimal specimens. Immediate reporting of deficiency, usually by phone, is the first step. Any negative or doubtful result on a poor specimen is to be prominently labeled "inadequate specimen." Provisions of instruction sheets for the clinical staff, including nurses and assistants, and another sheet for patients will assist in the achievement of proper specimens.

Successful culture requires getting the freshest possible specimens.

Sputum

Sterile 50-ml screw-capped centrifuge tubes, preferably of the one-use disposable type, are suitable containers. If acetyl-cysteine decontamination is used, it is desirable that the containers be graduated and the 10-ml volume be clearly marked, since this is the maximal amount of sputum which is desirable in this type of container. If it is desired to examine a larger volume, collection of two or more 10-ml specimens in separate tubes facilitates treatment. A good sputum specimen is 5 to 10 ml of recently discharged material from the bronchial tree, with minimal amounts of oral or nasal contaminants. Three such small specimens, kept refrigerated until processed, are better than a 24-h pooled specimen of equal total volume. Whether the specimen is obtained in early morning or at another time is unimportant although most patients are productive soon after rising in the morning.

Aerosol-induced sputum; gastric lavage

For patients who have neither cough nor spontaneous expectorations, suitable specimens may be obtained by inducing cough by inhalation of warm aerosolized, sterile 10% aqueous sodium chloride. Patients usually prefer such induction of sputum to aspiration of gastric contents. Induced sputum may be superior to gastric lavage for recovery of tubercle bacilli. An important advantage is that induced sputum is not contaminated with gastric contents. However, gastric lavage done 0.5 h after aerosol induction of sputum is profitable, especially in patients with minimal disease. The combination of induced sputum and gastric lavage will yield more positive results than either procedure alone (4). Time for sputum induction and gastric lavage is in the morning before meals.

Many commercially available nebulizers can be used for delivering a sterile warm aerosol of sodium chloride solution. Ultrasonic nebulizers are recommended (27). The equipment used for detection of cancer cells may be used, but propylene glycol should not be in the aerosol.

Since the objective in gastric lavage is to obtain swallowed sputum, the specimen should be obtained at least 8 h after the patient has eaten or taken oral drugs.

If processing of gastric lavage is to be delayed 1 day or longer, the collection bottle should contain sodium carbonate powder (about 100 mg) or other alkaline buffer salt. If delivered to the laboratory and processed promptly, buffer is not necessary and is not desirable, as it interferes with decontamination treatment.

Urine

The specimen of choice is the early morning, cleanly voided mid-stream portion. Multiple specimens of this kind are superior to a 24-h pooled specimen. Keep refrigerated prior to processing.

Pleural, spinal, joint, and other fluids, exudates, and tissues

These specimens should be submitted in sterile containers. If appropriate, add citrate or heparin anticoagulant. Large amounts of specimen are preferable. Small amounts of exudate may require moistening with sterile water. Examine while still fresh, or refrigerate.

Cerebrospinal fluid will be received in very small amounts, even less than 1 ml, and must be used sparingly for each of the several tests. Since any acid-fast organisms found can be assumed to be the etiological agent, and because of the urgency, extra consideration must be given to microscope examination. Smears prepared in several layers in an area of not more than 1 cm^2 allow examination of perhaps most of the preparation within 30 min.

Most samples of cerebrospinal fluid readily pass through a 0.45-μm pore size membrane filter, and this method may be used to collect all acid-fast bacilli in the specimen. The filter may then be placed on the surface of a moist, solid medium for growth of colonies.

MICROSCOPY: DETECTION OF ACID-FASTNESS

All clinical specimens submitted for determination of possible mycobacterial infection should be examined for acid-fast bacilli. The unique acid-fastness of mycobacteria makes microscopy of primary importance in the mycobacterial laboratory. Since the information obtained from the microscopic examination of smears is a major criterion for discharging tuberculous patients, the *utmost care* is strongly recommended. Whether the method used is the classic one represented by the Ziehl-Neelsen (Z–N) procedure or one of the fluorochrome procedures, the identical property is determined: bacterial retention of dye after exposure to acid alcohol. Fluorescence here is equivalent to acid-fastness. Microscopy provides help in detection of new cases of mycobacterial infection; serves as an adjunct to culture, for determining the acid-fastness of observed growth; indicates the appropriateness of direct drug susceptibility tests for given specimens and the appropriate dilution of the inocula; gives an indication of progress of disease in individual patients from whom a series of specimens is examined; and, rarely, contributes to species identification in instances when cellular morphology and arrangement may be somewhat distinctive.

Report forms should specify that a finding of acid-fast bacilli is indicative only of the presence of mycobacteria and that for species identification culture is required (" . . . report will follow").

Proper performance of microscopy for mycobacteria and interpretation of results require attention to the following considerations. (i) Occasionally, careful choice of selected portions of a specimen for smearing may result in a much better preparation than a concentrate. (ii) Many sputa or other specimens containing tubercle bacilli will be negative by smear examination because of the low sensitivity of the method. (iii) It is sometimes difficult to distinguish acid-fast artifacts from bacilli. Therefore, as a rule, one or only a few acid-fast "bodies" should be reported as "suspicious" together with a recommendation that further studies are indicated.

Occasionally, microscopy may be positive when subsequent culture is negative. This may result from inactivation of tubercle bacilli by drugs, or by too severe decontamination procedures.

Many sources of error which can lead to false-negative or false-positive reports must be guarded against. Insufficient destaining is a very common cause of poor preparations. Tubercle bacilli and other mycobacterial pathogens are strongly acid-fast and cannot easily be destained. Large portions of insufficiently destained material on a slide will make impossible the recognition of tubercle bacilli therein. If smears are too thick, they cannot properly be destained, and are prone to flake off. If only one or a very few acid-fast rods are found on a smear, another preparation should be examined.

Poor contrast also makes interpretation difficult. Stain and counterstain should be sharply contrasting; counterstain should be relatively weak so as not to hide acid-fast bacilli. Stains from different sources vary in dye content or brightness. Brilliant green counterstain may be better for the slightly color blind, although fluorochrome staining is much preferred.

Acid-fast organisms not originally in the specimen may come from tap water, from distilled water delivery tubes, or by transfer of material from specimen to specimen or slide to slide in the preparation of smears. Acid-fast bacilli may remain attached to glassware even through washing and autoclaving (use only new slides; use prolonged soaking of glassware in sulfuric acid-dichromate mixture). Transfer from a positive smear to others may occur by the vehicle of immersion oil (use cover glass or Diaphane). The flaking of smears from microscope slides is an important source of difficulty. Unwavering vigilance is required to minimize the possibility of cross-transfer of flakes. Observe the following precautions: make smears on new, clean slides, and fix thoroughly with heat; whenever possible, handle each slide separately, especially during washing, which must be gentle.

MICROSCOPY WITHOUT CULTURE

Note that this is perhaps the only mycobacterial laboratory procedure which is permissible without the use of a safety hood.

For physicians or small hospital laboratories lacking facilities for culture, microscopy remains a most valuable procedure. The specimen to be examined should initially be treated with an equal volume of 1% sodium hypochlorite (20% solution of commercial Clorox; see 44). This agent will cause disintegration of the bacilli if allowed to act too long, so smears should be examined promptly.

FLUORESCENCE MICROSCOPY WITH ULTRAVIOLET LIGHT SOURCE

The great advantages of fluorescence micros-

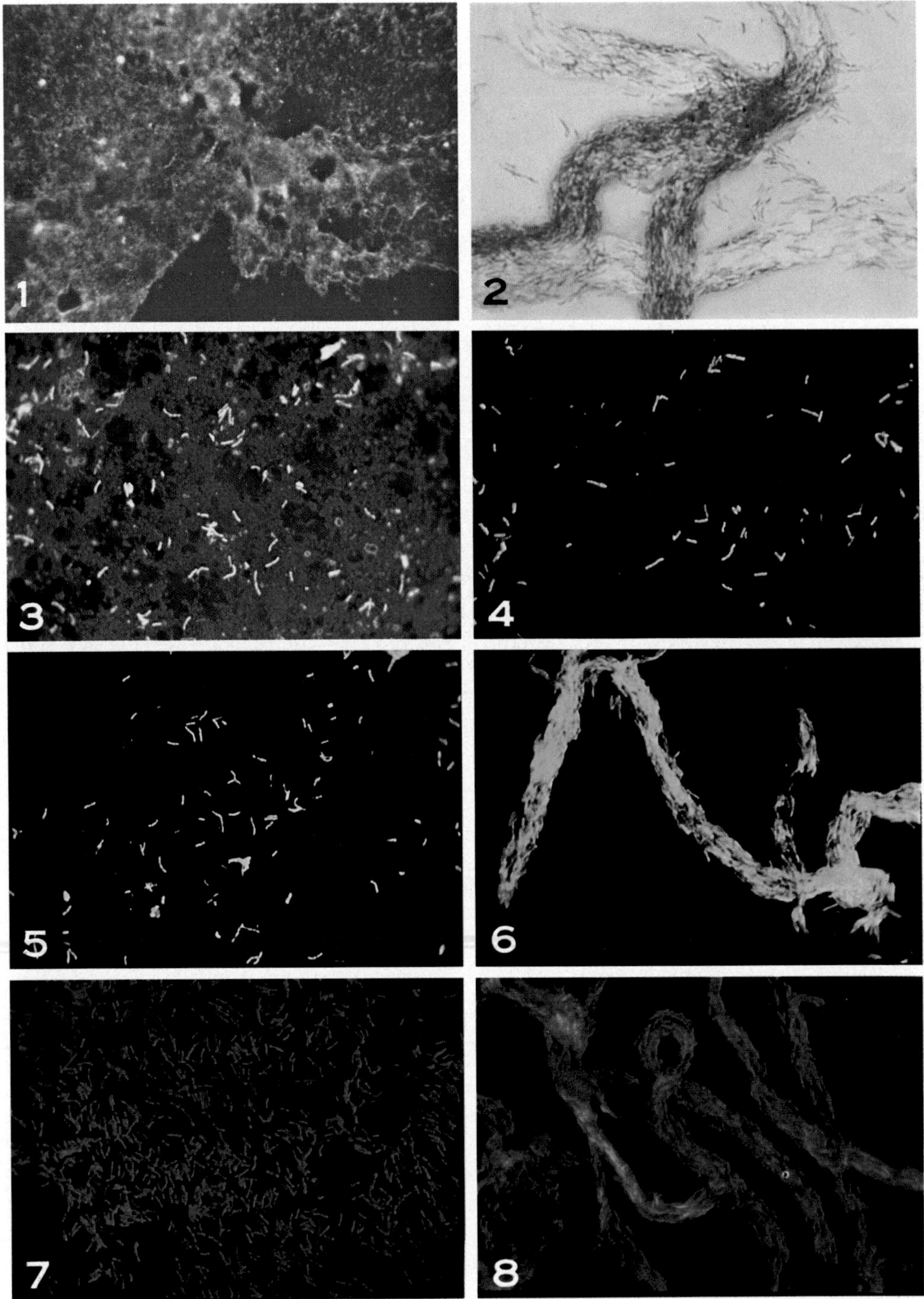

FIG. 1. *Fluorescence microscopy of Truant's auramine-rhodamine (A-R)-stained acid-fast preparations of Mycobacterium tuberculosis. The various Zeiss barrier filters (wavelengths of 410 to 530 nm) permit the rapid demonstration of the organisms in a variety of fluorescing color tones and morphological types (beading, etc.) at magnifications of ×900 to ×1200 (46). Acid-fast bacilli (AFB) were observed as follows:*

copy are in ease, speed, and thoroughness of observation. Low-power objectives may be used, permitting inspection of a large area in a short period of time. Other advantages are better contrast, minimal eye strain, and relative unimportance of the color acuity of microscopists. The well-established technique of Truant et al. (46) with auramine-rhodamine staining has been demonstrated to be highly satisfactory in many laboratories. AFB positive smears are interpreted according to Truant's illustrations shown in Fig. 1 (46).

Reagents. (i) Auramine-rhodamine stain: auramine, 1.5 g; rhodamine, 0.75 g; glycerol, 75 ml; phenol, 10 ml; distilled water, 50 ml. Clarify the solution by filtration through glass wool. Store at room temperature. (ii) Acid alcohol decolorizer: 0.5 ml of HCl in 100 ml of 70% ethyl alcohol. (iii) Counterstain: potassium permanganate, 0.5 g; distilled water, 100 ml. Store at room temperature in a dark bottle.

Staining procedure. Fix smears by heating on a slide warmer (65 C for 2 h; or overnight is acceptable). Fixing on an electric staining rack also is acceptable. Flood the smear with the fluorochrome stain solution and allow to stand for 15 to 20 min at room temperature (20 to 25 C); then rinse in tap water. Decolorize in 0.5% HCl in ethyl alcohol (acid alcohol), and again rinse thoroughly in tap water. Flood smears with counterstain and allow to stand 2 to 4 min. This functions to "quench" the background fluorescence of tissue debris. Excessive treatment with the counterstain (i.e., greater than 5 min) should be avoided as it may lower the intensity of fluorescence of stained bacilli. Rinse with water and air-dry. Microscope examination will demonstrate AFB in a variety of colors based on types of filters (see Fig. 1).

Equipment. Satisfactory filters are the Zeiss BG-12 or Corning 5113 primary (excitation light) filters, and the Corning OG-1 barrier filter. Although most fluorescence work is done with oil on the condenser, it is possible to obtain a dry dark-field condenser for some microscopes. This enables the microscopist to obtain a broader field of vision which is completely filled with light; of further benefit is the fact that with this combination it is possible to scan smears at a total magnification as low as 60 times. For magnification of 400 times with dry dark field, it is helpful to place a drop of immersion oil or glycerol over the smear and then cover with a cover slip.

FLUORESCENCE MICROSCOPY WITH BLUE LIGHT SOURCE

Excellent demonstration of fluorochrome-stained mycobacteria is obtained by use of a microscope equipped with a quartz-halogen illuminator and the proper combinations of primary (exciter) and secondary (barrier) filters. This system provides the same benefits as ultraviolet apparatus with the added advantages that the blue light apparatus does not require a special dark room (although subdued lighting is recommended), does not require oil on the condenser or slide, is simpler and more economical, and does not present radiation hazards. The following recommendations based on use of the Zeiss RA 38 microscope and attachments are applicable to other equipment having comparable features.

The equipment needed is a standard binocular microscope with an illuminator containing a collector lens and a 12-V, 100-W quartz-halogen lamp or high-intensity tungsten bulb, front-surface reflecting mirrors, bright-field condenser, low-power objectives (10× or 25×) for scanning and high dry (63×) planachromat (flat field; if the high dry objective is corrected for cover slip, then a cover slip must be placed, not mounted, over the smear), a 100× oil immersion objective for more critical examination of acid-fast (fluorescent) bodies, and 10× compensating eyepieces. A turret, or intermediate tube, with holder for secondary filters located in the tube body between the objectives and the eyepieces facilitates filter changing. The optics and light path must be precisely aligned to avoid loss of light intensity. The light source is adjusted for Koehler illumination by centering and focusing

Illustration	*Barrier filter wavelength (nm)*	*Color of AFB and description*
1	*410*	*Red and beaded in morphology*
2	*410*	*Red and white bacilli in cord formation*
3	*440*	*Predominantly white to colorless cells*
4	*470*	*Chiefly green bacilli*
5	*500*	*Predominantly yellow organisms*
6	*500*	*Cord formation in yellow fluorescence*
7	*530*	*Orange fluorescing bacilli*
8	*530*	*Cord formation in orange fluorescence*

the lamp filament on the closed iris diaphragm of the condenser. Maximal intensity is obtained by making small adjustments of the condenser while viewing an auramine-stained mycobacterial smear.

Combinations of primary and secondary filters are selected to provide good contrast between a dark background and the fluorescing, yellow bacillus (see Fig. 1). However, the background must be sufficiently light that nonfluorescing debris can be seen for maintaining focus while scanning the slide. A BG 12 primary filter transmitting only wavelengths less than about 500 nm (peak 404 nm) in combination with secondary filters which transmit only wavelengths above 500 nm or 530 nm, as Zeiss no. 50 or no. 53, respectively, provide satisfactory demonstration of fluorescing mycobacteria. The particular combination of complementary exciter and barrier filters determines the color of the background. The greater the overlap of transmission curves, the lighter the background is and vice versa. Therefore, the user should have on hand BG 12 filters of various thicknesses (1.0, 1.5, 2.0, 3.0 mm; obtainable from Fish-Schurman Corp., 70 Portman Road, New Rochelle, N.Y. 10802) for neutral density purposes and secondary filters having transmission cutoffs at 500, 515, and 530 nm to determine which combinations provide optimal background-contrast qualities. The following exciter and barrier filter combinations have been found to be excellent for demonstrating fluorochrome-stained mycobacteria: 3-mm BG 12 and no. 50—light green background; 4-mm BG 12 and no. 50—dark green; 3-mm BG 12 and no. 53—light brown; 3.5-mm BG 12 and no. 53—dark brown. Another primary filter, the fluorescein isothiocyanate (FITC) interference filter used in combination with a 3-mm BG 12 and a no. 50 or 53 barrier filter results in excellent dark green or dark red-brown backgrounds, respectively. The FITC laminated to a BG 38 (to reduce red transmission) and in combination with a 1.5-mm BG 12 produces a reddish-tinged gray background with the no. 50, and a pleasant red field with the no. 53.

Reagents. (i) Auramine O stain is prepared essentially as described by Richards and Miller (35). Completely dissolve 0.1 g of auramine O in 10 ml of 95% ethyl alcohol. Mix 3 ml of liquefied phenol in 87 ml of distilled water. Combine the alcoholic auramine O solution with the phenol-water. It is not necessary to filter the stain; turbidity develops upon standing but does not affect the staining reaction. Store at room temperature in amber bottles. (ii) Acid-alcohol: 0.5 ml of HCl in 100 ml of 70% ethyl alcohol. (iii) Potassium permanganate: 0.5% aqueous solution.

Staining procedure. Heat-fix smears of sputum or body fluids. Deparaffinize tissue sections and bring them down to water. Stain smears at room temperature for 15 min (tissues for 30 min); rinse with tap water. Decolorize smears for 2 min (tissues for 20 min) with acid-alcohol and rinse slides with tap water. Counterstain with potassium permanganate for 3 min. Rinse with water and air-dry.

Cover smear with cover slip of the correct thickness for the high dry objective to be used; however, noncorrected objectives are available for most microscopes, obviating the need for cover slips. Also, use of mounting medium with the cover slip is not absolutely necessary, but, if used, it must be nonfluorescing. Stained tissue sections should be mounted in the usual manner.

NONFLUORESCENCE MICROSCOPY

Ziehl-Neelsen stain

Reagents. (i) Carbolfuchsin: saturated solution of basic fuchsin (3 g of basic fuchsin in 100 ml of 95% ethyl alcohol), 10 ml; 5% aqueous solution of phenol, 90 ml. (ii) Acid alcohol: 3 ml of HCl with 95% ethyl alcohol to bring volume to 100 ml. (iii) Counterstain: methylene blue, water-soluble, 0.3% aqueous.

Staining procedure. Fix smears by gentle heating over a Bunsen flame (or on an electric slide warmer, 65 C for 2 h). Place a piece of filter paper, larger than the size of the smear, on the slide. Flood the slide with carbolfuchsin solution and heat to steaming with a Bunsen flame: allow to stand for 5 min without further heating. (If an electric staining rack is used, allow the slides to stain for 15 min.) Remove filter-paper strips and wash slides in tap water. Decolorize in several successive portions of acid alcohol until no more color appears in the washings (about 2 min; a longer time may be required for thicker smears). Wash with tap water. Beware of flakes from one smear settling on another. Counterstain with methylene blue for about 30 s. Wash with water and dry in the air or over gentle heat.

Kinyoun's acid-fast stain

Reagents. (i) Kinyoun's carbolfuchsin: basic fuchsin, 4 g; phenol, 8 g; alcohol (95%), 20 ml; distilled water, 100 ml. Dissolve fuchsin in alcohol. Add phenol and water. (ii) Acid alcohol; 3 ml of concentrated HCl in 97 ml of 95%

ethyl alcohol. (iii) Counterstain: malachite green (stock solution, 4 g of malachite green and 50 ml of 95% alcohol; working solution, 20 ml of stock solution and 180 ml of distilled water.

Staining procedure. Prepare smear; fix with gentle heat. Stain with Kinyoun's carbolfuchsin for 3 min (do not heat), and then wash gently in running water. Decolorize with acid alcohol until no more color appears in the washing (about 2 min); wash gently in running water. Counterstain with malachite green for 30 s, wash gently in running water, and dry in air.

Stain for tissue sections. For acid-fast bacilli in tissues, the Fite-Faraco stain is recommended (28), to be modified only by using hematoxylin as a counterstain rather than methylene blue. The tissue should be cut at 5 μm in thickness.

Observation of carbolfuchsin preparations

When conventional acid-fast stains are used, the search is done by oil immersion lens (900 to 1,000×), and mycobacteria are observed as red-stained bacilli against a blue or a green background, depending upon the counterstain used. The acid-fast organisms may be coccobacillary to long bacillary forms (from 0.5 to 5.0 by 0.2 to 0.6 μm). Occasionally, the microscopist will see bacilli whose shape is characteristic of a given species, such as *M. kansasii* (long, often broad, and banded cells) or *M. intracellulare* (pleomorphic, average cell very short). It is well to make note of these observations; indication of them to the clinician is warranted if good rapport is maintained.

GENERAL CONSIDERATIONS

The microscopist responsible for reading preparations stained with either fluorochrome or carbolfuchsin stains must make quantitative notations of the numbers of organisms observed per field or per slide. If the number of bacilli seen is only one or two per slide, make and examine another preparation. The preparation of inocula from digested, concentrated sputum specimens for direct drug susceptibility studies is based upon the numbers of bacilli observed by microscopy (see below, section on Drug susceptibility testing).

The following method of reporting is recommended by the American Thoracic Society of the American Lung Association (1969): if the number of organisms seen is 3 to 9, report as "rare"; 10 or more per slide, report as "few"; more than 1 per oil immersion field, report as "numerous." The same reporting scheme may be used for fluorescence microscopy, with one exception—namely, that the observation of greater than 2 bacilli per high dry field (630×) is reported as numerous.

PROCESSING AND CULTURE

Homogenization and decontamination

The best yield of tubercle bacilli may be expected to result from the use of the mildest digestion which gives sufficient control of contaminants. Agents which liquefy secretions may or may not also control contaminants. Sodium hydroxide, the most commonly used digestant, will serve both functions, but, like acids and some other digestants, is only somewhat less harmful to tubercle bacilli than it is to contaminating organisms. The stronger the alkali, the higher its temperature is, and especially the longer it is allowed to act, the greater is its killing action on *both* contaminants and mycobacteria.

Acetyl-cysteine and some enzyme preparations effectively liquefy tenacious sputum. Although these agents fail to inhibit contaminants, some evidence indicates that their use permits milder alkali treatment. Use of the wetting agent sodium lauryl sulfate with weak sodium hydroxide is advocated by several European investigators. Trisodium phosphate liquefies sputum rapidly, but requires long exposure for decontamination of the specimen when used alone. Benzalkonium chloride (Zephiran) as used with trisodium phosphate in a method here given shortens the required period and selectively destroys many contaminants, with little bactericidal action on tubercle bacilli.

Specimens differ greatly in their need of decontamination. The agent selected for this purpose ideally should reflect this and be modified in strength according to the nature and amount of troublesome contaminants. The freshness of a specimen and the adequacy of its refrigeration prior to processing very much affect the need for decontamination.

Some specimens may need no decontamination, and for these none should be used; aseptically obtained urine, surgical specimens, and spinal, synovial, or other internal body fluids; liver, lung, and kidney tissue may be contaminated. Tissues are conveniently handled by cutting them into pieces with sterile scissors and reducing the pieces to pulp in a glass-Teflon tissue grinder. Addition to 10 parts of water allows the development of a soupy fluid that can be transferred with a pipette. Clean surgical tissues do not require decontamination, but autopsy tissues usually do. Especially for specimens which are difficult or impossible to duplicate, it is good practice to hold a portion in a freezer pending results on the first portion cultured. Whenever doubt concerning contamination of a specimen exists, a portion of it may be planted without prior treatment in liquid medium (Dubos, Proskauer-Beck, or 7H9), and the remainder is kept refrigerated. Inspect the liquid culture daily, and if contamination develops subject both this culture and the remainder of the specimen to an appropriate decontamination procedure. If no contamination appears after 7 to 10 days, and no mycobacterial growth is apparent (by smear examination of the sediment), plant also the refrigerated portion of specimen without treatment. *Excessive contamination*, sometimes encountered in specimens from certain patients, from certain localities, or at certain times, may be a difficult problem. The following treatments are suggested. (It must be recognized that harsher treatments also are deleterious to tubercle bacilli and other mycobacteria.)

(i) Cautiously increase the strength, duration or temperature of alkali treatment; maximal limits are arbitrary, but 4% NaOH at 37 C for more than 60 min will probably kill most tubercle bacilli.

(ii) Add penicillin (50 to 100 units) and nalidixic acid (35 μg/ml) to egg medium before inspissation; mix with inoculum, or add to surface of slant (11). Polymyxin (20 to 25 μg/ml) may also be used. The commercially available Mycobactosel agar contains several agents to inhibit contaminants.

(iii) The oxalic acid method of Corper and Uyei (5) is reported to be superior to alkali for elimination of *Pseudomonas* and some other contaminants. Digest sputum with an equal volume of 5% oxalic acid. Agitate on a mixer, and then allow to stand at room temperature for 30 min with occasional shaking. Add sterile physiological saline. Centrifuge, decant the supernatant fluid, and bring the sediment to pH 7 with 4% NaOH containing a pH indicator.

(iv) Recourse to guinea pig inoculation may be advisable. Use a refrigerated portion of the specimen held in reserve, or another specimen.

Liquefaction, including viscosity reduction, in the presence or even in the absence of a digestant, is much facilitated by vigorous mixing achieved by use of a Vortex-type mixer. If properly used, aerosol production by such mixers is minimized. The tube should be held on the vibrating base in such a way that churning, splashing, and foaming of the mixture are avoided. Homogenization should occur not by vibratory agitation but by centrifugal swirling, and this should not be vigorous enough to permit material to rise to the cap. At least a 15-min waiting period after agitation should be allowed before opening. Any fine aerosol droplets possibly formed during the mixing will be eliminated during this period. Use of an effective mask as well as a safety transfer hood is, of course, appropriate here.

Concentration of bacilli by centrifugation

The success of centrifugation in achieving concentration of bacilli is affected by the adequacy of prior homogenization and reduction of viscosity of the specimen, the relative specific gravity of the bacilli and the suspending fluid, the centrifugal force employed, and the time of centrifugation. All of these factors can be controlled to some extent. Since the density of tubercle bacilli is usually only very little greater than that of the liquefied sputum, centrifugation should be at high speed and should be long continued within the limits of excessive exposure to the digestant; 2,000 $\times$ *g* for 30 min is good. (On a #2 IEC centrifuge, head radius 25 cm, 2,500 rpm gives 2,000 $\times$ *g*.) Because it is known that some bacilli actually are buoyant in centrifugation, the most thorough culture programs have included the planting of a portion of the supernatant fluid as well as the sediment. The advantage of this in routine practice has not been demonstrated.

For some fluids, use of bacteria-withholding filters may be an effective concentration procedure. Wayne found them useful only for spinal fluid (49).

Media for isolation of mycobacteria

Media selected should include both a tubed or bottled egg medium (such as Lowenstein-Jensen) and a clear agar medium (such as 7H11) for plates. Care should be exercised in preparing 7H11 media because excessive heat and/or light exposure may result in the release of toxic formaldehyde which will kill or inhibit mycobacteria (30). Both egg and agar media may be somewhat improved by enrichment. Use of an additional medium supplemented with 0.2% pyruvate is recommended when *M. bovis* is suspected (6). Addition to 7H11 of L-asparagine to 0.25 or 0.1% potassium aspartate (18) affords maximal production of niacin. Plate cultures, examined inverted on a low-power microscope, provide advantages of (i) earliest demonstration of growth, (ii) evidence of species (for example, a smooth-colony mycobacterium can be definitely and immediately recognized as not *M. tuberculosis;* characteristic colony forms aid in identification of several species), and (iii) early and definite recognition of contaminants (by colony selection and transfer, pure cultures often may readily be obtained). Although the clear agar media permit *earlier* detection of mycobacteria, on prolonged incubation Lowenstein-Jensen often yields a greater *number* of positive results (20). Therefore, use of *both* types of media gives optimal results in terms of speed and total yield.

CO_2 enrichment to 5 to 10% is *essential* for growth on 7H11 agar and is markedly stimulatory to growth on egg medium (1).

ACCEPTABLE DIGESTANT METHODS

Acetyl-cysteine-alkali procedure for sputum (22)

Reagents. (i) Acetyl-cysteine-alkali digestant: combine 50 ml of 2.94% trisodium citrate·$3H_2O$ (=0.1 M) with 50 ml of 4% NaOH. To this solution, add 0.5 g of powdered *N*-acetyl-L-cysteine (Mead Johnson Research Center, Evansville, Ind.; Sigma Chemical Co., St. Louis, Mo.) just before use. Discard after 24 or 48 h. If used for a 2-day period, the solution should be stoppered tightly and refrigerated. (ii) Phosphate buffer, 0.067 M, pH 6.8. (iii) Sterile 0.2% bovine albumin fraction V (Armour Pharmaceutical Co., Kankakee, Ill.; Pentex, Inc., Kankakee, Ill.) adjusted to pH 6.8.

Procedure. Note and, if requested, record the volume and nature of the specimen, i.e., purulent, mucopurulent, mucoid, serous, bloody, etc.

If the amount received is more than 10 ml, select with a pipette about 10 ml of choice portions, placing them in a sterile 50-ml aerosol-free screw-cap centrifuge tube. (Choice portions are those which may be bloody, cheesy, or purulent.) Add an equal volume of acetyl-cysteine-alkali digestant. Caution: digestant should be dispensed with a fresh, sterile pipette for each specimen. Take every precaution to avoid contaminating the digestant. Stopper tightly and mix for not more than 30 s on a Vortex-type test-tube mixer until liquefied. If liquefaction is not complete in this time, agitate at intervals during the following decontamination period. Avoid the kind of movement which causes aeration of the specimen since the acetyl-cysteine is readily inactivated by oxidation, and mucoid material may repolymerize.

Allow the mixture to stand for 15 min at room temperature (20 to 25 C) with occasional gentle shaking if needed; then fill the tube to within 1 or 2 cm of the top with sterile 0.067 M phosphate buffer (pH 6.8). Beware of cross-contamination: do not touch specimen containers with the buffer dispenser. Centrifuge at or near 2,000 $\times$ *g* for at least 15 min. Moisten the top of the tube with cotton or sponge soaked with 70% alcohol. Decant the supernatant fluid into a splash-proof discard-can containing 5% phenol or other germicide. Again, wipe the lip with alcohol.

Prepare smears on new microscope slides, for Ziehl-Neelsen or fluorochrome staining (see earlier section on Staining). Use either a sterile applicator stick or a flamed 3-mm bacteriological loop, smearing a portion of the sediment over an area about 1 by 2 cm. Note: if quantity of sediment is very small, delay making smears until after the next step, i.e., addition of albumin. Add to the sediment 1 ml of sterile 0.2% bovine albumin fraction V adjusted to pH 6.8.

Make a 1:10 dilution of 0.5 ml of the albumin suspension in sterile water. Occasionally, growth occurs only from this diluted inoculum. Inoculate appropriate media: seed each of the suspensions (diluted and not diluted) onto two tubes of an egg base medium (such as Lowenstein-Jensen) and onto a 7H11 agar plate. If "bi-plates" are used, both diluted and undiluted suspensions may be in the same plate. Inoculation may be made with disposable capillary pipettes delivering 3 drops to each medium. Use the remainder for planting drug-containing media as indicated below, or store in a refrigerator for further treatment if heavy contamination becomes evident.

Place all inoculated plate media into CO_2-permeable polyethylene bags to prevent drying and then into CO_2-enriched incubators. If a CO_2 incubator is not available, place cultures in CO_2-impermeable plastic bags, such as Mylar (Vac Pac Inc., Baltimore, Md.; 3-M Co., St. Paul, Minn.), and inflate by use of a compressed 5 to 10% CO_2-in-air mixture.

Sodium hydroxide procedure

Follow the same steps described for the acetyl-cysteine-alkali method, substituting sodium hydroxide, preferably not stronger than 2%, for the acetyl-cysteine-alkali digestant. In all NaOH procedures, timing must be rigidly controlled. If absolutely necessary to reduce excessive contamination, increase the NaOH concentration (e.g., to 3 or 4%) rather than increasing the time of exposure to the alkali.

Zephiran-trisodium phosphate digestion procedure (56)

Reagents. (i) Zephiran-trisodium phosphate (Z-TSP) digestant: dissolve 1 kg of trisodium phosphate ($Na_3PO_4 \cdot 12H_2O$) in 4 liters of hot distilled water. To this solution, add 7.5 ml of Zephiran concentrate (17% benzalkonium chloride, Winthrop Laboratories) and mix. (ii) Neutralizing buffer (Difco).

Procedure. To the specimen in a screw-capped jar or bottle, add an equal volume of Z-TSP digestant. Agitate vigorously for 30 min on a mechanical shaker. Permit the material to stand, without shaking, for an additional 30 min. Then transfer all or a portion thereof, under a safety hood, to a screw-capped 50 ml centrifuge tube. Centrifuge at 1,800 to 2,000 × *g* for 20 min. Decant the supernatant fluid to a splash-proof can, using precautions specified under the acetyl-cysteine-alkali method. Thoroughly resuspend the sediment in 20 ml of neutralizing buffer, and centrifuge again for 20 min. Tamol-N in the neutralizing buffer will serve to inactivate traces of Zephiran in the sediment (19).

Discard the supernatant fluid; there will be sufficient residual buffer to permit resuspension of the sediment. Using a disposable Pasteur pipette, inoculate 3 drops of the sediment to each of the media to be employed.

Sodium lauryl sulfate method (9, 43)

Reagents. (i) Lauryl sulfate-sodium hydroxide: dissolve 30 g of pure sodium lauryl sulfate in 1 liter of distilled water at about 60 C. Add 10 g of NaOH. Keep at 37 C. (ii) Sulfuric or phosphoric acid with bromocresol purple: to prepare 0.09% sulfuric acid with bromocresol purple, add 0.9 ml of concentrated H_2SO_4 to 1 liter of distilled water; add 2 ml of a 1:250 solution of bromocresol purple; autoclave. To prepare phosphoric acid with bromocresol purple, add 1.5 ml of *O*-phosphoric acid to 1 liter of distilled water; add bromocresol purple and autoclave as above.

Procedure. To one part of sputum, add three parts of the lauryl sulfate-sodium hydroxide reagent. (It may be preferable to add two parts of sputum to three parts of digestant.) Shake on a Vortex mixer three times at about 10-min intervals. At 10 min after the third shaking, centrifuge at 3,000 rpm for 30 min. Discard the supernatant fluid; neutralize the sediment with H_2SO_4 or H_3PO_4 containing bromocresol purple. Plant on egg-containing medium. (The lecithin in egg media is known to inactivate residues of lauryl sulfate which would otherwise interfere with mycobacterial growth.)

INCUBATION AND INSPECTION OF CULTURES

Tube or bottle cultures

Tube or bottle cultures should be examined weekly for 6 weeks. They may be held an additional 4 weeks; if they are still negative at that time, they may be discarded. Reports are made as soon as identification has been made, or at 6 weeks. If subsequently growth occurs, a corrected report must be issued.

As soon as growth is macroscopically evident on any cultures, make smears and examine for pigmentation (see below) and other properties.

Plate cultures

Plates should be in plastic waterproof bags (see under acetyl-cysteine method). Each plate may be in its own sealed bag. However, it is usually more convenient to place as many as 10 to 12 plates in a bag and to use rubber bands or tape to hold down the twisted and folded-over tops. Place the bagged plates so that no moisture condenses on the lids. Ordinarily, this will be achieved by having the plates upside down, heat rising from below; in some incubators or in some locations in a given incubator, conditions may require a different placement. Examine at 5 to 7 days and subsequently after 2 to 3 weeks using microscope with 100× magnification of the growth on plates inverted on the stage. This examination with transmitted light is much the most important. However, some microcolony features are better seen with reflected light and stereomicroscope.

PROPERTIES USEFUL FOR IDENTIFICATION OF MYCOBACTERIAL PATHOGENS

Most mycobacterial pathogens may be identified by rate of growth, pigmentation, colony morphology, and one or two other properties. However, one should never rely on the results of a single test for identification. From Table 1, and on the basis of the initial observations of the type of growth, selection of appropriate tests for establishing species may be made. Individual strains may deviate from the characteristics of the species. Where no entry is made in Table 1, the property does not contribute to identification, or insufficient information is available.

More complete characterizations are given in the following sections.

Although the properties characterizing nonpathogens are also included in Table 1, identification of these species in the clinical laboratory is usually unnecessary. It is helpful, however, to recognize the similarity of some of these to the disease agents.

Microscopy

Microscopy is the first step in species identification. In addition to examination of the smear made of the specimen or its concentrate, observation must be made of stained preparations of growth obtained on culture. This is for (i) confirmation that observed growth is mycobacterial, (ii) the determination of possible contamination of the culture, and, least important, (iii) some indication of species. Examine smears for acid-fastness and cell shape. Acid-fastness is usually 100% (as with *M. tuberculosis*) but may be as little as 5% (as with rapid growers). The following cell shapes may be observed: characteristic bacillus long, broad, and cross-banded (as with *M. kansasii, M. gordonae*); characteristic bacillus short, but some long, thin bacilli may also be seen (as with *M. intracellulare; M. scrofulaceum*); characteristic bacillus long, thin, curved (as with *M. xenopi*).

Growth in relation to temperature

In most cases, it is unnecessary to obtain more complete data regarding growth-temperature relations than will have been seen in the routine procedures for primary culture isolation. Digests from specimens obtained from external areas of the body (rather than, for example, sputum) should have been planted for culture at 24 C and preferably also at 32 C, as well as at 35 C in a CO_2 atmosphere (1). Evidence of rapidly growing mycobacteria will commonly be seen at the first of the weekly inspections of cultures, although some strains exhibit their characteristic growth rate only on subculture. When more definite and complete information for species identification is needed, prepare a barely turbid suspension of the bacilli. From a 10^{-2} dilution of this, inoculate equally subcultures for incubation at different temperatures, such as 24, 32, 37, and 45 C. Examine for initial appearance of grossly visible colonies.

Rapid growth (in <1 week) at 24 and 37 C. If growth occurs also at 45 C, the strain will usually be other than *M. fortuitum*; make arylsulfatase and MacConkey agar and iron uptake tests.

Slow growth (2 or more weeks). (i) Growth at 37 C, none at 24 or 45 C (*M. tuberculosis, M. bovis*). (ii) Growth at 37 and 45 C, none at 24 C (*M. xenopi*, some *M. avium*). (iii) Growth at 37 C, slower at 24 C, negative at 45 C (*M. kansasii*). (iv) Growth at 32 and 24 C in 2 weeks none or more slowly at 37 C (*M. marinum*). (v) Growth at 32 C in >3 weeks, not at 24 or 37 C (*M. ulcerans*).

The temperature-growth rate relationships are important in the identification of *M. marinum* and *M. ulcerans*, and are useful for *M. xenopi*.

Colonies

The characteristics of colonies here listed are as seen by transmitted light on plates inverted on the stage of a low-power microscope, and with stereomicroscopic observation of erect plates (37). For most species, growth is better on 7H11 than on corn meal-glycerol (CG) agar (glycerol, 3%), but some species differences may be more readily seen on CG agar. On CG agar, tubercle bacilli fail to grow; *M. kansasii* grows poorly unless seeded heavily; filamentous extensions from bacillary colonies are usually better developed and more persistent on CG.

The essence of roughness is the cohesion of bacteria, usually in cords or strands; these are commonly serpentine. With a regular microscope, curving strands are readily seen in thin colonies, but, if colonies become thicker, light is diffracted so much by the stranding that the colonies appear dark or opaque. Smooth colonies of comparable thickness have a homogeneous texture, permitting light transmission; hence, they are translucent.

Colony characteristics to be noted for species identification. Note that most strains will show more than one colony type, e.g., predominantly smooth strains may show a few rough colonies.

1. Roughness
   a. Amount (R, RS, SR, S)
   b. Kinds
      Stranding or cording; serpentine or other pattern
      Nonstranded roughness
2. Shape
   Thin, umbonate, domed; eugonic
3. Rhizodes
   Filamentous or more or less massive growth of the colony into medium from colony center, or dispersed.
4. Filamentous extensions
   Some of these are rhizodes; some on the surface of the medium; others may be short aerial hyphae; some may be branched.
5. Crystals or other extrabacillary formations

Pigmentation

Colonies of mycobacteria, if definitely colored, owe this principally to carotenoid pigments ranging in color from yellow to red. Scotochromogenic strains form pigment in the dark and also in the light; commonly, more pigment is produced if growth occurs in a lighted incubator. Photochromogenic strains are stimulated to produce pigment by light exposure and, ordinarily, show no yellow pigmentation unless exposed to light under proper conditions: during their early growth and with good aeration of culture surface (36, 52). *M. kansasii* becomes definitely yellow 6 to 12 h after 1 h of exposure to bright light. *M. szulgai* is rather unique, being scotochromogenic if grown at 37 C but photochromogenic when grown at 25 C. During routine examination of cultures, if the first colonies to appear are nonpigmented, leave the cultures close to a bright incandescent or fluorescent light in the laboratory for 1 h or more. During this period, smears may be made and examined. Return cultures with loosened caps to incubator and examine the colonies the next morning for yellow pigmentation, evidence of photochromogenicity.

Carotene crystals are regularly formed only by photochromogenic *M. kansasii* and by *M. marinum*. Crystals may be seen as early as 2 to 3 weeks if growth has been in continuous light. Use of 100× magnification, or somewhat lower, with a stereomicroscope, is required.

Properties related to pigmentation are as follows: none; weak, not definitely yellow (*M. tuberculosis*); scotochromogenic (Group II, some IV); photochromogenic (*M. kansasii*); crystalline β-carotene produced (*M. kansasii*); small colonies nonpigmented, older and larger colonies yellow, not light-induced (some strains of *M. intracellulare*); some strains pigmented, some not; variable (*M. smegmatis*); may become green on media containing malachite green (*M. fortuitum*).

Arylsulfatase, 3-day

The 3-day arylsulfatase test (24, 50) is used mainly for rapid growers. With few exceptions, only *M. fortuitum* (includes *M. chelonei*) splits phenolphthalein from tripotassium phenolphthalein sulfate within 3 days.

Cultures. Prepare a barely turbid suspension.

Reagents. (i) Substrate: incorporate 1 ml of glycerol and 65 mg of tripotassium phenolphthalein disulfate (Nutritional Biochemicals Corp., Cleveland, Ohio) in 100 ml of melted Dubos oleic agar base. Dispense in 2-ml amounts to 18 by 60 mm screw-capped vials. Autoclave. Permit to harden in an upright position. (ii) Na_2CO_3, 1 M (10.6 g in water to make 100 ml).

Procedure. Inoculate with one drop of the bacillary suspension. Incubate at 37 C for 3 days. Add 1 ml of Na_2CO_3 solution and observe for pink coloration, indicating free phenolphthalein.

Catalase, drop method

Essentially all mycobacteria are catalase-positive. The only exceptions are some isoniazid-resistant mutants of *M. tuberculosis*, *M. gastri*, and some nonpathogenic, isoniazid-resistant strains of *M. kansasii*. The catalase drop test is very useful for quick and easy determination of significant isoniazid resistance in *M. tuberculosis* which, of course, ordinarily reflects prior contact with this drug.

Cultures. Any (usually ones suspected or known to be *M. tuberculosis*) may be tested. Note that some *colonies* may be positive, others negative. Ordinarily, only colonies on medium without drugs are tested.

Reagents. A 1:1 mixture of 10% Tween 80 and 30% hydrogen peroxide (Superoxol; Merck & Co., Rahway, N.J.). Prepare a fresh mixture for each day's use.

Procedure. Add a drop of the reagent to growth on slant or plate. Observe for the formation of bubbles (O_2) around the colonies. By the rate and amount of bubble production, one may judge whether the strain is high, low, or negative (see also semiquantitative test below).

Catalase after 68 C heating

This test for catalase (23) has value in conjunction with the niacin test for recognition of tubercle bacilli. A positive test definitely indicates a species other than *M. bovis*, *M. tuberculosis*, *M. africanum*, or *M. gastri*. The latter species are always negative, but some other species (see Table 1) may rarely be negative.

Cultures. Strains which are niacin-negative and others. Include as controls a known positive, and a known negative (*M. tuberculosis*).

Reagents. (i) A 1:1 mixture of 10% Tween 80 and 30% hydrogen peroxide (freshly prepared). (ii) Phosphate buffer, 0.067 M, pH 7: 61.1 ml of 0.067 M disodium phosphate, Na_2HPO_4 (9.47 g/liter), 38.9 ml of 0.067 M potassium acid phosphate, KH_2PO_4 (9.07 g/liter).

Procedure. Suspend several colonies in 0.5 ml of pH 7 phosphate buffer (0.067 M) in a 16 by 125 mm screw-cap tube. Place the tube in a water bath at 68 C for 20 min. Cool the suspension to room temperature and add 0.5 ml of the Tween-peroxide mixture. Observe for bubbling and record as positive or negative. Hold tubes for 20 min before discarding as negative.

Catalase, semiquantitative

The semiquantitative test for catalase (21,

53) has proved valuable in the separation of some species of mycobacteria. Two subgroups of *M. kansasii* have been recognized: one produces less than 45 mm of bubbles, whereas those strains more commonly associated with disease produce more than 45 mm of bubbles. *M. marinum*, the *M. avium* complex, *M. gastri*, *M. xenopi*, and tubercle bacilli also produce less than 45 mm of bubbles, but other species usually produce more than 45 mm of bubbles.

Cultures. Prepare a dilute bacillary suspension. Activity is unimportant. Include uninoculated reagent control, a known strain of *M. tuberculosis* (<45 mm control), and a strain of *M. gordonae* (>45 mm control).

Reagent and medium. (i) Freshly prepared 1:1 mixture of 10% Tween 80 and 30% hydrogen peroxide. (ii) L-J butt tubes (available from Difco): dispense 5 ml of L-J medium in 20 by 150 mm screw-cap tubes. Inspissate with tubes in upright position in a water bath at 85 C for 60 min. Do not substitute agar medium. Remove tubes and incubate at 35 to 37 C overnight to check for sterility of medium.

Procedure. Inoculate L-J butt with 0.2 ml of the bacterial suspension. Incubate for 2 weeks at 35 to 37 C with the cap loose. Add 1 ml of the Tween-peroxide mixture to the L-J culture and measure the column of bubbles in millimeters after 5 min in an upright position at room temperature. Note the two categories: those that produce more and those that produce less than 45 mm of bubbles.

Iron uptake

In the iron uptake test (53), only rapid growers, such as *M. fortuitum* and *M. phlei*, are positive.

Cultures. L-J slants inoculated with one drop of barely turbid aqueous suspension of the strain to be tested.

Reagent. Aqueous ferric ammonium citrate, 20%. Dispense in small containers. Autoclave.

Procedure. Incubate the L-J slants at 37 C until definite growth appears. Add the sterile citrate solution, about one drop for each 1 ml of L-J medium. Incubate for a maximum of 21 days. Record the appearance of rusty-brown color in colonies and tan discoloration of the medium as positive.

MacConkey agar, growth test

Growth on MacConkey agar is used to distinguish the *M. fortuitum* complex from other species (13, 21). Only species of this complex grow within 5 days.

Cultures. Tween albumin broth (TAB) cultures 7 to 10 days old. Include known strains of *M. fortuitum* and *M. phlei* as positive and negative controls.

Medium. Prepare from dehydrated base; pour plates, about 15 ml each.

Procedure. Plant MacConkey plate with a 3-mm loopful of the TAB culture, streaking to obtain isolated colonies. Examine for growth after 5 and 11 days. Only strains of the *M. fortuitum* complex grow to the end of the streak. Some other mycobacteria may show some growth where the inoculum is very heavy.

Niacin test

The distinctiveness of abundant niacin production by the species *M. tuberculosis* has been widely demonstrated. Niacin is discharged from bacilli into the medium, and, if the medium is not liquid, an aqueous extract of the medium around the colonies is tested. If the test is negative, and other properties indicate *M. tuberculosis* (such as nitrate strongly reduced, catalase destroyed after heating at 68 C), the niacin test should be repeated with a more luxuriant culture. Niacin-negative *M. tuberculosis* strains are exceedingly rare. Also rare are positive niacin tests with strains of other mycobacterial species, except the photochromogenic *M. simiae* (*habana*). Most of these strains may be immediately recognized as other than tubercle bacilli (by rapid growth or by pigmentation). In a clinical laboratory, there is no advantage in doing niacin tests on strains which are scotochromogenic, photochromogenic (except *M. simiae* [*habana*]), or rapid growers. However, the possibility of individual strains of nonpigmented slow growers other than *M. tuberculosis* being niacin-positive must not be ignored.

Some avoid doing niacin tests because of the toxicity of one of the reagents: cyanogen bromide (tear gas). Its easily recognized odor is a warning. The less obvious danger of pipetting tubercle bacilli is probably greater. Both dangers are well controlled by use of an adequately ventilated safety hood. A paper-strip method for niacin determination has the advantages of simplicity and of much lessened exposure to tear gas (no handling of cyanogen bromide). The paper-strip method is fully dependable (16, 31, 57).

Acceptable niacin test methods

Cultures. Luxuriant growth on egg medium or on 7H11 enriched with L-asparagine, 0.25% (12), or 0.1% potassium aspartate (18). One- or two-week-old cultures in Proskauer-Beck (P-B) medium with 5% serum also are highly recommended. Include a known culture of *M. tuberculosis* and an uninoculated medium control.

Reagents. (i) Cyanogen bromide (CNBr), 10%. Working in a hood and wearing gloves, place about 2 tablespoons of pure CNBr in a tared Erlenmeyer flask. Weigh. Add enough water to make a 10% solution. When fully dissolved, transfer to a brown bottle and cap tightly. Include on the label a caution to avoid inhalation of fumes and contact with skin or mucous membranes. Keep both the solution and the stock bottle (solid) in refrigerator.

(ii) Aniline, 4%, in alcohol. Add 4 ml of aniline to 96 ml of 95% ethyl alcohol. Keep in a brown bottle in a refrigerator. If pure, this solution is clear and colorless. If it is brown or becomes so, discard it. Pure aniline may be obtained by redistillation.

Tube or spot-plate test (38, 39). Working in a hood, layer 0.5 to 1.5 ml of sterile water over the medium around the colonies. If growth is confluent, cut through it so that the water comes in contact with the underlying medium. Let stand at 36 C for 10 to 15 min (rarely an extended extraction time of 60 min may be necessary) and then remove a portion (0.5 ml or 2 drops) to a small test tube or to a porcelain spot plate. Add an equal volume of the aniline solution, and make note of any color; no yellow color should be evident. Add cyanogen bromide, same volume as of aniline. An immediately developing yellow color indicates niacin production. Add an excess of NaOH to eliminate toxicity before discarding the tests. The porcelain plate may be reconditioned by placing in boiling water for8a few minutes.

Test in P-B medium (14). Add 1 ml of aniline solution followed in 5 min by the addition of 1 ml of cyanogen bromide. If no yellow color develops in the 7-day-old culture, test a second culture which has incubated for 14 days. The yellow color of scotochromogens or photochromogens will not be mistaken for a positive niacin test because the pigment of these is not water-soluble.

Paper-strip method for niacin (57). Commercially available strips (niacin test strips available from General Diagnostics Division, Warner-Lambert Co., Morris Plains, N.J. [Pathotec-Niacin], or Difco Laboratories, Detroit, Mich. [Niacin Test Strips, TB]) may be used. Follow directions provided with the strips. Some investigators have found that a 2-h period for extraction of niacin (rather than the recommended 30 min) yields more strongly positive reactions for *M. tuberculosis* without causing false-positive reactions for other species.

Nitrate reduction

The nitrate reduction test (21, 22, 48) is valuable for the identification of *M. tuberculosis*, *M. kansasii*, *M. szulgai*, certain nonpathogens of Group III, and *M. fortuitum*, which are nitrate reductase-positive. *M. bovis*, *M. marinum*, *M. simiae* (*habana*), *the M. avium* complex, *M. xenopi*, *M. gastri*, and *M. chelonei* are negative or only very weakly positive.

Cultures. Should be 3 to 4 weeks old except rapid growers, which may be 2 to 4 weeks old. Include nitrate-positive culture (*M. kansasii*) and a reagent control without bacilli.

Reagents. (i) A 1:2 dilution of concentrated HCl; (ii) 0.2% aqueous solution sulfanilamide; (iii) 0.1% aqueous *N*-naphthylethylenediamine dihydrochloride; (iv) 0.01 M solution of $NaNO_3$ in 0.022 M phosphate buffer, pH 7 (Difco nitrate broth may be substituted); (v) powdered zinc.

Store solutions at room temperature. They remain stable for several weeks. If either reagent ii or iii changes in color, discard it and prepare a fresh solution.

Procedure. Place a few drops of sterile distilled water in a 16 by 125 mm screw-cap tube. Grind in one loopful or one spadeful of growth. Add 2 ml of $NaNO_3$ solution. Shake the mixture, and incubate it in a water bath at 37 C for 2 h. Add 1 drop of reagent i, 2 drops of reagent ii, and 2 drops of reagent iii. Examine immediately for development of a pink to red color contrasting with the reagent control. To all negative tubes, add a pinch of powdered zinc. This reduces nitrate to nitrite. Hence, formation of a red color here indicates that the negative reading was valid.

Color standards. If needed, color standards for the nitrate reduction test may be prepared (47).

Paper-strip method for nitrate reduction (34). Commercially available paper strips (Patho-Tec-Nitrate Reduction strips from General Diagnostics Division, Warner-Lambert Co., Morris Plains, N.J., or Nitrate Test Strips from Difco Laboratories, Detroit, Mich.) also are satisfactory for this test. Follow directions provided with the strips.

Sodium chloride tolerance

Of the slow growers, only *M. triviale* grows; of the rapid growers, only *M. chelonei* fails to grow in the presence of 5% NaCl (15, 21).

Cultures. Barely turbid suspension.

Substrate. American Thoracic Society (ATS) or Lowenstein-Jensen (LJ) medium containing NaCl, 5%. ATS or LJ medium without salt for control.

Procedure. Seed media with 0.1 ml of the bacterial suspension. Incubate at 37 C. Read for growth or no growth at 4 weeks.

Tellurite reduction

Reduction of colorless tellurite salt to black metallic tellurium within 3 to 4 days is the distinctive property of the *M. avium* complex strains (17, 21, 22). Of other mycobacteria tested, only rapid growers are also positive within this period.

Cultures. Cultures 7 days old, in 5 ml of Middlebrook 7H9 liquid medium in 20 by 150 mm screw-cap tubes. Should be fairly turbid, indicating active growth.

Reagent. A 0.2% aqueous solution (0.1 g in 50 ml of distilled water) of potassium tellurite. After dissolving the salt in water, dispense in 2- to 5-ml amounts and sterilize in an autoclave at 121 C for 10 min. To avoid contamination, use only one tube of tellurite solution for a series of tests performed on 1 day and discard the remainder.

Procedure. Add 2 drops of the tellurite solution to each culture and return the cultures to the incubator. Examine daily for 4 or more days.

Thiophene-2-carboxylic acid hydrazide

The thiophene-2-carboxylic acid hydrazide (T2H) test is used for distinguishing *M. bovis* from *M. tuberculosis* and other species. Only *M. bovis* is susceptible to low concentrations of this compound (3).

Substrate. Dubos oleic acid agar with albumin complex. Incorporate T2H (Aldrich Chemical Co., Milwaukee, Wis.), 10 μg/ml, into one portion. Dispense in 4-ml amounts as slants.

Procedure. Prepare a barely turbid suspension of the organisms to be tested in sterile water. Dilute this suspension 1:1,000 with sterile water. Plant 3 drops of the 1:1,000 suspension on the T2H and control media, and incubate at 37 C. Record the time when definite growth is observed on the control slant. Maintain the T2H-containing slant for an additional 3 weeks unless definite growth appears earlier. Record the organism as resistant if growth on the T2H medium is greater than 1% of the growth on the control. If the control slant has confluent growth, assume that this equals 10^4 organisms.

Tween hydrolysis

Enzymatic hydrolysis of Tween 80 (polyoxyethylene derivative of sorbitan monooleate) releases oleic acid, resulting in a change in color of neutral red (54). The test is important for mycobacteria of Groups II and III. Strains of these two groups which decompose Tween readily are of no clinical significance (rare exceptions). *M. scrofulaceum* strains are negative; *M. gordonae* strains, positive. *M. avium* complex and *M. xenopi* are negative; other members of Group III are positive.

Cultures. Actively growing, from solid medium. Include a strain of *M. kansasii* as positive control, and an uninoculated reagent control.

Reagents. (i) Phosphate buffer, 0.067 M, pH 7, 100 ml. (ii) Tween 80, 0.5 ml. (iii) Neutral red stock solution, 2 ml: 0.1% aqueous solution of actual dye content (e.g., if actual dye content is 85%, dissolve 0.1 g in 85 ml rather than 100 ml of water).

Mix the three reagents. Dispense in 4-ml amounts in 16 by 125 mm screw-cap tubes and autoclave at 121 C for 15 min. Incubate at 35 to 37 C overnight to check for sterility. Store in a refrigerator and protect from light. The substrate is not stable longer than 2 weeks at 4 to 10 C.

Procedure. Emulsify a 3-mm loopful of growth in a tube of substrate. Incubate at 35 to 37 C. Observe tubes for a color change from amber (straw) to red at 4 h, and at 5 and 10 days.

Interpretation. Record the number of days required for the first appearance of pink color. If this is less than 5 days, the test is positive; if 5 to 10 days, doubtful (±); if no change in color occurs by the 10th day, the test is negative.

Urease

Determination of ability of a culture to hydrolyze urea often helps in the characterization of mycobacterial strains which are aberrant in some other property. For example, *M. scrofulaceum* is urease-positive, whereas members of the *M. avium* complex are negative, and the urease test will be of help in recognizing the occasionally encountered pigmented strain of *M. intracellulare*. Similarly, *M. bovis* is urease-positive, and this test would help distinguish a drug-resistant *M. bovis* from an *M. avium* or *M. intracellulare*. The method described here is a modification of the procedure of Toda et al. (45).

Cultures. Actively growing, from solid medium. Include a strain of *M. kansasii* as a positive control, and an uninoculated reagent control.

Reagents. Mix 1 part of urea agar base concentrate (Difco) (or equivalent product) with 9 parts sterile water. Do *not* add agar. Dispense in 4-ml amounts to 16 by 125 mm screw-capped tubes and store in the cold.

Procedure. Emulsify the equivalent of a 3-mm loop of growth in a tube of substrate. Incubate at 35 to 37 C, observing for a color change from amber to pink or red. Discard after 3 days.

Interpretation. Change to pink or red within 3 days is recorded as a positive reaction.

IMMUNOLOGY—PHAGE SUSCEPTIBILITY

Fluorescent-antibody, double diffusion in gel, red cell or particle agglutination, and complement fixation tests all have been used with some success in differentiating species or in characterizing antibodies in patients' sera (or both), but no serological procedures for routine use in clinical laboratories have yet been standardized.

Simultaneously performed skin tests, using standardized purified protein derivatives from different mycobacterial species, have proved useful for identification of bacilli inoculated into guinea pigs (8, 26). In contrast to experimental animals, where single infecting agents can be documented, the possibility of multiple sensitizing infections in man often results in unpredictable cross-reactions which are difficult to interpret (33).

Agglutination tests with rabbit antisera are useful for differentiation of most strains of *M. kansasii*, *M. marinum*, *M. avium*, *M. intracellulare*, *M. scrofulaceum*, *M. szulgai*, some *M. gordonae*, *M. fortuitum*, and *M. chelonei* (40).

Many phages have been found to lyse various species of mycobacteria, but general application of this tool in the clinical laboratory has not been attained. As is true also for serotyping, phage typing may provide valuable information of epidemiological importance.

SPECIES IDENTIFICATION

Mycobacterium leprae, M. ulcerans, M. marinum

Any one of these three species may be present in specimens from a superficial body area. Since these bacteria rarely grow at 37 C or above, cultures planted with such specimens should be incubated at 32 ± 1 C, as well as (other cultures) at 37 C. *M. leprae* does not grow in vitro. Diagnosis of *M. leprae* is presumptive, dependent on correlation of typical leprosy lesions with their content of acid-fast bacilli. These are abundant in lepromatous tissue and very sparse in tuberculoid tissue (2). *M. leprae* may be present in discharges from mouth or nose. *M. ulcerans* or *M. marinum* are never to be expected in sputum or gastric lavage. *M. marinum* grows readily at 30 to 32 C on any medium commonly exployed for mycobacteria. *M. ulcerans* grows much more slowly, requiring 6 to 9 weeks on initial isolation, and may fail to grow on some media. All three species grow in footpads of mice, but the generation time for *M. leprae* is too long to make mouse inoculation of any significance in the clinical laboratory. Generation time of *M. ulcerans* is intermediate, being much longer than that of *M. marinum*, which causes swelling of footpads in <2 weeks. *M. marinum* resembles *M. kansasii* in photochromogenicity and in cell and colony morphology, but is easily distinguished by its source (superficial lesion), its more rapid growth at 31 C than at 37 C, or no growth at 37 C, and usually by its negative nitrate reduction test.

Mycobacterium tuberculosis

These bacilli are recognized by their slowly developing, rough, eugonic colonies (see Fig. 2) of characteristic buff tint, and by their production of niacin. On the most favorable media and with other optimal conditions, colonies are recognizable in less than 3 weeks, but some strains, especially drug-resistant ones and those growing on suboptimal media, may require 4 to 6 weeks or longer. Characteristic microcolonies may be readily recognized in less than a week by microscopic observation of growth on 7H11 plates (37). The variations seen in hue and texture of colonies of tubercle bacilli on a given medium are readily learned, but are difficult to describe. Similarity to the surface roughness, color, and texture of cauliflower has been noted. In preparation of smears from cultures, poor dispersability is recognized. Serpentine cord formation (as best seen in growth from liquid medium lacking a wetting agent) is typical, but it must be noted that rough strains of many mycobacterial species will exhibit stranding of bacilli (25, 37). If the niacin test is positive and other properties mentioned are in conformity, *M. tuberculosis* may be reported. If the niacin test is negative, a number of other tests should be made, including repetition of the niacin test on a more luxuriant culture. Other confirmatory properties: *M. tuberculosis* reduces nitrate, loses catalase activity after heating at 68 C, and usually is sensitive to streptomycin, *p*-aminosalicylic acid, and isoniazid, unless from long-treated patients. If a strain of *M. tuberculosis* is isoniazid-resistant, it may be found to be catalase-negative and have reduced or no virulence for guinea pigs.

Mycobacterium bovis

M. bovis grows poorly or not at all on some media favorable for *M. tuberculosis*. The Jensen modification of Lowenstein egg medium supports better growth of *M. bovis* than does 7H10 agar. Media most favorable for *M. bovis* contain pyruvate, as 0.2% $NaCO_2COCH_3$ (6). Poor or no growth on medium containing more than 1% glycerol is one of the distinguishing properties of *M. bovis*, especially on primary isolation. Colonies are colorless, low, small, and smooth-appearing on egg medium. On 7H11, colonies are very thin and often show little or no stranding, but, if pyruvate has been added to the medium, colonies show serpentine cords like eugonic *M. tuberculosis*. The following properties of *M. bovis* are useful for distinguishing it from *M. tuberculosis*. Nitrate is not reduced and the niacin test is usually negative. *M. bovis* is usually resistant to pyrazinamide but is susceptible to 1 μg of thiophene-2-carboxylic acid hydrazide per ml (unless it is isoniazid-resistant). Intravenous inoculation of rabbits with 0.01 mg (moist weight) of *M. bovis* (isoniazid-susceptible) results in progressive disease, leading to death in 8 to 10 weeks; *M. tuberculosis* in the same dosage produces only regressive disease. In contrast to *M. tuberculosis*, *M. bovis* is nicotinamidase-negative.

Mycobacterium kansasii

M. kansasii occurs in several forms: photochromogenic, high catalase; photochromogenic, low catalase; scotochromogenic; and nonchromogenic. All of these except the first are very rare in clinical specimens. Finding the very distinctive dependence upon light exposure for carotene formation, usually coupled with carotene crystal production (see Fig. 3C), in a strain having a growth rate similar to (or slightly more rapid than) that of *M. tuberculosis* at 37 C is sufficient for reporting *M. kansasii*. Additional properties: growth occurs at 25 C (cf. tubercle bacilli, no growth) but very slowly (cf. *M. marinum*, faster). Young cells are characteristically long, and some are broad and cross-banded (a structural evidence of utilization of fatty acid material of the medium). Colonies are characteristically intermediate between fully rough and fully smooth. The centers are elevated. In the thinner margins, curving strands of bacilli may usually be seen with a low-power microscope. Some strains, however, are almost fully smooth and others are completely rough. Nitrate is reduced; Tween 80, urea, and nicotinamide are hydrolyzed. The catalase activity of disease-related strains is vigorous: >45 mm in the semiquantitative test. Rarely, strains not related to disease may be encountered. These

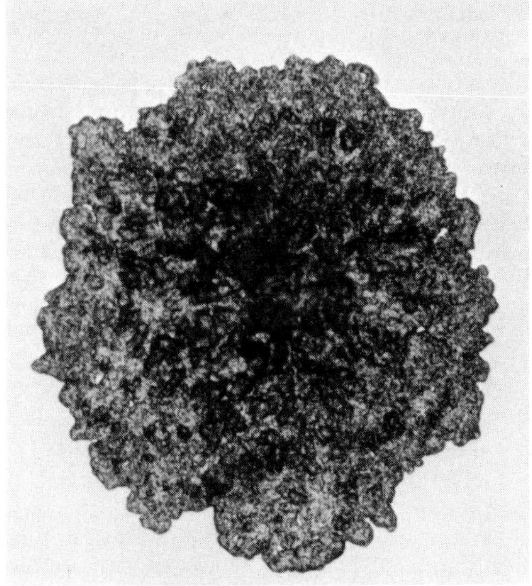

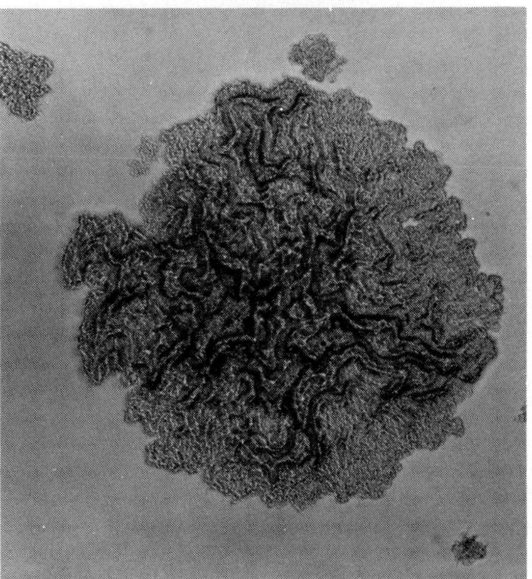

FIG. 2. *Mycobacterium tuberculosis. Mature (top) and immature (bottom) colonies, showing serpentine cording.* ×*10.*

have usually been found to be low in catalase activity (51).

The very rare scotochromogenic strains of *M. kansasii* (*M. kansasii* var. *aurantiacum*; 42) and those which fail to form pigment even if grown in the light (*M. kansasii* var. *album*) are characterized by all the properties of *M. kansasii* except pigmentation. Almost all strains of *M. kansasii* (not the fully rough ones) can be identified by specific agglutination (40); such strains also usually are susceptible to Redmond's AG1 phage.

Mycobacterium scrofulaceum, M. szulgai, and M. gordonae

Subdivisions of the slowly growing scotochromogens are not well defined. Some strains of the *M. avium* complex may be scotochromogenic, especially after prolonged incubation. The Tween 80 hydrolysis test provides initial separation of these organisms: *M. gordonae* is usually positive in 5 days and *M. szulgai* is slowly positive (usually >7 days), whereas *M. scrofulaceum* is not positive even after 10 days. *M. szulgai* is the only one of this group to give a positive nitrate reduction test. The urease test (45) will separate *M. scrofulaceum* both from *M. gordonae* and from occasional pigmented strains of the *M. avium* complex. *M. gordonae* is rarely, if ever, associated with disease. *M. scrofulaceum* is more commonly associated with disease, especially cervical adenitis in children, and *M. szulgai* has been associated with pulmonary disease, cervical adenitis, and olecranon bursitis (29). Both *M. gordonae* and *M. scrofulaceum* commonly occur as nonpathogens; however, less is known about the saprophytic characteristics of *M. szulgai*.

Mycobacterium intracellulare—Mycobacterium avium (M. avium complex)

These very similar species are not usually distinguished from one another, and need not be. They are characterized by slowly growing, thin, transparent, homogeneous, smooth colonies. A very small proportion of *M. intracellulare* colonies may be partially or fully rough (see Fig. 4C); for *M. avium*, the proportion of rough colonies may often be greater. After subculture, transformation to more eugonic-type colonies may occur, the centers becoming prominently domed (see Fig. 4A, B). Eventually, all colonies may be hemispherical. Usually nonpigmented, they may become yellow with age, particularly the dome-shaped colonies; rarely, others may be pigmented from the onset of detectable growth. Correlated with these colony variations are changes in other properties, notably of pathogenicity (7). Cells are commonly very short, although under certain conditions long, thin bacilli are seen. All strains are Tween-hydrolysis negative, and most reduce tellurite in 3 days. Although *M. intracellulare* may cause serious tuberculosis-like disease, most difficult to treat, it may also occur in clinical specimens as a nonpathogen.

Other species of slowly growing nonphotochromogens, not known as pathogens but encountered in the clinical laboratory, differ from the *M. avium* complex in hydrolyzing Tween in

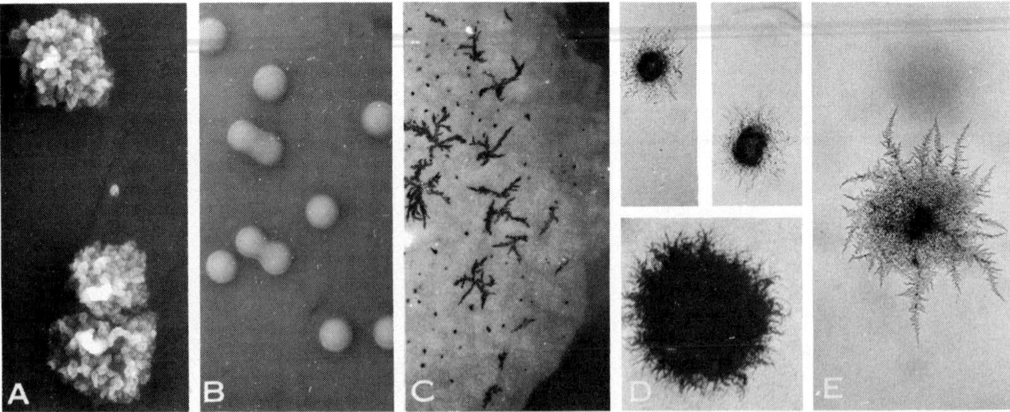

FIG. 3. (*A*) *Mycobacterium chelonei. Rough, serpentine-corded colonies of a rapid grower.* (*B*) *M. chelonei. Smooth colonies.* (*C*) *Crystals of β-carotene, lying on a colony of M. kansaii grown in continuous light (7H10). ×100. The crystals are dark red. The dark spots are other crystals embedded in the colony.* (*D*) *Colonies of two strains of M. xenopi, showing more or less matted filamentous extensions.* (*E*) *One colony of M. fortuitum on corn meal-glycerol-agar. Branching is commonly less extensive than that shown here, but is of the same character.* (*A and B, courtesy of Stottmeier and Bonicke.*)

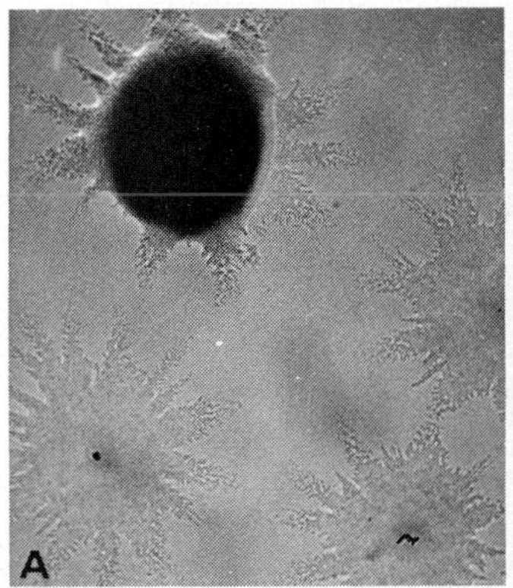

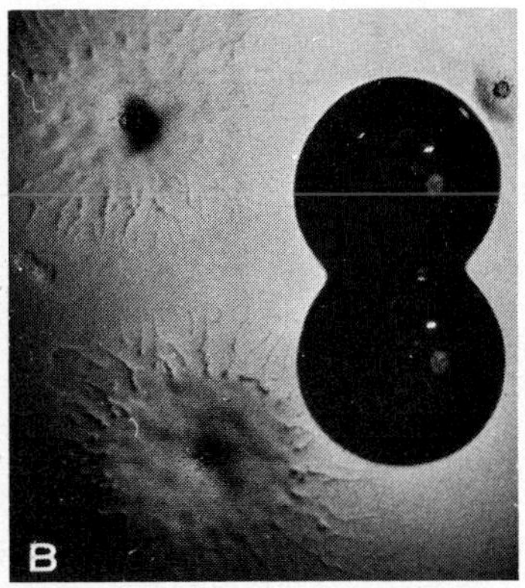

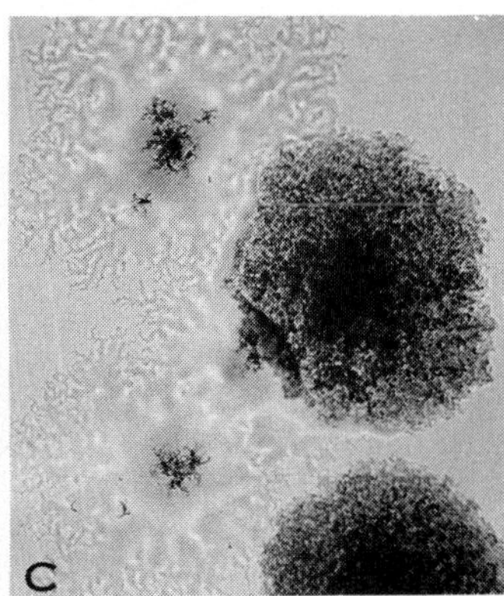

FIG. 4. *Colonies of Mycobacterium intracellulare (Battey bacilli) as seen with low power (50×) on plated media (7H10 or corn meal-glycerol-agar). In primary culture, all or almost all colonies are smooth, thin (T). On subculture, a variable proportion become thick, domed (D). Uncommonly, rough (R) colonies are seen. (A) T, asteroid colonies and one (TD) with a domed center (dark). (B) T and D colonies. (The latter, dark here, are white as seen by reflected light.) (C) T and R colonies. Dark markings in the centers of T colonies are nodular or filamentous colony extensions into the medium ("rhizodes").*

5 days or less, and in failure to reduce tellurite. Some of these nonpathogens have distinctive colonies. Strains of the *M. avium* complex and *M. triviale* may have colonies so rough as to be confused with tubercle bacilli, but these strains are niacin-negative, Tween-positive, and resistant to the tuberculosis drugs. Strains of *M. triviale* are distinguished from other nonphotochromogenic bacteria by their ability to grow in 5% sodium chloride. For other properties of the nonpathogenic species, including *M. gastri* and *M. terrae*, see Table 1.

Mycobacterium xenopi

This species will be recognized by its very slow growth, very small erect colonies, characteristic yellow color, failure to grow at 25 C, and greater susceptibility to drugs than is seen with other nontuberculosis mycobacteria, e.g., susceptibility to 1 μg of isoniazid per ml. Persistant branching filamentous extensions (as seen with a low-power microscope) around the circular colonies on CG agar or other plated media are very distinctive. Rough colonies usually exhibit aerial hyphae, as can be seen with a stereomicroscope. Growth is better at 41 C than at 37 C, and does not occur at 25 C. Occasional colonies are white, having no pigment.

Mycobacterium fortuitum, M. chelonei (M. fortuitum complex)

These species are recognized by rapid growth, rough or smooth colonies, absence of definitely yellow pigment (but sometimes green from malachite green dye in such media as Lowenstein-Jensen), positive 3-day arylsulfatase test, and growth on MacConkey agar. Very characteristic of *M. fortuitum* are branching filamentous extensions from colonies on CG agar, short aerial hyphae as seen with stereomicroscope on rough colonies, and full resistance to drugs which are regularly effective against *M. tuberculosis*. *M. chelonei* lacks filamentous extensions typical of *M. fortuitum* (37). Of further value, *M. fortuitum* is positive in nitrate reductase whereas *M. chelonei* is negative; most *M. fortuitum* strains are positive in iron uptake, whereas *M. chelonei* commonly is negative.

DRUG SUSCEPTIBILITY TESTING

Most newly diagnosed cases of tuberculosis will be treated with two or more of the five primary treatment drugs, isoniazid, streptomycin, *p*-aminosalicylic acid, ethambutol, and rifampin. Although it is desirable to test the susceptibility of a patient's bacilli to these drugs, it is not usually necessary to await the results of these tests to institute an *original* course of therapy. If the patient has received prior antituberculous chemotherapy, however, it is most important to determine the drug susceptibility pattern, as it is among *retreatment* cases that drug resistance is most commonly seen. In either case, if the drug regimen selected has not converted the patient's sputum to a negative status within a few months, there is the possibility that a drug-resistant organism is emerging, and susceptibility tests should be repeated.

Conventional diffusion techniques, in which

bacterial susceptibility to a given drug is measured in terms of a zone of inhibition surrounding a disk are not suitable for mycobacteria, because their very slow growth permits complete dispersal of the drug in the medium. As will be mentioned later, this fact has permitted development of a simplified method for preparation of drug-containing media.

The generally accepted methods for determining drug susceptibility of mycobacteria are based on growth on solid medium. Success depends on awareness of several aspects of this process.

(i) Medium composition must be such that minimal inactivation of drug occurs. Use of Middlebrook's 7H10 or 7H11 medium in place of Lowenstein or other egg media eliminates binding of drugs to large-molecule organic material, and also eliminates problems associated with inspissation.

(ii) Drugs vary in stability, and drug containing media may change potency on exposure to extremes of pH, temperature, prolonged storage, or drying out of the media. Drug-containing media should be stored in a refrigerator, shielded from light, and protected from evaporation, for no longer than 4 weeks after preparation. In view of the simplicity of preparing test media by the disk method to be described below, it should not be necessary to stockpile large amounts of prepared medium. Include a culture of well-established drug susceptibility as a control in every test to demonstrate the activity of drugs in the media used. The drug-susceptible *M. tuberculosis* strain H37Rv is satisfactory for this purpose.

(iii) Since the observed drug susceptibility result is a comparison of amounts of growth on control and drug-containing media, the inoculum for each culture must be of demonstrated uniformity. This may be shown by the amount of growth on two control cultures seeded with different dilutions of inoculum. Homogenization of the inoculum and avoidance of large clumps are essential. The inoculum must be heavy enough to result in at least 100 colonies on a control medium, thus providing for statistically significant data. The inoculum must not be so heavy that confluent growth covers the surfaces of both control cultures, for in this case even a very small proportion of drug-resistant bacilli ($<1\%$) may result in the presence of a large enough number of colonies on the drug-containing media to suggest more resistance than is actually present. It is useful to employ an inoculum which will permit the expression of resistance as less than or greater than 1% of the population of cells examined. This is because extensive experience has shown that when more than about 1% of a bacillary population has become resistant to a drug it does not continue to be useful; i.e., the 1% soon becomes the predominant form, nearly 100%. A native population contains far fewer than 1% of organisms resistant to any of the commonly employed drugs.

(iv) If susceptibility tests are made from cultures having discrete colonies, the inoculum must be prepared from a fully representative selection; all colony types seen, not just the large easily reached ones, should be sampled. The portion of a patient's population of bacilli which is drug-resistant may be slower to grow or may have smaller colonies.

(v) Since modification of the proportion of resistant bacteria may occur with in vitro subculture, direct susceptibility tests, made by use of the patients' (treated) specimens for inocula, are preferred whenever smear examination reveals acid-fast bacilli. Direct susceptibility tests also have the advantage of earliest possible reporting. However, the direct test may be unsatisfactory because of contamination or absence of growth.

(vi) Serious consequences may result from a false report of drug resistance, for it may lead to the substitution of secondary drugs which usually involve more discomfort and danger to the patient from drug toxicity, as well as greatly increased expense.

Drug media. In the past, it was necessary to prepare multiple batches of agar media and incorporate different concentrations of stock solutions of each of the drugs to be employed into these batches. This was both cumbersome and wasteful. The method of Wayne and Krasnow (55), in which disks containing standardized amounts of drugs are placed in individual quadrants of petri dishes, and measured amounts of drug-free 7H10 or 7H11 agar are pipetted over the disks, permits preparation of just the number of plates needed for immediate use. This technique also eliminates labeling errors, as the disks carry identification codes so the drug and concentration in a quadrant are apparent at a glance. The reliability of this method has been established (10; unpublished data), and the results have been shown to be comparable to those achieved by the older methods.

Paper disks containing appropriate concentrations of the primary antituberculous drugs are now commercially available. Dispense disks aseptically to individual sectors of *quadrant* petri dishes, centering the disks in the quadrants (see Table 2). Prepare 7H10 agar from 7H10 agar base and OADC (oleic acid, albumin, dextrose, and catalase) enrichment, taking care not to overheat the base during sterilization. A 50-ml amount of medium will be needed for the 10 quadrants to be used (note that quadrants III and IV of plate 3 receive no medium). Dispense 5.0 ml of medium to all four quadrants of plates 1 and 2, and to quadrants I and II of plate 3. Incubate the plates overnight to permit uniform diffusion of drug and to confirm sterility of medium. The medium may then be used immediately, or stored for a maximum of 4 weeks. Evaporation does occur, even on cold storage, resulting in some change in drug concentration, so it is best to use fresh medium whenever possible.

Inoculum for direct method. The direct method may be used if acid-fast bacilli are seen on the smear of the digest of the clinical specimen. Make dilutions of the sediment according to the schedule given in Table 3, and inoculate each quadrant with 0.1 ml.

Indirect method. In some cases, it will be necessary to perform susceptibility studies by inoculating from a previously grown culture. If the culture is fairly young or has not been stored for a long time, the inoculum may be prepared by scraping colonies from the surface of the medium, taking care to sample all parts of the cultures. Suspend the bacterial mass in about 4 ml of Dubos Tween albumin broth containing three or four sterile small glass beads, and place on a Vortex mixer for about 1 min, using precautions to obtain only swirling centrifugal mixing, not churning, which results in aerosol production. Let stand for 15 min or longer. Dilute the suspension in another portion of Tween albumin broth until it is just barely turbid. From this barely turbid suspension, prepare 10^{-2} and 10^{-4} dilutions. Plant 0.1 ml of the 10^{-2} dilution in control quadrant 1 and in each of the drug-containing quadrants. Plant 0.1 ml of the 10^{-4} dilution in control quadrant 2.

If the culture which is to be tested is quite old, it may be necessary to grow it in Dubos Tween albumin broth to prepare the inoculum, although it is undesirable to add this extra step if it can be avoided. Treat the culture in Dubos broth then as if it were a bacterial suspension as described above.

Incubation and reading. Incubate the plates at 37 C in an atmosphere of 5 to 10% CO_2, and read weekly for 3 weeks. Record the amount of growth as follows: innumerable to confluent, +++ to ++++; approximately 100 to 200 colonies, ++; 50 to 100 colonies, +; fewer than 50, actual count.

In most cases, it will be possible to estimate the proportion of resistant colonies as greater than or fewer than 1% of the control population when this schedule of inoculation and reading is employed. Thus, if growth on a drug quadrant *exceeds* the growth on the second dilution control (i.e., control no. 2), then more than 1% of the population is resistant. In only rare instances should there be an ambiguous result, and in such cases the tests should be repeated. *Report at 3 weeks*, or *earlier* if clearly recognizable growth occurs on drug-containing as well as on control media.

Secondary drug susceptibility testing

It is recommended that determination of resistance to secondary drugs (capreomycin, cycloserine, ethionamide, kanamycin, viomycin, pyrazinamide) be limited to a few reference laboratories. In general, the media and methods for testing susceptibility to the secondary drugs are the same as those employed for the primary drugs.

TABLE 2. *Distribution of drug-containing disks for susceptibility tests*

Plate no.	Quadrant no.	Drug	Amt (μg) per disk	Final drug concn (μg/ml)
1	I	(Control no. 1)	—	0
	II	Isoniazid	1	0.2
	III	Isoniazid	5	1.0
	IV	Ethambutol	25	5.0
2	I	(Control no. 2)	—	0
	II	Streptomycin	10	2.0
	III	Streptomycin	50	10.0
	IV	Rifampin	5	1.0
3	I	*p*-Aminosalicylic acid	10	2.0
	II	*p*-Aminosalicylic acid	50	10.0
	III	—	—	—
	IV	—	—	—

TABLE 3. *Dilution of concentrate for inocula*

No. of acid-fast bacilli per oil immersion field	Control quadrant 1	Control quadrant 2	Drug quadrants
Less than 1	Undiluted	10^{-2}	Undiluted
1–10	10^{-1}	10^{-3}	10^{-1}
More than 10	10^{-2}	10^{-4}	10^{-2}

In general, in performing susceptibility tests on mycobacteria other than *M. tuberculosis* or *M. bovis*, it is best to plant both dilutions of inoculum on drug as well as on control media, because of a tendency of heavily inoculated drug quadrants to yield heavy overgrowth, making it most difficult to interpret results.

ANIMAL TESTING

The guinea pig has virtually no resistance to infection with *M. tuberculosis* and *M. bovis*. Theoretically, one virulent bacillus will cause progressive, fatal disease. The guinea pig, moreover, tends to tolerate specimen commensals that are likely to contaminate cultures. It is possible, then, to employ for guinea pig inoculation a less severe decontamination procedure. This favors a higher survival rate of the mycobacteria in guinea pigs and may result in more positive results than are obtainable by culture. Decontamination with a final NaOH concentration of 0.25% is usually adequate preparation for diagnostic inoculation. Guinea pig inoculation is not recommended unless a source of dependably healthy animals and the special facilities required for controlled animal testing are available (see below). Ordinarily, guinea pig inoculation for diagnosis is not done except for specimens of unusual importance or for specimens having contamination such as to make culture unreliable.

Inoculation of contaminated specimens such as sputum or urine

Bring to a final concentration of 0.25% NaOH. Vortex mix or shake as for culture. Buffer the sediment and suspend it in albumin solution according to the acetyl-cysteine culture technique. Freeze a portion of sediment for reinoculation in case of premature animal death. Inoculate (in hood) up to 3 ml of sediment subcutaneously into lower right flank of a guinea pig with a Luer lock syringe and 18-gauge needle. To guard against loss of test by premature death of the animal, particularly if time is critical, inoculate two guinea pigs.

Inoculation of noncontaminated specimens

Included here are surgically resected tissues, fluids from enclosed spaces, and even clean-catch urine.

No pretreatment is required. Inoculate up to 20 ml distributed in right and left inguinal, abdominal, or thoracic sites, subcutaneously or intraperitoneally. Follow development of disease by inspection and palpation of the site of inoculation. Ulceration or large, firm lymph nodes strongly suggest tuberculosis and make the animal eligible for autopsy. (NB: tuberculosis ulcers are infectious; wear rubber gloves.)

From the site of inoculation, the organisms pass through lymphatic vessels to regional (inguinal or axillary) lymph nodes, thence to the chain of aortic lymph nodes, and thence into the venous blood stream. Some lodge in the lungs to produce disease, and some pass through the systemic circulation with seeding in all other organs and tissues. Drainage from lung lesions enters tracheobronchial lymph nodes.

Tuberculin test; time of autopsy

Skin test at 5 to 6 weeks, using 0.1 ml of 5% old tuberculin (OT) or second-strength purified protein derivative. A strongly positive reaction at 24 to 48 h (10 mm or more induration) indicates a diseased animal ready for autopsy. Otherwise, autopsy at 2 months.

Autopsy

Sacrifice animal with overdose of chloroform in covered container. (NB: avoid excessive inhalation of fumes.) Examine enlarged, firm lymph nodes (inguinal, iliac, portal, tracheobronchial) for granuloma or caseation. Prepare smears from softened caseous material for staining. Visceral tuberculosis is most pronounced in spleen with enlargement and bulging surface nodules (not to be confused with normal Malpighian bodies) or confluent cream-yellow caseous areas. Infarction sometimes results in a huge, smooth, dark-red spleen. The liver may be rough or granular, or may show tiny, angular, flat, gray places, or large regions of yellow caseation. Tuberculosis appears in the lungs as raised gray nodules or gray regions of solidification. The tracheobronchial lymph nodes may show disease when the lungs appear negative. Culture from inguinal nodes before the abdomen is opened may be done successfully without decontamination procedures.

Interpretation. It is arbitrarily assumed that guinea pig disease that looks like tuberculosis and that contains acid-fast bacilli is tuberculosis. A further assumption (confirmable by culture) is made that the bacilli are *M. tuberculosis* because of the rarity of human disease due to *M. bovis*. Finally, it is assumed that, with proper technique and the observed disease pattern, the guinea pig infection derived from the inoculated material. Visceral (lungs, liver, spleen) disease is required for a "positive" report. Local or lymph node disease only may be due to: (i) a very small inoculum of *M. tuberculosis*; (ii) *M. tuberculosis* of diminished virulence due to contact with isoniazid; or (iii) a mycobacterial species other than *M. tuberculosis* or *M. bovis*.

Other animal tests

Mice are useful (but unnecessary) for distinguishing *M. kansasii*, *M. marinum*, and *M. ulcerans*. *M. kansasii* produces disease only in internal organs, not in tail or footpads. The other two species, after intravenous or footpad inoculation, produce lesions in cooler parts of the mouse body, such as tail, footpad, nose, scrotum, etc. *M. ulcerans* is distinghished by the exceedingly slow development of disease as compared with that produced by *M. marinum*.

If specific skin test antigens are available, skin sensitivity of inoculated guinea pigs is very useful for identification of "atypical" strains (such as nonpigmented or scotochromogenic *M. kansasii*). Inoculate adult guinea pigs with 0.1 mg (wet weight) of actively growing bacilli subcutaneously in the back of the neck. Skin test with 0.1 ml of 25 TU strength purified protein derivatives at 3 weeks (see 8).

Facilities required

To prevent accidental infection of animals and personnel, use the following: vermin-proof quarters; small cages, e.g., 20 by 20 by 28 cm with ⅜-inch (7.6-mm) wire-mesh floor, over dropping trays containing disinfectant-soaked shavings or sawdust; phenol-soap disinfectant tank, and low-pressure (flowing) steam box for cage sterilization; daily phenolic-soap floor mopping; under-shielded ultraviolet irradiation of upper atmosphere; exhaust-ventilated inoculation and autopsy hoods; source of healthy animal stock; and vitamin C-containing food.

LITERATURE CITED

1. Beam, R. E., and B. P. Kubica. 1968. Stimulatory effects of carbon dioxide on the primary isolation of tubercle bacilli on agar containing medium. Amer. J. Clin. Pathol. **50**:395–397.
2. Binford, C. H. 1966. *In* W. A. D. Anderson (ed.), Pathology, p. 234. C. V. Mosby Co., St. Louis.
3. Bönicke, R. 1958. Die differenzierung humaner und boviner Tuberkelbakterien mit Hilfe von Thiophen-2-carbonsäure-hydrazid. Naturwissenschaften **46**:392.
4. Carr, D. T., A. G. Karlson, and G. G. Stilwell. 1967. A comparison of cultures of induced sputum and gastric washings in the diagnosis of tuberculosis. Mayo Clin. Proc. **42**:23–25.
5. Corper, H. J., and N. Uyei. 1930. Oxalic acid as a reagent for isolating tubercle bacilli and a study of the growth of acid-fast nonpathogens on different mediums with their reactions to chemical reagents. J. Lab. Clin. Med. **15**:348–369.
6. Dixon, J. M. S., and E. H. Cuthbert. 1967. Isolation of tubercle bacilli from uncentrifuged sputum on pyruvic acid medium. Amer. Rev. Resp. Dis. **96**:119–122.
7. Dunbar, F. P., I. Pejovic, R. Cacciatore, L. Peric-Golia, and E. H. Runyon. 1969. *Mycobacterium intracellulare*: maintenance of pathogenicity in relationship to lyophilization and colony form. Scand. J. Resp. Dis. **49**:153–162.
8. Edwards, L. B., L. Hopwood, and C. E. Palmer. 1965. Identification of mycobacterial infections. Bull W.H.O. **33**:405–412.
9. Engbaek, H. C., B. Vergmann, and M. W. Bentzon. 1967. The sodium lauryl sulfate method in culturing sputum for mycobacteria. Scand. J. Resp. Dis. **38**:268–284.
10. Griffith, M., M. L. Barrett, H. L. Bodily, and R. M. Wood. 1967. Drug susceptibility tests for tuberculosis using drug impregnated disks. Amer. J. Clin. Pathol. **47**:812–817.
11. Gruft, H. 1965. Nalidixic acid as a decontaminant in Löwenstein-Jensen medium. J. Bacteriol. **90**:829.
12. Hawkins, J. E., V. R. McClean, and N. Weinstock. 1967. The effect of asparagine in 7H10 medium on the niacin test and growth of mycobacteria. Transactions of the 26th Veterans Administration-Armed Forces Pulmonary Disease Research Conference, p. 26.
13. Jones, W. D. and G. P. Kubica. 1964. The use of MacConkey's agar for differential typing of *Mycobacterium fortuitum*. Amer. J. Med. Technol. **30**:187–195.
14. Karlson, A. G., J. K. Martin, Jr., and R. Harrington, Jr. 1964. Identification of *Mycobacterium tuberculosis* with one tube of liquid medium. Mayo Clin. Proc. **39**:410–415.
15. Kestle, D. G., V. D. Abbott, and G. P. Kubica. 1967. Differential identification of mycobacteria. II. Subgroups of Groups II and III (Runyon) with different clinical significance. Amer. Rev. Resp. Dis. **95**:1041–1052.
16. Kilburn, J. O., and G. P. Kubica. 1968. Reagent impregnated paper strips for detection of niacin. Amer. J. Clin. Pathol. **50**:530–532.
17. Kilburn, J. O., V. A. Silcox, and G. P. Kubica. 1969. Differential identification of mycobacteria. V. The tellurite reduction test. Amer. Rev. Resp. Dis. **99**:94–100.
18. Kilburn, J. O., K. D. Stottmeier, and G. P. Kubica. 1968. Aspartic acid as a precursor for niacin synthesis by tubercle bacilli grown on 7H-10 agar medium. Amer. J. Clin. Pathol. **50**:582–586.
19. Krasnow, I., and G. C. Kidd. 1965. The effect of a buffer wash of sputum sediments digested with Zephiran trisodium phosphate on the recovery of acid-fast bacilli. Amer. J. Clin. Pathol. **44**:238–240.
20. Krasnow, I., and L. G. Wayne. 1969. Comparison of method for tuberculosis bacteriology. Appl. Microbiol. **18**:915–917.
21. Kubica, G. P. 1973. Differential identification of mycobacteria. VII. Key features for identification of clinically significant mycobacteria. Amer. Rev. Resp. Dis. **107**:9–21.
22. Kubica, G. P., and W. E. Dye. 1967. Laboratory methods for clinical and public health mycobacteriology. U.S. Public Health Service Publication 1547 (available from Center for Disease Control, Atlanta, Ga. 30333).
23. Kubica, G. P., and G. L. Pool. 1960. Studies on the catalase activity of acid-fast bacilli. I. An attempt to subgroup these organisms on the basis of their catalase activities at different temperatures and pH. Amer. Rev. Resp. Dis. **81**:387–391.
24. Kubica, G. P., and A. L. Rigdon. 1961. The arylsulfatase activity of acid-fast bacilli. III. Preliminary investigation of rapidly growing acid-fast bacilli. Amer. Rev. Resp. Dis. **83**:737–740.
25. Lorian, V. 1968. Differentiation of *Mycobacterium tuberculosis* and Runyon Group III "V" strains on direct cord-reading agar. Amer. Rev. Resp. Dis.

97:1133–1135.

26. Magnusson, M. 1961. Specificity of mycobacterial sensitins. I. Studies on guinea pigs with purified "tuberculin" prepared from mammalian and avian tubercle bacilli, *Mycobacterium balnei* and other acid-fast bacilli. Amer. Rev. Resp. Dis. **83:**57–68.
27. Malik, S. K., and D. E. Jenkins. 1972. Alterations in airway dynamics following inhalation of ultrasonic mist. Chest **62:**660–664.
28. Manual of Histologic and Special Staining Technics. 1957. Armed Forces Institute of Pathology, Washington, D.C.
29. Marks, J., P. A. Jenkins, and M. Tsukamura. 1972. *Mycobacterium szulgai*—a new pathogen. Tubercle **53:**210–214.
30. Miliner, R. A., K. D. Stottmeier, and G. P. Kubica. 1969. Formaldehyde: a photothermal activated toxic substance produced in Middlebrook 7H-10 medium. Amer. Rev. Resp. Dis. **99:**603–607.
31. Morse, W. C., et al. 1968. Laboratory Report #317. Mycobacteriology Methods. U.S. Army Medical Research and Nutrition Laboratory. Fitzsimons General Hospital, Denver, Colo.
32. Nicholes, P. 1964. Comparative evaluation of a new surgical mask medium. Surg. Gynecol. Obstet. **118:**579–583.
33. Palmer, C. E., and L. B. Edwards. 1968. Identifying the tuberculous infected: the dual test technique. J. Amer. Med. Ass. **205:**167–169.
34. Prevorsek, M., D. P. Kronish, and B. Schwartz. 1968. Rapid presumptive identification of enterics with reagent impregnated paper strips. Amer. J. Med. Technol. **34:**271–286.
35. Richards, O. W., and D. K. Miller. 1941. An efficient method for the identification of tuberculosis bacteria with a simple fluorescence microscope. Amer. J. Clin. Pathol. Tech. Suppl. **5:**1–8.
36. Runyon, E. H. 1957. Photochromogenic mycobacterial pathogens. Transactions of the 16th Conference on the Chemotherapy of Tuberculosis, Veterans Administration, p. 278–281.
37. Runyon, E. H. 1972. Identification of acidfast pathogens utilizing colony characteristics, 3rd ed. Veterans Administration, Salt Lake City, Utah.
38. Runyon, E. H., A. P. Dufour, and J. E. Brisbay. 1960. Use of the niacin test for identification of *M. tuberculosis*: the spot test. Transactions of the 19th Conference on Chemotherapy of Tuberculosis, Veterans Administration-Armed Forces, p. 235.
39. Runyon, E. H., M. J. Selin, and H. W. Harris. 1959. Distinguishing mycobacteria by the niacin test. Amer. Rev. Tuberc. **79:**663–665.
40. Schaefer, W. B. 1968. Incidence of the serotypes of *Mycobacterium avium* and atypical mycobacteria in human and animal diseases. Amer. Rev. Resp. Dis. **97:**18–23.
41. Smith, C. R. 1968. Mycobactericidal agents. *In* C. A. Lawrence and S. S. Block (ed.), Disinfection, sterilization and preservation. Lea and Febiger, Philadelphia.
42. Tacquet, A., F. Tison, and B. Devulder. 1965. Les variétés scotochromogènes de *Mycobacterium kansasii*. Etudes bacteriologique et biochémique. Ann. Inst. Pasteur (Paris) **108:**514–525.
43. Tacquet, A., F. Tison, and B. Polspoel. 1965. L'utilisation des détergents pour l'isolement des mycobactéries a partir de produits pathologiques. Etude comparative —applications practiques. Ann. Inst. Pasteur (Lille) **16:**21–30.
44. Tarshis, M. S., and W. G. Lewis. 1949. Use of Clorox and trisodium phosphate in demonstration of acid-fast bacilli in sputum. Amer. J. Clin. Pathol. **19:**688–692.
45. Toda, T., Y. Hagihara, and K. Takeya. 1960. A simple urease test for the classification of mycobacteria. Amer. Rev. Resp. Dis. **83:**757–761.
46. Truant, J. P., W. A. Brett, and W. Thomas, Jr. 1962. Fluorescence microscopy of tubercle bacilli stained with auramine and rhodamine. Henry Ford Hosp. Med. Bull. **10:**287–296.
47. Vestal, A. L. 1973. Procedures for the isolation and identification of mycobacteria. Public Health Service Publication (available from Center for Disease Control, Atlanta, Ga. 30333).
48. Virtanen, S. 1960. A study of nitrate reduction by mycobacteria. Acta Tuberc. Scand. Suppl. **48:**1–119.
49. Wayne, L. G. 1957. The use of millipore filters in clinical laboratories. Amer. J. Clin. Pathol. **28:**565–567.
50. Wayne, L. G. 1961. Recognition of *Mycobacterium fortuitum* by means of the three-day phenolphthalein sulfatase test. Amer. J. Clin. Pathol. **36:**185–187.
51. Wayne, L. G. 1962. Two varieties of *Mycobacterium kansasii* with different clinical significance. Amer. Rev. Resp. Dis. **86:**651–656.
52. Wayne, L. G., and J. R. Doubek. 1964. The role of air in the photochromogenic behaviour of *Mycobacterium kansasii*. Amer. J. Clin. Pathol. **42:**431–435.
53. Wayne, L. G., and J. R. Doubek. 1968. Diagnostic key to mycobacteria encountered in clinical laboratories. Appl. Microbiol. **16:**925–931.
54. Wayne, L. G., J. R. Doubek, and R. L. Russell. 1964. Classification and identification of mycobacteria. I. Tests employing Tween 80 as substrate. Amer. Rev. Resp. Dis. **90:**588–597.
55. Wayne, L. G., and I. Krasnow. 1966. Preparation of tuberculosis susceptibility testing mediums by means of impregnated discs. Amer. J. Clin. Pathol. **45:**769–771.
56. Wayne, L. G., I. Krasnow, and G. C. Kidd. 1962. Finding the "hidden positive" in tuberculosis eradication programs. The role of the sensitive trisodium phosphate-benzalkonium (Zephiran) culture technique. Amer. Rev. Resp. Dis. **86:**537–541.
57. Young, W. D., Jr., A. Maslansky, M. S. Lefar, and D. P. Kronish. 1970. Development of a paper strip test for detection of niacin produced by mycobacteria. Appl. Microbiol. **20:**939–945.

Chapter 17

Aerobic Pathogenic *Actinomycetaceae*

MORRIS A. GORDON

The aerobic pathogenic actinomycetes are branched filamentous bacteria related to the mycobacteria and to saprophytic species of *Streptomyces*. Some species tend to fragment into bacillary and coccoid forms, and some form aerial chains of either conidia or arthrospores. They are gram-positive, but some tend to stain irregularly; some species are weakly and partially acid-fast. Their cell wall constitution is of type I, III, or IV, according to genus and species (4).

NOCARDIA, ACTINOMADURA, AND STREPTOMYCES

(*Nocardia asteroides*, *N. brasiliensis*, *N. caviae*, "*N. farcinica*," *Actinomadura madurae*, *A. pelletieri*, *A. dassonvillei*, *Streptomyces paraguayensis*, *S. somaliensis*.)

Characterization

These species form colonies varying from glabrous and waxy, raised or heaped, and variously pigmented to densely mycelial, white, tough, and moldlike. Growth rates are comparable to those of the rapidly growing mycobacteria; colonies of *N. asteroides* are usually apparent within 3 days, but others may take 1 week or more to develop. Optimal temperature for growth is 30 to 37 C, with a range of 10 to 50 C (varies with species). All species are nonencapsulated. All are catalase-positive. The species are differentiated biochemically by their action upon casein, tyrosine, xanthine, and starch agar plates, urea agar slants, and tubes of gelatin and bromocresol purple (BCP) milk (Table 1), and by whether they produce acid from certain sugars.

Cell wall analysis. The three genera in this group may be separated into cell wall types I, III, and IV by the presence in or absence from their cell walls of glycine, arabinose, galactose, and either of two isomeric forms of 2,6-diaminopimelic acid (3, 29; Table 1). (Mycobacteria have cell walls of type IV.)

Animal pathogenicity. Pathogenicity for laboratory animals varies with the species. Some are regularly lethal for guinea pigs on intraperitoneal injection, especially when the inoculum is mixed with hog gastric mucin; this property is useful in species identification.

Clinical significance

These agents may cause severe, suppurative pulmonary infection, often simulating tuberculosis (particularly *N. asteroides*); cutaneous and subcutaneous abscesses (*N. asteroides; N. brasiliensis*); blood stream invasion with secondary, often fatal involvement of meninges and brain, kidney, and other organs (*N. asteroides*); or actinomycetic mycetoma, i.e., swollen, indurated lesions which eventually involve the bone and which discharge granules in pus from sinuses. The organisms are found in clinical specimens, lesions of animals (e.g., bovine mastitis; 34), and soil, but probably are not maintained saprophytically on or in the human body. Transmission is by inhalation of contaminated dust or by direct, traumatic contact with contaminated soil or vegetation.

N. asteroides is in many cases an opportunistic pathogen. Pulmonary or generalized nocardiosis has become increasingly prevalent, especially in patients with severe underlying diseases, preponderantly neoplastic, who are receiving intensive medical therapy. Particularly implicated are steroids and antineoplastic drugs (40). In addition to lymphomas and leukemias, the predisposing conditions include pulmonary alveolar proteinosis, chronic pulmonary disease, chronic intestinal disease, cirrhosis of the liver, and severe wounds (5, 30). Although a recent review of the world literature (33) found nocardiosis associated with mycoses in 14 cases, the data show that almost all of the associated mycoses were themselves opportunistic infections (particularly candidiasis and aspergillosis); most of the patients suffered from neoplasms and other disorders mentioned above and had been treated with steroids or cytotoxic agents.

The respective species are not so geographically limited as some of their names imply. *N. brasiliensis* is most common in Mexico but is also found in the USA and elsewhere; *S.*

somaliensis has been found in Mexico as well as in Africa; *A. madurae* (see reference 16 for taxonomy) is cosmopolitan; and mycetomas, although traditionally considered tropical, occur in all parts of the world. There are several other so-called, but inadequately defined, species of *Nocardia* (9) which, along with most species of *Streptomyces*, are not known to incite human or animal disease and are not ordinarily found in clinical specimens. These species are not treated here. There is no general method for distinguishing disease-related from nonpathogenic species of the two genera.

Collection of specimens

Types of specimens. In pulmonary cases, fresh single (not cumulative) specimens of sputum or bronchial washings should be submitted in sterile screw-cap containers. All specimens should be adequate for both direct microscope examination and culture. Biopsy and autopsy specimens, exudate, pus, and scrapings from ulcers should be submitted in tightly stoppered, sterile vials, tubes, or bottles; desiccation of these specimens should be avoided. Swabs are not recommended; if there is no other recourse, they should be premoistened with sterile water and submitted in a sealed tube. They should not be coated with additives, such as charcoal, that may obfuscate direct examination. Spinal fluid or blood specimens for culture should be submitted in sterile sealed tubes.

Transport and storage. Specimens should be conveyed to the examining laboratory as quickly as possible. Specimens in storage or delayed in transit should be kept at a temperature of approximately 4 C. Preserving fluids are not recommended. If the laboratory is distant, isolation media are best inoculated locally and shipped as cultures.

Direct examination

Wet mount. Pus and other exudates from cases of suspected mycetoma should be diluted in sterile water if necessary and examined macroscopically for the presence of granules (microcolonies). These and other body fluids, including sputum, bronchial washings, and the centrifuged sediment from spinal fluid or urine, should be examined microscopically in an unstained wet mount between slide and cover slip, under greatly reduced light or phase contrast, for presence of branching filaments 1 μm or less in diameter. Differentiation of granules according to species is described in Table 2. Branched hyphal filaments may belong to any of these

TABLE 1. *Physiological characteristics of pathogenic Nocardia, Actinomadura, and Streptomyces species (12–14, 21, 24)*

Species	Cell wall type[a]	Decomposition[b] of							Acid from		Growth at 10 C
		Casein	Tyrosine	Xanthine	Starch	Gelatin	Bromocresol purple milk	Urea (12, 24)	Lactose	Xylose	
N. asteroides	IV	–	–	–	–[c]	–[d]	–[e]	+	–	–	
N. brasiliensis	IV	+	+	–	–[c]	+	+	+	–	–	
N. caviae	IV	–	–	+	–[c]	–	–[e]	+	–	–	
A. dassonvillei	III	+	+	+				± 35% +	–	+	–
A. madurae	III	+	+ 14% neg (12)	–	+	+	+	–	± 55% +	+	–
A. pelletieri	III	+	+	–	– 13% + (12)	+	+	–	–	–	
S. somaliensis	I	+	+	–	±	+	+	–	–	–	
S. paraguayensis	I	+	+	+	–	+	+	+			
Streptomyces spp. (nonpathogenic)	I	+ + –	+ + +	– + +	(+)[f]	(+)[f]	(+)[f]	± 50% +	+	+	+

[a] Cell walls of all actinomycetes contain glucosamine, muramic acid, glutamic acid, and alanine. In addition, major amounts of the following components are found in the respective groups: (I) LL-diaminopimelic acid (DAP) and glycine; (III) *meso*-DAP; (IV) *meso*-DAP, arabinose, and galactose (4).

[b] Within two weeks at 27 C.

[c] About 50% of strains positive by different method (14).

[d] Some strains reportedly liquefy certain gelatin media (8).

[e] Usually turns alkaline.

[f] Most species give positive tests.

TABLE 2. *Morphology and staining of pathogenic Nocardia and Streptomyces species*

Species	Appearance in host tissue (7, 21, 23)		Sabouraud dextrose agar culture, 27–37 C	Acid-fast
	Pus	Stained sections		
N. asteroides	Granules small (<1 mm), soft, white to yellowish, lobulated, sometimes clubbed; occurring only rarely, generally in mycetomas. Usually there are clumped or scattered, acid-fast branched filaments, undergoing fragmentation (Fig. 13).	Granules rare, irregularly oval, staining lightly with hematoxylin, often with a distinct eosinophilic periphery, fringed and sometimes clubbed; Gram stain gives a similar pattern (Fig. 5). More commonly there are either colonies made of a loose mycelium or scattered, fragmenting filaments sharply delineated by Grocott method (Fig. 4) but poorly or not at all by H & E.	Colonies orange, glabrous, heaped and folded (Fig. 6) to white or pink, raised and chalky with aerial hyphae (Fig. 7); crumbly or leathery and adherent. Hyphae fragment into bacillary and coccoid elements (Fig. 14). Chains of arthrospores (Fig. 16) occasionally form on aerial hyphae. Grows at 46 C.	+
N. brasiliensis	As above, but granules are common in mycetomas; branched filaments in cutaneous abscesses.		As above. No growth at 46 C	+
N. caviae	As in *N. brasiliensis*.		As above. Growth at 46 C variable.	+
A. dassonvillei	(Insufficient information; granules not reported; has been cultured from ulcerative and granulomatous lesions and especially from pulmonary sites; also from soil.)		Densely filamentous colonies (*Streptomyces*-like) with abundant aerial mycelium and long aerial chains of conidia (Fig. 15). Vegetative mycelium may fragment, to some extent, into rods. Growth (80% of strains) at 40 C; no growth at 45 C.	–
A. madurae	Large (1–5 mm), soft, white to yellowish or reddish granules, irregularly oval, serpiginous, or lobulated.	H & E: Center of granule is hollow or tenuous, surrounded by denser network staining dark purple; wide, dense, pink border with long fringes and usually clubs (Fig. 1).	Optimal temperature 37 C. Colonies are waxy, with folded center and flat periphery (Fig. 9), membranous and tough; white to tan, pale orange, pink or red. Nonfragmenting, but sparse aerial hyphae may form short chains of conidia.	–
A. pelletieri	Granules soft, small (300–500 μm), deep red, smooth-edged or finely denticulate, irregularly spherical, sometimes with large lobes.	H & E: Granules round, sharply delimited, characteristically fracturing into large segments; heavily and homogeneously purple, with a lighter purple peripheral band (Fig. 2).	Optimal temperature 37 C. Colony resembles a crushed cranberry, with areas of bright and dark red; slow-growing, heaped irregularly, and waxy-granular (Fig. 10). May have sparse aerial hyphae. Pigment soluble in mineral oil.	–
S. somaliensis	Hard, yellow to brown, round to oval granules, 1–2 mm diameter.	H & E: Granules both large and tiny, round, dense and homogeneous, but staining light purple and often partially pink in patches; tend to rupture into parallel strips; smooth, sharply defined, nonbanded border (Fig. 3).	Optimal temperature 30 C. Slow-growing, leathery, eventually heaped and folded; cream-colored to brown or black, glabrous or with whitish aerial hyphae (Fig. 12). Nonfragmenting; aerial hyphae may form chains of conidia characteristic of the genus.	–
S. paraguayensis	There is doubt as to the existence of this species as a distinct, pathogenic agent. It is associated with black-grained mycetoma. Cultures designated *N. paraguayensis* resemble saprophytic *Streptomyces* both morphologically (white or cream to gray, tough colonies with raised center [Fig. 11], often bearing short aerial hyphae) and physiologically (Table 1) and possess cell walls of type I (R. E. Gordon, personal communication).			–
Streptomyces spp.	Nonpathogenic.		Colonies tough; glabrous, velvety or (most often) chalky; of various colors, commonly white or grayish; often with earthy odor; nonfragmenting, but branches of aerial mycelium characteristically segment into medium to long, curved or spiral chains of conidia.	– (Spores often +)

three genera or to species of *Actinomyces*.

Gram stain. All forms of these species, whether filamentous, bacillary, or coccoid, are gram-positive; but *Nocardia* tends to stain irregularly, and its filaments are generally beaded (Fig. 14). Filamentous forms may not be differentiable from those of species of *Actinomyces*, and bacillary elements may resemble those of *Actinomyces*, *Mycobacterium*, or *Corynebacterium*. Intact granules reveal little detail and should be crushed before staining to expose the component filaments, which would distinguish them from microcolonies of *Staphylococcus* or other agents of botryomycosis.

Acid-fast stain. Acid-fastness is variable in *N. asteroides*, *N. brasiliensis*, and *N. caviae*, both in clinical specimens and in culture, but when observed it is very helpful in identifying these species. Individual filaments and fragments in a smear may vary from partially or completely acid-fast (Fig. 13) to entirely non-acid-fast. The usual Ziehl-Neelsen and Kinyoun staining procedures may be employed, but the period of decolorization with acid alcohol must not exceed 5 to 10 s.

Tissue sections. The various species may appear in sections of biopsy or autopsy specimens, generally within abscesses, either as granules (in mycetoma) or as radially dendritic colonies or scattered fine, branching filaments. Granules show up well in sections stained with hematoxylin and eosin (H & E; Fig. 1–3), but this stain often fails completely to demonstrate other morphological forms of *Nocardia*, even when they are shown by other stains to be present. The Grocott-Gomori silver-methenamine method also stains granules very well and is probably the best for disclosing dendritic colonies (Fig. 4) and individual filaments and fragments. The Gram-Weigert technique is effective for both granules (Fig. 5) and filaments if done properly, as are acid-fast stains for the appropriate species. Periodic acid-Schiff stains are not recommended. (See Table 2 for differentiation of species by morphological and staining characteristics of their granules or filaments.)

Culture and isolation

Specimens planted on duplicate or triplicate Sabouraud dextrose agar (SDA) slants (without antibiotics) and streaked on beef heart infusion-blood-agar plates are incubated aerobically at room temperature (preferably 25 to 27 C) and at 37 C, respectively. Beef infusion broth, to be incubated at 37 C, may be inoculated as an enrichment medium. Since *N. asteroides* grows well at 45 C, initial incubation at temperatures

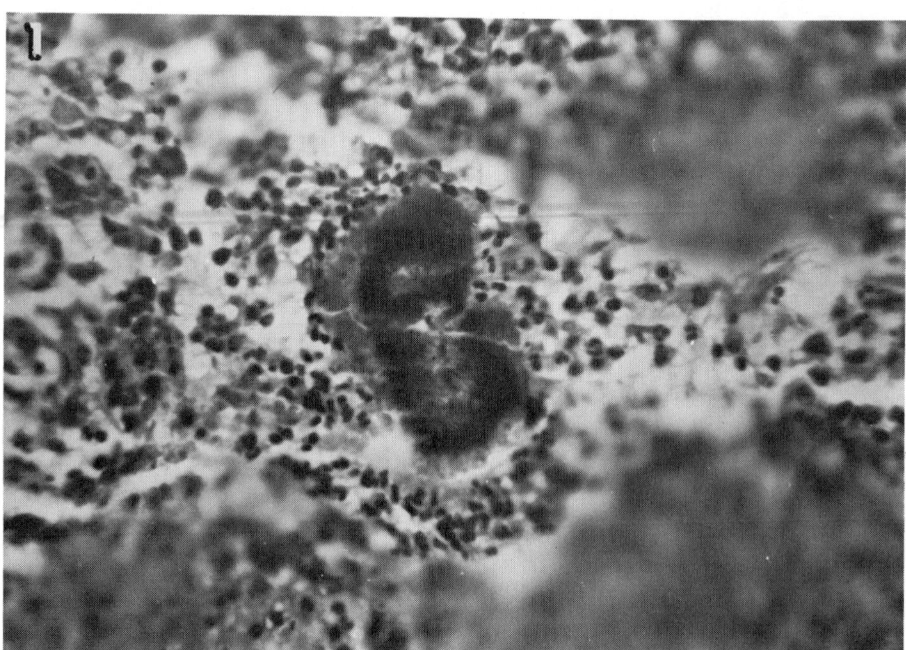

FIG. 1. *Actinomadura madurae: section from human mycetoma. Note tenuous center of granule, denser periphery stained with hematoxylin; wide, fringed, and clubbed eosinophilic border. Hematoxylin and eosin stain.* ×*378.*

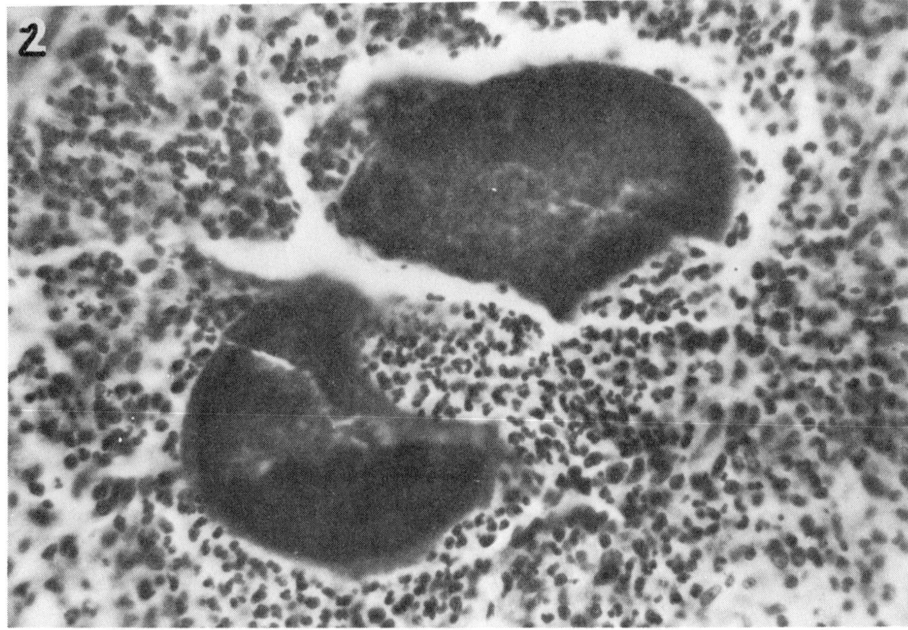

FIG. 2. *Actinomadura pelletieri: section from human mycetoma. Round granule, tending to break into large lobes; heavily hematoxylin-stained with somewhat lighter border. Hematoxylin and eosin stain. ×378.*

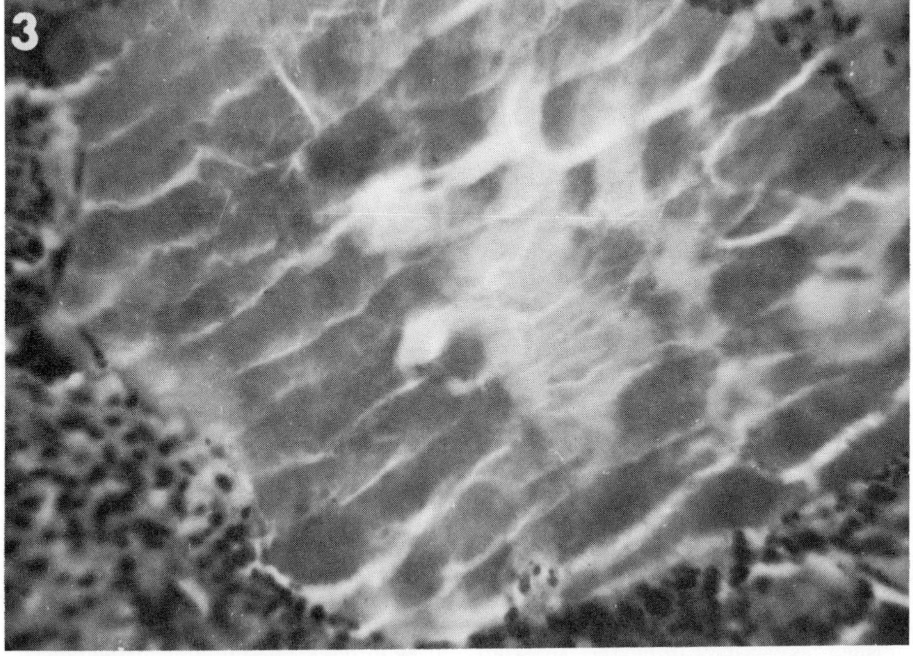

FIG. 3. *Streptomyces somaliensis: section from human mycetoma. Round, dense granule, lightly stained with hematoxylin; fracturing into strips. Hematoxylin and eosin stain. ×378.*

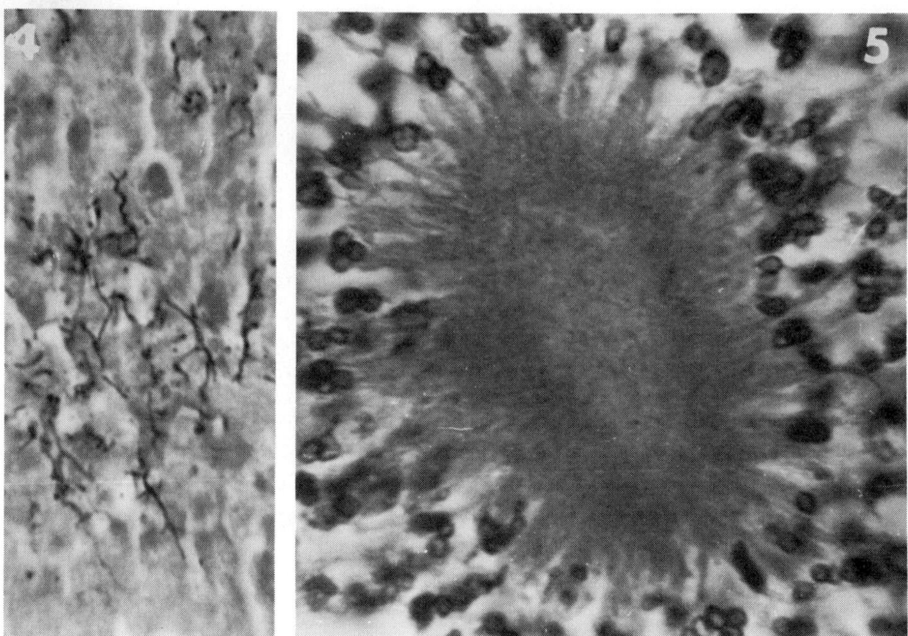

FIG. 4. *Nocardia asteroides colonies in section of human brain. Grocott stain. ×850.*
FIG. 5. *N. asteroides granule in section of abscessed omentum from experimentally infected guinea pig. Interior gram-positive; border fringed, clubbed, and gram-negative. Gram-Weigert stain. ×850.*

above 37 C may help to separate this species from other bacteria. Cultures are examined at intervals from 48 h to 2 weeks. *N. asteroides* often survives mycobacterial concentration procedures, including sodium hydroxide methods, and treatment of sputum with trisodium phosphate has been suggested (39). *Nocardia* species also grow well on mycobacterial isolation media, particularly Lowenstein-Jensen medium, on which they often appear moist and glabrous, similar to some species of mycobacteria. It is advisable to wash and crush granules for inoculation of media.

Identification

Cultural characteristics. Colonies of *Nocardia*, *Actinomadura*, and *Streptomyces* are, with few exceptions, readily differentiated from those of mycobacteria (Table 2; Fig. 6–12). In questionable cases, the presence of aerial hyphae in the actinomycetes may, if not obvious to the naked eye (Fig. 7), be observed by placing plate cultures of mature growth under a compound microscope, or by preparing special slide cultures (14) with Bennett's or Hickey and Tresner's (H-T) medium. Aerial hyphae may be distinguished as arising from the substrate hyphae and appearing wider, with a heavier, black outline (they are more refractile; Fig. 18). Their formation may be inhibited by exposure to light (20). Some strains elaborate a musty odor ("newly plowed earth") or the so-called tyrosinase reaction (clear brownish discoloration of the medium), or both, but these two properties are typical also of many saprophytic species of *Streptomyces*, generally with chalky colonies. Formation of pigment and spores is encouraged by growth on Czapek-Dox solution agar. Growth on liquid media, including BCP milk, occurs as a thick surface pellicle.

Since so-called *N. farcinica* apparently does not occur in the United States and is not known to cause human disease (it is known almost exclusively as isolates from bovine farcy in North Africa), and since its taxonomic status is much in doubt, it is not treated here in detail. Some isolates are thought to be referable to *N. asteroides* (14); and others, the so-called slow growers, have many characteristics in common with the mycobacteria. Rapidly growing mycobacteria may be distinguished from *Nocardia* species by their arylsulfatase activity and utilization of trimethylene diamine (38); on these bases, *N. farcinica* would be classified with the mycobacteria. (See also 36, 37.) *N. farcinica* has been differentiated from *N. asteroides* immunologically, as well (22).

Microscope examination of culture growth.

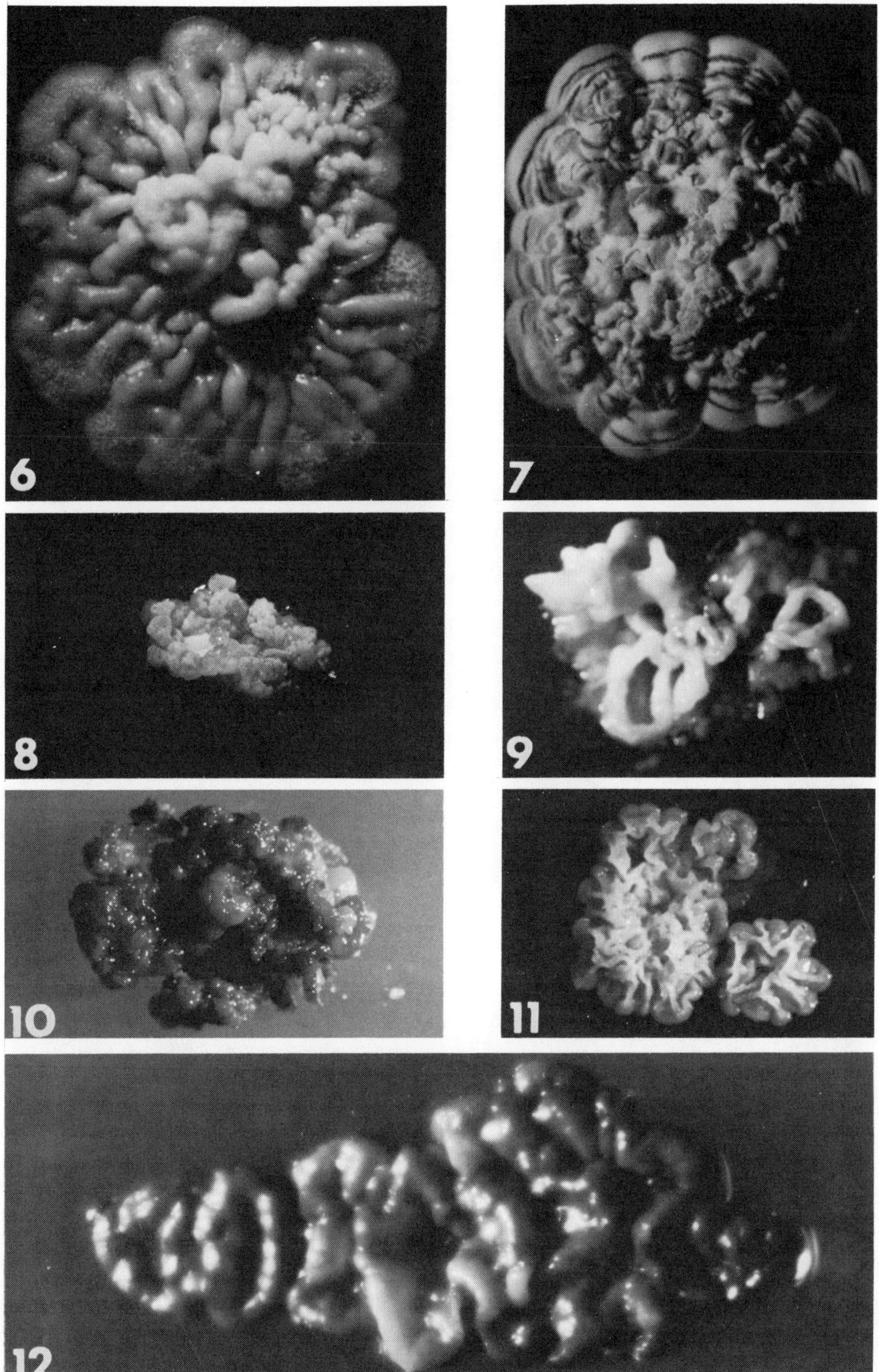

FIG. 6–11. *"Giant" colonies of various species on Sabouraud dextrose agar plates, 9 days at 27 C. ×6. Fig. 6: Nocardia asteroides, glabrous orange form. Fig. 7: N. asteroides, gypsoides (white, chalky) variety (N. brasiliensis and N. caviae are similar to N. asteroides). Fig. 8: N. farcinica. Fig. 9: Actinomadura madurae. Fig. 10: A. pelletieri. Fig. 11: Streptomyces paraguayensis.*

FIG. 12. *S. somaliensis, streaked heavily on blood-agar slant, 3 days at 27 C. ×6.*

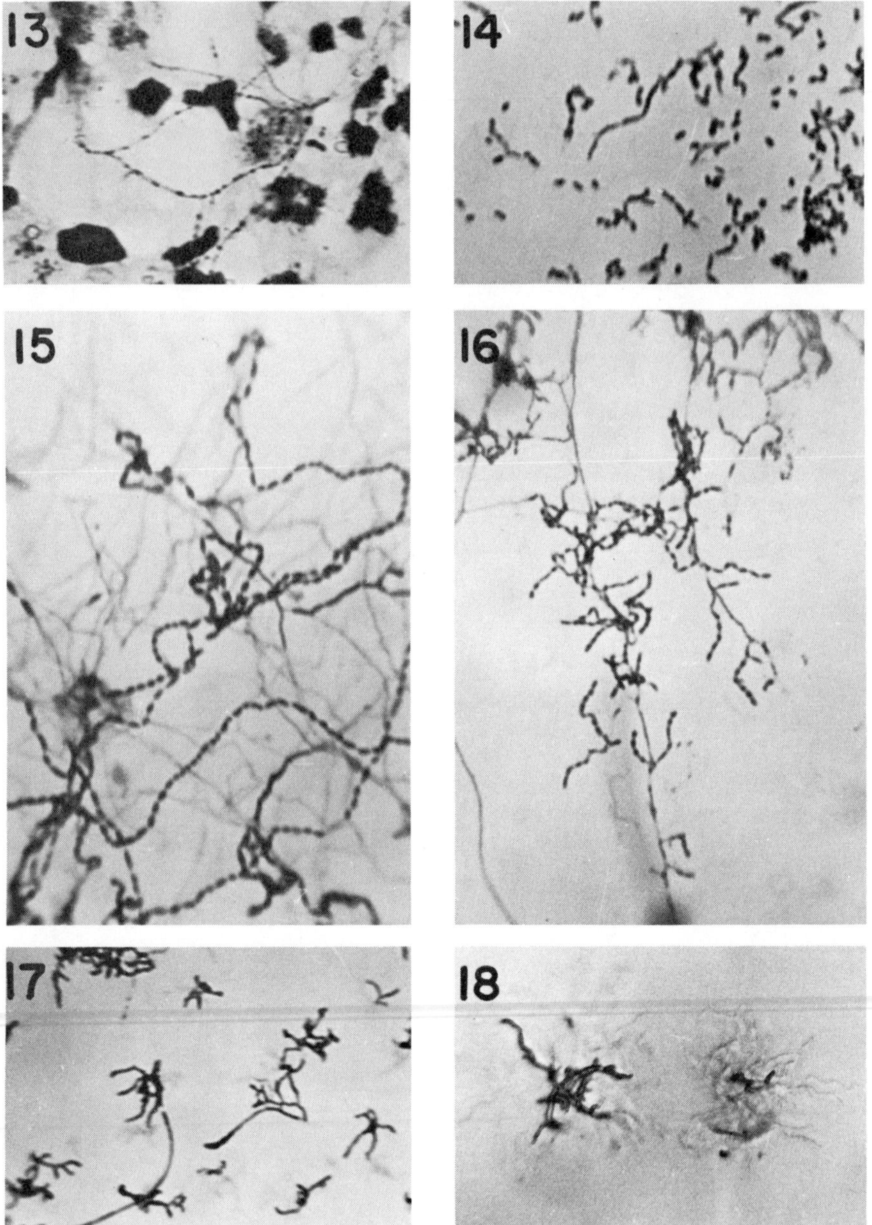

FIG. 13. *Nocardia asteroides in smear of abscessed omentum from experimentally infected guinea pig. Modified Kinyoun acid-fast stain.* ×972.

FIG. 14. *N. asteroides in smear from glabrous orange colony on Sabouraud dextrose agar, 3 weeks at 27 C; extensive fragmentation. Gram stain.* ×972.

FIG. 15. *Actinomadura dassonvillei, showing long chains of ovate conidia. Slide culture on Hickey and Tresner's medium, incubated 10 days at 25 C. Giemsa stain.* ×972.

FIG. 16. *N. asteroides, showing chains of aerial arthrospores. Slide culture on Hickey and Tresner's medium. Giemsa stain.* ×972.

FIG. 17. *A. pelletieri smear from colony on Sabouraud dextrose agar, 27 C; prepared in the manner of a blood film, causing moderate traumatic fragmentation. Gram stain.* ×972.

FIG. 18. *Pour-slide culture of N. asteroides on Hickey and Tresner's medium, 3 days at 27 C; photographed in situ with 43× objective to illustrate appearance of aerial (darker) as contrasted with substrate hyphae.* ×432.

Microscope examination of cultures, whether by wet mount, Gram stain, or acid-fast stain, reveals very fine branching filaments (less than 1 μm in diameter) with a tendency, in the acid-fast species, to fragment into bacillary and coccoid forms (Fig. 14). Acid-fastness is sometimes enhanced by prolonged growth on certain media, e.g., on BCP milk for 1 month. Species of *Actinomadura* (except *A. dassonvillei*) and the pathogenic *Streptomyces*, as well as saprophytic species of the latter, tend not to fragment; but the aerial mycelium of most saprophytic *Streptomyces* and of *A. dassonvillei* is characterized by medium to long chains of conidia (Fig. 15), often in spirals or whorls, which are sometimes acid-fast. Chains of aerial arthrospores may be seen in some pathogenic strains (Fig. 16) and conidia in others (Table 2). To detect spontaneous fragmentation, as distinct from breaking up of the mycelium during preparation of slides (Fig. 17), smears should be made with as little traumatization as possible.

Biochemical reactions. Media for the testing of biochemical reactions are incubated at 27 C and observed at 2-day intervals for 2 weeks or until good growth occurs. Reactions of the various species are given in Table 1.

Pathogenicity. There is some variation in virulence for guinea pigs among strains of *N. asteroides*, but the species is in general regularly pathogenic when tested in the following manner. All of the material on the surface of four SDA slants, each of which is at least half-covered with heavy growth, is finely emulsified in an equal volume of 5% hog gastric mucin by grinding with a mortar and pestle. Each of two guinea pigs, weighing 250 to 300 g, is injected intraperitoneally with 1 ml of the suspension. The animals generally die within 7 to 10 days and display more or less massive, often coalescing, caseous abscesses involving the organs of the abdominal cavity, particularly the omentum. If after this time the animals are not obviously ill, the abdomen should be palpated for adhesions or hard masses, the presence of which dictates sacrifice of the animal. If illness or death of the guinea pigs does not intervene, one is sacrificed at 2 weeks and the second at 4 weeks, and the omentum, abdominal viscera, and lungs are examined for lesions.

Smears should be prepared from pus, stained by both Gram and modified acid-fast methods, and examined for fragmenting, gram-positive, partially acid-fast, branching filaments (Fig. 13), which under the circumstances are diagnostic for one of the acid-fast species of *Nocardia*. Pus or diseased tissue should also be cultured on SDA at both room temperature and 37 C. A negative result, i.e., with no virulence for the guinea pig, does not rule out *N. asteroides*, since some strains are relatively avirulent under these conditions. Most of those strains, however, will display pathogenicity upon repetition of the test.

Strains of *N. caviae* and *N. farcinica* (26) and many strains of *N. brasiliensis* produce the same pathogenic effect in the guinea pig as *N. asteroides*. A suppurative orchitis is characteristic of *N. farcinica* infection. Species of *Actinomadura* and *Streptomyces* have been reported (21, 35) as nonpathogenic for guinea pigs.

Immunoserological diagnosis. Neither serology nor skin testing for nocardiosis has been generally standardized, and neither is in common use for diagnosis of this disease. However, both procedures are useful in distinguishing actinomycetoma from mycetoma caused by molds (27, 28).

Susceptibility to antimicrobial agents. In vitro testing of isolates of *N. asteroides* for antibiotic sensitivity is not a widespread routine procedure. Not only are there technical difficulties in performing the tests, but the in vitro sensitivities are difficult to relate to those in vivo. A recent report (2) gives results of in vitro testing of numerous strains of *N. asteroides* against 45 antimicrobial agents, in which the minimal inhibitory concentration of each antibiotic against different strains varied over a wide range. Minocycline was the most effective agent tested. Sulfonamides were found to be inactive against most strains with the method used, although they are generally considered the drug of choice for nocardiosis and have been remarkably successful in dealing with cases of this disease. Other investigators (30) have reached the conclusion that in vitro drug susceptibility tests are not accurate guides to the therapy of nocardiosis.

Essential criteria. Actinomycetes may be differentiated from fungi by the very fine diameter of their branching filaments, by cell wall composition, and by the absence of a nuclear membrane. They differ from mycobacteria in their more extensive filamentation, with true branching and usually aerial hyphae, in the tenacity of their colonies, and in being only weakly acid-fast or nonacid-fast. Mycobacteria have cell walls of type IV but differ from *Nocardia* in their mycolic acids (17).

Valuable presumptive tests. Presumptive identification of certain *Nocardia* species may be made, as suggested by Gordon and Mihm (14), as follows. An aerial hyphae-forming actinomycete that fails to dissolve casein, L-tyrosine, or xanthine may presumptively be identified as *N. asteroides*. An acid-fast culture with aerial hyphae which dissolves casein and tyrosine but not xanthine may safely be presumed to be *N. brasiliensis*. Aerial hyphae-forming strains that decompose xanthine but not casein or tyrosine may be presumed with reasonable safety to be *N. caviae*. Lack of demonstrable acid-fastness does not rule out any of these three species.

DERMATOPHILUS CONGOLENSIS

Characterization

D. congolensis and *Geodermatophilus obscurus* (18) are thus far the only recognized species in the family *Dermatophilaceae* (1, 10, 32; *Bergey's Manual*, 8th ed.) of the order *Actinomycetales*. Members of this family are unique among bacteria in forming more or less filamentous structures which segment transversely, as well as in at least two longitudinal planes, to form packets of coccoid cells which become motile spores. All stages of the complex life cycle are gram-positive and nonacid-fast; those of *D. congolensis* are encapsulated. Cell walls are of type III. Whole-cell hydrolysates of *D. congolensis* contain madurose; those of *G. obscurus* do not.

In *D. congolensis*, germination of the spore gives rise to a mycelium of narrow, tapering filaments with lateral branching at right angles. As longitudinal septa are laid down centrifugally, the filaments broaden from an initial diameter of 0.5 to 1.5 μm up to 5 μm, always tapering distally (Fig. 19). Formation of swarms of motile, coccoid spores completes the cycle (Fig. 20). Filamentation in *G. obscurus* is rudimentary or absent, the thallus often consisting of a muriform, tuber-shaped structure. The motile spores of *D. congolensis* are isodiametric with tufts of 5 to more than 50 flagella; those of *G. obscurus* are elliposoidal or bacillary with tufts of 1 to 4 flagella.

Clinical significance

D. congolensis is the etiological agent of streptotrichosis, an exudative, pustular dermatitis of worldwide distribution, affecting mainly cattle, sheep ("mycotic dermatitis," "lumpy wool," "strawberry foot rot"), and horses, but also goats and other domesticated and feral mammals and occasionally humans (6). Human infection, in the form of pustules, furuncles, or desquamative eczema of the hands or forearms, is acquired through contact with diseased animals. In animals, damage to hides and wool results from crusting and scab formation, and

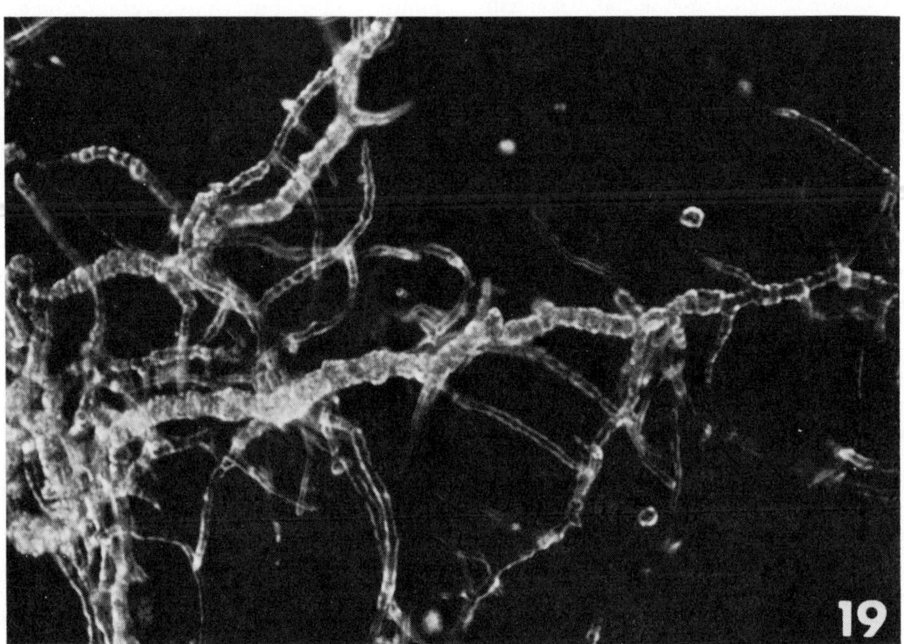

FIG. 19. *Dermatophilus congolensis, branched filaments, tapering from coarse multiseptate base to fine, nonseptate apical and lateral hyphae. Wet mount from broth culture; dark field.* ×*720. Reproduced with permission from the New York State Journal of Medicine.*

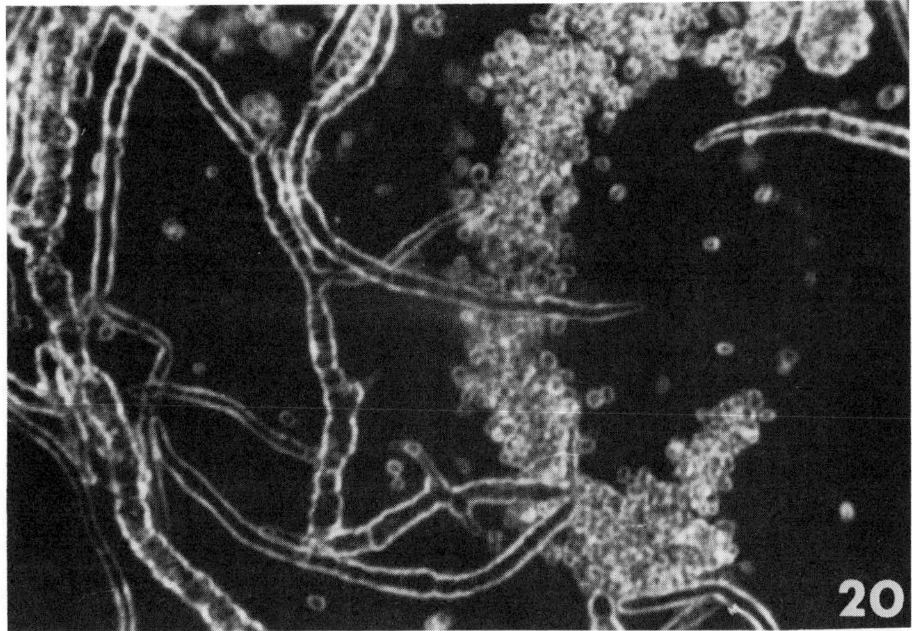

FIG. 20. *Dermatophilus congolensis, final transformation of mature hypha into an agglomeration of motile spores. Dark field.* ×*1,750. Reproduced with permission from the New York State Journal of Medicine.*

extensive infection often leads to fatalities in lambs and cattle (19), apparently through concurrent infection or cachexia. The microorganism has been isolated only from clinical specimens, although it may remain viable for prolonged periods in dried scabs.

Collection of specimens

D. congolensis may be isolated in pure culture from clinical materials by streaking the scrapings or exudate, preferably from unopened pustules, directly on blood-agar plates and incubating them at 37 C. Exudate should be submitted to the laboratory in sterile tubes or on swabs moistened with sterile water. These should be refrigerated if culturing is to be delayed. Scrapings, crusts, and scabs may be transmitted dry, in sterile tubes or jars, and stored at ambient temperature. Biopsy specimens for culture should be transmitted in sterile, screw-capped jars without preservative.

Direct examination

D. congolensis may be seen in any stage of its life cycle. The most diagnostic (and pathognomonic) stage is marked by the presence of branched filaments, 2 to 5 μm in diameter, dividing both transversely and longitudinally into packets of coccoid forms (Fig. 21). Smears and unstained wet mounts may be made from exudate, from the underside of crusts or the roofs of pustules, and from scabs ground and suspended in saline. Bacterial stains, particularly methylene blue, are effective in demonstrating the structures in smears, but the Gram stain tends to be too dark and obscures details. The Giemsa method is probably best. Giemsa and Grocott methenamine-silver stains are best for paraffin sections, which often reveal the microorganism abundantly in hair follicles, accompanied by large numbers of eosinophilic leukocytes (Fig. 21).

Culture and isolation

Clinical materials should be streaked, with the use of optimal isolation techniques, on beef infusion-blood-agar plates for aerobic incubation at 37 C. For highly contaminated specimens, animal passage (25), although uneconomical, is often effective. Crusts and scabs are ground and applied to the shaved and scarified skin of a rabbit; lesions appear in 2 to 7 days, and from these the organism is more readily isolated in pure culture (11, 31).

A method of concentrating the zoospores, based upon their chemotactic response (15), consists of immersing scab material in a bottle of distilled water for 3.5 h at room temperature, exposing it to CO_2 in a candle jar for 15 min, and streaking the surface film, to which the spores have migrated, on isolation media.

Identification

Cultural characteristics. When incubated on beef heart infusion-horse blood-agar plates for 24 h at 37 C, aerobically or with 5 to 10% CO_2, colonies are tiny (0.5 to 1.0 mm); round, square, or irregular; grayish-white; raised, rough, glabrous, hard, and adherent; and typically pitting the medium. In 2 to 5 days (Fig. 22), they characteristically develop orange pigment (more rapidly where colonies are crowded), but occasional variants remain white or gray. Beta-hemolysis, particularly prominent on horse blood, develops earliest in crowded areas. Isolated colonies grow to 4 to 6 mm in diameter in 1 week, and many become mucoid at the apex. At 27 C growth is similar but slower: pinpoint in size at 48 h and 1 to 2 mm, possibly up to 3 mm, at 1 week. Anaerobically (in a Brewer jar with platinum catalyst, using illuminating gas), colonies reach a diameter of 0.2 to 1 mm in 48 h but are less voluminous than aerobic colonies, white to translucent, and umbonate. Hemolysis develops later, if at all.

Heavy streak-inoculation of pure cultures onto brain-heart infusion (BHI) slants results, after 3 days, in confluent growth, which varies in color, according to the strain, from gray to orange and which may be granular or membranous. Growth is generally markedly adherent but often with a butyrous or caseous overlay. In beef infusion-peptone broth culture at 37 C, there is a thick sediment and clear supernatant fluid, occasionally with a surface ring. There is no growth on SDA or Czapek-Dox solution agar.

Microscope examination of culture growth. The characteristic microscopic appearance of *D. congolensis* is that of thickened, often branched filaments dividing both transversely and longitudinally (Fig. 23). However, there is extreme variation in morphology. Depending upon the strain and the age of the culture, one may see either a completely micrococcoid picture, with cocci arranged irregularly or in cubi-

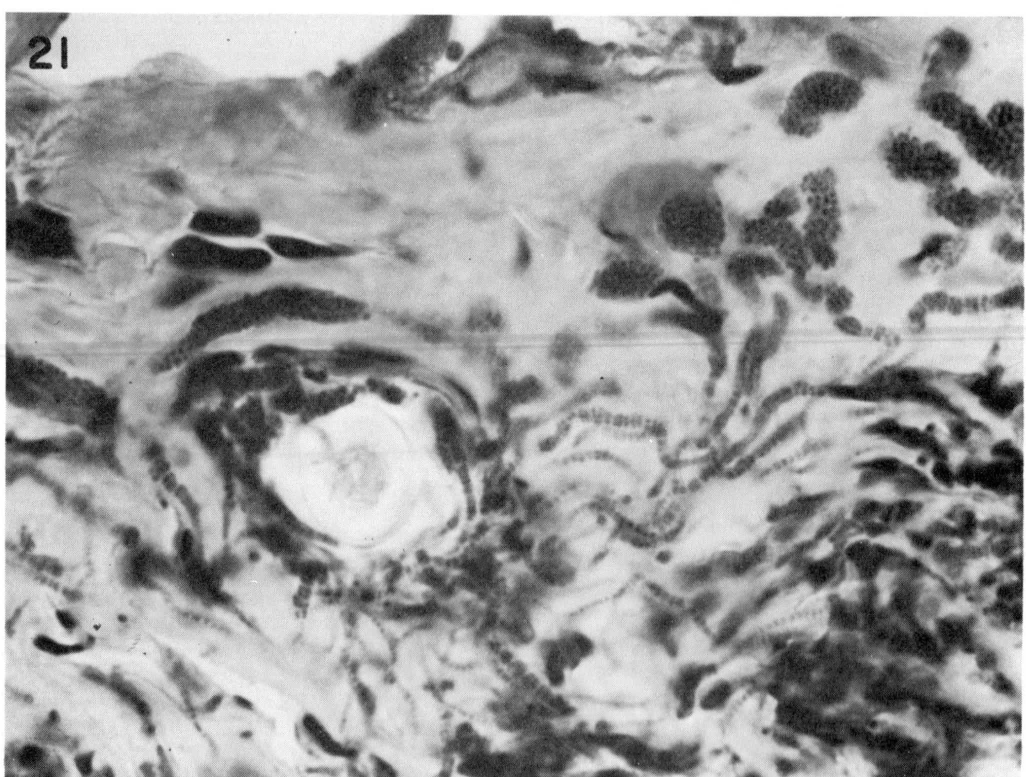

FIG. 21. *Dermatophilus congolensis; various developmental stages in section of mouse skin, concentrated around hair follicle. Hematoxylin and eosin stain. ×1,800. Reproduced with permission from the New York State Journal of Medicine.*

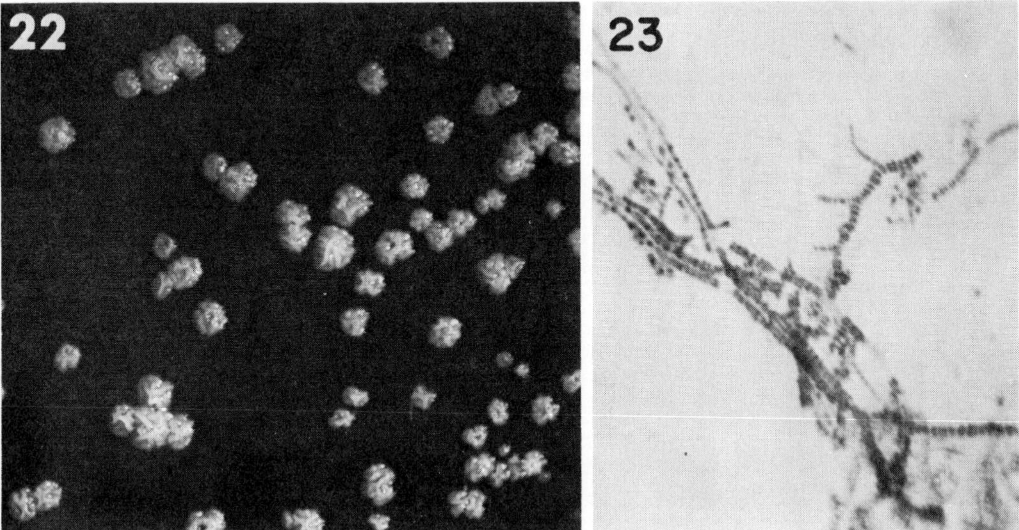

FIG. 22. *Colonies of Dermatophilus congolensis on blood-agar streak plate, 3 days at 37 C. ×3.6.*
FIG. 23. *D. congolensis; early segmentation stage from brain heart infusion agar, 3 days, 37 C. Methylene blue stain. ×972. Reproduced with permission from the Journal of Bacteriology.*

cal packets; or clusters of germinating spores; or branched filaments, segmenting or not. Motility is usually evident in recent isolates. If only cocci are seen and *D. congolensis* is suspected, cultures should be examined at an earlier age for hyphae.

Biochemical reactions. *D. congolensis* is catalase-positive as determined by a spot test. A half-loopful of growth from BHI agar (without blood, which itself gives a positive catalase test) is emulsified in a drop of 30% H_2O_2 and observed for effervescence. Other tests are incubated at 37 C and read at 48 h and at 5, 7, and 14 days. The urease test is regularly positive within 24 h. Casein and starch are hydrolyzed, but not tyrosine and xanthine. BCP milk is peptonized. Gelatin and Loeffler's coagulated serum medium are liquefied by almost all strains. Nitrate reduction, methyl red, and Voges-Proskauer tests are negative; indole is not produced. Acid but no gas is produced in proteose-peptone broth from glucose and fructose (in 48 h); it is produced transitorily from galactose (acid in 48 h, negative in 2 weeks), and, by some strains, belatedly (1 to 2 weeks) from maltose. No acid is produced from sucrose, lactose, xylose, dulcitol, mannitol, sorbitol, or salicin.

Pathogenicity. Demonstration of virulence for animals is not necessary for identification of *D. congolensis*, but infection is readily established in rabbits and may serve to differentiate this species from filamentous forms of *G. obscurus* (11). Experimental inoculation of abraded skin results in acute ulcerative pustular dermatitis involving principally the hair follicles (Fig. 21).

Essential criteria. The microscopic morphology of *D. congolensis* is unique among known microorganisms, and it can hardly fail to be recognized when seen in all of its manifestations, although *G. obscurus* resembles it in some respects. The typical biochemical properties serve as confirmatory characteristics.

ACKNOWLEDGMENTS

Thanks are due to F. Mariat for providing human mycetoma sections; to R. E. Gordon for cultures of *N. caviae*, *N. farcinica*, and *S. paraguayensis*; to the Center for Disease Control for several cultures; to the Department of Illustration and Photography of this Division for excellent photographic support; and to G. N. Little for technical assistance.

LITERATURE CITED

1. Austwick, P. K. C. 1958. Cutaneous streptothricosis, mycotic dermatitis, and strawberry foot rot. Vet. Rev. Annot. **4**:33–48.
2. Bach, M. C., L. D. Sabath, and M. Finland. 1973. Susceptibility of *Nocardia asteroides* to 45 antimicrobial agents in vitro. Antimicrob. Ag. Chemother. **3**:1–8.
3. Becker, B., M. P. Lechevalier, R. E. Gordon, and H. A. Lechevalier. 1964. Rapid differentiation between *Nocardia* and *Streptomyces* by paper chromatography of whole-cell hydrolysates. Appl. Microbiol. **12**:421–423.
4. Becker, B., M. P. Lechevalier, and H. A. Lechevalier. 1965. Chemical composition of cell-wall preparations

from strains of various form-genera of aerobic actinomycetes. Appl. Microbiol. **13:**236–243.

5. Cross, R. M., and C. H. Binford. 1962. Is *Nocardia asteroides* an opportunist? Lab. Invest. **11:**1103–1109.
6. Dean, D. J., M. A. Gordon, C. W. Severinghaus, E. T. Kroll, and J. R. Reilly. 1961. Streptothricosis: a new zoonotic disease. N.Y. State J. Med. **61:**1283–1287.
7. Emmons, C. W., C. H. Binford, and J. P. Utz. 1970. Medical mycology, 2nd ed. Lea and Febiger, Philadelphia.
8. Gonzalez-Mendoza, A., and F. Mariat. 1964. Sur l'hydrolyze de la gélatine comme caractère différentiel entre *Nocardia asteroides* et *N. brasiliensis*. Ann. Inst. Pasteur (Paris) **107:**560–564.
9. Goodfellow, M., D. E. Minnikin, P. V. Patel, and H. Mordarska. 1973. Free nocardomycolic acids in the classification of nocardias and strains of the 'Rhodochrous' complex. J. Gen. Microbiol. **74:**185–188.
10. Gordon, M. A. 1964. The genus *Dermatophilus*. J. Bacteriol. **88:**509–522.
11. Gordon, M. A., and U. Perrin. 1971. Pathogenicity of *Dermatophilus* and *Geodermatophilus*. Infect. Immunity **4:**29–33.
12. Gordon, R. E. 1966. Some criteria for the recognition of *Nocardia madurae* (Vincent) Blanchard. J. Gen. Microbiol. **45:**355–364.
13. Gordon, R. E., and A. C. Horan. 1968. *Nocardia dassonvillei*, a macroscopic replica of *Streptomyces griseus*. J. Gen. Microbiol. **50:**235–240.
14. Gordon, R. E., and J. M. Mihm. 1962. Identification of *Nocardia caviae* (Erikson) *Nov. comb.* Ann. N.Y. Acad. Sci. **98:**628–636.
15. Haalstra, R. T. 1965. Isolation of *Dermatophilus congolensis* from skin lesions in the diagnosis of streptothricosis. Vet. Rec. **77:**824–825.
16. Lechevalier, H. A., and M. P. Lechevalier. 1970. A critical evaluation of the genera of aerobic actinomycetes, p. 393–405. *In* H. Prauser (ed.), The *Actinomycetales* (The Jena International Symposium on Taxonomy, Berlin, Sept. 1968). VEB Gustav Fischer Verlag, Jena.
17. Lechevalier, M. P., A. C. Horan, and H. Lechevalier. 1971. Lipid composition in the classification of nocardiae and mycobacteria. J. Bacteriol. **105:**313–318.
18. Luedemann, G. M. 1968. *Geodermatophilus*, a new genus of the *Dermatophilaceae* (*Actinomycetales*). J. Bacteriol. **96:**1848–1858.
19. Macadam, I. 1964. The effects of ectoparasites and humidity on natural lesions of streptothricosis. Vet. Rec. **76:**354.
20. McClung, N. M., and I. Uesaka. 1961. Morphological studies in the genus *Nocardia*. VI. Aerial hyphal production and acid-fastness of *N. asteroides* isolates. Rev. Latinoamer. Microbiol. **4:**97–106.
21. Mackinnon, J. E., and R. C. Artagaveytia-Allende. 1956. The main species of pathogenic aerobic actinomycetes causing mycetomas. Trans. Roy. Soc. Trop. Med. Hyg. **50:**31–40.
22. Magnusson, M., and F. Mariat. 1968. Delineation of *Nocardia farcinica* by delayed type skin reactions on guinea pigs. J. Gen. Microbiol. **51:**151–158.
23. Mariat, F. 1962. Critères de détermination des principales espèces d'Actinomycètes aérobies pathogènes. Ann. Soc. Belg. Med. Trop. **4:**651–672.
24. Mariat, F. 1963. Activité uréasique des Actinomycètes aérobies pathogènes. Ann. Inst. Pasteur (Paris) **105:**795–797.
25. Mémery, G. 1961. La streptothricose cutanée. III. Bacteriologie. Rev. Elevage Med. Vet. **14:**141–163.
26. Mostafa, I. E. 1966. Bovine nocardiosis (cattle farcy). A review. Vet. Bull. **36:**189–193.
27. Murray, I. G., and E. S. Mahgoub. 1968. Further studies on the diagnosis of mycetoma by double diffusion in agar. Sabouraudia **6:**106–110.
28. Murray, I. G., and I. E. Moghraby. 1964. The value of skin tests in distinguishing between maduromycetoma and actinomycetoma. Trans. Roy. Soc. Trop. Med. Hyg. **58:**557–559.
29. Murray, I. G., and A. G. J. Proctor. 1965. Paper chromatography as an aid to the identification of *Nocardia* species. J. Gen. Microbiol. **41:**163–167.
30. Murray, J. F., S. M. Finegold, S. Froman, and D. W. Will. 1961. The changing spectrum of nocardiosis. Amer. Rev. Resp. Dis. **83:**315–330.
31. Pier, A. C., J. L. Richard, and E. F. Farrell. 1964. Fluorescent antibody and cultural techniques in cutaneous streptothricosis. Amer. J. Vet. Res. **25:**1014–1020.
32. Roberts, D. S. 1967. *Dermatophilus* infection. Vet. Bull. **37:**513–521.
33. Salfelder, K., M. Mendelovici, and J. Schwarz. 1973. Multiple deep fungus infections: personal observations and a critical review of the world literature. Curr. Top. Pathol. **57:**123–177.
34. Schalm, O. W., E. J. Carroll, and N. C. Jain. 1971. Bovine mastitis. Lea and Febiger, Philadelphia.
35. Soto, R. P. 1955. Contribución al estudio de la actinomicosis experimental. Rev. Biol. Trop. **3:**43–78.
36. Tanzil, H. O. K., and R. Bönicke. 1968. Über das vorkommen von diaminoxydasen im genus *Nocardia*. Zentralbl. Bakteriol. Parasitenk. Infektionskr. Hyg. Abt. I Orig. **209:**112–119.
37. Tanzil, H. O. K., and R. Bönicke. 1969. The significance of the phenolphthalein sulphatase test for the differentiation and identification of Nocardia species. Tubercle **50:**65–67.
38. Tsukamura, M. 1970. Relationship between *Mycobacterium* and *Nocardia*. Jap. J. Microbiol. **14:**187–195.
39. Uesaka, I. 1964. The tolerance of actinomycetes to acid, alkali, and malachite green as an aid to their classification and its application to the isolation of *Nocardia* from sputa. Preliminary report. Acta Tuberc. Jap. **14:**1–13.
40. Young, L. S., D. Armstrong, A. Blevins, and P. Lieberman. 1971. *Nocardia asteroides* infection complicating neoplastic disease. Amer. J. Med. **50:**356–367.

Chapter 18

Enterobacteriaceae

WILLIAM H. EWING AND WILLIAM J. MARTIN

INTRODUCTION

The system of classification of the family *Enterobacteriaceae* employed in this chapter is that proposed by one of us in 1963 (22) and subsequently emended and extended as required (18, 32). This system (Table 1) resulted from comparative studies of the biochemical reactions given by relatively large numbers of cultures of each of the genera and species (e.g., see references 18, 31, 38, 39, 42, 44). From the outset, the purpose of the above-mentioned investigations was to provide numerical and percentage data to be used to compare *all* of the reactions given by members of one genus or species with those of others, as well as to provide means for differentiation of the genera and species. Therefore, the genera *Escherichia* and *Shigella* are placed in the same tribe because biochemically these two genera are more closely related to each other than either is related to anything else in the family (Table 1). The genera *Salmonella*, *Arizona*, and *Citrobacter* are placed in the tribe *Salmonelleae* for the same reason, and so on throughout the family. We believe that classification of the microorganisms in this way, i.e., on the basis of overall similarities, is more logical and reasonable than classifications based upon one or two criteria.

At this point in time, it should be unnecessary to mention the so-called genus *Paracolobactrum* or "the paracolon group," since these have been dealt with by several investigators (e.g., reference 54). Suffice it to say that this genus or group does not exist as such. On the contrary, the microorganisms formerly labeled with these designations can and should be classified in the respective recognized genera and species to which they belong on the basis of their aggregate biochemical reactions and without regard to the speed with which they ferment lactose.

Investigations of the degree of relatedness of the deoxyribonucleic acids (DNAs) derived from representatives of the various genera and species of *Enterobacteriaceae* have, for the most part, confirmed the validity and usefulness of the classification of the family proposed earlier (5–7, 14), and have provided solutions to certain problems. For example, Brenner et al. (8) reported that the DNAs derived from strains of *Erwinia* and *Pectobacterium* generally are more closely related to each other than to other members of the family and that both of these genera belong in the family *Enterobacteriaceae*. These investigators proposed (8) maintenance of the tribe *Erwineae*, which would include the genera *Erwinia* (exemplified by *Erwinia amylovora*) and *Pectobacterium* (exemplified by *Pectobacterium carotovorum*). We have adopted these suggestions. Nevertheless, the biochemical reactions of strains of these two genera resemble those of members of the tribe *Klebsielleae* in many respects, and if a culture of either genus is isolated from a specimen of human origin or from a lower animal, differentiation from *Klebsiella*, *Enterobacter*, and *Serratia* still is required.

The following definition of the family *Enterobacteriaceae* Rahn has been in use for several years (18, 26).

> The family *Enterobacteriaceae* consists of gram-negative, aerobic, facultatively anaerobic, asporogenous, rod-shaped bacteria that grow well on artificial media. Some species are atrichous, and nonmotile variants of motile species also may occur. Motile forms are peritrichously flagellated. Nitrates are reduced to nitrites, and glucose is utilized fermentatively with formation of acid or of acid and gas. The indophenol oxidase test is negative, and alginate is not liquefied. Pectate is liquefied by members of only one genus (*Pectobacterium*).

Readers who are interested in other classifications or other definitions should consult references 18, 22, 31, and 65 and the several editions of *Bergey's Manual of Determinative Bacteriology* for information and additional citations.

PROCESSING OF SPECIMENS

From the standpoint of the effectiveness of the laboratory, nothing is more important than the adequacy and condition of the specimen received for examination. If specimens are not properly collected and handled or are not representative, the laboratory can contribute little or nothing to any investigation. This applies to specimens of all sorts (18, 23).

Specimens of extraintestinal origin

A schema that may be employed in the examination of specimens from extraintestinal sources is given in Fig. 1. This may be modified to suit the requirements of investigators in various kinds of laboratories and in accordance with the nature of a particular specimen. When colonies have been isolated on solid media, methods and procedures for further examination and identification of cultures of *Enterobacteriaceae* are very much the same, regardless of the nature of the specimen in which they originated. Therefore, with some modifications with respect to choice of primary plating media, the schemata given in Fig. 2 and 3 also may be used in the examination of specimens from extraintestinal sources. The use (Fig. 1) of lysine-iron-agar (LIA) and motility-indole-ornithine (MIO) media in conjunction with triple sugar-iron (TSI) or Kligler's iron (KI) agar is explained under the heading of Primary differentiation (below).

Blood cultures. Blood samples submitted for culture usually are derived from patients afflicted with febrile disease of unknown origin. If a clinician suspects bacteremia, it generally means that the patient involved is seriously ill. Therefore, it is imperative that blood culture techniques be carried out with design and care commensurate with the gravity of the clinical situation (see also chapter 6).

When possible, blood for culture should be collected during those times when the patient's temperature is rising or falling, since the maximal number of positive cultures may not be obtained from samples drawn at the peak of a temperature curve. Multiple specimens (two or three, drawn at 1- or 2-h intervals) should be collected when indicated. (In cases of suspected bacterial endocarditis, five or six blood specimens may be required.) Media and methods must be used that will support the growth of the more fastidious bacteria, such as brucellae or streptococci, as well as *Enterobacteriaceae*.

Since a specimen of blood from a bacteremia frequently may contain less than one microorganism per ml (57), it is advisable to inoculate 5 ml into 100 ml of glucose-phosphate broth and 5 ml into 100 ml of fluid thioglycolate medium. These amounts of blood and medium yielded a dilution of about 1:40 of noncellular elements of blood, which is sufficient to prevent clot formation and to inactivate complement and other constituents (78, 99). Blood contains no normal flora, hence enrichment media such as selenite broth are unnecessary. The cultures should be examined after 18 to 24 h of incubation at 35 to 37 C; if negative, they should be reincubated for 3 weeks, with examinations at frequent intervals (see also chapter 6). One of us (W.H.E.) has found it advantageous also to prepare pour plates with about 2 ml of patient's blood and an enriched infusion agar medium such as might be used for *Brucella*. When positive, such cultures yield valuable information at an early stage of investigation. However, this method should not be used in lieu of fluid blood cultures (above).

After incubation, blood cultures are streaked on media suitable for the isolation of *Enterobacteriaceae;* then the procedures outlined in Fig. 1 are followed.

In enteric fever caused by *Salmonella typhi*, *S. choleraesuis*, or *S. enteritidis* bioserotypes Paratyphi-A or Paratyphi-B, the microorganism often invades the bloodstream before it appears in large numbers in stools. For this reason, it is advisable to collect blood for culture early in the disease, since the bacteria may disappear from the blood after a short period. If blood cultures taken during the first week of enteric fever are negative, they should be repeated during the second and third weeks (82). This is particularly desirable in severe cases in which the temperature remains elevated for long periods (82).

Almost any enterobacterium (members of the

TABLE 1. *Classification of the family Enterobacteriaceae in outline*

Tribe	Genus
Escherichieae	*Escherichia* (1)[a]
	Shigella (4)
Edwardsielleae	*Edwardsiella* (1)
Salmonelleae	*Salmonella* (3)
	Arizona (1)
	Citrobacter (2)
Klebsielleae	*Klebsiella* (3)
	Enterobacter (4)
	Serratia (3)
Proteeae	*Proteus* (4)
	Providencia (2)
Erwineae	*Erwinia*[b]
	Pectobacterium[b]

[a] Number of species in genus (see also text and other tables).

[b] Several species are recognized in these genera (8).

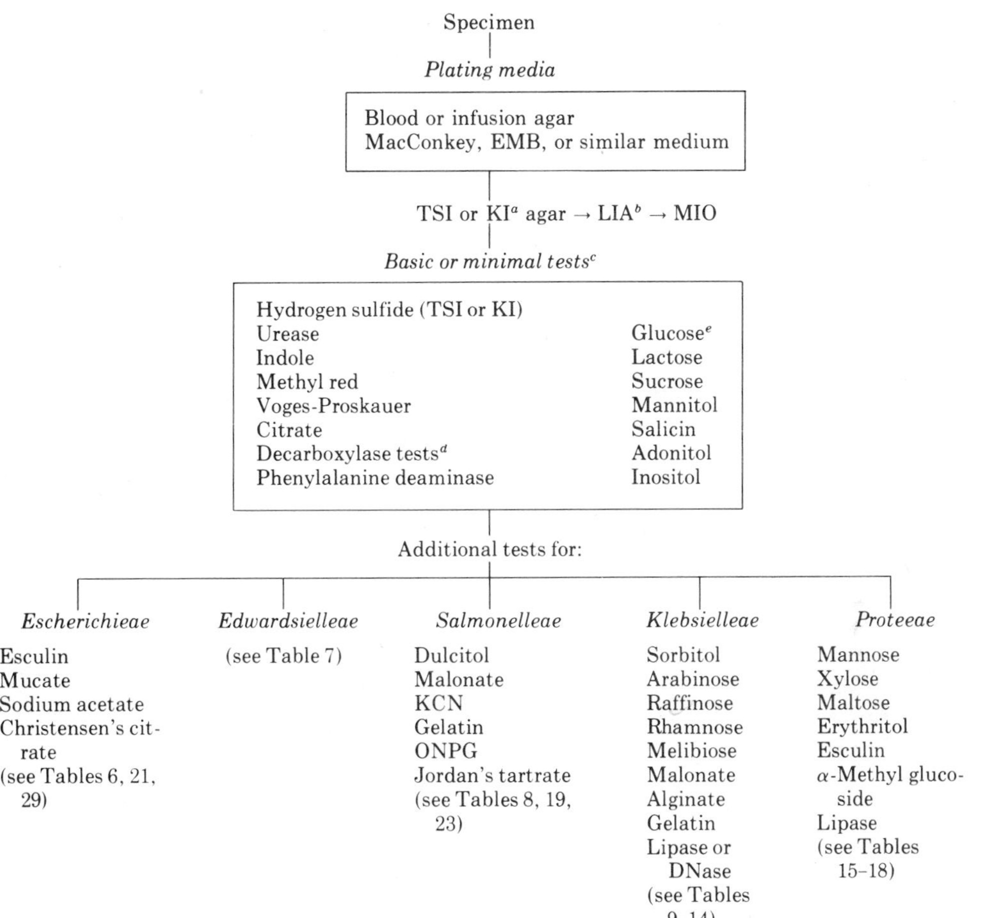

[a] Many workers use Kligler's iron (KI) agar for this purpose.
[b] Indole test papers may be suspended over lysine-iron agar (LIA) or motility-indole-ornithine (MIO) medium.
[c] Inclusion of media for oxidase and nitrate reduction tests is recommended.
[d] All three substrates and a control tube should be used.
[e] Insert tubes should be used in all fluid carbohydrate media.

FIG. 1. *Isolation and identification of Enterobacteriaceae from extraintestinal sources. Adapted from reference 32.*

first five tribes listed in Table 1, at least) may invade the bloodstream, and the occurrence of some species (e.g., *Escherichia coli* and *Klebsiella pneumoniae*) in that location is relatively frequent.

Urine cultures. Midstream specimens collected after thorough cleansing of the genitalia with soap should be selected for culture. Specimens should be examined as soon as possible after collection, since it is known that misleading results may be obtained if the bacteria are allowed to proliferate during the interval between specimen collection and the time of cultural examination. The number of *E. coli* cells, for example, in a urine sample held at 22 C may increase 100-fold within 4 h. (With this fact in mind, Amies and Corpas [2] developed a sodium chloride-polyvinylpyrrolidone preservative that can be used effectively for transport of urine specimens from the ward, service, or clinic to the laboratory. A marked improvement was demonstrated [1] in results obtained when the preservative was used. Samples so preserved may be used for several other tests, but not for specific gravity determinations [1].)

Specimens of urine should be inoculated directly onto plating media (Fig. 1). Blood-agar and a differential plating medium (e.g., MacConkey) are recommended for routine use (Fig. 1), but, if salmonellosis is suspected, a plate of bismuth sulfite agar also should be used.

Since quantification of the numbers of bacteria present usually is desirable, a loopful from a calibrated (0.01 or 0.001 ml) platinum-iridium

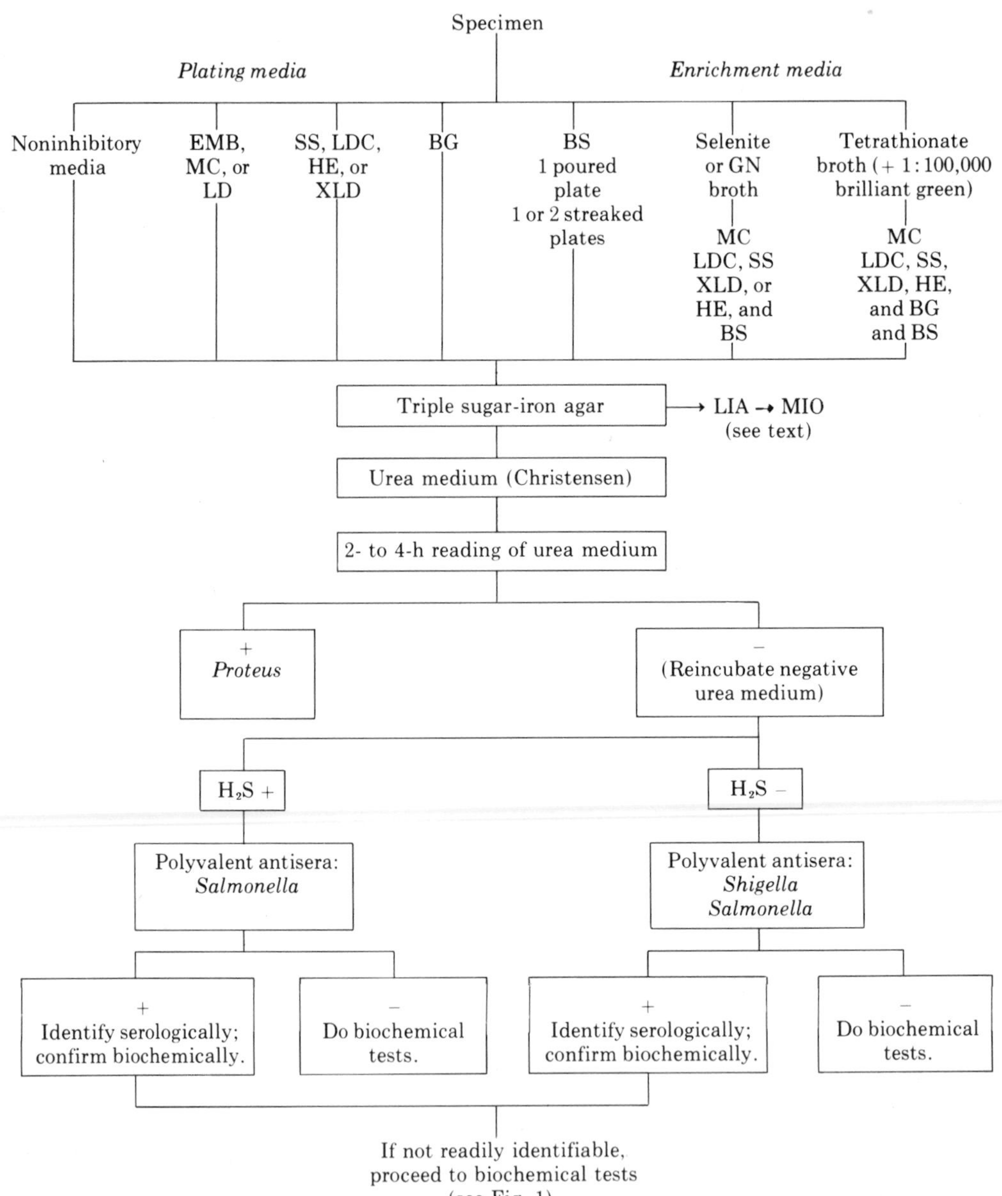

FIG. 2. *Isolation of Enterobacteriaceae from stool specimens. EMB, eosin-methylene blue agar; MC, MacConkey's agar; LD, Leifsen's deoxycholate agar; LDC, Leifsen's deoxycholate-citrate agar; SS, Salmonella-Shigella agar; BS, bismuth sulfite agar; BG, brilliant green agar; XLD, xylose-lysine-deoxycholate agar; HE, Hektoen enteric agar; LIA, lysine-iron-agar; MIO, motility-indole-ornithine medium. Modified from references 18 and 29.*

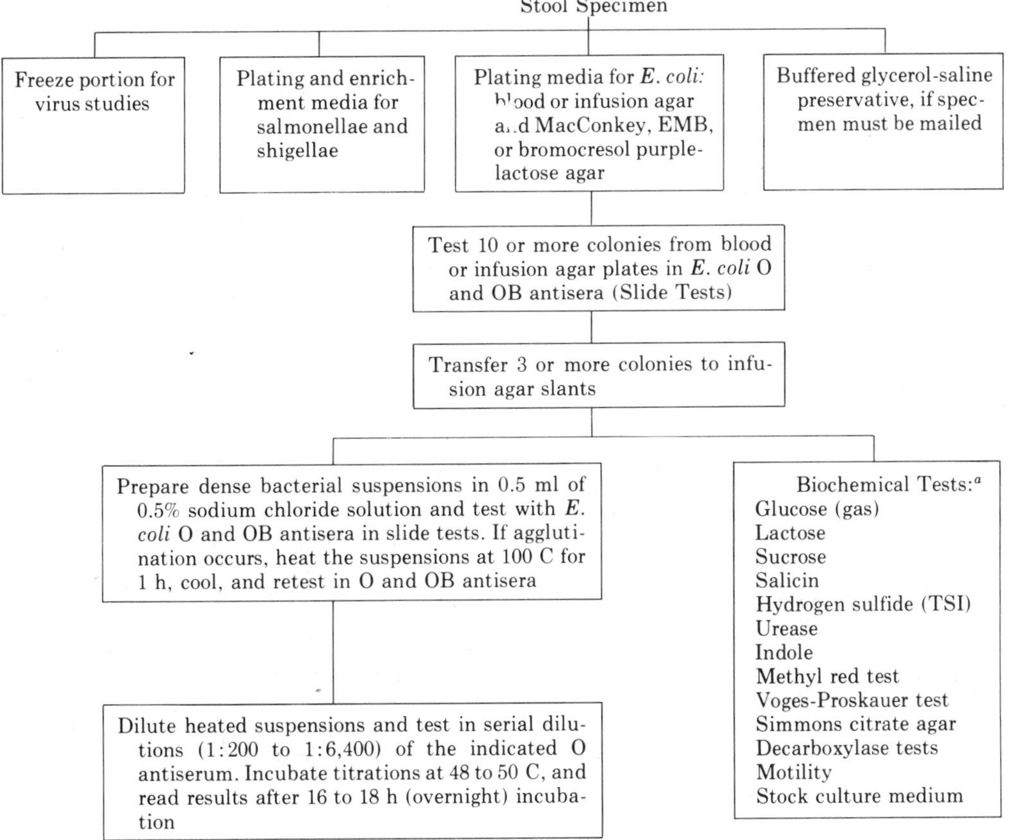

[a] See Fig. 1 and Tables. Modified from reference 28.

FIG. 3. *Methods for examination of stool specimens for Escherichia coli.*

wire loop may be used for inoculation. This permits an estimation of the numbers of bacteria in terms of light growth ($<10^4$ per ml), moderate growth (10^4 to 10^5 per ml), and heavy growth (100 or more colonies per plate or $>10^5$ per ml). If more exact quantitative procedures are required, decimal dilutions should be made and pour plates should be prepared from selected dilutions (see chapter 6 for details). When differential counts are desired, dilutions may be made and 0.05 ml of each is spread over the entire surface of plates of noninhibitory medium.

Specimens from other extraintestinal sources. In addition to examination of Gram stains, purulent material from wounds or abscesses, sediment from cerebrospinal fluid, sputa, nasopharyngeal swabs, exudates, and specimens from other sources should be examined by methods that may be expected to reveal the presence of any cultivatable microorganism. Blood-agar plates used in conjunction with differential plating media (Fig. 1) usually are sufficient for isolation of *Enterobacteriaceae*. However, in the examination of exudates from the pleural or peritoneal cavities, it is advisable to employ a plate of one of the selective media (see Fecal specimens, below, and Fig. 2) in addition to the general-purpose media listed above and in Fig. 1. Biopsy, necropsy, or surgical specimens such as liver, lymph nodes, portions of intestinal wall, or gall bladders should be ground aseptically and streaked on suitable plating media including blood agar, and a liberal portion should be placed in enrichment medium (Fig. 2). Duodenal drainage and bile are treated in the same manner that one would use to process a stool specimen.

If specimens of the sort mentioned above must be sent to another laboratory, the transport menstrua used for stool specimens (see below) generally can be used. Exudates, sediment from spinal fluid, macerated tissue, etc., may be collected on swabs, and these are placed in transport medium. In addition to the use of one of the transport media mentioned below, it is advisable to employ the chopped-meat medium commonly used for anaerobic bacteria. Various *Enterobacteriaceae* and other bacteria, as well as anaerobes, can be recovered from specimens transported in this medium (18).

Fecal specimens

Stools should be collected early in the course of enteric disease processes and before the initiation of antimicrobial therapy. Portions of the specimen are collected carefully and inoculated onto adequate plating and enrichment media as soon as possible after collection, since some etiological agents may decrease rapidly in numbers or may be overgrown by other microorganisms. If present, pathological constituents such as mucus should be selected for cultural work.

It is generally agreed that the specimen of choice in enteric disease is a freshly passed stool. Rectal swabs may be used in the examination of a sampling portion of those ill in an epidemic, but they should not be relied upon to yield the maximal number of positive cultures (69, 81, 91). Further, single rectal swabs are of little value in the examination of convalescent patients or in surveys for carriers.

Whenever possible, multiple specimens should be cultured. Many investigators have demonstrated the value of this procedure; for example, it was demonstrated at least as early as 1916 by Ten Broeck and Norbury (90). Similar data later were reported by others (e.g., see reference 18).

In the investigation of diarrheal diseases, the importance of obtaining specimens in the *acute* stage of the disease cannot be overemphasized. Usually the bacillary incitants of enteric disease are present in large numbers at that time and often are the predominant microorganism in the stool. As symptoms subside, the numbers of the causative agent rapidly decrease so that, in cultures taken after the acute stage of disease is past, the microorganisms responsible for the infection may be isolated only with difficulty or may not be found.

Transport solutions and media. Specimens that cannot be cultured very soon after collection should be placed in a transport solution or medium until they can be examined. A number of transport media have been described (see reference 18), and they all are designed to hold the bacterial population in a specimen more or less stationary, and to prevent, as much as possible, overgrowth of a particular microorganism by others that may be present. One of the oldest known, and probably still the most widely used, is the buffered glycerol saline solution described by Teague and Clurman (89) and modified by Sachs (80). The final pH of this solution should be 7.4, and if it becomes acid before use it should be discarded. Approximately 1 g of feces is added to 10 ml of solution and thoroughly emulsified in it.

Enrichment media. It always is advisable to employ enrichment media in the examination of various kinds of specimens, and their use is practically essential when dealing with fecal specimens from carriers or suspected carriers. Two such media have been employed extensively and may be recommended for general use. These are the tetrathionate medium of Muller (75) and the selenite F broth devised by Leifson (68). The combined enrichment medium of Kauffmann (63) is a modification of Muller's medium which contains bile and brilliant green. The efficacy of this medium for the enrichment of *Salmonella* is attested by the results of Kauffmann (64) and many others (18, 59, 69).

Tetrathionate base, which is Muller's medium with bile salts added, may be employed with all specimens, since salmonellae including *S. typhi* generally are greatly increased in numbers in this medium. Some shigellae also may be recovered from it. Tetrathionate medium with brilliant green added (1:100,000) is useful only for *Salmonella* other than *S. typhi.*

The selenite medium recommended by Leifson (68) for use with feces (selenite F) was designed for enrichment of *Salmonella* including *S. typhi*, not for shigellae. However, the selenite media available from most commercial sources have been modified slightly, and some shigellae may be recovered after plating from it.

Both selenite and tetrathionate media reportedly are toxic for *S. choleraesuis* and *S. enteritidis* serotype Abortus-ovis (83), whereas tetrathionate broth inhibits the growth of *S. enteritidis* bioserotype Paratyphi-A (3). Leifson reported the high toxicity of selenite for *S. choleraesuis* when he described the medium. The selenite F and tetrathionate media that are available in dehydrated form from several commercial outlets are quite efficient when prepared in exact accordance with the directions that accompany them, and these preparations can be recommended for use as outlined in the foregoing paragraphs.

Hajna (61) devised a broth medium (GN)

which is useful for enrichment. Increased numbers of salmonellae and shigellae were isolated with this medium. Croft and Miller (13) used GN broth successfully in the study of outbreaks of shigellosis, and Taylor and Schelhart (88) apparently found it useful for shigellae.

It is apparent that, if a single enrichment must be selected for general purposes, selenite broth probably is the medium of choice. When possible, a combination of media, such as selenite and GN, should be used. Enrichment media should be tubed in 8- to 10-ml amounts and inoculated with approximately 1 g (or 1 ml of fluid specimen) of feces. The inocula should be emulsified thoroughly in the medium. After incubation at 35 to 37 C (selenite, 12 to 16 h; tetrathionate, 18 to 24 h; GN 18 h), cultures in enrichment media should be streaked on plates of the same sort used for primary inoculation of specimens (Fig. 2). With noninhibitory and slightly inhibitory media, 1 loopful (3- to 4-mm loop) of inoculum should be used, but 2 or 3 loopsful may be streaked on moderately and highly selective media. In every instance, plates must be streaked carefully to assure growth of well-isolated colonies.

For additional information regarding the numerous varieties and modifications of enrichment media, readers should consult the publications cited above and references 18, 52, and 69.

Plating media. The media in general use for the isolation of various *Enterobacteriaceae* may be divided into a number of categories according to their selectivity (see chapter 95 or reference 18 for formulas and citations for authorship of plating media):

Noninhibitory media such as blood-agar, plain infusion agar, or nutrient agar.

Noninhibitory differential media, e.g., bromothymol blue-lactose (BTBL) and phenol red-lactose (PRL) agars.

Differential media with little selectivity as regards *Enterobacteriaceae.* These include MacConkey's, eosin methylene blue (EMB), and deoxycholate agars.

Differential, moderately selective media, such as *Shigella-Salmonella* (SS), deoxycholate-citrate, Hektoen enteric, and xylose-lysine-deoxycholate (XLD).

Highly selective media, which include bismuth sulfite agar and brilliant green agar. The latter may be called a one-purpose medium, particularly useful for the isolation of salmonellae. However, certain other bacteria (e.g., some pseudomonads and aeromonads) may grow on brilliant green agar and form pink colonies.

The results that may be expected when the above-mentioned agar plating media are properly prepared and used for the isolation of *Shigella*, *Salmonella typhi*, and other *Salmonella* species are shown in Table 2 (23). As might be expected, occasional strains of shigellae may not grow on MacConkey, SS, or deoxycholate-citrate agar, or a particular *Salmonella* strain may not appear on brilliant green agar. Therefore, it is advisable to use a variety of media whenever possible. The procedure to be followed in any laboratory is dictated by facilities, personnel, and the amount of time available for work of this sort. In any search for salmonellae, including *S. typhi*, bismuth sulfite agar always should be used, since it is the most efficient medium yet devised for the isolation of this microorganism. For the maximal number of isolations, many workers have found it advisable to use two plates. One plate should be streaked with feces or fecal suspension. The second is a poured plate, in which have been placed 5 ml of a suspension of feces. In the stools of typhoid patients in which *S. typhi* is present in large numbers, typical colonies usually will be found on the streaked plate. In specimens from carriers, where the bacteria may be present in small numbers, the organism frequently may be isolated from subsurface colonies in the poured plate. Subsurface colonies obviously must be restreaked on a medium such as MacConkey or EMB agar. The extreme variation in the numbers of *S. typhi* and *S. enteritidis* serotype Paratyphi-B excreted by different carriers is well illustrated by the work

TABLE 2. *Value of plating media for isolation of Shigella, Salmonella typhi, and other Salmonella species*

Organism	Agar medium					
	Infusion (etc.)	BTB[a] (etc.)	MacConkey (etc.)	SS[a] (etc.)	Bismuth sulfite	Brilliant green
Shigella	+	+	+	+	−	−
Salmonella typhi	+	+	+	+	+	−
Other *Salmonella* spp.	+	+	+	+	+	+

[a] BTB, bromothymol blue; SS, *Salmonella-Shigella*.

of Thomson (96), who recommended the addition of a very lightly inoculated plate in the examination of carriers. He obtained good results by streaking 0.02 ml of a 1:1,000 dilution of feces on deoxycholate-citrate agar. *S. typhi* frequently does not produce typical blackening of bismuth sulfite agar when the colonies are very numerous and crowded. For this reason, the use of two or more plates is advisable. Strains of other *Salmonella* usually grow well on bismuth sulfite agar, and it is a good medium for their isolation. However, on this medium, *Shigella* fails to develop except in very rare instances. Since bismuth sulfite agar is highly inhibitory, it is advisable to incubate plates for 48 h before they are discarded. Added reasons for the use of bismuth sulfite agar lie in the detection of members of the genus *Arizona* (19) and in the isolation of the rare strain of *Salmonella* that ferments lactose rapidly. For the isolation of shigellae, most workers prefer to use one plate of a purely differential or only mildly selective medium and one plate of a more highly selective preparation. MacConkey's, deoxycholate, or EMB agar can be used for the first, and deoxycholate-citrate or SS agar for the second. When possible, it is advisable to employ a variety of media, and XLD or Hektoen enteric agar media may be included (Fig. 2). Certain strains of *Shigella* grow very poorly on the more highly selective media, and for this reason one of the less inhibitory media should be included. For example, Wheeler and Mickle (100) demonstrated that *S. sonnei* form II does not grow well on selective media such as those just mentioned, and this form is prone to occur in convalescent patients and carriers (4). If XLD agar is used, it should be recalled that some shigellae ferment xylose.

In our experience, the best way to isolate the maximal number of shigellae is to inoculate several plates of plain infusion agar, each with small inocula, and pick a number of each colonial type that appears on each plate.

Salmonellae usually can be isolated from any of the above-mentioned media, but it is inadvisable to rely on only one plate of a single medium. On the contrary, at least one plate each of the slightly selective, selective, and the highly selective media such as bismuth sulfite agar should be employed.

Cultures in enrichment media should be inoculated onto the same kinds of plating media that are employed for fresh specimens. Isolation media should be inoculated in such a manner as to assure the maximal number of well-isolated colonies. All media employed for isolation should be freshly prepared in exact accordance with directions. One good plan is to prepare plating media one day and use it the next. With the exception of bismuth sulfite agar, the above-mentioned media may be kept in a refrigerator for about 3 days, provided that steps are taken to prevent evaporation. Bismuth sulfite agar should not be used after storage for 24 to 36 h. When this medium becomes green, it is too inhibitory, and good results cannot be expected.

Outlines of procedures for the isolation and preliminary identification of cultures of *Salmonella* and *Shigella* are given in Fig. 2. Members of other genera of *Enterobacteriaceae* also may be recovered and processed according to the procedures given in Fig. 2.

SELECTION AND ISOLATION OF COLONIES

In the examination of plates inoculated with feces or other specimens, either directly or from enrichment media, a *careful* search should be made for significant microorganisms. Cursory examination will not suffice. For example, *Shigella* and *Salmonella* usually produce typical colonies on the various plating media, but it must be remembered that colonial appearance may be altered by growth in close association with other bacteria. At times, these pathogens produce colonies of atypical appearance for reasons that are not entirely clear. Therefore, even persons of long experience in enteric bacteriology may be misled by colonial appearance. When searching for salmonellae or shigellae, it is advisable to pick at least two representatives of each type of colony, other than those of frank lactose fermenters, that appears on the plates. Examination of plates with a colony counter or magnifier may be helpful in distinguishing the various colony types.

Many kinds of microorganisms do not develop on selective media and viable bacteria that have not grown, or which may have produced only microscopic colonies, are present on the surface of the agar. Therefore, the greatest care must be exercised in picking colonies if pure cultures are to be obtained. It is advisable to use a straight wire and touch only the center of the selected colony. One should avoid touching the surface of the agar. Proper attention to this detail will result in fewer mixed cultures from plates inoculated with feces.

Primary differentiation

Bacteria from selected colonies should be transfered to tubes of triple sugar-iron (TSI) or

Kligler's iron (KI) agar. The butt of the medium first is stabbed to the bottom of the tube, and then the slant is streaked carefully over the entire surface. If good growth does not occur in the butt or on the slant of these media, atypical reactions may result. KI agar is recommended for use with specimens from extraintestinal sources, especially urine, since it is desirable to determine the species of isolates of *Proteus*. It always is advisable to mark and number each colony picked and to place the same number on the corresponding TSI or KI agar tube. A record of the nature of the colony should be kept (i.e., typical, atypical, etc.). If the reaction in TSI or KI agar medium after overnight (18 to 24 h) incubation deviates from what might be expected from the colonial appearance, the culture may be mixed. In such instances, the purity of the culture should be determined by replating on a differential medium. Gram stains also are helpful for determination of purity. The reactions given by various kinds of *Enterobacteriaceae* on TSI agar are recorded in Table 3.

Numerous complex media have been devised for the cultivation of colonies picked from isolation plates (see reference 18). A variety of biochemical and physiological properties may be determined in such media, some of which are tubed in two or even three layers, one superimposed upon another. Although not discounting the value of such media, nor detracting from their performance, we prefer to use TSI (or KI) agar in conjunction with lysine-iron agar (LIA) and motility-indole-ornithine (MIO) medium

TABLE 3. *Reactions of Enterobacteriaceae in triple sugar-iron (TSI) agar medium*[a]

Genus and species	Slant	Butt	Gas	H_2S
Escherichia	A (K)	A	+ (−)	−
Shigella	K	A	−	−
Salmonella typhi	K	A	−	+ (−)
Other *Salmonella* spp.	K	A	+	+++ (−)
Arizona	K (A)	A	+	+++
Citrobacter	K (A)	A	+	+++ (−)
Edwardsiella	K	A	+	+++
Klebsiella	A	A	++	−
Enterobacter	A	A	++	−
E. hafniae	K	A	+	−
Serratia	K or A	A	−	−
Proteus vulgaris	A (K)	A	+	+++
P. mirabilis	K (A)	A	+	+++
P. morganii	K	A	− (+)	−
P. rettgeri	K	A	−	−
Providencia	K	A	+ or −	−

[a] K, alkaline; A, acid. Modified from references 18 and 24. Symbols in parentheses indicate occasional reactions.

for the cultivation of colonies from isolation plates and to rely on conventional methods for determination of additional biochemical properties of isolants.

In the search for *Salmonella* or *Shigella* (Fig. 2), tubes of TSI agar that exhibit an acid butt and an alkaline slant should be planted immediately on the urea agar of Christensen (12). This medium is slanted so that the medium has a short slant and a deep butt. The medium is inoculated heavily on the slant only. Cultures of *Proteus* produce marked alkalinity in Christensen's urea agar after brief incubation. The cultures are examined after 2 to 4 h, and the negative tubes are reincubated. Cultures that belong to certain other genera produce various degrees of alkalinity in Christensen's medium after 24 or more h of incubation. If preferred, the rapid urease test of Stuart et al. (86) may be substituted for Christensen's medium.

For a number of years, we and our co-workers (24, 62) have used LIA and MIO medium (62) in conjunction with TSI or KI agar as aids in the examination of colonies picked from plating media. Others also have found the procedure helpful. With a straight wire, inoculum is taken carefully from a selected colony and transferred to TSI or KI medium in the usual way. Then, *without* going back to the colony, a tube of LIA is inoculated directly by stabbing the butt of the medium twice and streaking the slant. Inoculation of a tube of MIO medium (by stabbing to the bottom of the tube), in turn, also is helpful. The combinations of reactions obtained by means of this method yield a great deal of useful information early in the examination of a specimen. The use of a filter-paper strip previously impregnated with Kovacs' reagent, or that mentioned by Gillies (60), and dried furnishes additional valuable information, particularly when tests are positive. The paper strips may be suspended in tubes of LIA or MIO medium, being held in place by the closure. Negative tests obtained by this method should be retested by conventional means, especially when a negative test does not align itself with the results of other tests. The reactions given by members of the family *Enterobacteriaceae* in LIA are listed in Table 4. It should be emphasized that LIA is not considered a substitute for the standard (Moeller) method for determination of lysine decarboxylation. Although LIA and MIO are valuable media when used in the manner described, their use should be limited to preliminary work. Some cultures of *E. coli*, for example, may not yield evidence of lysine decarboxylation in the butt of LIA medium at

TABLE 4. *Reactions of Enterobacteriaceae in lysine-iron agar (LIA)*[a]

Genus and species	Slant	Butt	Gas	H_2S
Escherichia	K	K or N	− or +	−
Shigella	K	A	−	−
Salmonella	K	K or N	−	+ (−)
S. typhi	K	K[b]	−	+ or −
Paratyphi-A	K	A	+ or −	− or +
Arizona	K	K or N	−	+ (−)
Citrobacter	K	A	− or +	+ or −
Edwardsiella	K	K	− or +	+
Klebsiella	K or N	K or N	+ or −	−
Enterobacter cloacae	K or N	A	+ or −	−
E. aerogenes	K	K or N	+ (−)	−
E. hafniae	K	K or N	− or +	−
Serratia	K or N	K or N	−	−
Proteus vulgaris	R	A	−	− (+)
P. mirabilis	R	A	−	− (+)
P. morganii	K or R	A	−	−
P. rettgeri	R	A	−	−
Providencia	R	A	−	−

[a] K, alkaline; A, acid; R, red (oxidative deamination). An alkaline reaction in the *butt* of this medium indicates decarboxylation. Symbols in parentheses indicate occasional reactions. Adapted from references 18, 29, and 24.

[b] A rare culture of *S. typhi* may fail to decarboxylate lysine (51).

18 to 24 h, but may do so after 40 to 48 h (24).

Another system for the examination of colonies of gram-negative bacteria involves the use of TSI, LIA, Christensen's urea agar, Simmons' citrate, ornithine-motility, and peptone broth media. Material from a selected colony is inoculated into TSI medium, after which the other media are inoculated from the TSI agar. One of us (W.J.M.) has used this six-tube method for several years, and has found it to be advantageous since it permits identification of more than 90% of isolates from extraintestinal sources within 24 h (Laboratory procedures in clinical microbiology, J. A. Washington II [ed.], Little, Brown and Co., in press). This method, or slight modifications of it, is known to be employed in a number of well-established laboratories.

Several systems or devices are available that can be employed instead of the TSI (or KI)-LIA-MIO method mentioned above. The usefulness and accuracy of some of these, e.g., the Auxotab, the Enterotube, and the R-B System, have been evaluated extensively (70, 77, 84, 97, 98), and the authors of most of the evaluations have indicated that, if used and interpreted properly, the aforementioned systems or devices yield good results, particularly with typical cultures. In some instances, it was suggested that the addition of certain media, such as citrate and urea, enhanced the usefulness of the product (70). Another device that should be mentioned is the API (Analytab) system. However, this system should not be compared with those mentioned above, since it is composed of a series of about 20 tests and substrates. Hence, this system is a miniaturized version, more or less, of conventional methods. Evaluations have indicated (84, 98) that good results can be obtained with the API system. As with any method with which a laboratory worker is unfamiliar, there is an initial learning process regarding inoculation, interpretation of reactions, etc. involved with any of the above-mentioned systems.

BIOCHEMICAL REACTIONS OF ENTEROBACTERIACEAE

Application of the TSI (or KI)-LIA-MIO system (Fig. 1; or the six-tube method, above) to cultures of *Enterobacteriaceae* regardless of their source permits the laboratory to issue a preliminary or presumptive report regarding most isolates at 18 to 24 h. In some instances, specific identification can be made on the basis of the reactions in these three media. More often, however, it is necessary to employ the tests and substrates listed in Fig. 1 under the heading of basic or minimal tests together with those for differentiation within the several tribes. The species of many strains can be determined by means of the tests given in the basic list. For other isolates, these tests are sufficient to determine the tribe or genus and which of the additional substrates (Fig. 1) are required for accurate differentiation of species that belong to a particular genus. Finally, occasional cultures may yield atypical reactions in one or more tests; with these, it may be necessary to perform all known biochemical tests to be certain of the species to which they belong. This includes additional carbohydrate broths, alginate media, oxidation-fermentation tests, and performance of tests at 22 to 26 C.

We believe that any member of the family *Enterobacteriaceae* that is considered significant enough to warrant being picked from primary plating media is important enough to be identified to species. This is essential if one wishes to compile continuing data regarding patterns of susceptibility to antimicrobial agents and changes that occur over periods of time. It also is essential for epidemiological studies such as determination of nosocomial infections and their spread. Moreover, it is apparent that complete identification of strains to the species level is an integral part of any good bacteriological investigation.

It is recommended that oxidase and nitrate reduction tests be performed at an early stage in the identification of all isolates. If this is done, much time and labor can be saved, since all *Enterobacteriaceae* are oxidase-negative and all except a few reduce nitrate to nitrite but are not known to reduce nitrite. Members of several genera of bacteria, e.g., aeromonads, vibrios, most pseudomonads, and certain miscellaneous gram-negative microorganisms (chapter 24), are oxidase-positive, and the oxidase test alone differentiates these bacteria from *Enterobacteriaceae*. Cultures of some biogroups of *Enterobacter agglomerans* fail to reduce nitrate to nitrite (47–49), and members of the genus *Erwinia* are nitrate-negative in conventional tests. With rare exceptions, other *Enterobacteriaceae* (Table 1) reduce nitrate to nitrite (see tabular data in references 18 and 55), whereas strains of *Acinetobacter calcoaceticus* (chapter 24), for example, fail to do so. Other bacteria, e.g., some pseudomonads and some miscellaneous forms (chapter 24), reduce nitrate to gas or to an anaerogenic amine. The zinc dust test for unreduced nitrate should be done as indicated by the results of tests for nitrite.

The biochemical reactions given by members of the tribes of *Enterobacteriaceae* in differential tests are listed in Table 5. In addition, the reactions of members of various species in tests that are of particular value for differentiation are listed in Tables 6 to 19, with one exception (Table 14) in which the biochemical reactions of *E. agglomerans* are given in detail (see below). Judicious use of the data presented in Fig. 1 and Tables 6 to 19 should enable laboratory investigators to identify all except a very few of the *Enterobacteriaceae* encountered in daily practice, including some strains that may yield atypical results in one or more tests. Identification of the rare exception to this may require the use of additional tests and substrates. In such instances, the publications from which the data in Tables 6 to 19 were taken should be consulted; these publications are cited in the tables. Methods for preparation of media and performance of tests are given elsewhere (18, 35), and also are included in chapter 96. Unless otherwise indicated, the data in the tables were based upon results obtained with cultures incubated at 35 to 37 C.

With few exceptions (below), the information given in Tables 5 to 19 is self-explanatory. Means by which cultures of *E. coli* may be differentiated from members of the four species of *Shigella* are given in Table 6. Obviously, there is no difficulty in the differentiation of typical cultures of *E. coli* from shigellae. However, the anaerogenic, nonmotile forms, some of which are often referred to as Alkalescens-Dispar types, may require close examination before they can be classified definitely as *E. coli*. In attempting to classify a particular strain as *E. coli* or as a member of the genus *Shigella*, the biochemical reactivities should be considered as a whole. Shigellae are much less reactive than *E. coli*, and a culture that produces acid promptly (i.e., within 24 h) from all, or most, of a wide variety of carbohydrates, such as maltose, rhamnose, xylose, sorbitol, and dulcitol, probably is not a *Shigella* species.

Certain biotypes of *S. flexneri* 6 (the Newcastle and Manchester bioserotypes) produce gas from glucose; other shigellae do not. Cultures of

TABLE 5. *Differentiation of the tribes of Enterobacteriaceae by biochemical methods*[a]

Test or substrate	Tribes				
	Escherichieae	*Edwardsielleae*	*Salmonelleae*	*Klebsielleae*	*Proteeae*
Hydrogen sulfide (TSI)	−	+	+	−	+ or −
Urease	−	−	−	− or (+)	+ or −
Indole	+ or −	+	−	−	+ or −
Methyl red	+	+	+	−	+
Voges-Proskauer	−	−	−	+	−
Citrate (Simmons')	−	−	+	+	d
KCN	−	−	− or +	+	+
Phenylalanine deaminase	−	−	−	−	+
Jordan's tartrate	+ or −	−	d	+ or −	+ or −
Mucate	d	−	d	+ or −	−
Mannitol	+ or −	−	+	+	− or +

[a] *S. typhi*, *S. enteritidis* bioserotype Paratyphi-A, and some rare biotypes fail to utilize citrate. Cultures of *S. enteritidis* bioserotype Paratyphi-A and some rare biotypes may fail to produce hydrogen sulfide. Some strains of *P. mirabilis* may yield positive Voges-Proskauer tests. Symbols: +, 90% or more positive within 1 or 2 days; −, 90% or more no reaction; (+), delayed positive after 3 days or more; d, different biochemical reactions, +, (+), −; + or −, most cultures positive, some negative; − or +, most strains negative, some cultures positive. Adapted from references 18 and 32.

TABLE 6. *Differentiation within the tribe Escherichieae*[a]

Test or substrate	*Escherichia*		*Shigella*	
	Sign[b]	Percent positive[c]	Sign[b]	Percent positive[c]
Gas from glucose	+	90.7	–	2.1[d]
Lactose	+	90.8 (5.1)	–	0.3 (11.4)[d]
Sucrose	d	48.9 (5.6)	–	0.9 (31.1)[d]
Salicin	d	40 (14)	–	0
Motility	+ or –	69.1	–	0
Indole	+	99.2	– or +	37.8
Lysine decarboxylase	d	87.9 (1.2)	–	0
Arginine dihydrolase	d	17.2 (44.8)	d	7.6 (5.6)
Ornithine decarboxylase	d	63.4 (7.1)	– or +	20[d]
Esculin	d	30.9 (19.7)	–	0
Sodium acetate	+ or (+)	83.9 (9.7)	–	0[d]
Christensen's citrate	d	24.4 (21.2)	–	0
Mucate	+	91.6	–	0[d]

[a] Adapted from references 18, 30, 32, and 42.

[b] Sign: +, 90% or more positive within 1 or 2 days; (+), positive reaction after 3 or more days (decarboxylase tests: 3 or 4 days); –, no reaction (90% or more); + or –, most cultures positive, some strains negative; – or +, most strains negative, some cultures positive; + or (+), most reactions occur within 1 or 2 days, some are delayed; d, different reactions, +, (+), –.

[c] Figures in parentheses indicate percentages of delayed reactions (3 or more days).

[d] Cultures of *S. sonnei* usually ferment lactose and sucrose slowly, and strains of this species decarboxylate ornithine. Some cultures of *S. sonnei* are mucate-positive (weakly and slowly). Cultures of *S. flexneri* 4a (mannitol-negative biotype) grow on acetate medium.

S. sonnei ferment lactose and sucrose slowly and decarboxylate ornithine. Some strains of *S. sonnei* also utilize mucate slowly. Most cultures of the mannitol-negative bioserotype of *S. flexneri* 4a slowly utilize sodium acetate as a sole source of carbon, whereas other shigellae do not utilize it. Readers also are referred to Tables 26 and 29.

The biochemical reactions given by more than 1,800 cultures of *E. coli* are summarized in Table 29 (see section headed Examination of cultures of *Escherichia coli*). None of these strains produced hydrogen sulfide in TSI or peptone-iron (PI) agar. The occurrence of occasional isolates of certain bioserotypes (Alkalescens-Dispar) of *E. coli* that produce hydrogen sulfide in these media has been known for a long time (unpublished data, 1949 and 1950; reference 58), but cultures of this particular sort have not been seen in recent years. However, since about 1962 we have received some strains of *E. coli* that produce abundant hydrogen sulfide in TSI and PI agar. Such strains had not been seen for a long time, either by us or by other investigators (e.g., personal communication, 1970, I. Oerskov, State Serum Institute, Copenhagen, Denmark). It now is known (15, 67, 85) that hydrogen sulfide formation by isolates of *E. coli* is mediated by an episome or plasmid. Thus, the appearance of an atypical character in a culture that otherwise is typical may be explained, in many instances at least, by recombinations in which an episome or plasmid carrying genetic material for that character is involved (15, 67, 85). Darland and Davis

TABLE 7. *Differentiation of Escherichia and Edwardsiella*[a]

Test or substrate	*Escherichia*		*Edwardsiella*	
	Sign[b]	Percent positive[c]	Sign[b]	Percent positive[c]
Hydrogen sulfide (TSI)	–	0	+	99.7 (0.3)
Mucate	+	91.6 (1.4)	–	0
Jordan's tartrate	+	97.6	–	0
Sodium acetate	+ or (+)	83.8 (9.7)	–	0
Mannitol	+	97	–	0
Sorbitol	+	93.4 (0.5)	–	0.3
Rhamnose	d	81.8 (2.8)	–	0
Xylose	d	82.4 (6.7)	–	0
Trehalose	+	98.6 (1)	–	0.3

[a] Adapted from references 18, 42, and 50.

[b] Sign: +, 90% or more positive within 1 or 2 days; (+), positive reaction after 3 or more days (decarboxylase tests: 3 or 4 days); –, no reaction (90% or more); + or –, most cultures positive, some strains negative; – or +, most strains negative, some cultures positive; + or (+), most reactions occur within 1 or 2 days, some are delayed; d, different reactions, +, (+), –.

[c] Figures in parentheses indicate percentages of delayed reactions (3 or more days).

(15) studied 202 hydrogen sulfide-positive strains of *E. coli* received between 1966 and 1972. In the same period, 4,048 normal *E. coli* isolates were received; therefore, the incidence of hydrogen sulfide-positive cultures among this group of strains was 4.8%. However, we do not believe that the true incidence of such isolates among all *E. coli* strains is that high.

The biochemical reactions that are of particular value for differentiation of the three species

TABLE 8. *Differentiation of Salmonella, Arizona, and Citrobacter*[a]

Test of substrate	*Salmonella enteritidis*		*Arizona hinshawii*		*Citrobacter freundii*		*Citrobacter diversus*	
	Sign[b]	Percent positive[c]	Sign[b]	Percent positive[c]	Sign[b]	Percent positive[c]	Sign[b]	Percent positive[c]
Urease	–	0	–	0	d	69.4 (6.9)	d	77.9 (10.1)
KCN	–	0.1	–	8.7	+	96.2 (0.9)	–	0
Gelatin (22 C)	–	0.5	(+)	92	–	(0.9)		0 (2)
Lysine decarboxylase	+	99.4 (0.1)	+	100	–	0	–	0
Ornithine decarboxylase	+	100	+	100	d	17.2 (0.2)	+	100
Lactose	–	0.3	d	61.3 (16.7)	(+) or +	39.3 (50.9)	d	32.7 (51.4)
Sucrose	–	0.2	–	4.7	d	15.3 (9.4)	– or +	16.8
Dulcitol	+	97.7	–	0	d	59.8 (0.7)	+ or –	53.1
Adonitol	–	0	–	0	–	0	+	100
Inositol	d	43.8 (2)	–	0	–	3.3 (1.9)	–	0
Malonate	–	1 (0.1)	+	92.6 (0.7)	d	21.8 (0.7)	+ or –	88.5
Jordan's tartrate	d	84.2 (1)	–	5.3	+	100	+ or –	71.3
β-Galactosidase	–	2.1	+	92.8	+ or –	74.4	+	100[d]

[a] Adapted from references 18, 33, 36, 37, 45, and 72. N.B. Cultures of *C. diversus* do not produce hydrogen sulfide in TSI medium. The species *S. enteritidis* includes all salmonellae other than *S. choleraesuis* and *S. typhi*.

[b] Sign: +, 90% or more positive within 1 or 2 days; (+), positive reaction after 3 or more days (decarboxylase tests: 3 or 4 days); –, no reaction (90% or more); + or –, most cultures positive, some strains negative; – or +, most strains negative, some cultures positive; + or (+), most reactions occur within 1 or 2 days, some are delayed; d, different reactions, +, (+), –.

[c] Figures in parentheses indicate percentages of delayed reactions (3 or more days).

[d] Only lactose-negative cultures were tested.

TABLE 9. *Differentiation within the genus Klebsiella*[a]

Test or substrate	*K. pneumoniae*		*K. ozaenae*		*K. rhinoschleromatis*	
	Sign[b]	Percent positive[c]	Sign[b]	Percent positive[c]	Sign[b]	Percent positive[c]
Urease	+	95.4 (0.1)	d	14.8 (14.8)	–	0
Methyl red	– or +	11.3	+	97.7	+	100
Voges-Proskauer	+	93.7	–	0	–	0
Citrate (Simmons)	+	96.8 (0.6)	d	28.1 (32.4)	–	0
Malonate	+	92.5	–	6	+ or –	50
Mucate	+	92.8	– or +	25	–	0
Lysine decarboxylase	+	97.2 (0.1)	– or +	35.8 (6.3)	–	0
Gas from glucose	+	96	d	55.5 (9.4)	–	0
Lactose	+	98.7 (1)	d	26.2 (61.3)	d	6 (70)
Dulcitol	– or +	33	–	0	–	0

[a] Adapted from references 18, 32, and 55.

[b] Sign: +, 90% or more positive within 1 or 2 days; (+), positive reaction after 3 or more days (decarboxylase tests: 3 or 4 days); –, no reaction (90% or more); + or –, most cultures positive, some strains negative; – or +, most strains negative, some cultures positive; + or (+), most reactions occur within 1 or 2 days, some are delayed; d, different reactions, +, (+), –.

[c] Figures in parentheses indicate percentages of delayed reactions (3 or more days).

TABLE 10. *Differentiation of Klebsiella pneumoniae and Enterobacter cloacae*[a]

Test or substrate	*K. pneumoniae*		*E. cloacae*	
	Sign[b]	Percent positive[c]	Sign[b]	Percent positive[c]
Gas from				
Inositol	+	92.5 (1.5)	−	4.1 (1.5)
Adonitol	+ or −	84.4 (0.3)	− or +	21.7
Glycerol	+	92.2 (2.9)	d	5.5 (15)
Esculin	+	98.9 (1.1)	− or +	29.5
Lysine decarboxylase	+	97.2 (0.1)	−	0
Arginine dihydrolase	−	0.6	+	92.4 (2)
Ornithine	−	0	+	93.7 (1.3)
Gelatin (22 C)	−	1.9 (0.4)	(+)	0.6 (94.2)
Motility	−	0	+	92.4
Sodium alginate, synthetic	+ or (+)	88.5 (9.2)	−	0

[a] Adapted from references 18, 32, and 55.
[b] Sign: +, 90% or more positive within 1 or 2 days; (+), positive reaction after 3 or more days (decarboxylase tests: 3 or 4 days); −, no reaction (90% or more); + or −, most cultures positive, some strains negative; − or +, most strains negative, some cultures positive; + or (+), most reactions occur within 1 or 2 days, some are delayed; d, different reactions, +, (+), −.
[c] Figures in parentheses indicate percentages of delayed reactions (3 or more days).

TABLE 11. *Differentiation of Klebsiella pneumoniae and Enterobacter aerogenes*[a]

Test of substrate	*K. pneumoniae*		*E. aerogenes*	
	Sign[b]	Percent positive[c]	Sign[b]	Percent positive[c]
Urease	+	95.4 (0.1)	−	5[w]
Motility	−	0	+	91.7
Gelatin (22 C)	−	1.9 (0.4)	(+) or −	0 (77.3)
Ornithine decarboxylase	−	0	+	95.9 (0.8)
Sodium alginate, synthetic	+ or (+)	88.9 (8.9)	−	0

[a] Adapted from references 32 and 55.
[b] Sign: +, 90% or more positive within 1 or 2 days; (+), positive reaction after 3 or more days (decarboxylase tests: 3 or 4 days); −, no reaction (90% or more); + or −, most cultures positive, some strains negative; − or +, most strains negative, some cultures positive; + or (+), most reactions occur within 1 or 2 days, some are delayed; d, different reactions, +, (+), −; [w], weakly positive reaction.
[c] Figures in parentheses indicate percentages of delayed reactions (3 or more days).

TABLE 12. *Differentiation of Enterobacter cloacae and E. aerogenes*[a]

Test or substrate	*E. cloacae*		*E. aerogenes*	
	Sign[b]	Percent positive[c]	Sign[b]	Percent positive[c]
Urease	+ or −	74.6	−	5[w]
Lysine decarboxylase	−	0	+	97.5
Arginine dihydrolase	+	92.4 (2)	−	0
Jordan's tartrate	− or +	27.4	+ or −	78.3
Adonitol				
Acid	− or +	22.2	+	97.5
Gas	− or +	21.7	+	94.2 (0.8)
Inositol				
Acid	d	13 (12)	+	96.7
Gas	−	4.1 (1.5)	+	93.4 (0.8)
Glycerol				
Acid	d	43 (45)	+	99.1
Gas	d	5.5 (16)	+	94.4 (2.8)
Esculin	− or +	29.5	+	98

[a] Adapted from references 18, 32, and 55.
[b] Sign: +, 90% or more positive within 1 or 2 days; (+), positive reaction after 3 or more days (decarboxylase tests: 3 or 4 days); −, no reaction (90% or more); + or −, most cultures positive, some strains negative; − or +, most strains negative, some cultures positive; + or (+), most reactions occur within 1 or 2 days, some are delayed; d, different reactions, +, (+), −; [w], weakly positive reaction.
[c] Figures in parentheses indicate percentages of delayed reactions (3 or more days).

of *Klebsiella* are listed in Table 9, and those that are useful for differentiation of the species of *Enterobacter* (except *E. agglomerans*) are given in Tables 10 to 13.

The reactions of *E. agglomerans* are given in detail in Table 13 because these bacteria perhaps are less well known to medical bacteriologists than are some of the other species. Eleven biogroups of *E. agglomerans* are recognized; these are based upon the reactions of the strains in nitrate reduction, indole, and Voges-Proskauer tests (47–49). The majority of cultures of this species can be differentiated from members of the genera *Klebsiella* and *Enterobacter*, and most other *Enterobacteriaceae* as well, by their failure to decarboxylate any of the three amino acids, their production of yellow pigment (about 72%), and other reactions (Table 14). Space limitations do not permit inclusion of all of the tables of differential reactions for *E. agglomerans* that might be helpful. However, these are available in other publications (47–49).

TABLE 13. *Differentiation of Enterobacter aerogenes and E. hafniae*[a]

Test or substrate	*E. aerogenes*		*E. hafniae*	
	Sign[b]	Percent positive[c]	Sign[b]	Percent positive[c]
Gelatin (22 C)	(+) or –	0 (77.3)	–	0
Mucate	+	94.7	–	0
Adonitol	+	97.5	–	0
Inositol	+	96.7	–	0
Sorbitol	+	98.3	–	0
Raffinose	+	96.7	–	3.8 (1.1)
Salicin	+	99.2 (6.8)	d	11.2 (5.9)
α-Methyl glucoside	+	96 (2)	–	0
Esculin	+	98	–	6 (2)

[a] Adapted from references 18, 32, 46, and 55.

[b] Sign: +, 90% or more positive within 1 or 2 days; (+), positive reaction after 3 or more days (decarboxylase tests: 3 or 4 days); –, no reaction (90% or more); + or –, most cultures positive, some strains negative; – or +, most strains negative, some cultures positive; + or (+), most reactions occur within 1 or 2 days, some are delayed; d, different reactions, +, (+), –.

[c] Figures in parentheses indicate percentages of delayed reactions (3 or more days).

TABLE 14. *Summary of the biochemical reactions of Enterobacter agglomerans*[a]

Test or substrate	Sign[b]	Percent positive[c]	Test or substrate	Sign[b]	Percent positive[c]
Hydrogen sulfide	–	0	Arabinose	+	97.9 (0.4)
Urease	d	27.8 (8.4)	Raffinose	d	24.8 (3)
Indole	– or +	18.7	Rhamnose	+ or (+)	86.1 (4.3)
Methyl red	– or +	44.8	Malonate	+ or –	62
Voges-Proskauer	+ or –	67.9	Mucate	– or +	44.2
Citrate (Simmons)	d	66.6 (19.2)	Jordan's tartrate	–	1.3
KCN	– or +	34.2	Sodium acetate	d	32.4 (21)
Motility	+ or –	89.4	Sodium pectate	–	0
Gelatin (22 C)	d	3 (80.1)	Sodium alginate		
Lysine decarboxylase	–	0	Synthetic	–	0
Arginine dihydrolase	–	0	Nutrient	–	0
Ornithine decarboxylase	–	0	Lipase, corn oil	–	0
Phenylalanine deaminase	– or +	27.9	Maltose	+ or (+)	88.9 (4)
Glucose			Xylose	+	92.6 (3)
Acid	+	100	Cellobiose	d	56.2 (15.4)
Gas	– or +	21.1	Glycerol	d	18.7 (25.5)
Lactose	d	40.5 (11)	α-Methyl glucoside	–	6.7 (2.9)
Sucrose	d	77.1 (1.5)	Erythritol	–	0
Mannitol	+	100	Esculin	d	62 (22)
Dulcitol	– or +	12.2 (0.6)	Nitrate to nitrite	+ or –	85.9
Salicin	d	63.6 (18.8)	Oxidation-fermentation	F	100
Adonitol	–	6.7 (0.2)	Oxidase	–	0
Inositol	d	14.2 (4.8)	Cetrimide	–	2
Sorbitol	d	23.9 (0.4)	Pigment (yellow)	+ or –	71.6

[a] Adapted from reference 49.

[b] Sign: +, 90% or more positive within 1 or 2 days; (+), positive reaction after 3 or more days (decarboxylase tests: 3 or 4 days); –, no reaction (90% or more); + or –, most cultures positive, some strains negative; – or +, most strains negative, some cultures positive; + or (+), most reactions occur within 1 or 2 days, some are delayed; d, different reactions, +, (+), –; F, fermentative.

[c] Figures in parentheses indicate percentages of delayed reactions (3 or more days).

TABLE 15. *Differentiation of species of Serratia*[a]

Test or substrate	*S. marcescens*		*S. liquefaciens*		*S. rubidaea*	
	Sign[b]	Percent positive[c]	Sign[b]	Percent positive[c]	Sign[b]	Percent positive[c]
Voges-Proskauer	+	98.7	− or +	49.5	+	92
Lysine decarboxylase	+	99.6	+ or (+)	64.2 (31.2)	+ or (+)	61 (31)
Ornithine decarboxylase	+	99.6	+	100	−	0
Malonate	−	1.6	−	0.9	+ or −	86
KCN	+	98.9	+	91.7	− or +	22
Lactose	−	1.3 (4.6)	d	15.6 (21)	+	100
Adonitol	d	46.5 (13.8)	d	8.3 (5.5)	+ or (+)	88 (2)
Sorbitol						
Acid	+	99.1	+	97.3	−	8
Gas	−	0	d	57.8 (19.3)	−	0
Arabinose	−	0	+	97.3	+	100
Raffinose	−	1.2 (0.8)	+	90.8 (4.6)	+	96
Xylose	d	7.1 (17.2)	+	99.1 (0.9)	+	98
Glycerol						
Acid	+	97.2 (1.8)	+	92.2 (6.8)	d	29 (18)
Gas	−	0	d	39.8 (30.1)	−	0
Melibiose	−	0	d	73.8 (7.5)	+	96

[a] Adapted from references 32 and 39–41.

[b] Sign: +, 90% or more positive within 1 or 2 days; (+), positive reaction after 3 or more days (decarboxylase tests: 3 or 4 days); −, no reaction (90% or more); + or −, most cultures positive, some strains negative; − or +, most strains negative, some cultures positive; + or (+), most reactions occur within 1 or 2 days, some are delayed; d, different reactions, +, (+), −.

[c] Figures in parentheses indicate percentages of delayed reactions (3 or more days).

In our experience, about 95% of isolates of *Klebsiella* are *K. pneumoniae; K. ozaenae* occurs infrequently, and *K. rhinoschleromatis* is rare in the United States. Among the species of *Enterobacter*, about 69% of the strains examined have been *E. cloacae*, 26% have been *E. hafniae*, and about 5% have been *E. aerogenes* (55). Although 536 cultures of *E. agglomerans* were studied between 1949 and 1971 (47–49), the majority were received during the last 5 years of that period. Moreover, it is difficult to determine the influence on recognition of these bacteria that might have been engendered by the interest in their occurrence in nosocomial infections (73, 74).

Three species are recognized within the genus *Serratia: S. marcescens, S. liquefaciens*, and *S. rubidaea* (39–41). With rare exceptions, differentiation of these species can be accomplished with ease (Table 15 and references 40 and 41). Of 1,560 isolates of *Serratia* studied (39–41), about 90% were *S. marcescens*, 7% were *S.* liquefaciens, and 3% were *S. rubidaea*.

The data in the tables that deal with differentiation of *Proteus* and *Providencia* are self-explanatory. Further, the frequency of occurrence of members of these two genera is well known (e.g., see references 38, 44, 87).

TABLE 16. *Differentiation of Proteus vulgaris and P. mirabilis from P. morganii and P. rettgeri*[a]

Test or substrate	*P. vulgaris* and *P. mirabilis*		*P. morganii* and *P. rettgeri*	
	Sign[b]	Percent positive[c]	Sign[b]	Percent positive[c]
Hydrogen sulfide (TSI)	+	94.5	−	0
Gelatin (22 C)	+	91.6 (6.4)	−	0
Lipase (corn oil)	+ or (+)	89.6 (5.2)	−	0
Mannose	−	0	+	100
Swarm (2% agar)	+	94 (1)	−	0

[a] Adapted from references 18, 32, and 38.

[b] Sign: +, 90% or more positive within 1 or 2 days; (+), positive reaction after 3 or more days (decarboxylase tests: 3 or 4 days); −, no reaction (90% or more); + or −, most cultures positive, some strains negative; − or +, most strains negative, some cultures positive; + or (+), most reactions occur within 1 or 2 days, some are delayed; d, different reactions, +, (+), −.

[c] Figures in parentheses indicate percentages of delayed reactions (3 or more days).

PRELIMINARY SEROLOGICAL EXAMINATION OF CULTURES OF SALMONELLA AND SHIGELLA

Salmonella

The growing multiplicity of serotypes of

TABLE 17. *Differentiation of Proteus vulgaris and P. mirabilis*[a]

Test or substrate	*P. vulgaris*		*P. mirabilis*	
	Sign[b]	Percent positive[c]	Sign[b]	Percent positive[c]
Indole	+	91.4	−	3.2
Voges-Proskauer				
37 C	−	0	− or +	15.6
22 C	− or +	11.3	+ or −	51.6
Citrate (Simmons)	d	10.5 (14.1)	+ or (+)	58.7 (37.1)
Ornithine decarboxylase	−	0	+	98.4
Sucrose	+	94.7	d	18.9 (63.3)
Maltose	+	96.2 (1.9)	−	0.9 (0.4)
Salicin	d	58.2 (10.9)	d	0.8 (29.8)
α-Methyl glucoside	d	79.5 (5.1)	−	0
Esculin	d	59 (2.6)	−	(0.9)

[a] Adapted from references 18, 32, and 38.

[b] Sign: +, 90% or more positive within 1 or 2 days; (+), positive reaction after 3 or more days (decarboxylase tests: 3 or 4 days); −, no reaction (90% or more); + or −, most cultures positive, some strains negative; − or +, most strains negative, some cultures positive; + or (+), most reactions occur within 1 or 2 days, some are delayed; d, different reactions, +, (+), −.

[c] Figures in parentheses indicate percentages of delayed reactions (3 or more days).

Salmonella and the numerous antisera required for complete characterization of all of them make it impractical for the personnel of most laboratories to attempt complete serological typing of all salmonellae. However, this situation should not deter investigators in any laboratory, large or small, from making accurate identification of infections caused by salmonellae or from exact recognition of the serotypes that are of greatest importance in the epidemiology of salmonellosis. Exact recognition requires use of the best possible isolation procedures and adequate differential biochemical methods in addition to serological procedures, regardless of the extent to which the latter are pursued.

Various factors make it necessary for those in charge of each laboratory to decide how far work with salmonellae can be carried and how much time profitably can be devoted to it. In hospital laboratories, the census and its nature also are important factors to be considered in making this decision. Whatever the extent of the work may be, all work that is done should be performed with the greatest care and by the best methods.

Fortunately, there are a number of points at which more or less natural divisions can and should be made (18, 29). It is at one of these points or stages that work with the majority of cultures may be stopped in a particular laboratory. If serological identification of strains is not completed, they should be forwarded to a central or reference laboratory, together with the minimal required information regarding each isolate. (Identifying information: name, age, and sex of individual[s] involved. Source of specimen: feces, urine, blood, fluid, other [specify]. Clinical diagnosis: diarrheal disease, enteric fever, asymptomatic person, other [specify]. Epidemiological relationships of cases, when known.) The biochemical reactions of cultures should of course be determined

TABLE 18. *Differentiation of Proteus morganii and P. rettgeri*

Test or substrate	*P. morganii*		*P. rettgeri*	
	Sign[b]	Percent positive[c]	Sign[b]	Percent positive[c]
Citrate (Simmons)	−	0	+	95.6 (3.3)
Ornithine decarboxylase	+	95.7	−	0
Gas from glucose	d	84.9 (0.9)	− or +	12.2
Sucrose	−	1 (2.9)	d	13.3 (56.7)
Mannitol	−	0	+ or −	88.5
Adonitol	−	0	d	80.9 (5.6)
Inositol	−	0	+	93.3 (4.5)
Salicin	−	0	d	30 (6.6)
Erythritol	−	0	d	78.3 (6.5)
Esculin	−	0	d	30.4 (8.7)
Xylose	−	0	− or +	15.1

[a] Adapted from references 18, 32, and 38.

[b] Sign: +, 90% or more positive within 1 or 2 days; (+), positive reaction after 3 or more days (decarboxylase tests: 3 or 4 days); −, no reaction (90% or more); + or −, most cultures positive, some strains negative; − or +, most strains negative, some cultures positive; + or (+), most reactions occur within 1 or 2 days, some are delayed; d, different reactions, +, (+), −.

[c] Figures in parentheses indicate percentages of delayed reactions (3 or more days).

before they are forwarded to a reference laboratory. Moreover, strains should be inoculated into tubes of stock medium for shipment. *Neither TSI nor KI agar should be used for shipment of cultures.*

The first of these stages is complete identification of certain important species and serotypes of salmonellae. These are as follows:

S. typhi: 9, 12, Vi:d:-
S. enteritidis bioser Paratyphi-A:1,2,12:a:-
S. enteritidis ser Paratyphi-B:4,5,12:b:1,2
S. choleraesuis: 6,7:(c):1,5
S. enteritidis ser Typhimurium 4, 5, 12:i: 1, 2

The first three salmonellae listed above invade the blood stream and cause enteric fever. The fourth may produce enteric fever, particularly in children, but also may cause only primary gastroenteritis. These serotypes and species should be identified and a presumptive report should be sent to the physician as soon as possible so that appropriate treatment can be instituted. In addition, hospital authorities, including the hospital epidemiologist if one is available, should be notified so that appropriate control measures may be taken. The fifth microorganism (serotype Typhimurium) is listed because it occurs more frequently than any other serotype of *Salmonella* and should be identified. (Almost any serotype of *Salmonella* may invade the blood stream occasionally and produce enteric fever, and, infrequently, various serotypes may be isolated from other extraintestinal sources such as cerebrospinal fluid, bone marrow, etc. See reference 27 or 76.)

Clearly, only a few antisera are required for the first stage. These are a polyvalent antiserum, O antisera for serogroups A to E inclusive (the serogroup E antiserum referred to here is a mixed antiserum that agglutinates all members of E_1, E_2, E_3, and E_4), antisera for flagellar antigens a, b, c, d, i, and the 1 ... complex (mixed 1, 2; 1, 5; 1, 6; and 1, 7 antisera), single factor H antisera for factors 2 and 5, and a Vi antiserum produced with *Citrobacter* 029:Vi. These antisera permit complete characterization of several important salmonellae and partial characterization of many others. The addition of single-factor antisera for factors H6 and H7 permits complete characterization of a number of other serotypes.

The second stage is intermediate and should be useful to investigators in many laboratories. In this, the 50 or 60 commonly occurring serotypes of *S. enteritidis*, including bioserotype Paratyphi-A, and the species *S. choleraesuis* and *S. typhi* are identified completely. These species and serotypes belong to serogroups A to H, 18, 21, and 30, and comprise a list that may be regarded as an abbreviated antigenic schema (Table 20). The 50 serotypes and variants listed in Table 20 accounted for about 96% of salmonellae isolated from all sources in the United States (17, 66, 71). The same serotypes (Table 20) also were the most commonly occurring forms listed in other reports on incidence of serotypes (for citations and additional data, see references 27, 66, 76). Fifty-one unabsorbed and

TABLE 19. *Differentiation of Proteus morganii and Proteus rettgeri from Providencia alcalifaciens and Providencia stuartii*[a]

Test or substrate	*P. morganii*		*P. rettgeri*		*P. alcalifaciens*		*P. stuartii*	
	Sign[b]	Percent positive[c]	Sign[b]	Percent positive[c]	Sign[b]	Percent positive[c]	Sign[b]	Percent positive[c]
Urease	+	97.1 (0.5)	+	100	−	0	−	0
Ornithine decarboxylase	+	95.7	−	0	−	1.2	−	0
Gas from glucose	d	84.9 (0.9)	− or +	12.2	d	85.2 (0.6)	−	0
Mannitol	−	0	+ or −	88.5	−	1.9 (0.1)	d	11.8 (9.1)
Adonitol	−	0	d	80.9 (5.6)	+	94.3 (0.3)	− or +	12.4
Inositol	−	0	+	93.3 (4.5)	−	0.6	+	97.2 (2.8)
Erythritol	−	0	d	78.3 (6.5)	−	0	−	2.3
Esculin	−	0	d	30.4 (8.7)	−	0	−	0

[a] Adapted from references 18, 32, 38, and 44.
[b] Sign: +, 90% or more positive within 1 or 2 days; (+), positive reaction after 3 or more days (decarboxylase tests: 3 or 4 days); −, no reaction (90% or more); + or −, most cultures positive, some strains negative; − or +, most strains negative, some cultures positive; + or (+), most reactions occur within 1 or 2 days, some are delayed; d, different reactions, +, (+), −.
[c] Figures in parentheses indicate percentages of delayed reactions (3 or more days).

32 absorbed antisera are required for complete serological identification of the above-mentioned commonly occurring serotypes (17, 29). The antisera are listed in Table 21. Clearly, these antisera also permit complete serological identification of serotypes not listed in Table 20 and allow partial characterization of others.

The third stage is complete serological identification of all serotypes of *Salmonella*, including characterization of new serotypes. This work should be restricted to a relatively small number of laboratories which are equipped for the work and which may serve as reference centers.

Emphasis should be given to complete serological identification of the bacteria regardless of the stage that may be adopted. If the first stage is adopted, then the few species and serotypes mentioned should be identified completely. At least two additional stages should be mentioned. It is understood that there are many institutions in which the number of stool specimens submitted is so small that cultural examination is not warranted. In such instances, freshly collected specimens should be placed in transport medium and sent to a central laboratory together with pertinent information (see stage one). This procedure also should be followed in institutions in which the volume of specimens of other kinds is so large that time and technical assistance are unavailable for adequate work with stool specimens. Another possible stage might be applicable in institutions in which adequate cultural work can be done, but time or assistance may not be available for serological identification. In this situation, careful cultural examination of specimens should be made and isolates should be identified to the generic level by adequate biochemical tests. With few exceptions, cultures of *S. typhi* should be identified, at least presumptively (see below). Cultures of *Salmonella* and other significant isolates then should be sent to a central laboratory for serological identification. However, it is hoped that it will be feasible for the personnel of most laboratories to adopt stage one, two, or some modification of one of them, if this has not been done.

Polyvalent antisera and O group determinations. Cultures that yield reactions similar to those given by salmonellae on TSI, LIA, and urea agar media (Tables 3 and 4) should be tested in polyvalent antiserum for *Salmonella*. One of the simplest contains agglutinins for the O antigens of serological groups A through E and for Vi antigen. Approximately 95% of the serotypes of *Salmonella* isolated from man and lower animals belong to these few serogroups (27, 66, 76).

Suspensions for agglutination tests with polyvalent antiserum may be prepared by suspending a loopful of growth from a TSI, or infusion, agar slant in a few drops of phenol-treated (0.5%) physiological saline solution or mercuric iodide-saline solution. Such suspensions should be *dense*. A droplet of bacterial suspension is added to a droplet of properly diluted polyvalent antiserum on a slide, after which the slide is tilted back and forth several times. Positive tests are indicated by rapid, complete agglutination of the bacterial cells. If agglutination occurs, and the required antisera are available, serogrouping or complete serotyping may be done. If not, the biochemical reactions of the culture should be determined to make certain that the microorganism is of the genus *Salmonella*; then it may be forwarded to a reference laboratory for complete antigenic analysis. However, if typical agglutination is obtained, and the results of preliminary biochemical tests are characteristic (24- to 48-h readings), a report such as "*Salmonella*, serotype undetermined" may be issued. Strains that appear to be salmonellae with respect to their reactions on TSI and LIA media but fail to react with polyvalent antiserum may be encountered occasionally. Suspensions prepared from cultures of this sort should be heated in a beaker of boiling water for about 15 min, cooled, and retested in the antiserum. Some strains possess M antigens, which inhibit agglutination of living (unheated) suspensions. Further, suspensions that do not react in the polyvalent antiserum being used may belong to a serogroup (beyond E, for example) for which agglutinins are not represented in the polyvalent antiserum being used. The biochemical reactions of such a strain should be determined; if the results indicate that the culture probably is a *Salmonella*, it may be sent elsewhere for further examination.

A culture that is anaerogenic, produces an alkaline slant and acid reaction in the butt, forms only a small amount of hydrogen sulfide in TSI or KI agar medium (K/A^+), and fails to hydrolyze urea rapidly (i.e., within 1 or 2 h) should be considered as a possible strain of *S. typhi* and treated accordingly. A dense suspension prepared from such a culture first should be tested in the living (unheated) state in group D (*Salmonella*) antiserum and in Vi antiserum on a slide. After these tests are completed, the suspension should be heated in a beaker of boiling water for about 15 min, cooled, and retested in the same antisera (Table 22). Polyvalent antiserum, which contains Vi antibodies, also may be included in the above-mentioned

TABLE 20. *Abbreviated antigenic schema for Salmonella*[a]

Species and serotype	Group	Antigenic formula		
		O antigens	H antigens	
			Phase 1	Phase 2
S. enteritidis, bioser. Paratyphi-A	A	1,2,12	a	—
ser. Paratyphi-B	B	1,4,5,12	b	1,2
ser. Paratyphi-B, Odense	B	1,4,12	b	1,2
bioser. Java	B	1,4,5,12	b	[1,2]
ser. Stanley	B	4,5,12	d	1,2
ser. Schwarzengrund	B	1,4,12,27	d	1,7
ser. Saint Paul	B	1,4,5,12	e,h	1,2
ser. Reading	B	4,5,12	e,h	1,5
ser. Chester	B	4,5,12	e,h	e,n,x
ser. San Diego	B	4,[5],12	e,h	e,n,z_{15}
ser. Derby	B	1,4,5,12	f,g	—
ser. California	B	4,5,12	m,t	—
ser. Typhimurium	B	1,4,5,12	i	1,2
ser. Typhimurium, Copenhagen	B	1,4,12	i	1,2
ser. Bredeney	B	1,4,12	l,v	1,7
ser. Heidelberg	B	1,4,5,12	r	1,2
S. choleraesuis	C_1	6,7	c	1,5
S. choleraesuis, bioser. Kunzendorf	C_1	6,7	[c]	1,5
S. enteritidis, ser. Braenderup	C_1	6,7	eh	e,n,z_{15}
ser. Montevideo	C_1	6,7	g,m,s	—
ser. Oranienburg	C_1	6,7	m,t	—
ser. Thompson	C_1	6,7	k	1,5
ser. Infantis	C_1	6,7	r	1,5
ser. Bareilly	C_1	6,7	y	1,5
ser. Tennessee	C_1	6,7	z_{29}	—
ser. Muenchen	C_2	6,8	d	1,2
ser. Manhattan	C_2	6,8	d	1,5
ser. Newport	C_2	6,8	e,h	1,2
ser. Blockley	C_2	6,8	k	1,5
ser. Litchfield	C_2	6,8	l,v	1,2
ser. Tallahassee	C_2	6,8	z_4,z_{32}	—
ser. Kentucky	C_2	(8),20	i	z_6
bioser. Miami	D	1,9,12	a	1,5
S. typhi	D	9,12,Vi	d	—
S. enteritidis, ser. Berta	D	9,12	f,g,t	—
ser. Enteritidis	D	1,9,12	g,m	—
ser. Dublin	D	1,9,12	g,p	—
ser. Panama	D	1,9,12	l,v	1,5
ser. Javiana	D	1,9,12	l,z_{28}	1,5
bioser. Pullorum	D	9,12	—	—
ser. Anatum	E_1	3,10	e,h	1,6
ser. Meleagridis	E_1	3,10	e,h	l,w
ser. Give	E_1	3,10	l,v	1,7
ser. Newington	E_2	3,15	e,h	1,6
ser. Illinois	E_3	(3),(15),34	z_{10}	1,5

TABLE 20—*Continued*

Species and serotype	Group	Antigenic formula		
		O antigens	H antigens	
			Phase 1	Phase 2
ser. Senftenberg	E_4	1,3,19	g,s,t	—
ser. Simsbury	E_4	1,3,19	z_{27}	—
ser. Rubislaw	F	11	r	e,n,x
ser. Poona	G	13,22	z	1,6
ser. Worthington	G	1,13,23	z	l,w
ser. Cubana	G	1,13,23	z_{29}	—
ser. Florida	H	1,6,14,25	d	1,7
ser. Madelia	H	1,6,14,25	y	1,7
ser. Cerro	18	18	z_4,z_{23}	—
ser. Siegburg	18	6,14,18	z_4,z_{23}	—
ser. Minnesota	21	21	b	e,n,x
ser. Urbana	30	30	b	e,n,x

[a] Adapted from references 18, 25, 27, and 29. NOTE: Enclosure of the designation of an antigen in parentheses indicates that the complete antigen is not present, e.g., (8). Enclosure of an antigen designation in brackets indicates that the antigen or antigen complex may be present or absent, e.g., [1], [1, 2], etc.

tests. If the reactions of a culture are typical of *S. typhi* on TSI agar medium, if tests for urease are negative, and if a suspension reacts as shown in Table 22 (i.e., a reversal of the reactions in group D and Vi antisera after heat treatment), a presumptive report can, and should, be made at this point. Confirmatory biochemical tests (Tables 8, 23, 24) should be made, and the H (flagellar) antigens must be determined before a final report is issued.

Cultures that react in polyvalent antiserum for *Salmonella*, but fail to agglutinate in Vi antiserum should be tested in O grouping antisera (Table 25).

S. enteritidis bioserotype Paratyphi-A is relatively uncommon in the United States, but bacteriologists should be familiar with it since it sometimes is imported by tourists and others. The biochemical reactions of bioserotype Paratyphi-A are somewhat atypical as compared with salmonellae in general (see Tables 23 and 24). Hydrogen sulfide frequently is not formed in TSI or KI agar medium, but gas is formed from glucose; hence, the reactions in these media usually are K/Ag. Cultures that give this appearance in one or the other of these media and are urease-negative should be tested in O grouping antisera. If rapid and complete agglutination occurs in O serogroup A (1, 2, 12) antiserum (Table 25) and the confirmatory biochemical reactions obtained (20 to 24 h) are consistent with those given by bioserotype Paratyphi-A (Table 24), presumptive identification can be made and a preliminary report can be issued. The differential biochemical tests should be observed for a longer period, and the H antigens must be determined before a final report is made.

The reactions of the majority of salmonellae in TSI or KI agar medium are K/Ag^{+++} (Table 3). This is true of *S. choleraesuis*, bioserotype Kunzendorf, the most commonly occurring form of *S. choleraesuis*. Strains that yield this type of reaction in the above-mentioned primary differential media and are urease-negative first should be tested in polyvalent antiserum for *Salmonella* and then in O grouping antisera (Table 25). Confirmatory biochemical tests should be made, and the H antigens of such cultures must be determined before final reports can be made.

It is important to recall that strains of almost

TABLE 21. *Antisera needed for typing 50 commonly occurring Salmonella serotypes*[a]

O antisera		H antisera			
		Phase 1		Phase 2	
Unabsorbed	Absorbed	Unabsorbed	Absorbed	Unabsorbed	Absorbed
1,2,12	2	a	—	e,n,x	x
4,5,12	5	b	—	e,n,z_{15}	z_{15}
4,12,27	27	c	—	1,2	2
6,7	7	d	—	1,5	5
6,8	—	e,h	h	1,6	6
(8),20	20	f,g	f	1,7	7
9,12	—	g,m	m	z_6	z_6
3,10	10	g,m,s	m, and s		
3,15	15	g,p	p		
(3),(15),34	34	g,s,t	s, and t		
1,3,19	19	i	—		
11	—	k	—		
13,22	22	l,v	v		
1,13,23	23	l,w	w		
6,14,25	14, and 25	l,z_{13}	z_{13}		
18	—	l,z_{28}	28		
21	—	m,t	m, and t		
30	—	r	—		
		y	—		
Vi	—	z	—		
		z_4,z_{23}	z_{23}		
		z_4,z_{32}	z_{32}		
		z_{10}	—		
		z_{27}	—		
		z_{29}	—		
Totals (18 + Vi)	13	25	12	7	7

[a] Adapted from references 17, 18, and 29.

any serotype of *S. enteritidis*, as well as some cultures of *S. choleraesuis* and *S. typhi*, may fail to form detectable amounts of hydrogen sulfide in TSI, KI, or LIA media. Such cultures should not be discarded until it is certain that they are not salmonellae, or perhaps shigellae. In addition, members of other genera (e.g., *Arizona, Citrobacter, Escherichia*) may react in polyvalent antisera for salmonellae, particularly in the more comprehensive ones.

Phase reversal. Most serotypes of *Salmonella* are diphasic, and sometimes it is possible to identify both phases of a diphasic culture when it is first isolated or received for examination. More often, however, only one phase can be detected initially in diphasic cultures, especially when they are recently isolated from single colonies on plating media used in the recovery of salmonellae. A culture of serotype Typhimurium, for example, just picked from a single colony on isolation medium would be likely to react in i antiserum or in 1, 2 antiserum, but not in both. If the strain is in phase 1 (i), it is necessary to reverse the phases and isolate phase 2 (1, 2). Likewise, if only phase 2 is apparent, isolation of phase 1 is required.

TABLE 22. *Reactions of Salmonella typhi in slide agglutination tests*[a]

Suspension	Antisera		
	Salmonella polyvalent	*Salmonella* O group D (9,12)	Vi (*Citrobacter* 029)
Living	++++	–	++++
Heated	++++	++++	–

[a] Adapted from references 18, 25, and 29. Symbols: ++++, complete agglutination; –, no reaction.

If a culture suspected of being serotype Typhimurium is in phase 1 (i), it should be inoculated into semisolid phase reversal medium to which i antiserum has been added. A simple way of doing this is to add a 3-mm loopful of sterile i antiserum to 3 ml of melted and cooled (40 to 45 C) semisolid medium in a 13 by 100 mm tube. After thorough mixing, the semisolid medium is allowed to gel and is inoculated by just puncturing the medium at the surface (3 or 4 mm stab). The H agglutinins in the antiserum immobilize the homologous flagella (i in this instance) and, upon incubation, growth of the

TABLE 23. *Differentiation of species of Salmonella*[a]

Test or substrate	*S. choleraesuis*		*S. typhi*		*S. enteritidis*	
	Sign[b]	Percent positive[c]	Sign[b]	Percent positive[c]	Sign[b]	Percent positive[c]
Hydrogen sulfide (TSI)	+ or −	60	+[w]	94.4	+	98
Citrate (Simmons)	(+)	0 (90)	−	0	+	99.3 (0.7)
Ornithine	+	100	−	0	+	99
Gas from glucose	+	100	−	0	+	97.7
Dulcitol	d	5 (15)	d	6.2 (31.3)	+	98.3
Inositol	−	0	−	0	d	42.8 (1)
Trehalose	−	0	+	100	+	100
Arabinose	−	0	−	(6.3)	+	99.3
Rhamnose	+	100	−	0	+	95
Cellobiose	−	0	d	6[w] (31.3)	(+)	5 (92.8)
Erythritol	(+[w]) or −	0 (85)	−	0	−	0.6
Sodium acetate	− or (+[w])	0 (20)	−	0	+	92.4 (2.2)
Mucate	−	0	−	0	+ or −	88.3
Stern's glycerol fuchsin	−	0	−	0	+	98.2

[a] Adapted from references 18, 29, 32, 33, and 34. N.B. The species *S. enteritidis* includes all salmonellae other than *S. choleraesuis* and *S. typhi*.

[b] Sign: +, 90% or more positive within 1 or 2 days; (+), positive reaction after 3 or more days (decarboxylase tests: 3 or 4 days); −, no reaction (90% or more); + or −, most cultures positive, some strains negative; − or +, most strains negative, some cultures positive; + or (+), most reactions occur within 1 or 2 days, some are delayed; d, different reactions, +, (+), −; [w], weakly positive reaction.

[c] Figures in parentheses indicate percentages of delayed reactions (3 or more days).

TABLE 24. *Differentiation of Salmonella enteritidis bioserotype Paratyphi-A from other strains of S. enteritidis*[a]

Substrate or test	Bioserotype Paratyphi-A		*S. enteritidis*	
	Sign[b]	Percent positive[c]	Sign[b]	Percent positive[c]
Hydrogen sulfide (TSI)	− or +[w]	12.5	+	98
Citrate (Simmons)	− or (+)	0 (25)	+	99.3 (0.7)
Lysine decarboxylase	−	0	+	99.7
Jordan's tartrate	−	0	+	92.5
Inositol	−	0	d	42.8 (1)
Xylose	−	0	+	99
Cellobiose	d	12.5 (6.2)	(+)	5 (92.8)
Glycerol	(+)	0 (100)	d	5.7 (7.2)
Stern's glycerol fuchsin medium	−	0	+	98.2 (0.6)
Sodium acetate	−	(6.2)	+	92.4 (2.2)
Mucate	−	0	+ or −	88.3
Organic acids				
Citrate	−	0	+	96 (4)
D-Tartrate	−	0	+	92.3 (4)
i-Tartrate	−	0	d	4.7 (57.5)
l-Tartrate	−	0	d	11.8 (75.2)

[a] Adapted from references 18, 29, 32, and 34.

[b] Sign: +, 90% or more positive within 1 or 2 days; (+), positive reaction after 3 or more days (decarboxylase tests: 3 or 4 days); −, no reaction (90% or more); + or −, most cultures positive, some strains negative; − or +, most strains negative, some cultures positive; + or (+), most reactions occur within 1 or 2 days, some are delayed; d, different reactions, +, (+), −; [w], weakly positive reaction.

[c] Figures in parentheses indicate percentages of delayed reactions (3 or more days).

phase that is not immobilized spreads throughout the medium. After overnight incubation, the top portion of the medium is heated in a flame and the melted agar, including the point of inoculation, is poured from the tube. After the tube cools, a loopful of the spreading growth is transferred to infusion broth which is incubated overnight (or for 4 to 6 h in a water bath) and preserved by the addition of an equal volume of formalinized (0.6%) physiological saline solution. The desired phase may be obtained in this manner. Antisera to be added to phase reversal medium may be sterilized by addition of an excess of chloroform (add about 2 drops per ml, shake well, and refrigerate for 24 h). Ordinarily, a 3-mm loopful of glycerol-treated H antiserum diluted 1:5 or 1:6 (sterile) added to 3 ml of semisolid medium yields the desired result.

Some monophasic serotypes of *Salmonella* possess H antigens that also are present in many diphasic serotypes. Notable examples of this are bioserotype Paratyphi-A (1, 2, 12:a:-) and *S. typhi* (9, 12, Vi:d:-). The various combinations of O and H antigens of salmonellae may be determined by examination of the antigenic schema.

Only essential information regarding the serotyping of salmonellae is given in the foregoing paragraphs. Readers who are interested in pursuing the subject farther should consult references 18, 29, and 65.

Shigella

The examination of isolates of *Shigella* may be stopped at various points or stages analogous to those outlined for salmonellae. However, since serotyping of shigellae is dependent upon the determination of O antigens and O antigen factors, as H antigens are not involved, fewer antisera are required for complete serotyping of *Shigella* than for serotyping of *Salmonella*.

The genus *Shigella* is divided into four species, three of which are made up of a number of serotypes: *S. dysenteriae* (10 serotypes), *S. flexneri* (six serotypes and several subserotypes), *S. boydii* (15 serotypes), and *S. sonnei* (1 serotype). These species frequently are referred to as subgroups A, B, C, and D, respectively.

Polyvalent antisera. Isolates that are suspected of being shigellae should be tested for agglutination in polyvalent antisera for each of the four species (21). The antiserum for *S. sonnei* used at this point generally is a mixture of antisera for forms I and II. Dense suspensions prepared in physiological saline solution or mercuric iodide solution should be used for these slide tests. Since certain anaerogenic, nonmotile biotypes of *E. coli*, e.g., members of the "Alkalescens-Dispar (A-D) group," particularly A-D 01, occur frequently and resemble shigellae on TSI agar, the use of a polyvalent antiserum for these microorganisms also is recommended. Suspensions that are agglutinated rapidly and completely in one of the polyvalent antisera should be subjected to additional biochemical tests. If, after 18 to 24 h of incubation, the results of these tests are compatible with those given by shigellae, a preliminary report may be made indicating the presumptive identification. If a suspension fails to react in one or another of the aforementioned polyvalent antisera, it should be heated in a beaker of boiling water for about 15 min, cooled, and retested in the same antisera. Many shigellae possess envelope or capsular antigens that inhibit agglutina-

TABLE 25. *Agglutination reactions of salmonellae in O antisera (slide tests)*

O antigen suspensions	O antisera											
	1,2,12	4,5,12	4,12,27	6,7	(8)	(8),20	9,12	9,46	3,10	3,15	(3),(15), 34	1,3,19
1,12,12	++++	+	+	−	−	−	+	−	−	−	−	+
4,5,12	−	++++	++	−	−	−	+	−	−	−	−	−
4,12,27	−	++++	++++	−	−	−	+	−	−	−	−	−
6,7	−	−	−	++++	−	−	−	−	−	−	−	−
6,8	−	+	−	+	++++	++	−	−	−	−	−	−
(8),20	−	−	−	−	++	++++	−	−	−	−	−	−
9,12	+	+	+	−	−	−	++++	++++	−	−	−	−
(9),46	−	−	−	−	−	−	++++	++++	+	−	−	−
3,10	−	−	−	−	−	−	−	−	++++	++++	+	+
3,15	−	−	−	−	−	−	−	−	++++	++++	++++	+
(3),(15),34	−	−	−	−	−	−	−	−	−	++++	++++	−
1,3,19	++	−	−	−	−	−	−	−	+	+	−	++++

[a] Adapted from references 18, 25, and 29. The symbols +, ++, ++++ indicate degrees of agglutination.

tion of living (unheated) bacteria in O antisera. These antigens are inactivated by heat.

A suspension that is not agglutinated in any of the polyvalent antisera for *Shigella* or in the A-D polyvalent antiserum should be tested in polyvalent and grouping antisera for salmonellae. In particular, such a suspension should be tested in group D and Vi antisera (Table 22), since it may be a strain of *S. typhi* that fails to produce hydrogen sulfide.

Cultures that give the appearance of shigellae in TSI agar media, that are urease-negative, and that fail to agglutinate in any of the antisera for shigellae mentioned in the preceding paragraphs should be tested in antisera for serotypes not represented in the polyvalents and should be subjected to additional biochemical tests. Such strains may be shigellae, agglutinins for which are not contained in the polyvalent antisera, or they may be members of another genus.

Regardless of the outcome of serological tests, cultures suspected of being shigellae must be subjected to biochemical tests (Tables 6 and 26), since the O antigens of almost all of the serotypes of *Shigella* are identical with, or closely related to, those of various *E. coli* strains.

Cultures that are to be forwarded to a central or reference laboratory for additional study should be inoculated into stock culture medium, packed properly, and sent along with minimal information (as indicated above for *Salmonella*).

Identification of serotypes. As mentioned above, serotyping of shigellae is accomplished by determination of the O antigens and O antigen factors of the microorganisms. Some of the antisera may be used in the unabsorbed state, but the majority require absorption if definitive work is to be done.

Antisera for *S. dysenteriae* serotypes 1, 2, 8, and 10 must be absorbed. Antisera for the remaining serotypes of this species generally can be used without absorption, but this must be determined by adequate tests. Methods for production, evaluation, and absorption of antisera are given in reference 18.

Since there are extensive intraspecific relations among serotypes of *S. flexneri*, absorbed type-specific antisera must be used to identify them. Each *S. flexneri* type contains a specific or major antigen and a number of common group factors. These factors are responsible for the extensive cross-agglutination reactions exhibited by unabsorbed antisera. Similarly, the factor antisera employed for delineation of the subserotypes of *S. flexneri* (1a, 1b; 2a, 2b; etc.) must be absorbed to remove agglutinins for the type-specific antigens. The reactions that may be expected in properly absorbed typing fluids for *S. flexneri* are shown in Table 27.

Antisera for *S. boydii* 1, 4, 5, 6, 9, 10, 11, 12, 13, and 15 must be absorbed to render them type-specific. The remainder generally can be used in the unabsorbed state, but this must be determined by adequate tests.

Cultures of *S. sonnei* occur in two forms, I(S) and II(R), and it is necessary to employ antiserum that contains agglutinins for both forms for identification. *S. sonnei* form I(S) is the smooth form of the microorganism and form II(R) represents a stage in the degradation of the smooth toward the rough form. Transitional forms between I and II exist, and colonies of these transitional forms, as well as of *S. sonnei* I or II, may be encountered on primary isolation plates.

Experience has indicated that in acute infections caused by *S. sonnei* one may expect form I(S) colonies to be predominant, whereas in carriers form II(R) colonies or transitional forms predominate (4). By careful selection of colony forms I and II for antiserum production and by appropriate absorption of the antisera, it is possible to prepare antisera for differentiation of the two forms of *S. sonnei*. The rough antigens of *S. boydii* 6 are identical with those of *S. sonnei* II, and antisera for the former generally must be absorbed by the latter.

EXAMINATION OF CULTURES OF ESCHERICHIA COLI

The work of Kauffmann (see references 18, 28, 43, 53, 65) and his collaborators made possible the development of a system for serological typing of *E. coli* cultures and resulted in an antigenic schema in which the microorganisms may be classified. Interest in members of the genus *Escherichia* has been stimulated by association of certain serotypes with diarrheal disease, by studies on hospital-acquired infection, and by work on diseases of animals. As a result of this increased interest, the *E. coli* antigenic schema has been extended so that 157 O antigens, 93 K antigens, and 52 H antigens now are known. Further information relative to these antigens may be found in references 18 and 65. The O antigens of the bacteria are the somatic antigens not inactivated by heat at 121 C. K antigens are somatic antigens that occur as envelopes or as capsules. These antigens inhibit the agglutination of living bacteria in O antisera, but this inhibitory effect is

TABLE 26. *Biochemical reactions of species of Shigella*[a]

Test or substrate	*S. dysenteriae*		*S. flexneri* 1 to 5		*S. flexneri* 6		*S. boydii*		*S. sonnei*	
	Sign[b]	Percent positive[c]	Sign[b]	Percent positive[c]	Sign[b]	Percent positive[c]	Sign[b]	Percent positive[c]	Sign[b]	Percent positive[c]
Indole	− or +	43.7	+ or −	61.5	−	0	− or +	28.8	−	0
Arginine dihydrolase	d	1.5 (11.3)	−	0[d]	d	48.9 (10.3)	d	18.1 (31.9)	−	0.5 (5)
Ornithine decarboxylase	−	0	−	0	−	0	−	2.5[e]	+	99.4
Mucate	−	0	−	0	−	0	−	0	− or +	16.4
Jordan's tartrate	+ or −	78	−	0	−	0	− or +	13	+	100
Gas from glucose	−	0	−	0	− or +	18.1	−	0	−	0
Lactose	−	0 (1.6)[f]	−	0 (<0.1)	−	0	−	1	d	1.8 (88.1)
Sucrose	−	0 (4.2)	d	1.5 (41.9)	−	0	−	0	d	0.1 (85.4)
Mannitol	−	0	+	93.7	+ or −	82.5	+	97.6	+	98.9
Dulcitol	−	4.5 (0.5)	−	0	d	9.4 (72.2)	d	6.7 (10.4)	−	0 (1)
Sorbitol	d	29.2 (29.5)	d	30.6 (1.5)	(+) or +	30.2 (59.8)	d	41.8 (36.3)	−	1 (1)
Arabinose	d	43.6 (7.2)	d	65 (8.7)	+ or (+)	54.6 (39.3)	+	94.1	+	94.2 (2.9)
Raffinose	−	0	d	52.8 (28.4)	−	0	−	0	d	2.5 (81.5)
Rhamnose	d	32.4 (5.5)	d	6 (6.2)	−	1.6 (3.7)	−	0.2 (1.6)	+ or(+)	77.1 (21)
Maltose	d	12 (77)	d	28.4 (45.3)	(+) or +	16 (74.4)	d	16.6 (66)	+ or (+)	86.4 (6.8)
Xylose	d	3.9 (7.6)	−	1.8 (0.4)[g]	d	0.5 (18.2)	d	11.2 (57.2)	−	1
Trehalose	+ or (+)	89.8 (7.5)	+ or (+)	77.8 (12.2)	(+) or +	7.4 (92.6)	+ or (+)	85.2 (11.2)	+	100
Cellobiose	−	0	−	0	−	0	−	0	d	10.6 (1.8)
Glycerol	d	12.3 (72.5)	−	0	+ or (+)	60 (31.1)	+ or (+)	55.5 (34.8)	d	13 (32.7)
β-Galactosidase[h]	− or +	49.9	−	0.8	−	0	− or +	11.1	+	95

[a] Adapted from references 29 and 30.

[b] Sign: +, 90% or more positive within 1 or 2 days; (+), positive reaction after 3 or more days (decarboxylase tests: 3 or 4 days); −, no reaction (90% or more); + or −, most cultures positive, some strains negative; − or +, most strains negative, some cultures positive; + or (+), most reactions occur within 1 or 2 days, some are delayed; d, different reactions, +, (+), −.

[c] Figures in parentheses indicate percentages of delayed reactions (3 or more days).

[d] A few doubtful reactions occur, but these are regarded as negative.

[e] Only cultures of *S. boydii* 13 are positive.

[f] Some strains of *S. dysenteriae* 1 ferment lactose slowly; all are *o*-nitrophenyl-β-D-galactopyranoside-positive.

[g] Xylose is fermented by some cultures of the mannitol-negative bioserotype of *S. flexneri* 4.

[h] *o*-Nitrophenyl-β-D-galactopyranoside.

inactivated by heat at 100 or 121 C. The H, or flagellar, antigens are also inactivated by heat at 100 C. Antisera for O antigens are prepared by injection of smooth cultures that have been heated at 100 C for 2.5 h or at 121 C for 2 h to inactivate their K and H antigens. In the preparation of K antisera, Formalin-treated or living cultures of K forms selected from platings are used for injection into animals. Whenever possible, nonmotile strains should be used for K antiserum production. H antisera are produced with cultures of bacteria that have been passed through semisolid agar several times to enhance the development of H antigen. Detailed discussions of methods for the production and use of O, K, and H antisera may be found in reference 18.

The K antigens of *E. coli* cultures are a class composed of at least three varieties, designated L, A, and B. All varieties occur as sheath, envelope, or capsular antigens that inhibit agglutination of living bacteria in O antisera. One of the most important differences between L and B antigens is that the antibody-binding power of L antigen is inactivated by heat at 100 C, whereas the binding power of B antigen is not. A pure L antiserum may be prepared by absorption of an OL antiserum with a heated suspension of the homologous strain. Pure B antiserum cannot be prepared by this procedure because the antibody-binding power of B antigen is not inactivated by heat and, if OB antiserum is absorbed by a heated suspension of the homologous culture, both O and B agglutinins are removed from the antiserum.

Since complete serological typing of *E. coli* cultures is a time-consuming and somewhat involved procedure, it may properly be considered a function of a few centers and research institutions that are equipped for the work. The personnel of many laboratories may prefer to limit their activities to isolation and preliminary identification, and to forward selected strains to a center equipped for further study. However, it should be emphasized that, in addition to providing adequate means for the isolation of *E. coli* (Fig. 3), all laboratories should complete the following steps in the identification of serotypes of *E. coli*, whether or not the cultures are to be sent to a center: (i) determination of biochemical reactions, (ii) slide agglutination tests in which living suspensions are examined in both OB and O antisera prepared with serotypes that have been associated with diarrheal disease, (iii) slide tests in which heated suspensions are tested in the same OB and O antisera, and (iv) titration of heated suspensions in serial dilutions of the indicated O antisera for confirmation of the O antigen group (28).

Although there are more, certain serotypes of nine OB serogroups are generally accepted as etiological agents of diarrheal disease in infants and young children (0 to 2 or 2.5 years of age). The OB serogroups are as follows:

O26:K60(B6)
O55a:K59(B5)
O86a:K61(B7)
O111a,111b:K58(B4)
O119:K69(B14)
O125a,125b:K70(B15)
O125a,125c:K70(B15)
O126:K71(B16)
O127a:K63(B8)

TABLE 27. *Agglutination reactions of S. flexneri (slide tests)*[a]

Test antigens	Absorbed antisera								
	Type specific						Group factors		
	I	II	III	IV	V	VI	3.4	6	7.8
I:1,2,4,5,9 . . .	++++	–	–	–	–	–	++++	–	–(+)
I:1,2,4,5,6,9 . . .	++++	–	–	–	–	–	++(–)	++++	–
II:1,3,4 . . .	–	++++	–	–	–	–	++++	–	–
II:1,7,8,9 . . .	–	++++	–	–	–	–	–	–	++++
III:1,6,7,8,9 . . .	–	–	++++	–	–	–	–	++++	++++
III:1,3,4,6,7,8,9 . . .	–	–	++++	–	–	–	++	++++	++++
III:1,3,4,6 . . .	–	–	++++	–	–	–	++	++++	–
III:1,6 . . .	–	–	++++	–	–	–	–	++++	–
IV:1,3,4 . . .	–	–	–	++++	–	–	++++(–)	–	–(++)
IV:1,6 . . .	–	–	–	++++	–	–	–(++)	++++	–
V:1,5,7,9 . . .	–	–	–	–	++++	–	–	–	++++(–)
VI:1,2,4 . . .	–	–	–	–	–	++++	++(–)	–	–

[a] Adapted from references 18, 25, and 29. Degrees of agglutination: ++++, complete reaction; + to ++, relatively weaker reactions. Symbols in parentheses indicate occasional reactions.

O128a, 128b: K67(B12)
O128a, 128c: K67(B12).

According to the most recent data available to us (43), there are more than 130 serotypes that belong to the nine OB serogroups mentioned above. However, 20 serotypes were present in 81.7% of the cases. That is, 15% of the known serotypes were associated with 81.7% of the cases. These serotypes occurred very infrequently in materials from extraintestinal sources or in animals other than primates. When they occurred in animals, the animals usually were ill with enteritis. Thirteen of the above-mentioned 20 *E. coli* serotypes occurred in association with 75% of the cases of infantile diarrheal disease; these were

O26: K60(B6): NM
O26: K60(B6): H11
O55: K59(B5): NM
O55: K59(B5): H6
O55: K59(B5): H7
O111a, 111b: K58(B4): NM
O111a, 111b: K58(B4): H2
O111a, 111b: K58(B4): H12
O125a, 125c: K70(B15): H21
O126: K71(B16): NM
O126: K71(B16): H27
O127a: K63(B8): NM
O128a, 128c: K67(B12): H12.

E. coli cultures isolated from diverse sources or from animals without symptoms of diarrheal disease were, with few exceptions, serotypically different from the strains found frequently in association with infantile diarrheal disease.

Since about 1944 it has become apparent that certain serotypes of *E. coli*, usually different from those mentioned above, may be involved in diarrheal disease in children and adults (43). For example, strains of OB group 124: K(B17) have been isolated from patients involved in outbreaks of disease that is clinically indistinguishable from bacillary dysentery caused by *Shigella* (43). In other outbreaks, the disease may take the form of an enteritis, in which instances serotypes such as O148: K93: H may be involved (79). Several experimental models now are used to study the pathogenesis of various serotypes of *E. coli* (16).

Isolation

After incubation for 16 to 20 h, the primary plating media (Fig. 3) may be examined for colonies of *E. coli*. No specific directions can be given as to the selection of colonies for transfer because colonies of the various serotypes of *E. coli* all appear quite similar. Portions of 10 or more individual colonies that appear on the blood-agar or plain infusion agar plates should be tested directly in antisera. If strongly positive slide agglutination tests are obtained by this procedure, it may be considered presumptive evidence that one of the particular serotypes of *E. coli* is present in the specimen. This procedure not only affords a rough estimate of the presence or absence of serotypes for which antisera are available, but it also indicates the prevalence of a given serotype in the specimen. Examinations of this sort should be made with colonies on blood agar or infusion agar plates rather than with colonies from MacConkey agar plates, since it has been shown that the presence of bile salts may cause confusing agglutination reactions, which are not confirmed in subsequent work. Three or more entire, smooth, opaque, *Escherichia*-like colonies from each plating medium should be transferred to infusion agar slants (long slants prepared from plain infusion agar, without added sugar). Additional transfers should be made if possible. The slants should be inoculated over the entire surface to obtain maximal growth. After incubation, these slants are used for biochemical and serological studies.

Preliminary examination

A generous portion of the growth from each of the agar slant cultures should be emulsified in about 0.5 ml of 0.5% sodium chloride solution to make a very dense suspension. Droplets of the heavy suspensions may be tested for agglutination on slides with droplets of O and OB antisera for *E. coli*, first as living suspensions and again after being heated. Agglutinations of a living antigen in an OB antiserum and lack of a reaction in the corresponding O antiserum are indicative of the presence of B antigen in the

TABLE 28. *Preliminary examination of the K and O antigens of Escherichia coli (slide tests)*[a]

Antigen suspension	Antisera for *E. coli*							
	O26: B6	O26	O55: B5	O55	O111: B4	O111	O127: B8	O127
KO antigen (living)	–	–	–	–	++++	–	–	–
O antigen (100 C)	–	–	–	–	++++	++++	–	–

[a] Adapted from references 18 and 28. Symbols: ++++, complete agglutination; –, no reaction.

strain. If such a reaction occurs in one of the OB antisera, the suspension is heated at 100 C for 15 to 30 min, cooled, and retested in the indicated OB and O antisera. If the culture belongs to the O antigen group, the heated antigen may be expected to react in both OB and O antisera. An example of results that may be anticipated with freshly isolated cultures is given in Table 28. It is to be emphasized that, in slide agglutination tests with the unabsorbed antisera, *cognizance should be taken only of strong reactions*, and undue significance should not be attached to weak and delayed agglutination. If a living suspension reacts strongly in O antiserum as well as in the OB antiserum, the culture should be plated, and colonies that are inagglutinable in O antiserum should be selected for reexamination.

Suspensions prepared from agar slant cultures are diluted, heated at 100 C for 1 h, and titrated in serial dilutions (e.g., 1:200 to 1:6,400) of the indicated O antiserum. If desired, broth cultures that have been incubated for 4 to 6 h and then heated at 100 C for 1 h may be used in the titrations and, in the absence of O antisera, OB antiserum may be employed. Such tests are read after 16 to 18 h of incubation in a water bath at 48 to 50 C. If the results of slide agglutination tests performed in the first steps were clear-cut and the culture was inagglutinable in O antisera in the living state, confirmation by agglutination to or near the titer of the antiserum may be expected in the titrations. Other cultures of *E. coli*, however, are related to certain of the serotypes associated with infantile diarrhea through possession of common O antigenic fractions. A strain that belongs to one of these related O groups may be expected to cross-react in the titrations (18). It should be remembered also that living suspensions of cultures that belong to related O antigen groups may react in OB and O antisera in slide tests if they are O-agglutinable, and heated suspensions may be expected to cross-react. As an example, the O antigens of O group 25 strains are related to those of O 26, and an O group 25 suspension may react in O 26:B6 and O 26 antisera in slide tests, but, when tested by titration in O 26 antiserum, only a relatively low-titered reaction is obtained (18).

After preliminary serological tests are completed, the biochemical reactions of the cultures should be determined to make certain that they are *E. coli* (Tables 6 and 29). If all of the bacterial suspensions prepared with strains from a particular specimen are agglutinated by one of the antisera, one of these strains may be selected for biochemical studies. If the types of

TABLE 29. *Biochemical reactions of Escherichia coli*[a]

Test or substrate	Sign[b]	Percent positive[c]
Hydrogen sulfide (TSI)	–[d]	0
Urease	–	0
Indole	+	96.3
Methyl red	+	99.9
Voges-Proskauer	–	0
Citrate (Simmons)	–	0.2 (0.3)
KCN	–	2.6
Motility	+ or –	62.1
Gelatin (22 C)	–	0
Lysine decarboxylase	d	80.6 (1.5)
Arginine dehydrolase	d	16.3 (39.1)
Ornithine decarboxylase	d	57.8 (8)
Phenylalanine deaminase	–	0
Glucose		
Acid	+	100
Gas	+	92
Lactose	+	91.6 (4.2)
Sucrose	d	53.7 (5.5)
Mannitol	+	97.5
Dulcitol	d	49.3 (18)
Salicin	d	36 (12.3)
Adonitol	–	5.2 (0.4)
Inositol	–	0.9 (0.2)
Sorbitol	d	80.3 (1)
Arabinose	+	99.3 (0.5)
Raffinose	d	49.4 (2.1)
Rhamnose	d	83.5 (3.4)
Malonate	–	0
Mucate	+	91.6
Christensen's citrate	d	18.1 (22.6)
Jordan's tartrate	+	97.6
Sodium pectate	–	0
Sodium acetate	+ or (+)	83.8 (9.7)
Sodium alginate	–	0
Lipase, corn oil	–	0
Maltose	+	90.6 (2.4)
Xylose	d	82.8 (6.6)
Trehalose	+	98.2 (1.8)
Cellobiose	–	3.7 (6.1)
Glycerol	+ or (+)	89 (8.3)
α-Methyl glucoside	–	0
Erythritol	–	0
Esculin	d	30.0 (19.7)
Nitrate to nitrite	+	99.8 (0.2)
Oxidation-fermentation	F	100
Oxidase	–	0

[a] Adapted from references 18 and 42.

[b] Sign: +, 90% or more positive within 1 or 2 days; (+), positive reaction after 3 or more days (decarboxylase tests: 3 or 4 days); –, no reaction (90% or more); + or –, most cultures positive, some strains negative; – or +, most strains negative, some cultures positive; + or (+), most reactions occur within 1 or 2 days, some are delayed; d, different reactions, +, (+), –; F, fermentative.

[c] Figures in parentheses indicate percentages of delayed reactions (3 or more days).

[d] Some strains that produce hydrogen sulfide now are being seen (see text).

E. coli present in the specimens are not agglutinated by any of the antisera available, it is suggested that the biochemical reactions of three or more strains from each specimen should be determined. All strains that are examined biochemically also should be placed in stock culture medium.

Although any desired number of biochemical tests may be done (42), the tests listed in Fig. 3 are essential to determine whether a culture is *E. coli*. In many instances, it may be advantageous to determine whether the epidemic strain involved in a particular outbreak ferments sorbitol, dulcitol, salicin, adonitol, or other substrates.

When one of the OB groups of *E. coli* known to be associated with diarrheal disease is isolated, it is recommended that one or more cultures from each stool specimen be sent to a central laboratory with a request for confirmatory studies. Pertinent information regarding each case should be submitted with the cultures (as indicated above for *Salmonella*). In addition to confirmation of the O group, the B antigens, and biochemical characteristics, further studies should be made on the O antigen components of the cultures, and their H antigens should be determined (18, 43, 53). In attempts to trace the source of infection in an outbreak or in studies of intrahospital and interhospital spread of infection, determination of O antigenic components and of H antigens of the strains involved would seem to be essential, just as it is in the investigation of salmonellosis. These determinations also are necessary for the detection of other serotypes of the same O antigen group that may be introduced into a ward by newly admitted patients during the course of an epidemic and for the delineation of serotypes isolated from diverse sources. For a more complete discussion of the values of complete serotyping of selected *E. coli* strains, the reader should consult references 43 and 53.

If *Salmonella*, *Arizona*, *Shigella*, or serotypes of *E. coli* known to be associated with diarrheal disease are not isolated from patients in an outbreak, three or more cultures of the types of *E. coli* that are recovered from each patient should be forwarded to a central laboratory with a request for serological typing. Such cultures may belong to a serotype of *E. coli* previously found in association with diarrhea, or they may represent a serotype not hitherto recognized as being associated with the disease. In any event, additional information about the association of serotypes of *E. coli* with cases of diarrheal disease will become available as a result of the studies.

SEROLOGICAL ANALYSIS OF OTHER ENTEROBACTERIACEAE

Antisera for determining the capsule type of cultures of *Klebsiella* are available from commercial sources, and methods for their use are given elsewhere (18). An antigenic schema has been established in which members of the genus *Arizona* may be oriented (20, 56). However, antisera for serotyping these microorganisms are not generally available; hence the work must be done in central laboratories. Of necessity, such work must be limited to selected cultures or groups of cultures. Similarly, selected strains of *Citrobacter*, *Klebsiella*, *Serratia*, and *Providencia* may be examined in certain central laboratories when conditions warrant such examination and when prior arrangements are made. Antigenic schemata for most of the remaining genera of *Enterobacteriaceae* have been proposed by various investigators, but antisera for typing the bacteria are not available in this country. Work toward improvements of this situation has been begun primarily because of increased interest in the occurrence of these microorganisms in hospital-acquired infections, but a great deal of time will be required if this work ever is to be completed.

FLUORESCENT-ANTIBODY TECHNIQUES

The use of fluorescein-labeled antibodies has been advocated for identification of the etiological agents of a wide variety of infectious diseases. For excellent reviews of methods and applications, see Cherry and Moody (9) and Cherry and Thomason (10). Cherry et al. (11) reported the results obtained from a field evaluation of the use of fluorescent-antibody (FA) techniques for rapid presumptive identification of OB serogroups of *E. coli* in fecal smears. Evaluation of FA techniques for detection of *S. flexneri* and *S. sonnei* was reported by Thomason and co-workers (93), and Thomason and McWhorter (94) obtained good results in the detection of carriers of *S. typhi*. This work has been extended to the detection of salmonellae in feces, water, and foods (92, 95).

The literature cited above suggests that, with certain limitations, FA techniques are of value in the management and control of some diarrheal diseases in epidemic situations, as well as for detection of certain *Enterobacteriaceae* in water and foods. However, as pointed out by Cherry and Moody (9), FA techniques are not a substitute for isolation and definitive identification of the microorganisms. On the contrary, with *Enterobacteriaceae* they are designed for rapid, presumptive identification. As far as members of the family *Enterobacteriaceae* are concerned, no particular type can be *identified* by FA techniques alone, any more than it could be by means of slide agglutination tests alone. One has only to consider the known inter- and intrageneric antigenic relationships of members of the family to understand this.

LITERATURE CITED

1. Amies, C. R. 1973. Evaluation of a simple preservative for bacteriological tests on urine. Can. Med. Ass. J. **108**:469–471.
2. Amies, C. R., and A. Corpas. 1971. A preservative for urine specimens in transit to the bacteriological laboratory. J. Med. Microbiol. **4**:362–365.
3. Banwart, G. J., and J. C. Ayres. 1953. Effect of various enrichment broths and selective agars upon the growth of several species of *Salmonella*. Appl. Microbiol. **1**:296–301.
4. Branham, S. E., S. A. Carlin, and D. B. Riggs. 1952. A comparison of the incidence of phases I and II of *Shigella sonnei* in cultures from acute infections and carriers. Amer. J. Pub. Health **42**:1409–1413.
5. Brenner, D. J., and S. Falkow. 1971. Molecular relationships among members of the family *Enterobacteriaceae*. Advan. Genet. **16**:81–118.
6. Brenner, D. J., G. R. Fanning, K. E. Johnson, R. V. Citarella, and S. Falkow. 1969. Polynucleotide sequence relationships among members of the *Enterobacteriaceae*. J. Bacteriol. **98**:637–650.
7. Brenner, D. J., A. G. Steigerwalt, and G. R. Fanning. 1972. Differentiation of *Enterobacter aerogenes* from klebsiellae by deoxyribonucleic acid reassociation. Int. J. Syst. Bacteriol. **22**:193–200.
8. Brenner, D. J., A. G. Steigerwalt, G. V. Miklos, and G. R. Fanning. 1973. Deoxyribonucleic acid relatedness among Erwiniae and other *Enterobacteriaceae*: the soft-rot organisms (Genus *Pectobacterium* Waldee). Int. J. Syst. Bacteriol. **23**:205–216.
9. Cherry, W. B., and M. D. Moody. 1965. Fluorescent-antibody techniques in diagnostic bacteriology. Bacteriol. Rev. **29**:222–250.
10. Cherry, W. B., and B. M. Thomason. 1969. Fluorescent antibody techniques for *Salmonella* and other enteric pathogens. Pub. Health Rep. **84**:887–898.
11. Cherry, W. B., B. M. Thomason, A. Pomales-Lebron, and W. H. Ewing. 1961. Rapid presumptive identification of enteropathogenic *Escherichia coli* in fecal smears by means of fluorescent antibody. Bull. World Health Organ. **25**:159–171.
12. Christensen, W. B. 1946. Urea decomposition as a means of differentiating Proteus and paracolon cultures from each other and from Salmonella and Shigella types. J. Bacteriol. **52**:461–466.
13. Croft, C. C., and M. J. Miller. 1956. Isolation of *Shigella* from rectal swabs with Hajna "GN" broth. Amer. J. Clin. Pathol. **26**:411–417.
14. Crosa, J. H., D. J. Brenner, W. H. Ewing, and S. Falkow. 1973. Molecular relationships among the *Salmonelleae*. J. Bacteriol. **115**:307–315.
15. Darland, G., and B. R. Davis. 1973. Biochemical and serological characterization of hydrogen sulfide positive variants of *Escherichia coli*. Center for Disease Control, Atlanta, Ga.
16. DuPont, H. L., S. B. Formal, R. B. Hornick, M. J. Snyder, J. P. Libonati, D. G. Sheahan, E. H. LeBrec, and J. P. Kalas. 1971. Pathogenesis of *Escherichia coli* diarrhea. N. Engl. J. Med. **285**:1–9.
17. Edwards, P. R. 1962. Serologic examination of *Salmonella* cultures for epidemiologic purposes. Center for Disease Control, Atlanta, Ga.
18. Edwards, P. R., and W. H. Ewing. 1972. Identification of Enterobacteriaceae, 3rd. ed. Burgess Publishing Co., Minneapolis, Minn.
19. Edwards, P. R., and M. A. Fife. 1961. Lysine-iron agar in the detection of Arizona cultures. Appl. Microbiol. **9**:478–480.
20. Edwards, P. R., M. A. Fife, and W. H. Ewing. 1965. Antigenic schema for the genus *Arizona*. Center for Disease Control, Atlanta, Ga.
21. Ewing, W. H. 1950. *Shigella* grouping serums. J. Lab. Clin. Med. **36**:471–472.
22. Ewing, W. H. 1963. An outline of nomenclature for the family *Enterobacteriaceae*. Int. Bull. Bacteriol. Nomencl. Taxon. **13**:95–110.
23. Ewing, W. H. 1966. Isolation and identification of *Enterobacteriaceae:* principles and practice. Center for Disease Control, Atlanta, Ga.
24. Ewing, W. H. 1966. Differential reactions of *Enterobacteriaeceae*. Center for Disease Control, Atlanta, Ga.
25. Ewing, W. H. 1966. Preliminary examination of *Salmonella* and *Shigella*. Center for Disease Control, Atlanta, Ga.
26. Ewing, W. H. 1967. Revised definitions for the family *Enterobacteriaceae*. Center for Disease Control, At- Disease Control, Atlanta, Ga.
27. Ewing, W. H. 1969. Excerpts from: An evaluation of the *Salmonella* problem. Center for Disease Control, Atlanta, Ga.
28. Ewing, W. H. 1969. Isolation and preliminary identification of enteropathogenic serotypes of *Escherichia coli*. Pub. Health Lab. **27**:19–30.
29. Ewing, W. H. 1972. Isolation and identification of *Salmonella* and *Shigella*. Center for Disease Control, Atlanta, Ga.
30. Ewing, W. H. 1972. Biochemical characterization of *Shigella*. Pub. Health Lab. **30**:146–160.
31. Ewing, W. H. 1972. The nomenclature of *Salmonella*, its usage, and definitions of the three species. Can. J. Microbiol. **18**:1629–1637.
32. Ewing, W. H. 1973. Differentiation of *Enterobacteriaceae* by biochemical reactions. Revised. Center for Disease Control, Atlanta, Ga.
33. Ewing, W. H., and M. M. Ball. 1966. The biochemical reactions of the genus *Salmonella*. Center for Disease Control, Atlanta, Ga.
34. Ewing, W. H., M. M. Ball, and S. F. Bartes. 1970. The biochemical reactions of certain species and bioserotypes of *Salmonella*. J. Infect. Dis. **121**:288–294.
35. Ewing, W. H., and B. R. Davis. 1970. Media and tests for differentiation of *Enterobacteriaceae*. Center for Disease Control, Atlanta, Ga.
36. Ewing, W. H., and B. R. Davis. 1971. Biochemical characterization of *Citrobacter freundii* and *Citrobacter diversus*. Center for Disease Control, Atlanta, Ga.
37. Ewing, W. H., and B. R. Davis. 1972. Biochemical characterization of *Citrobacter diversus* (Burkey) Werkman and Gillen and designation of the neotype strain. Int. J. Syst. Bacteriol. **22**:12–18.
38. Ewing, W. H., and B. R. Davis. 1972. Biochemical characterization of the species of *Proteus*. Pub. Health Lab. **30**:46–57.
39. Ewing, W. H., and B. R. Davis. 1972. Biochemical characterization of *Serratia marcescens*. Pub. Health Lab. **30**:211–226.
40. Ewing, W. H., B. R. Davis, and M. A. Fife. 1972. Biochemical characterization of *Serratia liquefaciens* and *Serratia rubidaea*. Center for Disease Control, Atlanta, Ga.

41. Ewing, W. H., B. R. Davis, M. A. Fife, and E. F. Lessel. 1973. Biochemical characterization of *Serratia liquefaciens* (Grimes and Hennerty) Bascomb et al. (formerly *Enterobacter liquefaciens*) and *Serratia rubidaea* (Stapp) comb. nov. and designation of type and neotype strains. Int. J. Syst. Bacteriol. **23**:217–225.
42. Ewing, W. H., B. R. Davis, and W. J. Martin. 1972. Biochemical characterization of *Escherichia coli*. Center for Disease Control, Atlanta, Ga.
43. Ewing, W. H., B. R. Davis, and T. S. Montague. 1963. Studies of the occurrence of *Escherichia coli* serotypes associated with diarrheal disease. Center for Disease Control, Atlanta, Ga.
44. Ewing, W. H., P. R. Davis, and J. V. Sikes. 1972. Biochemical characterization of *Providencia*. Pub. Health Lab. **30**:25–38.
45. Ewing, W. H., and M. A. Fife. 1966. A summary of the biochemical reactions of *Arizona arizonae*. Int. J. Syst. Bacteriol. **16**:427–433.
46. Ewing, W. H., and M. A. Fife. 1968. *Enterobacter hafniae* (the "Hafnia group"). Int. J. Syst. Bacteriol. **18**:263–271.
47. Ewing, W. H., and M. A. Fife. 1971. *Enterobacter agglomerans*. The Herbicola-Lathyri bacteria. Center for Disease Control, Atlanta, Ga.
48. Ewing, W. H., and M. A. Fife. 1972. *Enterobacter* agglomerans (Beijerinck) comb. nov. (the Herbicola-Lathyri bacteria). Int. J. Syst. Bacteriol. **22**:4-11.
49. Ewing, W. H., and M. A. Fife. 1972. Biochemical characterization of *Enterobacter agglomerans*. Center for Disease Control, Atlanta, Ga.
50. Ewing, W. H., A. C. McWhorter, M. M. Ball, and S. F. Bartes. 1969. *Edwardsiella tarda:* biochemical reactions. Pub. Health Lab. **27**:129–141.
51. Ewing, W. H., A. C. McWhorter, G. A. Huntley, and G. J. Hermann. 1972. A lysine negative strain of *Salmonella typhi*. Pub. Health Lab. **30**:98–99.
52. Ewing, W. H., A. C. McWhorter, and T. S. Montague. 1966. Transport media in the detection of *Salmonella typhi* in carriers. Pub. Health Lab. **24**:63–65.
53. Ewing, W. H., H. W. Tatum, B. R. Davis, and R. W. Reavis. 1956. Studies on the serology of *Escherichia coli*. Center for Disease Control, Atlanta, Ga.
54. Fields, B. N., M. M. Uwaydah, L. J. Kunz, and M. N. Swartz. 1967. The so-called "paracolon" bacteria. A bacteriologic and clinical reappraisal. Amer. J. Med. **42**:89–106.
55. Fife, M. A., W. H. Ewing, and B. R. Davis. 1965. The biochemical reactions of the tribe *Klebsielleae*. Center for Disease Control, Atlanta, Ga.
56. Fife, M. A., and G. H. Hermann. 1973. Antigenic schema for the genus *Arizona*. Supplement III. Center for Disease Control, Atlanta, Ga.
57. Finegold, S. M., M. L. White, I. Ziment, and W. R. Winn. 1969. Rapid diagnosis of bacteremia. Appl. Microbiol. **18**:458–463.
58. Galton, M. M., and M. E. Hess. 1946. Hydrogen sulfide production by *Shigella alkalescens*. J. Bacteriol. **52**:143.
59. Galton, M. M., and M. S. Quan. 1944. *Salmonella* isolated in Florida during 1943 with the combined enrichment method of Kauffmann. Amer. J. Pub. Health **34**:1071–1075.
60. Gillies, R. R. 1956. An evaluation of two composite media for preliminary identification of *Shigella* and *Salmonella*. J. Clin. Pathol. **9**:368–371.
61. Hajna, A. A. 1955. A new enrichment broth medium for gram-negative organisms of the intestinal group. Pub. Health Lab. **13**:83–89.
62. Johnson, J. G., L. J. Kunz, W. Barron, and W. H. Ewing. 1966. Biochemical differentiation of the *Enterobacteriaceae* with the aid of lysine-iron-agar. Appl. Microbiol. **14**:212–217.
63. Kauffmann, F. 1930. Ein kombiniertes Anreicherungsverfahren für Typhus- und Paratyphusbazillen. Zentralbl. Bakteriol. Abt. I Orig. **119**:148–152.
64. Kauffmann, F. 1935. Weitere erfahrungen mit den kombinierten Anreicherungs verfahren für Samonellabazillen. Z. Hyg. Infektionskr. **117**:26–32.
65. Kauffmann, F. 1966. The bacteriology of Enterobacteriaceae. E. Munksgaard, Copenhagen.
66. Kelterborn, E. 1967. *Salmonella* species. Dr. W. Junk, The Hague, Netherlands.
67. Lautrop, H., I. Oerskov, and K. Gaarslev. 1971. Hydrogensulfide producing variants of *Escherichia coli*. Acta Pathol. Microbiol. Scand. Sect. B **79**:641–650.
68. Leifson, E. 1936. New selenite enrichment media for the isolation of typhoid and paratyphoid (*Salmonella*) bacilli. Amer. J. Hyg. **24**:423–432.
69. McCall, C. E., W. T. Martin, and J. R. Boring. 1966. Efficiency of cultures of rectal swabs and fecal specimens in detecting *Salmonella* carriers: correlation with numbers of salmonellae excreted. J. Hyg. **64**:261–269.
70. McIlroy, G. T., P. K. W. Yu, W. J. Martin, and J. A. Washington II. 1972. Evaluation of modified R-B system for identification of the family *Enterobacteriaceae*. Appl. Microbiol. **24**:358–362.
71. Martin, W. J., and W. H. Ewing. 1969. Prevalence of serotypes of *Salmonella*. Appl. Microbiol. **17**:111–117.
72. Martin, W. J., W. H. Ewing, A. C. McWhorter, and M. M. Ball. 1969. Biochemical reactions of *Salmonella* with emphasis on differentiation of this genus and the genera *Arizona* and *Citrobacter*. Pub. Health Lab. **27**:61–78.
73. Morbidity and Mortality Weekly Report. 1971. Nosocomial bacteremias associated with intravenous therapy-USA. Morbidity and Mortality Weekly Rep. **20**:110.
74. Morbidity and Mortality Weekly Report. 1973. Follow-up on septicemias associated with contamination of intravenous fluids-United States. Morbidity and Mortality Weekly Rep. **22**:124.
75. Muller, L. 1923. Un nouveau milieu d'enrichissement pour la recherche du bacille typhique et des paratyphiques. C. R. Soc. Biol. **89**:434–437.
76. Report, Committee on *Salmonella*. 1969. An evaluation of the *Salmonella* problem. Nat. Acad. Sci.-Nat. Res. Counc. Publ. 1683.
77. Rhoden, D. L., K. M. Tomfohrde, P. B. Smith, and A. Balows. 1973. Evaluation of the improved Auxotab 1 system for identifying *Enterobacteriaceae*. Appl. Microbiol. **26**:215–216.
78. Roome, A. P. C. H., and R. A. Tozer. 1968. Effect of dilution on the growth of bacteria from blood cultures. J. Clin. Pathol. **21**:719–721.
79. Rowe, B., J. Taylor, and K. A. Bettelheim. 1970. An investigation of travellers' diarrhoea. Lancet **1**:1–5.
80. Sachs, A. 1939. Difficulties associated with the bacteriological diagnosis of bacillary dysentery. J. Roy. Army Med. Corps **73**:235–239.
81. Shaughnessy, H. J., F. Friewer, and A. Snyder. 1948. Comparative efficiency of rectal swabs and fecal specimens in detecting typhoid and *Salmonella* cases and carriers. Amer. J. Pub. Health **38**:670–675.
82. Shaw, A. B., and H. A. F. MacKay. 1951. Factors influencing the results of blood culture in enteric fever. J. Hyg. **49**:315–323.
83. Smith, H. W. 1952. The evaluation of culture media for the isolation of salmonellae from faeces. J. Hyg.

50:21–36.

84. Smith, P. B., K. M. Tomfohrde, D. L. Rhoden, and A. Balows. 1972. API system: a multitest micromethod for identification of *Enterobacteriaceae*. Appl. Microbiol. **24**:449–452.
85. Stoleru, G. H., G. R. Gerbaud, D. H. Bouanchaud, and L. LeMinor. 1972. Étude d'un plasmide transférable determinant la production d'H_2S et la résistance a la tétracycline chez *Escherichia coli*. Ann. Inst. Pasteur Paris **123**:743–754.
86. Stuart, C. A., E. van Stratum, and R. Rustigian. 1945. Further studies on urease production by *Proteus* and related organisms. J. Bacteriol. **49**:437–444.
87. Suassuna, I. 1963. Estudos sôbre o gênero *Proteus*. Inst. Microbiol. University of Brazil, Rio de Janeiro, Brazil.
88. Taylor, W. I., and D. Schelhart. 1969. Isolation of shigellae. VII. Comparison of gram-negative broth with Rappaport's enrichment broth. Appl. Microbiol. **18**:393–395.
89. Teague, O., and A. W. Clurman. 1916. A method of preserving typhoid stools for delayed examination and a comparative study of the efficacy of eosin brilliant-green agar, eosin methylene-blue agar, and Endo agar for isolation of typhoid bacilli from stools. J. Infect. Dis. **18**:653–671.
90. Ten Broeck, C., and F. G. Norbury. 1916. *B. dysenteriae* as a cause of infectious diarrhea in infants. Boston Med. Surg. J. **174**:785–788.
91. Thomas, M. E. M. 1954. Disadvantages of rectal swabs in diagnosis of diarrhea. Brit. Med. J. **2**:394–396.
92. Thomason, B. M. 1971. Rapid detection of *Salmonella* microcolonies by fluorescent antibody. Appl. Microbiol. **22**:1064–1069.
93. Thomason, B. M., G. S. Cowart, and W. B. Cherry. 1965. Current status of immunofluorescence techniques for rapid detection of shigellae in fecal specimens. Appl. Microbiol. **13**:605–613.
94. Thomason, B. M., and A. C. McWhorter. 1965. Rapid detection of typhoid carriers by means of fluorescent antibody techniques. Bull. W.H.O. **33**:681–685.
95. Thomason, B. M., and J. G. Wells. 1971. Preparation and testing of polyvalent conjugates for fluorescent-antibody detection of salmonellae. Appl. Microbiol. **22**:876–884.
96. Thomson, S. 1955. The numbers of pathogenic bacilli in feces in intestinal diseases. J. Hyg. **53**:217–224.
97. Tomfohrde, K. M., D. L. Rhoden, P. B. Smith, and A. Balows. 1973. Evaluation of the redesigned Enterotube—a system for the identification of *Enterobacteriaceae*. Appl. Microbiol. **25**:301–304.
98. Washington, J. A., II, P. K. W. Yu, and W. J. Martin. 1971. Evaluation of accuracy of multitest micromethod system for identification of *Enterobacteriaceae*. Appl. Microbiol. **22**:267–269.
99. Waterworth, P. M. 1972. The lethal effect of tryptone-soya broth. J. Clin. Pathol. **25**:227–228.
100. Wheeler, K. M., and F. L. Mickel. 1945. Antigens of *Shigella sonnei*. J. Immunol. **51**:257–267.

Chapter 19

Yersinia

ALEX C. SONNENWIRTH

CHARACTERIZATION

The genus *Yersinia*, family *Enterobacteriaceae* (*Bergey's Manual*, 8th ed.) consists of the species *Y. pestis*, *Y. pseudotuberculosis* (both formerly included in the genus *Pasteurella*), and *Y. enterocolitica*.

The three species are primarily found in animals (zoonotic bacteria): *Y. pestis* in rodents and insect vectors, and the other two species in a wide variety of mammals and birds, where they may cause extensive epizootic outbreaks or may persist in healthy carriers.

In humans *Y. pestis* is the causative agent of plague, and *Y. pseudotuberculosis* and *Y. enterocolitica* are responsible for a variety of syndromes often (but semantically incorrectly) referred to as "pseudotuberculosis." The most common clinical infections due to these two species are *enterocolitis* and *acute mesenteric lymphadenitis* (often mimicking acute appendicitis); other manifestations are *erythema nodosum*, *typhoidal syndromes*, and *generalized septicemia*. *Y. enterocolitica* has also been isolated in meningitis (20), abscesses of the spleen, colon, and neck, local infection at indwelling catheter site, cholecystitis, eye infections, urine, and wounds (23). Occasionally, *Y. pestis* has been isolated from the throats of healthy carriers and *Y. enterocolitica* from the feces and lymph nodes of healthy humans.

Yersinia are relatively large (0.5 to 1.0 by 1 to 2 μm) coccobacillary, ovoid-, or rod-shaped gram-negative bacteria, nonmotile at 37 C; *Y. pseudotuberculosis* and *Y. enterocolitica* are motile at 22 to 25 C.

Growth. Aerobic; facultatively anaerobic. Grow on ordinary media, including MacConkey agar; *Y. enterocolitica* produces tiny translucent colonies on SS agar after 18 h. Temperature range said to be −2 to 45 C; recently, *Y. enterocolitica*, but not *Y. pestis* or *Y. pseudotuberculosis*, was shown to grow at 42 C (28). Optimal growth on isolation: 28 C for *Y. pestis*, 30 to 37 C for the other two species. Nonpigmented.

Biochemical characteristics. Major characteristics are identical with those of other *Enterobacteriaceae*: they are oxidase-negative, usually reduce nitrate to nitrite, and attack carbohydrates *fermentatively*; when present, flagella are peritrichous. Methyl red test positive; Voges-Proskauer negative at 37 C (*Y. enterocolitica* usually positive at 22 C). Lysine decarboxylase, arginine dihydrolase, phenylalanine deaminase, gelatin hydrolase, malonate utilization, tetrathionate reduction, and citrate utilization as sole source of carbon (Simmons citrate) negative. Catalase positive. Indole not produced by *Y. pestis* and *Y. pseudotuberculosis*.

Fermentations. Glucose, maltose, mannitol, trehalose, glycerol, xylose, and fructose fermented with acid, but no gas (*Y. enterocolitica* strains may produce very small amounts of gas when tested with a Durham tube). Lactose usually not fermented, but β-D-galactosidase produced. No fermentation of dulcitol, erythritol, fucose, inositol, glycogen, raffinose, and melezitose.

Differentiation from other Enterobacteriaceae. On initial isolation, *Yersinia* (especially *Y. enterocolitica*) strongly resemble certain other *Enterobacteriaceae* (especially anaerogenic "atypical coliforms," *Proteus rettgeri*, *P. morganii*, *Providencia*, and shigellae—all fermentative organisms) and are easily misdiagnosed (21, 22, 30). If triple sugar iron (TSI) agar is used for screening purposes, it can be employed in most instances in place of the oxidation-fermentation (OF) medium to establish the fermentative capability of the isolate.

With the combined use of TSI and lysine iron (LIA) agar slants (9, 10), *Yersinia* can be presumptively differentiated from a large number of other fermentative gram-negative bacilli, with further tests to be undertaken for definitive identification (see Table 1). TSI reactions: alkaline slant/acid butt, no gas (*Y. pestis*, *Y. pseudotuberculosis*); acid slant/acid butt, no gas (*Y. enterocolitica*, due to fermentation of sucrose; occasional *Y. pseudotuberculosis*). LIA reactions: alkaline slant/acid butt.

Any lactose-negative, gram-negative, fer-

TABLE 1. *Schema for the differentiation of catalase-positive, oxidase-negative, fermentative, gram-negative bacilli*[a]

Reactions observed in LIA slants	Reactions observed in TSI slants: K/A H_2S+	K/**a** H_2S+	K/**a**	K/A	A/**a** H_2S+	A/**a**	A/A
R/A		*P. vulgaris* (rare) *P. mirabilis*	*P. morganii* (rare) *Providencia*	*P. morganii* (rare) *P. rettgeri* *Providencia*	*P. vulgaris* *P. mirabilis* (rare)		*P. rettgeri* (rare)
K/K or N H_2S+	*S. typhi* (H_2S 1+) *Salmonella* (rare) *Arizona* (rare) *Edwardsiella* (rare)	*Salmonella* *Arizona* *Edwardsiella*	*Salmonella* (rare) *Arizona* (rare)	*S. typhi* (rare)	*Arizona* *Salmonella* (rare)		
K/K or N	*Salmonella* (rare)		*Enterobacter hafniae* *Klebsiella* *Serratia* (occasional)	*Serratia* *S. typhi* (rare) *Klebsiella* (rare) *Enterobacter hafniae* (rare)		*Klebsiella* *Enterobacter aerogenes* *liquefaciens* *E. coli*	*Serratia*
K/A H_2S+		*Citrobacter*			*Citrobacter*		
K/A			*E. agglomerans* *E. coli* *P. morganii* Paratyphi A *S. flexneri* 6-some biotypes (uncommon) *C. diversus*	*E. coli* (A–D) *Shigella* *P. morganii* *E. agglomerans* **Y. pseudotuberculosis** **Y. pestis** *A. actinomycetemcomitans* *C. violaceum*		*E. coli* (rare) *Citrobacter* (rare) *E. cloacae* *E. agglomerans* *H. aphrophilus*	*E. coli* *E. agglomerans* *C. diversus* (rare) *H. aphrophilus* **Y. enterocolitica** *C. violaceum* **Y. pseudotuberculosis** (occasional)

[a] Key: R = red, oxidative deamination of lysine; K = alkaline slant; A = acid slant; K = alkaline butt;/A = acid butt;/**a** = acid + gas in butt; H_2S+ = hydrogen sulfide production. From C. T. Hall, Bacteriology I, January 1973 Summary Analysis, Center for Disease Control, Atlanta, Ga.

mentative rod which is oxidase-negative, does not produce H_2S in TSI, is *motile only at room temperature*, and is *urease-positive* on Christensen urease agar in 3 to 24 h, but *phenylalanine-negative*, should be suspected of being *Y. enterocolitica* or *Y. pseudotuberculosis*, and its further identification should be pursued. Occasional strains of *Y. enterocolitica* ferment lactose; motility pattern should be helpful in differentiating such strains. *Y. pestis* is nonmotile at either 25 or 37 C and is usually urease-negative.

Differential characteristics of *Yersinia* are given in Table 2.

Additional sources of material are Goldenberg et al. (7), Wetzler (30), Sonnenwirth (21), Niléhn (18), and Winblad (32).

YERSINIA PESTIS

Clinical significance

Y. pestis is the causative agent of plague in man, rats, and ground squirrels; it is transmitted from rat to rat and from rat to man by the infected rat flea. In man, clinical forms are *bubonic* (commonest), *pneumonic*, and *septicemic* plague; rarely, meningitis occurs (19). Plague now occurs in Central and South Africa, South America, and Asia. In the United States, where it exists west of the 100th meridian, 38 cases were recognized in 1965–1970, all acquired from the reservoir of endemic sylvatic plague in wild rodents.

Material suspected of containing *P. pestis*

TABLE 2. *Differential characteristics of the genus Yersinia*

Characteristic[a]	*Y. pestis*	*Y. pseudotuberculosis*	*Y. enterocolitica*
Motility 22 C	−	+	+
37 C	−	−	−
Urease	−	+	+
Phenylalanine deaminase	−	−	−
Fermentation of:			
Glucose	A	A	A
Lactose	−	−	−, (L), (A)
Mannitol	A	A	A
Sucrose	−	−	A
Maltose	A	A	A (L)
Rhamnose	−	A	−
Salicin	A	A	−, (A)
Sorbitol	−	−	A
Xylose	A	A	A (L)
Cellobiose	−	−	A
Raffinose	−	−	−
Arabinose	A	A	A
Melibiose	−	A	−
Trehalose	A	A	A (L)
Adonitol	−	A (−)	−
Catalase	+	+	+
Oxidase	−	−	−
Citrate (Simmons)	−	−	−
H_2S (TSI)	−	−	−
β-Galactosidase	+	+	+
Nitrate reduction	+	+	+, (−)
Indole	−	−	+ or −
Methyl red	+	+	+
Voges-Proskauer 22 C	−	−	+, (−)
37 C	−	−	−
Lysine decarboxylase	−	−	−
Arginine dihydrolase	−	−	−
Ornithine decarboxylase	−	−	+
Esculin hydrolysis	+	+	−, (+)
Gelatin hydrolysis	−	−	−

[a] Reactions in italics important for differentiation both within the family and the genus. Results in parentheses occur infrequently. A = acid; L = late.

must be handled with extreme care; it is hazardous. Laboratory personnel may become infected via broken skin, mucous membranes, or the respiratory tract through laboratory accidents. Presumptive identification of *P. pestis* may be carried out at the clinical laboratory level, but suspicious cultures or specimens should be forwarded by the most expeditious means in proper containers to laboratories equipped to accomplish definitive and timely identification. In the case of suspected rodents, the whole carcass should be submitted. Suspect and/or confirmed cases should immediately be reported to the local health authority.

Specimens

The viability of *Y. pestis* is prolonged by use of Cary-Blair transport medium (2). Acute and (2 to 3 weeks later) convalescent serum should be collected for serological examination.

Aspirates from buboes, pus from infection (usually area of flea bite), heparinized or citrated blood (cultivable also in routine blood culture bottles), sputum, and throat swabs should be inoculated to blood-agar, MacConkey or deoxycholate agar, nutrient agar, and infusion broth. Autopsy material (i.e., spleen, liver, lymph nodes, lung, bone marrow) is also used. Highly contaminated specimens, as well as most specimens of rodent tissues and fleas, should be given a preliminary passage through experimental animals (if facilities are available) before cultural isolation is attempted, or they should be cultured on Knisely et al.'s selective medium (13).

Staining

Y. pestis is gram-negative. Bipolar staining ("safety-pin" appearance) is best demonstrated by use of Wayson's (carbol fuchsin-methylene blue) stain: air-dry smears, fix in absolute methanol for 2 to 5 min, and stain. With Wayson's stain (chapter 96), the polar bodies of *Y. pestis* are blue and the remainder is light blue to reddish. Bipolar staining is much more pronounced in tissue impressions, bubo aspirates, and pus than in smears of cultures. In broth cultures the organism appears predominantly in chains of 4 to 16 bacilli. Old cultures or those on media containing glycerol or 3% NaCl contain involution forms (filamentous, ring-shaped, pleomorphic organisms).

Cultivation

Optimal temperature is 28 C; range, 0 to 40 C. *Y. pestis* grows slowly on initial isolation. At 35 C in 18 to 24 h, colonies are pinpoint size on 5% blood-agar; isolated colonies become grossly visible after 2 days (1 to 2 mm). Broth cultures at 28 C after 24 h produce a flocculent type of growth, adhering to the side of the tube; if shaken, the growth settles on the bottom. With prolonged incubation, colonies continue to grow and assume a beaten copper surface. The center of the colonies is raised and the periphery is flat with an umbonate edge. Older colonies often assume a "fried egg" configuration. Growth on deoxycholate agar does not appear until the second day, when small, reddish, pinpoint colonies are observed. Blood cultures should be subcultured on solid media daily.

Identification

The organism is nonmotile at both 37 and 22 C, an important diagnostic feature. It does not utilize citrate (Simmons), does not grow in KCN, does not produce acid from lactose, sucrose, rhamnose, melibiose, or dulcitol, but ferments glucose, maltose, salicin, xylose, and mannitol (no gas). It is catalase- and esculin-positive; oxidase, indole, Voges-Proskauer, and urease are negative; no H_2S is formed in TSI agar; methyl red is positive; lysine and ornithine decarboxylase and arginine dihydrolase are negative, and β-D-galactosidase (ONPG) is positive.

For definitive identification, the following four tests are usually employed:

1. *Bacteriophage*. Strains of bacteriophage are available (not commercially) which lyse all known strains of *Y. pestis*. These phages also lyse *Y. pseudotuberculosis* but only at 37 C, not at 20 C (30). This is a fairly rapid and specific test.
2. *Agglutination test*. Specific *Y. pestis* antiserum can be used for the agglutination test with ether-methanol-glycerol-formalin-treated cells. No commercial antisera are presently available.
3. *FA test*. Fluorescent-antibody (FA) methods employing anti-*Y. pestis* hyperimmune serum globulins conjugated with fluorescein isothiocyanate are used for staining direct smear and tissues, but this test is less satisfactory for cultures. Because of the existence of cross-reactions, results of the FA test must be interpreted with caution (6). No commercial antisera are presently available.
4. *Animal inoculation*. Animal inoculation should be undertaken only where proper facilities are available. Guinea pigs or albino mice are used (inoculation by subcutaneous or intraperitoneal route). Autopsy of mice usually shows buboes and marked splenic enlargement with other nonspecific signs of generalized infection. In guinea pigs subcutaneous congestion, buboes in corresponding regional lymph nodes, enlargement of the spleen and liver with necrotic nodules, and pneumonic foci in the lungs are produced. *Y. pestis* is observed in abundance in direct smears from all tissues.

Tests for antibodies

A formalin-killed 1% suspension of a known *Y. pestis* strain, if available, can be used for agglutination procedures with patients' sera either by the tube or slide technique (7). The most sensitive test for *Y. pestis* antibodies is the indirect hemagglutination test with the specific Fraction I (envelope) antigen (4, 7, 33) of the plague bacillus. Fraction I is not available commercially.

Antibiotic susceptibility

Susceptibility testing of *Y. pestis* is misleading because it usually indicates susceptibility in vitro to penicillin, which is totally ineffective in practice. *Y. pestis* is susceptible, in addition, to streptomycin, tetracycline, and chloramphenicol. Tetracycline (or streptomycin) is the preferred therapeutic agent.

YERSINIA PSEUDOTUBERCULOSIS

Clinical significance

The organism is widespread in Europe among many species of mammals and birds (rabbits, cats, chickens, sheep, fox, raccoon). In the United States, it has been reported infrequently from turkeys, various rodents, sheep, goat, and cow (31). Until about 1955, the disease in humans was thought to occur only as a rare acute *septicemia*. Since then, however, several hundred cases have been recognized in Europe, mostly with *mesenteric lymphadenitis* suggesting appendicitis and some with *enteritis* or *erythema nodosum* (11, 15); the disease has been sporadically seen in the U.S. since 1938, and its recognition is slowly increasing (22, 29). The organism is excreted in the feces of infected animals and is likely spread by oral ingestion and possibly by skin contamination.

Specimens

Y. pseudotuberculosis can be isolated from blood (usually positive in generalized septicemia), mesenteric lymph nodes, effusions from serous cavities, organ specimens, and feces. For holding and selective enrichment, the specimen should be placed in isotonic saline with or without potassium tellurite (25 μg/ml) and promptly refrigerated (30).

Staining

On Gram stain, virulent *Y. pseudotuberculosis* appears as a relatively large (0.8 to 6.0 μm by 0.8 μm) gram-negative coccobacillus or rod. Wayson's stain reveals the bipolar appearance in most, but not all, isolates.

Cultivation

Y. pseudotuberculosis grows on blood-agar and various common media such as MacConkey, EMB, deoxycholate, or Endo agar, at both 22 and 37 C (more luxuriantly at the latter temperature than does *Y. pestis*). It grows well in tetrathionate broth. A selective plating medium was recommended by Morris (17). Colonies on blood-agar after 24 h reach 1 mm; on EMB or MacConkey agar, they are smaller and lactose-negative.

Identification

Y. pseudotuberculosis is facultatively anaerobic; grows well in air. It is motile at 22 to 25 C and nonmotile at temperatures greater than 28 C, an important diagnostic feature. TSI (overnight): alkaline slant/acid butt, no H_2S, no gas. LIA: alkaline slant/acid butt. Urease is positive, phenylalanine deaminase negative. Oxidase, indole, citrate, lysine and ornithine decarboxylase, and arginine dihydrolase are negative; catalase, esculin, methyl red, and β-D-galactosidase (ONPG) are positive. Carbohydrates are attacked fermentatively. No gas is produced. Fermentation occurs promptly with glucose, galactose, maltose, mannitol, levulose, mannose, rhamnose, melibiose, trehalose, and xylose. No fermentation occurs with lactose, sucrose, raffinose, dulcitol, inositol, and cellobiose.

Serology

Based on 15 somatic (O) antigens, six main serotypes with four subtypes have been established (24). Agglutination or hemagglutination tests can be used for antigenic analysis of the organism (30). Antibodies have been detected in the sera of acutely ill patients; these antibodies agglutinate live smooth strains and formalin- or phenol-killed organisms of the six serotypes, as well as erythrocytes coated with supernatant fractions of heat-killed or autoclaved cell suspensions. At present, no antigens or antisera are commercially available.

Animal pathogenicity

Y. pseudotuberculosis is virulent in mice, guinea pigs, gerbils, and white rabbits but not in white rats or hamsters.

Special methods

Tests for the following are not usually available in the clinical laboratory: (i) antisera containing antibodies against types I to VI agglutinate *Y. pseudotuberculosis* but not *Y. pestis* or *Y. enterocolitica;* (ii) *Y. pseudotuberculosis* phages lyse all strains but not *Y. pestis* or *Y. enterocolitica;* (iii) *Y. pestis* phage does not lyse *P. pseudotuberculosis* at 20 to 25 C.

Antibiotic susceptibility

Y. pseudotuberculosis is reported as being susceptible to chloramphenicol, kanamycin, streptomycin, and the tetracyclines. Some strains are resistant but others are susceptible to penicillin and/or ampicillin. Streptomycin, tetracycline, and kanamycin have been used as effective therapeutic agents.

YERSINIA ENTEROCOLITICA

The organism is closely related to *Y. pseudotuberculosis* when judged by morphological and cultural characteristics, but it differs from it in a number of biochemical reactions (demonstrable by standard techniques), antigenic composition, bacteriophage susceptibility, and virulence in laboratory animals.

Y. enterocolitica has been isolated in Europe from a variety of both sick and healthy animals (rabbit, swine, chinchilla, cow, horse, sheep, dog) and mostly from chinchilla and deer in the U.S. It has also been isolated from material likely to be contaminated by feces, such as milk and ice cream, and from water.

Clinical significance

Although human *Y. enterocolitica* infections were first recognized in the United States (1933–1947), the sharpest increase in their reported incidence occurred in Europe, where over 1,000 cases were diagnosed between 1964 and 1971 (16). No cases of human infection were recognized in the U.S. between 1947 and 1968, when a case of *Y. enterocolitica* meningitis and septicemia was reported from Missouri (20; A. C. Sonnenwirth, Bacteriol. Proc., p. 97, 1969). By mid-1973, about 50 culture-proven *Y. enterocolitica* infections were known to have occurred in the United States (8, 23, 27), and in Canada over 130 cases of gastroenteritis were observed in the period 1966–1972 (5, 14). Human *Y. enterocolitica* infections are now encountered, in addition, in the Congo, South Africa, and Japan.

The two most common forms of *Y. enterocolitica* infection (resembling those due to *Y. pseudotuberculosis*) are *enterocolitis* with usually nonbloody diarrhea and abdominal pain, occurring mainly in young children, and *mesenteric lymphadenitis* or *acute terminal ileitis* with symptoms suggesting acute appendicitis. Other manifestations include erythema nodosum, arthritis, Reiter's syndrome, septicemia, meningitis, panophthalmitis, indwelling catheter site infection, cholecystitis, and various abscesses (23). Hospital-acquired infections (25) as well as interfamilial outbreaks (8) occur. The portal of entry is probably the gastrointestinal tract, but the source of human infection is not yet known. Healthy animal and human carriers exist, but their role in transmission of the infection has not been elucidated.

Specimens

Y. enterocolitica can be isolated from mesenteric lymph nodes, blood, spinal fluid, urine, feces, eye, throat, wounds, and abscesses. Refrigeration in isotonic saline, with or without potassium tellurite (25 μg/ml), results in selective enrichment (30).

Staining

Y. enterocolitica is gram-negative and is generally coccobacillary, oval, or rod-shaped, measuring 0.8 to 3.0 μm by 0.8 μm. Many strains show little, if any, bipolarity with Wayson's stain.

Cultivation

Y. enterocolitica grows on blood-agar and such selective media as MacConkey agar, EMB agar, deoxycholate agar, and (most strains) Salmonella-Shigella (SS) agar. It grows somewhat slower at 35 to 37 C than other enteric pathogens, and at least 2 days of incubation is recommended before stool cultures are discarded as negative. On MacConkey agar the lactose-negative colonies are 0.5 to 1.0 mm in size after overnight incubation; on SS agar they are tiny, translucent, and homogeneous, with a hazy rim (5).

Identification

Y. enterocolitica is facultatively anaerobic; grows well in air. Like *Y. pseudotuberculosis*, it is motile when grown at 22 to 25 C (with peritrichous flagella) but nonmotile at temperatures above 30 C. TSI (overnight): acid slant/acid butt (because of sucrose fermentation), no H_2S, no gas. LIA: alkaline slant/acid butt. Urease is positive (3 to 48 h), but phenylalanine is negative. Oxidase, lysine decarboxylase, arginine dihydrolase, esculin, and citrate (Simmons) are negative. Indole is variable: the majority of human isolates in the U.S. are positive; most European human isolates are negative. Catalase, methyl red, β-D-galactosidase (ONPG), and ornithine decarboxylase are positive. Carbohydrates are attacked fermentatively. No gas is produced (small amounts of gas may be produced when tested with Durham tube). *Y. enterocolitica* ferments glucose, galactose, mannitol, maltose, and, in contrast to *Y. pseudotuberculosis*, sucrose, sorbitol, and cellobiose. It does not ferment rhamnose, adonitol (both fermented by *Y. pseudotuberculosis*), dulcitol, raffinose, lactose (occasional strain late, rarely prompt lactose fermenter), and salicin (most strains). Several tests are markedly temperature dependent: ONPG, maltose fermentation, VP, and motility tests are positive at 22 to 25 C and negative (or delayed) at 37 C.

Biotypes

Y. enterocolitica strains are biochemically heterogeneous and differ in a number of reactions. Wauters (26) divided the group into five biotypes, characteristics of which are given in Table 3.

Serology

Based on thermostable O antigens, 17 serotypes have been established (26). A simplified antigenic schema based on biochemical characteristics, containing six O groups, has recently been proposed (12). Agglutination or hemagglutination tests are used for antigenic analysis. Most isolates from patients in the United States are serotype 8 (not seen in Europe), some Canadian strains are type 3, and the most frequent European isolates are types 3 and 9. About 2.5% of normal individuals (in Sweden) possess significant *Y. enterocolitica* antibody titers. In frank infections antibody titers are demonstrable by agglutination or hemagglutination; usually absent at the onset, they rise rapidly within the first few days of illness, with

TABLE 3. *Biotypes of Yersinia enterocolitica (26)*

Characteristics	Biotypes				
	1	2	3	4	5
Lecithinase	+	–	–	–	–
Indole	+	(+) 29 C	–	–	–
Xylose, 48 h	+	+	+	–	–
Nitrate reduction	+	+	+	+	–
Trehalose	+	+	+	+	–
Ornithine decarboxylase	+	+	+	+	–
β-Galactosidase	+	+	+	+	–
Lactose *oxidation* (OF medium), 48 h	+	+	+	–	–

maximal titers obtained within 1 to 2 weeks, and then generally drop significantly within 1 to 2 months. Serological diagnosis is reliable only if performed by reference laboratories with a good collection of serotypes. Marked cross-agglutination reactions have been observed between *Brucella abortus* and *Y. enterocolitica* serotype 9. High brucella titers in some patients may possibly be due to infection with serotype 9 *Y. enterocolitica*. Antigens or antisera are presently not available from commercial sources.

Fluorescent-antibody staining

The organism has been detected in fecal smears stained with anti-*Y. enterocolitica* conjugated serum (3). The technique is not in general use.

Animal pathogenicity

In the usual laboratory animal (guinea pigs, mice, white rabbits), *Y. enterocolitica* is nonpathogenic by the intraperitoneal, intravenous, or subcutaneous route (unlike *P. pseudotuberculosis* which is pathogenic in all of these animals). One recent human isolate (1), however, is highly pathogenic in mice by intravenous and oral routes.

Bacteriophage

Strains of bacteriophage are available (not commercially) which allow grouping of *Y. enterocolitica* strains into nine phage types; type 10 consists of strains nontypable by phage.

Antibiotic susceptibility

Y. enterocolitica is reported as being susceptible in vitro to gentamicin, kanamycin, colistin, chloramphenicol, and streptomycin. Variable resistance to neomycin and ampicillin and resistance to cephalothin was noted.

LITERATURE CITED

1. Carter, P. B., C. F. Varga, and K. E. Keet. 1973. New strain of *Yersinia enterocolitica* pathogenic for rodents. Appl. Microbiol. **26:**1016–1018.
2. Cary, S. G., and E. B. Blair. 1964. New transport medium for shipment of clinical specimens. I. Fecal specimens. J. Bacteriol. **88:**96–98.
3. Cederberg, A. 1968. Demonstration of *Yersinia enterocolitica* by the fluorescent antibody technique. Acta Pathol. Microbiol. Scand. **73:**646–652.
4. Chen, T. H., and K. F. Meyer. 1954. Studies on immunization against plague. VII. A hemagglutination test with the protein fraction of *Pasteurella pestis*. J. Immunol. **72:**282–298.
5. Delorme, J., M. Laverdiere, B. Martineau, and L. Lafleur. 1974. Yersiniosis in children. Can. Med. Ass. J. **110:**281–284.
6. Goldenberg, M. I. 1968. Laboratory diagnosis of plague infection. Health Lab. Sci. **5:**38–45.
7. Goldenberg, M. I., B. W. Hudson, and L. Kartman. 1970. Pasteurella infections. 1. *Pasteurella pestis*, p. 422–439. *In* H. L. Bodily, E. L. Updyke, and J. O. Mason (ed.), Diagnostic procedures for bacterial, mycotic and parasitic infections, 5th ed. American Public Health Association Inc., New York.
8. Gutman, L. T., E. A. Ottesen, T. J. Quan, P. S. Noce, and S. Katz. 1973. An inter-familial outbreak of *Yersinia enterocolitica* enteritis. N. Engl. J. Med. **288:**1372–1377.
9. Hall, C. T. 1973. Bacteriology I, January 1973 Summary Analysis. Center for Disease Control, Atlanta, Ga.
10. Johnson, J. G., L. J. Kunz, W. Barron, and W. H. Ewing. 1966. Biochemical differentiation of the *Enterobacteriaceae* with the aid of lysine-iron-agar. Appl. Microbiol. **14:**212–217.
11. Knapp, W. 1958. Mesenteric adenitis due to *Pasteurella pseudotuberculosis* in young people. N. Engl. J. Med. **259:**776–778.
12. Knapp, W., and E. Thal. 1973. Die biochimische Charakteriesierung von *Yersinia enterocolitica* (syn. "Pasteurella X") als Grundlage eines vereinfachten O-Antigen Schemas. Zentralbl. Bakteriol. Parasitenk. Infektionskr. Hyg. Abt. I Orig. A **223:**88–105.
13. Knisely, R. F., L. M. Swaney, and H. Friedlander. Selective media for the isolation of *Pasteurella pestis*. J. Bacteriol. **88:**491–496.
14. Lafleur, L., B. Martineau, and L. Chicoine. 1972. *Yersinia enterocolitica*. Aspects biologiques, èpidèmiologiques et cliniques de 67 cas observés à l'Hôpital Saint-Justin (Montréal-Canada). Union Med. Can. **101:**2407–2413.
15. Mollaret, H. H. 1968. L'infection humaine et animale a *Bacille de Malassez et Vignal*, en France, de 1959 à 1967. Symp. Ser. Immunobiol. Stand. **9:**45–58.
16. Mollaret, H. H. 1971. L'infection humaine a *Yersinia enterocolitica* en 1970, a la lumière de 642 cas récents. Pathol. Biol. **19:**189–205.
17. Morris, E. J. 1958. Selective media for some *Pasteurella* species. J. Gen. Microbiol. **19:**305–311.
18. Niléhn, B. 1969. Studies on *Yersinia enterocolitica*—with special reference to bacterial diagnosis and occurrence in human acute enteric disease, p. 1–48. Acta Pathol. Microbiol. Scand., Suppl. 206.
19. Reed, W. P., D. L. Palmer, R. C. Williams, Jr., and A. Kisch. 1970. Bubonic plaque in the Southwestern United States. Medicine **49:**465–486.
20. Sonnenwirth, A. C. 1970. Bacteremia with or without meningitis due to *Yersinia enterocolitica*, *Edwardsiella tarda*, *Comamonas* and *Pseudomonas maltophilia*. Ann. N. Y. Acad. Sci. **174**(Art. 2)**:**488–502.
21. Sonnenwirth, A. C. 1970. Gram-negative bacilli, vibrios and spirilla, p. 1269–1352. *In* S. Frankel, S. Reitman, and A. C. Sonnenwirth (ed.), Gradwohl's clinical laboratory methods and diagnosis, 7th ed. C. V. Mosby Co., St. Louis.
22. Sonnenwirth, A. C. 1971. Human infection with *Pasteurella pseudotuberculosis* (Letter to Editor). Amer. J. Clin. Pathol. **56:**546.
23. Sonnenwirth, A. C., and R. E. Weaver. 1970. *Yersinia enterocolitica*. N. Engl. J. Med. **283:**1468.
24. Thal, E., and W. Knapp. 1971. A revised antigenic scheme of *Yersinia pseudotuberculosis*. Symp. Ser. Immunobiol. Stand. **15:**219–226. S. Karger, Basel.
25. Toivanen, P., A. Toivanen, L. Olkkonen, and S. Aantaa. 1973. Hospital outbreak of *Yersinia enterocolitica* infection. Lancet **1:**801–803.
26. Wauters, G. 1970. Contribution a l'étude de *Yersinia enterocolitica*. Thesis. Vander Ed., Louvain.

27. Weaver, R. E., and J. G. Jordan. 1973. Recent human isolates of *Yersinia enterocolitica*, p. 120–125. *In* S. Winblad (ed.), Contributions to microbiology and immunology, vol. 2. S. Karger, Basel.
28. Weaver, R. E., H. W. Tatum, and D. G. Hollis. 1972. The identification of unusual pathogenic gram-negative bacteria (Elizabeth O King). Center for Disease Control, Atlanta, Ga.
29. Weber, J., N. B. Finlayson, and J. B. D. Mark. 1970. Mesenteric lymphadenitis and terminal ileitis due to *Yersinia pseudotuberculosis*. N. Engl. J. Med. **283**:172–174.
30. Wetzler, T. F. 1970. Pseudotuberculosis, p. 449–468. *In* H. L. Bodily, E. L. Updyke and J. O. Mason (ed.), Diagnostic procedures for bacterial, mycotic and parasitic infections, 5th ed. American Public Health Association, Inc., New York.
31. Wetzler, T. F., and W. T. Hubbert. 1968. *Pasteurella pseudotuberculosis* in North America. Symp. Ser. Immunobiol. Stand. **9**:33–44. S. Karger, Basel.
32. Winblad, S. (ed.). 1973. *Yersinia*, *Pasteurella* and *Francisella*. Contributions to microbiology and immunology, vol. 2. S. Karger, Basel.
33. World Health Organization. 1970. Expert Committee on Plague, 4th report, p. 23–25. World Health Organ. Tech. Rep. Ser. No. 477.

Chapter 20

Aeromonas

WILLIAM H. EWING AND RUDOLPH HUGH

INTRODUCTION

Members of the genus *Aeromonas* are found in specimens from humans and lower animals, as well as in water, soil, foods, and other environmental sources (10, 14, 15, 29, 36, 40). When isolated, aeromonads must be differentiated from pseudomonads and vibrios and from *Enterobacteriaceae* and certain other fermentative bacteria. Three species are recognized: *A. hydrophila*, *A. shigelloides*, and *A. salmonicida*, the first two of which are known to be involved in human pathology.

There is, of course, a practical need to distinguish among gram-negative rod-shaped bacteria that utilize carbohydrates fermentatively, such as aeromonads, vibrios, and *Enterobacteriaceae*, those that acidify glucose or other carbohydrates oxidatively, e.g., pseudomoonads and *Acinetobacter calcoaceticus* var. *anitratus* (*Herellea*), and those that do not utilize carbohydrate by either method, such as *Alcaligenes*, *Acinetobacter calcoaceticus* var. *lwoffi* (*Mima*), and certain others (e.g., see chapter 24). Oxidation-fermentation (OF) medium was designed (22) specifically to detect small quantities of oxidative acidity and to distinguish fermentative acidity. In practice, it is advisable to inoculate two tubes of OF medium containing glucose and to seal one of the tubes with sterile stiff petrolatum. Oxidative microorganisms produce acid in the open tube only, fermentative bacteria yield acid or acid and gas in both tubes, and inactive (as regards carbohydrates) forms do not produce acid in either tube. In some instances, carbohydrate other than glucose must be used in OF medium (see chapters 23, 24 and 95). Other criteria that are helpful for differentiation of the above-mentioned groups of bacteria are the results of tests for production of indophenol oxidase (9), decarboxylation of amino acids (5), and growth on certain substrates (see below). Determination of flagellar anatomy (8, 23, 24) also is important and helpful. As is the case with any microorganism, identification of members of the genus *Aeromonas* should be made on the basis of their aggregate characteristics, not on the basis of one or two criteria.

Description of the genus

Members of the genus *Aeromonas* are gram-negative, asporogenous, rod-shaped bacteria, 1.0 to 3.5 μm long and 0.4 to 1.0 μm wide, with polar flagella when flagellated. They are heterotrophic and produce indophenol oxidase and catalase. Glucose and other carbohydrates are fermented with production of acid or acid and gas. Aeromonads are differentiated from *Enterobacteriaceae* by means of flagellar anatomy, production of indophenol oxidase, and other tests (see below). They are differentiated from *Pseudomonas* by fermentative rather than oxidative metabolism of glucose and other substrates in OF medium. Cultures of *Aeromonas* may be differentiated from vibrios in general by certain physiological characteristics and from most strains of *Vibrio cholerae* by their decarboxylase reactions and their failure to agglutinate in O group I antiserum for *V. cholerae* (5, 6, 21, 25).

Growth and isolation

Aeromonads are not fastidious in their requirements. Growth is abundant on nutrient agar medium, as well as blood-agar, and colonies often appear on differential and selective plating media such as MacConkey, eosin methylene blue, and *Shigella-Salmonella* (SS) agars. Some strains grow on brilliant green agar, in which instances the colonies resemble those of salmonellae. Strains of *Aeromonas* are fermentative and some isolates of *A. hydrophila* are aerogenic. Cultures that appear nonmotile or are sluggishly motile should be passaged serially through tubes of semisolid agar medium or on Gard (12) plates to enhance motility and flagellar development before an attempt is made to stain the flagella. Some isolates that are nonmotile and do not spread in semisolid agar medium may possess inactive flagella (8). Aeromonads may have numerous short lateral flagella in young (2 to 4 h) cultures, but a single polar flagellum or polar tuft of flagella is seen in older cultures (23). Reviews of the literature concerning members of the genus *Aeromonas* are available (2, 3, 8).

AEROMONAS HYDROPHILA

The type species of the genus *Aeromonas* is *A. hydrophila* (8, 26, 35). This species includes all aeromonads that have been described under various specific epithets (e.g., *liquefaciens*, *punctata*, *formicans*), except *A. shigelloides* and *A. salmonicida* (8). *A. hydrophila* has the attributes of the genus *Aeromonas* as described above.

Sources of isolation

A. hydrophila has been isolated from a wide variety of specimens of human origin including blood of febrile patients, exudates from wounds and ulcers, pus from osteomyelitis, throat swabs, urine, bile, and feces of persons with diarrheal disease and normal stools (8, 13, 14, 28, 40). It is found in water, food, sewage, and the feces of lower animals. *A. hydrophila* is pathogenic for fish, amphibians (e.g., frogs), and reptiles (e.g., snakes, turtles, and alligators). (See references 8, 28, 38, 39.)

Growth and isolation

A. hydrophila grows rapidly in nutrient and infusion broths at temperatures from about 18 to 38 C. Most cultures produce colorless colonies on media such as deoxycholate and MacConkey agars. A few strains promptly ferment lactose and yield colonies resembling *Escherichia coli* on these media. Surface colonies of some isolates on blood-agar are surrounded by a wide zone of completely hemolyzed erythrocytes. (Such hemolytic strains reportedly are virulent for mice when instilled intranasally [38].)

Morphology

A. hydrophila is a straight, rod-shaped bacterium, but some cells of a few cultures have a slight curve. With rare exceptions, it is polar monotrichous when flagellated, and the single polar flagellum generally has a wavelength of 1.7 μm. Cells with two flagella at one pole rarely are encountered in the predominantly monotrichous population. Nonmotile isolates are rare. In addition to the polar flagellum, cells in very young cultures (2 to 4 h) possess short lateral flagella which generally have a shorter wavelength (less than 1.7 μm) than the polar flagellum The typical flagellar morphology has been illustrated (8, 23, 24).

Biochemical reactions

The biochemical reactions given by cultures of *A. hydrophila* have been summarized by several investigators (3, 8, 21, 33, 34). The characteristics of 113 strains of this species are listed in Table 1. Unless otherwise indicated, the results given in Table 1 (and other tables in this chapter) are based on cultures incubated at 35 to 37 C. Means for differentiation of strains of *A. hydrophila* and *A. shigelloides* are provided in Table 2.

Serology

Some years ago, preliminary investigations were made of some of the O (somatic) and H (flagellar) antigens of *A. hydrophila*, but these studies were not continued (8, 10). We do not know of the existence of an antigenic schema in which these microorganisms may be oriented.

AEROMONAS SHIGELLOIDES

A. shigelloides possesses the attributes of the genus *Aeromonas* as given above. These bacteria originally were described independently as type C27 by Ferguson and Henderson (10) and as *Pseudomonas shigelloides* by Bader (1). Later, they were transferred to the genus *Aeromonas* (8). Others have suggested that these microorganisms should be reclassified as *Pleiseomonas shigelloides* (17) or as *Vibrio shigelloides* (18). Future studies on the degree of relatedness of the deoxyribonucleic acids (DNAs) of members of the genera *Aeromonas*, *Vibrio*, and other allied microorganisms may indicate that the above-mentioned taxonomic changes should be made. Until such data are available, we prefer to regard this species as a member of the genus *Aeromonas*. The work of Whang et al. (41) showed that cultures of *A. shigelloides* possess the common antigen of *Enterobacteriaceae*, whereas members of the other two species of *Aeromonas* do not.

Sources of isolation

A. shigelloides has been isolated from feces of humans and lower animals and from a variety of other specimens of human origin such as blood and cerebrospinal fluid (8). It has been found in association with shigellae in persons with dysentery. Further, members of this species have been incriminated as the etiological agent in two outbreaks of acute gastroenteritis (personal communication, I. G. T. Helliaratchy, Medical Research Institute, Columbo, Ceylon).

Growth and isolation

A. shigelloides grows well in nutrient and infusion broth media at 18 to 38 C. Most strains produce colorless colonies on plating media such as deoxycholate and MacConkey agars. Strains that ferment lactose promptly yield red or pink colonies on these media. Colonies often

TABLE 1. *Biochemical characteristics of Aeromonas hydrophila and A. shigelloides*[a]

Test or substrate	*A. hydrophila*		*A. shigelloides*	
	Sign[b]	Percent positive[c]	Sign[b]	Percent positive[c]
Hydrogen sulfide (TSI or KI agar)	−	0	−	0
Urease	−	4[w]	−	0
Indole	+ or −	87	+	100
Methyl red				
37 C	+	95	+	100
26 C	+ or −	57	+	100
Voges-Proskauer				
37 C	− or +	33	−	0
26 C	+ or −	66	−	0
Citrate (Simmons)	d	52 (26)	−	0
KCN (growth)	+ or −	58	−	2
Motility	+	98	+ or −	85
Gelatin, 22 C	+ or (+)	78 (21)	−	0
Gelatin, charcoal	+	99	− or (+)	0 (32)
Lysine decarboxylase	−	0	+	96 (4)
Arginine dihydrolase	d	75 (10)	+	93 (2)
Ornithine decarboxylase	−	0	+ or −	50
Phenylalanine deaminase	− or +[w]	25	− or +[w]	41
Glucose				
Acid	+	100	+	100
Gas	− or +	46	−	0
Lactose	d	9 (28)	+ or (+)	65 (26)
Sucrose	d	83 (4)	−	0 (6)
Arabinose	d	52 (2)	−	0
Mannose	+	93	d	4 (13)
Mannitol				
Acid	+	99	−	0
Gas	d	65 (1)	−	0
Dulcitol	−	0	−	0
Salicin	d	41 (22)	− or +	32
Adonitol	−	0	−	0
Inositol	−	0	+	100
Sorbitol	d	13 (1)	−	0
Raffinose	−	2[w]	−	0
Rhamnose	−	4	−	0
Maltose	+	98 (1)	+ or −	55
Xylose	−	0	−	0
Trehalose	+	100	+	96 (2)
Cellobiose	d	37 (2)	−	0
Glycerol	d	80 (9)	d	15 (68)
Esculin	+ or −	60	−	0
Melezitose	−	0	−	0
Melibiose	−	4 (2)	d	48 (9)
Malonate, mucate	−	0	−	0
Christensen's citrate	d	52 (26)	−	0
Sodium acetate	d	74 (8)	d	2 (33)
Lipase (corn oil)	+	98	−	0
Nitrate to nitrite	+	99	+	100
Nitrate to gas	−	0	−	0
Unreduced nitrate (Zn +)	−	1		
Oxidation-fermentation	F	100	F	100
Oxidase	+	100	+	98
Catalase	+	100	+	100
Cetrimide (growth)	−	2[w]	−	0
Tube hemolysis (sheep erythrocytes)	+ or −	53	− or +	13
Growth on MacConkey agar	+	100	+	91

TABLE 1—*Continued*

Test or substrate	*A. hydrophila*		*A. shigelloides*	
	Sign[b]	Percent positive[c]	Sign[b]	Percent positive[c]
Growth on SS agar	+ or −	85	+ or −	87
String test	−	10	−	0
Agglutination in O group I antiserum (*V. cholerae*)	−	0	−	0
Melaninlike pigment	−	2	−	0
No. of cultures	113		54	

[a] Adapted from data in references 8 and 21.

[b] Sign: +, 90% or more positive within 1 or 2 days; (+), positive reaction after 3 or more days (decarboxylase tests: 3 or 4 days); −, no reaction (90% or more); + or −, most cultures positive, some strains negative; − or +, most strains negative, some cultures positive; + or (+), most reactions occur within 1 or 2 days, some are delayed; d, different reactions, +, (+), −; F, fermentative; [w], weakly positive reaction.

[c] Figures in parentheses indicate percentages of delayed reactions (3 days or more).

are colorless or white after incubation for 24 h, but become pink, or colorless with red papillae, after continued incubation. Bacteria of this species grow well on SS and brilliant green media, and scantily on bismuth sulfite agar, when pure cultures are inoculated onto these media. Discernible pigment is not produced in ordinary media, and definite zones of complete hemolysis of erythrocytes do not appear around colonies of *A. shigelloides* on blood-agar plates.

Morphology

The species *A. shigelloides* is composed of rod-shaped bacteria that usually are motile, but nonmotile flagellated and nonmotile atrichous strains are known to occur When flagellated, members of this species produce one to five long polar flagella with an undulating wavelength which averages 3.5 to 4 μm. In young cultures (2 to 4 h), cells yield lateral flagella in addition to the polar flagellum or flagella. These lateral flagella definitely have a shorter wavelength (less that 1.7 μm) than the polar flagella. The typical flagellar morphology has been illustrated (8).

Biochemical reactions

The results of investigations into the biochemical reactions given by cultures of *A. shigelloides* have been reported by several workers (1, 8, 10, 17, 18). The characteristics of 54 strains of this species are summarized in Table 1, and means for differentiation of *A. shigelloides* and *A. hydrophila* are given in Table 2.

Serology

The O antigens of some strains of *A. shigelloides* are identical with those of *Shigella sonnei* form I (1, 4, 8, 10). It is known that several O antigen groups and a number of H antigens can be delineated among cultures of this species (8, 32), but the existence of an antigenic schema is not known to us.

AEROMONAS SALMONICIDA

A. salmonicida was classified in the genus *Aeromonas* by Griffin (see reference 8), but Smith (37) has suggested transfer of this species to the genus *Necromonas*. Until studies are made on the degree of relatedness of the DNAs of these microorganisms to aeromonads and certain other bacteria, we prefer to regard them as members of the genus *Aeromonas* (see above, under *A. shigelloides*).

Source of isolation

A. salmonicida produces epizootic furunculosis and bacteremia in fish, particularly *Salmonidae* (8, 15, 16). It has a wide geographic distribution in bodies of fresh water and is of considerable importance to the fish-rearing industry. To our knowledge, its isolation from specimens of human origin has not been reported. The microorganism is mentioned briefly because conceivably it might be isolated from humans at some time.

Growth and isolation

Cultures of *A. salmonicida* grow well in nutrient and infusion broth media at 18 to 25 C, the optimal temperature apparently being about 22 C. The microorganism does not grow or grows very poorly at 35 to 37 C; therefore, it is not likely to be recovered from plating media incu-

TABLE 2. *Differentiation of species of Aeromonas*[a]

Test or substrate	*A. hydrophila*		*A. shigelloides*	
	Sign[b]	Percent positive[c]	Sign[b]	Percent positive[c]
Indole	+ or −	87	+	100
Voges-Proskauer	− or +	33	−	0
Citrate (Simmons)	d	52 (26)	−	0
Gelatin, 22 C	+ or (+)	78 (21)	−	0
Lysine decarboxylase	−	0	+	96 (4)
Ornithine decarboxylase	−	0	+ or −	50
Lipase (corn oil)	+	98	−	0
Gas from glucose	− or +	46	−	0
Sucrose	d	83 (4)	−	0 (6)
Arabinose	d	52 (2)	−	0
Mannose	+	93	d	4 (13)
Mannitol	+	99	−	0
Inositol	−	0	+	100
Esculin	+ or −	60	−	0

[a] Based on data given in Table 1.

[b] Sign: +, 90% or more positive within 1 or 2 days; (+), positive reaction after 3 or more days (decarboxylase tests: 3 or 4 days); −, no reaction (90% or more); + or −, most cultures positive, some strains negative; − or +, most strains negative, some cultures positive; + or (+), most reactions occur within 1 or 2 days, some are delayed; d, different reactions, +, (+), −.

[c] Figures in parentheses indicate percentages of delayed reactions (3 days or more).

TABLE 3. *Differentiation of Aeromonas and Vibrio cholerae*[a]

Test or substrate	*A. hydrophila*		*A. shigelloides*		*V. cholerae*	
	Sign[b]	Percent positive[c]	Sign[b]	Percent positive[c]	Sign[b]	Percent positive[c]
Indole	+ or −	87	+	100	+	100
Citrate (Simmons)	d	52 (26)	−	0	(+) or −	0 (75)
Lysine decarboxylase	−	0	+	96 (4)	+	100
Arginine dihydrolase	d	75 (10)	+	93 (2)	−	0
Ornithine decarboxylase	−	0	+ or −	50	+	100
Phenylalanine deaminase	− or +[w]	25	− or +[w]	41	−	0
Gelatin, 22 C	+ or (+)	78 (21)	−	0	+	>99
Gas from glucose	− or +	46	−	0	−	0
Lactose	d	9 (28)	+ or (+)	65 (26)	(+)	(>99)
Sucrose	d	83 (4)	−	0 (6)	+	99
Arabinose	d	52 (2)	−	0	−	0
Mannose	+	93	d	4 (13)	+	100
Mannitol	+	99	−	0	+	100
Salicin	d	41 (22)	− or +	32	−	8
Inositol	−	0	+	100	−	0
Melibiose	−	4 (2)	d	48 (9)	−	0
Esculin	+ or −	60	−	0	−	0
Lipase (corn oil)	+	98	−	0	+	>99
Growth on SS agar	+ or −	85	+ or −	87	−	5
Agglutination in O group I antiserum for *V. cholerae*	−	0	−	0	+ or −	88[d]

[a] Based on data in Table 1 and references 8 and 19–21.

[b] Sign: +, 90% or more positive within 1 or 2 days; (+), positive reaction after 3 or more days (decarboxylase tests: 3 or 4 days); −, no reaction (90% or more); + or −, most cultures positive, some strains negative; − or +, most strains negative, some cultures positive: + or (+), most reactions occur within 1 or 2 days, some are delayed; d, different reactions, +, (+), −; [w], weakly positive reaction.

[c] Figures in parentheses indicate percentages of delayed reactions (3 days or more).

[d] Some cultures that are similar to *V. cholerae* are not agglutinated by O group I antiserum; some of these produce diarrheal disease (25, 30). See also chapter 32.

bated at those temperatures. Most strains produce soluble brown, melaninlike pigment, but this pigment is not formed in the absence of phenylalanine or tyrosine.

Morphology

A. salmonicida is a rod-shaped bacterium that is nonmotile and atrichous.

Biochemical reactions

Detailed descriptions of the biochemical characteristics of this very homogeneous species are given elsewhere (8, 16, 34, 37) and will not be repeated here. Suffice it to state that cultures of *A. salmonicida* can be differentiated from members of the other two species of *Aeromonas* by their lack of motility, failure to form indole, and failure to ferment lactose, by production by most strains of melaninlike pigment, and by other tests (8). A nonmotile, gram-negative, rod-shaped bacterium isolated from fish which produces brown pigment and indophenol oxidase may be identified presumptively as *A. salmonicida* (15).

DIFFERENTIATION OF AEROMONAS FROM MEMBERS OF CERTAIN OTHER GENERA

Cultures of *Aeromonas* can be differentiated from nonfermentative bacteria by their reactions in triple sugar iron (TSI) agar medium; strains that produce acid in the butt portion of this medium are fermentative, whereas bacteria that yield no change in the butt of TSI agar are nonfermentative. Subsequent use of sealed and unsealed tubes of OF medium containing glucose affords confirmation of reactions seen in TSI medium and permits differentiation of microorganisms that utilize glucose fermentatively, or oxidatively, or fail to catabolize it by either method.

Oxidative utilization of glucose by most pseudomonads (chapter 23), by *A. calcoacetius* var. *anitratus* (chapter 24), and by certain other bacteria (e.g., see chapter 24) permits their differentiation from aeromonads.

Vibrio cholerae and other vibrios are oxidase-positive (6, 9) and possibly might be misidentified as species of *Aeromonas*. Tests that are of

TABLE 4. *Differentiation of Aeromonas and Vibrio parahaemolyticus*

Test or substrate	*A. hydrophila*		*A. shigelloides*		*V. parahaemolyticus*	
	Sign[b]	Percent positive[c]	Sign[b]	Percent positive[c]	Sign[b]	Percent positive[c]
Indole	+ or −	87	+	100	+	100
Voges-Proskauer	− or +	33	−	0	−	0
Citrate (Simmons)	d	52 (26)	−	0	+	99.3 (0.3)
Lysine decarboxylase	−	0	+	96 (4)	+	100
Arginine dehydrolase	d	75 (10)	+	93 (2)	−	0
Ornithine decarboxylase	−	0	+ or −	50	+	96.3
Phenylalanine deaminase	− or +[w]	25	− or +[w]	41	−	0
Gas from glucose	− or +	46	−	0	−	0
Lactose	d	9 (28)	+ or (+)	65 (26)	+	96.3
Sucrose	d	83 (4)	−	0 (6)	−	5.6
Arabinose	d	52 (2)	−	0	− or +	19
Mannitol	+	99	−	0	+	92.9 (0.8)
Salicin	d	41 (22)	− or +	32	−	0.1
Inositol	−	0	+	100	−	0.2
Cellobiose	d	37 (2)	−	0	−	0
Growth on SS agar	+ or −	85	+ or −	87	− or +	26.2[w]
Growth in						
0% NaCl	+[d]				−	0.3
5 to 6% NaCl	−[d]				+	100
Sensitivity to vibrio-static agent 0/129	−	1			+	100

[a] Based on data in Table 1 and references 11, 27, and 31.

[b] Sign: +, 90% or more positive within 1 or 2 days; (+), positive reaction after 3 or more days (decarboxylase tests: 3 or 4 days); −, no reaction (90% or more); + or −, most cultures positive, some strains negative; − or +, most strains negative, some cultures positive; + or (+), most reactions occur within 1 or 2 days, some are delayed; d, different reactions, +, (+), −; [w], weakly positive reaction.

[c] Figures in parentheses indicate percentages of delayed reactions (3 days or more).

[d] Percentage data unavailable.

TABLE 5. *Differentiation of Aeromonas shigelloides and Escherichia coli*[a]

Test or substrate	*A. shigelloides*		*E. coli*	
	Sign[b]	Percent positive[c]	Sign[b]	Percent positive[c]
Gas from glucose	–	0	+	92
Sucrose	–	0 (6)	d	53.7 (5.5)
Mannitol	–	0	+	97.5
Dulcitol	–	0	d	49.3 (18)
Inositol	+	100	–	0.9 (0.2)
Sorbitol	–	0	d	80.3 (1)
Arabinose	–	0	+	99.3 (0.5)
Rhamnose	–	0	d	83.5 (3.4)
Mucate	–	0	+	91.6
Oxidase	+	100	–	0

[a] Based on data in Table 1 and in chapter 19.

[b] Sign: +, 90% or more positive within 1 or 2 days: –, no reaction (90% or more); d, different reactions, +, (+), –.

[c] Figures in parentheses indicate percentages of delayed reactions (3 days or more).

TABLE 6. *Differentiation of Aeromonas shigelloides and Shigella sonnei*[a]

Test or substrate	*A. shigelloides*		*S. sonnei*	
	Sign[b]	Percent positive[c]	Sign[b]	Percent positive[c]
Indole	+	100	–	0
Motility	+ or –	85	–	0
Lysine decarboxylase	+	96 (4)	–	0
Arginine dihydrolase	+	93 (2)	–	0.5 (5)
Phenylalanine deaminase	– or +[w]	41	–	0
Mannitol	–	0	+	98.9
Inositol	+	100	–	0
Oxidase	+	100	–	0

[a] Based on data in Table 1 and chapter 18.

[b] Sign: +, 90% or more positive within 1 or 2 days; (+), positive reaction after 3 or more days (decarboxylase tests: 3 or 4 days); –, no reaction (90% or more); + or –, most cultures positive, some strains negative; – or +, most strains negative, some cultures positive; d, different reactions, +, (+), –; [w], weakly positive reaction.

[c] Figures in parentheses indicate percentages of delayed reactions (3 days or more).

particular value for differentiation of *A. hydrophila*, *A. shigelloides*, and *V. cholerae* are listed in Table 3. (See also chapter 21.)

Means by which cultures of *Vibrio parahaemolyticus* may be differentiated from *A. hydrophila* and *A. shigelloides* are given in Table 4.

In the past, strains of *Aeromonas* have been misidentified as members of the family *Enterobacteriaceae*, and conversely. The indophenol oxidase test alone is sufficient to effect this differentiation (9), but flagellar anatomy (8, 21), decarboxylase reactions (5, 8), and other biochemical tests (6, 8, 9) also are helpful. Cultures of *A. hydrophila* that yield positive Voges-Proskauer (VP) reactions may be mistaken for VP-positive *Enterobacteriaceae*, particularly *Serratia* (9), and strains that are VP-negative may be mistaken for *E. coli* and similar microorganisms. However, the oxidase and other tests mentioned above should permit easy differentiation.

If the oxidase test is not done, cultures of *E. coli* may be misidentified as *A. shigelloides*. Some of the substrates that are of value for differentiation of members of these two species are listed in Table 5 (see also Table 1, chapter 19, and references 4 and 7–9). Similarly, if an isolate of *A. shigelloides* is agglutinated by antiserum for *S. sonnei*, it may be identified erroneously. There are many biochemical differences between these two microorganisms; some of them are listed in Table 6 (see also chapter 18 and reference 4).

LITERATURE CITED

1. Bader, R. E. 1954. Ueber die Herstellung eines agglutinierenden Serums gegen die Rundform von *Shigella sonnei* mit einem Stamm der Gattung *Pseudomonas*. J. Hyg. Infektionskr. **140:**450–456.
2. Caselitz, F. H. 1966. *Pseudomonas-Aeromonas* und ihre human-medizinische Bedeutung. Veb Gustav Fischer Verlag, Jena.
3. Eddy, B. P. 1961. Cephalotrichous fermentative gram-negative bacteria: the genus *Aeromonas*. J. Appl. Bacteriol. **23:**216–249.
4. Edwards, P. R., and W. H. Ewing. 1972. Identification of Enterobacteriaceae, 3rd ed. Burgess Publishing Co., Minneapolis, Minn.
5. Ewing, W. H., B. R. Davis, and P. R. Edwards. 1960. The decarboxylase reactions of *Enterobacteriaceae* and their value in taxonomy. Pub. Health Lab. **18:**77–83.
6. Ewing, W. H., B. R Davis, and W. J. Martin. 1966. Outline of methods for the isolation and identification of *Vibrio cholerae*. Center for Disease Control, Atlanta, Ga.
7. Ewing, W. H., B. R Davis, and W. J. Martin. 1972. Biochemical characterization of *Escherichia coli*. Center for Disease Control, Atlanta, Ga.
8. Ewing, W. H., R. Hugh, and J. G. Johnson. 1961. Studies on the Aeromonas group. Center for Disease Control, Atlanta, Ga.
9. Ewing, W. H., and J. G. Johnson. 1960. The differentiation of *Aeromonas* and C27 cultures from *Enterobacteriaceae*. Int. Bull. Bacteriol. Nomencl. Taxon. **10:**233–230.
10. Ferguson, W. W., and N. D. Henderson. 1947. Description of strain C27: a motile organism with the major antigen of *Shigella sonnei* phase I. J. Bacteriol. **54:**179–181.

11. Fishbein, M., I. J. Mehlman, and J. Pitcher. 1970. Isolation of *Vibrio parahaemolyticus* from the processed meat of Chesapeake Bay blue crabs. Appl. Microbiol. **20**:176-178.
12. Gard, S. 1938. Das Schwärmphänomen in der Salmonella Gruppe und seine praktische Ausnützung. Z. Hyg. Infektionskr. **120**:615-619.
13. Gilardi, G. L. 1967. Morphological and biochemical characteristics of *Aeromonas punctata (hydrophila, liquefaciens)* isolated from human sources. Appl. Microbiol. **15**:417-421.
14. Gilardi, G. L., E. Bottone, and M. Birnbaum. 1970. Unusual fermentative, gram-negative bacilli isolated from clinical specimens. II. Characterization of *Aeromonas* species. Appl. Microbiol. **20**:156-159.
15. Griffin, P. J., and S. F. Snieszko. 1951. A unique bacterium pathogenic for warm-blooded and cold-blooded animals. Fish. Bull. Fish Wildl. Serv. (U S.) **52**:187-190.
16. Griffin, P. J., S. F. Snieszko, and S. B. Friddle. 1953. A more comprehensive description of *Bacterium salmonicida*. Trans. Amer. Fish. Soc. **82**:129-138.
17. Habs, H., and R H. W. Schubert. 1962. Ueber die biochemischen Merkmal und die taxonomische Stellung von *Pseudomonas shigelloides* (Bader). Zentralbl. Bakteriol. Parasitenk. Infektionskr. Hyg. Abt. I. Orig. **186**:316-327.
18. Hendrie, M. S., J. M. Shewan, and M. Véron. 1971. *Aeromonas shigelloides* (Bader) Ewing et al.: a proposal that it be transferred to the genus *Vibrio*. Int. J. Syst. Bacteriol. **21**:25-27.
19. Hugh, R. 1965. A comparison of the proposed neotype strain and 258 isolates of *Vibrio cholerae* Pacini. Int. Bull. Bacteriol. Nomencl. Taxon. **15**:13-24.
20. Hugh, R. 1966. A comparison of the neotype strain and 119 isolates of *Vibrio eltor* Pribram 1933. Indian J. Med. Res. **54**:839-848.
21. Hugh, R. 1970. *Pseudomonas* and *Aeromonas*, p. 175-190. *In* J. E. Blair, E. H. Lennette, and J. P. Truant (ed.), Manual of clinical microbiology. American Society for Microbiology, Bethesda, Md.
22. Hugh, R., and E. Leifson. 1953. The taxonomic significance of fermentative versus oxidative metabolism of carbohydrates by various gram negative bacteria. J. Bacteriol. **66**:24-26.
23. Leifson, E. 1960. Atlas of bacterial flagellation. Academic Press Inc., New York.
24. Leifson, E., and R. Hugh. 1953. Variations in shape and arrangement of bacterial flagella. J. Bacteriol. **65**:263-271.
25. McIntyre, O. R., J. C. Feeley, W. B. Greenough III, A. S. Benenson, S. I. Hassan, and A. Saad. 1965. Diarrhea caused by noncholera vibrios. Amer. J. Trop. Med. Hyg. **14**:412-418.
26. Miles, E. M., and A. A. Miles. 1951. The identity of *Proteus hydrophila* Bergey et al. and *Proteus melanovogenes* Miles and Halnan, and their relation to the genus *Aeromonas* Kluyver and van Neil. J. Gen. Microbiol. **5**:298-306.
27. Molenda, J. R., W. G. Johnson, M. Fishbein, B. Wentz, I. J. Mehlman, and T. A. Dadisman, Jr 1972. *Vibrio parahaemolyticus* gastroenteritis in Maryland: laboratory aspects. Appl. Microbiol. **24**:444-448.
28. Nygaard, G. S., M. L. Bissett, and R. M. Wood. 1970. Laboratory identification of aeromonads from man and other animals. Appl. Microbiol. **19**:618-620.
29. Rahal, J. J., R. H. Meade, C. M Bump, and A. J. Reinauer. 1970. Upper respiratory tract carriage of gram negative bacilli by hospital personnel. J. Amer Med. Ass. **214**:754-756.
30. Sakazaki, R., C. Z. Gomez, and M Sebald. 1967. Taxonomical studies of the so-called NAG vibrios. Jap. J. Med. Sci. **20**:265-280.
31. Sakazaki, R., S. Iwanami, and H. Fukumi. 1963. Studies on the enteropathogenic, facultatively halophilic bacteria, *Vibrio parahaemolyticus*. I. Morphological, cultural and biochemical properties and its taxonomical position. Jap. J. Med. Sci. Biol. **16**:161-188.
32. Sakazaki, R., S. Namioka, R Nakaya, and H. Fukumi. 1959. Studies on so-called paracolon C27 (Ferguson). Jap. J. Med. Sci. Biol. **12**:355-363.
33. Schubert, R. H. W. 1967. The taxonomy and nomenclature of the genus *Aeromonas* Kluyver and van Neil 1936. I. Suggestions on the taxonomy and nomenclature of aerogenic *Aeromonas* species. Int. J. Syst. Bacteriol. **17**:255-259.
34. Schubert, R. H. W. 1967. The taxonomy and nomenclature of the genus *Aeromonas* Kluyver and van Neil 1936. II. Suggestions on the taxonomy and nomenclature of the anaerogenic aeromonads. Int. J. Syst. Bacteriol. **17**:273-279.
35. Schubert, R. H. 1971. Status of the names *Aeromonas* and *Aerobacter liquefaciens* Beijerinck and designation of a neotype strain for *Aeromonas hydrophila* Stanier Request for an opinion. Int. J. Syst. Bacteriol. **21**:87-90.
36. Simon, G., and A. von Graevenitz. 1969. Intestinal and water-borne infections due to *Aeromonas hydrophila*. Pub. Health Lab. **27**:159-162.
37. Smith, I. W. 1963. The classification of *Bacterium salmonicida*. J. Gen. Microbiol. **33**:263-274.
38. Thal, E., and Z. Dinter. 1953. Zur Pathogenität der Stammgruppe "455" (Enterobacteriaceae) für die Maus. Nord. Veterinaermed. **5**:855-858.
39. Vezina, R., and R. Desrochers. 1971. Incidence d' *Aeromonas hydrophila* chez la perche, *Perca flavescens* Mitchill. Can. J. Microbiol. **17**:1101-1103.
40. von Graevenitz, A., and A. H. Mensch. 1968. The genus *Aeromonas* in human bacteriology. N. Engl. J. Med. **278**:245-249.
41. Whang, H. Y., M. E. Heller, and E. Neter 1972. Production by *Aeromonas* of common enterobacterial antigen and its possible taxonomic significance. J. Bacteriol. **110**:161-164.

Chapter 21
Vibrio

JOHN C. FEELEY AND ALBERT BALOWS

INTRODUCTION

The genus *Vibrio* comprises a large and poorly characterized group of organisms which are abundant in the environment, especially in surface and marine waters. Many are halophilic.

The amended provisional description of the genus *Vibrio* Pacini 1854 recommended by the Subcommittee on Taxonomy of Vibrios, International Committee on Systematic Bacteriology (28), is as follows:

> "Gram-negative, asporogenous rods which have a single, rigid curve or which are straight. Motile by means of a single, polar flagellum. Produce indophenol oxidase and catalase. Ferment glucose without gas production. Acidity is produced from glucose by the Embden-Meyerhof glycolytic pathway. The guanine plus cytosine in the deoxyribonucleic acid of *Vibrio* species is within the range of 40 to 50 moles per cent."

This definition has been expanded by Hugh and Sakazaki (20) to include acid production from mannitol, positive lysine and ornithine decarboxylase reactions, and negative arginine dihydrolase activity.

Three species, *V. cholerae*, *V. parahaemolyticus*, and *V. alginolyticus*, are of consequence in clinical microbiology. *V. fetus*, a pathogen of animals and humans, is now classified in the genus *Campylobacter* (37; chapter 2).

VIBRIO CHOLERAE

V. cholerae, the causative agent of Asiatic cholera, is a gram-negative, slightly curved, motile, polar monotrichous, rod-shaped bacterium readily isolated from stools of patients with the disease. Epidemic strains can be identified only by agglutination in specific polyvalent antiserum in conjunction with biochemical and cultural tests.

Clinical significance

In its most severe form, Asiatic cholera is an acute diarrheal disease characterized by massive loss of fluid and electrolyte which, if untreated, may result in cardiovascular collapse and death in a single day. In reality, such cases are the exception rather than the rule, and epidemiological studies indicate that for each severe case there are 25 to 100 mild to asymptomatic infections. For the most part, significant propagating epidemics of cholera are limited to areas with poor sanitation, but the possible appearance of imported cases of cholera in countries with good sanitation is markedly enhanced by rapid air transportation and increases in tourism and other international travel. Since 1960, extension of the seventh pandemic of cholera westward from Southeast Asia across the Indian subcontinent, the Middle East, and into the African continent has involved many new countries, with outbreaks even in Europe.

It is now firmly established that the disease is produced by a heat-labile enterotoxin produced by *V. cholerae* multiplying in the small bowel (15). Infection follows the ingestion of water or food contaminated with human dejecta.

Collection, transport, and storage of specimens

Stool specimens should be collected early, preferably within the first 24 h of illness, and *before* the administration of any antimicrobial agents. Fluid stool, often "rice-water" in appearance, may be collected by inserting a petrolatum-lubricated soft rubber catheter into the rectum. Rectal swabs may also be employed; although highly efficient in the acute phase of illness, they probably are less satisfactory for culturing convalescent cases or suspected carriers. Administration of purgatives has been reported to increase the efficiency of detection of carriers (18).

Vomitus, if available, may also be collected for culture.

To provide a retrospective basis for diagnosis, acute-phase (within 72 h after onset) and convalescent-phase (10 days to 3 weeks after onset) sera should be obtained by venipuncture.

Transport. Whenever possible, stool or rectal swab specimens should be inoculated on isolation plates with minimal delay. Viability of *V.*

cholerae is well maintained in the alkaline milieu of "rice-water stool" but is unpredictable in formed stools. *V. cholerae* is very susceptible to desiccation; hence, specimens must not be allowed to dry.

When specimens cannot be cultured without delay, especially when they must be transported by courier, rectal swabs or stool material should be placed in the semisolid transport medium of Cary and Blair (7). The efficiency of this medium in maintaining viability of *V. cholerae* for up to 4 weeks has been verified by DeWitt et al. (10), who also found that buffered glycerol saline, often used in enteric bacteriology, was unsatisfactory even for short periods. Tellurite-taurocholate peptone broth has been extensively used with success as an "enrichment-transport" medium at the Cholera Research Laboratory in Dacca, Bangladesh, where specimens collected in the field are generally plated within 12 to 24 h (24). In the absence of available suitable transport media, strips of blotting paper may be soaked in rice-water stool and inserted into air-tight plastic bags. Specimens collected in this way may remain viable for up to 5 weeks (2).

Storage. Specimens in transport media may be shipped to the laboratory without refrigeration. Refrigeration, *but not freezing*, is preferable for delayed transportation of raw collected stool specimens.

Direct examination

Direct examination of stool material is not recommended for general purposes; however, dark-field examination of stool for characteristic darting motility of vibrios, especially after brief incubation in broth, has proven valuable in experienced hands (4).

Culture and isolation

Procedures for the isolation and preliminary identification of *V. cholerae* are outlined in Fig. 1. Rectal swabs or stool specimens should be inoculated lightly on nonselective media (taurocholate gelatin agar [TGA] *or* nutrient agar) and fairly heavily on selective media (thiosulfate-citrate bile salts [TCBS] agar *or* tellurite-taurocholate gelatin agar [TTGA]) and incubated at 35 C for 18 to 24 h. Swabs of stool material should also be inoculated for enrichment purposes into tellurite-taurocholate alkaline broth or, if this is unavailable, into alkaline peptone broth, pH 8.4 to 8.5. Enrichment cultures should be subcultured to a second set of selective and nonselective plates (as above), preferably after 6 to 8 h of incubation at 35 C, but if this is not feasible, after overnight incubation (16 to 18 h). Specimens received in transport media should be inoculated as above (direct plating and enrichment).

The bacteriologist should be aware that *V. cholerae* generally will not grow or grows poorly on common enteric media such as *Salmonella-Shigella* and eosin methylene blue, Brilliant Green, or bismuth sulfite agars. Most strains grow on MacConkey agar, with production of colorless colonies at 18 to 24 h.

Nutrient agar and TGA plates should be examined by low-magnification oblique light stereomicroscopy for typical lightly iridescent greenish to red-bronze finely granular colonies of *V. cholerae*, which are much less iridescent than neighboring colonies of *Enterobacteriaceae* (12, 16, 21). Colonies of *V. cholerae* on TGA are surrounded by cloudy zones because of strong gelatinase activity (36). On TCBS agar, *V. cholerae* produces yellow colonies (sucrose fermentation); on TTGA, colonies develop dark centers (tellurite reduction) and are surrounded by cloudy zones of gelatinase activity.

Well-isolated suspect colonies should be picked to Kligler's iron agar (KIA) slants (triple sugar iron [TSI] agar is less desirable since *V. cholerae* ferments sucrose) by stabbing and streaking in the usual manner. In picking colo-

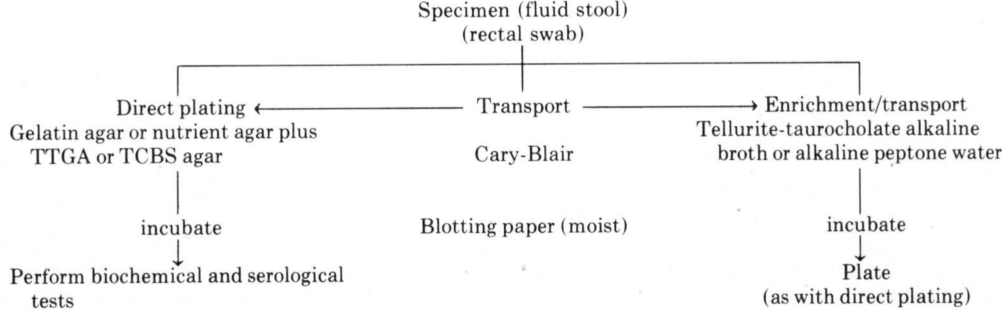

FIG. 1. *Schematic diagram of laboratory procedures for isolation and preliminary identification of* Vibrio cholerae. *TTGA = tellurite-taurocholate gelatin agar; TCBS agar = thiosulfate-citrate bile salts agar.*

nies from highly selective media, only the top central portion of the colony should be touched to minimize possible transfer of other inhibited but viable organisms. If available, lysine iron agar (LIA) should be inoculated by touching the point where the KIA slant is stabbed and transferring directly to a tube of LIA in which the butt is stabbed twice and the slant is streaked.

Identification

KIA slants should be examined after 18 to 24 h of incubation, and those which give reactions typical of *V. cholerae* [i.e., alkaline slant (K), acid butt (A) without gas, and absence of H_2S production (K/A$^-$)] should be examined further. TSI slants, if employed, will show acid slants, acid butt without gas, and absence of H_2S (A/A$^-$) with *V. cholerae*. If LIA is employed, expected reactions are as follows: alkaline slant, alkaline or neutral (N) butt (K/K$^-$ or K/N$^-$), since *V. cholerae* and most other *Vibrio* species decarboxylate lysine.

Isolates giving the above reactions should be tested by slide agglutination, with polyvalent antiserum against *V. cholerae*. (Antisera may be obtained from commercial sources or from H. L. Smith, Jr., Vibrio Reference Laboratory, Jefferson Medical College, Philadelphia, Pa.) A loopful of growth from the KIA or LIA slant should be thoroughly emulsified in a small amount of 0.85% NaCl (about 0.3 ml). A loopful (or droplet) of this suspension should be mixed with a loopful or droplet of antiserum on a divided slide. The slide should be rocked back and forth and examined with the naked eye for agglutination occurring within 1 min. Suitable controls should assure the absence of spontaneous agglutination and the reliability of the antiserum. Cultures agglutinating in polyvalent antiserum should be similarly tested with absorbed monospecific Ogawa and Inaba antisera to determine the serotype. This is best accomplished by sending the culture to a state or federal reference laboratory.

Under certain conditions, such as during a cholera outbreak, experienced workers may perform slide agglutination tests directly from isolation plates. Although this is expedient, it is not recommended for the novice, especially since growth from TCBS medium may fail to show typical rapid agglutination.

A *presumptive* report on any culture meeting these criteria should be issued at this point, pending completion of additional tests described below.

Cultures that resemble *V. cholerae* should be inoculated for performance of biochemical and other tests listed in Table 1, which contains a list of procedures regarded as more or less essential for differentiation of *V. cholerae*. Nutrient agar slants should also be inoculated to preserve the culture and for additional tests since viability is not well maintained on KIA. It is highly advisable to repeat slide agglutination test results from the growth thus obtained.

It should be emphasized that vibrios closely resembling *V. cholerae*, but which fail to agglutinate in cholera antiserum, may be isolated from stools and surface waters. In the past, these have been called "nonagglutinable" (NAG) or "noncholera" vibrios (NCV). These may or may not show minor biochemical differences from agglutinable strains (e.g., especially in fermentation of sucrose, mannose, and arabinose), and current taxonomic approaches based on numerical taxonomy and deoxyribonucleic acid base ratios and homology have been interpreted and support their inclusion in the species

TABLE 1. *Reactions of Vibrio cholerae in critical identification tests*[a]

Test or substrate	Sign[b]	Percent[c]
Indophenol oxidase	+	100
Indole	+	100
Methyl red (37 C)	+^{w}	95
Voges-Proskauer (37 C)	− or +	47.3
Simmons citrate	(+^{w}) or −	0 (74^w)
Urease	−	0
Glucose	+	100
Glucose, gas	−	0
Lactose	(+)	0 (100)
Sucrose	+	100
Mannose	+	100
Arabinose	−	0
Salicin	−	0
Lysine decarboxylase	+	100
Arginine dihydrolase	−	0
Ornithine decarboxylase	+	99.5
Decarboxylase control	−	0
Phenylalanine deaminase	−	0
Gelatinase	+	>96
Motility	+	96.5
Agglutination, O group I antiserum	+	100
"String" test	+	100

[a] Based on data in reference 11.

[b] Sign: +, 90% or more positive within 1 or 2 days; (+), positive reaction after 3 or more days (decarboxylase tests: 3 or 4 days); −, no reaction (90% or more); + or −, most cultures positive, some strains negative; − or +, most strains negative, some cultures positive; w, weakly positive reaction.

[c] Figures in parentheses indicate percentages of delayed reactions (3 days or more).

V. cholerae (8, 9, 31). This approach, which will be reflected in the 8th edition of *Bergey's Manual of Determinative Bacteriology*, will cause some confusion among medical bacteriologists, epidemiologists, and clinicians. Be that as it may, only agglutinable strains are currently regarded as significant epidemic threats. Nonetheless, vibrios resembling *V. cholerae*, but failing to agglutinate in cholera antiserum, have been strongly implicated as causative agents of both sporadically occurring cases and focal outbreaks of cholera-like diarrheal disease, as reviewed by Finkelstein (15). Therefore, their isolation and recognition is of importance.

Some useful cultural and biochemical tests which may be applied to differentiate *V. cholerae* (and related vibrios) from other organisms present in stool specimens are recorded in Table 2.

The indophenol oxidase test immediately eliminates all *Enterobacteriaceae*. Decarboxylase tests are of great value, as are tests for sensitivity to vibriostatic pteridine compound 0/129 (34) and the "string test" (35). The latter simple test is performed by emulsifying (with a *cool* loop) a small amount of growth from an agar slant or a plate in a drop of aqueous 0.5% sodium deoxycholate solution. In a positive reaction, a mucous-like "string" can be observed as the loop is lifted away from the slide. With typical agglutinable *V. cholerae*, the reaction is persistent for 45 to 60 s; with other vibrio strains, the reaction may be less persistent. Occasional cultures of *Aeromonas* may give transient positive reactions.

More detailed biochemical studies are advisable with randomly selected strains. Data on a variety of reactions have been summarized by Ewing et al. (11).

Agglutinable strains of *V. cholerae* may be differentiated into classical and El Tor biotypes. The latter biotype is so named because they were first recognized among Mecca pilgrims at the El Tor quarantine station on the Sinai Peninsula. The differentiation was made historically on the basis of the hemolytic properties of El Tor strains, and they were first thought incapable of producing serious epidemics, although small outbreaks were recognized in the 1930's in the Celebes (Indonesia). However, since 1960, there has been a far-reaching pandemic spread of cholera caused by El Tor strains westward across the Indian subcontinent, through the Middle East, and into the African continent with some outbreaks and a number of single important cases in Europe (15).

Technical difficulties with hemolysis tests have led to the development of other criteria for recognizing El Tor biotypes; some of the simpler, more reliable procedures are given in

TABLE 2. *Differentiation of vibrios from other organisms isolated from stool specimens*

Test	*Vibrio*	*Aeromonas*	*Plesiomonas*	*Pseudomonas*	*Enterobacteriaceae*
Indophenol oxidase	+[a]	+	+	+	–
Gelatinase	+	+	–	+	d
$NO_3^- \rightarrow NO_2^-$	+	+	+	+	+
$NO_3^- \rightarrow N_2$	–	–	–	d	–
Urease	–	–	–	–	d
Oxidation-fermentation test, glucose	F	F	F	O	F
Glucose, gas	–	– or +	–	–	+
Inositol	–	–	+	NC	d
Mannitol	+	+	–	NC	d
Lysine decarboxylase	+	–	+	NC	d
Arginine dihydrolase	–	+	+	+	d
Ornithine decarboxylase	+	–	+	NC	d
0/129 inhibition	+	–	– or +	–	–
"String" test	+[b]	–	–	–	–
Polar monotrichous flagella	+	+	+	+[c]	–

[a] Sign: +, 90% or more positive within 1 or 2 days; (+), positive reaction after 3 or more days (decarboxylase tests: 3 or 4 days); –, no reaction (90% or more); – or +, most strains negative, some cultures positive; d, different reactions, +, (+), –; F, fermentative; O, oxidative; NC, no change.

[b] Available data on *V. parahaemolyticus* and *V. alginolyticus* are contradictory; most strains apparently are negative or at best weakly positive.

[c] May have more than one flagellum per pole.

Table 3. Indeed, most strains isolated at present are only weakly hemolytic. Differentiation of biotypes should be made because of epidemiological differences, e.g., the higher ratio of mild cases and carriers to severe cases with El Tor strains (15). In severe cases, there is no clinical difference in illness caused by the two biotypes.

Immunoserological diagnosis

A retrospective diagnosis of cholera can be established with a high degree of certainty by titration of paired acute- and convalescent-phase sera by agglutination (6, 13, 19) or vibriocidal (3, 5, 13) antibody tests. Acute-phase sera should be collected 0 to 3 days, and convalescent-phase sera 10 to 21 days, after onset of illness. Paired sera should be submitted to laboratories familiar with these specialized tests (e.g., Center for Disease Control). Demonstration of a fourfold or greater rise in titer is diagnostic, provided recent (within 2 weeks) cholera immunization can be ruled out. Titration of single convalescent sera is usually not worthwhile, except that the absence of vibriocidal antibody would nearly exclude the diagnosis of cholera.

Susceptibility to antimicrobial agents

Therapy of cholera is primarily dependent on adequate intravenous and/or oral fluid and electrolyte therapy (25, 27). Oral tetracycline is the drug of choice as a useful adjunct to fluid therapy, resulting in more rapid elimination of *V. cholerae* from the gastrointestinal tract and a shortened period of diarrhea. Resistant strains are extremely rare and, since antimicrobial therapy is not essential, susceptibility tests are of largely academic interest.

Evaluation

Since cholera is a quarantinable disease under provisions of the *International Health Regulations*, prompt notification of isolation of *V. cholerae* should be made to the State Health Department concerned. Identification of the culture should be confirmed by the State Health Department, which will notify the Center for Disease Control. The Center for Disease Control, in turn, will advise the World Health Organization and initiate appropriate epidemiological studies.

VIBRIO PARAHAEMOLYTICUS AND VIBRIO ALGINOLYTICUS

V. parahaemolyticus (32) is a halophilic marine microorganism which is a major cause of gastroenteritis in Japan, where raw fish is frequently consumed. The organism is widely distributed in nature and has been isolated from seawater and a great variety of seafoods. It has been implicated as the cause of gastroenteritis in outbreaks associated, for example, with steamed crabs in Maryland (23) and boiled shrimp in Louisiana (1).

The Special Bacteriology Unit of the Bacteriology Branch, Center for Disease Control, has received several isolates of *V. parahaemolyticus* from a variety of extraintestinal infections, i.e., of the hands, feet, and ears. In these instances, the infection was localized and was associated with swimming or other contact in marine shore areas. Because of its ubiquitous distribution and the general unfamiliarity of laboratory personnel with its properties, it is likely underreported. *V. parahaemolyticus* must be differentiated from a similar organism, *V. alginolyticus* (29), which has not been implicated in gastroenteritis. *V. alginolyticus* and an unnamed halophilic *Vibrio* species have also been recovered from wounds and septicemias, and require further study (R. Weaver, Center for Disease Control, personal communication).

Procedures for isolation and identification of

TABLE 3. *Differentiation of classical and El Tor biotypes of Vibrio cholerae*[a]

Test	Classical		El Tor	
	Sign[b]	Percent +	Sign[b]	Percent +
Tube hemolysis	−	0	+ or −	71.3[c]
Phage IV susceptibility	+	100	−	0
Polymyxin B susceptibility (50 units)	+	100	−	0
Voges-Proskauer test, 22 C (48 h)	−	8.6	+	93.9
Chicken cell agglutination	− or +	18.1	+ or −	87.8

[a] Based on reference 14 with additional observations on polymyxin B susceptibility (Feeley, unpublished data).

[b] Sign: +, 90% or more positive; −, no reaction (90% or more); + or −, most cultures positive, some strains negative; − or +, most cultures negative, some strains positive.

[c] Many El Tor biotype strains isolated more recently than this study are weakly hemolytic or nonhemolytic in tube hemolysis tests.

V. parahaemolyticus and related vibrios have been reviewed recently (22, 23).

Collection, transport, and storage of specimens

Fecal specimens (rectal swabs or collected stool) and vomitus, if available, should be plated directly on TCBS agar or bromothymol blue-teepol (BTB-Teepol) agar plates.

If transport to a distance laboratory necessitates delay in plating, specimens may be placed in Cary-Blair transport medium (7, 26).

Specimens in transport media may be shipped without refrigeration. Refrigeration, *but not freezing*, is preferable for specimens not in transport media.

Direct examination

Direct microscope examination of stool specimens is not recommended.

Culture and isolation

Rectal swabs or stool specimens should be streaked heavily on TCBS or BTB-Teepol agar and incubated at 35 to 37 C for 18 to 24 h. Le Clair et al. (22) have reported that prior enrichment culture in 1% peptone water containing 3% NaCl (pH 7.2) incubated for 16 to 18 h increases the number of positive isolations over the direct plating technique.

Colonies of *V. parahaemolyticus* on TCBS and BTB-Teepol agar are round, 2 to 3 mm in diameter, and bluish-green in appearance. Colonies of *V. alginolyticus* are larger and are yellow because of sucrose fermentation; some strains of the latter species may exhibit *Proteus*-like spreading growth. Well-isolated suspect colonies should be picked to KIA or TSI agar slants (stab and streak in the usual manner).

Identification

KIA or TSI slants should be examined after 18 to 24 h of incubation. Typical reactions for *V. parahaemolyticus* on KIA or TSI are alkaline slant, acid butt without gas, and absence of H_2S production (K/A^-). *V. alginolyticus* yields K/A^- reactions on KIA but produces on acid slant, acid butt without gas, and no H_2S (A/A^-) on TSI medium.

Biochemical and cultural tests that are useful in the identification of *V. parahaemolyticus* and its differentiation from *V. alginolyticus* are recorded in Table 4. *V. parahaemolyticus* is readily differentiated from *V. cholerae* by failure to ferment sucrose, failure to agglutinate in cholera O group I antiserum, and by NaCl requirements. *V. alginolyticus* differs from *V. parahaemolyticus* by fermenting sucrose, by being Voges-Proskauer positive, and often by having higher NaCl tolerance. It also fails to agglutinate in cholera O group I serum. A detailed comparison of cultures of *V. parahaemolyticus* isolated in the United States and Japan has recently been published by Zen-Yoji et al. (38).

The taxonomic status of the very large number of possible halophilic marine vibrio species is poorly defined. Halophilic vibrios resembling *V. parahaemolyticus* are common from marine sources. A special test based on hemolysis of human or rabbit red blood cells, known as the Kanagawa phenomenon, is frequently of value, since most pathogenic strains isolated from gastroenteritis give a positive reaction (33). This test must be performed precisely with the use of Wagatsuma's agar containing washed human or rabbit erythrocytes. The agar surface is spot-inoculated and read for the presence or absence of clear (beta) hemolysis after 24 h of incubation at 35 C. Variations in technique upset this delicate test, and known positive and negative controls are essential.

Antigenic components designated as O, K, and H antigens have been described in cultures of *V. parahaemolyticus*. Serotyping based on O and K antigens has been employed by specialized laboratories (17, 38). Currently, 11 O antigens and 57 K antigens have been recognized. The value of serotyping remains unclear because several types have been isolated from single patients and these may not correlate with isolates from suspected seafood (1, 30).

Immunoserological diagnosis

Immunoserological diagnosis is not considered to be practical and is not of proven value.

Susceptibility to antimicrobial agents

The disease is generally self-limited. Antibiotic therapy has not been widely used and is not of proven efficacy. Le Clair et al. (22) have reported that the standard Kirby-Bauer method for determining in vitro antibiotic susceptibility patterns can be performed merely by incorporating 3% NaCl into the Mueller-Hinton agar used for testing. The high concentration of NaCl appears to have little or no effect on the most commonly employed antibiotics.

Evaluation

Suspected cases of gastroenteritis caused by *V. parahaemolyticus* should be brought to the attention of local or state health authorities,

TABLE 4. *Characteristics of Vibrio parahaemolytics and Vibrio alginolyticus*[a]

Test or substrate	*V. parahaemolyticus*			*V. alginolyticus*		
	No. of strains	Sign[b]	Percent positive[c]	No. of strains	Sign[b]	Percent positive[c]
H_2S	1,272	–	0	15	–	0
Urease	1,237	–	0	15	–	0
Indole	1,267	+	100	15	+ or –	86.7
Methyl red	120	+	99.2	15	–	0
Voges-Proskauer	120	–	0	15	+	100
Citrate (Simmons)	1,237	+	99.3 (0.3)	15	d	20 (46.7)
Motility	1,254	+	99.8	15	+	100
Gelatin	1,252	+	99.8	12	(+) or –	(83.5)
Lysine decarboxylase	27	+	100	15	+	100
Arginine dihydrolase	27	–	0	15	–	0
Ornithine decarboxylase	27	+	96.3	15	– or +	40
Glucose, acid	1,272	+	100	15	+	100
Glucose, gas	1,272	–	0	15	–	0
Lactose	1,272	–	0.4	15	–	0
Sucrose	126	–	5.6	15	+	100
Arabinose	480	– or +	19	ND		
Mannitol	126	+	92.9	15	+	100
Dulcitol	1,146	–	0	ND		
Salicin	1,163	–	0.1	ND		
Adonitol	1,218	–	0.2	ND		
Inositol	1,218	–	0.2	ND		
Sorbitol	1,202	–	0	ND		
Rhamnose	1,218	–	0.2	ND		
Maltose	1,272	+	99.8	9	+	100
Xylose	1,272	–	0	9	–	0
Cellobiose	56	–	0	ND		
Malonate	1,202	–	0	ND		
Mucate	1,146	–	0	ND		
D-Tartrate	1,146	+	100	ND		
Sodium acetate	100	+	94	ND		
Sodium alginate	1,146	–	0	ND		
Nitrate to nitrite	1,272	+	100	15	+	100
Oxidation-fermentation	1,146	F	100	15	F	100
Oxidase	1,272	+	100	15	+	100
Catalase	1,218	+	100	ND		
Sensitivity to 0/129	1,146	+	100	ND		
Agglutination, O-group I	?	–	0	15	–	0
Growth in broth						
0% NaCl	1,254	–	0.3	15	–	0
3–7% NaCl	1,254	+	100	15	+	100
10% NaCl	1,230	–	0.2	14	+ or –	50

[a] Based on data in references 17, 23, and 32 for *V. parahaemolyticus* and data from Harvey Tatum (Center for Disease Control, personal communication) for *V. alginolyticus*.

[b] Sign: +, 90% or more positive within 1 or 2 days; (+), positive reaction after 3 or more days (decarboxylase tests: 3 or 4 days); –, no reaction (90% or more); + or –, most cultures positive, some strains negative; – or +, most strains negative, some cultures positive; d, different reactions, +, (+), –; F, fermentative; ND, not determined.

[c] Figures in parentheses indicate percentages of delayed reactions (3 days or more).

since most cases are a result of improper food-handling methods. Cultures and suspected food, if available, should be transmitted to proper public health authorities.

LITERATURE CITED

1. Barker, W. H., Jr. 1974. *Vibrio parahaemolyticus* outbreaks in the United States. Lancet 1:551–554.
2. Barua, D. 1970. Laboratory diagnosis of cholera cases and carriers, p. 47–52. *In* Principles and practice of cholera control. Public Health Papers No. 40. World Health Organization, Geneva, Switzerland.
3. Barua, D., and R. B. Sack. 1964. Serological studies in cholera. Indian J. Med. Res. **52:**855–866.
4. Benenson, A. S., M. R. Islam, and W. B. Greenough III. 1964. Rapid identification of *Vibrio* cholerae by dark-field microscopy. Bull. W.H.O. **30:**827–831.
5. Benenson, A. S., A. Saad, and W. H. Mosley. 1968.

Serological studies in cholera. 2. The vibriocidal antibody response of cholera patients determined by a microtechnique. Bull. W.H.O. **38**:277–285.
6. Benenson, A. S., A. Saad, and M. Paul. 1968. *Vibrio* agglutinin response of cholera patients determined by a microtechnique. Bull. W.H.O. **38**:267–276.
7. Cary, S. G., and E. B. Blair. 1964. New transport medium for shipment of clinical specimens. I. Fecal specimens. J. Bacteriol. **88**:96–98.
8. Citarella, R. V., and R. R. Colwell. 1970. Polyphasic taxonomy of the genus *Vibrio:* polynucleotide sequence relationships among selected *Vibrio* species. J. Bacteriol. **104**:434–442.
9. Colwell, R. R. 1970. Polyphasic taxonomy of the genus *Vibrio:* numerical taxonomy of *Vibrio cholerae*, *Vibrio parahaemolyticus*, and related *Vibrio* species. J. Bacteriol. **104**:410–433.
10. DeWitt, W. E., E. J. Gangarosa, I. Huq, and A. Zarifi. 1971. Holding media for the transport of *Vibrio cholerae* from field to laboratory. Amer. J. Trop. Med. Hyg. **20**:685–688.
11. Ewing, W. H., B. R. Davis, and W. J. Martin. 1966. Outline of methods for the isolation and identification of *Vibrio cholerae*. Center for Disease Control, Atlanta, Ga.
12. Feeley, J. C. 1962. Isolation of cholera vibrios by positive-recognition plating procedures. J. Bacteriol. **84**:866–867.
13. Feeley, J. C. 1965. Comparison of vibriocidal and agglutinating antibody responses in cholera patients, p. 220–222. *In* Proceedings of the Cholera Research Symposium. Public Health Service Publication No. 1328. U.S. Government Printing Office, Washington, D.C.
14. Feeley, J. C. 1965. Classification of *Vibrio cholerae* (*Vibrio comma*), including El Tor vibrios, by infrasubspecific characteristics. J. Bacteriol. **89**:665–670.
15. Finkelstein, R. A. 1973. Cholera. CRC Crit. Rev. Microbiol. **2**:553–623.
16. Finkelstein, R. A., and C. Z. Gomez. 1963. Comparison of methods for the rapid recognition of cholera vibrios. Bull. W.H.O. **28**:327–332.
17. Fishbein, M., I. J. Mehlman, and J. Pitcher. 1970. Isolation of *Vibrio parahaemolyticus* from the processed meat of Chesapeake Bay blue crabs. Appl. Microbiol. **20**:176–178.
18. Gangarosa, E. J., H. Saghari, J. Emile, and H. Siadat. 1966. Detection of *Vibrio cholerae* biotype El Tor by purging. Bull. W.H.O. **34**:363–369.
19. Goodner, K., H. L. Smith, Jr., and H. Stempen. 1960. Serologic diagnosis of cholera. J. Albert Einstein Med. Cent. **8**:143–147.
20. Hugh, R., and R. Sakazaki. 1972. Minimal number of characters for the identification of *Vibrio* species, *Vibrio cholerae*, and *Vibrio parahaemolyticus*. J. Conf. Publ. Health Lab. Dir. **30**:133–137.
21. Lankford, C. E., and W. Burrows. 1965. Oblique light microscopy as an aid to rapid detection of enteric pathogens, p. 45–50. *In* Proceedings of the Cholera Research Symposium. Public Health Service Publication No. 1328. U.S. Government Printing Office, Washington, D.C.
22. Le Clair, R. A., H. Zen-Yoji, and S. Sakai. 1970. Isolation and identification of *Vibrio parahaemolyticus* from clinical specimens. J. Conf. Publ. Health Lab. Dir. **28**:82–92.
23. Molenda, J. R., W. G. Johnson, M. Fishbein, B. Wentz, I. J. Mehlman, and T. A. Dadisman, Jr. 1972. *Vibrio parahaemolyticus* gastroenteritis in Maryland: laboratory aspects. Appl. Microbiol. **24**:444–448.
24. Monsur, K. A. 1963. Bacteriological diagnosis of cholera under field conditions. Bull. W.H.O. **28**:387–389.
25. Nalin, D. R., and R. A. Cash. 1970. Oral or nasogastric therapy for cholera, p. 73–76. *In* Principles and practice of cholera control. Public Health Papers No. 40. World Health Organization, Geneva, Switzerland.
26. Neumann, D. A., M. W. Benenson, E. Hubster, and N. T. N. Tuan. 1972. Cary-Blair, a transport medium for *Vibrio parahaemolyticus*. Amer. J. Clin. Pathol. **57**:33–34.
27. Pierce, N. F., R. B. Sack, and D. Mahalanabis. 1970. Management of cholera in adults and children, p. 61–72. *In* Principles and practice of cholera control. Public Health Papers No. 40. World Health Organization, Geneva, Switzerland.
28. Report (1966–1970) of the Subcommittee on Taxonomy of Vibrios to the International Committee on Nomenclature of Bacteria. 1972. Int. J. Syst. Bacteriol. **22**:123.
29. Sakazaki, R. 1968. Proposal of *Vibrio alginolyticus* for the biotype 2 of *Vibrio parahaemolyticus*. Jap. J. Med. Sci. Biol. **21**:359–362.
30. Sakazaki, R. 1972. Recent trends of *Vibrio parahaemolyticus* as a causative agent of food poisoning. *In* Proceedings of the 8th International Symposium, The Microbiological Safety of Food, Reading, England.
31. Sakazaki, R., C. Z. Gomez, and M. Sebald. 1967. Taxonomical studies of the so-called NAG vibrios. Jap. J. Med. Sci. Biol. **20**:265–280.
32. Sakazaki, R., S. Iwanami, and H. Fukumi. 1963. Studies on the enteropathogenic, facultatively halophilic bacteria, *Vibrio parahaemolyticus*. I. Morphological, cultural and biochemical properties and its taxonomical position. Jap. J. Med. Sci. Biol. **16**:161–188.
33. Sakazaki, R., K. Tamura, T. Kato, Y. Obara, S. Yamai, and K. Hobo. 1968. Studies on the enteropathogenic, facultatively halophilic bacteria, *Vibrio parahaemolyticus*. III. Enteropathogenicity. Jap. J. Med. Sci. Biol. **21**:325–331.
34. Shewan, J. M., W. Hodgkiss, and J. Liston. 1954. A method for the rapid differentiation of certain non-pathogenic, asporogenous bacilli. Nature (London) **173**:208–209.
35. Smith, H. L., Jr. 1970. A presumptive test for vibrios: the "string" test. Bull. W.H.O. **42**:817–818.
36. Smith, H. L., Jr., R. Freter, and F. J. Sweeney, Jr. 1961. Enumeration of cholera vibrios in fecal samples. J. Infect. Dis. **109**:31–34.
37. Véron, M., and R. Chatelain. 1973. Taxonomic study of the genus *Campylobacter* Sebald and Véron and designation of the neotype strain for the type species, *Campylobacter fetus* (Smith and Taylor) Sebald and Véron. Int. J. Syst. Bacteriol. **23**:122–134.
38. Zen-Yoji, H., R. A. Le Clair, K. Ohta, and T. S. Montague. 1973. Comparison of *Vibrio parahaemolyticus* cultures isolated in the United States with those isolated in Japan. J. Infect. Dis. **127**:237–241.

Chapter 22

Pasteurella

GEORGE H. G. EISENBERG, JR., AND DAN C. CAVANAUGH

CHARACTERIZATION

Taxonomic status uncertain. Primarily animal pathogens but responsible for a variety of diseases in humans ranging from local abscesses to fatal septicemias.

Morphology. Coccobacilli to filamentous rods, gram-negative, non-acid-fast, marked bipolar staining, nonmotile, and nonsporeforming. May be encapsulated.

Growth. Facultative anaerobe: grows on ordinary media, but initiation of growth is facilitated by use of enriched media, such as blood- or serum-agar with increased CO_2 tension. Temperature range, 0 to 43 C; optimal temperature, 37 C. Nonpigmented.

Biochemical characteristics. Oxidase positive, catalase positive, citrate negative, gelatin not liquified, methylene blue reduced.

Carbohydrate fermentations. Glucose positive; adonitol, inulin, and starch negative. Generally anaerogenic, but gas-producing strains have been reported (6, 20).

Antibiotic susceptibility. Unusual among gram-negative bacteria in being susceptible to penicillin in vitro and in vivo, although there are reports of penicillin-resistant strains of *Pasteurella multocida* (18, 19).

PASTEURELLA MULTOCIDA

P. multocida is the type species for the genus *Pasteurella*. It is also known as *P. septica* (23). In early literature, the species designation depended on the animal from which the isolate was derived, such as *aviseptica* (fowl) *suiseptica* (pigs), *vituliseptica* (calves), *oviseptica* (sheep), *boviseptica* (cattle), *leptiseptica* (rabbits), and *muriseptica* (mice).

Clinical significance

Only recently has the frequency of *P. multocida* infections in humans been recognized (1, 3, 7, 9, 11, 12, 21, 22). The normal clinical patterns take three forms: local infections after cat scratch or animal bite; chronic pulmonary infections with *P. multocida* either the primary pathogen or in association with other organisms, such as *Histoplasma capsulatum;* and systemic infections with meningitis or bacteremia. Local infections due to transmission by animal bite or cat scratch into poorly vascularized areas are the most common of the clinical patterns seen with *P. multocida* (21). Within 18 to 24 h, the wound becomes extensively swollen, red, and very painful to the touch, with a gray-colored serous or sanguinopurulent discharge from puncture wounds. Regional adenopathy or evidence of toxicity may be present. If the synovial sheath or periosteum are punctured, osteomyelitis may occur (14, 21). Even with good antibiotic treatment, penicillin or tetracycline being the drugs of choice, granulation is delayed, healing is slow, and tissue damage may be extensive. In rare cases, septicemia may follow local infection (16, 21). Among those infections not related to animal bites, the most common are chronic bronchitis and bronchiectasis. These infections are most commonly found in ranchers, farmers, abattoir workers, and pet owners, people who have prolonged contact with animals or animal tissue processing. In these cases, *P. multocida* most certainly acts as an opportunistic pathogen, causing disease only when some damage has occurred in the bronchial tree that allows the bacteria to colonize and proliferate. Once the mucosa of the respiratory tract has been breached, menigitis, septicemia, sinusitis, and empyema may follow (1, 18). *P. multocida* has also been indicated as the causative agent in cases of abdominal abscesses, conjunctivitis, pyomyositis, and mouth ulcer (12).

Since neither clinical findings nor anatomical changes are pathognomonic, diagnosis of pasteurellosis is dependent on the isolation and identification of *P. multocida* from clinical specimens.

Types of specimens

Respiratory tract: early morning sputa, bronchial washing, or nasal swabs. Animal bite: purulent exudate. Meningitis: spinal fluid. Septicemia: repeated blood cultures.

Isolation procedures

Specimens for initial isolation of *P. multocida*, especially when inocula are small, should be plated directly on 5% blood-agar plates. Use of increased CO_2 tension during incubation may be helpful. Media containing bile are inhibitory.

Growth on agar plates

P. multocida produces no hemolysis on blood-agar plates. Medium may show brownish coloration after 48 to 72 h. Cultures have a distinctive odor, variously described as being musty or like semen or burning hair (1, 10). Three different colonial forms are recognized by 24-h growth on serum-agar at 37 C (23). Highly virulent strains, containing a type-specific polysaccharide capsular antigen, usually produce smooth (S) colonies, 1.0 to 1.5 mm in diameter, that are usually iridescent to obliquely transmitted light (9). Mucoid (M) strains are often isolated from the normal respiratory passages or from chronic infections. The colonies are large, reaching 2 to 3 mm in diameter. These isolates are generally of low virulence, possess a thick hyaluronic acid-containing capsule, but may or may not have the type-specific polysaccharide capsular antigen. The rough (R) strains are completely avirulent and have neither capsular nor mucoid antigens. The colonies are similar in appearance to S colonies, but are difficult to suspend in saline (5).

Growth in broth

Moderate growth, slight turbidity, slight powdery to viscous deposit after 24 h at 37 C.

Gelatin stab

Good filiform growth, confluent at surface and discrete below, extending to the bottom of stab line. No liquefaction.

Microscopic morphology

P. multocida cells are very small ellipsoidal rods 0.15 to 0.25 by 0.3 to 1.25 μm, arranged singly, in pairs, or in small bundles. *P. multocida* is gram-negative and non-acid-fast, and shows marked bipolar staining. It is nonsporeforming and nonflagellated. Mucoid and smooth virulent strains are capsulated in animal body and on media containing blood or serum at 37 C. Metabolism: aerobic, facultatively anaerobic. No hemolysins are formed. Optimal temperature, 37 C; temperature range, 0 to 43 C.

Biochemical characteristics

See Table 1. Though *P. multocida* is usually anaerogenic and lactose-negative, there is one report of a lactose-positive strain (10) and two reports noting observance of aerogenic strains (6, 20). Further, although Smith and Thal (19) use the oxidase reaction in their key to separate *Yersinia* (oxidase-negative) from *Pasteurella* (oxidase-positive), this reaction may be variable for *P. multocida* (1). However, the β-D-galactosidase (ONPG) reaction does seem to provide a clear separation of *P. multocida* (negative) from *Yersinia* (positive).

Recognition of pasteurellosis

From Table 1, it can be seen that carbohydrate fermentations, because of variability, are of little value in speciation. Further, because of its pleomorphism and the fact that *P. multocida* colonies on blood-agar often resemble colonies of enterococci, Gram-stained smears should be studied carefully for morphological identification, and this information should be

TABLE 1. *Biochemical characteristics of Pasteurella species*

Characteristic	*P. multocida*	*P. ureae*	*P. haemolytica*
Hemolysis	–	Green	Beta
Catalase	+	+	+
Oxidase	+	+	+
Urease	V	++	–
Indole	+	–	–
Methyl red	–	–	–
Voges-Proskauer	–	–	–
Citrate	–	–	–
Gelatin liquefaction	–	–	–
Growth on MacConkey agar	–	–	+
Methylene blue reduction	+	+	+
Requirement for X and V factors	–	–	–
Fermentation of:			
Glucose	+	+	+
Sucrose	+	+	+
Fructose	V	+	+
Lactose	–	–	V
Mannose	+	+	V
Mannitol	V	+	V
Maltose	V	+	+
Sorbitol	V	+	+
Xylose	V	–	V
Arabinose	V	–	V
Rhamnose	V	–	–
Dulcitol	V	–	–
Laboratory animal pathogenicity	+	–	–

coordinated with biochemical tests to prevent incorrect identifications as: *Haemophilus* (requirement for X and V factors); *Neisseria* (indole reaction); *Mima*, *Proteus*, and *Klebsiella* (growth in presence of bile); and enterococci (catalase reaction).

Antigenic structure

Five distinct serological types, A, B, C, D, and E, have been recognized (2). Standard agglutination tests are usually complicated by common somatic antigens or by the presence of a blocking capsular antigen in mucoid strains. Two methods, however, are available: the use of a slide agglutination test with young (6-h) cultures as the antigen, or the passive hemagglutination test (15). The soluble type-specific antigen can be extracted by heating a suspension of organisms to 56 C and can be absorbed onto human O erythrocytes, which then become specifically agglutinable by homologous antisera. Gel precipitin tests are of limited value because of the multiplicity of shared antigens among the various serotypes.

Agglutinins may be present in the sera of the patient with a generalized infection and can be detected by the hemagglutination test. Titers are usually not found in patients with localized infections.

Animal pathogenicity

Except for R forms, which are avirulent, *P. multocida* usually proves fatal for mice in 18 to 72 h, after a 24-h broth culture is injected either subcutaneously or intraperitoneally. Postmortem local edema and congestion with overwhelming septicemia are the only changes noted.

PASTEURELLA UREAE

First described in 1960 by Henriksen and Jyssum (8) as a variant of *P. haemolytica*, *P. ureae* is now being increasingly accepted as a separate species in the genus (19, 23).

Clinical significance

P. ureae is the only member of the genus for which no known animal host exists (13). At present, there is no conclusive proof of pathogenicity for humans. However, in one study it was isolated from 1% of routine sputum specimens and was either the predominant agent or present in large numbers in primary blood-agar plates from 17 patients suffering from chronic bronchitis and bronchiectasis. One strain has been isolated in pure culture from a patient with sinusitis (17), another has been indicated as the causative agent in a fatal case of endocarditis (4), and further isolations have been made together with known pathogens in cases of sinusitis and ozaena (8). Like *P. multocida*, *P. ureae* appears to be an opportunistic pathogen, requiring either trauma or primary invasion by some other pathogen to provide suitable conditions to produce disease.

Types of specimens

Respiratory tract: early morning sputa, bronchial washings, or nasal swabs. Septicemia: repeated blood culture.

Isolation procedures

Specimens should be plated on 5% blood-agar and incubated at 37 C under increased CO_2 tension. Media containing bile are inhibitory.

Growth

P. ureae is a facultative anaerobe. Colonies are mucoid in appearance and slightly translucent, being about 2 mm in diameter after 24 h of incubation. Serum or ascitic fluid must be provided in all media to enhance growth. Greening is seen on blood-agar, usually accompanied by partial hemolysis. Cultures have a faint fresh odor (8).

Microscopic morphology

P. ureae cells are pleomorphic gram-negative rods 0.5 to 0.7 μm wide, varying in length from short coccobacilli to long filaments. Some long forms have oval "vacuoles." *P. ureae* is nonsporeforming, nonmotile, and non-acid-fast, with bi-polar staining. A capsule is usually present.

Biochemical characteristics

See Table 1. One lactose-positive strain has been reported (4). Urease activity is exceptionally strong. Carbohydrate fermentations are anaerogenic.

Antigenic structure

Not elucidated at this time.

Animal pathogenicity

P. ureae has no known animal host. It is avirulent for mice, guinea pigs, and rabbits.

PASTEURELLA HAEMOLYTICA

Although no reports of infections in humans due to *P. haemolytica* have been found, increasing interest in infections due to members of the genus and the known pathogenic nature of this species in sheep and cattle indicate that isolation of this organism in human disease in the near future is probable. *P. haemolytica* is morphologically and biochemically similar to *P. multocida*. However, it is serologically distinct, and it is beta-hemolytic on blood-agar, bile resistant, avirulent for rabbits, and of low pathogenicity for other laboratory animals.

LITERATURE CITED

1. Branson, D., and F. Bunkfeldt. 1967. *Pasteurella multocida* in animal bites of humans. Amer. J. Clin. Pathol. **48:**552–555.
2. Carter, G. R., and R. V. S. Bain. 1960. Pasteurellosis (*Pasteurella multocida*). A review stressing recent developments. Vet. Rev. Annot. **6:**105–128.
3. Donaghue, M., and S. S. Raphael. 1971. Infection by *Pasteurella multocida*. Can. Med. Ass. J. **104:**1083.
4. Doty, G. L., G. N. Loomus, and P. L. Wolf. 1963. *Pasteurella* endocarditis. N. Engl. J. Med. **268:**830–832.
5. Dubos, R. J., and J. G. Hirsch (ed.). 1965. Bacterial and mycotic infections of man, 4th ed., p. 659–663. J. B. Lippincott Co., Philadelphia.
6. Gump, D. W., and R. A. Holden. 1972. Endocarditis caused by a new species of *Pasteurella*. Ann. Intern. Med. **76:**275–278.
7. Hawkins, L. G. 1969. Local *Pasteurella multocida* infections. J. Bone Joint Surg. **51A:**363–366.
8. Henriksen, S. D., and K. Jyssum. 1960. A new variety of *Pasteurella haemolytica* from the human respiratory tract. Acta Pathol. Microbiol. Scand. **50:**443.
9. Holloway, W. J., E. G. Scott, and Y. B. Adams. 1969. *Pasteurella multocida* infection in man. Report of 21 cases. Amer. J. Clin. Pathol. **51:**705–708.
10. Horne, W. I., and G. M. Berlyne. 1958. Empyema caused by *Pasteurella septica*. Brit. Med. J. **2:**896.
11. Hubbert, W. T. and M. N. Rosen. 1970. *Pasteurella multocida* infections. I. *Pasteurella multocida* infection due to animal bite. Amer. J. Pub. Health **60:**1103–1108.
12. Hubbert, W. T., and M. N. Rosen. 1970. *Pasteurella multocida* infections. II. *Pasteurella multocida* infection in man unrelated to animal bite. Amer. J. Pub. Health **60:**1109–1115.
13. Jones, D. M., and P. M. O'Connor. 1962. *Pasteurella haemolytica* var *ureae* from human sputum. J. Clin. Pathol. **15:**247–248.
14. Meyers, B. R., B. L. Berson, M. Gilbert, and S. Z. Hirschman. 1973. Clinical patterns of osteomyelitis due to gram-negative bacteria. Arch. Intern. Med. **131:**228–233.
15. Namioka, S., and M. Murata. 1961. Serological studies on *Pasteurella multocida*. I. A simplified method for capsule typing of the organism. Cornell Vet. **51:**498–507.
16. Normann, B., B. Nilehn, J. Rajs, and B. Karlberg. 1971. A fatal case of *Pasteurella multocida* septicaemia after cat bite. Scand. J. Infect. Dis. **3:**251–254.
17. Omland, T., and S. D. Henriksen. 1961. Two new strains of *Pasteurella haemolytica* var. *ureae* isolated from the respiratory tract. Acta Pathol. Microbiol. Scand. **53:**117–120.
18. Schmidt, E. C. H., L. V. Truitt, and M. L. Koch. 1970. Pulmonary abscess with empyema caused by *Pasteurella multocida*. Report of a fatal case. Amer. J. Clin. Pathol. **54:**733–736.
19. Smith, J. E., and E. Thal. 1965. A taxonomic study of the genus *Pasteurella* using a numerical technique. Acta Pathol. Microbiol. Scand. **64:**213–223.
20. Talbot, J. M., and P. H. A. Sneath. 1960. A taxonomic study of *Pasteurella septica*, especially of strains isolated from human sources. J. Gen. Microbiol. **22:**303–311.
21. Tindall, J. P., and C. M. Harrison. 1972. *Pasteurella multocida* infections following animal injuries, especially cat bites. Arch. Dermatol. **105:**412–416.
22. Torphy, D. E., and C. G. Ray. 1969. *Pasteurella multocida* in dog and cat bite infections. Pediatrics **43:**295–297.
23. Wilson, G. S., and A. A. Miles. 1964. Topley and Wilson's principles of bacteriology and immunity, vol. 1, 5th ed., p. 912–956. The Williams & Wilkins Co., Baltimore.

Chapter 23

Pseudomonas

RUDOLPH HUGH AND GERALD L. GILARDI

INTRODUCTION

Experience has demonstrated the practical need for distinguishing organisms, such as *Pseudomonas* and *Acinetobacter anitratus*, which oxidize carbohydrates, and organisms, such as *Enterobacteriaceae*, *Aeromonas*, and *Vibrio*, which ferment carbohydrates. Oxidative-fermentative medium (31; Difco OF basal medium at pH 6.8) was specially designed to detect small quantities of oxidative acidity and distinguish it from fermentative acidity. Carbohydrate oxidizers produce oxidative acidity which begins at the surface of OF medium, where most of the early growth is confined. Growth and acid production at the surface of this medium are expressions of the organism's demand for oxygen; oxygen, under these conditions, is essential for growth and for conversion of glucose (or other oxidizable carbohydrates) to acid. This conclusion can be substantiated by inoculating a duplicate tube of OF glucose medium and then layering it with sterile stiff petrolatum. Aerobic organisms grow and produce acid in the open tube, fail to produce acid from carbohydrate in OF medium sealed with petrolatum, and fail to grow, or at best grow very poorly, under the latter conditions. *P. aeruginosa* and *A. anitratus* are nonfermentative species which oxidize glucose. Pseudomonads which oxidize glucose have not been observed to produce acidity from glucose or other carbohydrates in OF basal media under a petrolatum seal. Some nonfermenters are unable to oxidize carbohydrates. *Alcaligenes faecalis* and *Comamonas terrigena* are strict aerobes which fail to oxidize or ferment glucose. Carbohydrate fermenters produce fermentative acidity throughout OF glucose medium, even under conditions where oxygen is excluded from the medium with a sterile stiff petrolatum seal. Facultative organisms grow and produce acid from carbohydrates in media sealed with petrolatum; they also grow and produce acid throughout the open tube. Fermentative organisms grow at the expense of glucose (and other fermentable carbohydrates) and produce acid in the absence of oxygen. *Escherichia coli* and *Salmonella typhi* are fermentative species with an anaerobic respiratory metabolism. Fermentative organisms may also oxidize carbohydrates. Gram-negative rods which fail to produce a sharp acid reaction in the butt of presumptive screening media, such as triple sugar iron agar and Kligler iron agar, should be inoculated to OF glucose medium to confirm that they are glucose nonfermenters.

Carbohydrate media, such as purple broth base (Difco), are very useful for the detection of fermentative acidity, but are not particularly suitable for the detection of small quantities of oxidative acidity produced by pseudomonads. There are several reasons why OF medium detects small quantities of oxidative acidity: (i) the acidity is detected in the presence of the small quantity of ammonia and other bases derived from the relatively small quantity of peptone present; (ii) the semisolid gel tends to localize and prevent mechanical dispersion of acidity; and (iii) the relatively high carbohydrate concentration (34, 37). OF basal medium, without added carbohydrate, should be inoculated with each nonfermentative organism under investigation.

A stiff petrolatum seal is a more effective oxygen deterrent than is an agar or a liquid mineral oil seal; it is especially desirable when cultures are incubated for prolonged periods. A liquid mineral oil seal is practical for aerogenic organisms inoculated to media containing a fermentable carbohydrate.

Although glucose and other carbohydrates may be oxidized to acids in OF media, they may not necessarily be suitable carbon and energy sources capable of supporting growth in a mineral base medium. Therefore, results based on acid production from carbohydrates in OF basal medium are not necessarily comparable with results based on detection of growth derived at the expense of carbohydrates in a mineral base medium. This discrepancy does not detract from the usefulness of OF basal medium for distinguishing nonfermentative bacteria.

Some fermentative and many nonfermentative gram-negative rods cannot be identified without knowledge of the flagellar anatomy. Flagella staining is an expedient and reliable procedure for determining the flagellar anatomy of the large number of strains of bacteria encountered daily in the clinical laboratory. It is an advantage to examine the flagellar anatomy of a great number of cells in a stained film, and it is a distinct virtue to exercise the option of reexamining the original stained film days, months, or years after the time of preparation. It is not mandatory to use an electron microscope, should one be conveniently available, to determine the presence or absence of bacterial flagella, or to establish the polar or peritrichous attachment of the flagellum or flagella on the bacterial soma.

A single taxonomic attribute, including susceptibility to antimicrobial agents, growth on MacConkey agar, synthesis of indophenol oxidase, growth factor requirements, and guanine plus cytosine content in the deoxyribonucleic acid, seldom enables one to predict invariably other characters of a strain. No character of a strain is immutable or a perfect basis for recognizing strains of a species or for differentiating species. A select combination of a few attributes with a known predictive capacity, rather than a single attribute, is a more reliable basis for recognizing and differentiating species. A species usually represents many strains; strains of a species are similar but not necessarily identical in all measurable attributes. Tests valuable for the identification of fermentative gram-negative rods are not necessarily useful for the recognition of nonfermentative gram-negative rods. Unfortunately, the minimal number and kinds of characters necessary for identification of some *Pseudomonas* species are not the same as those necessary for the identification of other nonfermentative gram-negative rods.

An experienced bacteriologist can accurately and expediently identify most field strains of bacteria encountered in clinical specimens on the basis of fewer than 25 characters of each strain. The quality and significance of the character measured are of greater importance than the quantity of characters measured for identification.

Bacillus subtilis, *Staphylococcus epidermidis*, *Serratia marcescens*, *Escherichia coli*, *Chromobacterium violaceum*, and *Alcaligenes faecalis* at one time were regarded as harmless, but each can be documented as the cause of life-threatening and fatal disease in humans. It is confusing, arbitrary, and misleading to divide bacterial species into categories such as pathogens (animal, human, and plant), nonpathogens, industrial, dairy, soil, marine, etc. There is extensive and significant overlapping among these categories. It appears that almost any bacterial species can produce disease in humans. Glucose-nonfermenting, gram-negative rods should not be regarded as harmless; they are often opportunistic agents of infections promoted by intravenous and antibiotic therapy, immunosuppressive agents, heroic medical and surgical procedures, instrumentation, trauma, and malignant diseases. Although *P. aeruginosa*, *A. anitratus*, and *P. maltophilia* appear to be the most frequently isolated glucose-nonfermenting gram-negative rods from clinical specimens, the clinical bacteriologist isolates an increasing number of species of nonfermentative gram-negative rods which cause serious human infections. The identification procedure should include a comparative study of the type, the neotype, or a recognized reference strain of the species concerned. This procedure assures that each laboratory will establish in-house standards for the identification of wild strains of species and is essential for correlating in-house observations with observations recorded in the literature. Table 1 contains a list of strains for this purpose.

PSEUDOMONAS SPECIES

The minimal characters necessary for the identification of most strains of *Pseudomonas* species are recorded in Table 2. Molecular oxygen is used to oxidize glucose and other carbohydrates to acid. Gas is not produced from carbohydrates. Some species do not produce acid from glucose. Energy is not obtained by fermentative or photosynthetic metabolism. Some species respire in the presence of nitrate and grow under anaerobic conditions in the presence of nitrate or arginine. They usually produce dense turbidity in neutral peptone broth in 18 to 24 h at 30 C and fail to grow in brain heart infusion broth at pH 4.5. Pseudomonads contain 57 to 70 moles percent guanine plus cytosine in the deoxyribonucleic acid (68).

Growth and isolation media

Pseudomonads are not fastidious in their growth requirements, although some may require certain vitamins or amino acids. They grow abundantly on nutrient-agar and blood-agar media. They often grow on selective-differential agar media such as deoxycholate, deoxycholate-citrate, MacConkey, and eosine methylene blue.

The attributes, expressed as frequency in percent positive, of glucose-oxidizing pseudomonads most frequently encountered in clinical

TABLE 1. *Type, neotype, and reference strains for identification of some nonfermentative gram-negative rods*

Organism	ATCC[a] no.	NCTC[b] no.	Status	Percent guanine + cytosine ratio
Pseudomonas aeruginosa	10145	10332	Neotype	
P. fluorescens	13525	10038	Neotype	
P. maltophilia	13637	10257	Type	67
P. pseudomallei		1691[c]	Neotype	
P. mallei	23344	3873	Neotype	69
P. cepacia	25416	10743	Type	67
P. stutzeri	17588		Neotype	65
P. putrefaciens	8071		Reference strain[d]	48
P. alcaligenes	14909	10367	Neotype	66
P. pseudoalcaligenes	17440		Type	63
P. pickettii	27511		Type	64
P. diminuta	11568	8545	Type	65
Comamonas terrigena	8461	1937	Neotype	65
Acinetobacter anitratus	19606		Type	41

[a] American Type Culture Collection, Rockville, Md.
[b] National Collection of Type Cultures, London, England.
[c] Ragaviah strains (71).
[d] Reference strains have no nomenclatural status.

TABLE 2. *Minimal characters for identification of strains of Pseudomonas species*

Character	Sign
Gram-negative, straight or slightly curved rod	+
Asporogenous	+
Polar monotrichous or polar tuft of flagella	+
Motility	usually +
OF glucose medium open, acid	+ or −
OF glucose medium sealed, acid	−
Glucose gas	−
Indophenol oxidase	+ or −
Catalase	+
Photosynthetic pigments	−
Indole, methyl red, and acetylmethylcarbinol	−

specimens are recorded in Table 3. The attributes of the polar flagellated, alkali-producing, gram-negative rods are recorded in Table 4. The results are based on cultures incubated at 30 C unless otherwise stated.

PSEUDOMONAS AERUGINOSA

Sources of isolation and relationship to disease

Metabolic, hematologic, and malignant diseases predispose patients to *P. aeruginosa* infections. Hospital-acquired infections occur in patients who have had prior instrumentation or manipulative procedures such as urethral catheterizations, tracheostomies, lumbar punctures, and intravenous infusions of medications and fluids. Patients become susceptible to *P. aeruginosa* infections after prolonged treatment with immunosuppressive agents, corticosteroids, antimetabolites, antibiotics, and radiation. *P. aeruginosa* often contaminates surgical wounds, decubitus ulcers, abscesses, burns, draining sinuses, ear infections, and lungs of patients treated with antibiotics. The primary etiological agents of these infections are eradicated by antibiotics, and *P. aeruginosa* can become the new infecting agent. *P. aeruginosa* cells in these sites serve as foci for hematogenous dissemination. *P. aeruginosa* is a cause of severe epidemic diarrhea of infants. Collaginase synthesized by *P. aeruginosa* in ocular infections is responsible for corneal perforation which may result in loss of the eye. *P. aeruginosa* infections are a major cause of deaths in patients with burns. *P. aeruginosa* is of increasing clinical importance as a result of its resistance to antibiotic therapy. Several literature reviews summarize the relationship of pseudomonads to human diseases (7, 16, 17, 20, 57, 76).

P. aeruginosa is a common inhabitant of soil and has a world-wide distribution. The normal human intestine does not appear to be a major habitat, but it is found in 1 of 10 normal stools. Feces and the anogenital region may serve as foci of epidemic infections and skin contamination. It has been isolated from benzalkonium chloride (Zephiran) solution, hexachlorophene soap, bedside water decanters, water faucets, forceps, brushes, oral thermometers, syringes, ward utensils, floors, baths, and sinks in the hospital environment. *P. aeruginosa* is encountered in clinical specimens more frequently than any other species of glucose-nonfermenting gram-negative rods.

Tests useful for identification of Pseudomonas aeruginosa

P. aeruginosa has the characters of the genus *Pseudomonas* as recorded in Table 2 and is the only *Pseudomonas* species known to excrete pyocyanin. Cyanomycin, produced by a *Streptomyces* species, is identical to pyocyanin. Pyocyanin is a water-soluble, nonfluorescent, blue, phenazine pigment that is soluble in chloroform. Pseudomonas agar P (Difco 0449)

TABLE 3. *Comparative value of tests used in the identification of certain glucose-oxidizing pseudomonads*[a]

Morphology, substrate, or test	*P. aeruginosa*	*P. fluorescens*	*P. putida*	*P. pseudomallei*	*P. mallei*	*P. cepacia*	*P. stutzeri*	*P. putrefaciens*	*P. maltophilia*
Polar monotrichous, fewer than three flagella per pole	93	0	0	0	0	0	100	100	0
Polar tuft, more than two flagella per pole	0	100	100	100	0	100	0	0	100
Atrichous	7	0	0	0	100	0	0	0	0
Motility	93	100	100	100	0	100	100	100	100
Glucose open	100	100	100	100	100	100	100	100 (d)	56 (44)
Glucose sealed	0	0	0	0	0	0	0	0	0
Maltose open	0	70	35	96 (4)	0 (100)	100	100	31 (d)	100
Maltose sealed	0	0	0	0	0	0	0	0	0
Adonitol	9 (3)	—	—	31 (58)	0 (67)	—	—	—	0
L-Arabinose	97 (3)	—	—	81 (19)	0 (83)	—	—	—	0
Cellobiose	12 (36)	—	—	100	33 (67)	—	—	—	10 (5)
Dulcitol	0	—	—	73 (23)	0	—	—	—	0
Ethyl alcohol, 3%	67 (29)	—	—	19 (65)	0	—	—	—	0 (5)
D-Fructose	69 (22)	97	99	92 (8)	50 (50)	100	100	44 (d)	59
D-Galactose	97 (2)	98	100	100	100	100	98	6 (d)	0 (10)
i-Inositol	12 (2)	—	—	96 (4)	50 (50)	—	—	—	0
Inulin	0	—	—	12	0	—	—	—	0
Lactose	0 (35)	26	28	100	17 (83)	100	0	19 (d)	0
D-Mannitol	81 (11)	94	19	100	0 (83)	100	89	0	0
D-Mannose	98 (1)	98	100	100	67 (33)	100	91	13 (d)	91 (3)
Melezitose	0	—	—	12 (4)	0	—	—	—	0
Melibiose	75 (22)	—	—	11 (8)	0	—	—	—	0 (15)
Raffinose	0	—	—	12	0	—	—	—	0 (5)
Rhamnose	6 (70)	84	63	0 (4)	0	0	71	18 (d)	0
D-Ribose	96 (4)	—	—	42 (58)	0	—	—	—	0
Salicin	0	—	—	12 (8)	0	—	—	—	25 (35)
D-Sorbitol	0	—	—	77 (23)	17 (83)	—	—	—	0
Sucrose	12 (3)	64	13	42	0	90	0	38 (d)	0
Trehalose	17 (43)	—	—	46 (54)	17 (83)	—	—	—	0
Xylose	98 (2)	98	96	27 (73)	0	100	100	6 (d)	0 (2)
OF base medium control, blue	100	100	100	100	100	100	100	100	100
Citrate, Simmons	100	—	—	96	0	—	—	—	32
Indophenol oxidase	100	100	100	100	67	90	100	100	0
Gelatin, charcoal	80 (19)	100	0	—	—	63	0	94	43 (57)
2-Ketogluconate	100	70	74	0	0	12	2	0	0
Lysine decarboxylase, ninhydrin	0	—	—	0	0	—	—	—	97
Nitrate to gas	94	2	0	85	0	0	100	0	0
Pyocyanin, chloroform-soluble pigment	58	0	0	0	0	0	0	0	0
Urease	23	40	51	35	17	33	27	25	0
L-Lysine decarboxylase	0	0	0	0	0	93	0	0	20 (43)
L-Arginine dihydrolase	96 (3)	98	97	100	83 (17)	0	0	0	0
L-Ornithine decarboxylase	0	0	0	0	0	29	0	100	0
Growth in brain heart infusion broth at 42 C	100	0	0	100	0	71	100	100	10
Growth at the expense of β-hydroxybutyrate	100	—	—	100	100	—	—	—	0
Sudan black granules	0	0	0	96	100	100	0	0	—
Growth at the expense of *p*-hydroxybenzoate	95	—	—	96	0	—	—	—	0
Ortho cleavage of protocatechuate	100	—	—	100	—	—	—	—	—
Growth on deoxycholate-agar	100	96	94	50	67	2	89	94	100

[a] Figures indicate percent positive within 2 days; those in parentheses indicate percent positive, delayed 3 or more days; (d) indicates reaction in some strains delayed 3 or more days; —, no test. Results are based on the following numbers of strains for each species: *P. aeruginosa*, 118; *P. fluorescens*, 50; *P. putida*, 72; *P. pseudomallei*, 26; *P. mallei*, 6; *P. cepacia*, 41; *P. stutzeri*, 45; *P. putrefaciens*, 16; *P. maltophilia*, 41.

TABLE 4. *Comparative value of tests used in the identification of polar flagellated alkali-producing gram-negative rods*[a]

Morphology, substrate, or test	*Pseudomonas alcaligenes* Biotype A	*Pseudomonas alcaligenes* Biotype B	*P. diminuta*	*Comamonas terrigena*
Polar monotrichous, fewer than three flagella per pole	100	100	100	0
Polar tuft, more than two flagella per pole	0	0	0	100
Motility	100	100	100	100
Adonitol, dulcitol, inulin, lactose, maltose, melezitose	0	0	0	0
L-Arabinose	0	7 (16)	0 (11)	0
Cellobiose	0	2	0	0
Glucose open	0	0	0	0
Ethyl alcohol, 3%	0 (42)	42 (56)	33	24 (14)
D-Fructose	0	49 (47)	22	1 (1)
D-Galactose	0	2 (4)	0	0
i-Inositol	0	0	11	0 (13)
D-Mannitol	0	4 (27)	0	0 (1)
D-Mannose	0	0 (2)	0	0
Melibiose, rhamnose	0	0	11	0
Raffinose, salicin, D-sorbitol, sucrose, trehalose	0	0	0	0
D-Ribose	0	9 (13)	22 (22)	1 (8)
Xylose	0	2 (22)	0	1 (4)
OF base medium control, blue	100	100	100	100
Citrate, Simmons	67	31	0	48
Indophenol oxidase, catalase	100	100	100	100
Gelatin, charcoal	0 (25)	0 (28)	0 (100)	0 (33)
Hydrogen sulfide, Kligler	0	0	0	0
Malonate	0 (17)	11	0	33 (3)
Nitrate to gas	0	4	0	1
Nitrate to nitrite	92	87	44	88
Zn dust test on negative nitrite tests	100	100	100	90
Phenylalanine deaminase	50	27	11	1
Pyocyanin, chloroform-soluble pigment	0	0	0	0
Urease	8	18	0	38
L-Lysine decarboxylase	0	0	0	0
L-Arginine dihydrolase	8 (25)	0 (20)	0 (33)	0
L-Ornithine decarboxylase	0	0 (2)	0 (11)	0
Growth in brain heart infusion at 42 C	0	100	50	36
Growth at the expense of β-hydroxybutyrate	100	100	25	86
Sudan black granules	0	80	25	100
Growth at the expense of *p*-hydroxybenzoate	0	0	0	54
Meta cleavage of protocatechuate	—	—	—	100
Growth at the expense of testosterone	—	—	0	15
Growth on deoxycholate-agar	92	98	33	90

[a] Figures indicate percent positive within 2 days; those in parentheses indicate percent positive, delayed 3 or more days; —, no test. Results are based on the following numbers of strains for each species: *P. alcaligenes* biotype A, 12; *P. alcaligenes* biotype B, 45; *P. diminuta*, 9; *Comamonas terrigena*, 80.

encourages pyocyanin synthesis. Although small quantities of pyocyanin may not perceptibly change the color of media, it can be detected by chloroform extraction. The neotype strain of *P. aeruginosa* (68) has been described (33). The minimal characters necessary for identification of most *P. aeruginosa* strains are recorded in Table 5. Most apyocyanogenic strains can be identified without determining the flagellar anatomy. Apyocyanogenic strains with aberrant biochemical character patterns and pyomelanogenic strains which fail to produce pyocyanin should be stained for flagella. Most cells of a strain of *P. aeruginosa* have only one flagellum per pole; a few cells may have two flagella per pole (33, 42). A few strains are atrichous. The uniformity of the morphological and biochemical character pattern of *P. aeruginosa* is remarkable, as is evident from a study of 354 strains (37) and from the 118 strains described in Table 3.

P. aeruginosa strains may synthesize various combinations of pyocyanin, pyoverdin (fluorescein), pyorubin, and pyomelanin. Pyocyanin

TABLE 5. *Minimal characters for identification of Pseudomonas aeruginosa strains*

Character	Sign	Percent positive[a]
Polar monotrichous, fewer than three flagella per pole	+	93
Motility	+	93
OF glucose medium open, acid	+	100
OF maltose medium, acid	−	0
OF xylose medium, acid	+	98 (2)
OF base medium control, blue	+	100
Citrate, Simmons	+	100
Indophenol oxidase	+	100
Nitrate to gas	+	94
L-Lysine decarboxylase	−	0
L-Arginine dihydrolase	+	96 (3)
L-Ornithine decarboxylase	−	0
Hydrogen sulfide, black butt in Kligler iron agar	−	0
Growth in brain heart infusion broth at 42 C	+	100

[a] Based on a study of 118 strains. Figures indicate percent positive within 2 days; those in parentheses indicate percent positive, delayed 3 or more days.

synthesis may be masked by other pigments. Fewer than 3% of the *P. aeruginosa* strains encountered in clinical specimens are pyomelanogenic (brown to black water-soluble pigment). Strains which produce pyomelanin or pyorubin are sometimes reluctant to produce acid from carbohydrates which are usually oxidized by the species (78).

P. aeruginosa grows in mineral base medium, without growth factors, containing ammonium ion as sole source of nitrogen and glucose as sole source of carbon and energy. The use of 146 organic compounds as carbon and energy sources available to 29 strains of *P. aeruginosa* has been recorded (70). The following universal features of pyocyanogenic strains are unreliable for the identification of apyocyanogenic strains: nitritase, gelatinase, caseinase, and lipase activity; production of 2-ketogluconate; triphenyltetrazolium chloride tolerance; and growth in mineral base medium with adipate, suberate, or acetamide as sole sources of carbon and energy (18, 21). Potentially useful phenotypic taxonomic tools for identifying *P. aeruginosa* and other pseudomonads include a comparison of the presence and relative amounts of cellular fatty acids (52) and investigation of nucleic acid reactions of intact cells (38).

Serological typing (23, 73, 77), a standardized bacteriophage typing system (72), and a system of typing by pyocin production (22) have been used independently and in combination (4, 13) as markers to trace the sources of infections to the epidemic foci. Changes in colonial morphology of descendants of a strain of *P. aeruginosa* are correlated with differences in bacteriophage pattern, antibiotic susceptibility, serology, and iridescence (80). There is no evidence that certain types of *P. aeruginosa* vary in their virulence for humans (4).

PSEUDOMONAS FLUORESCENS

Sources of isolation and relationship to disease

P. fluorescens has been isolated from wounds, sputum, pleural fluid, urine, and blood for transfusion. *P. fluorescens* is an environmental contaminant and rarely an opportunistic pathogen for humans (3, 20, 37, 57). *P. fluorescens* and other psychrophilic gram-negative rods multiply, autolyze, and release endotoxins in contaminated blood and blood products stored in a refrigerator. The biological effects of bacteria and bacterial products administered in blood transfusions are numerous. The pathogenic effects of the phospholipid moiety of endotoxin include irreversible shock.

Tests useful for identification of Pseudomonas fluorescens

P. fluorescens has the characters of the genus *Pseudomonas* as recorded in Table 2; the minimal characters necessary for identification of *P. fluorescens* strains are recorded in Table 6. The neotype strain of *P. fluorescens* (68) has been described (29).

Most *P. fluorescens* strains do not grow at 37 or 42 C (37), but they often withstand exposure to 37 C. Clinical specimens are usually incu-

TABLE 6. *Minimal characters for identification of Pseudomonas fluorescens strains*

Character	Sign	Percent positive[a]
Polar tuft of three or more flagella	+	100
Motility	+	100
OF glucose medium open, acid	+	100
OF maltose medium, acid	+ or −	70
OF xylose medium, acid	+	100
Indophenol oxidase	+	100
Pyocyanin	−	0
Pyoverdin (fluorescent pigment)	+	94
L-Arginine dihydrolase	+	98
Growth in brain heart infusion broth at 42 C	−	0

[a] Based on a study of 50 strains. Figures indicate percent positive within 2 days.

bated at 35 or 37 C; hence, the recovery rate of *P. fluorescens* is below what would be expected at lower incubation temperatures.

Although the number of flagella per cell varies from cell to cell in a *P. fluorescens* strain and the predominant type of flagellation may be one or two per pole with a range from zero to eight, the number of flagella per pole remains a valuable feature for distinguishing *P. aeruginosa* from *P. fluorescens*. Most *P. fluorescens* strains possess some cells with three or more flagella per pole, whereas it is uncommon for *P. aeruginosa* strains to have cells with three or more flagella per pole (29, 37, 43). Stained preparations illustrate the polar tuft of flagella (29) characteristic of *P. fluorescens*.

P. fluorescens is apyocyanogenic and some strains fail to produce the fluorescent pigment pyoverdin. Pseudomonas agar F (Difco 0448) encourages pyoverdin synthesis and suppresses pyocyanin synthesis. Pyoverdin is water-soluble, yellow, fluorescent, and not soluble in chloroform (11). Pseudomonads which produce modified phenazine pigments, such as phenazine α-carboxylic acid, chlororaphin, and oxychlororaphin, are considered biotypes of *P. fluorescens* (70).

P. fluorescens grows in mineral base medium, without growth factors, containing ammonium ion as sole source of nitrogen and glucose as sole source of carbon and energy.

There is some question whether *P. ovalis* and the nongelatinolytic *P. putida* can and should be distinguished from *P. fluorescens* (60, 61). The similarity and differences of 29 characters of 50 strains of *P. fluorescens* and 72 strains of *P. putida* are recorded in Table 3. *P. putida* and *P. ovalis* appear to be an integral part of a larger natural taxonomic group. Jessen (37) studied "505 unclassified fluorescent strains," not *P. aeruginosa*, and divided them into five groups and 81 biotypes. The majority of the strains of human origin were biotypes 11 and 63. Some workers (3, 18, 39, 40, 58, 70) distinguish *P. fluorescens* and *P. putida* on the basis of gelatinase, caseinase, and lecithinase production, and growth in mineral base media containing certain organic compounds as sole sources of carbon and energy. However, neither species has a broad homogeneous biochemical reaction pattern comparable to that found among *P. aeruginosa* strains. In spite of the numerous dissimilar physiological properties, it is possible and expedient to circumscribe non-phenazine-producing fluorescent pseudomonads by means of shared attributes.

PSEUDOMONAS MALTOPHILIA

Sources of isolation and relationship to disease

Although the habitat is obscure, *P. maltophilia* appears to have a wide geographic distribution and is recognized with increasing frequency. It has been isolated from stool, sputum, urine, blood, oropharyngeal swabs from normal adults, oropharyngeal swabs from patients with malignant diseases in various areas of the body, ascitic fluid, pericardial fluid, pleural fluid, cerebrospinal fluid, oviduct, lymph node, conjunctiva, leg ulcer, pus from various regions of the body, spleen, lung, brain abscess, and granulomatous tissue (74). It has been found in raw milk; well water; stagnant water; river water; sewage; tissue culture contaminant; frozen fish; feces of snakes, lizards, frogs, and rabbits; rotten eggs; streptomycin solution; and soil in petroleum zones. It has been recovered from the internal tissue of banana pseudostem, decaying banana sucker, cotton seed, bean pod, and tobacco seedlings. Thus, *P. maltophilia* appears to be a ubiquitous, free-living microbe that occasionally is an opportunistic pathogen for humans (17, 20, 57). The upper respiratory tract, wounds, blood, and urine appear to be the most frequent sources of *P. maltophilia* in clinical specimens.

Tests useful for identification of Pseudomonas maltophilia

P. maltophilia has the characters of the genus *Pseudomonas* as recorded in Table 2; the minimal characters necessary for identification of *P. maltophilia* strains are recorded in Table 7. The

TABLE 7. *Minimal characters for identification of Pseudomonas maltophilia strains*

Character	Sign	Percent positive[a]
Polar tuft of three or more flagella	+	99
Motility	+	99
OF glucose medium open, acid[b]	+	100
OF maltose medium open, acid[c]	+	100
OF maltose medium sealed, acid	−	0
OF mannitol medium, acid	−	0
Nitrate to gas	−	0

[a] Based on a study of 133 strains.

[b] Usually alkaline or neutral the first day; 56% become acid the second day; 44% become acid within 3 to 9 days.

[c] On the first day, 97% become acid; 3% become acid on the second day.

uniformity of the morphological and biochemical reaction pattern of *P. maltophilia* is evident in Tables 3 and 13. The type strain of *P. maltophilia* has been described, and stained preparations illustrate the polar tuft of flagella characteristic of the species (32, 35). It has a polar tuft of three or more flagella. Although the number of flagella per pole varies from zero to eight, each strain has some cells with tufts of three or more flagella.

OF basal medium (Difco) containing glucose may remain neutral or become weakly alkaline in 18 to 24 h; after continued incubation, it increases in acidity and becomes frankly acid. Oxidative acidity promptly accumulates in OF maltose medium. All strains produce extracellular deoxyribonuclease. The lysine decarboxylase reaction (Carlquist ninhydrin) is usually positive but is not an essential determinant for routine identification of strains in the clinical laboratory. *P. maltophilia* strains seldom produce a prompt alkaline reaction under a petrolatum seal in decarboxylase base Moeller (Difco 0890) containing lysine. Arginine dihydrolase is not produced.

P. maltophilia, *P. syringae*, and other phytopathogenic fluorescent pseudomonads do not produce indophenol oxidase (48, 65). These pseudomonads appear to lack cytochrome *c*, which may be necessary for the indophenol oxidase reaction (9, 70). Although methionine is an essential growth factor for most strains, peptone-containing culture media need not be supplemented with methionine to obtain good growth response. Some strains do not require methionine for growth. Some strains slowly produce a very faint yellow pigment which does not diffuse out of the colony into the agar medium; diffusible, water-soluble pigment (melanin) is not conspicuously produced around colonies growing on heart infusion agar (Difco 0045).

PSEUDOMONAS CEPACIA

Sources of isolation and relationship to disease

P. multivorans and *P. kingii* are junior synonyms for *P. cepacia* (27). *P. cepacia* causes onion bulb-rot. It has a wide geographic distribution and has been isolated from urine, wounds, blood, sputum, synovial fluid, ear, toe webs of troops with "foot rot," detergent solution, baby's thermometer, respirators, intravenous fluid, natural and tap water, rotting tree trunk, and soil. Patients are contaminated with the organism from the hospital environment. *P. cepacia* has been associated with endocarditis, septicemia, pneumonitis, wound infections, abscesses, and urinary tract infections.

TABLE 8. *Minimal characters for identification of Pseudomonas cepacia strains*

Character	Sign	Percent positive[a]
Polar tuft of three or more flagella	+	97
Motility	+	97
OF glucose medium open, acid	+	100
OF lactose, maltose, mannitol, and cellobiose, acid	+	100
Hydrogen sulfide, black butt in Kligler iron agar	−	0
Nitrate to gas	−	0
L-Lysine decarboxylase, ninhydrin	+	100
L-Arginine dihydrolase	−	0

[a] Based on a study of 32 strains. Figures indicate percent positive within 2 days.

Tests useful for identification of Pseudomonas cepacia

P. cepacia has the characters of the genus *Pseudomonas* as recorded in Table 2; the minimal characters necessary for identification of *P. cepacia* strains are recorded in Table 8. The type strain has been described (2). It is usually motile with a polar tuft of three to eight flagella, although some cells in the population may have only one flagellum at the pole. It grows abundantly in brain heart infusion broth at 30 C; some strains grow poorly at 37 C, and most grow very poorly or not at all at 42 C. Most, not all, grow on deoxycholate agar. Many strains produce a conspicuous sulfur-yellow, water-soluble nonfluorescent phenazine pigment which is readily seen in the colonies and in the surrounding agar medium after 48 h of incubation at 20 to 30 C. The colonies may be distinctly yellow on various media (also very distinctly pigmented on many other media including infusion agar); a few strains produce a purple pigment after several days of incubation at 20 C. Pigment synthesis is variable and some strains are nonpigmented.

Many strains fail to produce or produce a slow and very weak indophenol oxidase reaction. *P. cepacia* grows in mineral base medium, without growth factors, containing ammonium ion as sole source of nitrogen and glucose as sole source of energy and carbon. The strains are usually susceptible to chloramphenicol but not to antibiotics of the polymyxin group or gentamicin

(19, 27). A summary of the attributes of 41 strains of *P. cepacia* is recorded in Tables 3 and 13. It shares phenotypic and genetic similarities with *P. pseudomallei* and *P. mallei* (63).

PSEUDOMONAS PSEUDOMALLEI

Sources of isolation and relationship to disease

P. pseudomallei causes melioidosis, an endemic glanders-like disease of humans and animals, in Southeast Asia. Human melioidosis rarely occurs in the Western Hemisphere; it occurs in the United States among those who have returned from countries where it is known to exist. The organism may remain dormant and persist asymptomatically in humans for many years before the appearance of clinical infection. The incidence of asymptomatic infections in humans in endemic areas appears high. Pulmonary melioidosis is a relatively benign disease with good prognosis (69). Untreated septicemic melioidosis progresses rapidly and has a high mortality. The mortality rate of fulminant septicemia has dropped markedly with prompt appropriate antibiotic therapy.

P. pseudomallei has been isolated from soil and water in endemic areas. It appears to be a free-living soil organism which causes infection when contaminated water enters abrasions and lacerations of the skin. It is not transmitted from man to man. Because the host spectrum is broad and the clinical manifestation of melioidosis in humans is varied, diagnosis is dependent on isolation and identification of the etiological agent. Clinical diagnosis of the disease is usually delayed until the isolated organism reaches a bacteriologist actively working with *P. pseudomallei*. It can be isolated from sputum, urine, pus from cutaneous ulcers and abscesses, or blood, depending on the clinical situation.

Tests useful for identification of Pseudomonas pseudomallei

P. pseudomallei has the characters of the genus *Pseudomonas* as recorded in Table 2. Characters useful for the identification of *P. pseudomallei* are recorded in Table 9. The variation in colonial morphology reflects a dissociation similar to that of *P. aeruginosa*. *P. pseudomallei*, *P. mallei*, *P. aeruginosa*, and other pseudomonads may have wrinkled, rough, corrugated colonial variants. *P. pseudomallei* does not produce pyocyanin or pyoverdin. It has a polar tuft of three or more flagella per pole (44), and it oxidizes glucose, cellobiose, lactose, and maltose. It produces indophenol oxidase and arginine dihydrolase, and it grows at 42 C. It grows in mineral base medium, without growth factors, containing ammonium ion as sole source of nitrogen and glucose as sole source of energy and carbon. The agglutination and fluorescent-antibody reactions are useful for identification of *P. pseudomallei* (79). Antisera for serological identification are available from Difco. A summary of the attributes of 26 strains is recorded in Table 3; all of these strains produce alkali in open tubes of OF basal medium control (64).

PSEUDOMONAS MALLEI

Sources of isolation and relationship to disease

P. mallei is the etiological agent of glanders

TABLE 9. *Characters for the identification of Pseudomonas pseudomallei and P. mallei strains*[a]

Character	*P. pseudomallei*		*P. mallei*	
	Sign	Percent positive	Sign	Percent positive
Polar tuft of three or more flagella	+	100	−	0
Motility	+	100	−	0
OF glucose medium open, acid	+	100	+	100
OF cellobiose medium open, acid	+	100	+	33 (67)
OF maltose medium open, acid	+	96 (4)	+	0 (100)
OF dulcitol medium open, acid	+	73 (23)	−	0
Citrate, Simmons	+	96	−	0
Nitrate to gas	+ or −	85	−	0
L-Lysine decarboxylase	−	0	−	0
L-Arginine dihydrolase	+	100	+	83 (17)
Growth in brain heart infusion broth at 42 C	+	100	−	0

[a] Figures indicate percent positive within 2 days; those in parentheses indicate percent positive, delayed 3 or more days. Results are based on a study of 26 strains of *P. pseudomallei* and 6 strains of *P. mallei*.

(farcy), a natural disease primarily of equines. Occasionally, it is transmitted from equine hosts to humans by direct contact through abraded skin and inhalation. It can be transmitted from person to person. Glanders has been eradicated in the United States and Canada. The etiological agent of glanders in humans can be isolated from blood, sputum, or pus. *P. mallei* is thought to be the only highly adapted parasite of animals in the genus *Pseudomonas*.

Tests useful for identification of Pseudomonas mallei

P. mallei is a nonmotile species which has the characters of the genus *Pseudomonas* as recorded in Table 2. Characters useful for the identification of *P. mallei* strains are recorded in Table 9. It oxidizes glucose, produces arginine dihydrolase, does not produce pyocyanin or pyoverdin, and fails to grow at 42 C. The indophenol oxidase test, when positive, is often weak and develops slowly. It grows slowly in brain heart infusion broth when compared with *P. aeruginosa* and *P. pseudomallei*, and the cell crop yield is lower. Although *P. mallei* vigorously reacts with *P. pseudomallei* antiserum, the former is invariably nonmotile and produces scant growth in brain heart infusion broth in 24 h. *P. mallei* grows in mineral base medium, without growth factors, containing ammonium ion as sole source of nitrogen and glucose as the sole source of energy and carbon. A summary of the attributes of six strains of *P. mallei* is recorded in Table 3.

PSEUDOMONAS STUTZERI

Source of isolation and relationship to disease

P. stutzeri (*Bacillus denitrificans* II) is ubiquitous in soil and water. It has been found in manure, humus, straw, sewage, dung, stagnant water, baby formula, and animals (75). The organism has been recovered from clinical specimens on numerous occasions, including recovery from wounds, sputum, nose and throat, blood, cerebrospinal fluid, urine, ear, genitals, eye, and stool, but generally has not been directly associated with an infectious process. It is believed to live as a saprophyte in the human body. It is difficult to assess a pathogenic role for this organism, but *P. stutzeri* has been associated with otitis media, an old osteomyelitic lesion of the tibia, and with wounds after trauma (20).

TABLE 10. *Minimal characters for identification of Pseudomonas stutzeri strains*

Character	Sign	Percent positive[a]
Polar monotrichous, fewer than three flagella per pole	+	100
Motility	+	100
OF glucose medium open, acid	+	100
OF maltose and xylose media open, acid	+	100
OF lactose medium open, acid	−	0
Indophenol oxidase	+	100
Nitrate to gas	+	100
L-Arginine dihydrolase	−	0
L-Lysine, L-ornithine decarboxylase	−	0

[a] Based on a study of 45 strains. Figures indicate percent positive within 2 days.

Tests useful for identification of Pseudomonas stutzeri

P. stutzeri has the characters of the genus *Pseudomonas* as recorded in Table 2; the minimal characters necessary for identification of *P. stutzeri* strains are recorded in Table 10. It is a polar-monotrichous, nonfluorescent pseudomonad which produces rough wrinkled colonies with an intracellular brownish yellow pigment, resembling some strains of *P. pseudomallei*. It grows well on deoxycholate agar and grows at 42 C. Most strains are capable of active denitrification with the accumulation of large amounts of nitrogen gas. Oxidative acidity is produced from glucose, fructose, maltose, and mannitol. It is indophenol oxidase-positive and does not liquefy gelatin or produce 2-ketogluconate. Dihydrolase and decarboxylase activity for arginine, lysine, and ornithine are absent. Good growth is obtained in mineral base medium, without growth factors, containing ammonium ion as sole source of nitrogen and glucose as sole source of carbon and energy. The marked nutritional heterogeneity of this species is demonstrated by the relatively small number of organic compounds that serve as substrates for all strains (70).

P. stutzeri is differentiated from *P. pseudomallei* since the latter oxidizes lactose and sucrose, produces gelatinase and dihydrolase for arginine, and fails to grow on deoxycholate agar. A summary of the attributes of 45 strains of *P. stutzeri* is recorded in Tables 3 and 13.

A pseudomonad with similar features, *P. mendocina* (54), is differentiated from *P. stutzeri* since the former produces dihydrolase for arginine and fails to hydrolyze starch. Although *P. stutzeri* strains are often wrinkled, tough, and coherent, smooth variants are not uncommon. Colonies of *P. mendocina* are flat and smooth.

PSEUDOMONAS PUTREFACIENS

Sources of isolation and relationship to disease

P. putrefaciens is found in soil and water, and has a wide geographic distribution. It has been found in raw, sweet milk and cream, eggs, snake feces, sewage, stagnant and river water, tissue culture, oil emulsion, and natural gas and petroleum brines. It is responsible for putrid deterioration of butter, hydrogen sulfide spoilage in haddock fillets, and green discoloration of fresh meat, and it has been isolated from fresh, frozen, and stored cod fillets and frozen poultry carcasses. *P. putrefaciens* has been isolated from clinical specimens of human origin, e.g., blood culture, heart blood at autopsy, urine, feces, sputum, secretions from wounds, abscesses, ulcers, and otitis media, and throat swabs (27).

Tests useful for identification of Pseudomonas putrefaciens

P. putrefaciens has the characters of the genus *Pseudomonas* as recorded in Table 2; the minimal characters necessary for identification of *P. putrefaciens* strains are recorded in Table 11.

P. putrefaciens grows in brain heart infusion broth (Difco 0037), blood agar base (Difco 0045), and OF basal medium (Difco 0688). Many strains require 48 h of incubation for growth to appear on deoxycholate agar; others may fail to grow on this medium. Most strains produce a dense turbidity in neutral peptone broth and brain heart infusion broth in 18 to 24 h at 22 and 30 C; many strains fail to grow in these broths at 37 C. The growth may be reddish-tan or pink.

P. putrefaciens is a rod with a polar monotrichous flagellum. Some strains produce cells with lateral flagella which have a shorter wavelength than the terminal flagellum. It produces hydrogen sulfide and blackens the stabbed butt of Kligler iron agar and triple sugar iron agar media; for this reason, strains have been mistaken for salmonellae. National Collection of Industrial Bacteria strain 8615 (RH 2765) and National Collection of Dairy Organisms strain 1538 (Park 23, RH 1756) are *P. putrefaciens* strains (49).

P. putrefaciens fails to grow in standard mineral base medium containing *p*-hydroxybenzoate as the sole source of carbon; 15 of 16 strains grow in standard mineral base medium, without growth factors, at the expense of acetate as sole source of energy and carbon. Some strains fail to grow in brain heart infusion broth containing 6% sodium chloride, and others grow in nutrient broth containing 10% sodium chloride (62). A summary of the attributes of 16 strains of *P. putrefaciens* is recorded in Table 3. The name *P. putrefaciens* is used in this chapter without prejudice.

TABLE 11. *Minimal characters for identification of Pseudomonas putrefaciens strains*

Character	Sign	Percent positive[a]
Polar monotrichous, fewer than three flagella per pole	+	100
Motility	+	100
OF glucose medium open, acid	+, late +, or −	12 (38)
Indophenol oxidase	+	100
Deoxyribonuclease, extracellular	+	100
Hydrogen sulfide, black butt in Kligler iron agar	+	94
L-Ornithine decarboxylase	+	90 (6)

[a] Based on a study of 50 strains. Figures indicate percent positive within 2 days; those in parentheses indicate percent positive, delayed 3 or more days.

PSEUDOMONAS ALCALIGENES

Sources of isolation and relationship to disease

P. alcaligenes has been isolated from pond, river, swimming-pool, and turtle-aquarium water; raw milk; frozen fish; liver of piglet; and feces of rabbits, frogs, and humans. It is an opportunistic infectious agent that has been isolated from the blood of patients with pyrexia, urine, respiratory tract, and abscesses.

Tests useful for identification of Pseudomonas alcaligenes

This alkali-producing pseudomonad has the characters of the genus *Pseudomonas* as recorded in Table 2. *P. alcaligenes* (Monias 1928) does not produce acid from glucose in OF medium; it produces alkali in open tubes of OF glucose and OF basal media. The neotype strain, ATCC 14909, does not remove glucose from media (56). Many carbohydrates are not oxidized (see Table 4), and indophenol oxidase is produced. Pyocyanin, and lysine decarboxylase are not synthesized. It produces a dense turbidity, within 18 to 24 h at 21 and 37 C, in brain heart infusion broth and usually grows on deoxycholate agar.

The cells of most strains have no somatic curvature; some strains have a few cells which are distinctly curved. There is predominantly one polar flagellum per cell and only rarely two flagella per pole. The flagellar anatomy of the neotype strain is representative of the species; a stained preparation and an electron micrograph illustrate the unipolar attachment of the flagellum and the mean wavelength of 1.6 μm (30). The flagellar anatomy is similar to that of *P. aeruginosa*.

Many strains of this species are physiologically more active than others, and on this basis two biotypes are recognized in Table 4. Biotypes A and B are phenotypically heterogeneous (21, 54, 59), and biotype B appears to correspond to *P. pseudoalcaligenes* (70).

PSEUDOMONAS DIMINUTA

Sources of isolation and relationship to disease

P. diminuta has been isolated from stream and ditch water and from contaminated tissue culture. It has been isolated from the blood of a patient with endocarditis, respiratory tract, ascitic fluid, cerebrospinal fluid, urine, ear swab, and pus from maxillary sinus.

Tests useful for identification of Pseudomonas diminuta

This alkali-producing pseudomonad has the characters of the genus *Pseudomonas* as recorded in Table 2. It does not produce acid from glucose in OF basal medium; it produces alkali in open tubes of OF glucose and OF basal media. Most carbohydrates are not oxidized, and indophenol oxidase is produced. The attributes of nine strains of *P. diminuta* are recorded in Table 4.

Most cells of a strain of *P. diminuta* have one polar flagellum per cell. The flagellar anatomy of the type strain, ATCC 11568, illustrates the very short wavelength, 0.7 μm, characteristic of the species (44, 46).

One of four *P. dimunuta* strains grows in mineral base medium, without growth factors, containing ammonium ion as sole source of nitrogen and β-hydroxybutyrate as sole source of carbon and energy. Most strains require pantothenate, biotin, and cyanocobalamine (1).

COMAMONAS TERRIGENA

Sources of isolation and relationship to disease

C. terrigena has been recovered from blood; abscess; pleural and cerebrospinal fluids; catheterized urine; abdominal pus; respiratory tract; serum; feces of man, rabbit, turtle, frog, and cobra; sewer, ditch, river, and well water; fish aquarium water; raw milk; frozen shrimp; eye wash; and soil. *C. terrigena* has a wide geographic distribution and has been isolated in the United States, Australia, England, Italy, Japan, India, France, The Netherlands, and Java.

TABLE 12. *Minimal characters for identification of Comamonas terrigena strains*

Character	Sign	Percent positive[a]
Gram-negative, straight or slightly curved rod	+	100
Asporogenous	+	100
Polar tuft of three or more flagella	+	100
Motility	+	100
OF glucose medium open, alkaline	+	100
OF lactose and maltose media, alkaline	+	100
Indophenol oxidase	+	100
Hydrogen sulfide, black butt in Kligler iron agar	−	0

[a] Based on a study of 122 strains. Figures indicate percent positive within 2 days.

Tests useful for identification of Comamonas terrigena

C. terrigena is the type species, and only species, in the genus *Comamonas*. It is a gram-negative rod and is asporogenous. The majority of strains are populations of cells with no somatic curvature. An occasional cell of some cultures is distinctly curved. The cells are motile rods with a polar tuft of flagella. Catalase and indophenol oxidase are produced. *C. terrigena* does not produce acid from glucose in OF basal medium. Alkali is produced in open tubes of OF glucose and OF basal media. Glucose is not removed from media by comamonads (56). Most carbohydrates are not oxidized. Energy is not obtained by fermentative or photosynthetic metabolism. Indole, methyl red, and acetylmethylcarbinol tests are negative. Pyoverdin is not produced. The minimal characters necessary for identification of *C. terrigena* strains are recorded in Table 12. The attributes of 80 strains of *C. terrigena* are recorded in Table 4.

The number of flagella at one pole varies from one to six, with generally two to four flagella per pole. The strains usually contain some cells with tufts which possess three or more flagella. The tuft of flagella is located at one pole of the cell; cells with flagella at both poles appear to be dividing. The polar flagella have a mean wavelength of 3.1 μm and an amplitude of 1.08 μm. This distinctive flagellar morphology is illustrated in a photomicrograph published by Leifson and Hugh (45) and by photomicrographs in a publication by Leifson (44). Some strains produce variants with lateral flagella which have a shorter wavelength. A stable peritrichous mutant, ATCC 17758, has been isolated from the polar tufted neotype strain, ATCC 8461 (48). Variants with mixed flagella and the peritrichous mutant are illustrated in stained preparations (44, 45).

These aerobic organisms produce a dense turbidity in neutral peptone and brain heart infusion broths in 18 to 24 h at 30 and 37 C and fail to grow in brain heart infusion broth at pH 4.5. Comamonads are not fastidious in their growth requirements. They grow abundantly on nutrient- and blood-agar media. They generally, not universally, grow on selective-differential agar such as deoxycholate, MacConkey, and eosine methylene blue.

Eighty-five percent of 103 strains grow in standard mineral base medium at the expense of β-hydroxybutyrate; all strains which use β-hydroxybutyrate as sole source of carbon and energy accumulate Sudan black granules. Sixty percent of 103 strains grow on mineral base medium, without growth factors, at the expense of *p*-hydroxybenzoate; all strains which use *p*-hydroxybenzoate as the sole source of energy cleave protocatechuate at the *meta* position. Only a small number of strains use testosterone as the sole source of carbon and energy. Strains which fail to grow in standard mineral base media at the expense of *p*-hydroxybenzoate, testosterone, or β-hydroxybutyrate may do so if the media are supplemented with one or more growth factors such as amino acids, niacinamide, pantothenate, and pteroylglutamate. It is apparent that standard mineral base medium containing β-hydroxybutyrate, without growth factors, is an unsatisfactory enrichment and isolation medium for many wild strains of *C. terrigena*.

Although comamonads do not produce indole, some strains produce anthranilic acid and kynurenine in tryptone broth; these and other tryptophan derivatives cause Kovacs' reagent to become orange (R. Hugh and J. D. Welch, Bacteriol. Proc., p. 148, 1969).

A neotype strain, ATCC 8461, for *C. terrigena* was designated (24) in accordance with the provisions of the International Code of Nomenclature of Bacteria (ICNB), and it has the characteristics which Gunther attributed to *Vibrio terrigenus*. *V. terrigenus* (Gunther 1894) is an older name for *Vibrio percolans* (Mudd and Warren 1923), and therefore the specific epithet *terrigena* is retained in the name applied to these organisms (26). Bacteria which have a polar tuft of flagella and which fail to ferment glucose are excluded from the genus *Vibrio* as defined by the ICNB Subcommittee on Taxonomy of Vibrios (28, 36). Numerous names, including *Pseudomonas terrigena*, have been applied to this organism (10, 24, 26, 27, 55, 70) during the past 79 years. The curved soma, flagellar morphology, and physiology of *C. terrigena* indicate a relationship to spirilla. The somatic and flagellar morphology of filamentous comamonads resembles certain spirilla. Comamonads should be included in the family *Spirillaceae*.

Pseudomonas testosteroni and *Pseudomonas acidovorans* are included in and are a segment of *C. terrigena*. Strains of *C. terrigena* which use testosterone have been designated *P. testosteroni;* strains which use ethanol and mannitol have been designated *P. acidovorans*. Other pseudomonads (41) and fungi also can oxidize testosterone.

Flagellar morphology remains a very useful criterion for the delineation of motile, alkali-producing gram-negative rods, i.e., *P. alcaligenes*, *P. diminuta*, *C. terrigena*, *Alcaligenes faecalis*, and *Bordetella bronchicanis* (30). Flagella staining is the most expedient procedure for determining the flagellar anatomy of a large number of strains of bacteria which are encountered daily in the clinical diagnostic laboratory. Many species of bacteria cannot be identified without knowledge of the flagellar morphology. The salient biochemical and morphological features of pseudomonads have been reviewed in a study of over 400 strains (21) and with the 543 strains described in Table 13.

AEROMONAS SPECIES

Aeromonas species are gram-negative, asporogenous rods 1.0 to 3.5 μm in length and 0.4 to 1.0 μm in width, with polar flagella when flagellated. The morphology and gram-reaction of *Aeromonas* and *Pseudomonas* species are similar. They are expediently differentiated by their manner of glucose metabolism: *Aeromonas* species ferment glucose; *Pseudomonas* species fail to ferment glucose although they may oxidize it. The major practical methods of differentiating *Aeromonas* species from genera of *Enterobacteriaceae*, which they resemble physiologically, are synthesis of indophenol oxidase and polar attachment of flagella by aeromonads. Although *Aeromonas hydrophila* and *Serratia* produce extracellular deoxyribonuclease, they can be differentiated because *Serratia* fails to synthesize indophenol oxidase. *Vibrio* species are anaerogenic fermenters; *Vibrio cholerae*, *Aeromonas hydrophila*, and *Aeromonas shigelloides* can be distinguished by the lysine decarboxylase, arginine dihydrolase, and ornithine decarboxylase reactions recorded in Table 14 and by other characters (12, 25, 36, 66, 67; chapter 20). *V. cholerae* strains can be grouped into serotypes and lysotypes. Serotype I strains are usually agglutinated by Gardner and Venkatraman O group I antiserum, may be hemolytic or nonhemolytic, and are the principal cause of human cholera. (See also chapters 20 and 21.)

METHODS

The methods described here are peculiar and essential to this chapter. Other media and methods mentioned in this chapter are given elsewhere.

Flagellar morphology

Formalin-treated 18-h peptone broth cultures incubated at 18 to 20 C are centrifuged, washed in distilled water, and stained for flagella by Leifson's technique (43, 44).

Motility medium

Motility medium contains: Casitone, 10 g; yeast extract, 3 g; sodium chloride, 5 g; agar, 3 g; and distilled water, 1,000 ml; pH 7.2. Suspend the ingredients in water and heat to boiling to dissolve the agar. Dispense 4 ml in 13 by 100 mm tubes. Autoclave at 121 C for 15 min.

Motility media containing higher concentrations of agar produce gels through which many motile organisms cannot spread. Ability of organisms to spread in semisolid agar is a substitute for microscope examination of wet-mount preparations. Spreading in semisolid medium is judged by macroscopic examination of the medium for a diffuse zone of growth emanating from the line of inoculation. Many aerobic pseudomonads fail to grow deep in semisolid medium in a test tube. Organisms possessing "paralyzed" flagella are nonmotile and cannot spread in the medium. Some filamentous organisms spread in or on semisolid medium but are nonmotile and nonflagellated. Although cultures may grow at 37 C or higher temperatures, the flagellar proteins of some organisms are not synthesized optimally at this temperature; hence, motility medium should be incubated at temperatures near 18 to 20 C.

The significance of the appearance of growth in motility medium requires judicious interpretation and to some extent limits the validity of the concept as the sole taxonomic criterion for differentiating species.

Strains which appear nonmotile, appear sluggishly motile, or possess very few motile cells in the total population should be inoculated into a shallow layer of motility medium, 18 to 20 ml in a 100-mm diameter petri dish (15). The medium is inoculated in the center, and motile descendants which have spread through the semisolid agar are fished from the periphery of the giant colony. Descendants selected from the periphery contain cells with a high proportion of vigorously motile cells.

2-Ketogluconate medium

2-Ketogluconate medium contains: potassium phosphate, monobasic, 5.4 g; potassium nitrate, 2 g; potassium gluconate, 20 g; and distilled water, 1,000 ml; pH 6.5. Sterilize the medium by filtration, and dispense it aseptically in 1-ml quantities in sterile 13 by 100 mm tubes. Inoculate with a loopful of a 24-h broth culture and incubate for 18 to 24 h. Add 0.3 ml of double-strength Benedict's solution to each tube. Place the tubes in a boiling-water bath for 10 min. Oxidation of gluconate to 2-ketogluconate is indicated by the presence of red-brown copper-colored precipitate (51).

Lysine decarboxylase-ninhydrin test

Use Carlquist ninhydrin base (6) available from Difco. This procedure has its greatest value in the recognition of *P. maltophilia* and *P. cepacia*.

Nitrate reduction

Combine: Casitone, 10 g; yeast extract, 3 g; potassium nitrate, 2 g; and distilled water, 1,000 ml; pH 7.1. Dispense the broth in 4-ml quantities in 13 by 100 mm test tubes containing Durham vials for the collection of gas, and autoclave at 121 C for 15 min. Cultures are inoculated, incubated at 30 C, and examined after 24 and 48 h for the reduction of nitrate to nitrogen gas, which accumulates in the Durham tube. The culture is tested for the presence of nitrite after 2 days by the addition of 0.5 ml each of reagents A and B (see below). The development of a red color indicates the presence of nitrite, provided the uninoculated control medium is negative. Cultures which fail to reduce nitrate to nitrite are detected by the addition of zinc dust to the medium to convert unreduced nitrate to nitrite.

TABLE 13. *Salient features for the identification of pseudomonads*[a]

Test, substrate or morphology	*P. aeruginosa*, 55[b]	*P. fluorescens*, 50	*P. putida*, 72	*P. pseudomallei*, 6	*P. cepacia*, 41	*P. acidovorans*, 21	*P. testosteroni*, 7	*P. alcaligenes*, 15	*P. pseudoalcaligenes*, 14	*P. stutzeri*, 45	*P. putrefaciens*, 16	*P. maltophilia*, 195	*P. diminuta*, 6
Acid													
Glucose, 1% (OFBM)	+ (100)[c]	+ (100)	+ (100)	+ (100)	+ (100)	$+^{w}$ (95)	− (0)	− (0)	$+^{w}$ (93)	+ (100)	+/(+) (100)	$+/+^{w}$ (100)	− (0)
D-Fructose	+ (96)	+ (96)	+ (99)	+ (100)	+ (100)	+ (100)	− (0)	− (0)	+ (100)	+ (100)	−/+/(+) (44)	+ (99)	− (0)
Xylose	+/− (87)	+ (98)	+ (96)	+ (100)	+ (100)	− (0)	− (0)	− (0)	−/+ (29)	+ (100)	− (6)	+/− (53)	− (0)
Lactose	− (0)	−/+ (26)	−/+ (28)	+ (100)	+ (100)	− (0)	− (0)	− (0)	− (0)	− (0)	−/+/(+) (19)	+ (90)	− (0)
Maltose	− (0)	+/− (70)	−/+ (35)	+ (100)	+ (100)	− (0)	− (0)	− (0)	−/+ (14)	+ (100)	−/+/(+) (31)	+ (100)	− (0)
D-Mannitol	+/− (71)	+ (94)	−/+ (19)	+ (100)	+ (100)	+ (100)	− (0)	− (0)	− (0)	+/− (89)	− (0)	− (0)	− (0)
Lactose, 10% (PAB)	−/+ (20)	+/− (56)	−/+ (40)	+ (100)	+ (100)	− (0)	− (0)	− (0)	− (0)	− (0)	− (6)	− (0)	− (0)
ONPG	− (0)	− (4)	− (1)	− (0)	+ (90)	− (0)	− (0)	− (0)	− (0)	− (0)	− (0)	+ (95)	− (0)
Pyoverdin	+/− (89)	+ (94)	+/− (83)	− (0)	− (0)	− (0)	− (0)	− (0)	− (0)	− (0)	− (0)	− (0)	− (0)
Hydrogen sulfide (KIA)	− (0)	− (0)	− (0)	− (0)	− (0)	− (0)	− (0)	− (0)	− (0)	− (0)	+ (100)	− (0)	− (0)
Denitrification	+/− (60)	− (2)	− (0)	+ (100)	− (0)	− (0)	− (0)	− (0)	− (0)	+ (100)	− (0)	− (0)	− (0)
Indophenol oxidase	+ (100)	+ (100)	+ (100)	$+/+^{w}$ (100)	$+/+^{w}$ (90)	+ (100)	+ (100)	+ (100)	+ (100)	+ (100)	+ (100)	− (1)	+ (100)
Arginine dihydrolase (DBM)	+ (98)	+ (98)	+ (97)	+ (100)	− (0)	− (0)	− (0)	− (0)	−/+ (14)	− (0)	− (0)	− (0)	− (0)
Lysine decarboxylase	− (0)	− (0)	− (0)	− (0)	+ (93)	− (0)	− (0)	− (0)	− (0)	− (0)	− (0)	+ (100)	− (0)
Ornithine decarboxylase	− (0)	− (0)	− (0)	− (0)	−/+ (29)	− (0)	− (0)	− (0)	− (0)	− (0)	+ (100)	− (0)	− (0)
Esculin hydrolysis	− (0)	− (0)	− (0)	+/− (67)	+/− (85)	− (0)	− (0)	− (0)	− (0)	− (0)	−/+ (25)	+ (99)	− (0)
Starch hydrolysis	− (0)	− (0)	− (0)	− (0)	− (0)	− (0)	− (0)	− (0)	− (0)	+/− (89)	− (0)	− (0)	− (0)
Deoxyribonuclease	−/+ (15)	− (0)	− (0)	− (0)	− (0)	− (0)	− (0)	− (0)	− (0)	− (4)	+ (100)	+ (100)	+ (100)

Lecithinase	−/+ (13)	+ (98)	− (0)	+ (100)	−/+ (46)	− (0)	− (0)	− (0)	− (0)	− (9)	− (0)	− (0)	− (0)
Gelatin hydrolysis	+/− (60)	+ (100)	− (0)	+ (100)	+/− (63)	− (0)	− (0)	− (6)	− (0)	− (0)	+ (94)	+ (100)	+ (100)
6.5% NaCl tolerance	− (6)	− (6)	− (7)	− (0)	− (0)	− (0)	− (0)	− (0)	− (0)	+ (100)	+ (94)	− (0)	− (0)
*p*H 5.6 tolerance (SGA)	+ (95)	+ (98)	+ (100)	+ (100)	+ (100)	+ (100)	+ (100)	+ (100)	+/− (71)	− (0)	− (0)	+ (100)	+ (100)
Cetrimide tolerance (PA)	+ (98)	+ (98)	+/− (89)	− (0)	+/− (71)	− (0)	− (0)	−/+ (12)	+/− (79)	− (4)	− (0)	− (2)	− (0)
Growth on SS agar	+ (93)	+ (98)	+ (100)	− (0)	− (2)	+ (90)	− (0)	− (0)	+/− (86)	+/− (89)	+ (94)	− (0)	− (0)
Growth at 42 C	+ (100)	− (0)	− (0)	+ (100)	+/− (71)	−/+ (29)	− (0)	+/− (82)	+ (93)	+ (100)	+ (100)	+/− (76)	+ (100)
Polymyxin-susceptible	+ (100)	+ (100)	+ (100)	− (0)	− (0)	+/− (81)	− (0)	+/− (88)	+ (93)	+ (100)	+ (100)	+/− (86)	− (0)
Growth in MBM + acetate	+ (100)	+ (100)	+ (100)	+ (100)	+ (98)	+ (100)	+ (100)	+/− (88)	+ (100)	+ (100)	+ (94)	− (4)	− (0)
Wrinkled colonies	− (0)	− (0)	− (0)	+/− (83)	− (0)	− (0)	− (0)	− (0)	− (0)	+ (100)	− (0)	− (0)	− (0)
Sudan black granules[d]	−	−	−	+	+	+	+	−	−/+	−	−	−	
No. of flagella[e]	1	>1	>1	>1	>1	>1	>1	1	1	1	1	>1	1

[a] Except where indicated, cultures were incubated at 35 C. *P. aeruginosa* strains were apyocyanogenic. Abbreviations: OFBM, OF basal medium; PAB, purple agar base; ONPG, *o*-nitrophenyl-β-D-galactopyranoside; KIA, Kligler iron agar; DBM, decarboxylase base Moeller; SDA, Sabouraud dextrose agar; PA, Pseudosel agar; MBM, mineral base medium.

[b] Number of strains.

[c] Sign: +, 90% or more positive within 2 days; −, no reaction (90% or more); +/(+), most reactions occur within 2 days, some are delayed; +/−, most cultures positive, some strains negative; −/+, most strains negative, some cultures positive; −/+/(+), most strains negative, some reactions occur within 2 days, some are delayed; $+^{w}$, weakly positive. The numbers in parentheses show the percent positive.

[d] Not all strains were tested; the results are based on the fraction of strains examined.

[e] Not all strains were examined; the results are based on the fraction of strains examined; 1, polar monotrichous; >1, polar tuft of flagella.

TABLE 14. *Differentiation of Aeromonas hydrophila, A. shigelloides, and Vibrio cholerae*

Character	*A. hydrophila*[a]		*A. shigelloides*[b]		*V. cholerae*[c]	
	Sign	Percent positive	Sign	Percent positive	Sign	Percent positive
Gram-negative, asporogenous rod	+	100[d]	+	100	+	100
Motility	+	99	+	84	+	99
Indophenol oxidase	+	100	+	100	+	100
Glucose, acid under petrolatum seal	+	100	+	100	+	100
Glucose, gas	d[e]	71	−	0	−	0
D-Mannitol, acid	+	99	−	3	+	99
i-Inositol, acid	−	1	+	100	−	0
L-Lysine decarboxylase	−	0	+	100	+	100
L-Arginine dihydrolase	+	90	+	97	−	0
L-Ornithine decarboxylase	−	0	+	100	+	99

[a] Based on a study of 163 strains, polar monotrichous.
[b] Based on a study of 31 strains, polar tuft of flagella.
[c] Based on a study of 429 strains, polar monotrichous.
[d] Figures indicate percent positive within 2 days.
[e] Different biochemical types.

Nitrite reagent A. Dissolve 4 g of sulfanilic acid in 100 ml of 5 N acetic acid.

Nitrite reagent B. Dissolve 3 ml of dimethyl-alphanaphthylamine in 100 ml of 5 N acetic acid.

Peptone broth for indole production

Combine: tryptone or Casitone, 10 g; sodium chloride, 5 g; and distilled water, 1,000 ml; pH 7.1. Dispense the broth in 4-ml quantities in 13 by 100 mm test tubes and autoclave at 121 C for 15 min. Inoculate, incubate for 48 h, and test for indole production by the addition of 0.5 ml of modified Kovacs' indole reagent (14).

Indole reagent. Kovacs' reagent, modified by Gadebusch and Gabriel (14), contains: isoamyl alcohol (isobutyl carbinol), 75 ml; hydrochloric acid, concentrated, 25 ml; and *p*-dimethylaminobenzaldehyde, 5 g. Dissolve the light-yellow crystals of *p*-dimethylaminobenzaldehyde in alcohol; then add the hydrochloric acid. Alcohols resulting in indole reagents which become deep brown in color should not be used. The above-mentioned reagent is stable at room temperature and has a light yellow color.

Standard mineral base containing β-hydroxybutyrate (70)

The composition is as follows: Na_2HPO_4 + KH_2PO_4 (1 M; pH 6.8), 40 ml; concentrated vitamin-free mineral solution, 20 ml; $(NH_4)_2SO_4$, 1.0 g; DL-β-hydroxybutyrate, 5 g; and distilled water to 1,000 ml. Dispense 4 ml into 13 by 100 mm test tubes. Autoclave at 121 C for 15 min. The copious precipitate which forms during autoclaving redissolves at room temperature to form a water-clear solution. The medium is inoculated with a needle. Smears are prepared for turbid cultures which develop in 1 to 3 days and are stained with Sudan black.

Concentrated vitamin-free mineral solution (8)

The composition is as follows; nitrilotriacetic acid, 10.0 g; $MgSO_4$, 14.45 g; $CaCl_2 \cdot 2H_2O$, 3.335 g; $(NH_4)_6MO_7O_{24} \cdot 4H_2O$, 0.0093 g; $FeSO_4 \cdot 7H_2O$, 0.099 g; concentrated metals solution, 50 ml; and distilled water to 1,000 ml. Dissolve and neutralize nitrilotriacetic acid with potassium hydroxide, about 7.3 g. Add the remaining ingredients and adjust the pH to 6.8 before making up to the final volume.

Concentrated metals solution (8)

Concentrated metals solution contains: ethylenediaminetetraacetic acid, 2.5 g; $ZnSO_4 \cdot 7H_2O$, 10.95 g; $FeSO_4 \cdot 7H_2O$, 5.0 g; $MnSO_4 \cdot H_2O$, 1.54 g; $CuSO_4 \cdot 5H_2O$, 0.392 g; $Co(NO_3)_2 \cdot 6H_2O$, 0.248 g; $Na_2B_4O_7 \cdot 10H_2O$, 0.177 g; sulfuric acid to retard precipitation, a few drops; and distilled water to 1,000 ml.

Sudan black B fat stain (5)

Dissolve 0.3 g of Sudan black B in 100 ml of 70% ethyl alcohol. Shake the solution and allow it to stand overnight before use. Dry and fix the smear with heat. Stain the slide with Sudan black for 10 min, drain, and blot dry. Wash and clear the smear with xylol. Counterstain with 0.5% aqueous solution of safranine for 10 to 15 s. The cells stain red, and the highly refractile poly-β-hydroxybutyrate granules are blue-black.

Standard mineral base containing p-hydroxybenzoate (70)

Combine: Na_2HPO_4 + KH_2PO_4 buffer (1 M; pH 6.8), 40 ml; concentrated vitamin-free mineral base, 20 ml; $(NH_4)_2SO_4$, 1 g; *p*-hydroxybenzoate, 5 g; Ionagar No. 2, 10 g; and distilled water to 1,000 ml. Autoclave at 121 C for 15 min. Cool to 45 C and pour into petri dishes. Each test must be controlled by inoculating the above medium without *p*-hydroxybenzoate.

Cleavage of protocatechuate

Growth harvested from standard mineral base containing *p*-hydroxybenzoate is suspended in 2 ml of Tris buffer. Add 4 drops of toluene and 0.1 ml of 3% protocatechuate solution. Mix the suspension. The suspension turns bright yellow within a few minutes if *meta* cleavage occurs.

The tubes which fail to produce *meta* cleavage are incubated at 30 C for 1 h and tested for the presence of β-keto groups of β-ketoadipate. Keto groups are detected by the nitroprusside test (Rothera reaction). Add 0.5 to 1 g of ammonium sulfate to each tube, followed by 2 drops of concentrated ammonium hydroxide and 2 drops of 5% sodium nitroprusside solution. Mix the suspension. A positive *ortho* cleavage reaction becomes purple.

Tris buffer

Tris buffer contains: tris(hydroxymethyl)aminomethane, 2.24 g; and distilled water to 1,000 ml; pH 8.0.

Standard mineral base containing testosterone

Mix the following ingredients in distilled water and dissolve by boiling: Na_2HPO_4 + KH_2PO_4 (1 M; pH 6.8), 40 ml; concentrated vitamin-free mineral solution, 20 ml; $(NH_4)_2SO_4$, 1 g; Ionagar No. 2, 10 g; and distilled water to 1,000 ml. Autoclave the solution at 121 C for 15 min.

Disperse 2 g of testosterone in 50 ml of distilled water by treatment for 30 min in a 9-kc, 50-W Raytheon sonic oscillator (50). Add this testosterone suspension to the hot standard mineral base. Cool to 45 C and pour into petri dishes. Each test should be controlled by inoculating the above medium without testosterone.

Organisms which use testosterone as the sole source of carbon and energy clear the agar medium of suspended testosterone around the colonies.

LITERATURE CITED

1. Ballard, R. W., M. Doudoroff, R. Y. Stanier, and M. Mandel. 1968. Taxonomy of the aerobic pseudomonads: *Pseudomonas diminuta* and *P. vesiculare*. J. Gen. Microbiol. **53**:349–361.
2. Ballard, R. W., N. J. Palleroni, M. Doudoroff, R. Y. Stanier, and M. Mandel. 1970. Taxonomy of the aerobic pseudomonads: *Pseudomonas cepacia*, *P. marginata*, *P. alliicola*, and *P. caryophylli*. J. Gen. Microbiol. **60**:199–214.
3. Blazevic, D. J., M. H. Koepcke, and J. M. Matsen. 1973. Incidence and identification of *Pseudomonas fluorescens* and *Pseudomonas putida* in the clinical laboratory. Appl. Microbiol. **25**:107–110.
4. Bobo, R. A., E. J. Newton, L. F. Jones, L. H. Farmer, and J. J. Farmer III. 1973. Nursery outbreak of *Pseudomonas aeruginosa*: epidemiological conclusions from five different typing methods. Appl. Microbiol. **25**:414–420.
5. Burdon, K. L. 1946. Fatty material in bacteria and fungi revealed by staining dried, fixed slide preparations. J. Bacteriol. **52**:665–678.
6. Carlquist, P. R. 1956. A biochemical test for separating paracolon groups. J. Bacteriol. **71**:339–341.
7. Caselitz, F. H. 1966. Pseudomonas-Aeromonas und ihre human-medizinische Bedeutung. Veb Gustav Fischer Verlag, Jena.
8. Cohen-Bazire, G., W. R. Sistrom, and R. Y. Stanier. 1957. Kinetic studies of pigment synthesis by non-sulfur purple bacteria. J. Cell. Comp. Physiol. **49**:25–68.
9. d'Aubert, S. 1963. Richerche sulle ossidasi degli schizomiceti. Ann. Microbiol. Enzimol. **13**:85–92.
10. Davis, G. H. G., and R. W. A. Park. 1962. A taxonomic study of certain bacteria currently classified as *Vibrio* species. J. Gen. Microbiol. **27**:101–119.
11. Elliott, R. P. 1958. Some properties of pyoverdine, the water-soluble fluorescent pigment of the pseudomonads. Appl. Microbiol. **6**:241–246.
12. Ewing, W. H., R. Hugh, and J. G. Johnson. 1961. Studies on the *Aeromonas* group. CDM Monograph, Center for Disease Control, Atlanta, Ga.
13. Farmer, J. J., III, and L. G. Herman. 1969. Epidemiological fingerprinting of *Pseudomonas aeruginosa* by the production of and sensitivity to pyocin and bacteriophage. Appl. Microbiol. **18**:760–765.
14. Gadebusch, H. H., and S. Gabriel. 1956. Modified stable Kovacs' reagent for the detection of indole. Amer. J. Clin. Pathol. **23**:1373–1375.
15. Gard, S. 1938. Das Schwärmphänomen in der Salmonella-Gruppe und seine praktische Ausnützung. Z. Hyg. Infektionskr. **120**:615–619.
16. Gardner, P., W. B. Griffin, M. N. Swartz, and L. J. Kunz. 1970. Nonfermentative gram-negative bacilli of nosocomial interest. Amer. J. Med. **48**:735–749.
17. Gilardi, G. L. 1969. *Pseudomonas maltophilia* infections in man. Amer. J. Clin. Pathol. **51**:58–61.
18. Gilardi, G. L. 1971. Characterization of nonfermentative nonfastidious gram negative bacteria encountered in medical bacteriology. J. Appl. Bacteriol. **34**:623–644.
19. Gilardi, G. L. 1971. Antimicrobial susceptibility as a diagnostic aid in the identification of nonfermenting gram-negative bacteria. Appl. Microbiol. **22**:821–823.
20. Gilardi, G. L. 1972. Infrequently encountered *Pseudomonas* species causing infection in humans. Ann. Intern. Med. **77**:211–215.
21. Gilardi, G. L. 1973. Nonfermentative gram-negative bacteria encountered in clinical specimens. Antonie van Leeuwenhoek J. Microbiol. Serol. **39**:229–242.
22. Gillies, R. R., and J. R. W. Govan. 1966. Typing of

Pseudomonas pyocyanea by pyocyine production. J. Pathol. Bacteriol. **91:**339–345.
23. Homma, J. Y., K. S. Kim, H. Yamada, M. Ito, H. Shionoya, and Y. Kawabe. 1970. Serological typing of *Pseudomonas aeruginosa* and its cross-infection. Jap. J. Exp. Med. **40:**347–359.
24. Hugh, R. 1962. *Comamonas terrigena* comb. nov. with proposal of a neotype and request for an opinion. Int. Bull. Bacteriol. Nomencl. Taxon. **12:**33–35.
25. Hugh, R. 1965. A comparison of the proposed neotype strain and 258 isolates of *Vibrio cholerae* Pacini. Int. Bull. Bacteriol. Nomencl. Taxon. **15:**13–24.
26. Hugh, R. 1965. A comparison of *Pseudomonas testosteroni* and *Comamonas terrigena*. Int. Bull. Bacteriol. Nomencl. Taxon. **15:**125–132.
27. Hugh, R. 1970. A practical approach to the identification of certain nonfermentative gram-negative rods encountered in clinical specimens. J. Conf. Public Health Lab. Directors **28:**168–187.
28. Hugh, R., and J. C. Feeley. 1972. International Committee on Systematic Bacteriology Subcommittee on Taxonomy of Vibrios. Int. J. Syst. Bacteriol. **22:**189–190.
29. Hugh, R., L. Guarraia, and H. Hatt. 1964. The proposed neotype strains of *Pseudomonas fluorescens* (Trevisan) Migula 1895. Int. Bull. Bacteriol. Nomencl. Taxon. **14:**145–155.
30. Hugh, R., and P. Ikari. 1964. The proposed neotype strain of *Pseudomonas alcaligenes* Monias 1928. Int. Bull. Bacteriol. Nomencl. Taxon. **14:**103–107.
31. Hugh, R., and E. Leifson. 1953. The taxonomic significance of fermentative versus oxidative metabolism of carbohydrates by various gram negative bacteria. J. Bacteriol. **66:**24–26.
32. Hugh, R., and E. Leifson. 1963. A description of the type strain of *Pseudomonas maltophilia*. Int. Bull. Bacteriol. Nomencl. Taxon. **13:**133–138.
33. Hugh, R., and E. Leifson. 1964. The proposed neotype strains of *Pseudomonas aeruginosa* (Schroeter 1872) Migula 1900. Int. Bull. Bacteriol. Nomencl. Taxon. **14:**69–84.
34. Hugh, R., and R. Reese. 1967. Designations of the type strain for *Bacterium anitratum* Schaub and Hauber 1948. Int. J. Syst. Bacteriol. **17:**245–254.
35. Hugh, R., and E. Ryschenkow. 1961. *Pseudomonas maltophilia*, an Alcaligenes-like species. J. Gen. Microbiol. **26:**123–132.
36. Hugh, R., and R. Sakazaki. 1972. Minimal number of characters for the identification of *Vibrio* species, *Vibrio cholerae*, and *Vibrio parahaemolyticus*. J. Conf. Public Health Lab. Directors **30:**133–137.
37. Jessen, O. 1965. *Pseudomonas aeruginosa* and other green fluorescent pseudomonads. A taxonomic study. E. Munksgaard, Copenhagen.
38. Klein, M. M., and D. J. Blazevic. 1972. Nucleic acid enzyme studies of nonfermentative gram-negative bacteria using thin-layer chromatography. Appl. Microbiol. **23:**276–279.
39. Klinge, K. 1960. Die Bedeutung der Oxydase-Reaktion für die Identifizierung von *Pseudomonas aeruginosa*, *Pseudomonas fluorescens* und *Pseudomonas putida*. Arch. Hyg. Bakteriol. **144:**263–276.
40. Klinge, K., and W. Gräf. 1959. Hämolyse, Eigelb-Reaktion und Amöbenauflösung durch *Pseudomonas fluorescens*. Zentralbl. Bacteriol. Parasitenk. Infektionskr. Hyg. Abt. Orig. **174:**243–252.
41. Kundsin, R. B., R. H. Underwood, and L. I. Rose. 1972. *Pseudomonas* sp. ATCC 27330 with 17-dehydrogenase activity: a contaminant in an endocrine laboratory. Appl. Microbiol. **24:**665–666.
42. Lautrop, H., and O. Jessen. 1964. On the distinction between polar monotrichous and lophotrichous flagellation in green fluorescent pseudomonads. Acta Pathol. Microbiol. Scand. **60:**588–598.
43. Leifson, E. 1951. Staining, shape, and arrangement of bacterial flagella. J. Bacteriol. **62:**377–389.
44. Leifson, E. 1960. Atlas of bacterial flagellation. Academic Press Inc., New York.
45. Leifson, E., and R. Hugh. 1953. Variation in shape and arrangement of bacterial flagella. J. Bacteriol. **65:**263–271.
46. Leifson, E., and R. Hugh. 1954. A new type of polar monotrichous flagellation. J. Gen. Microbiol. **10:**68–70.
47. Leifson, E., and M. Mandel. 1966. The DNA base composition of a flagellar mutant of *Comamonas terrigena* ATCC 8461. Antonie van Leeuwenhoek J. Microbiol. Serol. **32:**57–59.
48. Lelliott, R. A., E. Billing, and A. C. Hayward. 1966. A determinative scheme for the fluorescent plant pathogenic pseudomonads. J. Appl. Bacteriol. **29:**470–489.
49. Levin, R. E. 1972. Correlation of DNA base composition and metabolism of *Pseudomonas putrefaciens* isolates from food, human clinical specimens, and other sources. Antonie van Leeuwenhoek J. Microbiol. Serol. **38:**121–127.
50. Marcus, P. I., and P. Talalay. 1956. Induction and purification of alpha- and beta-hydroxysteroid dehydrogenase. J. Biol. Chem. **218:**661–674.
51. Moore, H. B., and M. J. Pickett. 1960. The Pseudomonas-Achromobacter group. Can. J. Microbiol. **6:**35–42.
52. Moss, C. W., S. B. Samuels, and R. E. Weaver. 1972. Cellular fatty acid composition of selected *Pseudomonas* species. Appl. Microbiol. **24:**596–598.
53. Palleroni, N. J., and M. Doudoroff. 1972. Some properties and taxonomic subdivisions of the genus *Pseudomonas*. Annu. Rev. Phytopathol. **10:**73–100.
54. Palleroni, N. J., M. Doudoroff, and R. Y. Stanier. 1970. Taxonomy of the aerobic pseudomonads: the properties of the *Pseudomonas stutzeri* group. J. Gen. Microbiol. **60:**215–231.
55. Park, R. W. A. 1962. A study of certain heterotrophic polarly flagellate water bacteria: *Aeromonas*, *Pseudomonas*, and *Comamonas*. J. Gen. Microbiol. **27:**121–133.
56. Park, R. W. A. 1967. A comparison of two methods for detecting attack on glucose by pseudomonads and achromobacters. J. Gen. Microbiol. **46:**355–360.
57. Pedersen, M. M., E. Marso, and M. J. Pickett. 1970. Nonfermentative bacilli associated with man. III. Pathogenicity and antibiotic susceptibility. Amer. J. Clin. Pathol. **54:**178–192.
58. Pickett, M. J., and M. M. Pedersen. 1970. Characterization of saccharolytic nonfermentative bacteria associated with man. Can. J. Microbiol. **16:**351–362.
59. Pickett, M. J., and M. M. Pedersen. 1970. Salient features of nonsaccharolytic and weakly saccharolytic nonfermentative rods. Can. J. Microbiol. **16:**401–409.
60. Rhodes, M. E. 1959. The characterization of *Pseudomonas fluorescens*. J. Gen. Microbiol. **21:**221–263.
61. Rhodes, M. E. 1961. The characterization of *Pseudomonas fluorescens* with the aid of an electronic computer. J. Gen. Microbiol. **25:**331–345.
62. Riley, P. S., H. W. Tatum, and R. E. Weaver. 1972. *Pseudomonas putrefaciens* isolates from clinical specimens. Appl. Microbiol. **24:**798–800.
63. Rogul, M., J. J. Brendle, D. K. Haapala, and A. D. Alexander. 1970. Nucleic acid similarities among *Pseudomonas pseudomallei*, *Pseudomonas multivorans*, and *Actinobacillus mallei*. J. Bacteriol. **101:**827–835.
64. Rogul, M., and S. R. Carr. 1972. Variable ammonia production among smooth and rough strains of *Pseudomonas pseudomallei*: resemblance to bacteriocin production. J. Bacteriol. **112:**372–380.

65. Sands, D. C., F. H. Gleason, and D. C. Hildebrand. 1967. Cytochromes of *Pseudomonas syringae*. J. Bacteriol. **94:**1785–1786.
66. Schubert, R. H. W. 1967. The taxonomy and nomenclature of the genus *Aeromonas* Kluyver and Van Niel 1936. I. Suggestions on the taxonomy and nomenclature of the aerogenic *Aeromonas* species. Int. J. Syst. Bacteriol. **17:**23–37.
67. Schubert, R. H. W. 1967. The taxonomy and nomenclature of the genus *Aeromonas* Kluyver and Van Niel 1936. II. Suggestions on the taxonomy and nomenclature of the anaerogenic aeromonads. Int. J. Syst. Bacteriol. **17:**273–279.
68. Shewan, J. M., and W. C. Haynes. 1967. Report of the Subcommittee on *Pseudomonas* and related organisms (1962–1966). Int. J. Syst. Bacteriol. **17:**255–259.
69. Spotnitz, M., J. Rudnitzky, and J. J. Rambaud. 1967. Melioidosis pneumonitis. J. Amer. Med. Ass. **202:**950–954.
70. Stanier, R. Y., N. J. Palleroni, and M. Doudoroff. 1966. The aerobic pseudomonads: a taxonomic study. J. Gen. Microbiol. **43:**159–271.
71. Stanton, A. T., W. Fletcher, and S. L. Symonds. 1927. Melioidosis in a horse. J. Hyg. **26:**33–35.
72. Sutter, R. L., V. Hurst, and J. Fennell. 1965. A standardized system for phage typing *Pseudomonas aeruginosa*. Health Lab. Sci. **2:**7–16.
73. Verder, E., and J. Evans. 1961. A proposed antigenic schema for the identification of strains of *Pseudomonas aeruginosa*. J. Infect. Dis. **109:**183–193.
74. von Graevenitz, A. 1965. Uber die Isolierung von *Pseudomonas maltiphilia* aus klinischem Untersuchungsmaterial. Med. Welt. **3:**177–178.
75. von Graevenitz, A. 1965. *Pseudomonas stutzeri* isolated from clinical specimens. Amer. J. Clin. Pathol. **43:**357–360.
76. von Graevenitz, A., and J. Weinstein. 1971. Pathogenic significance of *Pseudomonas fluorescens* and *Pseudomonas putida*. Yale J. Biol. Med. **44:**265–273.
77. Yabuuchi, E., N. Miyajima, H. Hotta, and Y. Furu. 1971. Serological typing of 31 achromogenic and 40 melanogenic *Pseudomonas aeruginosa* strains. Appl. Microbiol. **22:**530–533.
78. Yabuuchi, E., and A. Ohyama. 1972. Characterization of "pyomelanin"-producing strains of *Pseudomonas aeruginosa*. Int. J. Syst. Bacteriol. **22:**53–64.
79. Zierdt, C. H., and H. H. Marsh, III. 1971. Identification of *Pseudomonas pseudomallei*. Amer. J. Clin. Pathol. **55:**596–603.
80. Zierdt, C. H., and P. J. Schmidt. 1964. Dissociation in *Pseudomonas aeruginosa*. J. Bacteriol. **87:**1003–1010.

Chapter 24

Miscellaneous Gram-Negative Bacteria

HARVEY W. TATUM, WILLIAM H. EWING, AND ROBERT E. WEAVER

INTRODUCTION

The named and unnamed bacteria described in this chapter represent only a small part of the total collection assembled by the late Elizabeth O. King and her successors. It was through the continued efforts of Miss King over many years that these microorganisms were characterized and placed in groups or genera according to their similarities. It is evident from the numbers of cultures received that both the named and unnamed bacteria pose problems of identification in many laboratories.

The bacteria discussed in this chapter are gram-negative rod-shaped microorganisms, but cellular morphology varies considerably among members of the different genera and groups. These microorganisms also are asporogenous, and none yields a positive Voges-Proskauer test. Major similarities end here, however, and, since some do not produce acid from carbohydrates either oxidatively or fermentatively, others are oxidative, and some are fermentative, the groups and genera must be discussed separately.

MATERIALS AND METHODS

In the 24-year period between 1949 and 1973, 35,000 cultures were received for identification by Miss King and her successors. Of these, 4,489 (about 13%) belonged to the named and unnamed genera and groups of bacteria discussed in this chapter. The following is a list of these particular microorganisms. The figures in parentheses indicate the number of each species or group that was received during the above-mentioned period. These numbers should afford a general idea of the frequency of occurrence of the bacteria.

1. *Eikenella corrodens* (595)
2. *Acinetobacter calcoaceticus* var. *anitratus* (1,139)
   Acinetobacter calcoaceticus var. *lwoffi* (646)
3. *Alcaligenes faecalis* (73)
   Alcaligenes odorans (75)
   Alcaligenes denitrificans (48)
   Group IVe (29)
4. *Achromobacter xylosoxidans* biotype IIIa (118)
   Achromobacter xylosoxidans biotype IIIb (120)
   Achromobacter species biotype 1 (46)
   Achromobacter species biotype 2 (25)
5. *Pseudomonas*-like:
   Group IIk biotype 1 (127)
   Group IIk biotype 2 (41)
   Group Va biotype 1 (38)
   Group Va biotype 2 (47)
   Group Ve biotype 1 (19)
   Group Ve biotype 2 (35)
6. Group IIf (78)
   Group IIj (36)
7. *Flavobacterium meningosepticum* (187)
   Flavobacterium species group IIb (170)
   Group TM-1 (93)
   Group M-1 (*Moraxella kingii*) (29)
   Cardiobacterium hominis (25)
   Group HB-5 (38)
   Group EF-4 (93)
8. *Moraxella lacunata* (25)
   Moraxella bovis (5)
   Moraxella nonliquefaciens (100)
   Moraxella osloensis (170)
   Moraxella phenylpyruvica (62)
   Group M-3 (23)
   Group M-4 (27)
   Group M-4f (41)
   Group M-5 (41)
   Group M-6 (33)

The methods outlined here are sufficient for identification of the bacteria discussed in this chapter. Since these microorganisms comprise a heterogeneous collection, methods for their study and identification must be included in the chapter.

The following recommended methods have been devised, modified, and revised over a period of years and now may be regarded as more or less standard for the identification of these microorganisms. Basic, uniform procedures are employed in the examination of all cultures, but these basic procedures must be extended at times to include additional tests or substrates that may be necessary for accurate identification of particular isolates. The laboratory worker must exercise judgement in the choice of additional substrates or tests and in instances when the addition of enrichment to media, the use of increased carbon dioxide tension, or incubation at temperatures other than 35 to 37 C may be required. The tabular data and figures presented should be helpful in this regard.

Ordinarily, these miscellaneous gram-negative rod-shaped bacteria are isolated on blood, chocolate, MacConkey, or eosin methylene blue agar, or on other media used for plating of specimens. Gram stains and the oxidase tests (see below) may be done from colonies on some of these media (e.g., blood-agar plates). Isolates selected for further study and ultimate identification should be replated on heart infusion agar containing 5% defibrinated rabbit blood. The plates are streaked in a manner so as to obtain well-isolated colonies and the agar is stabbed several times. This procedure provides information pertaining to action on blood cells not only of surface colonies but also of subsurface growth. Plates are incubated for 18 to 24 h at 35 to 37 C in an initial atmosphere of about 3% carbon dioxide (a candle jar is satisfactory). Growth on the plates is examined with a 12× dissecting microscope or a hand lens, and data regarding colonial morphology, pigment, and action on blood cells are recorded. The oxidase test is performed by adding one or two drops of reagent (0.5% aqueous solution of tetramethyl-*p*-phenylenediamine dihydrochloride) on the growth on a portion of a plate held in a slightly tilted position. This test also may be performed by the method of Kovacs (17). The latter method is very sensitive and final readings of tests are made at 10 s.

A well-isolated colony is picked to a tube of slanted heart infusion agar, heart infusion broth, and to a tube of triple sugar iron agar (TSI; see Fig. 1). The TSI medium is inoculated over the entire surface of the slant, and the butt of the medium is stabbed to the bottom of the tube. A lead acetate paper strip is suspended over the slant of TSI agar medium. These three tubes are incubated overnight (18 to 24 h), and a record is made of characteristics such as growth, pellicle formation, pigmentation, hydrogen sulfide formation, etc. Gram stains made of growth from heart infusion agar and heart infusion broth cultures are prepared and examined.

Preliminary information as to whether a microorganism utilizes carbohydrate fermentatively or is nonfermentative is obtained from reactions in TSI medium. Acidity in the butt of TSI medium indicates that a bacterium is fermentative, whereas an alkaline or neutral slant and a neutral pH in the butt in TSI agar is characteristic of a nonfermenter. Acidity of the slant portion of TSI medium may be observed with *Pseudomonas pseudomallei* and an occasional strain of *Acinetobacter calcoaceticus* var. *anitratus* (*Herellea*), both of which utilize carbohydrate oxidatively. Differentiation of fermentative and nonfermentative bacteria on the basis of their reactions in TSI agar compares favorably with results obtained by use of open and sealed tubes of oxidation-fermentation (O-F) medium containing 1% glucose. Therefore, the reactions in TSI agar may be used as a

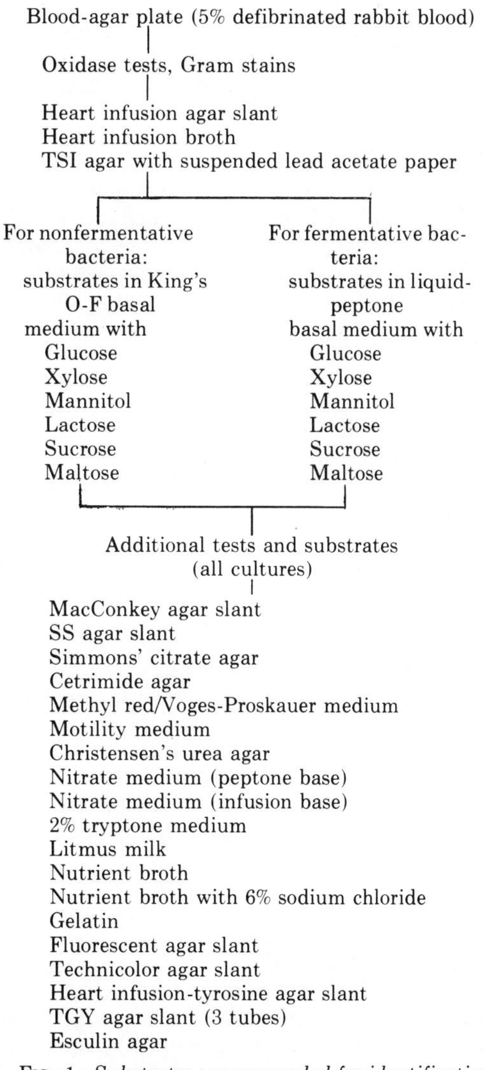

Blood-agar plate (5% defibrinated rabbit blood)

Oxidase tests, Gram stains

Heart infusion agar slant
Heart infusion broth
TSI agar with suspended lead acetate paper

For nonfermentative bacteria: substrates in King's O-F basal medium with	For fermentative bacteria: substrates in liquid-peptone basal medium with
Glucose	Glucose
Xylose	Xylose
Mannitol	Mannitol
Lactose	Lactose
Sucrose	Sucrose
Maltose	Maltose

Additional tests and substrates (all cultures)

MacConkey agar slant
SS agar slant
Simmons' citrate agar
Cetrimide agar
Methyl red/Voges-Proskauer medium
Motility medium
Christensen's urea agar
Nitrate medium (peptone base)
Nitrate medium (infusion base)
2% tryptone medium
Litmus milk
Nutrient broth
Nutrient broth with 6% sodium chloride
Gelatin
Fluorescent agar slant
Technicolor agar slant
Heart infusion-tyrosine agar slant
TGY agar slant (3 tubes)
Esculin agar

FIG. 1. *Substrates recommended for identification of miscellaneous gram-negative bacteria.*

guide in the selection of which of two sets of media (below and Fig. 1) to use with a particular microorganism. Many of the more fastidious or dysgonic bacteria grow poorly on or in TSI medium, however, and in such circumstances the laboratorian must make a more or less arbitrary decision as to which course to take leading to final identification. It perhaps is better to proceed as if such a microorganism were fermentative and to use enrichment (see below and tables) until certain.

Either of two basic sets of media for determination of carbohydrate reactions is used depending upon whether a bacterium is nonfermentative or fermentative (Fig. 1). The set for nonfermentative microorganisms consists of six substrates in the semisolid O-F medium of King (14) with phenol red indicator. The set used for fermentative bacteria is made up of six substrates in liquid peptone basal medium with Andrade's indicator. There are instances in which it is necessary to enrich this basal medium by the addition of two drops of rabbit serum to each tube to assure or enhance growth of fastidious microorganisms such as *Cardiobacterium hominis*. All media are incubated for 48 h in an ordinary incubator or in a candle jar depending upon which is considered optimal for the particular microorganism under investigation. In addition to the carbohydrate media mentioned above, each of the sets include media and test procedures which permit determination of the most important characteristics of the bacteria discussed in this chapter, and which provide sufficient data for identification of the majority of them at 48 h. These additional tests are listed in Fig. 1.

Tests for nitrate reduction and indole production are made after 48 h of incubation. The Durham inserts in the nitrate medium should be examined carefully for evidence of gas formation. Tests for indole are made by extracting the tryptone water cultures with xylol before addition of Ehrlich-Boehme reagent. Extraction is a prerequisite because many of these bacteria produce minute quantities of indole. Heart infusion broth cultures also may be used for indole determinations, especially with dysgonic microorganisms.

Methyl red and Voges-Proskauer tests are performed only with fermentative bacteria. The methyl red test is done after 4 to 5 days of incubation. The Coblentz method is recommended for detection of acetoin (acetylmethylcarbinol). Two tubes of nutrient broth are included in each set of biochemical tests (Fig. 1). These are used when needed to determine sodium chloride requirements or tolerances of various microorganisms. One of the tubes of nutrient broth contains 6% sodium chloride in which such species as *Vibrio parahaemolyticus* and *V. alginolyticus* (both of which are fermentative) may be expected to grow. Another microorganism that requires sodium chloride but is oxidative is a biotype of *Pseudomonas putrefaciens*. None of these three grows in plain nutrient broth.

The three tryptone-glucose-yeast extract (TGY) agar slants (Fig. 1) are incubated at 25, 35 to 37, and 42 C, respectively, to determine the optimal growth temperature. Occasionally, it is necessary to inoculate additional TGY agar slant cultures and incubate them at 5 C or at 50 to 65 C to determine whether a particular isolate is psychrophilic or thermophilic. The catalase test is performed by flooding the surface of the slant of the TGY agar culture that exhibits optimal growth with 3% hydrogen peroxide.

In some instances, additional tests and substrates must be used for accurate identification. These include tests for decarboxylase activities (Moeller method), production of 2-ketogluconate or 3-ketolactonate, *nitrite* reduction, and for production of phenylalanine deaminase. When necessary for definitive identification, bacteria are stained (Leifson method) to determine the arrangement of flagella.

A key to the identification of these miscellaneous gram-negative bacteria is given in Fig. 2.

EIKENELLA CORRODENS

Jackson and Goodman (11) proposed the name *Eikenella corrodens* for the microorganism originally described by Eiken (7) as *Bacteroides corrodens*. Comparison of microaerophilic bacteria designated HB-1 by King and Tatum (16) with the type strain of *B. corrodens* (ATCC 23834, NCTC 10696) indicated that these microorganisms are biochemically and serologically identical (23).

E. corrodens is a gram-negative, straight, uniformly staining, rod-shaped bacterium that does not exhibit branching. It is nonmotile and nonsaccharolytic. The microorganism is microaerophilic and exhibits optimal growth under increased carbon dioxide tension (about 3%). A slight green discoloration is produced by growth in the stabbed areas of a blood-agar plate after 24 h of incubation at 35 to 37 C. The odor elicited is characteristic; it is similar to that of hypochlorite bleach. Colonies on blood-agar plates after 24 h usually are minute to not more than 0.5 mm in diameter. Observation by oblique light reveals that colonies frequently are

INACTIVE (carbohydrates not utilized oxidatively or fermentatively)
- MacConkey negative
  - Oxidase positive
    - Catalase negative
      - Nonproteolytic: *Eikenella corrodens* (Table 1)
      - Proteolytic: *Moraxella bovis* (Tables 14, 15)
    - Catalase positive
      - Indole positive: Groups IIf, IIj (Tables 10, 11)
      - Indole negative: *Moraxella bovis, Moraxella lacunata, Moraxella osloensis, Moraxella nonliquefaciens, Moraxella phenylpyruvica* (Tables 14, 15)
- MacConkey positive
  - Oxidase negative: *Acinetobacter calcoaceticus* var. *lwoffi* (Tables 2, 3)
  - Oxidase positive
    - Nonmotile: *Moraxella osloensis, Moraxella phenylpyruvica*, Groups M-3, M-4, M-4f, M-5, M-6 (Tables 14, 15)
    - Motile: *Alcaligenes faecalis, Alcaligenes odorans, Alcaligenes denitrificans*, Group IVe (Tables 4, 5)

GLUCOSE (WEAK) OXIDIZER
- MacConkey positive
  - Oxidase positive
    - Motile: *Achromobacter xylosoxidans* biotypes IIIa, IIIb (Tables 6, 7)

GLUCOSE OXIDIZERS
- MacConkey negative
  - Oxidase positive: Group IIk biotype 1
  - Oxidase negative: Group IIk biotype 1 (Tables 8, 9)
- MacConkey positive
  - Oxidase negative
    - Nonpigmented: *Acinetobacter calcoaceticus* var. *anitratus* (Tables 2, 3)
    - Yellow pigmented: Group Ve biotypes 1, 2 (Tables 8, 9)
  - Oxidase positive
    - Motile (polar): Groups IIk biotype 2, Va biotypes 1, 2 (Tables 8, 9)
    - Motile (peritrichous): *Achromobacter* species biotype 1, 2 (Tables 6, 7)

QUESTIONABLE OR WEAK FERMENTERS
- MacConkey negative
  - Oxidase positive: Group M-1 (*Moraxella kingii*), Group TM-1, Group IIb *Flavobacterium* species (Tables 12, 13)
- MacConkey positive
  - Oxidase positive: *Flavobacterium meningosepticum*, IIb *Flavobacterium* species (Tables 12, 13)

FERMENTERS
- MacConkey negative
  - Oxidase positive: *Cardiobacterium hominis*, Groups EF-4, EF-5 (Tables 12, 13)
  - Oxidase negative: Group HB-5 (Tables 12, 13)
- MacConkey positive
  - Oxidase positive: Groups EF-4, HB-5 (Tables 12, 13)
  - Oxidase negative: Group HB-5 (Tables 12, 13)

FIG. 2. *Key to identification of miscellaneous gram-negative bacteria.*

situated in a shallow pit or crater in the agar, and upon continued incubation, for 3 or 4 days, colonies increase in size and fill the depressions. Colonies develop umbonate morphology with translucent peripheries. Some colonial variation may occur: some may not exhibit any pitting (above), whereas others may appear mottled. Growth is butyrous and pigmented (pale yellow). All cultures examined were oxidase-positive.

Growth of *E. corrodens* in broth media usually is granular, and the granules adhere to the sides of the glass tubes. Lysine and ornithine are decarboxylated. The biochemical reactions of 595 isolates that we examined were uniform with rare exceptions (Table 1). For example, only 2 strains failed to reduce nitrate, 5 grew very slightly on MacConkey agar after 5 to 7 days, and 54 yielded trace to weak (1+) catalase reactions. Pits or craters in agar media were observed in 270 (45%) of the cultures.

Of the above-mentioned 595 isolates, 255 (43%) were recovered from abscesses of the face and neck or from chest fluids and the lungs, and 98 (16%) were isolated from the abdomen, including the peritoneal cavity. Among the remaining 40%, 26 were from blood cultures, 7 were from brain abscesses, 3 were from spinal fluid, and 206 were from miscellaneous anatomical sources.

For additional information regarding *E. corrodens*, the reader should consult references 11 and 12. The microorganism discussed here should not be confused with the strictly anaerobic form presently called *Bacteroides corrodens*. The taxonomic position and nomenclature of the latter microorganism are under investigation by the Subcommittee on *Bacteroidaceae* of the American Society for Microbiology.

ACINETOBACTER

The genus *Acinetobacter* includes microorganisms previously known by a wide variety of names and designations (see the first edition of this *Manual*, p. 191, for synonyms), of which *Herellea*, *Mima*, and *Bacterium anitratum* perhaps are the best known in the western hemisphere. The members of the International Subcommittee on the Taxonomy of *Moraxella* and Allied Bacteria (20) concluded that the genus *Acinetobacter* should consist of a single species, *Acinetobacter calcoaceticus*, and that this species should include the microorganisms previously known by the specific epithets *anitratum* and *lwoffi*. We accept the species name *A. calcoaceticus*, but for practical reasons, and without prejudice, we recognize two varieties or subspecies: *A. calcoaceticus* var. *anitratus* (corresponding to *Herellea vaginicola* and *B. anitratum*) and *A. calcoaceticus* var. *lwoffi* (*Mima polymorpha*, oxidase-negative forms). A proposal has been made to designate ATCC culture 23055 as the type strain of *A. calcoaceticus* (Beijerinck) Baumann et al. (1).

TABLE 1. *Biochemical characteristics of Eikenella corrodens (595 cultures)*

Test or substrate	Sign[a]	Percent +[b]
Oxidase	+	100
Catalase	–	9[w]
Growth on MacConkey agar	–	0.8
SS agar	–	0
Cetrimide agar	–	0
Hydrogen sulfide TSI agar	–	0
Pb ac papers	(+) or –	0 (64)
Oxidation-Fermentation	I	100
Urease	–	0
Indole	–	0
Methyl red/Voges-Proskauer	–	0
Citrate (Simmons') K	–	0
Motility	–	0
Gelatin	–	0
Glucose, xylose	–	0
Mannitol, lactose	–	0
Sucrose, maltose	–	0
Esculin	–	0
Nitrate to nitrite only	+	99.7
Pigment (pale yellow)	+	100

N.B. See text for other characteristics

[a] Sign: + = 90% or more positive in 1 or 2 days.
– = no reaction (90% or more).
(+) or – = most strains positive after 3 or more days, some cultures negative.
I = Inactive
K = Alkaline reaction.
w = Weakly positive reaction.

[b] Figures in parentheses indicate percentage of delayed reactions (3 days or more).

Both varieties of *A. calcoaceticus* grow well and may be recovered on simple media without supplements or enrichment. Several types of reaction may be observed on blood-agar plates with 5% defibrinated rabbit blood after 24 h of incubation at 35 to 37 C. An occasional strain of either variety (*anitratus* or *lwoffi*) may fail to exhibit any action on red blood cells, but the majority of cultures of both varieties produce indeterminate, partial lysis of the cells rather than clear, sharp, well-defined zones of beta-type hemolysis (Table 2). Of 775 isolates of *A. calcoaceticus* var. *anitratus*, 678 (87.4%) yielded indeterminate, partial lysis, and 97 (12.5%) gave well-defined zones of beta-type hemolysis (Table 2). Similarly, of 277 cultures of var. *lwoffi*, 243 (87.7%) exhibited partial lysis, and 34 (12.5%) were beta-hemolytic (Table 2). It is characteristic that the majority of beta-hemolytic strains of either variety grow on *Salmonella-Shigella* (SS) agar medium, liquefy gelatin, and peptonize litmus milk, whereas most strains that produce partial lysis of red cells usually are not proteolytic and do not grow on SS agar (Table 2).

The colony size of *A. calcoaceticus* var. *anitratus* after 18 to 24 h of aerobic growth on blood-agar plates averages 2.0 to 3.0 mm in diameter; strains of var. *lwoffi* usually produce smaller colonies of 1.0 to 1.5 mm. Many strains of both varieties have a very unpleasant odor. An occasional strain of var. *anitratus* yields a fruity odor reminiscent of that of a pared apple. Colonies of both varieties are circular, convex, smooth, glossy, butyrous, uniformly creamy to grayish-white, and opaque, with entire edges. Strains may be encountered that are rough or very mucoid. Rough forms grow with a heavy flocculent sediment and thick pellicle in heart infusion broth, and the mucoid strains are stringy when picked and grow with a moderately thick, ropy sediment in broth. Mucoid forms are encapsulated. Colonies of the two varieties are not pigmented, but a few isolates of either exhibit a tan to slight brown soluble pigment in heart infusion agar and semisolid motility medium (Table 2).

The typical cellular morphology of both varieties of *A. calcoaceticus* consists of coccoid, diplococcoid, and plump bacillary forms. Occasional strains exhibit extreme pleomorphism, showing long, thick, wavy filaments with large

TABLE 2. *Characteristics of cultures of Acinetobacter calcoaceticus*[a]

Test or substrate	*Acinetobacter calcoaceticus* (1,002 cultures)							
	var. *anitratus (Herellea)* (775 cultures)				var. *lwoffi (Mima)* (277 cultures)			
	Indeterminate partial hemolysis (678 cultures)		Beta-like hemolysis (97 cultures)		Indeterminate partial hemolysis (243 cultures)		Beta-like hemolysis (34 cultures)	
	Number	Percent	Number	Percent	Number	Percent	Number	Percent
MacConkey agar								
Growth	678	100	97	100	227	94.5	34	100
No growth	0		0		16	6.5	0	
SS agar								
Growth	67	10	75	77	15	6	19	56
No growth	607	90	22	23	228	94	15	44
Christensen's urea agar								
Positive, 1-5 days	229	44.1	9	9	38	16	6	17
Negative, 7 days	377	55.9	88	91	205	84	28	83
Simmons' citrate agar								
Alkaline	636	94	86	89	97	40	34	100
No change	42	6	11	11	146	60	0	
Litmus milk								
Acid	300	44	15	16	0		0	
Alkaline	98	15	13	13	85	35	22	65
Acid clot	80	12	36	37	0		0	
Indicator reduction	57	8	1	1	0		0	
Peptonization	8	1	19	20	1	0.5	4	12
No change	132	19	13	13	157	64.5	8	23
Gelatin								
Liquefaction, 1-14 days	16	2	64	66	1	0.5	10	29
No liquefaction	622	92	31	32	242	99.5	24	70
Not tested	40	6	2	2				
Nitrate reduced to nitrite								
Positive	5	0.5	0		0		0	
Negative	673	99.5	97	100	243	100	34	100
Tan to brown soluble pigment								
Produced	17	2.5	0		26	11	2	6
Not produced	661	97.5	97	100	217	89	32	94

[a] See also Table 3.

swollen areas. The Gram reaction is negative; however, there is a tendency toward retention of the crystal violet stain by some cells in most cultures.

The two varieties of *A. calcoaceticus*, *anitratus* and *lwoffi*, have many characteristics in common. Both are strictly aerobic, oxidase-negative, nonmotile, and asporogenous, and are incapable of accumulating poly-β-hydroxybutyrate as a cellular reserve material. Indole, hydrogen sulfide, and acetoin are not produced and phenylalanine is not deaminated. Lysine, arginine, and ornithine are not decarboxylated. Both varieties produce strongly positive catalase reactions. Neither grows on cetrimide agar or hydrolyzes esculin. Only eight strains of var. *anitratus* have been encountered which reduced nitrate to nitrite in plain nitrate broth. In a study of six of these strains, Juni (13) confirmed their ability to reduce nitrate to nitrite and further verified their generic status as acinetobacters by deoxyribonucleic acid relatedness studies. All other strains of var. *anitratus* as well as all of the cultures of var. *lwoffi* failed to reduce nitrate (Table 2).

The utilization of various carbohydrates oxidatively with resulting acid production is the main differential characteristic between the two varieties of *A. calcoaceticus*. This reaction is more discernible in O-F medium than in liquid peptone medium. Variety *anitratus* forms acid from glucose and 10 of 27 other substrates (see Table 3 and p. 193, first edition of this *Manual*). Variety *lwoffi* does not produce acid from any of these substrates except ethyl alcohol (3%).

Cultures of var. *lwoffi* produce an alkaline reaction on the slant (K/N) of TSI agar after 24 h of incubation. Of 775 strains of *anitratus* examined in TSI agar, 758 exhibited an alkaline slant with no change in the butt of the medium after 24 h. Five cultures showed no change on either the slant or in the butt of TSI medium after 7 days of incubation, although good growth occurred on the slant. Twelve isolates exhibited weak to pronounced acid reactions on the slant of TSI medium with no change in the butt after 1 to 7 days. Strains of *Acinetobacter* do not produce hydrogen sulfide in TSI agar nor darken lead acetate papers within 24 h; however, a few cultures may produce enough hydrogen sulfide to discolor lead acetate papers slightly after about 7 days (Table 3).

Most cultures of *Acinetobacter* grow well and produce an alkaline reaction on Simmons' citrate within 24 h (Table 2). A few strains of each variety yield delayed alkaline reactions (48 h to

7 days), and occasional isolates grow sparsely on this medium but fail to alkalinize it (Table 2). Hydrolysis of urea in Christensen's medium by strains of either variety of *A. calcoaceticus* is delayed when it occurs, but most cultures are negative (Table 2).

Members of the genera *Acinetobacter* and *Moraxella* are considered to be rod-shaped. However, at times they may appear coccoid and may resemble species of *Neisseria* and *Branhamella* (4, 5), which are true cocci. The oxidase test readily differentiates the genus *Acinetobacter* from the other three genera named.

Thorough studies by Baumann et al. (1), Samuels et al. (24), and Juni (13) of a large number of oxidase-negative aerobes previously classified under different generic names give ample evidence for their classification in the genus *Acinetobacter*.

Members of the species *A. calcoaceticus* are widely distributed in nature and have been recovered from almost every conceivable source on or within the human body, including feces. Their occurrence in urine, blood, and spinal fluid has been reported. Further, they have been isolated from lower animals and from food and water.

ALCALIGENES SPECIES

Microorganisms that belong to several genera have been misidentified as species of *Alcaligenes*. This probably occurred because of the lack of an adequate definition of the genus *Alcaligenes* or because of inadequate determination of the properties of the microorganisms. We believe that a definition of this genus should include the following basic characteristics: gram-negative rod-shaped bacteria, motile with peritrichous flagellation, oxidase-positive, nonsaccharolytic, and urease-negative. The positive oxidase reaction and motility are sufficient for the differentiation of *Alcaligenes* and *Acinetobacter calcoaceticus* var. *lwoffi*. The nonsaccharolytic character of members of the genus *Alcaligenes* serves to differentiate them from the oxidizing species of peritrichously flagellated *Achromobacter*. Inability to hydrolyze urea in Christensen's medium distinguishes *Alcaligenes* from *Bordetella bronchiseptica*, which also is peritrichously flagellated and nonsaccharolytic.

Only three species of *Alcaligenes* are considered to be of sufficient importance to be included in this chapter. These are *A. faecalis*, *A. denitrificans* (19), and *A. odorans* (21).

Cultures of *A. faecalis* and *A. denitrificans* produce varying reactions on blood-agar medium after 24 h. These reactions range from indeterminate lysis to a greenish-brown discoloration. Isolates of *A. odorans* usually produce a pronounced dark green color on this medium (Table 4). No particular odor can be ascribed to *A. faecalis* or *A. denitrificans*, but *A. odorans* produces a sweetish odor reminiscent of pared apples. There are differences in the size of colonies of the three species after 24 h of incubation. Colonies of *A. faecalis* usually are about 1.0 mm in diameter, whereas *A. denitrificans* produces colonies of about 0.5 mm. Those of *A. odorans* are 1.0 to 1.5 mm with a characteristic flat, spreading periphery.

TABLE 3. *Biochemical characteristics of Acinetobacter calcoaceticus*[a]

Test or Substrate	var. *anitratus (Herella)*		var. *lwoffi (Mima)*	
	Sign[b]	Percent +[c]	Sign	Percent +
Oxidase	–	0	–	0
Catalase	+	100	+	100
Hydrogen sulfide: TSI agar	–	0	–	0
Pb ac paper	–	0	–	0
Oxidation-fermentation	O	100	I	100
Indole	–	0	–	0
Methyl red/Voges-Proskauer	–	0	–	0
Motility	–	0	–	0
Glucose	+	100	–	0
Xylose	+	100	–	0
Mannitol	–	0	–	0
Lactose	(+)	0 (100)	–	0
Sucrose	–	0	–	0
Maltose	(+) or –	0 (76)	–	0

[a] See also Table 2.
[b] Sign: + = 90% or more positive in 1 or 2 days.
– = no reaction.
(+) = 90% or more positive after 3 days or more.
d = different biochemical reactions [+, (+), –].
I = inactive.
O = oxidative
[c] Figures in parentheses indicate percentage of delayed reactions (3 days or more).

TABLE 4. *Characteristics of species of Alcaligenes and an unnamed group*[a]

Substrate or character	*A. faecalis*	*A. odorans*	*A. denitrificans*	Group IVe
Action on blood:[b] lysis	Indeterminate[c]	Indeterminate	Indeterminate	0 to Indeterminate
color[d]	Green to brown	Green to brown	Green	0
Carbon dioxide (2-4%) required	0	0	0	0
Pigment	0	0	0	0
Pronounced odor	0	Fruity	0	0
Flagellation	Peritrichous	Peritrichous	Peritrichous	Polar and long lateral flagella
Enrichment[e]	0	0	0	0
TSI agar	K/N or K/K	K/N or K/K	K/N	K/N
Litmus milk (peptonization)	–	–	–	–

[a] See also Table 5.
[b] Heart infusion agar with 5% rabbit blood.
[c] See text.
[d] Discoloration of medium around colonies.
[e] About 3% sterile rabbit serum added.
0 = None or not required.
– = Not peptonized.
K = Alkaline.
N = Neutral.

Members of the three species of *Alcaligenes* are gram-negative rod-shaped bacteria, which exhibit little variation in cellular morphology. They are oxidase-positive, grow well (heavily) on MacConkey agar, and alkalinize Simmons' citrate medium (Tables 4 and 5). All cultures of each species are nonsaccharolytic and nonproteolytic (Tables 4 and 5). They produce an alkaline slant (K/N) in TSI agar after 24 h, and the butt of this medium becomes alkaline (K/K) after 5 to 7 days. Hydrogen sulfide is not produced in the butt of TSI medium (Table 5). Most strains of *A. faecalis* and *A. denitrificans* fail to yield evidence of hydrogen sulfide production on lead acetate papers, but some isolates produce trace to moderate (2+) discoloration of the papers upon prolonged incubation (5 to 7 days). The lead acetate papers are consistently negative with cultures of *A. odorans*, even after 5 to 7 days (Table 5).

Members of the genus *Alcaligenes* do not form indole, and methyl red and Voges-Proskauer tests both are negative (Table 5). Urea is not hydrolyzed, but an occasional strain may produce an equivocal slight pink color after 5 to 7 days. Twenty-four of 73 isolates of *A. faecalis* reduced nitrate to nitrite without gas formation, whereas 49 cultures failed to reduce nitrate (Table 5). All strains of *A. denitrificans* reduced nitrate and nitrite to gas. This reduction usually was complete after 48 h of incubation, but some isolates revealed incomplete reduction of nitrite (Table 5). This is interpreted as a quantitative rather than a qualitative difference. Cultures of *A. odorans* do not reduce nitrate, but members of this species reduce nitrite to gas (Table 5). Additional reactions are given in Tables 4 and 5.

We compared the type strain (NCTC 10416) of *A. odorans* (21) with the type strain (NCTC 10388) of *A. odorans* var. *viridans* (22) and found them to be identical.

In our experience, the most frequent individual sources of *A. faecalis* cultures were as follows: the ear, 13; urine, 11; blood, 4; thoracic fluid, 3; and spinal fluid, 2. With *A. denitrificans*, these sources were blood (six cultures), ear (five), spinal fluid (five), and urine (four). In the case of *A. odorans* the most frequent individual source was urine (33 cultures). Two cultures of *A. odorans* were from ear infections, and one was isolated from spinal fluid. The sources of the remaining isolates of each of the three species of *Alcaligenes* were similar, i.e., various wounds and abscesses, as well as feces, lower animals, soil, and milk.

Group IVe

Members of this unusual group resemble species of *Alcaligenes* in some respects, and for that reason they are discussed at this point. This group is composed of gram-negative bacteria, the cellular morphology of which is coccoid, rod-shaped, or filamentous. At 24 h, growth on blood-agar plates is light, and the action on blood cells is negligible to indeterminate partial lysis in areas where growth is heaviest. Colonies are minute to 0.5 mm. Growth after 48 h is moderate, and blood cells in the entire plate may be lysed; colonies are 1.0 mm in diameter, convex, circular with an entire edge, whitish-opaque, smooth, and butyrous in consistency. Growth is more luxuriant at 35 to 37 C than at 25 C. No growth occurs at 42 C.

Cultures of group IVe are oxidase-positive (Table 5). The catalase test also is positive, but the intensity of the reactions varies from weak (1+) to strong (4+) with different strains. An alkaline reaction occurs on the slant of TSI agar (K/N) after 24 to 48 h of incubation; this is followed by alkalinization (K/K) of the butt of the medium after 5 to 7 days. Evidence of hydrogen sulfide is not seen in TSI agar, but the majority of cultures slightly darken lead acetate paper strips suspended over TSI agar cultures (Table 5).

The three most outstanding characteristics of group IVe isolants, other than their source (see below), are their rapid urease reactions, nitrate reduction, and flagellar arrangement (Tables 4 and 5). All cultures exhibit almost immediate hydrolysis of urea in Christensen's medium when the medium has been warmed from refrigerator to room temperature prior to use (Table 5). When tested after 5 days of incubation, strains of this microorganism yield a variety of nitrate reactions (Table 5). The zinc dust test for unreduced nitrate is performed as required.

Most cultures of group IVe bacteria grow lightly to moderately on MacConkey agar, but only 1 of 23 isolates grew on SS agar. The microorganisms are nonsaccharolytic, and growth is light in liquid peptone media with various carbohydrates. Growth in O-F media with added carbohydrates is very light. Indole is not produced, the methyl red and Voges-Proskauer tests are negative, and gelatin is not liquefied. The reactions obtained with other substrates and tests are summarized in Tables 4 and 5.

Frequently, it is difficult to detect motility in strains of group IVe in semisolid motility media. Motile cells sometimes are detected in wet preparations when there is no indication of motility in semisolid medium. Stained preparations made from motile cultures exhibit polar and long lateral flagella with long wavelength

TABLE 5. *Biochemical characteristics of Alcaligenes and an unnamed group*[a]

Test or substrate	*Alcaligenes faecalis* (77 cultures)		*Alcaligenes odorans* (73 cultures)		*Alcaligenes denitrificans* (50 cultures)		Group IV[e] (26 cultures)	
	Sign[b]	Percent +[c]	Sign	Percent +	Sign	Percent +	Sign	Percent +
Oxidase	+	95	+	100	+	100	+	100
Catalase	+	100	+	100	+	94	+	100
Growth on MacConkey agar	+	100	+	100	+	100	(+) or +	38 (57)
SS agar	+ or –	83	+	93	+ or –	58	–	0
Cetrimide agar	– or +^{w}	27	d	47 (11)	d	20 (8)	–	0
Hydrogen sulfide TSI agar	–	0	–	0	–	0	–	0
Pb ac paper	– or (+^{w})	0 (39)	–	0	or (+^{w})	0 (46)	d	43^w (24^w)
Oxidation-fermentation	I	100	I	100	I	100	I	100
Urease (Christensen's agar)	–	0	–	0	–	0	+[d]	100
Indole	–	0	–	0	–	0	–	0
Methyl red/Voges-Proskauer	–	0	–	0	–	0	–	0
Citrate (Simmons') K	+	94	+	99	+	92 (6)	d	10 (28)
Motility	+	91	+ or –	84	+	100	d	24 (5)
Gelatin	–	0	–	0	–	0	–	0
Glucose	–	0	–	0	–	0	–[e]	0
Xylose	–	0	–	0	–	0	–	0
Mannitol, lactose	–	0	–	0	–	0	–	0
Sucrose, maltose	–	0	–	0	–	0	–	0
Esculin, glycerol	–	0	–	0	–	0	–	0
Nitrate reduction								
Nitrate to nitrite only	– or +	33	–	0	–	0	–	8
Nitrate to nitrite and gas	–	0	–	0	–	5	– or +	27
Nitrate to amine, no gas	–	0	–	0	–	0	– or +	12
Nitrate to gas	–	0	–	0	+	100	– or +	54
Nitrite to gas	–	0	+	100	+	100	– or +	81
Unreduced nitrate (Zn+)	+ or –	67	+	100	–	0	–	5
Pigment	–	0	–	0	–	0	–	0

[a] See also Table 4.

[b] Sign:
+ = 90% or more positive in 1 or 2 days.
– = no reaction (90% or more).
+ or – = most cultures positive, some strains negative.
– or + = most strains negative, some cultures positive.
(+) or + = most reactions delayed, some occur within 1 or 2 days.
d = different biochemical reactions [+, (+), –].
w = weakly positive reaction.
I = inactive.
K = alkaline.

[c] Figures in parentheses indicate percentage of delayed reactions (3 days or more).

[d] Rapid hydrolysis of urea (see text).

[e] Frequently no growth in carbohydrate media.

TABLE 6. *Characteristics of Achromobacter*[a]

Substrate or character	*Achromobacter xylosoxidans*		*Achromobacter* species	
	Group IIIa	Group IIIb	Biotype 1	Biotype 2
Action on blood:[b] lysis	0 to indeterminate[c]	0 to indeterminate	0 to indeterminate	0 to indeterminate
color[d]	0	0	0	0
Carbon dioxide (2-4%) required	0	0	0	0
Pigment	0	0	0	0
Pronounced odor	0	0	0	0
Flagellation	Peritrichous	Peritrichous	Peritrichous	Peritrichous
Enrichment[e]	0	0	0	0
TSI agar	K/N	K/N	K/N	K/N
Litmus milk (peptonization)	–	–	–	–

[a] See also Table 7.
[b] Heart infusion agar with 5% rabbit blood.
[c] See text.
[d] Discoloration of medium around colonies.
[e] About 3% sterile rabbit serum added.
0 = none or not required.
– = not peptonized.
K = alkaline.
N = neutral.

and low amplitude.

Of 26 cultures available, 23 were from urine specimens: 10 from males, 4 from females, and 9 from humans whose sex is unknown to us. The sex of the persons from whom the remaining three strains were isolated is not known to us, nor is the anatomical source of the isolates.

ACHROMOBACTER

The generic term *Achromobacter* was introduced in *Bergey's Manual of Determinative Bacteriology* in 1923. Since then many microorganisms have been misidentified as members of this genus. Perhaps this occurred because of lack of an adequate, unambiguous definition of the genus and lack of a designated type of neotype strain of the type species (presently *Achromobacter liquefaciens*).

We believe that the genus *Achromobacter* should include only gram-negative rod-shaped, peritrichously flagellated bacteria, which are oxidase-positive, are strictly aerobic, attack carbohydrates oxidatively, and fail to produce 3-ketolactonate. The four biogroups discussed below under *Achromobacter xylosoxidans* and *Achromobacter* species possess the aforementioned characteristics. A neotype culture of *A. liquefaciens* should possess the above-mentioned characteristics and, in addition, should liquefy gelatin. However, we never have seen such a culture. A search for it should continue, but eventually it may be necessary to designate another species (gelatin-negative) as the type culture of the redefined genus.

Achromobacter xylosoxidans

Members of group IIIb (Tables 6 and 7) were named *A. xylosoxidans* by Yabuuchi and Ohyama (27), but this species is divisible into two variants or biotypes designated groups IIIa and IIIb. The bacteria of these groups differ only in the extent to which they reduce nitrate: cultures of group IIIa reduce nitrate to nitrite only, whereas strains of IIIb reduce nitrate to gas. We induced reduction to gas in about 20% of group IIIa isolates by serial transfer in the nitrate medium of Stanier et al. (26); therefore, group IIIa is regarded as a variant or biotype of *A. xylosoxidans*.

The general characteristics of cultures of *A. xylosoxidans* IIIa and IIIb are summarized in Tables 6 and 7. The bacteria of both groups are gram-negative and are noticeably barred when stains are made from broth cultures. At 24 h, growth on blood-agar is moderate with an indeterminate lysis of the blood cells. Colonies are usually less than 1.0 mm in diameter and are convex, circular, smooth, glossy, butyrous, and with an entire edge.

The oxidase and catalase tests are positive, and growth on MacConkey, SS, and cetrimide agar media is moderate to heavy. After incubation for 18 to 24 h, the slant of TSI agar is alkalinized (K/N), but hydrogen sulfide and indole are not produced. The methyl red and Voges-Proskauer tests are negative and 3-ketolactonate is not produced (Table 7). Xylose is oxidized in O-F medium within 18 to 24 h of incubation, whereas oxidation of glucose is delayed 5 to 7 days (Table 7). The other carbohydrates listed in Table 7 are not oxidized.

The most frequent individual sources of *A. xylosoxidans* IIIa were spinal fluid (14 cultures), blood (13), bronchial washings (12), and urine (11), and in the case of *A. xylosoxidans* IIIb the most frequent individual sources were blood (19), urine (12), spinal fluid (8), and wounds (7). The remainder of strains of each group were recovered from specimens from humans and lower animals and from water.

Achromobacter species

The bacteria designated *Achromobacter* species (Tables 6 and 7) differ from *A. xylosoxidans*, but a name has not been applied to them. The original group designated Vd was subdivided into two biotypes which are characterized and differentiated by means of their oxidative metabolism of certain carbohydrates (Table 7).

These microorganisms are thin, uniformly staining gram-negative rods, the general characteristics and biochemical reactions of which are similar (Tables 6 and 7): The action on blood-agar varies with different strains from none to an indeterminate lysis of the blood cells, often with a slight greening or browning of the medium.'

Differentiation of the two biotypes is made on the basis of reaction in mannitol, sucrose, and maltose media (Table 7). After incubation for 18 to 24 h, the slant of TSI agar medium is alkalinized (K/N). A rare strain of either biotype may produce a trace hydrogen sulfide reaction on the slant of TSI agar, but not in the butt of the medium. Moderate to strong (2+ to 4+) reactions are apparent on lead acetate paper strips. Urea is hydrolyzed after 24 to 48 h. Nitrate is reduced to gas. Further details are given in Table 7.

The most frequent individual sources of strains of *Achromobacter* species biotype 1 were respiratory tract (14), blood (9), urogenital tract and urine (6), wounds (3), and feces (3). In the case of isolates of biotype 2, the most frequent individual sources were blood (6), respiratory tract (5), urogenital tract and urine (5), and feces (1). The remaining cultures of each biotype were isolated from miscellaneous anatomical locations.

TABLE 7. *Biochemical characteristics of Achromobacter*[a]

Test or substrate	*Achromobacter xylosoxidans*				*Achromobacter* species			
	Group IIIa (25 cultures)		Group IIIb (25 cultures)		Biotype 1 (46 cultures)		Biotype 2 (25 cultures)	
	Sign[b]	Percent +[c]	Sign	Percent +	Sign	Percent +	Sign	Percent +
Oxidase	+	100	+	100	+	100	+	100
Catalase	+	100	+	100	+	100	+	100
Growth on MacConkey agar	+	100	+	100	+	100	+	100
SS agar	+	100	+	100	+	100	+	100
Cetrimide	+ or (+)	88 (12)	+	96	–	0	–	0
Hydrogen sulfide TSI agar	–	0	–	0	–	0	–	0
Pb ac paper	– or (+^{w})	0 (12)	–	0	(+)	0 (100)	(+)	0 (100)
Oxidation – fermentation	O	100	O	100	O	100	O	100
Urease (Christensen's agar)	–	0	–	0	+	100	+	100
Indole	–	0	–	0	–	0	–	0
Methyl red/Voges-Proskauer	–	0	–	0	–	0	–	0
Citrate (Simmons') K	+	92 (8)	+	96 (4)	+ or –	72	+	100
Motility	+	96	+	100	+	100	+	100
3-ketolactonate	–	0	–	0	–	0	–	0
Gelatin	–	0	–	0	–	0	–	0
Glucose	(+^{w})	0 (100)	(+^{w})	0 (100)	+	100	+	100
Xylose	+	96 (4)	+	100	+	100	+	100
Mannitol	–	0	–	0	–	0	+	100
Lactose	–	0	–	0	–	0	–	0
Sucrose	–	0	–	0	–	0	+	100
Maltose	–	0	–	0	–	0	+	100
Esculin	–	0	–	0	NT		NT	
Raffinose, melibiose	–	0	–	0	–	0	–	0
Nitrate reduction								
Nitrate to nitrite only	+	96						
Nitrate to nitrite and gas	–	0	+	100	+	100	+	100
Nitrate to amine, no gas	–	0	–	0	–	0	–	0
Unreduced nitrate (Zn +)	–	4	–	0	–	0	–	0
Pigment	–	0	–	0	–	0	–	0

[a]See also Table 6.
[b]Sign: + = 90% or more positive in 1 or 2 days.
– = no reaction (90% or more)
(+) = 90% or more delayed.
+ or – = most cultures positive, some strains negative.
– or + = most strains negative, some cultures positive.
+ or (+) = most reactions occur within 1 or 2 days, some are delayed.
– or (+) = most are negative, some reactions delayed.
w = weakly positive reaction.
K = Alkaline.
NT = Not tested.
[c] = Figures in parentheses indicate percentage of delayed reactions (3 days or more)

TABLE 8. *Characteristics of Pseudomonas-like bacteria*[a]

Substrate or character	Group IIk (1)	Group IIk (2)	Group Va (1)	Group Va (2)	Group Ve (1)	Group Ve (2)
Action on blood[b]: lysis	0 to indeterminate[c]	0 to indeterminate	0 to indeterminate	0 to indeterminate	indeterminate	indeterminate
color[d]	slight green	slight green	0	0	green to lavender-green	green
Carbon dioxide (2-4%) required	0	0	0	0	0	0
Pigment in growth	deep yellow	0 to slight yellow	0	0	yellow	yellow
Pronounced odor	0	0	0	0	0	0
Flagellation	1 polar	1 polar	1 polar	1 polar	Polar tuft > 3	1 polar
Enrichment required	0	0	0	0	0	0
TSI agar	N/N or K/N	N/N or A/N	K/N	K/N	K/N	K/N
Litmus milk (peptonization)	− or +	− or +	−	−	− or +	−

[a]See also Table 9.
[b]Heart infusion agar medium with 5% rabbit blood.
[c]See text.
[d]Discoloration of medium around colonies.
NB The name *Pseudomonas pickettii* was proposed recently for the bacteria of Group Va, biotype 2 (E. Ralston et al., Int. J. Syst. Bacteriol. **23**:15-19, 1973).

0 = None or not required.
K = Alkaline.
A = Acid.
N = Neutral.
− or + = Most strains do not peptonize milk, some do.
− = Not peptonized.

PSEUDOMONAS-LIKE BACTERIA

The bacteria included in this section are divided into three groups, IIk, Va, and Ve, each of which is subdivided into two biotypes for purposes of discussion and for differentiation (Tables 8 and 9). All of these microorganisms are polarly flagellated and their metabolism of carbohydrates generally is oxidative. Members of two groups (IIk and Ve) produce yellow pigment. At present, the taxonomic position of these bacteria is undecided, but their characteristics are such that they may be considered to be members of the genus *Pseudomonas*, or possibly of the genus *Xanthomonas*.

Group IIk

This group is composed of gram-negative bacteria that grow well on blood-agar and yield minute colonies after 24 h of incubation. After 48 to 72 h of incubation, the colonies are usually 1.0 mm in diameter, circular with entire edge, convex, and glossy. Colonies of biotype 1 are deep yellow pigmented while those of biotype 2 are usually pale to light yellow. Members of group IIk may exhibit no action on red blood cells, or indeterminate lysis may occur with slight green discoloration of the medium (Table 8).

The reactions given by cultures of group IIk in TSI medium are varied (Table 8). Most strains alkalinize the slant of this medium (K/N), but some yield an acid reaction on the slant (A/N). In both instances the butt of the TSI medium remains unchanged. A few isolates produce acid throughout TSI medium, which is indicative of a fermentative microorganism. Some of the latter yield equivocal results even when inoculated into O-F medium containing glucose and sealed with petrolatum. It is questionable whether these particular strains are oxidizers or latent fermenters. However, most cultures of group IIk yield unequivocal reactions in O-F medium; therefore, it is advisable to employ O-F medium for determination of the method of substrate utilization as well as for determination of which carbohydrates are utilized. Strains of group IIk yield no evidence of hydrogen sulfide production in TSI agar medium itself, but trace to strong (4+) reactions occur on lead acetate paper strips (Table 9).

Members of group IIk do not grow on SS or cetrimide agar media and do not produce indole. Lysine, arginine, and ornithine are not decarboxylated, phenylalanine is not deaminated, and 2-ketogluconate is not produced (Table 9). Some cultures are oxidase-negative. A few strains alkalinize Simmons' citrate medium, liquefy gelatin, and peptonize milk (Tables 8 and 9).

Since results of tests for motility of group IIk microorganisms in semisolid agar medium may be equivocal, wet preparations should be used. Flagella stains (Leifson's method) reveal the presence of a single polar flagellum.

The major differential characters of biotypes

TABLE 9. *Biochemical characteristics of Pseudomonas-like bacteria*[a]

Test or Substrate	Group IIk				Group Va				Group Ve			
	Biotype 1 (100 cultures)		Biotype 2 (40 cultures)		Biotype 1 (9 cultures)		Biotype 2 (14 cultures)		Biotype 1 (16 cultures)		Biotype 2 (11 cultures)	
	Sign[b]	Percent +[c]	Sign	Percent +	Sign	Percent +	Sign	Percent +	Sign	Percent +	Sign	Percent +
Oxidase	+ or –	75	+	100	+	100	+	100	–	0	–	0
Catalase	+	100	+	100	$+^w$	100	$+^w$ or –	79	+	100	+	100
Growth on MacConkey agar	d	4 (19)	+	100	+	100	+	100	+	100	+	100
SS agar	–	0	–	0	–	0	–	0	d	56 (19)	d	9 (18)
Cetrimide agar	–	0	–	0	–	0	–	0	–	0	+ or (+)	55 (36)
Hydrogen sulfide TSI agar	–	0	–	0	–	0	–	0	–	0	–	0
Pb ac paper	(+)	0 (100)	(+)	0 (100)	$+^w$ or –	56	– or $(+^w)$	0 (14)	–	$0 (6^w)$	$(+^w)$ or –	0 (55)
Oxidation-fermentation	0 or F	91 O,9F	0	100	0	100	0	100	0	100	0	100
Urease (Christensen's agar)	–	0 (4)	+	100	+	100	+	100	+ or (+)	81 (19)	+ or (+)	73 (18)
Indole	–	0	–	0	–	0	–	0	–	0	–	0
Methyl red/Voges-Proskauer	–	0	–	0	–	0	–	0	–	0	–	0
Citrate (Simmons') K	– or (+)	0 (17)	– or (+)	0 (30)	+	100	+ or (+)	86 (14)	+	100	+	100
Motility	–	0 (7)	–	0 (5)	+ or –	78[d]	+ or –	50[d]	+	94	+	100
Gelatin	–	0 (4)	– or (+)	0 (10)	–	0	– or (+)	0 (14)	(+) or –	0 (56)	–	0
Moeller's decarboxylase media												
Lysine	–	0	–	0	–	0	–	0	–	0	–	0
Arginine	–	0	–	0	–	0	–	0	+	100	–	0
Ornithine	–	0	–	0	–	0	–	0	–	0	–	0
2-ketogluconate	–	0	–	0	–	0	–	0	– or +	12	+ or –	88
Glucose	+	100	+	100	+ or (+)	89 (11)	+	100	+	100	+	100
Xylose	+	100	+	100	+	100	+	100	+	100	+	100
Mannitol	–	0	–	0	–	0	–	0	$+^w$	100	$(+^w)$ or +	$45 (55^w)$
Lactose	+	100	+	100	+ or (+)	56 (44)	–	0	–	0 (6)	– or (+)	0 (18)
Sucrose	+	100	+	100	–	0	–	0	–	6	d	$18 (18^w)$
Maltose	+	100	+	100	+ or (+)	56 (44)	–	0	+	100	+	100
Esculin	+ or (+)	50 (43)	+ or (+)	50 (43)	–	0	–	0	+	100	–	0
Glycerol	– or +	23	– or +	38	+ or (+)	78 (22)	+	100	(+)	0 (100)	+ or (+)	82 (18)
Salicin	+ or –	66	+	90	–	0	–	0	+	100	–	0
Sorbitol	–	1	–	0	–	0	–	0	–	0	+	100
Glycogen	–	97	+ or –	88	–	0	–	0	–	0	–	0
Inulin	– or +	12	+	90	–	0	–	0	–	0	–	0
Starch	–	0	+ or –	88	–	0	–	0	–	0	–	0
Nitrate reduction												
Nitrate to nitrite	–	5	– or +	38	+	100	+	100	+ or –	63	–	0
Nitrate to nitrite and gas	–	0	–	0	+ or –	56	+ or –	50	–	0	–	0
Nitrate to amine, no gas	–	0	–	0	–	0	–	0	–	0	–	0
Unreduced nitrate (Zn+)	+	95	+ or –	87	–	0	–	0	– or +	37	+	100
Pigment (yellow)	+	92	+ or –	70	–	0	–	0	+	100	+	100

[a] See also Table 8.

[b] Sign:
+ = 90% or more positive in 1 or 2 days.
– = no reaction (90% or more).
(+) = 90% or more delayed.
+ or – = most cultures positive, some strains negative.
– or + = most strains negative, some cultures positive.
+ or (+) = most reactions occur within 1 or 2 days, some are delayed.
(+) or – = most reactions are delayed, some are negative.
d = different biochemical reactions [+, (+), –].
K = Alkaline.
O = Oxidative.
w = weakly positive reaction or light growth.

[c] Figures in parentheses indicate percentage of delayed reactions (3 days or more).

[d] Very sluggishly motile in semisolid agar medium.

1 and 2 follow. Cultures of biotype 1 are made up predominantly of long rod-shaped bacteria, which produce deep yellow pigment, usually do not grow on MacConkey agar, do not hydrolyze urea in Christensen's medium, and which do not oxidize glycogen, inulin, or starch (Tables 8 and 9). Biotype 2 strains are comprised of coccoid forms and short rod-shaped bacteria, which usually are nonpigmented or produce pale yellow pigment, grow on MacConkey agar, hydrolyze urea, and oxidize glycogen, inulin, and starch. Additional reactions given by these biotypes are summarized in Tables 8 and 9.

Cultures of group IIk bacteria have been isolated, in descending order of frequency, from blood, environmental sources, spinal fluid, urine, and various wounds and abscesses.

Group Va

This group is divisible into two biotypes, which are similar but which can be differentiated by their utilization of certain substrates. Cultures of both biotypes are composed of gram-negative, short to medium length, rod-shaped bacteria. Pigment is not produced. It is characteristic that these microorganisms tend to become nonviable after 72 to 96 h in artificial media.

Cultures of group Va grow lightly on blood-agar plates during 18 to 24 h of incubation. Their action on red blood cells usually is a slight indeterminate lysis. Colonies are minute to 0.5 mm in diameter, mottled, and mucoid in consistency.

Members of group Va are oxidase-positive, usually produce weakly positive catalase reactions, and are not pigmented (Table 8). Growth does not occur on SS agar medium, esculin is not hydrolyzed, and lysine, arginine, and ornithine are not decarboxylated (Table 9). Moderate growth occurs on MacConkey agar. Alkalinization of Simmons' citrate medium and hydrolysis of urea in Christensen's medium usually are weak at 24 h, but these reactions progress and are more pronounced after 48 h of incubation (Table 9). Nitrate is reduced to nitrite or to nitrite and gas during 48 h, but a residue of unreduced nitrite is left even after 5 to 7 days of incubation (by this time, however, the cultures may have become nonviable). Reduction of nitrite by cultures that do not produce gas can be demonstrated by serial passage in the nitrate medium of Stanier et al. (26).

The major differential characters of biotypes 1 and 2 (see footnote NB, Table 8) of group Va follow. Cultures of biotype 1 oxidize glucose, xylose, lactose, and maltose, but not sucrose or mannitol (Table 9). Of these six substrates, strains of biotype 2 oxidize only glucose and xylose (Table 9). However, isolates of group Va may be encountered that yield as many as five different oxidation patterns which differ from those just described. These are intermediate or constitute additional biotypes and emphasize the fact that group Va is heterogeneous.

Members of group Va are motile when examined by means of a wet preparation made from a broth culture. Cells possess a single polar flagellum (Leifson's method).

Cultures that belong to group Va have been recovered from diverse specimens of human origin, including wounds, abscesses, and sputa. They have been isolated from environmental sources such as dialysis fluid, nebulizers, paper mill effluent, teething rings, and water.

Group Ve

This group also is divisible into two biotypes that possess distinct differential characters. Microorganisms of this group are oxidase-negative and produce yellow pigment (Tables 8 and 9). They are gram-negative, and the cells are short to medium length and slightly thickened with tapered ends; hence, they often appear to be spindle-shaped. Cells stain irregularly and frequently appear to contain vacuoles.

Growth is heavy on blood-agar plates after incubation for 24 h, and the colony size is approximately 1.0 mm in diameter. Colonies may be wrinkled or semirough in appearance. Lysis is indeterminate and the medium usually is discolored green or lavender-green (Table 8). The slant of TSI medium is alkalinized (K/N) during 24 h of incubation, there being no change in the butt of the medium. Evidence of hydrogen sulfide production is not apparent in TSI medium, but some strains produce slight discoloration of lead acetate paper strips (Table 9).

The major differential characteristics of the two biotypes follow. Cultures of biotype 1 oxidize salicin but not sorbitol, hydrolyze esculin, and dihydrolyze or decarboxylate arginine; the cells possess multitrichous polar flagella. Nitrate reduction, gelatin liquefaction, and peptonization of litmus milk also are differential when positive (Tables 8 and 9). Strains of biotype 2 oxidize sorbitol but not salicin and do not hydrolyze esculin or arginine; the cells possess a single polar flagellum. Nitrate is not reduced, gelatin is not liquefied, and milk is not peptonized. We believe that there are sufficient differences between these biotypes to warrant their acceptance as separate species.

Microorganisms of group Ve have been re-

TABLE 10. *Characteristics of bacteria of groups 2f and 2j*[a]

Substrate or character	Group IIf	Group IIj
Action on blood:[b] lysis	0	indeterminate[c]
color[d]	lavender-green	lavender-green
Carbon dioxide (2-4%) required	0	0
Soluble pigment	tan to brown	tan to brown
Pronounced odor	0	0
Flagellation	Atrichous	Atrichous
Enrichment required[e]	0	0
TSI agar	K/N	K/N
Litmus milk (peptonization)	+	− or +

[a] See also Table 11.
[b] Heart infusion agar medium with 5% rabbit blood.
[c] See text.
[d] Discoloration of medium around colonies.
[e] About 3% sterile rabbit serum added.
0 = None or not required.
\+ = Milk peptonized.
− or + = Most strains do not peptonize, some do.
K = Alkaline.
N = Neutral.

covered from specimens from a variety of anatomical sources in the human; however, the most frequent source is wounds and abscesses.

GROUPS IIf AND IIj

Gram-negative microorganisms in groups IIf and IIj possess unusual characteristics; they produce indole, but are nonsaccharolytic. However, indole production is weak, and the indole must be extracted before tests are made with Ehrlich-Boehme reagent. The microorganisms are nonmotile.

Group IIf

Bacteria of this group are eugonic and grow heavily on blood-agar medium within 18 to 24 h; there is production of lavender-green discoloration of the blood cells (Table 10). Colonies are 1.0 to 1.5 mm in diameter, convex with entire edges, yellowish-opaque, and very moist. If the upper portion of an agar slant is inoculated, the growth frequently flows down to the bottom of the slant within 24 h. When growth from a heart infusion agar culture is examined, the microorganisms appear as coccoid forms and short rod-shaped bacteria; from a broth culture, they appear as rods of medium length together with filaments.

Members of group IIf alkalinize the slant of TSI medium (K/N) within 18 to 24 h (Table 10). There is no evidence of hydrogen sulfide production in the butt of TSI medium, but slight discoloration (1+ to 2+ reactions) occurs on lead acetate paper strips (Table 11).

Group IIf bacteria produce tan or amber to brown soluble pigment, are oxidase-positive, and yield moderately strong (1+ to 2+) catalase reactions (Tables 10 and 11). Growth does not occur in nutrient broth that contains 6% sodium chloride, nor does it occur on SS, cetrimide, or Simmons' citrate media (Table 11). A few strains grow slowly on MacConkey agar. Good growth occurs in O-F medium with various carbohydrates, but acid is not formed (Table 11). Gelatin is liquefied and milk is peptonized (Tables 10 and 11).

Of 76 isolates of IIf bacteria, 56 (74%) were recovered from human females: urine, 26; cervix, 11; vagina, 12; cyst of Bartholian gland 1; blood, umbilical stump, and ear, 1 each. Only five cultures (6.6%) were isolated from males: urethra, three; spinal fluid, one, and blood, one. The sex of 11 patients was unknown to us, but seven of the strains were from urine, and one each was from the abdominal cavity, a pelvic inflammation, spinal fluid, and the mastoid process. The sources of four cultures were unknown.

Group IIj

The microorganisms of this group yield moderate growth on blood-agar plates after 24 h of incubation. Colonies are usually no more than 0.5 mm in diameter, convex, circular with entire edges, translucent, smooth, glossy, and butyrous. Some cultures have no action on red blood cells, whereas others produce slight green to pronounced lavender-green discoloration of the cells within 24 h. The cellular morphology is that of medium length to long, thin rods. Often, pleomorphic cells may be observed which have bulbous ends and thin centers, giving the appearance of the cell being stretched or pulled apart.

Bacteria of group IIj produce tan to brown soluble pigment, are oxidase-positive, and yield moderately strong (1+ to 2+) catalase reactions. The slant of TSI medium is alkalinized (K/N), but the reaction generally is delayed 48 h or more. There is no evidence of hydrogen sulfide production in TSI agar, but weak to moderate (1+ to 2+) discoloration of lead acetate paper strips occurs. Growth does not occur in nutrient broth that contains 6% sodium chloride, nor does it occur on MacConkey, SS, cetrimide, or Simmons' citrate media (Table 11). When inoculated heavily on Christensen's medium, urea is hydrolyzed rapidly.

Growth usually does not occur in O-F media and nitrate is not reduced (Table 11). Gelatin is liquefied, but only 4 of 36 cultures peptonized milk (Tables 10 and 11).

Of 36 cultures of group IIj bacteria, 17 were recovered from infected lesions that resulted from bites or scratches of dogs or cats. Eleven other strains were isolated from humans, but it is not known whether there was a history of a bite or scratch; these were isolated from various anatomical sources such as spinal fluid, blood, and sputa. Seven isolates were from lower animals, including dogs and cats.

FLAVOBACTERIUM AND OTHER FERMENTATIVE BACTERIA

Flavobacterium

F. meningosepticum, characterized by King (15), and the unnamed species of *Flavobacterium* labeled group IIb have characteristics in common, but are sufficiently different (Tables 12 and 13) to permit easy identification. The flavobacteria are fermentative, but may appear to be inert during the first 24 or 48 h of incubation. When inoculated into O-F medium containing glucose and sealed with petrolatum, acid production is minimal and may be delayed several days. Since reactions in liquid peptone media with carbohydrates often are delayed as long as 14 to 21 days, it is advisable to treat flavobacteria as oxidizers and employ O-F media (unsealed) for determination of carbohydrate reactions.

Flavobacteria are long, thin, rod-shaped gram-negative bacteria, which usually exhibit slightly bulbous ends. A lavender-green discoloration of the red blood cells occurs in

TABLE 11. *Biochemical characteristics of groups 2f and 2j*[a]

Test or substrate	Group IIf (78 cultures)		Group IIj (36 cultures)	
	Sign[b]	Percent +[c]	Sign	Percent +
Oxidase	+	100	+	94
Catalase	+	99	+	100
Growth on MacConkey agar	– or (+)	0 (10)	–	0
SS agar	–	0	–	0
Cetrimide agar	–	0	–	0
Hydrogen sulfide TSI agar	–	0	–	0
Pb ac paper	+[d]	97	+[w]	97
Oxidation – fermentation	I	100	I or NG	100
Urease (Christensen's agar)	– or (+[w])	0 (32)	+[e]	100
Indole	+	100	+	100
Methyl red/Voges-Proskauer	–	0	–	0
Citrate (Simmons') K	–	0	–	0
Motility	–	0	–	0
Gelatin	+	100	+	94
Glucose, xylose	–	0	–[f]	0
Mannitol, lactose	–	0	–	0
Sucrose, maltose	–	0	–	0
Esculin, glycerol	–	0	–	0
Nitrate to nitrite	–	0	–	0
Unreduced nitrate (Zn +)	+	100	+	100
Pigment (tan or amber to brown)	+	100	+	94

[a] See also Table 10.

[b] Sign:
+ = 90% or more positive in 1 or 2 days.
– = no reaction (90% or more).
– or (+) = most are negative, some are positive delayed.
K = Alkaline.
I = Inactive.
NG = No growth.
w = Weakly positive reaction.

[c] Figures in parentheses indicate percentage of delayed reactions (3 days or more).

[d] Trace to 3+ reaction.

[e] Rapid hydrolysis of urea (see text).

[f] Frequently no growth in carbohydrate media.

TABLE 12. *Characteristics of Flavobacterium, Cardiobacterium, and other fermentative bacteria*[a]

Substrate, character, or morphology	Questionable or weakly fermentative				Fermentative		
	Flavobacterium meningosepticum	*Flavobacterium* species Group IIb	Group TM-1	Group M-1 (*Moraxella kingii*)	*Cardiobacterium hominis*	Group HB-5	Group EF-4
Action on blood:[b] lysis	0	indeterminate[c]	0 to indeterminate	Beta-like	0	0 to indeterminate	0 to indeterminate
color[d]	lavender-green	lavender-green	0	0	0	0 to slight green	0 to slight green
Carbon dioxide (2-4%)	0	0	Preferred	Preferred	Preferred	Preferred	Preferred
Pigment in growth	slight yellow	yellow	0	0	0	0	0
Pronounced odor	0	0[e]	0	0	0	0	0
Flagellation	atrichous	atrichous	atrichous	atrichous	atrichous	atrichous	atrichous
Enrichment[f]	0	0	required	usually required	required	0	0
TSI agar	K/N	K/N	K/N or N/N	N/N or A/N[c]	A/A	A/A	K/A or K/N
Litmus milk (peptonization)	+	+	–	+ or –	–	–	–

[a]See also Table 13.
[b]Heart infusion agar with 5% rabbit blood.
[c]See text.
[d]Discoloration of medium around colonies.
[e]Some strains (about 8%) produce a fruity odor.
[f]About 3% sterile rabbit serum added.
0 = None or not required.
+ = Milk peptonized.
– = Not peptonized.
K = Alkaline.
N = Neutral.
A = Acid.

blood-agar medium during 18 to 24 h of incubation on blood-agar plates, indicative of their proteolytic nature (Table 12).

Colonies of *F. meningosepticum* after 18 to 24 h of incubation are about 1.0 mm in diameter, circular with an entire edge, convex, smooth or slightly mottled, glistening, and butyrous, and produce a slightly yellow pigment (Table 12). Colonies of group IIb bacteria are similar but there is a definite yellow pigment (Table 12).

The above-mentioned flavobacteria produce oxidase and catalase and grow heavily in nutrient broth; however, growth does not occur in nutrient broth containing 6% sodium chloride. The slant of TSI medium usually is alkalinized (K/N) after 18 to 24 h of incubation. Some strains of group IIb produce acid on the slant of TSI medium (A/N). Production of hydrogen sulfide is not evident in TSI agar, but reactions on lead acetate papers are moderate to strong (2+ to 4+). The cells are nonmotile and do not grow on SS or cetrimide agar media (Table 13). Indole is produced, but the amount formed is small. Therefore, extraction with xylol is necessary. Gelatin is liquefied and milk is peptonized (Tables 12 and 13).

Of 185 cultures of *F. meningosepticum* studied, 96% grew on MacConkey agar, whereas 64% of group IIb strains did so (see also Table 13). Growth on this medium may be light or moderate and may be delayed 5 to 7 days. With few exceptions, strains of *F. meningosepticum* are urease-negative, but many isolates of group IIb bacteria are urease-positive (Table 13). Nitrate is not reduced by isolates of *F. meningosepticum* nor by most strains of group IIb. However, some cultures of the latter bacteria reduce both nitrate and nitrite to an anaerogenic amine (Table 13). Other differential characteristics are given in Tables 12 and 13. Tests made with 10 cultures each of *F. meningosepticum* and group IIb bacteria indicated that isolates of the former species are β-galactosidase-positive and nonlipolytic in corn oil medium, whereas strains of the latter (IIb) are β-galactosidase-negative and lipolytic.

The aforementioned flavobacteria are free-living microorganisms, and their natural habitat apparently is soil and water. However, *F. meningosepticum* has high virulence and selectivity for infants with a predilection for prematures. This microorganism has been involved in several episodes of meningitis in hospital nurseries, in which the mortality rates were high. It has been isolated from the nipples of nursing bottles, sink traps, and hoses attached to faucets in delivery rooms. This subject was reviewed by Brody et al. (see 15), King (15), and Eeckles et al. (6). Group IIb bacteria have been isolated from a variety of specimens of human origin, but are not known to have been incriminated in a nursery outbreak.

Group TM-1

The bacteria of this group, which was characterized and designated TM-1 by Hollis et al. (10), superficially resemble *Eikenella corrodens*, members of groups M-1 (*Moraxella kingii*)

TABLE 13. *Biochemical characteristics of Flavobacterium, Cardiobacterium, and other fermentative bacteria*[a]

Test or Substrate	Questionable or weakly fermentative								Fermentative					
	Flavobacterium meningosepticum (25 cultures)		*Flavobacterium* species Group IIb (25 cultures)		Group TM-1 (24 cultures)		Group I (*Moraxella kingii*) (28 cultures)		*Cardiobacterium hominis* (25 cultures)		Group HB-5 (34 cultures)		Group EF-4 (85 cultures)	
	Sign[b]	Percent +[c]	Sign	Percent +	Sign	Percent +	Sign	Percent +	Sign	Percent +	Sign	Percent +	Sign	Percent +
Oxidase	+	100	+	96	+	100	+	100	+	100	$+^{w}$ or –	59	+	100
Catalase	+	100	+	100	– or +	13	–	0	–	0	–	3^{w}	+	100
Growth on MacConkey agar	+ or (+)	60 (32)	(+) or –	0 (64)	–	0	–	0	–	0	$(+^{w})$ or –	0 (68)	$(+^{w})$ or –	0 (65)
SS agar	–	0	–	0	–	0	–	0	–	0	–	0	–	$0 (4^{w})$
Cetrimide	–	0	–	0	–	0.	–	0	–	0	–	0	–	0
Hydrogen sulfide TSI agar	–	0	–	0	–	0	–	0	–	0	–	0	–	0
Pb ac paper	+	100	+	100	$(+^{w})$ or –	0 (71)	– or $+^{w}$	43	$+^{w}$ or –	84	(+)	0 (94)	(+)	0 (96)
Oxidation-fermentation	F^{w}	100	F^{w}	100	(F^{w})[a]	0 (100)	F^{w}[a]	36 (57)	F	100	F	100	F	100
Urease (Christensen's agar)	–	3	d	8 (56)	–	0	–	0	–	0	–	0	–	0
Indole	+	100	+	96	–	0	–	0	+	96	+	100	–	0
Methyl red	–	0	–	0	–	0	–	0	(+) or –	0 (84)[d]	–	0	– or $(+^{w})$	0 (11)
Voges-Proskauer	–	0	–	0	–	0	–	0	–	0	–	0	–	0
Citrate (Simmons') K	–	0 (4)	–	0 (4)	–	0	–	0	–	0	–	0	–	0
Motility	–	0	–	0	–	0	–	0	–	0	–	0	–	0
Gelatin	+ or (+)	84 (16)	(+) or –	0 (88)	–	0	–	0	–	0	–	0	– or (+)	0 (25)
Glucose	+	100	+ or (+)	52 (48)	(+)	0 (100)	$(+^{w})$ or $+^{w}$	36 (57)	+ or (+)	68[e] (32)[e]	+[f]	97 (3)	+ or (+)	82 (18)
Xylose	–	0	– or (+)	0 (40)	–	0	–	0	–	0	–	0	–	0
Mannitol	+	92 (8)	– or (+)	0 (16)	–	0	–	0	d	24 (64)	–	0	–	0
Lactose	d	12 (36)	–	0	–	0	–	0	–	0	–	0	–	0
Sucrose	–	0	– or (+)	0 (20)	–	0	–	0	(+) or +	36 (60)	–	0	–	0
Maltose	+	92 (8)	(+) or –	44 (52)	–	0	$+^{w}$ or $(+^{w})$	61 (36)	+ or (+)	64 (32)	–	0	–	0
Esculin	(+)	0 (96)	(+) or –	0 (84)	–	0	–	0	–	0	–	0	–	0
Nitrate reduction														
Nitrate to nitrite	–	0	–	4			– or $+^{w}$	11	–	0	+	100	– or +	26
Nitrate to nitrite and gas	–	0	–	0	+	100							+ or –	55
Nitrate to amine, no gas	–	0	– or +	19	–	0							– or +	15
Unreduced nitrate (Zn+)	+	100	+ or –	68	–	0	+ or –	89	+	100			–	4
Pigment (yellow)	+	100	+	100	–	0	–	0	–	0	–	0	–	0

[a] See also Table 12 and text.
[b] Sign: + = 90% or more positive in 1 or 2 days.
(+) = 90% or more positive after 3 or more days.
– = no reaction (90% or more).
– or + = most strains negative, some cultures positive.
+ or (+) = most reactions occur within 1 or 2 days, some are delayed.
(+) or – = most reactions delayed, some are negative.
K = Alkaline
F = Fermentative
(F) = Fermentative reaction delayed 3 or more days.
w = Weakly positive reaction or light growth.
[c] Figures in parentheses indicate percentage of delayed reactions (3 days or more).
[d] Methyl red tests positive after 5 days.
[e] Some strains produce only weakly acid reactions in carbohydrate media.
[f] Small volumes (bubble to 10%) of gas are produced after 3 or more days.

and EF-4, and *Neisseria* with respect either to cellular or colonial morphology, as well as some biochemical characteristics. They can be differentiated easily, however.

Group TM-1 is composed of gram-negative, coccoid to short, straight rod-shaped bacteria. Pairs and short chains may be observed and occasionally a long rod-shaped bacterium is seen. This microorganism has been isolated most frequently on Thayer-Martin (TM) selective medium inoculated with pharyngeal swabs collected during surveys for carriers of meningococci. The colonies, after 24 h of incubation on blood-agar, are usually no more than 0.5 mm in diameter, circular, low convex, and semitranslucent. Some strains of group TM-1 bacteria exhibit pitting of agar media comparable to that given by cultures of *Eikenella corrodens*. The colonial morphology of strains of TM-1 that do not pit agar is similar to that of *Neisseria gonorrhoeae* and *N. lactamica*. However, cellular morphology is sufficient to differentiate *Neisseria*.

The TM-1 bacteria are oxidase-positive, catalase-negative, nonproteolytic, and nonmotile (Tables 12 and 13). The red cells in blood-agar medium usually are unaffected, but occasionally a slight green discoloration may be seen. Alkaline reactions on the slant of TSI medium (K/N) are delayed; no doubt this is the result of the dysgonic nature of the microorganisms. Often there is no pH change in the slant or the butt (N/N) of this medium (Table 12).

Acid is produced slowly in liquid peptone medium with added carbohydrates (Table 13), and addition of a few drops of rabbit serum to each tube may be necessary to assure adequate growth of some strains. Acid is not produced from xylose, mannitol, lactose, sucrose, or maltose. Indole is not produced, and decarboxylation of lysine, arginine, or ornithine does not occur. Nitrate is reduced to nitrite and gas (Table 13).

Means for differentiation of TM-1 bacteria from allied bacteria (e.g., members of group EF-4) are given in Table 13. For example, the EF-4 bacteria are catalase-positive and do not grow on TM medium. Moreover, arginine is dihydrolyzed or decarboxylated by strains of EF-4.

Group M-1

Members of this group, so designated by King (14), subsequently were named *Moraxella kingii* (8). However, since they are saccharolytic, we do not believe that the group M-1 bacteria should be classified in the genus *Moraxella*. Furthermore, the members of the Subcommittee on *Moraxella* and Allied Bacteria (20) do not recognize these microorganisms as *Moraxella*.

The cellular morphology of group M-1 microorganisms is similar to that presented by moraxellae (see below). Colonies on blood-agar plates produce beta-like hemolysis, and the bacteria are oxidase-positive and catalase-negative. After 24 h of incubation on blood-agar, the colonies are usually 0.5 mm in diameter, increasing to approximately 1.0 mm after 48 h. They are low convex, nonpigmented, semiopaque, glossy, and smooth. Many strains exhibit pitting in the agar.

About 35% of group M-1 bacteria do not grow on TSI medium, about 25% grow but do not change the indicator in the slant or the butt of the medium (N/N), about 10% produce acid on the slant only (A/N), and the remainder alkalinize the slant (K/N). Rarely, a strain produces acid throughout (A/A) in TSI agar (Table 12). Most isolates do not discolor lead acetate paper strips but some produce trace to weak (1+) reactions. About 10% of cultures grow very lightly on MacConkey agar; growth does not occur on SS, cetrimide, or Simmons' citrate media (Table 13). Moreover, group M-1 bacteria do not grow in nutrient broth.

Acid is produced from glucose and maltose in liquid peptone medium, but xylose, mannitol, lactose, and sucrose are not utilized. About 80% of group M-1 cultures peptonize milk. Gelatin is not liquefied, urea is not hydrolyzed, and nitrate is reduced to nitrite only rarely (Tables 12 and 13).

Of 27 strains belonging to group M-1, 12 were recovered from blood and 9 were isolated from throats. The remainder originated in specimens from various anatomical sites. None was from spinal fluid.

Cardiobacterium hominis

Members of this species were designated group IId by King (14) and were named by Slotnick and Dougherty (25). This species is composed of gram-negative rod-shaped bacteria, which are pleomorphic with bulbous ends, and which have a tendency to retain some of the crystal violet stain. Frequently, the cells occur in clusters that resemble a rosette.

Cultures of *C. hominis* do not hemolyze red cells when cultivated on agar plates that contain 5% rabbit blood (Table 12). Colonies on blood-agar after 24 h of incubation are minute but attain a size of 1.0 mm after 48 h. They are convex, circular with entire edges, smooth, glossy, and butyrous. Recommended conditions of incubation are 35 to 37 C with increased carbon dioxide tension (about 3%).

C. hominis is fermentative and produces acid throughout TSI medium (A/A), but there is no evidence of hydrogen sulfide production in this medium. Most strains yield trace to moderate (2+) reactions on lead acetate paper strips (Table 13). However, many strains fail to discolor such papers.

These microorganisms are oxidase-positive, catalase-negative, nonproteolytic, and nonmotile. They do not grow on MacConkey, SS, cetrimide, or Simmons' citrate media. Urea is not hydrolyzed and nitrate is not reduced (Tables 12 and 13). Indole is formed, but the amount produced within 48 h is small, and extraction with xylol generally is necessary for its demonstration.

Since the bacteria are fermentative, acid is produced in both open and sealed tubes of O-F medium containing glucose. Carbohydrate utilization may be determined in liquid peptone medium to which about two drops of rabbit serum per tube have been added to insure adequate growth. Various degrees of acidity are produced from glucose, mannitol, sucrose, and maltose within 2 to 7 days. Xylose and lactose are not fermented (Table 13).

C. hominis undoubtedly is a significant etiological agent of endocarditis in humans (25). Of 25 cultures studied, 22 were isolated from blood, and single isolates were recovered from specimens of sputum, thoracic fluid, and spinal fluid.

Group HB-5

This arbitrary designation is applied to a group of fermentative microorganisms which are quite uniform in their biochemical characteristics. The group is composed of gram-negative, coccoid to rod-shaped bacteria of medium length.

Recommended conditions for growth are incubation for 18 to 24 h under increased carbon dioxide tension (about 3%). Under such conditions, colonies on blood-agar plates usually are 0.5 to 1.0 mm in diameter and smooth, entire, and convex in appearance. Sometimes colonies are mottled. The red cells in this medium are not hemolyzed and usually are not discolored. Occasionally, however, there is slight green discoloration of the cells, particularly in stabbed areas.

HB-5 bacteria are fermentative and produce acid throughout (A/A) in TSI medium. Some strains produce a small amount of gas in the butt of this medium. There is no evidence of hydrogen sulfide production in TSI agar, but trace to moderate (2+) reactions are seen on lead acetate paper strips. Most cultures do not grow in O-F medium containing glucose.

The microorganisms are oxidase-positive, although about 40% of strains produce weakly positive reactions. They are catalase-negative and nonproteolytic. About 68% grow lightly on MacConkey medium after 5 to 7 days, but growth does not occur on SS, cetrimide, or Simmons' citrate medium (Table 13). Urea is not hydrolyzed, and lysine, arginine, and ornithine are not decarboxylated. HB-5 strains grow moderately well in nutrient broth but not in the same medium with 6% sodium chloride added. Indole is produced in small amounts (Table 13); hence, extraction with xylol is necessary before tests are made. Nitrate is reduced to nitrite.

Fermentation tests are made in liquid peptone medium with added carbohydrate and enriched by the addition of sterile rabbit serum. Glucose, fructose, and mannose are fermented with production of small volumes (10% or less of Durham insert) of gas. Some isolates also ferment galactose and glycerol, but acid production is weak. Twenty-two other carbohydrate substrates (see list, p. 193, first edition of this *Manual*) are not attacked.

In our experience, most (53%) cultures of HB-5 bacteria originated in specimens from human females (vagina and labia, three; urine, three; placenta, three; Bartholian gland, two; rectal abscess, two; infected fingers, two; and one each from cervix, amniotic fluid, lochia, and blood). Fourteen strains were isolated from males (urine, four; penile lesions, two; urethral exudates, two; rectal abscess, two; and one each from scrotal abscess, leg abscess, fistula, and surgical incision). The sex of patients from whom three cultures were recovered is unknown to us, but one originated in a urine specimen and two were from blood.

Group EF-4

This group of microorganisms is composed of gram-negative, short, rod-shaped bacteria. Small coccoid forms, long rods, and chains of four to seven cells also may be observed. These bacteria are eugonic and their metabolism of carbohydrates is fermentative.

Bacteria of group EF-4 may have no effect on the cells in blood-agar plates or may produce an indeterminate reaction. A slight green discoloration of the blood cells in this medium may occur (Table 12). After 24 h of incubation, the colonies average 1.0 mm in diameter and are convex, entire, circular, semi-opaque, and smooth. The slant of TSI medium is alkalinized after 24 to 48 h of incubation, and most cultures produce acid in the butt of the medium (K/A). However, some strains fail to acidify the butt portion of this medium (K/N). There is no evidence of hydrogen sulfide production in TSI medium, but trace to moderate (2+) reactions occur on lead acetate papers (Table 13).

Members of this group are nonmotile, are oxidase- and catalase-positive, and produce a soluble yellow to tan pigment. About 64% of strains grow lightly and slowly (5 to 7 days) on MacConkey medium, but they do not grow on SS, cetrimide, or Simmons' citrate media (Table 13). Urea is not hydrolyzed in Christensen's medium and indole is not formed. About 60% of cultures dihydrolyze or decarboxylate arginine, but lysine and ornithine are not decarboxylated. Milk is not peptonized and only about 33% of isolates liquefy gelatin (5 to 15 days). When tests are made after 48 h of incubation, a variety of nitrate reactions are observed (Table 13). The reduction of nitrate and nitrite without gas recorded in Table 13 occurred in infusion-base medium, not in peptone-base medium. Good growth occurs in nutrient broth, but EF-4 bacteria do not grow in nutrient broth containing 6% sodium chloride.

Cultures of EF-4 produce acid in open and sealed tubes of O-F medium containing glucose. Most strains ferment glucose within 24 h in liquid peptone medium, but some isolates required 5 to 7 days (Table 13). Other carbohydrates (see list, p. 193, first edition of this *Manual*) are not fermented.

Of 85 strains of EF-4 microorganisms, 32 were isolated from wounds in humans who had been bitten by dogs or cats. Thirty-four other isolates were recovered from wounds in humans, but in these instances it is not known whether the wounds resulted from bites of animals. A few cultures were isolated from other extraintestinal sources in humans. Eleven were isolated from dogs: gums, mandible, lung, etc.

MORAXELLA

Five species of *Moraxella* are recognized by the International Subcommittee on *Moraxella* and Allied Bacteria (20); these are *M. lacunata*, *M. bovis*, *M. nonliquefaciens*, *M. phenylpyruvica*, and *M. osloensis*. The microorganisms formerly called *M. liquefaciens* are indistinguishable from *M. lacunata* and have been incorporated into the latter species (9). The type species is *M. lacunata*.

The species of *Moraxella* are composed of gram-negative, deep-staining, short rod-shaped or coccoid bacteria which occur singly, in pairs, or in short chains. Some strains exhibit filamentous forms and some contain elements that have a tendency to retain the crystal violet stain. All species of *Moraxella* are nonmotile, nonsaccharolytic, indole-negative, and oxidase-positive. All species are susceptible to penicillin. Two species, *M. lacunata* and *M. bovis*, are proteolytic and digest blood serum in Loeffler's medium, liquefy gelatin, and peptonize litmus milk (Tables 14 and 15). The other three species are not proteolytic. Cultures of *M. bovis* produce betalike hemolysis, whereas members of the other four species have no effect on red blood cells or produce only indeterminate reactions on blood-agar medium.

Moraxella lacunata and M. bovis

Members of these species usually alkalinize the slant of TSI medium, but some cultures of *M. lacunata* fail to grow on this medium (Table 14). Members of these two species are more fastidious than the other species of *Moraxella*, and usually it is necessary to add about two drops of rabbit serum to each of the various media to assure adequate growth. Cultures of *M. lacunata* and *M. bovis* may be differentiated from each other by hemolysis and by their catalase and nitrate reactions, and from the other species by proteolysis and several other reactions (Tables 14 and 15).

The majority of the cultures of *M. lacunata* in our collection were isolated from the eyes of humans, but a few originated in the respiratory tract and one was recovered from a blood culture. The *M. bovis* strains all were isolated from conjunctivitis in cattle.

Moraxella nonliquefaciens and M. osloensis

Members of these two species resemble each other in many of their characteristics, but differ in some of their reactions (Tables 14 and 15). Cultures of *M. nonliquefaciens* do not grow on MacConkey medium, whereas about 50% of strains of *M. osloensis* do so (Table 15). This seems to indicate that *M. nonliquefaciens* is slightly more fastidious than *M. osloensis*. Members of the former species reduce nitrate to nitrite, but only about 28% of cultures of *M. osloensis* do so (Table 15). Furthermore, many isolates of *M. osloensis* grow on Simmons' citrate medium, but do not alkalinize it. According to Bovre and Henriksen (3), cultures of *M. osloensis* grow in Koser's citrate medium and in Audureau's medium with ethyl alcohol as the sole source of carbon. Moreover, these investigators reported (3) that *M. nonliquefaci-*

ens and *M. osloensis* differ in their resistance to heat, in the base composition of their deoxyribonucleic acids, and in genetic compatibility as measured by streptomycin resistance transformation. They also reported that some strains of *M. nonliquefaciens* and *M. osloensis* hydrolyze urea when freshly isolated, but lose this property when subcultured for a time.

Bovre and Henriksen (3) stated that, in their experience, *M. nonliquefaciens* occurs more frequently in the respiratory tract than any of the other species of *Moraxella*. We can confirm this. Of 53 cultures of *M. nonliquefaciens* studied, 21 were recovered from the nasopharynx and 19 were from throats, sputa, and lung. Of 68 strains of *M. osloensis*, only 8 were isolated from throats, sputa, and lungs, whereas 16 were from blood, 4 were from urine, 3 were from spinal fluid, and the remainder were from a variety of sources other than the respiratory tract.

Moraxella phenylpyruvica

This name was proposed (2) to replace *Moraxella polymorpha* Flamm. The outstanding characteristics of members of this species are hydrolysis of urea and deamination of phenylalanine or tryptophan (Table 15). Bovre and Henriksen (2) compared their strains of *M. phenylpyruvica* with the original culture of *M. polymorpha* Flamm and found them to be the same except that the latter isolate failed to hydrolyze urea. We have observed strains of this sort and also have encountered cultures that hydrolyzed urea but failed to deaminate phenylalanine. It is possible that variants of the latter sort may be strains of *M. osloensis* that have retained their ability to hydrolyze urea (see above). The occurrence of an occasional atypical member of any species of bacteria is not rare.

The 62 cultures of *M. phenylpyruvica* that we studied were recovered from urine (12), blood (9), spinal fluid (4), urethra (4), vagina (3), and a variety of other sources in humans. A few strains originated in lower animals.

BACTERIA THAT RESEMBLE MORAXELLA

There are five groups of unnamed bacteria that resemble members of the genus *Moraxella* in many of their characteristics. These groups are composed of gram-negative, rod-shaped bacteria, which may appear to be coccoid or diplococcoid. Filamentous forms are seen occasionally, and some elements have a tendency to retain the crystal violet stain. Members of these groups are nonmotile, nonsaccharolytic, and

TABLE 14. *Characteristics of species of Moraxella and certain unnamed bacteria*[a]

Substrate or character	*M. lacunata*	*M. bovis*	*M. nonliquefaciens*	*M. osloensis*	*M. phenylpyruvica*	Group M-3	Group M-4	Group M-4f	Group M-5	Group M-6
Action on blood:[b] lysis	0 to indeterminate[c]	Beta-like	0 to indeterminate	0 to indeterminate	0 to indeterminate	0	0 to indeterminate	0	0 to indeterminate	0
color[d]	0	0	0	0	0	0	0	lavender-green	0	0
Carbon dioxide (2-4%)	Preferred	0	0	0	0	0	0	0	0	0
Pigment	0	0	0	0	0	0	0	light yellow	slight yellow	0
Pronounced odor	0	0	0	0	0	0	0	Fruity	0	0
Flagellation	Atrichous	Atrichous	Atrichous	Atrichous	Atrichous	Atrichous	Atrichous	Atrichous	Atrichous	Atrichous
Enrichment[e]	Required	0	0	0	0	0	0	0	0	0
TSI agar	NG or K/N	K/N	K/N or N/N	K/N	K/N	N/N, K/N or NG	K/N	K/N	K/K or K/N	K/K, K/N or N/N
Litmus milk (peptonization)	+	+	–	–	–	–	–	+	–	–

[a]See also Table 15.
[b]Heart infusion agar medium with 5% rabbit blood.
[c]See text.
[d]Discoloration of medium around colonies.
[e]About 3% sterile rabbit serum added.
0 = None or not required.

– = Not peptonized.
\+ = Peptonized.
K = Alkaline.
N = Neutral.
NG = No growth.

TABLE 15. *Biochemical characteristics of Moraxella and certain unnamed bacteria*[a]

Test or substrate	*Moraxella lacunata* (25 cultures)		*Moraxella bovis* (5 cultures)		*Moraxella nonliquefaciens* (54 cultures)		*Moraxella osloensis* (68 cultures)		*Moraxella phenylpyruvica* (61 cultures)		Group M-3 (22 cultures)		Group M-4 (27 cultures)		Group M-4f (41 cultures)		Group M-5 (41 cultures)		Group M-6 (32 cultures)	
	Sign[b]	Percent +[c]	Sign	Percent +	Sign	Percent +	Sign	Percent +	Sign	Percent	Sign	Percent +	Sign	Percent +	Sign	Percent +	Sign	Percent +	Sign	Percent +
Oxidase	+	100	+	100	+	100	+	100	+	100	+	100	+	100	+	98	+	100	+	100
Catalase	$+^w$	100	–	1	$+^e$	98	$+^w$	97	$+^w$	90	$+^w$ or –	86	+	100	+	100	+	100	–	6^w
Growth on MacConkey agar	–	0	–	0	–	0	$+^w$ or –	50	d	77^w (10^w)	+	100	+	100	+	95	+ or –	85	+ or –	50
SS agar	–	0	–	0	–	0	–	0	–	0	–	0	–	0	d	46 (7)	–	0	–	0
Cetrimide agar	–	0	–	0	–	0	–	0	–	0	–	0	–	0	–	0	–	0	–	0
Hydrogen sulfide TSI agar	–	0	–	0	–	0	–	0	–	0	–	0	–	0	–	0	–	0	–	0
Pb ac paper	– or $+^w$	28	$+^w$	100	$+^w$ or –	78	$+^w$ or –	76	– or $+^w$	49	– or $+^w$	32	–	0	– or $+^w$	17	$+^w$	93	$+^w$	97
Oxidation-fermentation	I	100	I	100	I	100	I	100	I	100	I or NG	100	I	100	I	100	I	100	I or NG	100
Urease (Christensen's agar)	–	0	–	0	–	0	–	0	+	95	–	0	–	0	+	100	–	0	–	0
Indole	–	0	–	0	–	0	–	0	–	0	–	0	–	0	–	0	–	0	–	0
Methyl red/Voges-Proskauer	–	0	–	0	–	0	–	0	–	0	–[d]	0	–	0	–	0	–	0	–	0
Citrate (Simmons') K	–	0	–	0	–	0	–	0	–	0	–	0	+	100	–	0	–	0	–	0
Phenylalanine deaminase	NT		NT		–	0	–	0	+ or –	70	NT		–	0	+	100	NT		–	0
Motility	–	0	–	0	–	0	–	0	–	0	–	0	–	0	–	0	–	0	–	0
Gelatin	+	92 (4)	(+) or +	20 (80)	–	0	–	0	–	0	–	0	–	0	+ or (+)	88 (10)	–	0	–	0
Glucose, xylose	–	0	–[d]	0	–	0	–	0	–	0	–[d]	0	–	0	–	0	–	0	–	0
Mannitol, lactose	–	0	–	0	–	0	–	0	–	0	–	0	–	0	–	0	–	0	–	0
Sucrose, maltose	–	0	–	0	–	0	–	0	–	0	–	0	–	0	–	0	–	0	–	0
Esculin, glycerol	NT		NT		–	0	–	0	–	0	–	0	–	0	–	0	–	0	–	0
Nitrate, reduction																				
Nitrate to nitrite	+	100	–	0	+	100	– or +	28	+ or –	64	–	0	–	0	–	0	–	0	–	0
Nitrate to amine, no gas	–	0	–	0	–	0	–	0	–	0	–	0	–	0	–	0	–	0	+	100
Nitrite to amine or to gas	–	0	–	0	–	0	–	0	–	0	–	0	–	0	+	100	–	0	–	0
Unreduced nitrate (Zn +)	–	0	+	100	–	0	+ or –	72	– or +	36	+	100	+	100	+	100	+	100	–	0
Pigment (yellow)	–	0	–	0	–	0	–	0	–	0	–	0	–	0	+	93	+ or –	44	+ or –	16

[a]See also Table 14 and text.

[b]Sign:
- \+ = 90% or more positive in 1 or 2 days.
- – = no reaction (90% or more).
- \+ or – = most cultures positive, some strains negative.
- – or + = most strains negative, some cultures positive.
- \+ or (+) = most reactions occur within 1 or 2 days, some are delayed.
- (+) or + = most reactions delayed, some occur in 1 or 2 days.
- d = different biochemical reactions [+, (+), –].
- K = alkaline.
- I = inactive.
- NT = not tested.
- NG = no growth.
- w = weakly positive reaction or light growth.

[c]Figures in parentheses indicate percentage of delayed reactions (3 days or more).

[d]Frequently no growth in carbohydrate media.

[e]Trace to 4+ reactions.

indole-negative; all are oxidase-positive. There is no evidence of hydrogen sulfide production in TSI medium by any of these microorganisms, but many cultures yield weak reactions on lead acetate papers. The bacteria of groups M-3, M-4, M-5, and M-6 are susceptible to penicillin, whereas members of group M-4f are resistant. The characteristics of members of these groups are given in Tables 14 and 15.

Group M-3

Members of this group are fastidious and do not grow in O-F medium or in liquid peptone medium unless it is enriched by addition of serum. It is characteristic that the M-3 bacteria yield light to moderate growth on MacConkey agar medium, although they usually fail to grow on most other unenriched media. Urea is not hydrolyzed and nitrate is not reduced (Tables 14 and 15).

About 50% of the M-3 strains that we studied were recovered from blood specimens. The remainder were isolated from a variety of sources in humans, including spinal fluid.

Group M-4

This group is made up of a portion of the species formerly called *Mima polymorpha* var. *oxidans* DeBord. The strains of this species that fail to alkalinize Simmons' citrate medium now are classified as *M. osloensis*, whereas the isolants that alkalinize Simmons' medium have not been named or incorporated into any species. The latter bacteria are designated group M-4 herein.

Colonies of M-4 bacteria generally are more opaque than those of the recognized species of *Moraxella*. The microorganisms grow moderately to heavily on MacConkey agar medium, but not on SS or cetrimide agar media. The slant of TSI medium is alkalinized (K/N), and growth occurs in nutrient broth containing 6% sodium chloride. Urea is not hydrolyzed and nitrate is not reduced (Table 15). M-4 bacteria grow well in O-F medium containing various carbohydrates; however, the carbohydrate substrates are not acidified (Table 15). The majority of strains alkalinize Simmons' citrate medium within 48 h and all do so within 7 days.

Sixteen of our cultures of M-4 bacteria were isolated from the genitourinary tract of females, whereas six strains were from males. Among others, Lautrop et al. (18) reported the isolation of bacteria of this sort.

Group M-4f

Members of this group are proteolytic and produce a lavender-green discoloration of the red cells in blood-agar medium (Table 14). They peptonize milk and liquefy gelatin (Tables 14 and 15). Colonies of M-4f bacteria are pale yellow, and a tan soluble pigment also is formed (Tables 14 and 15). A fruity odor is produced which is similar to that given off by cultures of *Alcaligenes odorans*. The cellular morphology is similar to that presented by the recognized moraxellae, but curved forms sometimes are seen and filaments frequently occur.

The M-4f bacteria grow moderately well to heavily on MacConkey agar medium, but only about half of the cultures are able to grow on SS agar (Table 15). The slant of TSI medium is alkalinized (K/N), and only a few strains produce discoloration of lead acetate paper strips (Tables 14 and 15). Simmons' citrate medium is not alkalinized and the M-4f bacteria are not lipolytic. Urea is hydrolyzed in Christensen's medium after 18 to 24 h of incubation, and phenylalanine (and tryptophan) is deaminated (Table 15). These microorganisms grow well in O-F medium, but they do not acidify carbohydrate substrates (Table 15). Nitrate is not reduced, but nitrite is reduced to gas (40% of cultures) or to an anaerogenic compound (60% of cultures). Cultures that gave the latter result were tested with zinc dust to be certain that nitrification had not occurred; all such tests were negative for nitrate.

Of 40 cultures of M-4f bacteria studied, 23 were isolated from urine specimens, 12 were recovered from wounds and cutaneous ulcers, and 5 were from lower animals.

Group M-5

Members of this group produce little or no change in the red cells in blood-agar medium, but a slight green discoloration sometimes is seen. The cells are thin to medium in width, may be short or long, and occur in pairs and chains. Occasionally, a filamentous form may be seen. A slight yellow to tan soluble pigment is produced by most cultures.

The majority of strains of M-5 bacteria grow lightly or moderately well on MacConkey agar medium after 3 to 7 days, but growth does not occur on SS, cetrimide, or Simmons' citrate media (Table 15). The slant of TSI agar is alkalinized (K/N). The M-5 bacteria are urease-negative and nonproteolytic, and they do not reduce nitrate. Catalase is produced and the reactions are strong (3+ to 4+). The microorganisms grow well in O-F medium but carbohydrates are not acidified (Table 15).

Group M-5 bacteria resemble cultures of *M. osloensis* in their aggregate reactions. However, the former may be differentiated by their atypical cellular morphology and their failure to grow on Simmons' citrate medium. Further, the apparent association of M-5 microorganisms with canines may be of some help (see below).

Of 41 cultures that we studied, 25 were isolated from infected wounds that resulted from dog bites, 4 were from dogs (tongue, gums, and trachea), and 12 were recovered from wounds in humans, details of which were not known to us.

Group M-6

Members of this group produce little or no effect on the red cells in blood-agar medium (Table 14). The cellular morphology is similar to that of group M-5 strains (above). About 50% of cultures grow lightly on MacConkey agar medium after about 5 days (Table 15), but growth does not occur on SS, cetrimide, or Simmons' citrate media (Table 15). The slant of TSI medium usually is alkalinized (K/N or N/N). Weak to moderate reactions (1+ to 2+) occur on lead acetate paper strips (Table 15). Group M-6 strains are nonproteolytic, do not hydrolyze urea, are catalase-negative, and reduce nitrate and nitrate without gas formation within 48 h. These microorganisms grow poorly in O-F medium and do not produce acid from carbohydrates (Table 15).

The 32 isolates of group M-6 bacteria that we studied were recovered from human sources: throat and sputum, 19; feces, 4; and the remaining specimens from a number of sites.

LITERATURE CITED

1. Baumann, P., M. Doudoroff, and R. Y. Stanier. 1968. A study of the *Moraxella* group. J. Bacteriol. **95**:1520–1541.
2. Bovre, K., and S. D. Henriksen. 1967. A revised description of *Moraxella polymorpha* Flamm 1957, with a proposal of a new name, *Moraxella phenylpyruvica* for this species. Int. J. Syst. Bacteriol. **17**:343–360.
3. Bovre, K., and S. D. Henriksen. 1967. A new *Moraxella* species, *Moraxella osloensis*, and a revised description of *Moraxella nonliquefaciens*. Int. J. Syst. Bacteriol. **17**:127–135.
4. Catlin, B. W. 1970. Transfer of the organism named *Neisseria catarrhalis* to *Branhamella gen. nov*. Int. J. Syst. Bacteriol. **20**:155–159.
5. Catlin, B. W. 1971. Report (1966–1970) of the Subcommittee on the Taxonomy of the *Neisseriaceae* to the International Committee on Nomenclature of Bacteria. Int. J. Syst. Bacteriol. **21**:154–155.
6. Eeckels, R., J. Vandepitte, and V. Seynhaeve. 1965. Neonatal infections with *Flavobacterium meningosepticum*. Report of two cases and a review. Belg. Tijdschr. Geneesk. **21**:244–256.
7. Eiken, M. 1958. Studies on an anaerobic, rod-shaped Gram-negative microorganism: *Bacteroides corrodens* N. sp. Acta Pathol. Microbiol. Scand. **43**:404–416.
8. Henriksen, S. D., and K. Bovre. 1968. *Moraxella kingii* sp. nov., a haemolytic saccharolytic species of the genus *Moraxella*. J. Gen. Microbiol. **51**:377–385.
9. Henriksen, S. D., and K. Bovre. 1968. The taxonomy of the genera *Moraxella* and *Neisseria*. J. Gen. Microbiol. **51**:387–392.
10. Hollis, D. G., G. L. Wiggins, and R. E. Weaver. 1972. An unclassified gram-negative rod isolated from the pharynx on Thayer-Martin medium (selective agar). Appl. Microbiol. **24**:772–777.
11. Jackson, F. L., and Y. E. Goodman. 1972. Transfer of the facultatively anaerobic organism *Bacteroides corrodens* Eiken to a new genus, *Eikenella*. Int. J. Syst. Bacteriol. **22**:73–77.
12. Jackson, F. L., Y. E. Goodman, F. R. Bel, P. C. Wong, and R. L. S. Whitehouse. 1971. Taxonomic status of facultative and strictly anaerobic "corroding bacilli" that have been classified as *Bacteroides corrodens*. J. Med. Microbiol. **4**:171–184.
13. Juni, E. 1972. Interspecies transformation of *Acinetobacter:* genetic evidence for a ubiquitous genus. J. Bacteriol. **112**:917–931.
14. King, E. O. 1964. The identification of unusual pathogenic Gram-negative bacteria. Center for Disease Control, Atlanta, Ga.
15. King, E. O. 1959. Studies on a group of previously unclassified bacteria associated with meningitis in infants. Amer. J. Clin. Pathol. **31**:241–247.
16. King, E. O., and H. W. Tatum. 1962. *Actinobacillus actinomycetemcomitans* and *Haemophilus aphrophilus*. J. Infect. Dis. **111**:85–94.
17. Kovacs, N. 1956. Identification of *Pseudomonas pyocyanea* by the oxidase reaction. Nature (London) **178**:703.
18. Lautrop, H., K. Bovre, and W. Frederiksen. 1970. A *Moraxella*-like microorganism isolated from the genitourinary tract of man. Acta Pathol. Microbiol. Scand. **78**:255–256.
19. Leifson, E., and R. Hugh. 1954. *Alcaligenes denitrificans n. sp.* J. Gen. Microbiol. **11**:512–513.
20. Lessel, E. F. 1971. International Committee on Nomenclature of Bacteria. Subcommittee on the Taxonomy of *Moraxella* and Allied Bacteria. Int. J. Syst. Bacteriol. **21**:213–214.
21. Malek, I., M. Radochova, and O. Lysenko. 1963. Taxonomy of the species *Pseudomonas odorans*. J. Gen. Microbiol. **33**:349–355.
22. Mitchell, R. G., and Suzanne K. R. Clarke. 1965. An *Alcaligenes* species with distinctive properties isolated from human sources. J. Gen. Microbiol. **40**:343–348.
23. Riley, P. S., H. W. Tatum, and R. E. Weaver. 1973. Identity of HB-1 of King and *Eikenella corrodens* (Eiken) Jackson and Goodman. Int. J. Syst. Bacteriol. **23**:75–76.
24. Samuels, S. B., B. Pittman, H. W. Tatum, and W. B. Cherry. 1972. Report on a study set of moraxellae and allied bacteria. Int. J. Syst. Bacteriol. **22**:19–38.
25. Slotnick, I. J., and M. Dougherty. 1964. Further characterization of an unclassified group of bacteria causing endocarditis in man: *Cardiobacterium hominis gen.* et *sp. N.* Antonie van Leeuwenhoek J. Microbiol. Serol. **30**:261–272.
26. Stanier, R. Y., N. J. Palleroni, and M. Doudoroff. 1966. The aerobic pseudomonads: a taxonomic study. J. Gen. Microbiol. **43**:159–271.
27. Yabuuchi, E., and A. Ohyama. 1971. *Achromobacter xylosoxidans n. sp.* from human ear discharge. Jap. J. Microbiol. **15**:477–481.

Chapter 25

Brucella

W. J. HAUSLER, JR., AND F. P. KOONTZ

CHARACTERIZATION

Parasites occurring in animals and producing infections in animals and humans. Cause epizootic abortions in a variety of animals and septicemic febrile illness or localized infection of bone, tissue, or organ systems in humans. Isolated from unpasteurized dairy products from infected animals and from clinical specimens such as blood, tissues, and occasionally abscesses which occur in organs.

Reported cases of human brucellosis have decreased markedly in the 20-year period from 1953 to 1972 from slightly in excess of 2,000 cases in 1953 to slightly less than 200 reported in 1972 (20). This significant decrease in human infections is directly related to extremely effective disease eradication efforts, particularly in bovines and swine. Most reported human cases are now due to occupational exposures in the abattoir. During the past few years, several episodes of human brucellosis have been traced to canines. In most instances the organism responsible was *Brucella canis* (3, 4); however, at least one report of *B. suis* transmitted via a dog bite has been recorded (16). The rare episode of food-associated brucellosis has occurred in two of the last three years. In both instances the organism responsible was *B. melitensis* and the vehicle was Mexican goat cheese (17, 21).

Small, nonmotile, nonsporing, gram-negative rod, usually coccobacillary; 0.4 to 1.5 μm in length; occurring singly, in pairs, and rarely in short chains. Capsules, if present, are small.

Growth. Aerobic, often enhanced by CO_2, but no growth under strict anaerobic conditions. Grow slowly on ordinary media or may require special media. Optimal temperature, 37 C; temperature range, 10 to 42 C. Nonpigmented, characteristic colonies produced. *B. abortus* requires 10% CO_2 for primary isolation. Do not consider certain primary cultures (blood, cerebrospinal fluid, etc.) negative until after 21 days of incubation.

Biochemical characteristics. Catalase positive, oxidase usually positive (*B. neotomae* and *B. ovis* are oxidase-negative). Urea hydrolyzed to a variable extent. Gelatin not liquefied. Production of H_2S and resistance to thionin and basic fuchsin help to differentiate the species. Specific biotype or strain differentiation is accomplished by oxidative metabolism studies (10, 12, 13, 19).

Sugar fermentations. Sugar reactions are of little value in speciation unless special media are employed (15).

Serological identification. Genus-specific antisera are available with known cross-reactions to tularemia, cholera, and *Yersinia enterocolitica* (6, 7). Monospecific antiserum produced by absorption differentiates *B. melitensis* from *B. abortus* and *B. suis*. The latter two species cannot be differentiated serologically. Fluorescent-antibody techniques useful for genus identification only (2).

Animal inoculation. Healthy, male guinea pigs inoculated. Usually intraperitoneally, occasionally subcutaneously. Characteristic lesions of spleen, liver, and genitalia produced.

RECOGNITION OF BRUCELLA

The *Brucella* group are, with rare exceptions, slow-growers that require special media and techniques. They are either dependent on or enhanced by an increased CO_2 atmosphere. Isolation of the etiological agent leaves no question as to diagnosis, whereas the serological procedures are open to interpretive errors. Species identification also provides valuable epidemiological and therapeutic information to the clinician. The isolation of *Brucella* is not overly difficult if the specimen is collected and treated properly.

COLLECTION AND HANDLING OF SPECIMENS

Blood

Several types of collection outfits are suitable for the culture of whole blood (see chapter 6).

In laboratories which handle specimens taken under varying conditions and shipped through the mail, contaminated cultures can be controlled by adding 1.4 ml of 0.1% aqueous crystal violet (certified) per liter of broth before sterilization. It should be noted, however, that this concentration of crystal violet may inhibit small numbers of *B. suis*. Cultures of *B. melitensis* may be similarly inhibited. The medium proposed by Weed (22) for potentially contaminated specimens is also recommended. If Weed's medium or any other medium containing inhibitors is utilized, it is good practice to include the basal medium without inhibitors. In this manner, *Brucella* species sensitive to inhibitors are not overlooked. Incubate at 35 C under 10% CO_2 tension for at least 72 h, and examine daily for growth. Subculture every 3 days or when evidence of growth appears. Retain cultures for 21 days before reporting them as negative.

Since small numbers of *Brucella* cells may be present in pleural and cerebrospinal fluid, it is necessary to inoculate guinea pigs with centrifuged sediment and proceed as outlined below in the section on Animal Inoculation.

Bone marrow and exudates

Spread material over culture media, and inoculate guinea pigs.

Occasionally, the microbiologist must attempt to identify the organism in the infected animal. This may be accomplished by observing the organisms on Gram-stained smears of clinical specimens or by isolation of the *Brucella* species, or by both methods.

Cerebrospinal, joint, and peritoneal fluids

If a fibrinous clot of pellicle is present, remove it aseptically and grind in a mortar, in the presence of sterile sand. Add this ground material to the fluid portion, allow sand to settle, decant, centrifuge, and inoculate media and guinea pigs. Incubate and observe as described for blood cultures.

Urine

Collect 50 to 100 ml of catheterized urine. Centrifuge at 3,000 rpm for 30 min. Spread the sediment over the surface of two tryptose-agar plates, or agar plates prepared from other commercially dehydrated media, containing 1.4 ml of 0.1% aqueous crystal violet (certified) per liter added before sterilization, or use the medium recommended by Weed (22). Incubate plates under 10% CO_2 tension at 35 C for 48 h. Reincubate an additional 4 days and subculture daily. Identify suspected colonies as directed in the section on Cultural Examination.

DIRECT MICROSCOPIC EXAMINATION

Three possible staining procedures (see below) can be used to detect *Brucella* in heavily infected tissue specimens. The brucellae, which are usually located inside the cells, retain the primary stain in both procedures. The smear can be made by swab method or tissue impression, depending upon the type of tissue to be examined. Swab smears can be made from the fetal membranes, the fetal stomach contents, or the vagina of the aborting animal or human. If tissues are obtained at necropsy, impression smears may produce better results with the fluorescent-antibody technique. After the smears have dried, they are fixed and stained by either the modified Ziehl-Neelsen or the modified Koster method or are observed by the fluorescent-antibody method.

Vibrio fetus, *Listeria monocytogenes*, and other organisms causing abortion in animals can usually be differentiated from *Brucella* by morphological criteria, even though they also will retain the primary stain.

CULTURAL EXAMINATION

Primary culture

Incubate at 37 C under 10% CO_2 tension. If a transport culture outfit containing CO_2, similar to that described in chapter 6, has been used, no additional CO_2 need be furnished. Other cultures should be placed in sealed incubating chambers or jars and provided with increased CO_2 tension.

Incubate for 4 to 5 days before making first transfer unless visible growth appears. Reincubate primary culture, renewing CO_2 if it has been dissipated, and make subsequent transfers every 4 days. The primary culture should be incubated for at least 21 days before the specimen is designated as negative. The high humidity which develops in sealed chambers or jars under these conditions promotes rapid growth of molds; these may contaminate and render valueless many cultures if the moisture is not controlled. A layer or tray of dry $CaCl_2$ placed in the bottom of the chamber or jar will help to control humidity.

Subcultures

Use freshly prepared slants or plates of tryptose-agar or Trypticase soy agar. Some fastidious strains of *Brucella* require more elaborate media such as serum-dextrose-agar or Tween-dextrose-agar for subculture isolation. Gently mix primary culture. Aseptically withdraw 0.5 ml and use as an inoculum to streak an entire agar plate, or transfer several drops to an agar slant. Incubate under 10% CO_2 tension for 4 days at 37 C.

Examination of culture plates

Examine plates for signs of growth during the 4-day incubation period. *Brucella* colonies are 2 to 7 mm in diameter, spheroidal in shape, moist, slightly opalescent in appearance, and translucent. These characteristics may vary somewhat with available pH and moisture. Do not consider a blood culture negative for *Brucella* until the final subculture at 21 days has failed to yield the organism.

Study of suspected colonies

Transfer isolated colonies to several tryptose-agar slants or slants prepared from commercial dehydrated media, and incubate under 10% CO_2 tension at 37 C for 48 h. If sufficient growth has not been obtained, reincubate for another 24-h period. *Brucella* species yield a fine, clear, translucent growth with a slight amber tinge. Gram stain and examine for gram-negative pleomorphic coccobacilli. Since brucellae take the counterstain poorly, apply counterstain for 1 to 3 min instead of the usual 30 s. A presumptive identification of *Brucella* can then be made by the judicious use of fluorescent-antibody methods (2) or standard serological procedures, or both. If *B. suis* is suspected, a rapid presumptive test is to inoculate heavily a small area of a urea-agar slant. A rapid change in the indicator, due to hydrolysis of urea, indicates that the isolate is probably *B. suis*. A spot slide-agglutination test may be made with *Brucella* antiserum in suitable dilution (usually not less than 1:10). However, one should control for pseudoagglutination by noting smoothness of emulsion of the growth in a drop of isotonic saline.

Differentiation of Brucella species

The most common tests used for the differentiation of the species of the genus *Brucella* are (i) the need for increased CO_2, especially on primary isolation; (ii) the production of H_2S for a period of 4 to 5 days; (iii) the bacteriostatic action of basic fuchsin and thionin in solid media; (iv) agglutination in monospecific sera; and (v) the urease test, which is useful in the differentiation of *B. suis* from other *Brucella* species.

This differentiation is primarily quantitative rather than qualitative. However, a majority of the strains can be identified as belonging to one of the three classical species (Table 1).

It should be emphasized that certain strains will deviate from the classical differentiation presented in Table 1.

The isolation of any species of *Brucella* from human or animal tissues, fluids, or products constitutes conclusive evidence of infection. However, negative cultures do not necessarily rule out brucellosis. Repeated negative cultures combined with repeated negative agglutination tests are indicative but not conclusive evidence for the absence of brucellosis.

Differential culture methods

Thionin-tryptose-agar. To prepare, melt previously sterilized tryptose-agar. Adjust the medium while hot to pH 6.6 to 6.8. Heat a small amount of 1% aqueous thionin (certified) in a boiling-water bath for 20 min, and then add approximately 0.1 ml while hot to each 100 ml of medium. (The actual amount added is dependent upon the bacteriostatic action and dye content of each lot of dye.) Mix, pour plates or slants, and use within 48 h. The surface of the plates or slants must be dry before inoculation, which may be accomplished by placing them in an incubator for 24 to 48 h. Known *Brucella* cultures should be included as a medium control.

Basic fuchsin-tryptose-agar. To prepare, melt previously sterilized tryptose-agar. Heat a small amount of 1% aqueous basic fuchsin (certified) in a boiling-water bath for 20 min, and then add approximately 0.1 ml while hot to each 100 ml of medium, as for the thionin-tryptose-agar. Mix, dispense, and use within 48 h. The medium should be dark rose-red in color; 1% basic fuchsin solution older than 2 months may deteriorate, yielding lighter plates not suitable for use. Always store basic fuchsin solution in the dark. Known *Brucella* cultures should be included as a medium control.

From each pure culture and the control strains, streak a thionin-tryptose-agar plate or slant and a basic fuchsin-tryptose-agar plate or slant. Four cultures may be tested on each plate, one in each quadrant. Use a moderately heavy inoculum, streaking one small area at the top of each plate heavily and streaking off onto the rest of the plate or quadrant. Incubate plates under 10% CO_2 at 37 C for 72 h. Examine and record the presence or absence of distinct growth. Do not confuse heavy inoculum with growth, but look for distinct growth on the streaked portions of the plate.

TABLE 1. *Differentiation of Brucella species and their biotypes*[a]

Species and biotype	CO_2 required	H_2S produced	Growth on dyes[b]					Agglutination by		
			Basic fuchsin		Thionin			Monospecific sera[c]		Anti-rough serum
			II	III	I	II	III	A	M	
B. melitensis										
1	−	−	+	+	−	+	+	−	+	−
2	−	−	+	+	−	+	+	+	−	−
3	−	−	+	+	−	+	+	+	+	−
B. abortus										
1	±	+	+	+	−	−	−	+	−	−
2	+	+	−	−	−	−	−	+	−	−
3	±	+	+	+	+	+	+	+	−	−
4	±	+	+	+	−	−	−	−	+	−
5	−	−	+	+	−	+	+	−	+	−
6	−	±	+	+	−	+	+	+	−	−
7	−	±	+	+	−	+	+	+	+	−
8	+	−	+	+	−	+	+	−	+	−
9	±	+	+	+	−	+	+	−	+	−
B. suis										
1	−	+	−	−	+	+	+	+	−	−
2	−	−	−	−	−	+	+	+	−	−
3	−	−	+	+	+	+	+	+	−	−
4	−	−	+	+	+	+	+	+	+	−
B. neotomae	−	+	−	−	−	−	+	+	−	−
B. ovis	+	−	+	+	+	+	+	−	−	+
B. canis	−	−	−	−	+	+	+	−	−	+

[a] From World Health Organ. Tech. Rep. Ser. No. 464, 1971, p. 71.

[b] Species differentiation is obtained on tryptose-agar with the following graded concentrations of dyes: 1:25,000 (I), 1:50,000 (II), 1:100,000 (III).

[c] A = abortus; M = melitensis.

Tests for CO_2 requirement and H_2S production. Inoculate two tryptose-agar slants from each pure culture. Suspend a lead acetate strip directly over, but not touching, the inoculated surface of one of the slants for the detection of H_2S production. Incubate the plain slant aerobically and the one for H_2S production under 10% CO_2 at 37 C for 4 days. Examine daily for both growth and H_2S production, replacing the lead acetate strip with a fresh strip each day. Record H_2S produced as "none" (0), "trace" (±), and "moderate to marked" (+).

Pickett and Nelson (15) used sugar fermentation differences to assist in delineation of the species and major biotypes of *Brucella*. Some workers have incorporated these fermentative characteristics into their differential scheme.

Certain strains of *Brucella* will deviate from the classical identification scheme, and two methods have been developed to speciate these aberrant strains. These methods include the use of brucellaphage and oxidative metabolism.

The Subcommittee on Taxonomy of *Brucella* presented the following differential characteristics of the three species and their biotypes in its report to the 8th International Congress for Microbiology in 1962 (19). At present, there is a difference of opinion whether *B. canis* and *B. ovis* should be recognized as separate species or included as biotypes of previously recognized species. These differences are primarily based on deoxyribonucleic acid homology, gel immunodiffusion, and gas chromatographic studies (5, 8, 9, 11, 14).

DIFFERENTIAL CHARACTERISTICS OF BRUCELLA SPECIES

Brucella melitensis (reference strain B. melitensis 16M)

Aerobic. Produce no H_2S or no more than a trace on ordinary media. Usually grow in the presence of basic fuchsin and thionin. Usually have M antigen predominant. Oxidize L-alanine, D-alanine, L-asparagine, and L-glutamic acid. Do not oxidize L-arabinose, D-galactose, D-ribose, D-xylose, L-arginine, DL-citrulline, DL-ornithine, or L-lysine. Not lysed by brucellaphage Tbilisi (Tb) at routine test dilution.

Usually pathogenic for goats and sheep but can also affect other species. including cattle and humans.

Brucella abortus (reference strain B. abortus 544)

Usually require added CO_2 for growth, especially on primary isolation. Usually produce moderate amounts of H_2S but may be negative. Usually grow in presence of basic fuchsin but are inhibited by thionin. Usually have A antigen predominant. Oxidize L-alanine, D-alanine, L-asparagine, L-glutamic acid, L-arabinose, D-galactose, and D-ribose; do not oxidize D-xylose, L-arginine, DL-citrulline, DL-ornithine, or L-lysine. Cultures in the smooth or smooth-intermediate phase are lysed by brucellaphage Tb at routine test dilution. Usually pathogenic for cattle, causing abortion, but can also affect other species, including humans.

Brucella suis (reference strain B. suis 1330)

Aerobic. Produce large amounts of H_2S or none at all. Grow in the presence of thionin but are usually inhibited by basic fuchsin. Usually have A antigen predominant. Oxidize L-alanine, D-alanine, L-glutamic acid, L-arabinose, D-galactose, D-ribose, D-xylose, L-arginine, DL-citrulline, DL-ornithine, and L-lysine. Do not oxidize L-asparagine. Not lysed by brucellaphage Tb at routine test dilution. Usually pathogenic for pigs, but can also affect hares and other species, including humans.

Oxidative metabolic tests are cumbersome and time-consuming, and require apparatus and materials which are expensive and are not routinely found in modern diagnostic laboratories. Only those laboratories which have trained personnel and necessary equipment should attempt to differentiate the biotypes within a species. Therefore, it is suggested that if conventional tests and bacteriophage typing do not permit a culture to be identified satisfactorily it should be sent to a laboratory proficient in performing these tests.

SEROLOGICAL CONFIRMATION

Serological identification of members of the genus *Brucella* is not utilized to the same degree as with *Salmonella*, where every serotype is designated as a species. In fact, confirmatory serology of *Brucella* isolates is used predominantly at the genus level, as indicated in earlier discussion. When an isolate is suspected to be *Brucella*, known antiserum is utilized to confirm the suspicion. The antiserum may be conjugated with a fluorescent dye such as fluorescein isothiocyanate (see chapter 4), and the isolate is then examined by the fluorescent-antibody technique (2). Unconjugated serum can be used for simple agglutination procedures of either the tube or slide type. A positive reaction, in the presence of a negative antigen control (isolate in isotonic saline), indicates that the isolate is indeed a member of the genus *Brucella*.

To differentiate *B. melitensis* from *B. abortus* and *B. suis*, monospecific sera produced by antibody absorption procedures must be employed. Predominant brucella antigens are frequently referred to as "M antigen" (melitensis) or "A antigen" (abortus-suis complex).

A good reactive heterologous antiserum is divided into two parts. One part is absorbed with *B. melitensis* (strain 16M) cells until all of the common antibodies are removed. This will yield a serum specific for *B. abortus-B. suis* complex (monospecific serum A). (*B. abortus* cannot be differentiated antigenically from *B. suis.*) The other portion of heterologous antiserum is absorbed with *B. abortus* (strain 544) cells until all of the common antibodies are removed, yielding a serum specific for *B. melitensis* (monospecific serum M). These specific absorbing strains should be used in the production of monospecific antisera, and of course it is obviously essential that they be in the smooth colony form.

Absorption technique

The absorbing antigen is harvested with isotonic saline and heated at 60 C for 1 h. Care must be taken to ascertain that at least 99% of the colonies are of the smooth type. Phenol is added for a final concentration of 0.5%, and the suspensions are stored in the cold until used.

A 1-ml amount of packed absorbing cells is resuspended in 10 ml of the antiserum to be absorbed, and the mixture is placed in a water bath at 37 C for 2 h. The suspension should be shaken every 15 min during incubation. The suspension is then centrifuged, and the supernatant fluid is used to resuspend a second 1 ml of packed cells, incubated as above, and centrifuged. This procedure is followed until agglutination is no longer visible.

The monospecific antisera obtained can then be stored in small portions in a freezer, or, after the addition of phenol to a final concentration of 0.5%, they can be stored at 4 C or lyophilized.

Slide test

For the serological confirmation of *Brucella*, a drop of homologous serum is placed on a slide, and a small portion of the culture to be tested is mixed into the serum with a loop. The serum should be diluted at least 1:10 for the test. It is recommended that a control serum without brucella agglutinins also be tested to rule out false-positive reactions known to occur with some other gram-negative organisms.

The same basic procedure is employed when testing with the monospecific antisera. However, all four sera (heterologous, two monospecific, negative control) are tested simultaneously. Care must be exercised to be sure that the suspensions are equal and not too dense. The testing sera are diluted to a level where known control strains will agglutinate in the monospecific serum within 1 min without being visibly agglutinated by the heterologous serum in that time. If agglutination occurs with both monospecific antisera, the culture should be retested by the tube method.

Tube method

To confirm an isolate as *Brucella*, the heterologous antiserum and a known negative control serum are placed in appropriate tubes and diluted at least 1:10; an equal amount of the suspected culture suspension is added. The tubes are then incubated at 37 C for 24 h and read.

The culture suspension is prepared by harvesting a fresh slant culture with phenolized saline. The harvest is then heated at 60 C for 1 h, diluted, and standardized to 78% light transmission at a wavelength of 650 nm in an electrophotometer.

The monospecific tube test is performed in duplicate, i.e., one set of tubes for each of the monospecific sera. The serum is diluted just beyond its known titer by the double-dilution method, starting at 1:5. An equal amount of the antigen suspension, prepared as above, is then added to each tube plus the saline control. The tubes are incubated for 24 h at 37 C and read. Usually the strain being studied will be agglutinated by one of the sera to its known titer but not at all by the other serum. Some strains are agglutinated by both monospecific sera at varying titers. *B. melitensis* biotype 3 and *B. abortus* biotype 7 produce this type of result (1).

There is one other facet of serological examination that warrants mention in this chapter, i.e., the febrile agglutination procedure. The patient's serum is tested against known *Brucella* antigen. At times, the patient with chronic brucellosis will be repeatedly culture-negative but will show a marked rise in brucella agglutinins. The test can be performed by either a slide or a tube method. Since this is a standard technique, we will not go into detail, but the reader is referred to Spink et al. (18) for the preparation of the antigen for febrile agglutinations and for the techniques for performing the test. Numerous commercial antigens with their appropriate techniques are also readily available; however, it has been the experience of many qualified laboratories that these products provide variable results.

ANIMAL INOCULATION

Use healthy male guinea pigs with a body weight of 300 to 600 g. Animals should be prebled to determine presence or absence of brucella antibody. If material which has been prepared for inoculation is likely to contain many contaminating organisms, inoculate the animals subcutaneously; otherwise, inoculate them intraperitoneally. Inject 2 ml into each animal, using at least two animals per specimen. Six weeks after inoculation, bleed each animal and test for brucella agglutinins. Post those animals that react, and examine each organ for characteristic changes as follows.

Spleen. Enlarged, sometimes five or six times; usually with nodules that are at first hemorrhagic, later becoming encapsulated, gray, and discrete, and occasionally having necrotic centers; occasionally abscesses (usually *B. suis*).

Liver. Gray, glistening, discrete nodules (0.5 to 2.0 mm in diameter) just below surface on the capsule; occasionally abscesses (usually *B. suis*).

Genitalia. Sometimes abscessed in testes and epididymes (sublumbar lymph nodes may also be involved).

Cultures should be made from suspected lesions by rubbing the cut surface of the tissue over a culture medium surface. Incubate, transfer colonies, and identify organisms as previously directed. Fluorescent-antibody procedures may be employed by preparing impression smears of the cut surface of the suspect lesion. With the use of standard techniques for fluorescence microscopy, *Brucella*, if present, will be easily identifiable (2). Post at 8 weeks those animals with negative agglutination tests at 6 weeks.

LITERATURE CITED

1. Alton, G. G., and L. M. Jones. 1967. Laboratory techniques in brucellosis. W.H.O. Monogr. Ser. No. 55. Ser. No. 55.
2. Biegeleisen, J. Z., Jr., M. D. Moody, B. B. Marcus, and J. W. Flynt. 1962. The use of fluorescein-labeled anti-*Brucella suis* globulin for demonstrating *Brucella* antigen in animal tissues. Amer. J. Vet. Res. **23**:592–595.
3. Center for Disease Control. 1974. Brucellosis surveillance,

annual summary 1972 (issued February 1974). Center for Disease Control, Atlanta, Ga.

4. Faigel, H. C. 1969. Beagle fever (canine brucellosis). Clin. Pediat. **8**:59.
5. Hoyer, B. H., and N. B. McCullough. 1968. Homologies of DNA from *Brucella ovis*, canine abortion organism and other *Brucella* species. J. Bacteriol. **96**:1783–1790.
6. Hurvell, B. 1972. Serological cross-reactions between different *Brucella* species and *Yersinia enterocolitica*. Immunodiffusion and immunoelectrophoresis. Acta Vet. Scand. **13**:472–483.
7. Hurvell, B., P. Ahvonen, and E. Thal. 1971. Serological cross-reactions between different *Brucella* species and *Yersinia enterocolitica*. Agglutination and complement fixation. Acta Vet. Scand. **12**:86–94.
8. Jones, L. M., M. Zanardi, D. Leong, and J. B. Wilson. 1968. Taxonomic position in the genus *Brucella* of the causative agent of canine abortion. J. Bacteriol. **95**:625–630.
9. McCullough, N. B. 1968. DNA homology relationships within the genus *Brucella*. Proc. U.S. Livestock Sanit. Ass. **72**:79–82.
10. Meyer, M. E. 1961. Metabolic characterization of the genus *Brucella*. III. Oxidative metabolism of strains that show anomalous characteristics by conventional determinative methods. J. Bacteriol. **82**:401–410.
11. Meyer, M. E. 1969. *Brucella* organisms isolated from dogs: comparison of characteristics of members of the genus *Brucella*. Amer. J. Vet. Res. **30**:1751–1756.
12. Meyer, M. E., and H. S. Cameron. 1961. Metabolic characterization of the genus *Brucella*. I. Statistical evaluation of the oxidative rates by which type I of each species can be identified. J. Bacteriol. **82**:387–395.
13. Meyer, M. E., and H. S. Cameron. 1961. Metabolic characterization of the genus *Brucella*. II. Oxidative metabolic patterns of the described biotypes. J. Bacteriol. **82**:396–400.
14. Mitruka, B. M., and M. Alexander. 1970. Differentiation of *Brucella canis* from other *Brucella* by gas chromatography. Appl. Microbiol. **20**:649–650.
15. Pickett, M. J., and E. L. Nelson. 1955. Speciation within the genus *Brucella*. IV. Fermentation of carbohydrates. J. Bacteriol. **69**:333–396.
16. Robertson, M. G. 1973. Brucella infection transmitted by dog bite. J. Amer. Med. Ass. **225**:750–751.
17. Seyffert, W. A., and J. A. Bernard. 1969. Brucellosis—report of six cases. Tex. Med. **65**:46–52 (April).
18. Spink, W. W., N. B. McCullough, L. M. Hutchings, and C. K. Mingle. 1954. A standardized antigen and agglutination technic for human brucellosis. Report no. 3 of the national research council committee on public health aspect of brucellosis. Amer. J. Clin. Pathol. **24**:496–498.
19. Stableforth, A. W. and L. M. Jones. 1963. Report of the Subcommittee on taxonomy of the genus *Brucella*. Speciation in the genus *Brucella*. Int. Bull. Bacteriol. Nomencl. Taxon. **13**:145–158.
20. U.S. Department of Health, Education, and Welfare (Public Health Service). 1973. Morbidity and mortality weekly report. Annual supplement. Summary 1972. **21**:(no. 53).
21. U.S. Department of Health, Education, and Welfare (Public Health Service). 1973. Morbidity and mortality weekly report. **22**:193–194. Publication No. (CDC)74-8017.
22. Weed, L. A. 1957. The use of a selective medium for isolation of brucella from contaminated surgical specimens. Amer. J. Clin. Pathol. **27**:482–485.

Chapter 26

Haemophilus

VIOLA M. YOUNG

CHARACTERIZATION

Members of the genus *Haemophilus* are strict parasites characteristically requiring accessory factors for in vitro growth. These microorganisms are minute (0.2 to 0.5 by 0.3 to 2.0 μm) gram-negative rods, often coccobacillary; formation of threadlike filaments and pleomorphism are common. Bipolar staining is frequent. They are nonmotile and nonsporulated. Capsules are present in many strains. Smooth colonies which are hemolytic must be differentiated from the dew-drop colonies of beta-hemolytic streptococci. Rough colonies may be flat, slightly wrinkled, granular, and cohesive.

Haemophilus ducreyi is notably difficult to grow in vitro. *Haemophilus aphrophilus* shares some characteristics with *Actinobacillus actinomycetemcomitans* and can be confused with this organism when it occurs in active mycotic lesions (17, 20). *Haemophilus influenzae* is antigenically related to *Diplococcus pneumoniae* (1), *Staphylococcus aureus*, *Staphylococcus epidermidis*, group A beta-hemolytic streptococci, *Streptococcus viridans*, *Bacillus* spp., *Escherichia coli*, and diphtheroids (3).

CLINICAL SIGNIFICANCE

Although most *Haemophilus* spp. are normal inhabitants of the upper respiratory tract of humans, they may become primary or secondary invaders (4). *H. influenzae* type b is responsible for up to 95% of infection caused by *Haemophilus* spp. in children from 6 months to 3 years of age (24); above that age, other serotypes increase in frequency. Infections include meningitis, acute epiglottitis, acute obstructive laryngotracheal infection, pharyngitis, sinusitis, pneumonia, otitis media, and bacteremia. Subacute bacterial endocarditis and septic arthritis are occasionally caused by these organisms. Less frequent are similar infections in adults (15, 24) with alcoholism or immune deficiencies as predisposing factors. In adults, disease of the upper respiratory tract caused by *H. influenzae* as a secondary invader usually follows influenza which is viral in origin. In fact, it was recovered so regularly from patients during influenza pandemics that it was considered for some time to be the causal agent. Infections due to *H. aphrophilus* are rare, occur in adults as often as children, and include most of the aforementioned diseases (22). *H. parainfluenzae* (2, 12, 18) and *H. haemoglobinophilus* (canis; 10) are very rarely encountered. *H. aegyptius* (Koch-Weeks Bacillus) causes occasional cases of acute conjunctivitis. Soft chancre or chancroid, caused by *H. ducreyi*, was reported to occur at a rate of 0.6 per 100,000 population in 1973 (23).

The seven species of *Haemophilus* which usually are found in humans are listed in Table 1 together with the sources from which they are most often recovered.

COLLECTION OF SPECIMEN

Care should be exercised to assure that adequate sputum samples are obtained and that they are contaminated as little as possible with oral cavity flora. As *Haemophilus* spp. are normal inhabitants of the upper respiratory tract, the importance of obtaining a sample which reflects with accuracy the predominant flora, to enable the physician to make clinical decisions based on correct data, cannot be overemphasized. Any method which bypasses the oral cavity, such as bronchial washings, transtracheal aspiration, etc., is preferable for sampling. Swabs for nose and throat cultures, etc., should be moistened in broth before the sample is taken and kept moist during transport to the laboratory to prevent loss due to drying. Similarly, scrapings from the conjunctiva or chancroid lesions should not be allowed to dry. Media should be inoculated immediately on arrival of the sample in the laboratory.

H. influenzae does not survive well in sputum samples sent to the laboratory by mail. Approximately half of the organisms die within 24 to 30 h after collection in samples which are posted and cultured later (19). The pH of the sputum does not appear to be a major factor influencing survival. There is some indication that these microorganisms survive better in samples kept at room temperature rather than 4 or 37 C,

TABLE 1. *Sources of the seven species of Haemophilus commonly isolated from humans*

Specimens	Species
Throat swabs, sputum, bronchial washings, etc.	*H. influenzae* *H. parainfluenzae* *H. haemolyticus* *H. parahaemolyticus* *H. aphrophilus*
Cerebrospinal fluid, blood[a], pus	*H. influenzae*
Conjunctival swabs or scrapings	*H. aegyptius*
Chancroid scrapings	*H. ducreyi*

[a] Isolated cases of several other *Haemophilus* species in the blood have been reported.

though a carefully controlled study of this parameter apparently has not been made.

DIRECT EXAMINATION

Gram-stained smears of sputum or swabs are useful only to determine the presence of gram-negative rods and to rule out pneumococci, which may cause similar clinical syndromes. However, smears of normally sterile material, such as cerebrospinal fluid, pleural fluid, etc., particularly in the age group wherein *H. influenzae* is a common pathogen, are a useful guideline. Likewise, smears of conjunctival scrapings or chancroid lesions, although not diagnostic, are a clinically useful aid. Such smears should be made of the purulent material in sputum, of spinal fluid, or of the sediment obtained by centrifugation of spinal fluid samples that exceed 2 ml. In preparation of the Gram stain, care should be exercised in decolorization, particularly of the heavier portions of sputum smears, as the coccobacillary forms of *Haemophilus* somewhat resemble pneumococci in morphology. Also, if they exhibit bipolar staining, as they occasionally do, with the rest of the organism being very pale in appearance, they could mistakenly be considered gram-positive. The organisms usually are seen as minute gram-negative rods, coccobacillary in form. The strains which are pleomorphic or filamentous in form are nonencapsulated.

The encapsulated strains are recovered more frequently from disease processes in children, but the nonencapsulated strains appear to cause otitis media (13) and disease in adults as often as those which form capsules. If a sufficient number of organisms are present in an exudate or spinal fluid and *Haemophilus* infection is suspected, it is useful to attempt a direct capsular swelling test with *H. influenzae* typing sera (see section below on Immunoserological diagnosis). Most cerebrospinal or blood stream invasions, as well as acute upper respiratory disease in children caused by *H. influenzae*, are due to serotype b. Nonencapsulated strains are, of course, nontypable by this method.

CULTURE AND ISOLATION

Sputum, spinal fluid, purulent exudate, and swabs from nose, throat, or wounds should be inoculated directly (or in the case of swabs, carefully rolled) onto the surface of rabbit, guinea pig, or horse blood-agar plates or on chocolate-agar, and the streaking should be performed as described in chapter 6. Fresh human and sheep bloods contain heat-labile inhibitors of *H. influenzae* and should not be used for the preparation of blood-agar plates, but are useful for preparation of the chocolate-agar as these inhibitors are destroyed by the heating process. However, if the sample has been streaked to sheep or human blood-agar plates for the growth of other organisms, it is useful to compare this plate with growth observed on the rabbit or horse blood-agar or chocolate-agar plates. If microorganisms have been observed in the cerebrospinal fluid or other samples which morphologically resemble *Haemophilus* spp. and/or the case is clinically congruous with *Haemophilus* infection, Levinthal's or Filde's enrichment agar (see chapter 95) is recommended and will yield *Haemophilus* colonies which are larger and easier to observe.

The accessory growth factors required by members of the genus *Haemophilus* for in vitro growth are the heme portion of hemoglobin, necessary for the synthesis of respiratory enzymes, which is known as the "X" factor, and nicotinamide adenine dinucleotide, a coenzyme called the "V" factor. Various methods have been utilized to ascertain the presence of these factors in sufficient quantity in the primary plating media, and the requirement for one or both of these factors for in vitro growth is an aid in differentiation of the species. Both factors are available commercially (Difco) and can be added directly to the media according to the manufacturer's recommendation. Another common device utilized to supply accessory growth factors is the staphylococcus satellite method (6), in which a strain of *Staphylococcus aureus* is counterstreaked to the surface of a blood-agar plate which has been previously streaked with the sample. *Haemophilus* colonies which require V factor will grow more luxuriantly near the staphylococcal colonies.

Particular care must be exercised that isolated colonies are obtained from cultures of mixed flora. Under these circumstances *Haemophilus* cells may be readily overgrown or their growth may be inhibited. Various substances have been utilized to suppress the growth of other organisms; in my experience, the addition of 300 μg of bacitracin to an additional chocolate-agar plate (14) sharply increases the yield of *Haemophilus* in such mixed flora samples. Incubation under 10% CO_2 enhances or is necessary to the growth of some strains, particularly on primary isolation. Although growth is usually apparent in 24 h, the plates should be re-examined after 48 h of incubation at 37 C.

Scrapings from chancroids suspected of being caused by *H. ducreyi* should be inoculated onto freshly prepared meat infusion plates to which 3% agar and 20 to 30% defibrinated rabbit blood have been added. Better results have been reported by some investigators for initiation of growth of this fastidious organism by inoculating freshly clotted rabbit blood, incubating at 37 C, and subculturing daily to rabbit blood-agar until growth is detected.

IDENTIFICATION

Type-specific colonies of *H. influenzae* on blood-agar are "dew-drop" in appearance, are very small, and have a bluish sheen in obliquely transmitted light. Other species of *Haemophilus* are similar in appearance with the exception that *H. aegyptius* may grow more slowly. *H. parainfluenzae* and *H. aphrophilus* tend to be more opaque, and *H. parahaemolyticus* colonies are generally larger. *H. haemolyticus* and *H. parahaemolyticus* produce zones of hemolysis on horse and rabbit blood. *H. ducreyi* is only slightly hemolytic. Zinnemann has proposed a new species of hemolytic *Haemophilus*, *Haemophilus paraphrohaemolyticus* (25) which prefers CO_2 and is V factor-dependent.

Differentiation of *Haemophilus* species is largely based on ability to hemolyze, accessory growth factor requirements, and enhancement of growth under CO_2 (Table 2). *H. influenzae*, *H. aegyptius*, and *H. haemolyticus* require both X and V factors; *H. parainfluenzae* and *H. parahaemolyticus* require only V factor; *H. aphrophilus* requires X factor only in air containing CO_2; and *H. ducreyi* requires X factor. Determination of these requirements may be tested by different means. The simplest method is to place paper strips containing X factor, V factor, and both X and V factors (Difco and BBL) on Trypticase soy agar or brain heart infusion agar previously inoculated with the test organism. The inoculum should be diluted (1:100 of a 16- to 24-h culture is usually satisfactory) to prevent carry-over of X factor. Plates should be incubated aerobically at 37 C. In those few instances when equivocal results are obtained or no growth factor appears to be required, tests should be repeated after further subculture of the *Haemophilus* strain. Duplicate plates should be incubated under atmospheric O_2 and in the presence of 10% CO_2 and read after 24 and 48 h of incubation. Peptone agar, which has no accessory growth factor, streaked across with a *Staphylococcus aureus* strain to supply V factor, and peptone agar containing autoclaved blood (X factor) also can be used to determine growth requirements. Peptone broth medium, to which X factor in a final concentration of 1:250,000 or V factor to a final concentration of 1:10,000,000 (commerically available) has been added, can be similarly used, singly and in combination. Whenever feasible, known control strains should be cultured on the media utilized.

TABLE 2. *Growth factor requirements and hemolytic activity of Haemophilus species*

Organism	Growth factor		Hemolysis
	X	V	
H. influenzae	+	+	−
H. parainfluenzae	−	+	−
H. haemolyticus	+	+	+
H. parahaemolyticus	−	+	+
H. aphrophilus	+	−	−
H. aegyptius	+	+	−
H. ducreyi	+	−	Slight

Many strains of *H. aphrophilus* will not grow in the absence of moisture. Further tests of some differential value are indole production, nitrate reduction, and sugar fermentation. Growth factors added to indole medium allow growth for detection of indole production. Eveland (9) reported that *H. influenzae* capsular types a, b, c, and f give indole-positive reactions, whereas types d and e do not and nonencapsulated strains give a plus-minus reaction. Indole is not produced by *H. aegyptius*, *H. aphrophilus*, and *H. ducreyi*, and is usually not produced by the remaining strains. Sugar reactions can be demonstrated on agar slants containing Andrade indicator and 1% of the carbohydrate to be tested. Acid is produced from glucose by all species and with a small amount of gas by *H. aphrophilus*. Mannitol is not fermented; polysaccharides are fermented only by *H. aphrophilus*, *H. parainfluenzae*, and *H. parahaemolyticus*. All species of *Haemophilus* reduce nitrates to nitrites. Catalase production by *A. actinomycetemcomitans* is a useful means of differentiating this organism from *H. aphrophilus*, which does not produce catalase. This test can be performed by dropping 3% H_2O_2 on growth on an agar surface (not containing blood) and observing for bubbles of gas. Also, *H. aphrophilus* ferments lactose with the production of gas, but does not ferment mannitol or xylose whereas *A. actinomycetemcomitans* does not ferment lactose, but does ferment mannitol and xylose. *H. haemoglobinophilus*, a species of *Haemophilus* which is normally found in dogs, has been reported from human infection (10) and has characteristics similar to X-dependent strains of *H. aphrophilus*. However, *H. haemoglobinophilus* produces indole and also does not ferment lactose but does ferment mannitol and xylose.

Type-specific strains of *Haemophilus* tend to produce fluffy colonies in liquid media, whereas non-type-specific strains are usually granular. Most other species of *Haemophilus* give granular growth in broth with the exceptions of *H. aphrophilus*, which produces fluffy colonies that cling to the sides of the tube, and *H. aegyptius*, the granular growth of which often develops a fluffy outgrowth.

The correct taxonomic status of an organism recovered from the human genital tract described by Gardner and Dukes in 1955 (11) and designated *Haemophilus vaginalis* has been disputed. Dunkelberg et al. (8) and Zinnemann et al. (25) have called it *Corynebacterium vaginale;* others favor the theory that it is a biological variant of lactobacilli. Evidence exists for a causal relationship of this organism to vaginitis including production of vaginitis by inoculation from culture (7). Gram staining results and the need for X and V factors are also disputed. On direct microscope examination of Gram-stained vaginal discharge, these organisms appear as small gram-negative to gram-variable coccobacillary bacteria, numbers of which may attach to the surface of epithelial cells ("clue cells"). Cultures obtained on sterile swabs and placed on blood agar (preferably Casman's agar, Difco, enriched with blood), or on chocolate agar, yield very small, gray, slightly convex colonies generally with a narrow zone of green discoloration. The presence of CO_2 improves initial growth. Age of culture and media utilized effect the Gram staining reaction. They grow as small "puff-ball" aggregations in thioglycolate broth enriched with serum and are reported to be catalase and indole negative and to reduce nitrates to nitrites. They must be differentiated from "other" *Corynebacterium* and *Haemophilus* species.

IMMUNOSEROLOGICAL DIAGNOSIS

Type-specific strains of *Haemophilus* should be selected for all serological testing procedures. Antisera are commercially available (Difco) only for typing of *H. influenzae*, which has six known serological types, a, b, c, d, e, and f. Serological identification is performed by slide agglutination procedures or by the capsular swelling (Quellung) reaction. The manufacturer's recommendations for slide agglutination tests should be followed, and care should be exercised that a heavy suspension of the organism is utilized. The Quellung reaction (chapter 9) is rapid and accurate, and has the added advantage that it can be used for direct typing of microorganisms in the cerebrospinal fluid, exudates, etc. If the test is to be performed on organisms that have been cultured, young cultures, preferably in the log phase of growth, should be utilized.

For those laboratories which have the equipment and trained personnel, the direct fluorescent-antibody technique is also rapid and reliable. It too can be used for direct typing of *H. influenzae* present in samples as well as for cultured organisms. Direct typing procedures offer the great advantage of giving prompt information to the physician treating a patient with an infection such as meningitis. Fluorescent antibody for this procedure is commercially available (Difco).

Precipitin tests are less frequently used for serological diagnosis, but can be utilized for confirmation of identification. To perform the test, use a capillary tube to draw up a 1-cm column of broth culture (or spinal fluid supernatant fraction) onto an equal quantity of antiserum. Place it upright in Plasticine placed on a wooden or plastic block or other convenient base. Observe for cloudiness at the interface of the two fluids. Incubation at 37 C may hasten the reaction, and the test should be allowed to stand as long as 2 h before being considered negative.

H. influenzae type b is usually found in cerebrospinal fluid and blood, and organisms recovered from these sources should be first tested against type b antiserum. Type-specific antigens of *H. influenzae* cross-react as previously mentioned. The most important of these are the cross-reactions with *Diplococcus pneumoniae;* i.e., *H. influenzae* type a cross-reacts with *D. pneumoniae* subgroup 6, *H. influenzae* type b cross-reacts with *D. pneumoniae* groups 15A and 35B as well as with subgroups 6 and 29, and *H. influenzae* type c, with *D. pneumoniae* 11 (1).

Antibody response to infections with *H. influenzae* is erratic, particularly in infants and young children, and has not been used as a diagnostic tool. Whether this is due to immune paralysis or immaturity of the response mechanisms has not been determined (21). However, high precipitin titers have been used as evidence that this organism plays a role in chronic bronchitis, bronchiectasis, etc., in adults, and the presence of a high titer of *Haemophilus*-specific antibodies demonstrable by immunoelectrophoresis has been recommended as an objective criterion for the inclusion of a patient in a chemotherapeutic trial for these disorders (5). Agglutination, hemagglutination, bactericidal tests, and complement-fixation tests have also been used to study the antibody response.

SUSCEPTIBILITY TO ANTIMICROBIAL AGENTS

Most *H. influenzae* strains are susceptible to penicillin and its derivatives, to sulfonamides, and to the tetracycline group, and these antibiotics have been extensively used to treat *Haemophilus* infection. Chloramphenicol is also effective, but potential aplasia, although rare, limits its usefulness. One hundred percent of *Haemophilus* strains are inhibited by achievable blood levels of ampicillin (16), and this drug is most commonly used today along with tetracycline (24). The inoculum should be grown in Levinthal's broth or brain heart infusion plus 5% Fildes enrichment (chapter 95) and diluted 10-fold before inoculation of chocolate-agar plates for disk susceptibility tests (chapter 46); the plates are then incubated under 10% CO_2. Broth dilution susceptibility test (chapter 45) should utilize 10^5 to 10^6 viable microorganisms/ml as an inoculum, and meat infusion broth containing enrichment factors should be used as the test medium.

EVALUATION

The report to the physician should state the species of *Haemophilus* recovered from the sample, and the serotype if the strain is type-specific and recovered from an infant or from an apparently pathogenic process. As these organisms constitute part of the normal flora of the upper respiratory tract, interpretation of the results is dependent upon clinical observation. Evaluation of significance based upon abundance of *H. influenzae* organisms recovered from areas of mixed flora is hazardous because of the well-known stimulation by *S. aureus* and other organisms occasionally present, as well as the suppression or overgrowth by *D. pneumoniae* or alpha-hemolytic streptococci. Encapsulated strains are more invasive, but a majority of strains causing otitis media are nonencapsulated. Increasing numbers of the latter are being found to cause disease in adults with impaired host defenses.

LITERATURE CITED

1. Alexander, H. E., G. Leidy, and C. MacPherson. 1946. Production of types a, b, c, d, e, and f *H. influenzae* antibody for diagnostic and therapeutic purposes. J. Immunol. **54**:207–211.
2. Bradshaw, J., and C. Phillips. 1970. *Hemophilus parainfluenzae* meningitis in a 4 year old boy. Pediatrics **45**:856.
3. Bradshaw, M. W., R. Schneerson, J. C. Parke, Jr., and J. B. Robbins. 1971. Bacterial antigens cross-reactive with the capsular polysaccharide of *Haemophilus influenzae* type b. Lancet **1**:1095–1096.
4. Burnett, G. W., and H. W. Scherp. 1968. Oral microbiology and infectious diseases. The Williams & Wilkins Co., Baltimore.
5. Burns, M. W., and J. R. May. 1967. *Haemophilus influenzae* precipitins in the serum of patients with chronic bronchul disorders. Lancet **1**:354–358.
6. Cooper, R. G., and I. D. Attenborough. 1968. An indicator method for the detection of bacterial X and V factor dependence. Aust. J. Exp. Biol. Med. Sci. **46**:803–805.
7. Criswell, B. S., C. L. Ladwig. H. L. Gardner, and C. D. Dukes. 1969. *Haemophilus vaginalis:* vaginitis by inoculation from culture. Obstet. Gynecol. **33**:195–199.
8. Dunkelberg, W. E., Jr., R. Skaggs, and D. S. Kellogg, Jr. 1970. A study and new description of Corynebacterium vaginale (*Haemophilus vaginalis.*) Amer. J. Clin. Pathol. **53**:370–377.
9. Eveland, W. C. 1970. *In* Diagnostic procedures for bacterial, mycotic and parasitic infections, 5th ed. American Public Health Association, Inc., New York. p. 129.
10. Frazer, J., and K. B. Rogers. 1972. The isolation of an X-dependent strain of *Haemophilus* from otitis media identified as *H. haemoglobinophilus* (canis). J. Clin. Pathol. **25**:179–180.
11. Gardner, H. L., and C. D. Dukes. 1955. *Haemophilus vaginitis*. A newly defined specific infection classified "nonspecific" vaginitis. Amer. J. Obstet. Gynecol. **69**:962–976.
12. Gullekson, E., and M. Dumoff. 1966. *H. parainfluenzae* meningitis in a new-born. J. Amer. Med. Ass. **198**:1221.
13. Halsted, L., M. L. Lepow, N. Balassanian, J. Emmerich, and E. Wolinsky. 1968. Otitis media. Clinical observations, microbiology and evaluation of therapy. Amer. J. Dis. Child. **115**:542–551.
14. Hovig, B., and E. H. Aandahl. 1969. A selective method for the isolation of *Haemophilus* in material from the respiratory tract. Acta Pathol. Microbiol. Scand. **77**:677–684.
15. Johnstone, J. M., and H. S. Larry. 1967. Acute epiglottitis in adults due to infection with *Haemophilus influenzae* type b. Lancet **2**:134–136.
16. Kahn, W., S. Ross, and E. A. Zaremba. 1967. Comparative inhibition of *Haemophilus influenzae* by eight antibiotics. Antimicrob. Ag. Chemother. 1966, p. 393–396.
17. King, E. O., and H. W. Tatum. 1962. *Actinobacillus actinomycetemcomitans* and *Hemophilus aphrophilus*. J. Infect. Dis. **111**:85–94.
18. Krishnaswami, R., J. Schwartz, and W. Boodish. 1972. Pathogenicity of *H. parainfluenzae*. Pediatrics **50**:498–499.

19. May, J. R., and D. M. Delves. 1964. The survival of *Haemophilus influenzae* and pneumococci in specimens of sputum sent to the laboratory by post. J. Clin. Pathol. **17**:254–256.
20. Page, M. I., and E. O. King. 1966. Infection due to *Actinobacillus actinomycetemcomitans* and *Hemophilus aphrophilus*. N. Engl. J. Med. **275**:181–188.
21. South, M. A. 1972. Lack of immune response to *Hemophilus influenzae:* immune paralysis or immaturity? J. Pediatrics **80**:348–350.
22. Sutter, V. L., and S. M. Finegold. 1970. *Haemophilus aphrophilus* infections: clinical and bacteriologic studies. Ann. N.Y. Acad. Sci. **174**:468–487.
23. V.D. Fact Sheet. 1973. Dept. of Health, Education & Welfare Publication No. (CDC) 74-8195. PHS, Ed. 30, Table 3.
24. Weinstein, L. 1970. Type B *Haemophilus influenzae* infections in adults. N. Engl. J. Med. **4**:221–222.
25. Zinnemann, K., K. B. Rogers, J. Frazer, and S. K. Devaraj. 1971. A haemolytic V-dependent CO_2-preferring *Haemophilus* species (*Haemophilus paraphrohaemolyticus* nov. spec.). J. Med. Microbiol. **4**:139–143.
26. Zinnemann, K., and G. C. Turner. 1963. The taxonomic position of "*Haemophilus vaginalis*" (*Corynebacterium vaginale*). J. Pathol. Bacteriol. **85**:213–219.

Chapter 27

Bordetella

B. PITTMAN

CHARACTERIZATION

The three species of the genus *Bordetella* belong to the family *Brucellaceae*. *Bordetella pertussis*, the etiological agent of pertussis, commonly called whooping cough, was isolated by Bordet and Gengou (5) in 1906. It is a small gram-negative coccobacillus that is encapsulated, grows aerobically, is relatively inert biochemically, and requires the addition of blood, charcoal, or ion-exchange resins to neutralize inhibitors in the medium (21, 29–31). Growth occurs in phases I-IV, with the first phase being smooth and antigenically competent. One of the outstanding properties of this organism is its ability to vary culturally and serologically with alterations in the medium. This characteristic has proven to be a problem from time to time in the production of potent vaccines (29). *B. pertussis* contains a number of cellular components that are important in infection and vaccine production, such as heat-labile dermonecrotic toxin, lipopolysaccharide (endotoxin), agglutinogens and serotype antigens, sensitizing substances including histamine-sensitizing factor, lymphocytosis-promoting factor, protective and adjuvant factors, hemagglutinin, and hemolysin (29).

There are other species of the genus *Bordetella* which cause a pertussis-like syndrome. *B. parapertussis*, formerly classified as *Haemophilus parapertussis*, was found by Lautrop (22) to be as widespread as pertussis, but the rate of clinical to subclinical infection was 3 to 4% in parapertussis as compared to 75% in pertussis. *B. bronchiseptica*, formerly classified as *Brucella bronchisepticum*, is not uncommonly isolated from the respiratory tract of animals. It is isolated from humans only after close contact with rabbits, guinea pigs, cats, and other domestic animals (6).

The antigenic relationships of the *Bordetella* species are based on heat-labile agglutinogens (called factors) held in common (13). Serotyping of *B. pertussis* is important in the epidemiology of pertussis because it is important to know what serotypes must be included to produce a vaccine that will give adequate protection (32). To date, however, the mouse protection test is the most reliable means of selecting cultures for pertussis vaccine production (18, 29). A summary of antigenic factors is presented in Table 1.

CLINICAL SIGNIFICANCE

The importance of the recognition of pertussis cannot be too strongly emphasized, for in the first year of life it causes more deaths than infectious hepatitis, scarlet fever, poliomyelitis, chicken pox, and mumps combined (6). There have been several reports of a pertussis syndrome in which *B. pertussis* was not isolated but in which adenoviruses were isolated or implicated by rises in antibody titer (8, 9, 20). The significance of these findings is not yet understood.

Though the morbidity and mortality due to pertussis have steadily declined over the years, it is still a very serious disease. A summary of reported cases and deaths in the USA for 1950–1972 is presented in Fig. 1.

The clinical course of pertussis follows three distinct phases:

(i) The catarrheal phase, which lasts about 2 weeks, is characterized by rhinorrhea, low-grade fever, a nonproductive and progressive cough that frequently becomes nocturnal, a lymphocytosis which may account for 60 to 80% of the total count, and the decline of lymphocytes, which usually coincides with the disappearance of *B. pertussis*. Hypoglycemia is observed also.

(ii) The paroxysmal phase, which lasts 2 to 4 weeks, is characterized by an inspiratory whoop at the end of a long paroxysm of coughing, usually followed by the expulsion of thick and tenacious mucus. Vomiting often occurs and the patient may become malnourished. This whoop is characteristic, but may be absent, particularly in very young infants, and in older children and adults who may have been immunized early in life (26). The cause of the paroxysmal cough and whoop has not yet been precisely defined, but current information on

B-adrenergic blockage in mice by pertussis vaccine supports the hypothesis that it is neurologic in origin (16, 29).

(iii) The convalescent period lasts 2 to 3 weeks and is characterized by a gradual subsiding of the cough as the patient returns to normal.

The natural habitat of the organism is the mucous membranes of the respiratory tract. Recovery of the organisms from the respiratory tract by culturing is highest during the first week of infection, when approximately 95% of the cultures may be positive. By the fourth week, the number of positive cultures decreases to about 50% or less. Rarely is there a positive finding in the fifth week, even though the patient may still be whooping (11). The finding of positive smears by fluorescent-antibody (FA) staining closely parallels the appearance of positive cultures. Antibiotic therapy affects the rate of isolation and FA detection, even during the early acute state of infection. Isolations are seldom made after antibiotic treatment of 48-h duration, although positive FA results may be obtained with dead cells that can still be recovered from the respiratory tract (35). The organisms are not isolated from the blood.

The carrier state in pertussis has not been completely demonstrated, since only rarely have specimens from asymptomatic persons been cultured. Studies have shown that, although transient carriers may exist among contacts of patients, they are of no known epidemiological significance. It is believed that incubationary and unrecognized cases rather than carriers are probably the significant factors in the spread of pertussis (1, 24).

TABLE 1. *Antigenic factors of the Bordetella species*

Species	Species-specific factor	Other factors present
B. pertussis	1	2, 3, 4, 5, 6, and 7[a]
B. parapertussis	14	8, 9, 10, and 7[a]
B. bronchiseptica	12	8, 9, 10, 11, and 7[a]

[a] Factor 7 is held in common by all *Bordetella* species.

COLLECTION, TRANSPORT, AND STORAGE OF SPECIMENS

Since many laboratories are not equipped for cultural isolation for *B. pertussis*, specimens must be collected and transported to a central laboratory where this service is offered. If carefully followed, the procedures presented here can provide successful cultural and/or FA identification of *B. pertussis*.

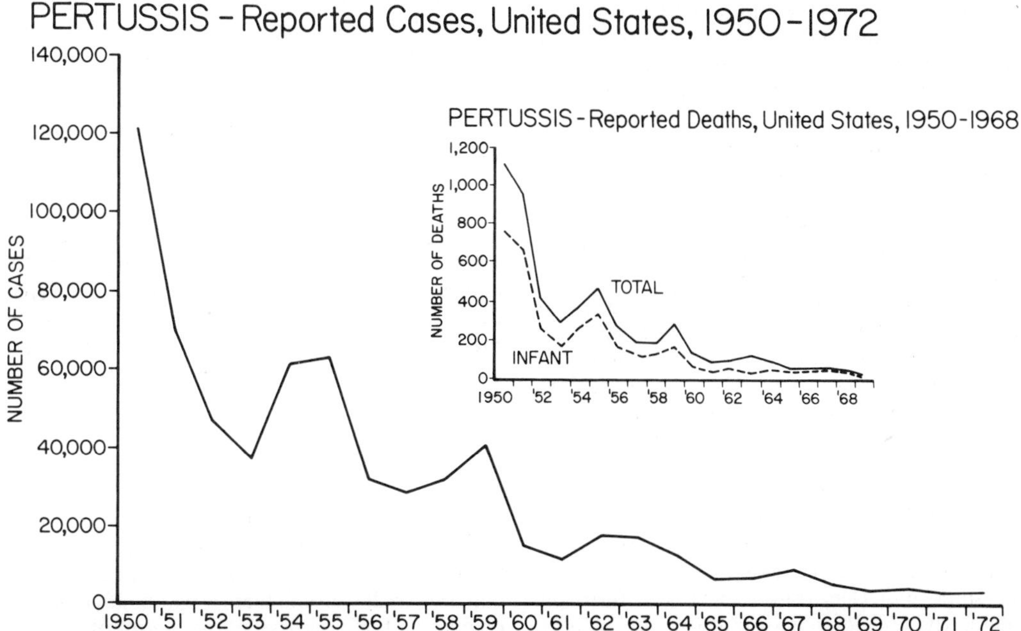

FIG. 1. *Morbidity and mortality due to pertussis in the USA. Taken from the CDC Morbidity and Mortality Annual Supplement, Summary 1972, published by U.S. Department of Health, Education, and Welfare, Publication No. (CDC) 74-8241.*

Method of collection

A nasopharyngeal swab is the specimen of choice. The swab should be small and flexible, and in no way inhibitory to the organisms. The most satisfactory swab for this purpose is one made of Teflon tubing to which a small wad of cotton has been securely attached (B. Pittman and W. B. Cherry, Bacteriol. Proc., p. 51, 1965). Other swabs that have been used are ones prepared by wrapping a small wad of cotton tightly on a flexible wire (17) and the commercially prepared Calgiswab marketed by Colab Laboratories, Inc.

To take the specimen, immobilize the patient's head and gently pass the swab through the nostril into the nasopharynx. If resistance is met in the passageway, do not force entry because the patient may have a deviated septum or large turbinate. Try the other nostril. If the swab cannot be passed through either nostril, enter through the mouth. A coughing paroxysm is usually evoked by the taking of the swab. This increases the discharge of organisms, thus increasing the chances for isolation.

Transport

The transportation of clinical specimens can severely limit the successful identification of *B. pertussis*. Once the swab has been taken, it is imperative that it be streaked immediately on Bordet-Gengou agar, or maintained in the "status quo" no longer than is absolutely necessary for transport to the laboratory. This may be accomplished by placing the swab in 0.25 to 0.5 ml of sterile 1% Casamino Acids solution, pH 7.2, and holding for no longer than 2 h, since *B. pertussis* tends to die off and other organisms present overgrow it. If the swab used is attached to a metal wire, the oligodynamic effect of the metal ions causes an increased die-off of organisms.

If the time required from the taking of the specimen until its placement on Bordet-Gengou plates is greater than about 2 h, an adequate transportation method must be employed. Various transport media, particularly Stuart's (34), have been used successfully to maintain the viability of a variety of organisms in clinical specimens which must be mailed to a central laboratory for identification. Antonis (4) found that, when swabs were placed in Stuart's transport medium and processed in the laboratory the same day that they were taken from patients, they yielded an isolation rate of 30%. Repeated culturing of 20 swabs kept overnight at room temperature yielded 19 positive isolations, although all swabs showed a reduction in the number of colonies. One culture was negative; only six colonies were present originally. He concluded that Stuart's transport medium was of value in the diagnosis of whooping cough. Gästrin et al. (14) described a modification of Stuart's medium, called SBL. This medium was enclosed in nitrogen-filled glass ampoules which were opened just prior to use. Using pure cultures, they found that *B. pertussis* decreased only 0.2 log after storage in this medium for 72 h at room temperature; the decrease with Stuart's medium was 2.3 to 3.0 logs. When the storage time was increased to 96 h, the decrease was 1.5 logs in the SBL medium and 5 logs in Stuart's medium.

Jones and Kendrick (15) described the use of a blood-free medium for the transport and growth of *B. pertussis*. The medium is a modification of Mishulow's charcoal agar (25), in which heart infusion broth was substituted for fresh beef heart, the agar content was reduced to 2%, charcoal (Norit FQP) was added, and penicillin was added after the medium had been autoclaved. The medium was dispensed in short, wide, screw-cap bottles that would withstand mailing and allow adequate surface area of the slant for the development of isolated colonies. Simulated specimens were inoculated onto this medium, mailed to a given address, and returned for examination. The results showed that the modified charcoal agar not only maintained viability but also supported some growth of *B. pertussis* while in transit. In addition, these cultures can be incubated for growth without subculture to another medium. An early identification may be made by taking a sweep of growth from the slant when it is received and staining with FA. This medium has had limited field evaluation but should be used more extensively, for it holds promise as a good transport medium for *B. pertussis* (17). Jones and Kendrick (15) also found a rapid die-off of *B. pertussis* in Stuart's transport medium, and they consider it unsatisfactory for the routine transport of specimens containing *B. pertussis*.

Storage

There are few reports in the literature of storage of clinical specimens. Pittman and Cherry (Bacteriol. Proc., p. 51, 1965) used pure cultures to determine factors which affected the recovery of *B. pertussis*; they presented data from this study on the storage of swabs under several conditions. Multiple sets of three kinds of swabs—untreated bronze wire, Saran-tipped wire, and Teflon tubing, all of which had a small wad of cotton securely attached—were inoculated with a known concentration of a *B. pertussis* culture. One set of swabs was kept in dry tubes, one set was placed in 0.5 ml of 1% Casamino Acids solution, pH 7.2 to 7.4, and the third set was placed in 2 ml of Stuart's transport medium. The swabs were either held at room temperature (21 to 24 C) or placed in a refrigerator (4 to 10 C). Viability of the cells was checked immediately, at 6, 24, and 72 h, and after 2 weeks of storage, by streaking directly onto Bordet-Gengou plates and counting colonies. FA smears were also prepared and stained at these time intervals. Consistently higher counts were obtained with the Teflon tubing than with the other two types of swabs used. No *B. pertussis* survived on any of the swabs after 72 h at room temperature. A summary of these data is presented in Table 2. FA staining was generally satisfactory for all conditions tested, although few cells could be found. A reading of 3 to 4+ was obtained for all specimens up to 72 h, after which the fluorescence decreased. Donaldson and Whitaker (10) reported collecting a series of direct smears over a period of about 6 months and storing them at room temperature in airtight cans over anhydrous calcium sulfate. No change in staining was indicated. I have had clinical smears that gave FA positive staining 2 weeks after smears were prepared and mailed. The smears had received no special treatment and were in transit at ambient temperature.

CULTURE AND ISOLATION

Recommended procedure for primary isolation

Emulsify the specimen on the nasopharyngeal swab in 0.25 to 0.5 ml of Casamino Acids solution so that the same inoculum will be available for culturing and FA smears. Using the swab or an inoculation loop, streak a plate of Bordet-Gengou agar (Difco) containing 15 to 20% rabbit, sheep, or horse blood and another Bordet-Gengou plate which also contains 0.5 unit of penicillin/ml of medium. Incubate the plates aerobically at 35 C and examine daily for growth. Molds or other spreading colonies may develop within 24 h and may overgrow the plate. Remove such colonies by cutting out with a sterile needle or scalpel the agar supporting and surrounding them. Growth of *B. pertussis* usually occurs by the 4th day, and plates may be discarded after 6 days. These organisms grow best in a moist medium; to help keep them from drying out, place plates in a candle jar (do not light) for incubation.

Other cultural methods

B. pertussis may adapt to other media such as blood, chocolate, or brain-veal infusion agar, but these should not be used because the organisms tend to dissociate from smooth to rough and show antigenic differences.

When a large amount of growth is required, as

TABLE 2. *Colony counts of Bordetella pertussis from three types of swab materials under various storage conditions*

Swab	Time and temp of testing				
	Immediate[a] (room)	6 h		24 h	
		Refrigerator	Room	Refrigerator	Room
Untreated bronze wire swabs					
Dry	95	67	—	1	—
CAS[b]	96	14	—	—	—
Stuart	58	49	11	15	2
Saran-tipped bronze wire swabs					
Dry	127	35	—	8	—
CAS	77	19	29	51	—
Stuart	58	39	21	63	13
Teflon swabs					
Dry	534	152	394	293	217
CAS	620	110	283	116	57
Stuart	576	181	248	98	42
Culture control[c]	400–600	400–600	400–600	400–600	400–500

[a] Plating was done within 1 h.
[b] Casamino Acids solution, 1%, pH 7.3.
[c] A 0.1-ml amount of a 10^{-4} dilution of *B. pertussis* 8319.

for vaccine production, Cohen-Wheeler broth (7) or Bordet-Gengou agar (5) containing added peptone (BBL) is used. Peptone has an inhibitory effect on growth and requires a large inoculum to overcome this effect. This medium (BBL) therefore should not be used as a primary isolation medium (33) since clinical specimens may have relatively few *B. pertussis* cells present.

IDENTIFICATION

Cultural characteristics

In reflected light, the colonies of *B. pertussis* appear as droplets of mercury or half pearls, smooth, raised, transparent, and glistening; they have an entire circular edge, and usually are not over 1 mm in diameter. *B. parapertussis* colonies are usually larger than *B. pertussis*, and the surface is, as a rule, somewhat more dull; a slight brownish color may be present. *B. bronchiseptica* colonies look very much like *B. pertussis* colonies but can become considerably larger with continued incubation. All three species produce zones of hemolysis. The nature and degree of hemolysis depends upon the blood used, its concentration, and the length and temperature of incubation.

Microscope examination

Bordetella organisms are small gram-negative bacilli which occur singly, in pairs, or in clumps and are usually 1.0 by 0.3 to 0.5 μm in size. Because of the rather slow uptake of the counter-stains used in the Gram stain, a longer period of time for this step may be desired (23). In older cultures, the cells become very pleomorphic and may have threadlike filaments or thick bacillary forms. *B. parapertussis* is typically the most rod-shaped and can, to a limited degree, appear in palisade arrangements. *B. bronchiseptica* is motile by peritrichous flagella; the others are not motile. *Bordetella* organisms are nonsporeforming, and capsules can be demonstrated by staining but not by capsular swelling (33).

Biochemical reactions

Bordetella cells are relatively inert biochemically. They do not ferment sugars; gelatin is not liquefied; indole and acetyl methylcarbinol are not produced; H_2S is not produced; most strains are catalase-positive; and litmus milk is rendered alkaline. The production of an alkaline reaction in most media is also characteristic. Urease is rapidly produced (4 h) by *B. bronchiseptica*.

A summary of differential characteristics of the *Bordetella* species is presented in Table 3. A typical brownish coloration is produced by *B. parapertussis* on blood-free peptone agar. The pigment is of the melanine type and is believed to be formed by the action of tyrosinase on tyrosine, which is present in the medium. Care must be taken to maintain an aerobic state, because the pigment is not produced under anaerobic conditions (23).

Serological methods

Slide agglutination tests can be performed with specific antiserum as soon as growth is apparent on Bordet-Gengou plates. Suspend a loopful of growth in saline, and adjust the turbidity to 20 billion cells/ml, using a National Institutes of Health opacity standard, or to 10 billion cells, using a McFarland no. 3 turbidity standard (19). On one end of a clean glass slide, place a drop of the cell suspension. On the other end, place several small drops of antipertussis serum at the appropriate dilution and mix. Clumping of cells indicates a positive reaction. Controls should include a known *B. pertussis* culture and a negative control containing cells suspended in saline only. *B. pertussis* characteristically suspends well in saline after a momentary clumping effect which disappears with slight agitation (19). Anti-*Bordetella* sera are commercially available, but must be checked for specificity before use.

For serotyping *Bordetella*, specifically absorbed antisera are used in the tube agglutination test (13). Serotyping has been limited to epidemiological studies and to selecting cultures for vaccine production. These sera are presently not commercially available.

Eldering et al. (12) observed certain discrepancies in the results of *B. pertussis* agglutination tests and FA reactions. The results they obtained suggested that the antibodies responsible for these two reactions may be different.

TABLE 3. *Differential characteristics of the Bordetella species*[a]

Characteristic	*B. pertussis*	*B. parapertussis*	*B. bronchiseptica*
Growth on blood-free peptone agar	−	+	+
Browning of peptone agar	−	+	−
Produces urease	−	+	+ 4 h
Reduces nitrate	−	−	+
Motility	−	−	+

[a] Reactions: −, negative; +, positive.

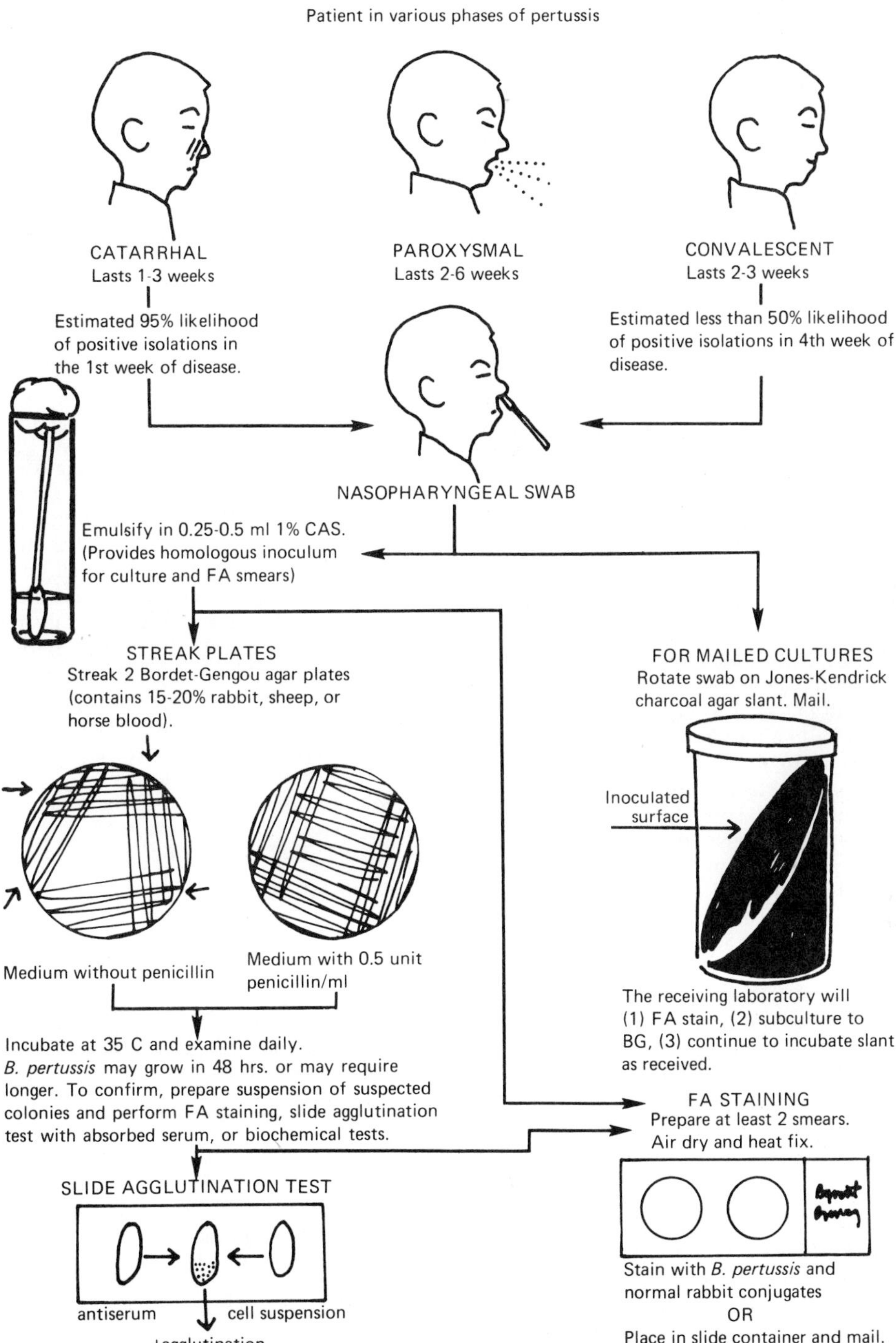
Patient in various phases of pertussis
CATARRHAL
Lasts 1-3 weeks
PAROXYSMAL
Lasts 2-6 weeks
CONVALESCENT
Lasts 2-3 weeks
Estimated 95% likelihood of positive isolations in the 1st week of disease.
Estimated less than 50% likelihood of positive isolations in 4th week of disease.
NASOPHARYNGEAL SWAB
Emulsify in 0.25-0.5 ml 1% CAS. (Provides homologous inoculum for culture and FA smears)
STREAK PLATES
Streak 2 Bordet-Gengou agar plates (contains 15-20% rabbit, sheep, or horse blood).
FOR MAILED CULTURES
Rotate swab on Jones-Kendrick charcoal agar slant. Mail.
Inoculated surface
Medium without penicillin
Medium with 0.5 unit penicillin/ml
The receiving laboratory will (1) FA stain, (2) subculture to BG, (3) continue to incubate slant as received.
Incubate at 35 C and examine daily. B. pertussis may grow in 48 hrs. or may require longer. To confirm, prepare suspension of suspected colonies and perform FA staining, slide agglutination test with absorbed serum, or biochemical tests.
FA STAINING
Prepare at least 2 smears.
Air dry and heat fix.
SLIDE AGGLUTINATION TEST
antiserum
cell suspension
+agglutination
Stain with B. pertussis and normal rabbit conjugates
OR
Place in slide container and mail.

FIG. 2. *Flow chart for the identification of Bordetella pertussis.*

IMMUNOSEROLOGICAL DIAGNOSIS

FA procedures are not a substitute for cultural isolation, but they do offer diagnostic aid to those laboratories not prepared to culture for *B. pertussis* (28). Smears of exudate may be stained locally or mailed to a laboratory equipped to perform this service. It is possible to have a tentative diagnosis of pertussis within 1 h after the swab is taken.

Chapters 3 and 4 deal with the preparation of reagents and equipment for successful diagnosis by FA methods.

Procedure for direct fluorescent-antibody staining

Obtain a nasopharyngeal swab and emulsify as previously described. If the smear is to be made from a culture, sweep through the growth and emulsify. Make two smears on a slide with a loopful or small drop of the emulsified material. Allow to air-dry; heat-fix by gently passing through a flame three times. Place on a flat surface and add a small drop of the appropriate dilution of *B. pertussis* and normal rabbit conjugates, and spread to cover the smear completely. Leave under a moist chamber for 30 min. Tap off excess conjugate and rinse in one container of phosphate-buffered saline, pH 7.6; then transfer to another container and leave for 10 min. Allow to air-dry or very gently blot with bibulous paper. Place a drop of mounting fluid on the smear and add a cover slip. Examine under the fluorescence microscope. Look for very small, brightly stained organisms that may occur singly or in small groups. There should be no staining with the normal rabbit conjugate. (Animals used to prepare anti-*Bordetella* sera or normal serum conjugates should be examined for the natural occurrence of *B. bronchiseptica* antibodies. A rabbit with an agglutination titer of 1 : 10 or less should be satifactory to use.)

Serological tests to demonstrate circulating antibodies in patients' serum are of limited diagnostic help since they occur late in the infection. These tests, however, are used to evaluate the responses of children to vaccination (1).

The Analytical Bacteriology Section of the Center for Disease Control (CDC) has been receiving mailed nasopharyngeal smears and cultures for *B. pertussis* identification by FA staining since 1964. To date (September 1973), there have been 169 specimens submitted, 49 of which have given positive FA reactions. Since November 1957, the Clinical Bacteriology Section of the CDC has received only 38 cultures for confirmation as *B. pertussis*. It is apparent that more diligent efforts must be made to promote the submitting of specimens when pertussis infections are suspected. Figure 2 is a flow chart summarizing the steps necessary for the identification of *B. pertussis*.

SUSCEPTIBILITY TO ANTIMICROBIAL AGENTS

The efficacy of antimicrobial therapy for pertussis is doubtful since it does not seem to alter the course of the disease or relieve symptoms (27). Ames et al. (3) compared the effects of streptomycin, chloramphenicol, rabbit antiserum, and human immune serum without showing convincing proof of therapeutic value for any of the specific agents. At one time, secondary bacterial pneumonia was a frequent complication of pertussis, but since the advent of antibiotics it has become rare.

Two recent reports (3, 27) have suggested that ampicillin or tetracycline therapy for 5 days is effective in the eradication of *B. pertussis* from the nasopharynx. However, in another study (2) it was found that 10 days of ampicillin and 7 days of tetracycline therapy may not be effective. Apparently, these antibiotics may be of some use in shortening the period of communicability of *B. pertussis*, but further controlled studies must be conducted to establish this fact. A patient should not be assumed to be noncontagious after therapy, and appropriate cultures are necessary to determine whether nasopharyngeal carriers exist.

LITERATURE CITED

1. Abbott, J. D., N. W. Preston, and R. I. Mackay. 1971. Agglutinin response to pertussis vaccination in the child. Brit. Med. J. **1**:86–88.
2. Adasek, P. J., M. N. Meyer, and C. G. Ray. 1969. Antibiotics and their effect on *Bordetella pertussis* in the nasopharynx. Pediatrics **44**:606–609.
3. Ames, R. G., S. M. Cohen, A. E. Fischer, J. Kohn, A. Z. McPherson, J. Marlow, J. Rutzky, and H. E. Alexander. 1953. Comparison of the therapeutic efficacy of four agents in pertussis. Pediatrics **11**:323–337.
4. Antonis, A. H. 1970. Isolation of *Bordetella pertussis* from pernasal swabs stored in Stuart's medium. J. Med. Microbiol. **3**:184–186.
5. Bordet, J., and O. Gengou. 1906. L'endotoxine coquelucheuse. Ann. Inst. Pasteur Paris **23**:415–419.
6. Brooksaler, F., and J. D. Nelson. 1967. Pertussis: a reappraisal and report of 190 confirmed cases. Amer. J. Dis. Child. **114**:389–396.
7. Cohen, S. M., and M. W. Wheeler. 1946. Pertussis vaccine prepared with phase I cultures grown in fluid medium. Amer. J. Pub. Health **36**:371–376.
8. Collier, A. M., J. D. Connor, and W. R. Irving, Jr. 1966. Generalized type 5 adenovirus infection associated with the pertussis syndrome. J. Pediat. **69**:1073–1078.
9. Connor, J. D. 1970. Evidence for an etiologic role of adenoviral infection in pertussis syndrome. N. Engl. J. Med. **283**:390–394.
10. Donaldson, P., and J. A. Whitaker. 1960. Diagnosis of pertussis by fluorescent antibody staining of nasopharyngeal smears. Amer. J. Dis. Child. **99**:423–427.

11. Eldering, G. 1968. Some laboratory aspects of a pertussis surveillance program, p. 91–95. *In* Proceedings of 5th Annual Immunization Conference, San Diego. U.S. Department of Health, Education, and Welfare, Atlanta, Ga.
12. Eldering, G., W. C. Eveland, and P. L. Kendrick. 1962. Fluorescent antibody staining and agglutination reactions of *Bordetella pertussis* cultures. J. Bacteriol. **83**:745–749.
13. Eldering, G., C. Hornbeck, and J. Baker. 1957. Serological study of *Bordetella pertussis* and related species. J. Bacteriol. **74**:133–136.
14. Gästrin, B., L. O. Kallings, and A. Marcetic. 1968. The survival time for different bacteria in various transport media. Acta Pathol. Microbiol. Scand. **74**:371–380.
15. Jones, G. L., and P. L. Kendrick. 1959. Study of a blood-free medium for transport and growth of *Bordetella pertussis*. Health Lab. Sci. **6**:40–45.
16. Keller, K. F., and C. W. Fishel. 1967. In vivo and in vitro manifestations of adrenergic blockade in *Bordetella pertussis*-vaccinated mice. J. Bacteriol. **94**:804–811.
17. Kendrick, P. L. 1969. Transport media for *Bordetella pertussis*. Pub. Health Lab. **27**:85–92.
18. Kendrick, P. L., G. Eldering, M. K. Dixon, and J. Misner. 1947. Mouse protection tests in the study of pertussis vaccine: a comparative series using intracerebral route for challenge. Amer. J. Pub. Health **37**:803–810.
19. Kendrick, P. L., G. McL. Lawson, and J. J. Miller. 1950. *Hemophilus pertussis*, p. 136–155. *In* Diagnostic procedures and reagents, 3rd ed. American Public Health Association, Inc., New York.
20. Klenk, E. L., J. V. Gaulney, and J. W. Bass. 1972. Bacteriologically proved pertussis and adenovirus infection. Amer. J. Dis. Child. **124**:203–207.
21. Kuwajima, Y., T. Matsui, and M. Kishigami. 1957. The growth-supporting effect on some anion exchange resins for Phase I *Haemophilus pertussis*. Jap. J. Microbiol. **1**:375–381.
22. Lautrop, H. 1971. Epidemics of parapertussis: 20 years' observation in Denmark. Lancet **1**:1195–1198.
23. Lautrop, H., and B. W. Lacey. 1960. Laboratory diagnosis of whooping cough or *Bordetella* infections. Bull. W.H.O. **23**:15–35.
24. Linnemann, C. C. 1968. Pertussis carrier study in Louisiana, p. 95–97. *In* Proceedings of 5th Annual Immunization Conference, San Diego. U.S. Department of Health, Education, and Welfare, Atlanta, Ga.
25. Mishulow, L., L. S. Sharpe, and L. L. Cohen. 1952. Beef-heart charcoal agar for the preparation of pertussis vaccines. Amer. J. Pub. Health **43**:1466–1472.
26. Morse, S. I. 1972. Whooping cough, p. 303–307. *In* P. D. Hoeprich (ed.), Infectious diseases. Harper and Row, Publishers. Hagerstown, Md.
27. Nelson, J. D. 1969. Antibiotic treatment of pertussis. Pediatrics **44**:474–476.
28. Nelson, J. D., B. Hempstead, R. Tanaka, and F. P. Pauls. 1964. Fluorescent antibody diagnosis of infections. J. Amer. Med. Ass. **188**:1121–1124.
29. Pittman, M. 1970. *Bordetella pertussis*: bacterial and host factors in the pathogenesis and prevention of whooping cough, p. 239–269. *In* S. Mudd (ed.), Infectious agents and host reactions. W. B. Saunders Co., Philadelphia.
30. Pollock, M. R. 1947. The growth of *Hemophilus pertussis* on media without blood. Brit. J. Exp. Pathol. **28**:295–307.
31. Powell, H. M., C. G. Culbertson, and P. W. Ensminger. 1951. Charcoal agar culture medium for preparing *Hemophilus pertussis* vaccine. Pub. Health Rep. **66**:346–348.
32. Preston, N. W. 1963. Type specific immunity against whooping cough. Brit. Med. J. **2**:279–296.
33. Rowatt, E. 1957. Some factors affecting the growth of *Bordetella pertussis*. J. Gen. Microbiol. **17**:279–296.
34. Stuart, R. D. 1956. Transport problems in public health bacteriology: the use of transport media and other devices to maintain the viability of bacteria in specimens. Can. J. Pub. Health **47**:114–122.
35. Whitaker, J. A., P. Donaldson, and J. D. Nelson. 1960. Diagnosis of pertussis by the direct fluorescent antibody method. N. Engl. J. Med. **263**:850–851.

Chapter 28

Francisella tularensis

HENRY T. EIGELSBACH

CHARACTERIZATION

Although *Francisella tularensis*, originally named *Bacterium tularense* in 1911, was designated *Pasteurella tularensis* in the 7th edition (1957) of *Bergey's Manual of Determinative Bacteriology*, confusion and disagreement concerning its classification continued. Upon the recommendation of USA and USSR investigators, it will be listed in the 8th edition under "Part 7, Gram Negative, Aerobic Rods and Cocci, Genera of Uncertain Affiliation, Genus Francisella" to honor the late Edward Francis and the U.S. Public Health Service for pioneering investigations on tularemia and its etiological agent. United Kingdom investigators generally refer to this microorganism as *Brucella tularensis* because of cross-reactions with agglutinating antigens of the genus *Brucella*.

F. tularensis is a particularly small, singly occurring, nonmotile, nonencapsulated, nonsporulating, poorly staining, bipolar, aerobic rod that requires special media for isolation and growth. In young cultures (propagated for 18 to 24 h on solid medium), morphology is relatively uniform, but older cultures exhibit pleomorphism. It is distinguished from other bacteria by its small size (0.3 to 0.5 by 0.2 μm), faint bipolar staining with aniline dyes, inability to grow on ordinary media, obligate requirement for cystine or cysteine, solubility in sodium ricinoleate, fluorescent-antibody reaction, and by agglutination with specific antiserum.

Biochemical characterization is of little value in identification. Only one serotype has been described. In the agglutination test, no difficulty should be encountered in distinguishing the high-titer homologous reaction from low-titer (usually <1:20) cross-reactions that occur with heterologous antigens of the *Brucella* species.

CLINICAL SIGNIFICANCE

Human tularemia in North America is an acute, usually moderately severe, febrile, granulomatous, infectious, zoonotic disease. The clinical picture and severity vary appreciably according to the route of infection and the virulence of the organism. In North America, before the advent of antibiotic therapy, glandular, ulceroglandular, and oculoglandular tularemia in untreated patients resulted in a case mortality rate of approximately 5%. A substantially higher mortality, approximately 30%, resulted from pulmonary (inhalational) tularemia or from the "typhoidal"-type infection (characterized by the absence of an obvious portal of infection and usually resulting from ingestion of contaminated water or undercooked infected meat). Some lung involvement may occur in all forms of tularemia and is attributed to a transient bacteremia. Severe pulmonary disease initiated by other than inhalation of the organism is termed secondary pneumonia. Mortality rates in Eurasia are lower for all clinical types (averaging less than 1%) because of the innate lower virulence of strains common to that area.

Tularemia is transmitted to humans by a variety of animals, including wild rabbits, muskrats, beavers, squirrels, woodchucks, sheep, and game birds, or by biting insects (usually ticks or deer flies). Infection follows handling of infected animal carcasses, insect bites, ingestion of improperly cooked meat or contaminated water, or inhalation of airborne organisms. Bites or scratches by resistant wild or domestic carnivores whose mouth parts have been contaminated by eating infected animals may also result in human infection. Although humans of all ages, sexes, and races are susceptible, man-to-man transmission is extremely rare. The incubation period in humans is usually 3 to 4 days but ranges from 2 to 10 days dependent primarily on dose. Most cases are characterized by the formation of a slightly tender, erythematous papule at the site of entry of the organism that progresses to pustule formation and then to a focal ulcer with surrounding erythema. Regional lymph nodes become enlarged, tender, and ofter suppurate. These local manifestations accompany or precede the sudden onset of the usual constitutional reactions that consist of fever, chills, severe headache, myalgia, malaise, anorexia, nausea, and sometimes prostration. Secondary pneumonia may occur and is usually accompanied by substernal chest pain, cough and dyspnea. The clinical diagnosis can be confirmed by isolation of *F. tularensis* from local lesions, regional lymph nodes, sputum, gastric aspirates, or nasopharyngeal washings. In oculoglandular tularemia, conjunctival scrapings frequently yield the organism. *F. tularensis* is rarely recovered from the blood except during the first few days after infection and in untreated fulminating disease.

COLLECTION, TRANSPORT, AND STORAGE OF SPECIMENS

Although blood samples only infrequently yield isolates of *F. tularensis*, it is suggested nonetheless that at least 3 ml of blood, without anticoagulant, be cultured on either of the recommended agar media subsequently described. A primary lesion and/or enlarged draining regional lymph nodes usually contain sufficient *F. tularensis* cells to ensure abundant growth. The pustule or crusted sites of draining lymph nodes and areas immediately surrounding the ulcer are cleansed with 70% alcohol and allowed to dry; the pustule should be incised with a sterile scalpel. A drop or more of fluid is gently expressed and is collected in a sterile capillary tube fitted with a rubber bulb; single samples usually suffice. In oculoglandular tularemia, conjunctival scrapings may be obtained by traversing the area with a sterile swab under gentle pressure. A portion of each of these clinical specimens should be inoculated, at bedside, directly onto culture medium; the remainder should be expressed into a small tube containing 0.5 ml of sterile nutrient broth (BBL 11478, Bacto 0003, or equivalent) at approximately neutral pH and frozen for further reference. If no primary lesion is present or if the organism is not isolated from the primary lesion, enlarged intact lymph nodes may be injected with 2 ml of sterile saline and the material is withdrawn and cultured; as subsequently described, a portion of the sample should be frozen and stored. Biopsy specimens can be cultured directly; however, excision of enlarged lymph nodes, even during therapy, may cause a severe constitutional reaction (8). Viable *F. tularensis* may be isolated from sputum, gastric aspirates, and pharyngeal washings during the systemic phase of tularemia regardless of the type of clinical disease; culturing these materials as well as pleural fluid and bronchial secretions is recommended primarily when "typhoidal" or pulmonary tularemia is suspected. Sputum, gastric aspirates, and pharyngeal washes are obtained in the early morning before the patient drinks water or brushes his teeth. To secure pharyngeal washes, the patient is requested to gargle about 15 ml of sterile nutrient broth and expectorate into a sterile container with cover. If possible, several daily samples should be examined. More consistent isolation has been obtained from sputum samples and gastric aspirates than from pharyngeal washes (6).

After collection, specimens must be kept at a temperature of 10 C or lower to prevent overgrowth by normal flora; procedures for isolation should be performed immediately or as soon as possible. It must be anticipated that direct culture procedures might fail; therefore, a portion of the clinical specimens should be held at −30 to −70 C. The rate of freezing is unimportant, but thawing should be accomplished rapidly at 37 C (5). The size of the container should limit the volume of air as much as is practical. Specimens for transmittal to another laboratory for testing should be packaged with dry ice in a container that conforms to postal regulations.

DIRECT EXAMINATION

Direct or indirect fluorescent-antibody techniques are considered to be the best tools for rapid and specific identification of *F. tularensis* in exudates, tissue impressions, and tissue sections; even preparations preserved in Formalin or paraffin may be employed (chapter 4). Ordinary light microscope examination of dye-stained clinical specimens is unproductive.

CULTURE AND ISOLATION

When enriched with defibrinated rabbit blood or outdated, packed, human blood cells, commercially prepared glucose cysteine agar with thiamine or cystine heart agar is satisfactory for growth of *F. tularensis* from most clinical specimens. Incorporation of antibiotics (penicillin, polymyxin B, and cycloheximide) is required when clinical specimens containing normal flora are cultured for *F. tularensis*. Formulas for the recommended media will be found in Chapter 95. Occasionally a marginal lot of medium can be improved to yield more rapid and abundant growth by addition of 0.5 g of ferrous sulfate per liter of medium. Every precaution should be observed to restrict formation of surface moisture on plates, a condition that is deleterious to the growth of *F. tularensis*. Each lot of media should be quality control tested by inoculation with avirulent *F. tularensis* NIH B-38 (American Type Culture Collection no. 6223), a strain with more fastidious growth requirements than virulent strains.

It is mandatory that laboratory personnel utilize a syringe (needle removed) or a pipette fitted with a safety suction device to transfer potentially highly infectious material to the medium. The volume of inoculum should not exceed 0.2 to 0.3 ml per plate. Clinical specimens that are relatively small in volume with a potentially high concentration of *F. tularensis* organisms as well as normal flora (ulcer, draining lymph nodes, conjunctival scrapings) should be streaked with a wire loop to ensure that isolated colonies are obtained. Gastric aspirates, pharyngeal washes, pleural fluid, lymph node perfusions, or excised tissue (processed in Ten Broeck grinders with 2 ml of sterile saline) should be transferred to the surface of the medium at the center of the plate and thoroughly spread with a sterile U-shaped glass rod. At least 3 ml of gastric aspirates or pharyngeal washes should be cultured because of the relatively low concentration of *F. tularensis* cells. Plates are inverted and incubated at 37 C. Increased CO_2 is not required but is not harmful.

Direct culture of adequate amounts of clinical specimens on appropriate growth medium is usually sufficient for isolation of *F. tularensis* and has the advantages of being more rapid and less hazardous than inoculation of laboratory animals. However, if adequate facilities (including restricted entry with regard to personnel and the use of clear plastic cages fitted with filter tops to be opened only in a vented hood) are available for the housing of highly infectious animals, appropriate samples of clinical specimens that fail to yield isolates on direct culture can be inoculated intraperitoneally into guinea pigs. The presence of one to five viable cells of *F. tularensis* usually results in death within 5 to 10 days; the spleen pathology is pathognomonic of tularemia (enlargement four to five times normal and studding with numerous, minute, gray foci of necrosis). Moribund animals should be cultured immediately; *F. tularensis* can be readily isolated from heart blood, spleen, and liver.

IDENTIFICATION

Clinical specimens containing massive numbers of viable *F. tularensis* cells or tissues from infected guinea pigs will yield confluent, smooth, gray growth within 18 h when cultured on recommended media. When relatively few organisms are present, pinpoint colonies may appear as early as 24 h after inoculation and develop into 1.0- to 1.5-mm, smooth, gray colonies within 48 h. Incubation for 72 to 96 h results in colonies 3 to 4 mm in diameter. The medium immediately surrounding confluent growth or colonies is characteristically green in appearance. A Gram stain of the growth will usually reveal closely aligned but individual, faintly staining, minute, gram-negative, coccoidal forms. Closer inspection of well-separated organisms at the periphery of the stained area will demonstrate that the coccoidal forms are actually the bipolar components of the rod-shaped organism separated by an even more faintly staining central area. Characteristic morphology is more readily observed in Giemsa-stained preparations. Specific identification can be made with direct or indirect fluorescent-antibody techniques.

F. tularensis ferments glucose, maltose, mannose, and fructose with the production of acid but no gas; H_2S is produced in media containing cysteine or cystine; however, biochemical characterization is not necessary or recommended for identification. Glycerol fermentation and possession of a citrulline ureidase system (4) serve to distinguish strains fully virulent for humans and rabbits from those of lower virulence for these species.

Serological confirmation is routinely and rapidly accomplished by slide agglutination. A small loop of suspect confluent or colony growth is suspended uniformly in 0.5 ml of saline containing 0.5% Formalin. A drop of suspension is placed into each of two wells or waxed enclosures on a slide. To one well or enclosure an equal quantity of specific antiserum (commercially available) is added, and the other receives the same amount of normal serum; the contents of each combination are mixed with separate applicator sticks. Gentle rocking of the slide increases speed of agglutination. In a positive reaction, clumping occurs almost immediately and is observed macroscopically over a slit light source or preferably with a dissecting microscope. All strains of *F. tularensis* agglutinate with specific antiserum. Commercially available concentrated antigen can be used undiluted to prepare a positive control; the negative control should show no clumping. Cross-reactions are rare and are characterized by slow and incomplete clumping.

Animal inoculation is not required or recommended for routine identification of *F. tularensis* isolates.

IMMUNOSEROLOGICAL DIAGNOSIS

The agglutination test is standard and reliable, and usually becomes positive early in the second week of infection. In the absence of a previously known infection, a titer of 1:40 is considered diagnostic, but diagnosis must be confirmed by a rising agglutinin titer. By the third week, titers usually range to 1:320 or higher. Antibiotic therapy, initiated prior to serological confirmation of the diagnosis, does not prevent development of a diagnostic titer.

Sera from patients with tularemia or brucellosis may show minor cross-reactions; therefore, a control with *Brucella* antigen should be included. Serum that agglutinates both organisms to the same or similar titer should be subjected to agglutinin absorption tests (2).

SUSCEPTIBILITY TO ANTIMICROBIAL AGENTS

Streptomycin is actively bactericidal for *F. tularensis* and remains the drug of choice for treatment of tularemia; tetracycline is bacteriostatic but offers the convenience of oral administration (7). Kanamycin is also bactericidal but provides no advantage over streptomycin; chloramphenicol is as effective as tetracycline but is not usually recommended because of potential hematological toxicity. All naturally occurring strains are susceptible to these antibiotics, and development of antibiotic resistance during treatment has not been reported. Patients administered bacteriostatic broad-spectrum drugs (tetracycline or chloramphenicol) sometimes relapse; reinstitution of the same therapy is invariably followed by prompt clinical recovery. Routine susceptibility testing is accomplished with one of the special media described for the growth of *F. tularensis* and the disk agar diffusion method described in chapters 44 and 46. Readings are made after overnight incubation at 37 C.

EVALUATION

Valuable guides for laboratory diagnosis of tularemia include the following differential criteria: absence of growth on ordinary media and little or no growth on blood-enriched media that lack added cysteine or cystine, relatively slow colony growth on special media, distinctive bacteriological morphology and staining properties, specific fluorescent-antibody reaction, slide agglutination with specific antiserum, and a rise in agglutinin titer during transition of the patient from acute to convalescent phase of illness. If the isolate meets the cultural and morphological criteria indicated above and the organisms are agglutinated by specific antiserum, it should be reported as *F. tularensis*. Serologically, even in the absence of other data, rising agglutinin titers in successive tests are diagnostic. If acute-phase serum is not available but relatively high agglutinin titers are obtained during convalescence and a negative history of previous tularemia infection or vaccination is ascertained, data are reported as indicative of tularemia.

Although numerous laboratory infections have occurred in nonvaccinated laboratory personnel routinely working with high concentrations of *F. tularensis* in cultures and in tissues, trained technicians using reasonable precautions and readily available safety equipment can perform diagnostic procedures with minimal risk. It is mandatory that precautions be taken to prevent creation of aerosols and contamination of the skin. All work with potentially infectious clinical materials and cultures of *F. tularensis* should be performed in a vented hood; surgical gloves should be worn to prevent skin contact with the organism. Also, special care must be observed in housing animals inoculated with clinical specimens and in examination of their tissues.

An innocuous but highly effective live vaccine has been developed for immunization of individuals at risk, including laboratory animal caretaker personnel (1, 3). The live vaccine is not directly available commercially but can be obtained by consultation with the Center for Disease Control, Attention: Immunobiologics Activity, Atlanta, Ga. 30333.

LITERATURE CITED

1. Eigelsbach, H. T., R. B. Hornick, and J. J. Tulis. 1967. Recent studies on live tularemia vaccine. Med. Ann. D.C. **36**:282–286.
2. Francis, E., and A. C. Evans. 1926. Agglutination, cross agglutination and agglutinin absorption in tularemia. Pub. Health Rep. **41**:1273–1295.
3. Hornick, R. B., and H. T. Eigelsbach. 1966. Aerogenic immunization of man with live tularemia vaccine. Bacteriol. Rev. **30**:532–538.
4. Marchette, N. J., and P. S. Nicholes. 1961. Virulence and citrulline ureidase activity of *Pasteurella tularensis*. J. Bacteriol. **82**:26–32.
5. Mazur, P., M. A. Rhian, and B. G. Mahlandt. 1957. Survival of *Pasteurella tularensis* in sugar solutions after cooling and warming at sub-zero temperatures. J. Bacteriol. **73**:394–397.
6. Overholt, E. L., W. D. Tigertt, P. J. Kadull, and M. K. Ward. 1961. An analysis of forty-two cases of laboratory-acquired tularemia. Amer. J. Med. **30**:785–806.
7. Perkins, R. L. 1973. Tularemia, p. 72–73. *In* Howard F. Conn (ed.), Current therapy. W. B. Saunders Co., Philadelphia.
8. Saslaw, S., H. T. Eigelsbach, H. E. Wilson, J. A. Prior, and S. Carhart. 1961. Tularemia vaccine study. I. Intercutaneous challenge. Arch. Intern. Med. **107**:689–701.

Chapter 29

Actinobacillus

AARON D. ALEXANDER

CHARACTERIZATION

Members of the genus *Actinobacillus* cause acute septicemia or localized purulent granulomatous lesions or abscesses in cattle, horses, swine, and sheep, and occasionally in humans and other animals. Isolated from lesions; also frequently found in the mouth and gastrointestinal tract of normal natural hosts.

Coccobacillary organisms; 0.3 to 0.5 by 0.5 to 1.5 μm; occur singly, in pairs, and in short chains; pleomorphic coccal, long rod, or filamentous forms occur. Gram-negative. Nonmotile. No spores.

Growth. Aerobic; facultatively anaerobic. Grows best in 10% serum-agar or blood-agar; growth of fresh isolates on nutrient media favored in an atmosphere of 10% CO_2. Optimal temperature, 37 C. Grows best in slightly alkaline media.

Biochemical characteristics. Nitrites produced from nitrates. Urease test positive. Gelatin: growth but no liquefaction. Indole not produced. H_2S (lead acetate strip) produced feebly or not at all. Litmus milk slowly acidified. Methylene blue weakly reduced. Voges-Proskauer test negative. Hemolysis variable. Sodium citrate not utilized.

Sugar reactions. Fermentative reactions; acid, but no gas, from glucose, sucrose, maltose, and usually, but not invariably, from lactose, fructose, galactose, and zylose. Dulcitol, rhamnose, inositol, and sorbitol usually not fermented. Variable reactions with other sugars.

Serological identification. Serologically heterogeneous group. Types have not been adequately defined to permit identification by conventional tube or plate agglutination test.

Animal pathogenicity. Avirulent for usual laboratory animals.

RECOGNITION OF ACTINOBACILLUS INFECTIONS

Actinobacillus infections have been attributed preponderantly to *A. lignieresii* and *A. equuli* strains. The characteristics of the two designated species are indistinguishable. The clinical manifestations of actinobacillosis are not pathognomonic. Diagnosis is contingent on the isolation and identification of the causative organism. The organisms are present in the purulent discharge of lesions. They may, however, be encased in small granules which should be macerated prior to culture. Isolation is best accomplished in slightly alkaline nutrient media enriched with 5% blood or 10% serum. Growth of fresh isolates in ordinary peptone media is usually poor or absent, but may occur if cultures are placed in an atmosphere of 10% CO_2.

DIRECT EXAMINATION

A. lignieresii and *A. equuli* organisms stain easily with aniline dyes. They are gram-negative, do not contain spores, and are nonmotile. Organisms are coccobacilli measuring 0.3 to 0.5 by 0.5 to 1.5 μm, and occur singly, in pairs, and in short chains. However, they may present pleomorphic coccal, long bacillary, and filamentous forms.

Stained films of pus or crushed granules from lesions contain numerous organisms. The small granules frequently found in lesions consist of radially disposed clublike bodies emanating from a center occupied by organisms.

CULTURAL EXAMINATION

Cultural isolation of *A. lignieresii* and *A. equuli* strains succeeds best in blood-agar or 10% serum media. The addition of antibiotics —oleandomycin, 20 μg/ml, plus neomycin, 1.5 μg/ml (14), or oleandomycin, 1 μg/ml, plus nystatin, 200 μg/ml (9)—has been used to provide a more selective medium. Rough and smooth types of colonies are formed; the former type occurs more commonly in primary cultures. After 24 h of incubation, the rough colonies are 0.5 to 1.0 mm in diameter, slightly raised, grayish, opaque, convex, tenacious, and firmly adherent to the medium. The surface appears dry and dull; edges are entire or undulate. The colony size increased to a diameter of 3 to 4 mm in 72 h. On continued incubation, slightly effuse, semiopaque or translucent margins appear.

Smooth colonies are the same size as those of rough forms. They are small, discrete, convex, and semiopaque, with entire edges and glistening surfaces. The colonies appear gray but may have a blue to yellowish hue when viewed by transmitted light. After 4 or 5 days of incubation, effuse peripheral growth is evident, giving the colony a domed appearance when examined microscopically. The formation of smooth colony variants is favored on continued subculture. Dwarf colony forms are frequently seen in agar plate cultures.

Inoculated broth cultures containing serum usually produce granular growth along the sides and bottom of culture tubes after 24 h of incubation. Granular growth, particularly in ordinary nutrient broth, may be preceded by a uniform turbidity. A surface film and a heavy tenacious sediment may appear in old broth cultures. Cultures tend to die out quickly in nonbuffered culture media.

The identification of selected colonies as *A. lignieresii* and *A. equuli* can be established by the following reactions.

Nitrates. Reduced to nitrites.

Urease test. Positive.

Indole test. Negative.

H_2S. Negative on triple sugar-iron-agar, but frequently weakly positive when lead acetate-impregnated paper strips are placed in tubes of liver-agar slant cultures.

Methylene blue. Weakly reduced.

Litmus milk. Slow acidification, usually after 5 days of incubation, with formation of a chalky precipitate.

Gelatin. Growth but no liquefaction.

Voges-Proskauer test. Negative.

Sodium citrate. Not utilized.

Sugar reactions. Utilization of carbohydrates is best determined in phenol red broth base with 10% horse serum and 1% carbohydrate solution. Acid, but no gas, from glucose, sucrose, and maltose, and usually from lactose, fructose, galactose, and xylose. Dulcitol, rhamnose, and inositol not attacked. Variable reactions with other sugars.

pH. No growth at pH 5.6 to 6.5. Growth at pH 7.6.

Hemolysis of sheep red blood cells. Variable; isolates from swine, and occasionally from horses, sheep, and cattle, produce clear hemolysis on blood-agar. This attribute may be transient.

Potato slants. No growth.

Differential enteric media. No growth on *Salmonella-Shigella* or eosin-methylene blue-agar; slight or no growth on MacConkey agar.

SEROLOGICAL EXAMINATION

Strains of *A. equuli* and *A. lignieresii* are serologically heterogeneous, intergrading in antigenic relationships (4, 6, 11, 15, 17). There appears to be some host specificity in the distribution of serological types. Suitable antigens for agglutination tests can be prepared from *Actinobacillus* strains and may provide additional means for their identification if tested with an array of type-specific antisera. However, serological types have not been adequately defined nor studied for routine use of serological methods for identification of cultures.

Tests for serological diagnosis of patients are unsatisfactory because of the high percentage of nonspecific reactions in normal hosts and seronegative reactions in proven cases (8, 10).

DISCUSSION

Two species, *A. lignieresii* and *A. equuli*, are recognized for the genus *Actinobacillus* in the 8th edition of *Bergey's Manual*.

Cited differential criteria for *A. equuli* are sedimented growth in broth, failure to reduce methylene blue, hydrolysis of sodium hippurate, gelatinase activity, and fermentation of raffinose and trehalose. Gelatinase activity for *A. equuli* was not detected by other investigators (3, 6, 15, 17). Variable findings with other cited criteria limit their usefulness for differentiating the two species. Mraz (6) differentiated the two species primarily on the basis of host origin, relative speed of lactose fermentation, and guanine plus cytocine ratios of their deoxyribonucleic acid (42.0 moles % for *A. lignieresii* versus 40.6 moles % for *A. equuli*). The separate speciation of *A. lignieresii* and *A. equuli* has been validly questioned (17).

Also listed in *Bergey's Manual* as "Species incertae sedis" are *Bacterium actinomycetemcomitans*, *Bacillus actinoides*, *A. capsulatus*, *A. suis*, van Dorssen and Jaartsveld, and *A. suis*, Zimmermann. *Bacterium actinomycetemcomitans* has been primarily associated with human infections. Superficially, strains of this species resemble *A. lignieresii* in cultural characteristics. However, King and Tatum (5) found that those strains were more closely related to *Haemophilus aphrophilis*.

B. actinoides was originally isolated from cases of calf pneumonia in 1917 and 1918 by Theobald Smith (13). *B. actinoides* was never validly described or compared with type strains of *Actinobacillus* to justify separate speciation. Smith (13) left it for "future investigators to determine whether it [*B. actinoides*] is specifically identical with Lignieres actino-bacillus or not." The original isolates may no longer be existent.

A. capsulatus (1) was isolated from granulomatous lesions in rabbits but was not compared with representative strains of *Actinobacillus*, which it superficially resembles.

A. suis was independently proposed by van Dorssen and Jaartsveld (16) and Zimmermann (18) for hemolytic variants of *Actinobacillus* isolated from blood or tissues of diseased swine. Such strains were classified as hemolytic variants of *A. equuli*, by Mraz (6), whereas Wetmore et al. (17) proposed that hemolytic swine isolates as well as nonhemolytic *A. equuli* be grouped under *A. lignieresii*. Ross et al. (12) isolated from sow vagina hemolytic organisms which appeared to be antigenically related to but distinct from other *Actinobacillus* strains. The isolate also differed from other *Actinobacillus* strains in spectrum of carbohydrate fermentations and in patterns of cell proteins separated by electrophoresis.

A. seminis (2) associated with cases of swine epididymitis differs significantly from other strains of *Actinobacillus* in its poor saccharolytic activity, failure to reduce nitrates, and negative urease activity.

Mraz (7) suggested that *Pasteurella hemolytica* be transferred to the genus *Actinobacillus* on the basis of guanine and cytocine base ratios of deoxyribonucleic acid and cultural, biochemical and antigenic characters. It differs principally from *Actinobacillus* strains in production of urease. The taxonomic relationship of proposed *Actinobacillus* species to each other and to other members of the family *Brucellaceae* needs further study.

LITERATURE CITED

1. Arseculeratne, S. N. 1962. *Actinobacillosis* in joints of rabbits. J. Pathol. Bacteriol. **79**:331–336.
2. Baynes, I. D., and G. C. Simmons. 1960. Bovine epididymitis caused by *Actinobacillus seminis*, n. sp. Aust. Vet. J. **36**:454–459.
3. Edwards, P. R. 1931. Studies on *Shigella equirulis* (*Bact. viscosum equi*). Kentucky Agr. Exp. Sta. Bull. No. 320, p. 291–330.
4. Edwards, P. R. 1932. Serologic characteristics of *Shigella equirulis* (*B. nephritides-equi*) J. Infec. Dis. **51**:268–272.
5. King, E. D., and H. W. Tatum. 1962. *Actinobacillus actinomycetemcomitans* and *Hemophilus aphrophilus*. J. Infec. Dis. **111**:85–94.
6. Mraz, O. 1968. Reevaluation of original strains *Actinobacillus suis* and haemolytic strains *Actinobacillus lignieresii* isolated from the organs of diseased pigs. Acta Univ. Agr. Brno Fac. Vet. **37**:277–290.
7. Mraz, O. 1969. Vergleichende Studie der Arten *Actinobacillus lignieresii* and *Pasteurella haemolytica*. III. *Actinobacillus haemolyticus* (Newsom and Cross, 1932) Comb. nov. Zentralbl. Bakteriol. Parasitenk. Infektionskr. Hyg. Abt. I Orig. **209**:349–364.
8. Pathak, R. C., and M. Ristic. 1962. Detection of an antibody to *Actinobacillus lignieresii* in infected human beings and the antigenic characterization of isolates of human and bovine origin. Amer. J. Vet. Res. **23**:310–314.
9. Phillips, J. E. 1964. Commensal actinobacilli from the bovine tongue. J. Pathol. Bacteriol. **87**:442–444.
10. Phillips, J. E. 1965. The incidence of agglutinating antibodies to *Actinobacillus lignieresii* in the sera of normal and infected cattle. J. Pathol. Bacteriol. **90**:557–566.
11. Phillips, J. E. 1967. Antigenic structure and serological typing of *Actinobacillus lignieresii*. J. Pathol. Bacteriol. **93**:463–475.
12. Ross, R. F. 1972. Characterization of an *Actinobacillus* isolated from the sow vagina. Int. J. Syst. Bacteriol. **22**:39–46.
13. Smith, T. 1918. A pleomorphic bacillus from pneumonic lungs of calves simulating *Actinomyces*. J. Exp. Med. **28**:333–344.
14. Till, D. H., and F. P. Palmer. 1960. A review of actinobacillosis with a study of the causal organism. Vet. Rec. **72**:527–534.
15. Vallee, A., P. Thibault, and L. Second. 1963. Contribution a l'etude d'*A. lignieresii* et d'*A. equuli*. Ann. Inst. Pasteur (Paris) **104**:108–114.
16. Van Dorssen, C. A., and F. H. J. Jaartsveld. 1962. *Actinobacillus suis* (novo species), een by ket vasken voorkomende bacterie Tijdschr. Diergeneesk. Memo. **27**:450–458.
17. Wetmore, P. W., J. F. Thiel, Y. F. Herman, and J. R. Harr. 1963. Comparison of selected *Actinobacillus* species with a hemolytic variety of *Actinobacillus* from irradiated swine. J. Infec. Dis. **113**:186–194.
18. Zimmermann, T. 1964. Untersuchungen uber die Actinobazillose des Schweines 1. Mitteilung: Isolierung und Charakterisierung der Erreger. Deut. Tieraerztl. Wochenschr. **71**:457–461.

Chapter 30

Calymmatobacterium granulomatis

DOUGLAS S. KELLOGG, JR.

CHARACTERIZATION

Calymmatobacterium granulomatis is in the family *Brucellaceae*. Responsible for granuloma inguinale, a chronic, specific infection manifested clinically by ulcerating granulomatous lesions involving, in the majority of cases, the skin and subcutaneous tissues. Secondary involvement of the bones and joints has occurred. Associated infections with pyogenic organisms, Vincent's organisms, and especially the other venereal diseases are common. Isolation has been accomplished from granulating tissues of lesions and the fluids of pseudobubos.

Coccobacilli; 0.5 to 1.5 × 1 to 2 μm. Gram-negative, nonmotile, encapsulated, no spores.

Growth. Microaerophilic to anaerobic. Do not grow on ordinary laboratory media, simple or complex. Grow in special media and egg yolk sacs. Optimal temperature, 37 C. Nonpigmented.

Serological identification. A complement-fixation procedure with bacterial antigens or boiled-medium filtrate antigens has been used for the detection of antibodies against this organism in human sera.

Animal pathogenicity. Not pathogenic for laboratory animals; the disease characteristics have been reproduced in man through subcutaneous inoculation of volunteers with lesion pus (18), tissue fragments (6), and yolk sac cultures (7). Lesions typical of granuloma inguinale appear 40 to 45 days after inoculation. Numerous mononuclear cells containing the characteristic "Donovan bodies" are observed.

COLLECTION OF SPECIMENS

Lesions containing *C. granulomatis* are always replete with numerous other bacteria. To reduce these populations and remove tissue debris, swab such lesions with sterile saline-soaked gauze sponges. Use a biopsy punch to secure a small piece of clean granulation tissue from the active, growing periphery of the lesion, and make films with this tissue. Use the clean under-surface of this tissue to make smears. Obtain an inoculum for cultural examination by cutting a small piece of cleansed granulation tissue and mincing it into small particles. The in vitro cultivation of *C. granulomatis* requires a low oxidation-reduction potential and a factor, or factors, found in egg yolks.

DIRECT EXAMINATION

Direct examination of stained smears or tissue sections has been the most effective means of establishing the presence of *C. granulomatis* in lesion material (4). The Wright stain has been most widely used, although the Giemsa stain is a good alternative.

To obtain optimal stain distinction with Wright stain, allow the dye to remain on the smear for 1.5 min before diluting with pH 6.4 phosphate buffer (5). With the Wright stain, a positive specimen will exhibit large mononuclear cells in which the cytoplasm contains small, straight or curved dumbbell-shaped rods that are blue to deep purple and surrounded by pink capsules. Prominent polar granules are characteristically seen with these organisms, and account for the "safety pin" description given by some authors. Large and well-defined capsules are easily demonstrable in infected cells containing few organisms; however, capsules may not be stained when numerous organisms are within infected cells.

In another effective staining procedure pinacyanole dye is used (19). Place a 1% solution of pinacyanole dye in methanol on the specimen for 1.5 to 2 min. Dilute the stain with an equal volume of sterile distilled water and leave it on the smear for 1.5 to 2 min. With pinacyanole staining, the organisms stain a dark blue and the capsules stain a purplish pink.

Extracellular atypical forms (nonencapsulated forms appearing as small diplococci or rod forms with metachromatic staining) are suggestive of granuloma inguinale and indicate the need for additional specimens and examinations. Several authors (5, 19, 21) emphasize the unreliability of the clinical aspects of the disease and the need for repeat specimens when negative findings are obtained. Only intracellular forms compatible with the described characteristics should be reported as positive findings.

CULTURAL EXAMINATION

Cultivation of primary isolates of *C. granulomatis* has been accomplished only in some form of liquid medium. The most frequently used method of isolation culture is the inoculation of the yolk sacs of 5-day-old chicken embryos followed by incubation for 72 h at 37 C (1, 2). Examination of the yolk sac fluid reveals large numbers of encapsulated organisms consistent with the morphology of the Donovan bodies as seen in lesions.

Another successful cultural procedure has employed coagulated egg yolk slants known as "Dulaney slants" (9, 16). Add approximately 0.2 ml of lesion material to the slant, and then add sufficient Locke's solution to cover three-fourths of the slant. Close the tubes and incubate them in an upright position for 48 to 72 h. Viability is maintained in such cultures for at least 10 weeks. Research has indicated that nonfertile yolk from chickens, ducks, geese, and turkeys is satisfactory (16). The same author states that egg yolk from range-fed birds was effective, whereas that from defined diet-fed birds was inadequate.

Good growth of *C. granulomatis* laboratory strains has been obtained in a semisynthetic medium (12). Four strains of *C. granulomatis* were transferred more than 100 times on this medium and shown to be antigenically very similar to the same strains cultured in the yolk sacs of 5-day embryonic eggs or in the fluid of "Dulaney slants." Sodium azide (0.4 mg/ml) and brilliant green (0.2 mg/ml), included in this semisynthetic medium, were used to isolate from feces (13) an organism identical with *C. granulomatis*. Several strains of *C. granulomatis* have been adapted to growth on other media (5, 11, 16, 26), but these are of interest primarily for the routine maintenance of stock strains or for studies of metabolic characteristics.

Two factors of importance in the cultivation of *C. granulomatis* are (i) the maintenance of a low oxidation-reduction potential and (ii) the requirement for a factor or factors found in egg yolk, phytone, and lactalbumin hydrolysate. Various media do not influence the morphology of *C. granulomatis* grown in vitro (26). Encapsulation is not generally seen in vitro, except in yolk sac cultivation; however, the medium fluid does become sticky, thereby indicating that the capsular material may have diffused away from the cells.

SEROLOGICAL EXAMINATION

There is no uniform serological procedure for either detecting antibodies against *C. granulomatis* in human sera or identifying the organism as an isolate; however, antibodies can be detected in human sera by complement-fixation procedures (3, 9, 10–13, 17). The methodology varied with the researcher, and the antigens used included pus from granuloma inguinale lesions, whole or ruptured *C. granulomatis*, and boiled or extracted egg yolk medium after growth of *C. granulomatis*. An average of 85% of sera from smear-positive cases of granuloma inguinale were reactive with the different procedures and antigens. The percentage of sera from smear-positive cases of granuloma inguinale having reactivity in a complement-fixation procedure rose to a peak in patients who had the disease for 1 to 3 months (17). Normal sera, sera from patients with chronic ulcerous conditions, and sera from patients with tuberculosis were nonreactive. Patients with other venereal diseases, particularly lymphogranuloma venereum or syphilis, demonstrated reactivity in 10 to 30% of their sera, the rate being dependent upon the antigen used in the test (9–11, 24). Studies with human sera (25) and rabbit sera (13, 23) indicated that *C. granulomatis* shares antigens with several members of the tribe *Escherichieae*.

DISCUSSION

In the final analysis, the detection and differentiation of *C. granulomatis* rest with smear examinations. A serological procedure could probably be developed that would be sensitive enough to assist in the diagnosis of the disease. However, the increased sensitivity may cause a serious problem with specificity. There is good evidence that *C. granulomatis* is antigenically very similar to, but not identical with, *Klebsiella rhinoscleromatis* and *K. pneumoniae*.

Several characteristics of *C. granulomatis* cast doubt on its taxonomic assignment. According to *Bergey's Manual of Determinative Bacteriology* (7th ed.), *C. granulomatis* is classified in the family *Brucellaceae*, although morphologically and antigenically this organism resembles members of the genus *Klebsiella*. It is a nonobligate intracellular parasite, apparently of low-grade infectivity, which has been cultured only under microaerophilic to anaerobic conditions. It is considered a venereal disease agent; however, an organism identical with it has been isolated from feces (13). In one study less than 1% of the marital partners of patients having granuloma inguinale contract the disease. Male homosexuals who practice passive sexual intercourse have anal lesions exclusively (15, 22). However, support for sexual transmission is found in a recent paper in which conjugal infection was demonstrated in 52% of 50 marital partners in addition to concurrent syphilis in 45% of all cases studied (21). Researchers generally support the contention that this disease is not venereal in the usual sense of the term, but is more consistent with the characteristics of a fecal organism that has the capability of becoming a pathogen or at the least a secondary invader (14). Differing sexual practices in various parts of the world may account for the apparent disparity in transmission character. For example, ano-rectal intercourse is not exclusively a homosexual practice and heterosexual relations could result in the introduction of fecal microorganisms into the vaginal canal.

Two textbooks (8, 27) have placed this organism in the family *Enterobacteriaceae*, in association with the genus *Klebsiella*. Chronic lesions of the anal area or adjacent to the genitalia, especially when accompanied by poor personal hygiene, should raise a suspicion of granuloma inguinale. A recent review adequately covers the epidemiology, clinical studies, and treatment regimens of granuloma inguinale (20).

LITERATURE CITED

1. Anderson, K. 1943. The cultivation from granuloma inguinale of a microorganism having the characteristics of Donovan bodies in the yolk sac of chick embryos. Science **97**:560–561.
2. Anderson, K., W. A. DeMonbreun, and E. W. Goodpasture. 1944. An etiologic consideration of *Donovania granulomatis* cultivated from granuloma inguinale (three cases) in embryonic yolk. J. Exp. Med. **81**:25–40.
3. Anderson, K., E. W. Goodpasture, and W. A. DeMonbreun. 1944. Immunologic relationship of *Donovania granulomatis* to granuloma inguinale. J. Exp. Med. **81**:41–50.
4. Cannefax, G. R. 1948. The technique of the tissue spread method for demonstrating Donovan bodies. J. Vener. Dis. Info. **29**:201–204.
5. Dienst, R. B. 1948. Laboratory diagnosis of granuloma inguinale and studies on the cultivation of the Donovan body. Amer. J. Syph. Gonor. Vener. Dis. **32**:301–306.
6. Dienst, R. B., R. B. Greenblatt, and C. H. Chen. 1950. Experimental transfer of chemoresistant granuloma inguinale. Amer. J. Syph. Gonor. Vener. Dis. **34**:189–190.
7. Dienst, R. B., C. R. Reinstein, H. S. Kupperman, and R. B. Greenblatt. 1947. Studies on the causal agent of granuloma inguinale. Amer. J. Syph. Gonor. Vener. Dis. **31**:614–617.
8. Dubos, R. J., and J. G. Hirsch. 1965. Bacterial and mycotic infections of man, 4th ed. J. B. Lippincott Co., Philadelphia.
9. Dulaney, A. D., K. Guo, and H. Packer. 1948. *Donovania granulomatis:* cultivation, antigen preparation, and immunological tests. J. Immunol., **59**:335–340.
10. Dulaney, A. D., and H. Packer. 1947. Complement-fixation studies with pus antigen in granuloma inguinale. Proc. Soc. Exp. Biol. Med. **65**:254–256.
11. Dunham, W., and G. Rake. 1948. Cultural and serologic studies on granuloma inguinale. Amer. J. Syph. Gonor. Vener. Dis. **32**:145–149.
12. Goldberg, J. 1959. Studies on granuloma inguinale. IV. Growth requirements of *Donovania granulomatis* and its relationship to the natural habitat of the organism. Brit. J. Vener. Dis. **35**:266–268.
13. Goldberg, J. 1962. Studies on granuloma inguinale. V. Isolation of a bacterium resembling *Donovania granulomatis* from the faeces of a patient with granuloma inguinale. Brit. J. Vener. Dis. **38**:99–102.
14. Goldberg, J. 1964. Studies on granuloma inguinale. VII. Some epidemiological considerations of the disease. Brit. J. Vener. Dis. **40**:140–145.
15. Goldberg, J., and R. Bernstein. 1964. Studies on granuloma inguinale. VI. Two cases of perianal granuloma inguinale in male homosexuals. Brit. J. Vener. Dis. **40**:137–139.
16. Goldberg, J., R. H. Weaver, and H. Packer. 1953. Studies on granuloma inguinale. I. Bacteriologic behavior of *Donovania granulomatis*. Amer. J. Syph. Gonor. Vener. Dis. **37**:60–70.
17. Goldberg, J., R. H. Weaver, H. Packer, and W. G. Simpson. 1953. Studies on granuloma inguinale. II. The complement-fixation test in the diagnosis of granuloma inguinale. Amer. J. Syph. Gonor. Vener. Dis. **37**:71–76.
18. Greenblatt, R. B., R. B. Dienst, E. R. Pund, and R. Torpin. 1939. Experimental and clinical granuloma inguinale. J. Amer. Med. Ass. **113**:1109–1116.
19. Greenblatt, R. B., R. B. Dienst, and R. M. West. 1951. A simple stain for Donovan bodies for the diagnosis of granuloma inguinale. Amer. J. Syph. Gonor. Vener. Dis. **35**:291–293.
20. King, A. 1964. Recent advances in venerology, p. 334–351. Little, Brown and Co., Boston.
21. Lal, S., and C. Micholas. 1970. Epidemiological and clinical features in 165 cases of granuloma inguinale. Brit. J. Vener. Dis. **46**:461–463.
22. Marmell, M. 1959. Donovanosis of the anus in the male, an epidemiological consideration. Brit. J. Vener. Dis. **35**:213–218.
23. Packer, H., and J. Goldberg. 1950. Studies of the antigenic relationship of *D. granulomatis* to members of the tribe Escherichieae. Amer. J. Syph. Gonor. Vener. Dis. **34**:342–350.
24. Rake, G. 1948. The antigenic relationships of *Donovania granulomatis* (Anderson) and the significance of this organism in granuloma inguinale. Amer. J. Syph. Gonor. Vener. Dis. **32**:150–158.
25. Rake, G. 1948. A further note on the antigenic relationships of Donovania granulomatis (Anderson). J. Bacteriol. **55**:865–867.
26. Rake, G., and J. J. Oskay. 1948. Cultural characteristics of Donovania granulomatis. J. Bacteriol. **55**:667–675.
27. Smith, D. T., N. F. Conant, and J. R. Overman. 1964. Microbiology (Zinsser), 13th ed., p. 608–609. Meredith Publishing Co., New York.

Chapter 31

Streptobacillus moniliformis and *Spirillum minor*

MORRISON ROGOSA

STREPTOBACILLUS MONILIFORMIS

Pathogenesis and epidemiology of rat-bite fever caused by Streptobacillus moniliformis

Infections due to *Streptobacillus moniliformis* are usually acquired following the bite of a rat, mouse, or other rodent (3, 4, 6, 20, 26, 38). The nasopharynx and infected middle ears of wild rats and mice (40) very frequently harbor the organism, and epizootic incidents characterized by naturally occurring polyarthritis have occurred in laboratory mice (13). Isolations have also been made from the tendon sheath and sternal bursa of arthritic turkeys (5, 44) and from cervical abscesses in guinea pigs. Human cases from the ingestion of milk to which rats had access have been reported as Haverhill fever or erythema arthriticum epidemicum (16, 30, 33, 34, 39). Infrequently, there is no history of a rodent bite or animal contact, and the disease may appear following traumatic injury (16, 27, 39).

Although there may be some inflammation (3, 4, 6) following a bite wound, there is usually normal healing without induration. Unlike the lesion of Sodoku, there is no subsequent reactivation of the initial lesion or uncomplicated lymphadenitis (3, 20, 21). The incubation period is usually less than 10 days followed by abrupt prostrating illness with chills, fever, vomiting, and severe headache. Alternate remissions and febrile incidents may persist for weeks or months. Usually, there is an accompanying cutaneous eruption (rubellaform, morbilliform, or petechial). Arthritic symptoms are frequent with excess joint fluid and painful swellings (3, 20). Reported mortality varies from 0 to 10% in untreated cases (3, 6, 20, 37). Endocarditis or pneumonia may be serious sequelae (3, 15, 32, 36, 37). *S. moniliformis* has been recovered from blood, joint fluids, the cutaneous eruptions (3, 6, 36, 37), and a brain abscess (29).

Bacterial-phase infections have been successfully treated with penicillin (1, 18, 37). Penicillin-resistant infections have been effectively treated with streptomycin (27, 37, 39). Two cases of L-phase variant infections (where the organisms are resistant to penicillin) were eliminated by chlortetracycline (10).

Otherwise normal patients with bacterial-phase infections have been successfully treated with daily penicillin doses varying from 60,000 to 1,700,000 units over periods of 4 to 19 days of therapy (37). However, because there is a good correlation between drug dosage and response to therapy, and also because penicillin-resistant transitional and L-forms are not uncommon, it is wise to prescribe daily penicillin dosages of at least 1,000,000 units combined with 1-g daily doses of streptomycin for a period of at least 7 days. In successful therapy, a dramatic drop to body temperature, accompanied by signs of returning well-being, occurs within 1 to 2 days (37). Exposed patients with underlying heart disease (rheumatic fever, valvular heart disease, etc.) are especially susceptible to endocarditis. *S. moniliformis* endocarditis should be treated as if for streptococcal endocarditis, i.e., daily doses of 12 to 15 million units of penicillin plus 0.5 to 1 g of streptomycin for 3 to 4 weeks.

Characteristics of Streptobacillus moniliformis

Synonyms of *S. moniliformis* are listed in *Bergey's Manual* and *Index Bergeyana* (7). The 7th edition of *Bergey's Manual* placed the genus *Streptobacillus* in the strictly anaerobic family *Bacteroidaceae;* however, the 8th edition places the genus in "Part VIII, Gram negative, facultatively anaerobic rods" in a group containing eight "Genera of uncertain affiliation."

Rods, nonsporing, less that 1 μm wide by 1 to 5 μm long, with rounded or pointed ends, are highly pleomorphic, forming long, curved, and looped filaments as long as 100 to 150 μm. In young cultures, filaments are relatively homogeneous, appearing to consist of single cells. As the culture ages, fine granules and alternate light and dark bands often appear in the filaments, and fragmentation into irregular, coccobacillary elements occurs. The filaments may consist of a series of oval to elongated bulbous swellings, 1 to 3 μm in diameter, giving the appearance of a string of beads, and may contain numerous granules randomly distributed. True branching does not occur. Also, cell membrane-associated and extracellular oil-like, ether-soluble droplets containing cholesterol and other lipids are very characteristic (25, 31, 35). Morphology is influenced considerably by media, cultural conditions, and age of culture. Under favorable conditions, such as in young cultures in favorable media, smears from pathological blood, joint fluids, etc., cells generally appear to be more rodlike and uniform with occasional short filaments randomly arranged. There is considerable irregularity in retention of stains; the monilia-like swellings stain more intensely than the filaments. *S. moniliformis* is not acid-fast by Ziehl-Neelsen techniques and is gram-negative. Giemsa or Wayson stains may be more satisfactory for demonstrating the organisms than the Gram stain.

Growth. *S. moniliformis* is aerobic and facultative. Although growth occurs at reduced partial pressures of oxygen, in candle jars, etc., such closed environments are not strictly anaerobic but supply increased CO_2 and conserve essential moisture at the surface of agar media. Blood, serum, or ascitic fluid is required for growth. However, growth on Loeffler's serum-agar slants is poor. Growth does not occur or cannot be sustained in infusion, nutrient, and other broths and agars, unless supplemented with one of these body fluids. The pH optimum is 7.4 to 7.6 with a range of 7.0 to 8.0. Colonies generally 1 to 2.5 mm in diameter develop within 3 days on serum-agar at 35 to 37 C and may be viable for as long as 1 week. There is no growth at 23 C. Bacterial-phase colonies tend to be round with a discrete edge, low-convex or slightly raised, and glistening, and have a butyrous consistency; smaller granular and rougher colonies intermediate in size between the first type and L_1 colonies are sometimes seen. Within, beneath, or adjacent to the primary colonies, microscopic L-form colonies may be found. The L-phase colonies are embedded in the agar and have a "fried egg" configuration with a relatively dark center surrounded by a translucent zone containing swollen bodies and what appear to be oil globules. Thus, the spontaneously appearing L-phase variant colonies of *S. moniliformis* are indistinguishable from other L-phase, pleuropneumonia, or *Mycoplasma* colonies (2, 9, 11, 12, 14, 22–24, 28) and must be examined by the same microscopic methods (see chapter 32 in this *Manual*). Bacterial-phase cells have normal cell walls and are susceptible to penicillin (1- or 10-unit disks), whereas L-phase cells lack a cell wall (28, 35) and are resistant to potassium penicillin G (1,000 units or more/ml). The latter have varying revertant tendencies in the absence of penicillin. Incorporation of penicillin in media stabilizes the culture in the L-phase if such cells are present. In fluid culture containing 10% blood, growth generally appears as fluffy balls resembling bread crumbs and may be confined to the bottom portion of the tube or on the surface of sedimented cells and stroma.

Media. Bacterial-phase organisms have been isolated and maintained on a number of common basal media enriched with 15% sterile defibrinated rabbit blood. However, it is preferable to employ a clear medium which will enhance the isolation and maintenance of the more fragile and nutritionally fastidious L-phase variants (9). The following recommended medium is very useful because it favors the growth of a wide variety of L-phase and bacterial-phase nutritionally fastidious organisms (2, 9): dissolve 40 g of dehydrated Heart Infusion Agar (Difco) in 850 ml of deionized, distilled water; adjust the pH to 7.6 with 5 N NaOH; dispense in 85-ml volumes into screw-cap bottles; sterilize by autoclaving for 15 min at 121 C; just before pouring plates add 10 ml of sterile horse serum (previously heated for 30 min at 56 to 60 C) and also add 5 ml of sterile 10% (wt/vol) solution of yeast extract (Oxoid, Difco, or BBL) previously adjusted to pH 7.0 and sterilized by filtration through a Seitz-type pad (0.01-μm pore size) or through a Millipore or similar filter (0.45-μm pore size); pour plates in sterile disposable 60 $\times$ 15 mm plastic petri dishes (Falcon Plastics, Los Angeles, Calif.).

A similar broth medium containing 25 g of dehydrated Heart Infusion Broth (Difco) instead of 40 g of dehydrated Heart Infusion Agar (Difco), but with all other ingredients and medium preparation identical with the agar medium, is recommended.

Laboratory diagnosis of Streptobacillus moniliformis infections

A blood specimen is citrated by adding 10 ml of blood to 10 ml of sterile 2.5% sodium citrate in a small sterile flask and is mixed as usual. Prepare three separate films, and stain with Gram, Wayson, and Giemsa stains. Centrifuge for 30 to 45 min to pack the cells. Discard the supernatant fluid. Use the sedimented cells to inoculate one freshly poured solidified agar plate and two tubes of broth. Take an estimated 0.1 ml of sedimented cells and mix with 0.1 ml of broth; inoculate 0.1 ml of the mixed suspended cells on the surface of an agar plate and distribute the inoculum by gently tilting the plate in a number of directions. Use the remaining cells to inoculate the two cotton-plugged tubes of broth. Place tubes and plates upright in a wide-mouth screw-cap glass jar, include a lighted candle, tighten the screw-cap cover, and incubate at 35 to 37 C. Incubate plates for 2 to 3 days. Examine tubes daily for the appearance of characteristic fluff balls, particularly on the surface of sedimented cells. Use a good light for this inspection and do not shake or disturb the tubes. If no growth is apparent, transfer daily 1 ml to fresh broth tubes for at least 3 successive days. If growth is observed, remove a fluff ball by pipette for subsequent transfer. Also, transfer a small drop to three separate clean slides, spread, dry, fix gently, and stain with Gram, Giemsa, and Wayson stains. Examine for characteristic microscopic morphology.

Joint fluids should also be citrated by mixing equal volumes of fluid and 2.5% citrate. Otherwise, joint fluids may often clot. Stain smears with Gram, Giemsa, and Wayson stains. Inoculate two tubes of recommended broth with 1 or more ml of fluid per tube (as much as the sample volume will permit). Also, inoculate 0.1 ml on fresh agar plates and distribute the inoculum by carefully tilting the plate in a number of directions. Incubate and examine in the same way as blood cultures.

Pus or exudate from a wound, cutaneous eruption, or an abscess should be smeared, stained, and examined microscopically. Also, inoculate one tube of broth and one agar plate (by swabbing, if the sample is limited). Incubate and examine as already described.

For transfer of L-phase colonies, a small agar block is cut out with a sterile spade or spatula from an area of dense growth (9, 22). Invert this on a fresh agar plate so that the growth area contacts the agar plate surface. Push the agar block gently half way across the surface with a sterile spatula, taking care to leave the agar block in the same inverted position. Incubate plates as already described.

An entire "fluff ball" or "bread crumb" of growth should be removed from broth by appropriate pipette for replating. Deposit one or two drops containing heavy growth on a fresh agar plate, spread the inoculum, and incubate as previously described.

In purification and transfer procedures, a wire needle or loop should never be used. Large inocula by agar block cutouts from plates or by pipette transfers (10%, vol/vol) from broth are essential (9, 22, 26). This is often the case with fastidious organisms.

A laboratory specimen may contain several species of L-phase variants because they are naturally occurring or because of previous antibiotic therapy. L-phase variants of coryneform bacteria are not uncommon (43), and some of these may have been mistaken in the past for *S. moniliformis*. Some incorrect earlier literature statements that *S. moniliformis* is gram-positive in young broth cultures and an attempt to classify *S. moniliformis* as *Actinobacillus muris* (42) or *Asterococcus muris* (17) may stem from this confusion. It is therefore important to purify these cultures by replating colonies on the maintenance or isolation agar medium by the agar block technique. The purification procedure should be repeated, if necessary, until there is reasonable assurance of culture purity before biochemical tests are performed.

In isolated pure cultures, a marked decrease of pH in broth cultures occurs in 1 to 2 days and cultures easily become nonviable. It is therefore necessary to subculture daily. However, young broth cultures and organisms in infected tissues and body fluids frozen at −20 to −70 C remain viable for several years. Cells are killed when held at 55 to 56 C for 30 min.

Agglutinins in patient serum may be demonstrated in infections with *S. moniliformis*. A titer of 1:80 is regarded as diagnostic, and titers of 1:5,120 have been reported (6, 36). Two or more serum specimens at intervals of 5 days should be tested, especially if the titer of the initial sample is 1:80. The antigen of the bacillary-phase culture may be difficult to prepare because of clumping of cells. However, if glycerol (final concentration 3%) is added to broth media before inoculation, this tendency to agglutinate spontaneously may be overcome (36). Cultures are killed with Formalin (1.2 ml per 10-ml tube), centrifuged, washed three times with 0.85% NaCl, and resuspended in saline to an optical density of approximately 0.5. Perform standard agglutination procedures. Incubate tubes at 56 C overnight, then refrigerate tubes for 3 h, and read the results as usual. In addition to the usual controls, a normal human and known agglutinating rabbit antiserum should be included for security of diagnosis. Strain ATCC 14647 may be used in the preparation of agglutinogen in the agglutination test and for antigen in preparing rabbit antisera. Consistent low titers of approximately 1:80 are not diagnostic of a recent infection because titers in this range may persist for at least 2 years (6).

The L-phase variant shares a common antigen with the bacillus but lacks a second antigen present in the bacillary form (24). L-phase antisera protect against challenge with homologous L-phase antigen but do not protect against the bacillus (14).

Wasserman tests in *S. moniliformis* infections have been reported positive. However, this does not now appear to be correct. In the past, this disease may have been clinically confused with Sodoku where about 50% of sera have given positive Wasserman reactions (20).

Biochemical characteristics of S. moniliformis

This section is based largely on the studies of Aluotto et al. (2) and Cohen et al. (9), and on the description of *Streptobacillus* in the 8th edition of *Bergey's Manual*. The basal medium is the same as the agar medium described for isolation and maintenance except that, for each liter of complete test agar, the basal constituents are dissolved in only 750 ml of water to allow for the addition of test solutions without diluting the strength of basic components. For phenylalanine deamination and esculin hydrolysis tests only, the respective substrates and reagents for testing the reactions are incorporated in the basal medium before autoclaving. The remaining test substrate solutions are added aseptically after being sterilized by filtration through Swinnex-25 plastic filter units fitted with 25-mm diameter, 0.22-μm pore size MF-Millipore, type GS membrane filters (Millipore Corp., Bedford, Mass.). Table 1 outlines the protocol of substrates and reagent quantities used in a variety of tests.

The basal agar is dispensed in 19-ml volumes into 2-oz (59-ml) prescription bottles. Just be-

TABLE 1. *Concentrations of substrates, indicators, and reagents employed in tests for biochemical reactions*

Test	Substrate	Indicator or reagent	Stock solution (%, w/v)	Final concn (%, w/v)	Amt added per 25 ml of medium
Oxidase activity		*N,N*-dimethyl-*p*-phenylenediamine hydrochloride	1.0		
Catalase activity		Hydrogen peroxide	30		
Phosphatase activity	Phenolphthalein diphosphate Na salt		1.0	0.01	0.25 ml
		NaOH	20		
Oxidation-fermentation	Glucose		10	1.0	2.5 ml
		Phenol red[a]	0.25	0.0025	0.25 ml
Phenylalanine	DL-phenylalanine			0.2	0.05 g
		Ferric chloride	10		
Esculin hydrolysis	Esculin			0.1	0.025 g
		Ferric citrate		0.05	0.0125 g
Arginine hydrolysis	L-Arginine hydrochloride		10	1.0	2.5 ml
		Phenol red	0.25	0.0025	0.25 ml
Urea hydrolysis	Urea		20	2.0	2.5 ml
		Phenol red	0.25	0.0025	0.25 ml
Nitrate reduction	Potassium nitrate		1.0	0.1	2.5 ml
		Sulfanilic acid[b]	0.8		
		α-Naphthylamine[b]	0.5		
Tetrazolium reduction	2,3,5-Triphenyltetrazolium chloride		1.0	0.005	0.125 ml
Tellurite reduction	Potassium tellurite		1.0	0.005	0.125 ml
AMC production	Glucose		10	0.5	1.25 ml
		Creatine	1.0		
		Potassium hydroxide	40		
Carbohydrate breakdown	Inulin and salicin		5	0.5	2.5 ml
	All other carbohydrates		10	1.0	2.5 ml
		Phenol red	0.25	0.0025	0.25 ml

[a] Prepared by dissolving 0.25 g of phenol red in 70.5 ml of 0.1 N NaOH and then bringing the volume to 100 ml with water.

[b] In 5 N acetic acid.

Reproduced from Cohen, Wittler, and Faber (9) with the permission of the American Society for Microbiology and the courtesy of the authors.

fore pouring plates, add 2.5 ml of heated horse serum and 1.2 ml of 10% (wt/vol) yeast extract to each bottle of molten agar held at 50 C. Since horse serum contains an active maltase, rabbit serum must be used *only* in maltose test plates. Also, add the individual sterile substrates, reagent, or indicator stock solutions to separately prepared bottles of media (see Table 1). Test controls must include an uninoculated plate containing substrate and an inoculated plate in which distilled water is substituted for substrate solution.

Prepare bacterial-phase inocula by swabbing off a single culture plate and suspending the swab in 2 ml of 0.85% NaCl; use 1 drop to inoculate each test plate. L-phase variants are inoculated on test plates by the agar block method as already described. All cultures are incubated in candle jars (see previous description).

The pH of plates containing phenol red can be estimated by using indicator standards (LaMotte Chemical Products Co., Baltimore, Md.). Incubate media containing carbohydrate for 3 weeks, if necessary. Reactions may be considered positive if the pH is reduced throughout the plate by 0.4 unit greater than controls. Changes in pH of less than 0.4 unit or localized changes confined to areas of heavy growth only are weak reactions. The other tests listed in Table 1 are performed and evaluated as described by Aluotto et al. (2) and Cohen et al. (9).

Comprehensive studies of the biochemical activities of *S. moniliformis* are few (9; *Bergeys Manual*, 8th ed.). The following reactions are negative: gelatin liquefaction, casein or serum digestion, indole and acetylmethylcarbinol production, phenylalanine deamination, urea hydrolysis, nitrate reduction, oxidase, catalase, and benzidine reactions, and gluconate oxidation. Esculin may be hydrolyzed slightly, and H_2S may be produced in slight amounts. Alkaline phosphatase is produced, methylene blue is reduced anaerobically, potassium tellurite and 2,3,5-triphenyl tetrazolium chloride are reduced aerobically and anaerobically. Phosphatase and tetrazolium reduction tests may be weakly positive.

The following carbohydrates and polyols are not attacked: adonitol, cellobiose, dulcitol, glycerol, inositol, inulin, mannitol, melezitose, melibiose, raffinose, rhamnose, sorbitol, sorbose, and trehalose (9; *Bergey's Manual*, 8th ed.). There may be variable acid production from arabinose, lactose, salicin, sucrose, and xylose. Acid without gas is produced from dextrin, fructose, galactose, glucose, glycogen, maltose, mannose, and starch. Galactose, maltose, and mannose fermentations may be weak.

Glucose is catabolized fermentatively. The most reliable of the tests (i.e., reproducible under the test conditions) are those for oxidase, catalase, phosphatase, glucose oxidation or fermentation, phenylalanine deamination, esculin hydrolysis, nitrate, tetrazolium and tellurite reduction, and carbohydrate utilization (2, 9). Variable results are sometimes obtained in the arginine, urea, and acetylmethylcarbinol tests, because of probably marginal sensitivities of the demonstrating reactions (9). The characteristics of *S. moniliformis* are summarized by Wittler and Cary in the 8th edition of *Bergey's Manual* now in press.

The moles percent of guanine plus cytosine in the deoxyribonucleic acid of an L-phase variant was a remarkably low 23.9% as determined by thermal denaturation (41).

SPIRILLUM MINOR

Pathogenesis and epidemiology of Sodoku rat-bite fever caused by Spirillum minor

Much of the earlier literature has referred to the disease of *Soduku* (sic) and the organism as *Spirillum minus* (see previous edition of this *Manual* and included citations). However, because *Sodoku* more nearly reproduces Japanese phonetics and *Spirillum minor* (8; *Bergey's Manual*, 8th ed.) is correct, these are the presently employed terms. The organism can be transferred to mice, rats, guinea pigs, and monkeys. Usually infection follows the bite of a rat, mouse, or other rodents, or of a cat, weasel, or other rodent-ingesting animal (3, 8, 19–21, 38). The incubation period is about 2 weeks. The major clinical features differentiating *Sodoku* from *S. moniliformis* infections are: (i) a recrudescence of the initial wound with inflammation, induration, and an occasional chancre-like ulceration; (ii) associated lymphangitis and regional lymphadenitis; (iii) a different rash appearing as a maculopapular, erythematous, or dark purple eruption spreading from the initial lesion; (iv) occasional palpable liver; and (v) failure to cultivate the etiological agent (3). The remaining major clinical signs are indistinguishable in *S. minor* and *S. moniliformis* infections (3).

Mortality appears to be 6 to 10% (20, 37). The disease has been successfully treated with streptomycin (20, 21, 37) and also with penicillin (20, 37).

Characteristics of Spirillum minor

Although Roughgarden (37) cites two claims that *S. minor* has been cultivated in laboratory media, these claims have never been confirmed and it seems safe to say that *S. minor* has not been cultivated in vitro (*Bergey's Manual*, 8th ed.). The cells are gram-negative. They appear short and thick and may vary in dimensions but are generally 0.5 μm in diameter and 1.7 to 5 μm in length; two to six spirals, and bipolar tufts of flagella are present with active motility.

Laboratory diagnosis of Spirillum minor

In humans, microscopic demonstration of *S. minor* should be attempted in exudates from the initial lesion, in adjacent lymph nodes, in cutaneous eruptions, or in blood. Wet mounts should be examined by dark-field or phase-contrast microscopy. Care should be taken not to confuse numerous fibrils and stroma with *S. minor*. Blood films should also be stained with Giemsa or Wright stains.

Cultural studies are sufficient to make a laboratory diagnosis of *S. moniliformis* infections, and animal inoculations are not necessary. But in suspected Sodoku, there is no other recourse than animal studies when initial microscopy fails to demonstrate *S. minor*.

Before inoculating laboratory animals, blood should be examined for naturally occurring organisms resembling *S. minor*. Such organisms are sometimes present, and these animals should not be employed. Four mice should be injected intraperitoneally with 1 ml of patient blood, and one guinea pig should be injected with 2 ml of blood by the same route. In mice, the organism is most abundant in blood within 2 to 3 weeks. Wet mounts and smears of mouse peritoneal fluid should be examined weekly for 4 weeks. Guinea pig blood should be defibrinated and lightly centrifuged, and the fibrin-free supernatant blood should be examined in wet mounts by dark-field or phase-contrast microscopy. Slide films should also be stained and examined by usual light microscopy. *S. minor* is usually most numerous in infected guinea pig blood 1 to 3 weeks after injection. As controls, an equivalent number of animals should be injected with a patient blood specimen previously heated to 52 C for 1 h and examined as already described.

Often, when organisms are scarce or not demonstrable in the peritoneal fluid or blood of inoculated animals, impression films of the heart muscle may reveal numerous cells (5 to 50 per microscopic field). The heart of a dead or sacrificed animal is sliced in half, and a clean glass microscope slide is passed with pressure across the cut surface. Dry, fix, and flood the slide with a dilute Giemsa stain. This consists of 1 drop of Giemsa spirochete stain (Hynson, Westcott, and Dunning, Inc.) added to 1 ml of distilled water. After 20 min, the slide is drained and rinsed with acetone for about 15 s (21). In these cases, heart tissue sections stained by silver impregnation methods also reveal the organism. Impression smears of crushed heart tissue preparations may also be stained with Thedan blue solution T-5 (Allied Chemical Co., New York, N.Y.). The saponin present in this stain destroys erythrocytes and many blood elements, and *S. minor* is stained within 3 min (19).

Live organisms in a fresh preparation have been immobilized by immune serum. However, this test has been questioned (19) and is not routinely used. An active lytic principle is present in immune sera from rabbits and monkeys. An infectious suspension of mouse heart is neutralized within 3 h at 35 C and protects inoculated mice from infection. Human sera have not been evaluated in this mouse protection test (19). Complement fixation tests for syphilis with patient serum have been reported positive (3, 19, 20). Sera from rabbits infected with *S. minor* have given positive Weil-Felix reactions with *Proteus* OX strains (19).

LITERATURE CITED

1. Altemeier, W. A., H. Snyder, and G. Howe. 1957. Penicillin therapy in rate bite fever. J. Amer. Med. Ass. **127**:270–273.
2. Aluotto, B. B., R. G. Wittler, C. O. Williams, and J. E. Faber. 1970. Standardized bacteriologic techniques for the characterization of *Mycoplasma* species. Int. J. Syst. Bacteriol. **20**:35–58.
3. Anderson, W. A. D. 1961. Pathology, 4th ed., p. 285–286. The C. V. Mosby Co., St. Louis, Mo.
4. Blake, F. G. 1916. The etiology of rat-bite fever. J. Exp. Med. **23**:39–60.
5. Boyer, C. I., Jr., D. W. Bruner, and J. A. Brown, 1958. A streptobacillus, the cause of tendo-sheath infection in turkeys. Avian Dis. **2**:418.
6. Brown, T. McP., and J. C. Nunemaker. 1942. Rat-bite fever: a review of the American cases with reevaluation of etiology: report of cases. Bull. Johns Hopkins Hosp. **70**:201–328.
7. Buchanan, R. E., J. G. Holt, and E. F. Lessel, Jr. 1966. Index Bergeyana. An annotated alphabetic listing of names of the taxa of bacteria, p. 1068–1069, p. 1035. The Williams & Wilkins Co., Baltimore.
8. Carter, H. V. 1888. Note on the occurrence of a minute blood-spirillum in an Indian rat. Sci. Mem. Med. Offrs. Army India Part **3**:45–48.
9. Cohen, R. L., R. G. Wittler, and J. E. Faber. 1968. Modified biochemical tests for characterization of L-phase variants of bacteria. Appl. Microbiol. **16**:1655–1662.

10. Dolman, C. E., D. E. Kerr, H. Chang, and A. R. Shearer. 1951. Two cases of rat-bite fever due to *Streptobacillus moniliformis*. Can. J. Pub. Health **42:**228–241.
11. Edward, D. G. 1953. A difference in growth requirements between bacteria in the L-phase and organisms of the pleuro-pneumonia group. J. Gen. Microbiol. **8:**256–262.
12. Fabricant, J., and E. A. Freundt. 1967. Importance of extension and standardization of laboratory tests for the identification and classification of mycoplasma. Ann. N.Y. Acad. Sci. **143:**50–58.
13. Freundt, E. A. 1956. *Streptobacillus moniliformis* infection in mice. Acta Pathol. Microbiol. Scand. **38:**231–245.
14. Freundt, E. A. 1956. Experimental investigations into the pathogenicity of the L-phase variant of *Streptobacillus moniliformis*. Acta Pathol. Microbiol. Scand. **38:**246–258.
15. Hamburger, M., and H. C. Knowles, Jr. 1953. *Streptobacillus moniliformis* infection complicated by acute bacterial endocarditis; report of a case in a physician following bite of laboratory rat. Arch. Intern. Med. **92:**216–220.
16. Hazard, J. B., and R. Goodkind. 1932. Haverhill fever (erythema arthriticum epidemicum); a case report and bacteriologic study. J. Amer. Med. Ass. **99:**534–538.
17. Heilman, F. R. 1941. A study of *Asterococcus muris* (*Streptobacillus* moniliformis). I. Morphologic aspects and nomenclature. J. Infect. Dis. **69:**32–44.
18. Heilman, F. R., and W. E. Herrell. 1944. Penicillin in the treatment of experimental infections with *Spirillum minus* and *Streptobacillus moniliformis* (rat-bite fever). Proc. Staff Meet. Mayo Clin. **19:**257–264.
19. Jellison, W. L. 1963. Soduku, p. 640–641. *In* A. H. Harris and M. B. Coleman (ed.), Diagnostic procedures and reagents. American Public Health Association, Inc., New York.
20. Jellison, W. L. 1963. Rat-bite fever (Soduku and Haverhill fever), p. 652–667. *In* T. G. Hull (ed.), Diseases transmitted from animals to man, 5th ed. Charles C Thomas, Publisher, Springfield, Ill.
21. Jellison, W. L., P. L. Eneboe, R. R. Parker, and L. E. Hughes. 1949. Rat-bite fever in Montana. Pub. Health Rep. (U.S.) **64:**1661–1665.
22. Klieneberger, E. 1935. The natural occurrence of pleuropneumonia-like organisms in apparent symbiosis with *Streptobacillus moniliformis* and other bacteria. J. Pathol. Bacteriol. **40:**93–105.
23. Klieneberger, E. 1938. Pleuropneumonia-like organisms of diverse provenance: some results of an enquiry into methods of differentiation. J. Hyg. **38:**458–476.
24. Klieneberger, E. 1942. Some new observations bearing on the nature of the pleuropneumonia-like organism known as L_1 associated with *Streptobacillus moniliformis*. J. Hyg. **42:**485–497.
25. Knipp, L. H., and J. R. Sokatch. 1969. The chemical composition of the cell envelope of *Streptobacillus moniliformis*. Can. J. Microbiol. **15:**665–669.
26. Levaditi, C., S. Nicolau, and P. Poincloux. 1925. Sur le rôle étiologique de *Streptobacillus moniliformis* (nov. spec.) dans l'érythème polymorphe aigu septicémique. C. R. Acad. Sci. Paris **180:**1188–1190.
27. Levey, J. S., and S. Levey. 1948. Chemotherapy of joint involvement in mice produced by *Streptobacillus moniliformis*. Proc. Soc. Exp. Biol. Med. **68:**314–317.
28. McGee, A. A., and R. G. Wittler. 1969. The role of L-phase and other wall-defective microbial variants in disease, p. 697–720. *In* L. Hayflick (ed.), The *Mycoplasmatales* and the L-phase of bacteria. Appleton-Century-Crofts, New York.
29. Oeding, P., and H. Pederson. 1950. *Streptothrix muris ratti* (*Streptobacillus moniliformis*) isolated from a brain abscess. Acta Pathol. Microbiol. Scand. **27:**436–442.
30. Parker, F., Jr., and N. P. Hudson. 1926. The etiology of Haverhill fever (erythema arthriticum epidemicum). Amer. J. Pathol. **2:**357–379.
31. Partridge, S. M., and E. Klieneberger. 1941. Isolation of cholesterol from the oily droplets found in association with the L_1 organism separated from *Streptobacillus moniliformis*. J. Pathol. Bacteriol. **42:**219–223.
32. Peterson, E. S., N. B. McCullough, C. W. Eisele, and J. M. Goldinger. 1950. Subacute bacterial endocarditis due to *Streptobacillus moniliformis*. J. Amer. Med. Ass. **144:**621–622.
33. Place, E. H., and L. E. Sutton. 1934. Erythema arthriticum (Haverhill fever). Arch. Intern. Med. **54:**659–684.
34. Place, E. H., L. E. Sutton, and O. Willner. 1926. Erythema arthriticum epidemicum; preliminary report. Boston Med. Surg. J. **194:**285–287.
35. Razin, S., and C. Boschwitz. 1968. The membrane of the *Streptobacillus moniliformis* L-phase. J. Gen. Microbiol. **54:**21–32.
36. Robinson, L. B. 1963. *Streptobacillus moniliformis* infections, p. 642–651. *In* A. H. Harris and M. B. Coleman (ed.), Diagnostic procedures and reagents, 4th ed. American Public Health Association, Inc., New York.
37. Roughgarden, J. W. 1965. Antimicrobial therapy of rat bite fever; a review. Arch. Intern. Med. **116:**39–54.
38. Schottmüller, H. 1914. Zur Ätiologie und Klinik der Bisskrankheit (Rattin-, Katzen-, Eichhörnchen-Bisskrankheit). Dermatol. Wochenschr. **58**(Suppl.)**:**77–103.
39. Sprecher, M. W., and J. R. Copeland. 1947. Haverhill fever due to *Streptobacillus moniliformis*. J. Amer. Med. Ass. **134:**1014–1016.
40. Strangeways, W. I. 1933. Rats as carriers of *Streptobacillus moniliformis*. J. Pathol. Bacteriol. **37:**45–51.
41. Williams, C. O., R. G. Wittler, and C. Burris. 1969. Deoxyribonucleic acid base compositions of selected Mycoplasmas and L-phase variants. J. Bacteriol. **99:**341–343.
42. Wilson, G. S., and A. A. Miles. 1964. Topley and Wilson's principles of bacteriology and immunity, 5th ed., p. 518–520. The Williams & Wilkins Co., Baltimore.
43. Wittler, R. G., W. F. Malizia, P. E. Kramer, J. D. Tuckett, H. N. Pritchard, and H. J. Baker. 1960. Isolation of a corynebacterium and its transitional forms from a case of subacute bacterial endocarditis treated with antibiotics. J. Gen. Microbiol. **23:**315–333.
44. Yamamoto, R., and G. T. Clark. 1966. *Streptobacillus moniliformis* infection in turkeys. Vet. Rec. **79:**95–100.

Chapter 32

Mycoplasma

GEORGE E. KENNY

CHARACTERIZATION

Members of the *Mycoplasmatales*. Previously termed pleuropneumonia-like organisms (PPLO). *Mycoplasma pneumoniae* is a major cause of primary atypical pneumonia (3). *M. hominis*, a common cervical isolate, can be isolated from the upper female reproductive tract and the blood stream, indicating that it is an opportunist. The possible role of T strains in nonspecific urethritis is controversial, but these organisms could have some role as opportunists. They can be recovered from the vagina and urethra in the absence of disease, but appear to be spread sexually. *M. salivarium* is a common inhabitant of the gingival crevice and is not observed in edentulous persons; its etiological role in periodontal disease is presently uncertain. *M. pharyngis* (*M. orale* type I), *M. orale* type II, and *M. orale* type III are recovered from the mouth and throat and are considered normal flora. *M. fermentans* is a rare isolate from the genitourinary tract. *Acholeplasma laidlawii* (previously *Mycoplasma laidlawii*) is occasionally isolated from throat swabs and has been recovered from burns. A considerable number of other species are distributed in the animal kingdom and cause, primarily, respiratory diseases, genital infections, and arthritis.

Membrane-bounded cells appear as coccoid bodies, filamentous, and star-shaped forms. Although the morphology is variable, some species exhibit unique morphologies, and the size of individual organisms can be approximated as spheres of 0.3 to 0.5 μm in diameter. Cells do not Gram stain but can be stained (poorly) with Giemsa. Cells are best observed in broth cultures by dark-field or phase-contrast microscopy.

Growth. Organisms form small colonies, 10 to 100 μm in diameter, on enriched medium. Colonies frequently show "fried-egg" appearance (colony will show a dark center where organisms have grown into agar). Very faint turbidity is produced in broth culture, though some species may show presence of spherules (floating colonies). Complex medium is required for growth and ordinarily contains, in addition to peptones, both yeast extract and serum.

Taxonomy. Although all species commonly isolated from humans are currently classified in genus *Mycoplasma*, it is clear that the heterogeneity observed far exceeds that of a genus. Serologically, the species that infect humans can be divided into four groups (Table 1). Species are presently identified by inhibition of growth on agar by disks impregnated with antiserum (2).

Biochemical characteristics. The groups of species can be most clearly separated by the following biochemical characteristics (Table 1): glucose fermentation, arginine hydrolysis, urea hydrolysis, and aerobiasis.

Nomenclature. The correct trivial name in biological nomenclature for organisms in genus *Mycoplasma* is mycoplasmata, though the term mycoplasmas, the English common name, has been more widely used. The T strains have not yet been specifically named; however, it appears that a new genus name other than *Mycoplasma* will be proposed. If reclassification continues, it is possible that none of the organisms listed in Table 1 will be classified in the genus *Mycoplasma*. Certainly *M. pneumoniae* will be reclassified into a new and separate genus in due time.

RECOGNITION OF MYCOPLASMIC INFECTIONS

Three groups of organisms are commonly sought in mycoplasmic infections: *M. pneumoniae*, *M. hominis*, and T strains. *M. pneumoniae* will ordinarily be sought from the respiratory tract of patients with bronchitis and pneumonia. *M. hominis* and T strains will be sought from infections of the upper female reproductive tract; both of these organisms are common inhabitants of the vagina and cervix. Specimens ordinarily submitted will be swabs from internal organs and blood cultures. The etiological role of the other organisms is uncertain, although a variety of species (including species of animal origin) may be found as contaminants in animal cell cultures.

TABLE 1. *Biochemical characteristics of mycoplasmata isolated from humans*

Characteristic	Serological group[a]						
	Group 1			Group 2, *M. fermentans*	Group 3, *Acholeplasma laidlawii*	Group 5, *M. pneumoniae*	Group ?, T strains
	Mycoplasma hominis	*M. salivarium*	*M.*[b] *pharyngis* (*orale* 1)				
Glucose fermentation	−	−	−	+	+	+	−
Arginine hydrolysis	+	+	+	+	−	−	−
Urea hydrolysis	−	−	−	−	−	−	+
Atmospheric conditions for isolation							
Air	++[c] (1–3)	−	−	?[d] (2–10?)	?[d] (1–4)	++++[c] (5–10)	−
Microaerophilic[e] (95% N_2, 5% CO_2)	+++	++++ (2–4)	++	?	?	+	+++ (1–3)
Hydrogen-CO_2[f]	++++	++++	++++ (2–4)	?	?	±	++

[a] Groups are divided serologically. Organisms inside a group show common antigens, whereas organisms in different groups do not cross-react in double immunodiffusion testing with the use of hyperimmune sera. Numbering of the groups is arbitrary and is similar to that shown in the review by Kenny (5), where ***M. gallisepticum*** (an avian organism) was classified in group 4.

[b] The properties of *M. orale* types II and III are similar to *M. orale* I.

[c] Growth ranges from −, no growth, to ++++, maximal growth. Figures in parentheses indicate the usual time in days when colonies appear from wild isolates under the indicated conditions on the recommended media.

[d] Ideal atmosphere for isolation of wild strains unknown, prototype organisms grow well both aerobically and microaerophilically.

[e] An atmosphere of 95% N_2-5% CO_2 where oxygen is removed by flushing.

[f] H_2-CO_2 atmosphere where oxygen is removed catalytically (GasPak method).

SPECIAL CONSIDERATIONS FOR CULTURE OF MYCOPLASMATA

Colonies of organisms in the *Mycoplasmatales* are minute (10 to 100 μm, Fig. 1) and grow imbedded in the agar. Consequently, organisms will not transfer when picked with a bacteriological loop. To transfer organisms, individual colonies should be excised from the plate with a metal loop or scalpel. The resultant agar block can be rubbed "face down" on a new agar plate, emulsified in broth and then streaked on a plate, or grown up in broth and then transferred to a plate to produce new colonies. A stereoscopic microscope with oblique lighting is employed at 20 to 60× magnification for observing colonies because it provides the best working distance and resolution for observing the colonies on the agar surface through the bottom of the plate without opening the plate. This method of observation is rapid and avoids contamination of the agar surface not only with bacteria but also with mycoplasmata during the repeated observations necessary to detect growth. Except for specialized stains for the T strains, colonies of individual species cannot be definitively distinguished. Individual colonies can be studied in greater detail by use of Dienes staining technique (9), although this method does not assist identification. A major concern is the isolation of cell wall-deficient bacteria (see chapter 33) on medium intended for isolation of mycoplasmata. These organisms ordinarily form large fried-egg colonies which transfer poorly, and they usually revert to bacteria on penicillin-free bacteriological medium. Fortunately, these

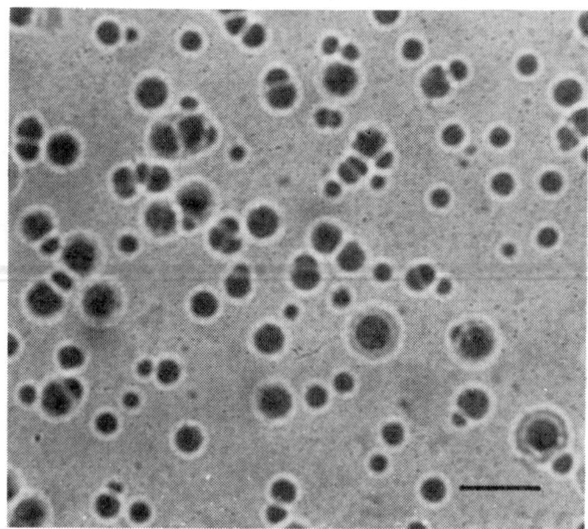

FIG. 1. *Colonies of Mycoplasma pneumoniae (strain AP-164) on E agar, 10 days of incubation. Bar = 100 μm.*

organisms are rarely isolated on the recommended mycoplasmic medium, and they cannot be typed by disk inhibition as mycoplasmic species.

Selection of type of species to be isolated can be accomplished by the relative aerobiasis of the incubation. *M. pneumoniae* is aerobic, whereas nearly all oral species, except *M. hominis*, are better isolated on the media recommended under microaerophilic or anaerobic conditions. *M. hominis* can be separated from T strains by aerobic incubation, and the growth of *M. hominis* in mixed cultures of *M. hominis* and T strains can be suppressed by the inclusion of lincomycin in the medium (10). Mycoplasmic species can be specifically identified by inhibition of colonial growth by specific antiserum. The method ordinarily used (2) employs the inhibition of colonial growth in a zone around a disk soaked with specific antiserum (the zone of inhibition is analogous to that produced with bacteria around an antibiotic-containing disk). Several colonies should be grown up for serotyping since mixed cultures occur. The isolation of T strains is unique in several respects: the organisms are inhibited by ordinary agar (purified agars such as agarose are necessary); they grow best at acid pH (6.0); and they are inhibited by thallium acetate, which is ordinarily used to suppress bacterial growth (10).

A major consideration in embarking on isolation of mycoplasmata lies in the wide variation of peptones, sera, and agar in isolation efficiency for mycoplasmata. Additionally, prototype strains are selected for growth on agar medium and may grow on medium which will not effectively isolate wild organisms. Accordingly, laboratories embarking on isolation of mycoplasmata should accumulate wild mycoplasmic isolates to evaluate the sensitivity of their cultural media. Otherwise negative results may have little significance. An annoying artifact in isolation of mycoplasmata is the formation of pseudocolonies on agar media (4). Pseudocolonies are whorls of material which appear on the surface of agar plates. Interestingly, these "crystals" propagate in that they can be transferred and will form new "pseudocolonies." However, utilization of glucose, arginine, or urea will not be observed in broth cultures, and the formation of pseudocolonies cannot be inhibited with tetracycline. Tissue cells and other material in cultures may strikingly resemble mycoplasmic colonies; however, these will not transfer. Similarly, large amounts of cellular material may produce acid from glucose; again, this effect will not be transferable. Because of these artifacts, positive culture results should only be reported for transferable entities.

Penicillin is ordinarily employed in mycoplasmic medium to inhibit bacterial overgrowth of the slowly growing mycoplasmic species. Thallium acetate is also employed to inhibit bacterial growth but should be avoided in T strain isolation attempts.

COLLECTION OF SPECIMENS

Specimens collected on swabs should be placed into transport medium; 2 ml of Trypticase soy broth with 0.5% bovine albumin has been used satisfactorily. Mycoplasmata are remarkably sensitive to drying; thus, specimens on swabs should be placed in transport medium or tested promptly. Penicillin is usually incorporated in transport medium to suppress bacterial overgrowth; however, other antibiotics such as aminoglycosides and tetracyclines should not be used because they inhibit mycoplasmic growth. Tissues and sputum specimens can be submitted directly. Although storage conditions have not clearly been worked out for all strains and species, it appears that both T strains and *M. pneumoniae* survive storage at 4 C for several days and at −80 C for years with little loss in viability. The picture is less clear for *M. hominis* since positive specimens may become negative upon storage.

ISOLATION OF MYCOPLASMA PNEUMONIAE

Specimens from the respiratory tract are usually examined. A 0.1-ml amount of transport medium (in which the swab has been extracted) should be inoculated both into diphasic broth and onto an E-agar plate. Sputum, body fluids, and disrupted tissue materials should be diluted 1:10 and 1:100 before being used to inoculate broth and plates to reduce the amount of inhibiting substances normally present in tissues. The agar plates should be incubated at 37 C aerobically in a sealed container, and the plates should be examined microscopically at 2, 5, 10, 15, 25, and 30 days for presence of typical colonies. Diphasic cultures should be examined microscopically by looking at the broth through the side of the tube for presence of "spherules" (fluid medium colonies), which will appear as early as 5 days. Diphasic cultures should also be observed for decrease in pH as judged by the phenol red indicator. Diphasic cultures should be transferred to E plates at 21 days, and these cultures should be observed for 21 days. Most positive specimens will show typical small colonies on agar and will show spherule production and acid production in fluid medium by 10 to 12 days, although some specimens may turn positive only after longer intervals (up to 30 days). These three factors allow a tentative identification of *M. pneumoniae* which can be verified by a hemolysis test (1) done on the original isolation plate if sufficient colonies exist. The only other organisms isolated from the respiratory tract under the recommended conditions are *M. hominis*, which grows rapidly and forms large colonies, and rarely *A. laidlawii*, which will also hemolyze guinea pig red blood cells. The hemolysis test is carried out by overlaying the colonies with a thin layer of 8% guinea pig red blood cells in saline-agar. Incubation is carried out overnight at 37 C, and a zone of hemolysis will be observed surrounding the colonies. At this point, specimens may be reported as positive for an organism with cultural characteristics resembling *M. pneumoniae*. Absolute identification can be accomplished by inhibition of colonial growth with specific antiserum. One-tenth-milliliter aliquots of serial 10-fold dilutions of the broth culture (1:1, 1:10, 1:100) are spread uniformly over E agar plates and allowed to absorb; then paper disks (2 to 3 mm) soaked with antiserum (available commercially) are placed on the plates. Incubation is carried out for 4 to 6 days aerobically, and plates are examined for zones of inhibition of colonial growth. The test is quite sensitive to excess organisms (2).

M. pneumoniae is relatively easy to isolate since patients carry the organism for 2 to 3 months after infection and isolation is little hampered by antibiotic therapy (3). However, the slowness of isolation greatly hampers the diagnostic utility of testing for the organism but is useful epidemiologically and in family infections (3). Althought the *M. orale* strains and *M. salivarium* are abundant in throat swabs, E medium is selective in that these organisms will rarely be recovered aerobically. Other media are less selective, and 0.002% methylene blue has been employed in both agar and broth medium to inhibit these organisms (7).

ISOLATION OF MYCOPLASMA HOMINIS AND T STRAINS

Since *M. hominis* and T strains are ordinarily sought from the genital tract, isolation of these organisms will be considered together. Specimens in collection medium should be inoculated in 0.1-ml amounts onto E agar, onto Mes agar, and into urea broth. Agar plates must be incubated in at least a microaerophilic atmosphere. This may be achieved by placing the plates in a sealable container such as a glass desiccator, evacuating this chamber to −600 mm (−24 inches) of Hg, and replacing the atmosphere with 95% N_2-5% CO_2 to −100 mm of Hg. This procedure should be repeated three times and the container should be incubated at 37 C. Before opening the container, its pressure should be tested; a negative pressure assures that a leak has not occurred. Broth cultures can be incubated aerobically. Plates should be observed at 1, 2, 4, and 10 days for presence of small colonies under 60× magnification. The urea broth should be observed twice daily (early morning and late evening) for pH increase. Broth cultures should be transferred immediately to a new urea broth and an agar plate if a pH change is observed (T strains die rapidly both on plates and on agar). Colonies of T strains can be differentiated from *M. hominis* colonies by the rapid single-reagent urease test of Shepard (11). One drop of reagent is added to the agar plate with colonies and the plate is immediately observed. T strain colonies immediately turn brown, whereas *M. hominis* colonies are unaffected. Isolates which form typical T strain colonies are considered to be confirmed if they prove to be transferable entities which utilize urea. Although present data suggest that the T strains are comprised of a number of serotypes (8), practical simple means are not yet available for typing of T strains. Isolates may be tentatively identified as *M. hominis* if they utilize arginine and produce typical large colonies. Their identity can be verified by disk inhibition in a manner similar to that for *M. pneumoniae*.

Isolation of T strains and *M. hominis* from blood has been accomplished; however, specific medium formulations have not been extensively evaluated. Diphasic cultures should be prepared, the fluid phase of which is 20-fold the volume of the sample of blood to be cultured, and medium should contain penicillin but not thallium acetate. Blood should be collected without anticoagulant and directly inoculated into the medium. Cultures should be subcultured to agar and T agar at daily intervals for 1 week and observed for typical colonies.

Unless isolated from blood, isolations of *M. hominis* and T strains may have little significance if the specimen has been contaminated by urethral or vaginal materials in the obtaining of the specimen. As mentioned earlier, the role of either organism in urethritis is controversial.

ISOLATION OF MYCOPLASMATA FROM CELL CULTURES

Clinical laboratories engaging in mycoplasmic isolation are frequently asked to monitor cell cultures from virology laboratories for mycoplasmic contamination (5). The optimal specimen is dispersed cells, and these should be inoculated onto E agar and into diphasic broth. One plate should be incubated aerobically, another microaerophilically, and, if available, a third plate under strict anaerobiasis (such as the GasPak method). One diphasic culture should also be incubated under strict anaerobiosis. Cultures should be observed at 2-day intervals, and subculture from broth should be made to agar plates on the fourth day. Although the dispersed animal cells may look much like mycoplasmic colonies, they will not transfer. The microscopic morphology of the animal cells can be assessed by observing the plates immediately after the inoculum has been absorbed. Mycoplasmata are considered to have been isolated if a transferable entity with typical colonial morphology is obtained.

SEROLOGICAL DIAGNOSIS OF MYCOPLASMIC INFECTIONS

The difficulties and slow isolation of the *Mycoplasmatales*, and *M. pneumoniae* in particular, indicate that serological diagnosis might be more efficient and simpler for laboratories not wishing to place a major investment in mycoplasmic technology. Although effective serological tests for antibodies to *M. hominis* and T strains are still in the developmental stage, in large part because of the antigenic heterogeneity of these organisms, detection of antibodies to *M. pneumoniae* is relatively simple. Fortunately, the major antigen of *M. pneumoniae* is heat-stable because of its lipid nature (6), and thus antigens can be readily stored for long periods of time. Whole organism antigens can be purchased from commerical sources and can be used in complement fixation tests in the conventional manner. Several factors are important: antigens are frequently anticomplementary and are low titered. The antigen can be made more sensitive and less anticomplementary by extraction of the active lipid principle with chloroform-methanol (6), a relatively simple procedure. Sera for testing should be collected as close to onset as possible and 3 weeks later. Fourfold antibody rises are considered indicative of recent infections. High titers are not useful because significant antibody titers may persist for 1 or more years after infection. Approximately two-thirds of those with *M. pneumoniae* isolates will show fourfold antibody rises (3). Similarly, two-thirds of those with fourfold antibody rises will yield isolates of the organism. The comparison of serology and isolation results provides an excellent check on the sensitivity of both assay methods.

LITERATURE CITED

1. Clyde, W. A. 1963. Hemolysis in identifying Eaton's pleuropneumonia-like organism. Science **139**:55.
2. Clyde, W. A. 1964. Mycoplasma species identification based upon growth inhibition by specific antisera. J. Immunol. **92**:958–965.
3. Grayston, J. T., H. M. Foy and G. E. Kenny. 1969. The epidemiology of Mycoplasma infections of the human respiratory tract, p. 651–682. *In* L. Hayflick (ed.), The Mycoplasmatales and L-phase of bacteria. Appleton-Century-Crofts, New York.
4. Hayflick, L. 1965. Tissue cultures and mycoplasmas. Tex. Rep. Biol. Med. **23**:285–303.
5. Kenny, G. E. 1973. Contamination of mammalian cells in culture with mycoplasmata, p. 107–129. *In* J. Fogh (ed.), Contamination in tissue culture. Academic Press Inc., New York.
6. Kenny, G. E., and J. T. Grayston. 1965. Eaton PPLO (*Mycoplasma pneumoniae*) complement fixing antigen: extraction with organic solvents. J. Immunol. **95**:19–25.
7. Kraybill, W. H., and Y. E. Crawford. 1965. A selective medium and color test for *Mycoplasma pneumoniae*. Proc. Soc. Exp. Biol. Med. **118**:965–970.
8. Lin, J. S., and E. H. Kass. 1973. Serotypic heterogeneity in isolates of human genital T-mycoplasmas. Infect. Immunity **7**:499–500.
9. Madoff, S. 1960. Isolation and identification of PPLO. Ann. N.Y. Acad. Sci. **79**:383–392.
10. Shepard, M. C. 1967. Cultivation and properties of Mycoplasma associated with non-gonococcal urethritis. Ann. N.Y. Acad. Sci. **143**:505–514.
11. Shepard, M. C. 1973. Differential methods for the identification of T-mycoplasmas based on demonstration of urease. J. Infect. Dis. **127**:S22–S25.

Chapter 33

Cell Wall-Defective Bacteria

THOMAS R. CATE

CHARACTERIZATION

Since the pioneering work of Dienes and Weinberger (7) and Klieneberger-Noble (18), much has been learned about the behavior of cell wall-defective bacteria, as evidenced by several recent books and review articles (4, 9, 13, 15, 19, 23, 24, 28). Cell walls of gram-positive and gram-negative bacteria differ both in their staining characteristics and in their appearance on electron micrographs, but both have a rigid mucopeptide skeleton and variable amounts of other substances which may serve as identifying antigens, toxins, inhibitors of phagocytosis, etc. Subjacent to the cell wall is the delicate, selectively permeable, cytoplasmic membrane which maintains the characteristically hypertonic internal milieu of bacteria. The encasing cell wall maintains the distinctive shape of the organism and protects it against osmotic lysis which might otherwise occur in media having the tonicity of human serum.

Several materials can cause bacteria to have defective cell walls. Penicillins and cephalosporins have interference with synthesis of cell walls as their major mechanism of action. Lysozyme can hydrolyze the glycosidic linkages of the mucopeptide, making the cell wall nonrigid, but preceding damage to the bacterial surface by something such as ethylenediaminetetraacetate, lipase, or antibody plus complement may be necessary for lysozyme to gain access to the mucopeptide. Lysostaphin can lyse mucopeptide cross-linkages of staphylococci. Glycine and D-amino acids can also apparently reverse cross-linking of the mucopeptide of many bacteria.

Properties of cell wall-defective bacterial variants differ from those of the parent bacterium in many important respects. Lacking a rigid encasement, cell wall-defective variants are pleomorphic and prone to lysis if not in an osmotically protective medium. Variants originating from gram-positive bacteria may be gram-variable in staining, or may become gram-negative with further loss of cell wall material. Orderly bacterial division is no longer possible without the cell wall. Penicillins and cephalosporins are not active against cell wall-defective variants, but these organisms may exhibit increased susceptibility to antibiotics with other mechanisms of action, indicating that cell wall interference with access of the antibiotic to the membrane or intracellular sites can be an important mechanism of resistance.

Transitions between the various cell wall-defective bacteria are represented in the Fig. 1 (16, 22, 24). Transitional phase variants have damaged cell walls and are gram-variable and pleomorphic; they are unstable in culture with frequent reversion to the parent bacterium or transition to the L-phase. Most cell wall-defective organisms recovered from clinical specimens are probably in the transitional phase. Protoplasts may be distinguished from spheroplasts by demonstration of the complete absence of cell wall in the former; these variants are of a rather uniform size similar to or larger than the parent bacterium, spheroidal, gram-negative, and unable to undergo serial replication without reversion to the parent or transition to the L-phase. L-phase variants are gram-negative and can have variable amounts of cell wall material on their surface like spheroplasts, but, in contrast to the latter, they are pleomorphic and variable in size from "large bodies" larger than the parent bacterium to "small bodies" as small as the larger viruses. L-phase variants may become less susceptible to osmotic lysis than the other cell wall-defective variants and are also unique in their ability to replicate serially with production of characteristic, "fried-egg," L-form colonies. Those L-phase variants which can be reverted to the parent bacterium are referred to as "unstable," while those which resist this reversion are called "stable." It should be noted that all of the cell wall-defective variants retain the genetic material of the parent bacterium and may secrete toxins characteristic of the parent.

L-phase bacterial variants can closely resemble mycoplasmas in their ultrastructure and colony forms; however, the structural configuration of groups of mycoplasma organisms on electron microscopy may be sufficiently distinc-

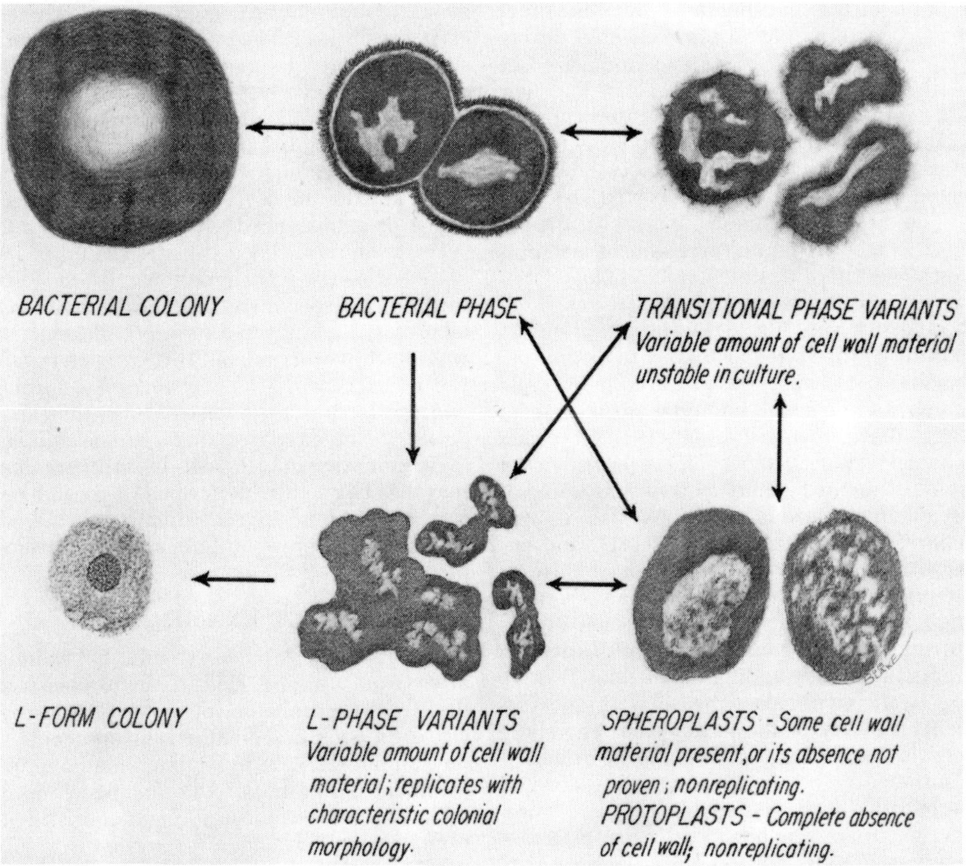

FIG. 1. *Representation of transitions between vegetative bacteria and various cell wall-defective variants (16, 22, 24). Drawings of the individual organisms are magnified approximately 2,000-fold relative to drawings of the colony forms.*

tive to be of use differentially if special attention is paid to the details of preparation (5). Differences between parasitic mycoplasmas and L-phase variants also include a sterol requirement for growth of mycoplasmas, and the production of cell wall components and osmotic fragility of many L-phase variants. Nevertheless, it may be extremely difficult to differentiate an L-phase variant from a mycoplasma without a history of the derivation of the organism or reversion of the L-phase variant back to the parent bacterium.

CLINICAL SIGNIFICANCE

A variety of techniques have been utilized in attempts to demonstrate the importance of cell wall-defective bacteria in infectious processes. These include: (i) recovery of organisms in enriched, hypertonic media but failure to recover them in normal media; (ii) recovery of an increased number of organisms on hypertonic media as opposed to isotonic media; (iii) ability to culture organisms from specimens after passage through a 0.45-μm filter which should remove ordinary bacteria but pass some of the cell wall-defective variants; (iv) reduction in the number of organisms recoverable after submitting the specimen to osmotic shock; and (v) ability of the organism to grow on penicillin-containing, hypertonic medium. Problems involved in interpretation of the data include: artifacts which can resemble L-form colonies; contaminants which can fluorish in the enriched medium; mistaking mycoplasmas for L-phase variants; fastidious organisms (either saprophytic or pathogenic) which preferentially grow on enriched medium but are not cell wall-defective; and conversion of organisms to cell wall-defective variants in the culture medium or in blood, urine, or discharge while the true pathogen in the local site of infection is the parent organism. Nevertheless, cell wall-defective forms of not only bacteria, but also fungi and mycobacteria, have been recovered during a wide variety of infections as summarized in several reviews (4, 9, 13, 19, 21, 22), and new reports continue to appear in the literature.

Results of cultures for cell wall-defective bacteria in consecutive clinical specimens from selected sites have also been reported (1, 8, 10, 29). The special techniques, expensive media, low percentage yield, and problems of interpretation suggest that a clinical microbiology laboratory should limit attempts to recover cell wall-defective variants to special situations in which the cultures are most likely to be productive and clinically useful. For example, one role that cell wall-defective bacterial variants seem likely to play in causing disease is to serve as a mechanism of persistence of the organism in spite of therapy; this may lead to continuing or subsequently relapsing infections such as pyelonephritis (6, 12), osteomyelitis (11), and endocarditis (26, 30), even though routine cultures appropriately turn negative during therapy. Although the clinician may suspect that such is occurring in a particular patient and institute a therapeutic trial by adding an antibiotic which might be effective against the cell wall-defective variant, recovery of the variant and antibiotic susceptibility testing could clearly be of aid.

Another example in which cultures for cell wall-defective organisms could be clinically useful is the patient who has an apparent infection but whose routine cultures have been consistently negative (3, 20). While recognizing that recovery of an organism from any clinical specimen only on enriched, osmotically protective medium does not necessarily prove that a cell wall-defective phase of the organism is responsible for the disease, nevertheless such recoveries can be the key to diagnosis and therapy. Of course, cultures for fungi, mycobacteria, nocardia, and anaerobic organisms may also be indicated depending on the clinical setting.

COLLECTION OF SPECIMENS

Samples to be examined for cell wall-defective organisms should be collected from as close a proximity to the site of infection as possible and in such a way as to minimize the possibility of contamination with saprophytic organisms. These are general principles applicable to the recovery of most pathogens, but they assume added importance in the present instance for attempting to determine whether transition to cell wall-defective organisms is occurring only after the organism is shed, for avoiding confusing recoveries of fastidious saprophytes, and for avoiding saprophytic overgrowth of slowly replicating cell wall-defective variants. Preferred specimens are tissues and body fluids which should normally be sterile.

A satisfactory transport medium for swabs, for mixing in equal portions with liquid specimens (cerebrospinal fluid, pleural fluid, urine, etc.), and for biopsy specimens (avoid use of saline or a "balanced" salt solution) is a 20% sucrose solution. Blood cultures should be inoculated directly into hypertonic broth culture medium. All specimens must be delivered to the laboratory and cultured promptly if fragile, cell wall-defective organisms are to be recovered. Preceding consultation between the physician and the laboratory is necessary so that appropriate, freshly prepared media can be available.

Examination for cell wall-defective organisms may also be usefully performed on routine broth cultures which appear slightly turbid, but which fail to grow on subculture to ordinary media.

DIRECT EXAMINATION

Smears of specimens should be examined after Gram staining. Heat-fixing of smears may destroy the morphology of some cell wall-defective organisms, and air-dried smears should also be examined (2). Individual or small clumps of pleomorphic, gram-variable organisms may be seen, but these may be difficult to distinguish from debris. Phase microscopy can be useful for detecting the pleomorphic variants in broth cultures. In the research setting, electron microscopy and fluorescent staining (if the identity of the organism is known or correctly surmised) can also be useful for demonstrating cell wall-defective organisms.

CULTURE AND ISOLATION

Media for culture of cell wall-defective organisms are not well standardized, although formulas have been published for preparing media that will grow variants of diverse bacteria likely to be found in clinical specimens (2, 25, 27).

Useful agar and broth media for recovery of cell wall-defective organisms can be prepared by use of Difco PPLO agar and broth with subsequent supplementation just prior to use. Unsupplemented media are prepared according to the manufacturer's directions (results in 5.0% beef heart for infusions, 1.0% peptone, 0.5% sodium chloride, with or without 1.4% agar) with the addition of 20% sucrose and 0.2% $MgSO_4 \cdot 4H_2O$, and adjustment of pH to 7.6 to 7.8. The unsupplemented media may be distributed in appropriate samples, autoclaved, and stored at 4 to 5 C for up to several months. The agar is melted in boiling water and cooled to 50 C for final preparation of media.

To 7 parts of the above unsupplemented media, 2 parts of horse serum and 1 part of yeast extract are added for final preparation of the supplemented media. The horse serum is not inactivated. The serum used should at least be shown to support growth of mycoplasmas (e.g., horse serum for mycoplasma growth, Microbiological Associates, Inc.) if there is not an opportunity to test it with cell wall-defective organisms. Agamma horse serum can help in reduction of pseudocolony formation. The yeast extract may also be purchased (e.g., Microbiological Associates, Inc.), or prepared as follows: add 1 part of active dry bakers' yeast (Fleischmann 20–40) to 4 parts of distilled water (wt/vol); boil; filter by gravity through medium-porosity paper; adjust the pH to 8.0 with sodium hydroxide; distribute in appropriate portions; and autoclave. The yeast extract may be stored at −20 C for up to a few months, and one should avoid using the precipitate which usually forms.

Some of the variations in the media include: using an unsupplemented base of beef heart infusion broth rather than the PPLO broth, and adding 1.0 to 1.2% Special Agar Noble (Difco) for solid medium; reduction of sucrose to 10% in agar media; substitution of 5% NaCl (add 4.5% to PPLO broth or agar) for the sucrose; heat inactivation (56 C, 30 min) of the horse serum; reduction of the horse serum supplement to 10%; and reduction of the yeast extract supplement to 1.0%.

Specimens cultured for cell wall-defective organisms should be cultured on routine as well as hypertonic media, and control hypertonic media should be processed simultaneously. Solid specimens may be minced for inoculation into broth, or ground in 20% sucrose solution for inoculation into broth and onto agar. Liquid specimens may be inoculated in fairly large volumes directly into broth (for example, 5 to 10 ml of blood into 50 ml of broth), or in small volumes onto agar media so as to not obscure colonies on subsequent microscope examination or leave excess free fluid on the agar. With specimens having a high risk of contamination by saprophytes, it may be desirable to culture with and without prefiltration through a 0.45-μm filter, recognizing that the latter may remove some cell wall-defective forms but may also prevent saprophytic overgrowth.

Cultures are incubated at 37 C in a moist 5% CO_2-in-air atmosphere; anaerobic incubation is indicated when anaerobic organisms are suspected. Broth cultures are examined by Gram stain of a smear or by phase microscopy two to three times weekly, and are subcultured to hypertonic agar media weekly or when growth is seen. Agar media are examined two to three times weekly with the aid of a low-power microscope and oblique lighting. "Fried-egg" colonies are subcultured to hypertonic agar medium by cutting out a block of agar with a colony, inverting it on a fresh plate, and pushing. Pseudocolonies caused by calcium and magnesium soaps in the enriched medium can closely resemble L-form and mycoplasma colonies, and can appear to replicate on subculture; Dienes' stain can help in differentiation by failing to stain pseudocolonies, by giving initial staining of bacterial and L-form colonies which subsequently fades, and by permanently staining mycoplasma colonies (14). Bacterial colonies are subcultured by loop transfer to ordinary media. Cultures should be observed for 1 month before being called negative.

IDENTIFICATION

The key to identification of cell wall-defective organisms is their reversion to the parent organism which can then be identified by standard methods. Spontaneous reversion may occur quickly or after prolonged incubation in hypertonic media, but reversion may also require many passages with gradual reduction in the percent serum supplement (e.g., 20, 15, 10, 5%) and periodic subculture to ordinary media. If reversion attempts fail and the organism is not an identifiable mycoplasma species, further attempts at identification will require techniques such as biochemical characterization (L-phase organisms should retain many, but not necessarily all, of the biochemical reactions of the parent organism), serological tests with antiserum against the suspected parent organism or its products, determination of the guanine plus cytosine ratio, or deoxyribonucleic acid hybridization studies (31). L-phase variants have been successfully stored for future study in hypertonic broth medium at −70 C or colder, but significantly lower storage temperatures may not result in survival (16).

IMMUNOLOGICAL DIAGNOSIS

Detection of an increasing antibody titer to the parent organism or its products by standard techniques for that organism is a useful way of proving the significance of cell wall-defective variants from clinical specimens, particularly when the variants are the only form of the organism recovered. Various serum inhibitory tests similar to those for mycoplasmas may also be performed with L-phase variants (16), but caution is necessary because of the occurrence of nonspecific inhibitory factors in some sera (17).

SUSCEPTIBILITY TO ANTIMICROBIAL AGENTS

Tests for susceptibility to antimicrobials may be performed in hypertonic medium by standard techniques, but comparison tests with organisms of known susceptibility should be performed in the same medium as an aid to interpretation.

EVALUATION

The techniques described are aimed primarily at recovering organisms as an aid to diagnosis and therapy rather than proving a pathogenetic role for cell wall-defective organisms. However, when organisms are recovered in hypertonic media, there still remains a problem of interpretation (22). Reversion of a variant to an organism known to have been present previously may serve as presumptive evidence for the clinical significance of the variant. The problem is more difficult when cell wall-defective variants are the only potential pathogens recovered from a patient. The importance of having negative control cultures of all media is self-evident. Contamination with saprophytes should be avoided so far as possible, and the reverted organism should be one with the potential capability of producing the disease. Visual demonstration of the variants in specimens, repeated recovery of the same variant, and detecting an antibody response to the reverted organism are important evidence that the variant may be playing a role in the disease. Further evidence for clinical significance and justification of the effort required to recover the variants would be improvement of the patient with eradication of the organisms.

LITERATURE CITED

1. Bhattacharyya, T. K., Y. N. Mehra, and S. C. Agarwal. 1972. Incidence of bacteria, L-form and mycoplasma in chronic sinusitis. Acta Oto-Laryngol. **74:**293–296.
2. Charache, P. 1968. Atypical bacterial forms in human disease, p. 484–494. *In* L. B. Guze (ed.), Microbial protoplasts, spheroplasts, and L-forms. The Williams & Wilkins Co., Baltimore.
3. Charache, P., T. M. Bayless, W. M. Shelley, and T. R. Hendrix. 1966. Atypical bacteria in Whipple's disease. Trans. Ass. Amer. Physicians **79:**399–408.
4. Clasener, H. 1972. Pathogenicity of the L-phase of bacteria. Annu. Rev. Microbiol. **26:**55–84.
5. Clyde, W. A., Jr. 1969. Biophysical characteristics of the mycoplasmas, p. 349–363. *In* L. Hayflick (ed.), The mycoplasmatales and the L-phase of bacteria. Appleton-Century-Crofts, New York.
6. Crowe, C. C., and K. K. Koblasz. 1971. Isolation of L-forms in recurrent urinary tract infections. Amer. J. Med. Technol. **37:**367–370.
7. Dienes, L., and H. J. Weinberger. 1951. The L forms of bacteria. Bacteriol. Rev. **15:**245–288.
8. Dominque, G. J., and J. U. Schlegel. 1970. The possible role of microbial L-forms in pyelonephritis. J. Urol. **104:**790–798.
9. Feingold, D. S. 1969. Biology and pathogenicity of microbial spheroplasts and L-forms. N. Engl. J. Med. **281:**1159–1170.
10. Gnarpe, H., J. Wallin, and A. Forsgren. 1972. Studies in venereal disease. I. Isolation of L-phase organisms of *N. gonorrhea* from patients with gonorrhea. Brit. J. Vener. Dis. **48:**496–499.
11. Gordon, S. L., R. B. Greer, and C. P. Craig. 1972. Recurrent osteomyelitis: report of four cases culturing L-form variants of staphylococci. J. Bone Joint Surg. **53:**1150–1156.
12. Gutman, L. T., M. Turck, R. G., Petersdorf, and R. J. Wedgewood. 1965. Significance of bacterial variants in urine of patients with chronic bacteriuria. J. Clin. Invest. **44:**1945–1952.
13. Guze, L. B. (ed.). 1968. Microbial protoplasts, spheroplasts and L-forms. The Williams & Wilkins Co., Baltimore.
14. Hayflick, L. 1965. Tissue cultures and mycoplasmas. Tex. Rep. Biol. Med. **23:**285–303.
15. Hayflick, L. (ed.). 1969. The mycoplasmatales and the L-phase of bacteria. Appleton-Century-Crofts, New York.
16. Hijmans, W., C. P. A. Van Boven, and H. A. L. Clasener. 1969. Fundamental biology of the L-phase of bacteria, p. 67–143. *In* L. Hayflick (ed.), The mycoplasmatales and the L-phase of bacteria. Appleton-Century-Crofts, New York.
17. Kalmanson, G. M., E. G. Hubert, J. Z. Montgomerie, and L. B. Guze. 1968. Serum bactericidal activity against protoplasts, p. 293–305. *In* L. B. Guze (ed.), Microbial protoplasts, spheroplasts and L-forms. The Williams & Wilkins Co., Baltimore.
18. Klieneberger-Nobel, E. 1962. Pleuropneumonia-like organisms (PPLO): Mycoplasmataceae. Academic Press Inc., New York.
19. Kundsin, R. B. (ed.). 1970. Unusual isolates from clinical material. VII. L-forms. Ann. N.Y. Acad. Sci. **174:**880–931.
20. Louria, D. B., T. Kaminski, M. Grieco, and J. Singer. 1969. Aberrant forms of bacteria and fungi found in blood or cerebrospinal fluid. Arch. Intern. Med. **124:**39–48.
21. McGee, Z. A., and R. G. Wittler. 1969. The role of L-phase and other wall-defective microbial variants in disease, p. 697–720. *In* L. Hayflick (ed.), The mycoplasmatales and the L-phase of bacteria. Appleton-Century-Crofts, New York.
22. McGee, Z. A., R. G. Wittler, H. Gooder, and P. Charache. 1971. Wall-defective microbial variants: terminology and experimental design. J. Infect. Dis. **123:**433–438.
23. Madoff, S. (ed.). 1971. Mycoplasma and the L-forms of bacteria. Gordon and Breach Science Publishers, New York.
24. Martin, H. H. 1963. Bacterial protoplasts—a review. J. Theor. Biol. **5:**1–34.
25. Mattman, L. H. 1968. L-forms isolated from infections, p. 472–483. *In* L. B. Guze (ed.), Microbial spheroplasts, protoplasts and L-forms. The Williams & Wilkins Co., Baltimore.
26. Neu, H.C., and B. Goldreyer. 1968. Isolation of protoplasts in a case of enterococcal endocarditis. Amer. J. Med. **45:**784–788.

27. Nimmo, L. N., and D. J. Blazevic. 1969. Selection of media for the isolation of common bacterial L-phase organisms from a clinical specimen. Appl. Microbiol. **18:**535–541.
28. Smith, P. F. 1964. Comparative physiology of pleuropneumonia-like and L-type organisms. Bacteriol. Rev. **28:**97–125.
29. Swierczewski, J. A., and P. Reyes. 1970. Isolation of L-forms in a clinical microbiology laboratory. Appl. Microbiol. **20:**323–327.
30. Wittler, R. G., W. F. Malizia, P. E. Kramer, J. D. Tuckett, H. N. Pritchard, and J. J. Baker. 1960. Isolation of a corynebacterium and its transitional forms from a case of subacute bacterial endocarditis treated with antibiotics. J. Gen. Microbiol. **23:**315–333.
31. Wittler, R. G., Z. A. McGee, C. O. Williams, C. Burris, R. L. Cohen, and R. B. Roberts. 1968. Identification of L-forms: problems and approaches, p. 333–339. *In* L. B. Guze (ed.), Microbial protoplasts, spheroplasts and L-forms. The Williams & Wilkins Co., Baltimore.

Section III

SPIROCHETES

Chapter 34

Leptospira

AARON D. ALEXANDER

CHARACTERIZATION

Members of the genus *Leptospira* are serologically heterologous. Basic taxon is the serotype. Recognition of two species, *L. interrogans* and *L. biflexa*, has been proposed, respectively, for the so-called "pathogenic" and "saprophytic" leptospires (Minutes of Leptospira Subcommittee Meeting, International Committee on Systematic Bacteriology, Jerusalem 1973, to be published). The "saprophytic" or "water" leptospires are found predominantly in fresh surface waters, are found less frequently in seawater, and are rarely associated with mammalian infections. Pathogenic leptospires occur naturally in a wide variety of wild and domesticated mammals throughout the world, and cause acute, febrile, systemic disease of humans and other mammals. They are isolated from clinical specimens, carriers, and natural waters.

Helicoidal flexible organisms, usually 6 to 20 μm in length and approximately 0.1 μm in diameter; semicircular hooked ends (occasionally, ends are straight; (Fig. 1). Motile. Electron microscopy reveals a cylindrical body helicoidally wound about two flagellum-like components (axial filaments), each of which is inserted subterminally at each end of the helicoidal body with its free end extending towards the middle of the cell (Fig. 2). A common external sheath covers both structures. Faintly colored after staining with aniline dyes. Invisible by bright-field but readily seen by dark-ground microscopy.

Growth. Aerobic. Grows in medium containing 10% serum (preferably rabbit) or serum albumin plus fatty acids at pH 6.8 to 7.8. Optimal temperature, 30 C. Incubation time for optimal growth ranges from a few days to 4 weeks or longer (usually 6 to 14 days).

Biochemical characteristics. Leptospires within species are not distinguishable on the basis of biochemical characteristics.

Serological identification. Serotypes are identified by microscopic-agglutination and agglutinin-adsorption tests with serotype-specific rabbit antiserum. Serotypes with major antigenic affinities as disclosed in cross-agglutination tests are arbitrarily assembled into serogroups (not a taxonomic subdivision).

Animal pathogenicity. Pathogenic leptospires produce lethal to subclinical infections in hamsters, guinea pigs, gerbils, and weanling rabbits on intraperitoneal inoculation.

RECOGNITION OF LEPTOSPIROSIS

Etiological agents of leptospirosis comprise approximately 150 different serotypes (the basic taxon) determined on the basis of their agglutinogenic properties (30). The pathogenic serotypes are otherwise indistinguishable morphologically and by biochemical activity. Natural reservoirs of infection are rodents and a large variety of other feral and domestic animals. Many serotypes occur predominantly in select mammalian hosts. The distribution of a specific serotype in a select host is not exclusive. The same species may be a primary reservoir for several different serotypes and may also carry types occurring primarily in other mammals.

The nesting site for leptospires in natural hosts is the lumen of nephritic tubules, from whence they are shed into the urine. The persistence and intensity of leptospiruria may vary with the host and serotype infection. The Norway rat infected with serotype *icterohaemorrhagiae* sheds profuse numbers of leptospires for the remainder of its natural life. Strains of serotype *canicola* are apparently less efficient in persisting in the kidneys of rats. Shedding in infected dogs, cattle, and swine may be heavy for only a few months after infection and is usually sparse or absent after 6 months (25).

Infections are incurred by contact with urine of carriers or indirectly by contact with streams, ponds, swamps, or wet soils contaminated with urine of carriers. Pathogenic leptospires can survive for 3 months or longer in neutral or slightly alkaline waters but do not persist in brackish or acid waters. Organisms enter hosts through abrasions of the skin or through mucosal surfaces of the nasopharynx or esophagus, or the eye.

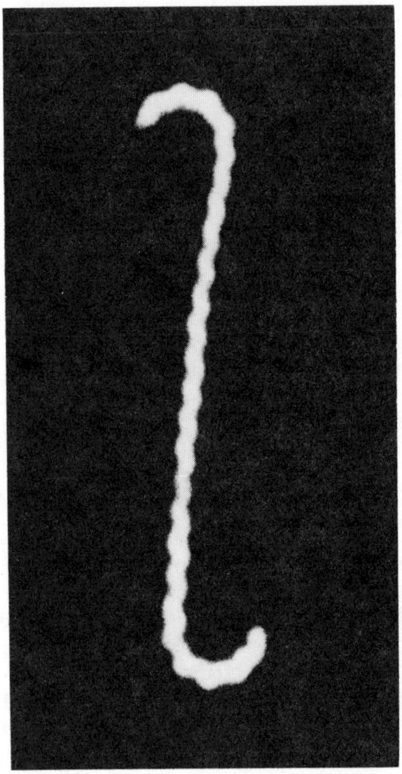

FIG. 1. *Leptospira. Dark-ground illumination. ×1,250. Courtesy of C. D. Cox, Department of Microbiology, University of Massachusetts, Amherst.*

Leptospirosis in humans is primarily associated with occupational exposure. Work with animals or in rat-infested surroundings poses infection hazards (e.g., veterinarians, dairymen, swineherds, abattoir workers, miners, fish and poultry processors). In various parts of the world, leptospirosis occurs sporadically or in epidemic proportions in agricultural workers engaged in the raising of rice, cane, flax, and vegetables, in rubber plantation workers, and in soldiers exposed to natural environments contaminated by animal carriers. The potential infection hazards of bathing or swimming in ponds or streams about which livestock are pastured have been demonstrated repeatedly (5, 14).

The clinical manifestations of leptospirosis in humans and animals are variable, ranging from mild catarrh-like illness to icteric disease with severe kidney and liver involvement. Diagnosis can only be established in the laboratory by demonstration of the organisms or by serological tests. A variety of procedures are available for laboratory diagnosis. Selection and use of appropriate tests are contingent on the understanding of the course of leptospiral infections.

The incubation period ranges from 3 to 30 days, but is usually 10 to 12 days. Leptospiremia occurs at time of disease onset and persists for approximately 1 week. During this acute phase, leptospires may also be present in cerebrospinal fluid and in milk of lactating animals. Detectable antibodies appear by the sixth to tenth day of disease, reaching maximal levels at the third or fourth week of disease. Thereafter, antibody levels gradually recede but may be detectable for years (28).

In humans and domestic animals, leptospires may be found in the urine after the first week of disease. Urinary shedding may persist for 2 to 3 months in a large proportion of cases. In some cases, intermittent shedding may occur for longer periods of time. Infection in pregnant livestock during the latter half of gestation may result in abortion several weeks later, at which time the dam may have detectable antibodies and may be a urinary shedder.

DIRECT EXAMINATION

The concentration of leptospires in blood and cerebrospinal fluid of naturally occurring cases is small, and organisms are difficult to demonstrate by direct microscopy. The chances of

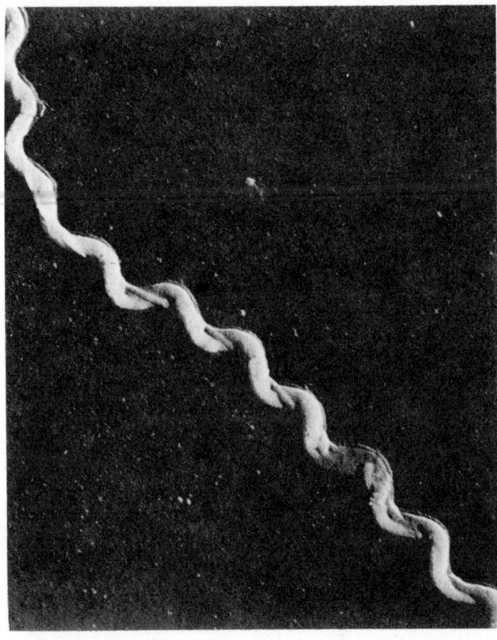

FIG. 2. *Electron micrograph of a portion of a leptospira. Courtesy of Armed Forces Institute of Pathology, Washington, D.C.*

demonstrating leptospires may be increased by centrifuging blood treated with sodium oxalate or heparin at low speed to remove cellular elements, then at high speed to concentrate, and examining the remaining elements in the plasma (28). Although the method may be valuable in establishing a rapid diagnosis, it frequently results in misdiagnosis by mistaken identification of fibrils, extrusions from cells, as spirochetes. Therefore, direct dark-field examination of blood is not recommended as a single diagnostic procedure (24).

Direct dark-field examination may be of value for examination of specimens in which there is a high concentration of leptospires, e.g., blood, peritoneal fluid, or liver suspension of hamsters or guinea pigs infected with clinical material, or urine or kidney suspensions of wildlife, and frequently of swine, dogs, and other domestic animals.

The examination of blood or other fluids and tissue suspensions is conducted on a minute drop, distributed in a thin layer between a glass slide and cover slip. It is important to disperse cellular particles; otherwise, too much light may be refracted and may interfere with detection of leptospires. The typical morphology and motility of leptospires should be evident before a presumptive diagnosis is made. *The failure to detect leptospires does not rule out their presence. Diagnosis by microscope examination should be confirmed by cultural or serological tests.*

Staining techniques for demonstration of leptospires in films of blood, urine, and tissue preparations have been described (6, 21, 22). These procedures have the same limitations as those in dark-field microscopy and are not routinely used. Use of a silver-deposition technique (22) to demonstrate organisms in tissue section may be of value when cultural and serological procedures are not possible. Fluorescent-antibody (FA) techniques have been used to demonstrate leptospires in urine and tissues from animals (9, 13, 22). The potential usefulness of FA techniques as routine diagnostic tools requires further evaluation (30).

CULTURAL EXAMINATION

During the first week of disease, the most reliable means of detecting leptospires is by direct culturing of blood on appropriate media (see chapter 95). Fletcher's semisolid and Stuart's liquid media (chapter 95) containing rabbit serum will grow most strains of leptospires (28). A few strains are more readily cultivated in media (chapter 95) containing albumin and fatty acid in lieu of serum (12, 15). Media are dispensed in approximately 5-ml amounts in 16 by 125 mm test tubes (preferably screw-capped). Prepared media can be stored for months at room temperature. It is advisable to use at least four tubes of media from two different types or lots of medium for each sample. Repeated daily blood cultures with the use of 1 to 2 drops of blood per 5 ml of medium during the first week of disease are recommended. The use of minimal inocula, particularly after the fourth day of disease, serves to minimize the effect of growth-inhibitory substances that may be present in the blood. If media are not available at the time blood is collected, the blood may be defibrinated or mixed with anticoagulants (heparin or sodium oxalate; citrate solutions may be inhibitory) and subsequently cultured. Alternatively, clotted blood may be triturated and cultured. If spinal fluid is obtained during the acute phase of disease, leptospires may also be recovered by culture.

After the first week of disease, blood cultures are rarely successful. However, at this time and for several months thereafter, the urine may contain leptospires, which may be isolated by culturing or animal inoculation. In human cases, the concentration of leptospires in the urine is low; shedding may be intermittent. Therefore, repeated isolation attempts should be made. Isolation attempts should be made as soon as possible after collection. Leptospires may not survive in acid urine for more than a few hours. Urine obtained aseptically, e.g., by perforation of the bladder—a technique used for infected dogs—may be cultured directly (13). The undiluted urine may contain growth-inhibiting substances. Therefore, both undiluted urine and a 10-fold dilution of urine are recommended for culture, with the use of 1 to 2 drops of inocula. Direct cultural isolation is also possible for midstream urine samples carefully collected from cleansed genitalia. The samples may be cultured directly in medium containing added 5-fluorouracil (5-FU) in a concentration of 200 μg/ml. The pyrimidine analogue does not inhibit the growth of leptospires but may serve to prevent the growth of contaminating microorganisms. For cultures of aseptically derived material, 5-FU media should be used in conjunction with conventional media, as growth of some leptospires may be slowed in the presence of 5-FU. Pasteur pure culture techniques—culturing of serial 10-fold dilutions of voided urine—have been used for the recovery of leptospires from domestic animals (13). The addition to rabbit serum medium of neomycin (5 to 25 mg/liter) either singly or in combination with sulfathiazole (50 mg/liter) and cycloheximide (0.5 mg/liter) has also been recommended to inhibit growth of contaminating microorganisms (10, 18). Higher concentrations (300 mg/liter) of neomycin were recommended for use in albumin-fatty acid media because of the presence of substances which inhibit the actions of the antibiotics (18).

In fatal cases, leptospires may be present in various tissues as well as in the blood. Liver and kidney are the tissues of choice for recovery of organisms. Tissues are triturated in glass grinders or by the use of sand and mortar and pestle, and are suspended in nine parts of physiological salt solution or media. The 10% suspension, and 1:10 and 1:100 dilutions thereof, are cultured as in the method for urine. The higher dilutions of tissue suspensions are cultured to limit effects of growth-inhibitory substances that may be present. Alternatively, especially under field conditions (for example, in culturing kidneys of trapped small animals), 0.5 to 1.0 g of kidney can be expressed through the barrel of a 2- or 5-ml syringe (without needle) directly into media, which can then be diluted further and subcultured. For culturing kidneys of large domestic animals, a representative sample can be obtained by scraping the cortex with sterile metal bottle caps with grated surfaces. The grated surface is prepared by punching out holes with a nail. The ground tissue is collected on the undersurface of the bottle cap. Portions of tissue punched out with a capillary pipette can also be cultured directly into media as in blood cultures. The use of 5-FU or antibiotic media in cultivation of tissues may increase the chances of isolation if specimens are contaminated with other microorganisms. If tissues cannot be processed immediately, they can be collected aseptically in sterile bottles, rapidly frozen, and stored at dry-ice temperatures. The addition of a cryoprotective agent such as glycerol (1 part to 20 parts of tissue) prior to freezing may minimize the deleterious effects of freezing on leptospires.

Cultures are incubated at 30 C or in the dark at room temperature. Most pathogenic strains are detected in culture after 6 to 14 days of incubation. In some cases, leptospires may first be seen as early as the third day or as late as 4 or 5 weeks after incubation. There are a few strains, e.g., serotype *hardjo* found in cattle, that are difficult to isolate and maintain in culture media (4). At time of optimal growth, the concentration of leptospires may be 10^8 to 4 $\times$ 10^8 organisms per ml. Cultures should be examined at 5- to 7-day intervals and discarded if negative after 6 weeks of incubation.

Growth in tubes of semisolid media occurs in the form of a linear disk located 1 to 3 cm below the surface. The absence of a disk does not necessarily rule out the absence of leptospires. Fluid media inoculated with leptospires become faintly turbid. For examination of cultures for growth, a minute drop is obtained a few centimeters below the surface of fluid cultures or from the ringed area of growth in semisolid media. The drop is placed on a slide, covered with a cover slip, and examined by dark-ground microscopy, first at low (150 times) and then at high dry magnification (450 times). Leptospires are recognized by their characteristic motility as well as morphology. In fluid media, leptospires oscillate or rotate rapidly on their longitudinal axis, moving backward and forward. The motility is characteristic because of the spinning hooked ends. In semisolid medium or in a more viscous milieu, serpentine as well as boring and flexing movements occur.

Positive cultures should be transferred to fresh medium. The inoculum should comprise 5 to 10% of the volume of subculture. Stock cultures are best maintained in semisolid medium, such as Fletcher's. After ringed growth occurs, cultures can be stored at room temperature. Transfers are usually made at 6- to 8-week intervals. Cultures maintained in fluid medium should be transferred more frequently, at 3- to 6-week intervals. For long-term preservation, cultures of leptospires can be stored by liquid nitrogen refrigeration with the use of glycerol or dimethylsulfoxide as a cryoprotective agent (3).

Contaminated cultures may be purified by passage in 5-FU medium with the use of small inocula. If cultures are heavily contaminated, it may be advisable to use three or more serial 10-fold dilutions for inoculating subcultures. Cultures may also be purified by filtration through bacteriological filters with average pore sizes ranging approximately from 0.22 to 0.45 μm. Animal inoculation methods may be used. Weanling hamsters or young guinea pigs are inoculated intraperitoneally with 0.5 to 1.0 ml of the contaminated culture. After 10 to 15 min, blood is obtained from the heart and cultured. It may be possible to purify some cultures by subculturing on solid plating medium (16, 27) containing 1% agar. Not all strains form colonies readily in plating media (16). Leptospires form subsurface colonies and may be picked for transfer with a sterile capillary pipette.

ANIMAL INOCULATION

Animal inoculation methods are particularly useful for isolation of strains from tissues or body fluids containing contaminating bacteria.

For material that can be obtained aseptically, animal inoculation techniques provide no greater chances of isolation than direct cultural methods, except for rare instances where strains are not cultivated easily but can be demonstrated in animals (4).

The choice laboratory animals for leptospirosis are weanling hamsters and young guinea pigs. Species of *Meriones* (25) and weanling rabbits (26) have also been used. Selected laboratory animals should be known to be free from natural infections. The course of disease in laboratory animals varies with different serotypes or even with different strains of the same serotype, and may be inapparent to lethal. Material is inoculated intraperitoneally preferably in at least three animals. Heart blood for culture and microscope examination is obtained whenever signs of disease are present; otherwise, samples are taken on the 4th and 6th days and then at 3- to 4-day intervals up to the 20th day after inoculation. Kidney cultures should also be done if animals are alive at the time of the last bleeding.

SEROLOGICAL EXAMINATION

Detection of antibodies

The microscopic-agglutination test is the procedure most often used. It is highly sensitive and specific, and can be used to test animal as well as human sera for diagnostic as well as epidemiological purposes. It is highly serotype-specific. To insure detection of antibodies which may be produced by any of the large number of different serotypes, it is necessary to employ a battery of different antigens encompassing most of the known cross-reactions of leptospires. The following 15 serotypes have been recommended (1) for use in microscopic-agglutination tests: *copenhageni*, *poi*, *canicola*, *castellonis*, *pyrogenes*, *grippotyphosa*, *wolffi*, *borincana*, *szwajizak*, *djatzi*, *autumnalis*, *bratislava*, *pomona*, *tarassovi*, and *patoc*. The following serotypes were recommended for supplementary tests: *shermani*, *panama*, *celledoni*, *djasiman*, *cynopteri*, and *louisiana*. Serotype *patoc*, a biflexa-type leptospire, is used because of the frequent occurrence of cross-reactions with this antigen in sera from human leptospirosis patients. The proposed list of antigens may be modified according to local experience and needs. Substitution of local isolates of the same or related type could provide a more sensitive test.

Antigens used in microscopic-agglutination tests may be live or Formalin-treated. Live antigens consist of 4- to 7-day-old cultures in fluid medium (e.g., Stuart's). Cultures for use as antigens are examined microscopically for homogeneity, purity, and density. Small clumps of cells (e.g., microcolonies), if present, may be removed by centrifugation at 1,500 to 2,000 × *g* for 15 to 30 min. The recommended density of cultures is 2×10^8 organisms per ml (30). It can be determined nephelometrically or by microscope counts in a Petroff-Hausser chamber. Density can also be estimated by microscope examination of a measured drop under a 22 by 22 mm cover slip. A count of 100 to 200 leptospires per high dry field (450 times) for a 0.01-ml drop will provide an antigen of satisfactory density. Too dense antigens can be diluted with media or physiological salt solution.

Formalin-fixed antigens are prepared by addition of reagent-grade, neutral Formalin to a final concentration of 0.3% by volume to 4- to 7-day-old cultures previously checked for purity, density, and homogeneity. The antigen is allowed to stand for 1 to 2 h; then it is centrifuged for 10 min at 1,000 to 1,500 × *g* to remove aggregated cells. Formalin-treated antigen (also live antigen) may be tested further for suitable sensitivity by titration against standard homologous antisera with the use of a twofold dilution scheme. Formalin-treated antigen is usually stable for 1 or 2 weeks if stored at 4 C. Stored antigens should be checked microscopically for appearance and homogeneity before each use.

A fourfold dilution scheme is used for test sera to provide final dilutions of 1:100 to 1:6,400 after addition of antigen. Physiological salt solution (some laboratories use phosphate-buffered, pH 7.4, isotonic solution) is used as diluent. The initial serum dilution of 1:50 is prepared by adding 0.2 ml of serum to 9.8 ml of dilution, from which sequential dilutions of 1:200, 1:800, and 1:3,200 are prepared. Each dilution is added in 0.2-ml amounts to a series of agglutination tubes or wells in plastic trays; then 0.2 ml of antigen is added to each tube or well in the serum dilution series. The tubes or trays are shaken, incubated for 2 to 3 h at 30 C, shaken again, and examined. To read the reactions, place small drops from the respective dilutions on a slide with a dropper or loop, spread to flatten, and examine microscopically (10× objective and 15× ocular) by darkground illumination. Reactions are graded on the following basis: 4+, 75% or more of cells agglutinated; 3+, 50 to 75% of cells agglutinated, many clumps present in each field; 2+, 25 to 50% of cells agglutinated, at least one specific clump in each field; 1+, occasional small clumps or small stellate aggregations.

The microscopic-agglutination test has been adapted for use with microtitration techniques with considerable savings in time and reagents (8). Dilutions are prepared in microdilution plates with flat-bottom wells with the use of 0.025- or 0.050-ml microdiluters. Antigens are added in equivalent volume with disposable microtiter pipettes. Reactions in wells may be examined directly under a microscope by use of a dry dark-field condenser and long-working-distance 10× objective.

Two types of reactions are manifested by positive sera with live antigens: agglutination and so-called "lysis." Agglutinated cell clumps are spherical in shape; occasionally, some antigens may agglutinate along their longitudinal axis, giving a "frayed-rope" appearance. When "lysis" occurs, there are few leptospires or rare freely moving leptospires, and small refractile granules are present. The refractile granules are tightly packed clumped cells.

When Formalin-treated antigens are used, "lysis" does not occur; clumps are larger and irregular in outline, and have a lacy or frayed-rope appearance. Compared with live antigens, fixed antigens are generally less sensitive and tend to cross-react more broadly with diverse serotypes, although the overall specificity is similar. Positive and negative control sera should be included in each test. Reference to reactions of controls is helpful in determining the degree of agglutination and also in distinguishing agglutinated clumps from microcolonies, when the latter are present. Prozone phenomena may occur, particularly with high-titer positive serum.

The recommended end-point reaction (30) is defined "as the highest final dilution of serum in the serum-antigen mixture in which 50% or more of the cells are agglutinated" (e.g., 3+ reaction). Titers of 1:100 or greater are considered to be specific. Since leptospiral agglutinins may persist for a considerable period of time after infection, the presence of leptospiral antibodies in a single serum may indicate past or current infection. Generally, a titer of 1:1,600 or greater in single specimens provides strong presumptive evidence of recent infection, Preferably, tests should be done on paired acute and convalescent serum samples. A fourfold or greater rise in titer is considered to be significant.

The laboriousness of microscopic-agglutination tests limits its usefulness for the small diagnostic laboratory. A variety of other serological procedures have been proposed (23). Two procedures that have been widely used in lieu of microscopic-agglutination tests are the macroscopic-agglutination (slide or plate) test (13, 19), and a "genus-specific" hemolytic (or erythrocyte-sensitizing substance) test (11).

Antigens used in slide or plate tests consist of Formalin-treated washed cells suspended to a standard concentration in a suitable buffer. Antigens are prepared from 12 or more diverse serotypes and are used singly or are pooled in groups of three. The test is conducted on a glass plate or slide by mixing a drop of serum to a drop of antigen. After being shaken for a few minutes, the mixtures are examined for agglutination. Pooled antigens are usually stable for 9 months or longer. Older preparations may give nonspecific reactions. It is important to use positive and negative control sera in the application of this test. The test is simple to perform and has good sensitivity and specificity for detecting antibodies in humans and animals with current or recent illness. It is not as sensitive as the microscopic-agglutination test for detecting antibodies in retrospect, e.g., in serological surveys (29). Paired acute and convalescent sera can be tested with pooled antigens or with individual antigens to demonstrate titer conversions. The titers, however, are not as high as those elicited in microscopic-agglutination tests. Macroscopic-agglutination antigens are now available commercially in the United States.

The hemolytic test is conducted with one antigen consisting of a 50% ethyl alcohol-insoluble, 95% ethyl alcohol-soluble extract from leptospiral cells. *L. biflexa* strains (e.g., serotype *codice*, strain CDC) are commonly used as a source of antigen. It can be stored for years in the freeze-dried state without loss of activity. The antigen is very light. Human albumin in a concentration of 2% is added to stock solutions as a binder prior to freeze-drying. A predetermined optimal dilution of antigen is used to sensitize sheep red blood cells. The sensitized cells are washed and resuspended to a concentration of 1%, and then are added together with guinea pig complement to serial dilutions of sera. A positive reaction is manifested by lysis of sensitized erythrocytes. The test can be done by microtiter techniques. It can detect antibodies in human sera irrespective of the infecting serotypes. It may lack sensitivity for detecting antibodies in animal sera, and its use for this purpose is not recommended. Its potential usefulness as a serological survey tool requires further study. The hemolytic test is particularly useful for diagnosis of cases in endemic areas of multiple leptospirosis and for testing large numbers of samples. The test is relatively laborious for testing few samples. The test has been simplified by the use of sensitized sheep erythrocytes preserved with glutaraldehyde in an indirect hemagglutination procedure (7). The fixed antigen reportedly remained stable in appearance and reactivity at 4 C for over 2 years.

A complement-fixation test in which a fixed *L. biflexa* antigen is used has been advantageously used for the diagnosis of human cases, but it lacks sensitivity when used with animal sera (20).

Culture typing

Microscopic-agglutination techniques are used for culture typing. An isolate employed as antigen is first screened with a select group of 12 or more serotype antisera to determine its serogroup relationship. Isolates are then tested with different serotypes of one or more selected serogroups to determine further antigenic relationships. On the basis of observed cross-reactions, representative strains of serotypes are chosen for reciprocal agglutinin-adsorption tests. "Two strains are considered to belong to different serotypes if, after cross-absorption with adequate amounts of heterologous antigen, 10% or more of the homologous titer regularly remains in at least one of the two antisera in repeated tests" (30). Procedures for conduct of definitive culture typing have been described in detail (2, 28). Antigenic factor analysis has been used for classification of strains (17), but single-factor sera for such tests are not generally available.

Definitive typing of strains is usually done in leptospirosis reference laboratories. In the United States, such tests are done at the WHO/FAO Leptospirosis Reference Laboratory, Walter Reed Army Institute of Research, Washington, D.C., and at the Leptospirosis Reference Laboratory, Center for Disease Control, Atlanta, Ga. Presumptive serogroup or serotype identification can usually be made in diagnostic laboratories by cross-agglutination tests with antisera of strains used for serological diagnosis. Antisera are prepared in rabbits by injecting successive doses of 0.5, 1.0, 2.0, and 4.0 ml of live cultures into the marginal ear vein at 5- to 7-day intervals. Five- to seven-day-old cultures in Fletcher's medium are commonly used as a source of inoculum. Seven days after the last injection, a blood sample is obtained and the serum therefrom is tested with homologous antigen. If the titer is 1:6,400 or greater, blood is removed by cardiopuncture. The separated serum is distributed into vials and stored at −20 to −30 C. Alternatively, it can be stored in the freeze-dried state or can be preserved by the addition of an equal volume of glycerol or by the addition of Merthiolate (concentration 1:10,000).

DISCUSSION

Unequivocal laboratory diagnosis of current cases of leptospirosis can be established by isolation of the organism from the blood or cerebrospinal fluid, or by the demonstration of significant rises in antibody titer in two or more properly timed serum samples.

Direct cultural procedures are relatively simple and within the capabilities of the ordinary diagnostic laboratory. Repeated blood culture attempts during the final week of disease usually are successful. The use of replicate culture tubes is particularly important. Isolation of leptospires from only one of four or more tubes inoculated is not unusual. Recognition of isolated organisms as leptospires is based on their morphology, motility, and cultural characteristics. The cultural isolation of strains also allows their identification by culture typing tests, which may have epidemiological or forensic importance, as in occupational diseases.

The definitive identification of isolates can be established only by recovery and subsequent typing tests. The microscopic-agglutination test, which is highly serogroup- and serotype-specific, may provide clues to the identity of the infecting serotype. However, determination of serotypes on the basis of patient's serological response has the following limitations: the agglutinins may be cross-reacting antibodies initiated by a type not included among the test antigens; higher titers may occur against serologically heterologous but antigenically related strains as well as against unrelated serologically heterologous strains ("paradoxical reactions"); complex serological responses may occur in repeated or simultaneous infections.

From the clinician's viewpoint, the management and treatment of leptospirosis does not depend on the infecting serotype; thus, a laboratory diagnosis of leptospirosis per se serves as confirmation of clinical diagnosis. In this respect, the macroscopic-agglutination test with pooled antigens and the hemolytic test may suffice. Unfortunately, the current serological tests and isolation procedures rarely provide a rapid laboratory confirmation of infection before the first week of disease. The current methods for identification of leptospires in blood and other body fluids by microscope examination have pitfalls that obviate their usefulness as laboratory confirmatory tests.

LITERATURE CITED

1. Abdussalam, M., A. D. Alexander, B. Babudieri, K. Bogel, C. Borg-Petersen, S. Faine, E. Kmety, C. Lataste-Dorolle, and L. H. Turner. 1972. Research needs in leptospirosis. Bull. W.H.O. **47:**113–122.
2. Alexander, A. D., L. B. Evans, A. J. Toussiant, R. Marchwicki, and F. R. McCrumb. 1957. Leptospirosis in Malaya. II. Antigenic analysis of 110 leptospiral isolates and other serologic studies. Amer. J. Trop. Med. Hyg. **6:**871–889.
3. Alexander, A. D., E. F. Lessel, L. B. Evans, E. Franck, and S. S. Green. 1972. Preservation of leptospiras by liquid-nitrogen refrigeration. Int. J. Syst. Bacteriol. **22:**165–169.
4. Alexander, A. D., H. G. Stoenner, G. E. Wood, and R. J. Byrne. 1962. A new pathogenic *Leptospira*, not readily cultivated. J. Bacteriol. **83:**754–760.
5. Alston, J. M., and J. C. Broom. 1958. Leptospirosis in man and animals. E. and S. Livingstone, Edinburgh.
6. Babudieri, B. 1961. Laboratory diagnosis of leptospirosis. Bull. W.H.O. **24:**45–58.
7. Baker, L. A., and C. D. Cox. 1973. Quantitative assay for genus-specific leptospiral antigen and antibody. Appl. Microbiol. **25:**697–698.
8. Cole, J. R., Jr., C. R. Sulzer, and A. R. Pursell. 1973. Improved microtechnique for the leptospiral microscopic agglutination test. Appl. Microbiol. **25:**976–980.
9. Cook, J. E., E. H. Coles, F. M. Garner, and L. G. Luna. 1971. Using scrapings from formalin-fixed tissues to diagnose leptospirosis by fluorescent-antibody technics. Stain Technol. **46:**271–274.
10. Cousineau, J. G., and J. A. McKiel. 1961. In vitro sensitivity of Leptospira to various antimicrobial agents. Can. J. Microbiol. **7:**751–758.
11. Cox, C. D. 1957. Standardization and stabilization of an extract from *Leptospira biflexa* and its use in the hemolytic test for leptospirosis. J. Infect. Dis. **101:**203–209.
12. Ellinghausen, H. C., Jr., and W. B. McCullough. 1965. Nutrition of *Leptospira pomona* and growth of 13 other serotypes: fractionation of oleic albumin complex and a medium of bovine albumin and polysorbate 80. Amer. J. Vet. Res. **26:**45–51.
13. Galton, M. M., R. W. Menges, E. B. Shotts, Jr., A. J. Nahmias, and E. W. Heath, Jr. 1962. Leptospirosis. Epidemiology, clinical manifestation in man and animals and methods in laboratory diagnosis. Communicable Disease Center, Atlanta, Ga.
14. Heath, C. W., Jr., A. D. Alexander, and M. M. Galton. 1965. Leptospirosis in the United States. Analysis of 403 cases in man 1949–1961. N. Engl. J. Med. **273:**857–864, 915–922.
15. Johnson, R. C., and V. G. Harris. 1967. Differentiation of pathogenic and saprophytic leptospires. I. Growth at low temperatures. J. Bacteriol. **94:**27–31.
16. Kirschner, L., and L. Graham. 1959. Growth, purification and maintenance of leptospira on solid media. Brit. J. Exp. Pathol. **40:**57–60.
17. Kmety, E. 1967. Factorenanalyse von Leptospiren der Icterohaemorrhagiae und Einiger Verwandter Serogruppen. Edition of Scientific Committees for General and Special Biology of the Slovak Academy of Science, vol. 13, no. 3. Bratislava.
18. Myers, D. M., and V. M. Varela-Díaz. 1973. Selective isolation of leptospiras from contaminated material by incorporation of neomycin to culture media. Appl. Microbiol. **25:**781–786.
19. Stoenner, H. G., and E. Davis. 1967. Further observations on leptospiral plate antigens. Amer. J. Vet. Res. **28:**259–266.
20. Sturdza, N., M. Elian, and G. Tulpan. 1960. Diagnosis of human leptospirosis by the complement-fixation test with a single antigen. Arch. Roum. Pathol. Exp. **19:**572–582.
21. Sturdza, N., and D. Safiresco. 1964. Sur la colorabilité des leptospires et des triponèmes. Arch. Roum. Pathol. Exp. Microbiol. **23:**927–938.
22. Thompson, S. W. 1966. Selected histochemical and histopathological methods. Charles C Thomas, Publisher, Springfield, Ill.
23. Turner, L. H. 1968. Leptospirosis. II. Serology. Trans. Roy. Soc. Trop. Med. Hyg. **62:**880–899.
24. Turner, L. H. 1970. Leptospirosis. III. Maintenance, isolation, and demonstration of leptospires. Trans. Roy. Soc. Trop. Med. Hyg. **64:**623–646.
25. Van der Hoeden, J. 1954. The pathogenicity of leptospiras to field rodents in Israel (a new test animal for use in Leptospira research). J. Infect. Dis. **95:**213–219.
26. Varfolomeeva, A. A. 1958. Young rabbits as a laboratory model for leptospirosis, p. 18–21. *In* Leptospirae and leptospirosis in man and animals. Problem Session Series of Polish Academy of Sciences XIX, Warsaw.
27. Wannon, J. S. 1958. Isolation of leptospiras from contaminated cultures by plating. Aust. J. Sci. **20:**239.
28. Wolff, J. W. 1954. The laboratory diagnosis of leptospirosis. Charles C Thomas, Publisher, Springfield, Ill.
29. Wolff, J. W., and H. J. Bohlander. 1966. Evaluation of Galton's macroscopic slide test for the serodiagnosis of leptospirosis in human serum samples. Ann. Soc. Belg. Med. Trop. **46:**123–132.
30. World Health Organization. 1967. Current problems in leptospirosis. Report of a World Health Organization Expert Group. World Health Organ. Tech. Rep. Ser. No. 380.

Chapter 35

Borrelia

RICHARD T. KELLY

CHARACTERIZATION

Members of the *Treponemataceae*.

Filamentous, spiral-shaped organisms, 0.2 to 0.5 by 10 to 20 μm. Spirals are much broader and more flexible than treponemes or leptospires; they can be observed with light microscopy if stained with aniline dyes. In infected blood they are highly motile with corkscrew movements, which may suddenly be reversed.

Growth. Tick-borne *Borrelia* species indigenous to the USA, *B. hermsi*, *B. parkeri*, and *B. turicatae*, can be grown in Kelly's (8) medium A (see chapter 95). They are microaerophilic, ferment glucose, and exhibit helical rotation and twisting motion. *B. recurrentis*, the louse-borne agent of relapsing fever, has not been grown and subcultured in vitro.

Serological identification. Serological classification of tick-borne borrelia has not been successful because of marked antigenic instability of the organism.

CLINICAL SIGNIFICANCE

Borreliae are the causative agents of an acute, febrile illness in man, relapsing fever, which is transmitted by an infected arthropod. Relapsing fever is a severe febrile septicemic illness with a rapid onset after an incubation period of 2 to 15 days. The fever persists from 3 to 7 days and is followed by an afebrile interval of several days to several weeks after which a relapse occurs as a result of antigenic variation. The number of relapses in untreated cases is variable, ranging from none to an average of three to five. Detailed clinical descriptions of the disease are given by Bryceson et al. (1).

Relapsing fever borreliae are subdivided into louse- and tick-borne varieties. *B. recurrentis*, the sole etiological agent of louse-borne relapsing fever, is transmitted from person to person by the human body louse, *Pediculus humanus*. Infection is acquired by crushing infected lice during scratching. Borreliae released from the lice enter the body at the site of the louse bite or through skin abraded by scratching. Lice become infected by feeding on humans with *B. recurrentis* infection and remain infectious for life although, in contrast to tick-borne relapsing fever, the organisms are not transmitted congenitally. *B. recurrentis* infection, once worldwide in distribution, is at present confined primarily to Eastern Africa.

There are many species of tick-borne relapsing fever organisms, each of which is named after the species of *Ornithodoros* tick transmitting the infection. They are endemic in nature with a wide variety of rodents serving as the natural reservoir of infection. Borreliae are transmitted transovarianly in ticks with the result that a large percentage of the offspring are also infective. Human infection occurs when an infected tick feeds on man. Tick-borne relapsing fever organisms are found in many areas of the world. The principal species found in the United States are *B. hermsi*, *B. parkeri*, and *B. turicatae*.

COLLECTION OF SPECIMENS

Venous blood is drawn with a syringe containing 3.8% sodium citrate (1 volume of citrate to 9 volumes of blood) and mixed with the anticoagulant. Culture medium is then inoculated or the blood is used for animal inoculation. Specimens may be safely stored at 4 C for up to 48 h in completely filled screw-cap tubes. When it is necessary to ship the specimen to another laboratory for identification, the blood specimen is centrifuged at 1,000 × *g* for 10 min. The supernatant plasma containing the organisms is removed, and glycerol is added to a final concentration of 10%. The specimen is then placed in dry ice and shipped. Borreliae may be maintained in the laboratory for several years by adding glycerol as described above to either plasma or culture media and storing at −70 C or in liquid nitrogen.

DIRECT EXAMINATION

In severely ill patients, borreliae usually are found without difficulty either in stained blood smears or in wet mounts examined by dark-field microscopy. Borreliae are readily stained by a large number of aniline dyes. Common laboratory stains such as Wright or Giemsa are usually employed, and prolonged staining is helpful (Fig. 1). Felsenfeld's method of counterstaining blood films with 1% crystal violet for 30 s after initially staining with Giemsa or Wright strain is recommended (2).

For dark-field examination, a small drop of blood is placed on a slide, a cover slip is placed over the blood, and the edges of the cover slip are sealed with either lanolin or liquid paraffin. The slide is examined at a magnification of about 400× (high dry). The presence of the organisms is frequently first detected by observing movement of erythrocytes which are disturbed as the organisms move about. When these areas are focused upon, the characteristic large spirochetes are readily seen. A microhematocrit concentration technique has recently been described for detecting the presence of borreliae in blood from lightly infected patients (6).

CULTURE

Tubes of borreliae culture medium are inoculated with 0.1 ml of citrated blood and incubated at 35 C. At 2-day intervals, a drop of medium is removed and examined by dark-field microscopy for the presence of borreliae. Organisms are usually seen within 2 to 6 days, but cultures are held for 14 days before being discarded as negative. The density of growth in positive cultures reaches 10^7 organisms/ml before growth is limited by acid production. Borreliae should be subcultured to new media when the phenol red indicator begins to change to orange-yellow.

ANIMAL INOCULATION

In lightly infected patients or during afebrile intervals, the number of organisms in the blood may be insufficient to be detected by microscopic methods. If culture medium is not available, animal inoculation may be helpful in establishing a diagnosis of relapsing fever. The susceptibility of various animal species to infection with the different species of borreliae is variable. For tick-borne *Borrelia* species found in the United States, the animals of choice are mice. Young mice (10 to 12 g) are inoculated via the intraperitoneal route with 1 ml of blood. At daily intervals, the end of the tail is snipped and blood is examined by dark-field microscopy or in stained smears. Spirochetes are usually demonstrable within 2 or 3 days, but on occasion may not be seen for up to 7 days. Mice tolerate infection well, and it is not uncommon to find the blood of an apparently normal animal teeming with borreliae.

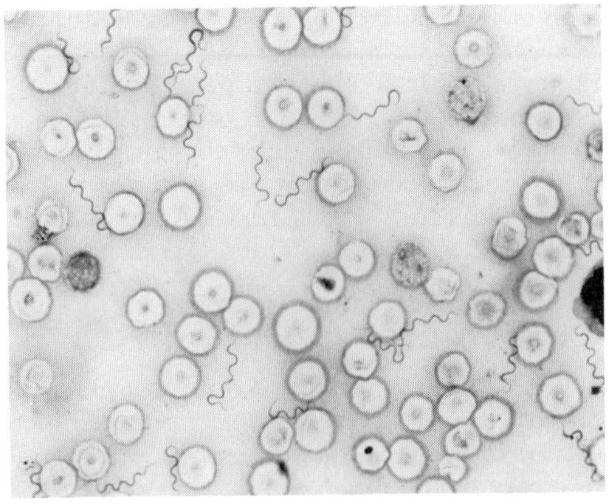

FIG. 1. *Borrelia hermsi in blood. ×1,000. Wright stain with 1% crystal violet counterstain, 30 s.*

The strain of *B. recurrentis* currently seen in Eastern Africa does not infect mice or other small animals, but infection can be established in monkeys.

IDENTIFICATION

At present, *Borrelia* isolates cannot be speciated by either biochemical reactions or serological methods. The laboratory can only report the presence of borreliae as demonstrated in blood, cultures, or inoculated animals.

Few biochemical studies of the characteristics of borreliae have been reported. Because of the previous inability to culture any of the organisms, most studies have been done with organisms isolated from infected blood. Fulton and Smith demonstrated the presence of the glycolytic pathway in *B. duttoni* (4), and in a subsequent study Smith characterized several enzymes in the pathway (9). Felsenfeld et al. (3) showed that extracts of *B. turicatae* contain cholesterol, lecithin, and several other uncharacterized lipids. Ginger demonstrated the presence of muramic acid in material prepared from *B. duttoni*, thus supporting the classification of borreliae as bacteria rather than protozoa (5). In a study of lipid metabolism in three species of tick-borne relapsing fever borreliae grown in vitro, Pickett and Kelly (in press) found that the organisms required fatty acids for growth. These are obtained by hydrolysis of lysolecithin by lysolecithinase (phospholipase B). Lipase or lecithinase activity was not detected. *B. hermsi*, *B. parkeri*, and *B. turicatae* have been grown in vitro with a variety of different carbohydrates to determine whether differences in fermentation patterns could be detected. Differentiation of species was not possible since all three species fermented the same carbohydrates and had similar biochemical reactions (7).

SEROLOGICAL IDENTIFICATION

Serological classification of tick-borne *Borrelia* species has not been successful because of the marked antigenic instability of the organisms. The present classification based on the species of tick harboring the organisms thus may be quite artificial. Additional studies are needed to determine whether organisms isolated from various species of *Ornithodoros* ticks or from patients bitten by the ticks are sufficiently different to justify individual speciation.

IMMUNOSEROLOGICAL DIAGNOSIS

Although a number of tests have been reported for the serodiagnosis of *Borrelia* infection, they are of questionable value and reagents are not commercially available. Transiently positive tests for reagin are seen in a small percentage of patients. In some cases of relapsing fever, rising agglutination titers to *Proteus* OX-K or OX-19 have been observed during the course of the disease.

ANTIMICROBIAL SUSCEPTIBILITY

Borreliae are susceptible to a number of antibiotics. The drug of choice for treatment is tetracycline. After administration of the drug, a severe Jarisch-Herxheimer reaction may take place (1).

EVALUATION

The demonstration of spirochetes in the blood by staining techniques is sufficient to establish a firm diagnosis of relapsing fever. Spirochetes associated with other disease processes may on occasion be present in blood, but they cannot be made visible by conventional stains.

LITERATURE CITED

1. Bryceson, A. D. E., E. H. O. Parry, P. L. Perine, D. A. Warrell, D. Vukotich, and C. S. Leithead. 1970. Louse-borne relapsing fever. Quart. J. Med. **39**:129–170.
2. Felsenfeld, O. 1971. Borrelia, p. 121. W. H. Green, Inc., St. Louis.
3. Felsenfeld, O., W. J. Decker, J. A. Wohlhieter, and A. Rafyi. 1965. Studies on borreliae. II. Some immunologic, biochemical, and physical properties of antigenic components of *Borrelia turicatae*. J. Immunol. **94**:805–817.
4. Fulton, J. D., and P. J. C. Smith. 1960. Carbohydrate metabolism in *Spirochaeta recurrentis*. 1. The metabolism of spirochaetes *in vivo* and *in vitro*. Biochem. J. **76**:491–499.
5. Ginger, C. D. 1963. Isolation and characterization of muramic acid from two spirochaetes: *Borrelia duttoni* and *Leptospira biflexa*. Nature (London) **199**:159.
6. Goldsmid, J. M., and K. Mahomed. 1972. The use of the microhematocrit technic for the recovery of *Borrelia duttonii* from the blood. Amer. J. Clin. Pathol. **58**:165–169.
7. Holdeman, L. V., and W. E. C. Moore (ed.). 1972. Anaerobe laboratory manual, p. 96–97. Virginia Polytechnic Institute Anaerobe Laboratory, Blacksburg.
8. Kelly, R. 1971. Cultivation of *Borrelia hermsi*. Science **172**:443–444.
9. Smith, P. J. C. 1960. Carbohydrate metabolism in *Spirochaeta recurrentis*. 2. Enzymes associated with disintegrated cells and extracts of spirochaetes. Biochem. J. **76**:500–508.

Chapter 36

Treponema

RICHARD T. KELLY

CHARACTERIZATION

Members of the *Treponemataceae*.

Pathogenic treponemes are thin, filamentous, 6 to 10 μm in length, and less than 0.2 μm in width; they are not stained with ordinary staining techniques. They contain 6 to 14 spirals (Fig. 1) and are actively motile, rotating about their long axis. Electron microscope studies have demonstrated that treponemal cells are composed of an external envelope, fibrils, cytoplasmic membrane, and cytoplasm. The fibrils are wound in helical coils around the cytoplasmic membrane and run the length of the cell.

Growth. Only saprophytic, nonpathogenic treponemes are cultivatable. They are anaerobic, ferment glucose or amino acids, and require serum bovine albumin or volatile fatty acids for growth.

Pathogenic treponemes cannot be grown in vitro but will survive for several days under anaerobic conditions in media containing bovine serum ultrafiltrate, pyruvate, albumin, and a sulfhydryl compound. In vitro survival of organisms in suspension prepared from infected rabbits, incubated with serum and complement, is the basis of the *Treponema pallidum* inhibition test for the serodiagnosis of syphilis (4).

CLINICAL SIGNIFICANCE

Three species of treponemes pathogenic for humans are recognized. Infection with *T. pallidum*, the etiological agent of syphilis, is usually acquired through venereal contact. The disease is classically divided into three stages: primary, secondary, and tertiary syphilis. In primary and secondary syphilis, the organisms may be demonstrated in specimens from patients, whereas in tertiary syphilis organisms are rarely seen except at autopsy. The primary lesion of syphilis, or chancre, appears on an average of 3 weeks after exposure. Usually, only a single, firm, nontender, ulcerated lesion is present. Organisms can be observed in exudate from the lesion by dark-field microscopy. In primary syphilis, serological tests for syphilis are positive in only 25% of patients at the time of the initial appearance of the chancre. Secondary syphilis develops on an average of 6 to 8 weeks after the primary lesion, which has usually healed in the interim. Although clinically variable, secondary syphilis usually presents as a rash involving both skin and mucous membranes. The lesions are highly infectious, and treponemes can be seen in wet mounts prepared from abraded skin, especially from the moist lesions. Serological tests are positive. The clinical manifestations of tertiary or late syphilis, which are quite diverse, develop in about one-third of nontreated patients. Individuals with tertiary syphilis are not infectious for others, and organisms usually cannot be demonstrated. A diagnosis of tertiary syphilis is made when various clinical findings are seen in association with positive, specific serological tests for syphilis in serum or cerebrospinal fluid.

T. pertenue and *T. carateum*, the etiological agents, respectively, of yaws and pinta, are morphologically and serologically indistinguishable from *T. pallidum*. Yaws is a disease of skin and bone which is acquired primarily by children through direct, nonvenereal contact. At present, the disease is chiefly limited to areas in South America, Africa, and India. Pinta, a chronic cutaneous treponematosis of children, is endemic to regions of South and Central America. Lesions are confined to skin and may appear red or blue in color initially; they later become depigmented. Infection is acquired by contact with infected persons or possibly by the bite of insects acting as vectors.

COLLECTION AND DIRECT EXAMINATION OF SPECIMENS

Treponemes are extremely delicate organisms and are quite sensitive to drying, changes in osmotic pressure, oxygen, and temperature. Under adverse conditions, morphological alterations may occur and globular or ball-shaped organisms are seen. Because of the lability of the organisms, specimens taken for diagnostic purposes should be examined without delay.

A diagnosis of syphilis can be established by the demonstration of characteristic organisms

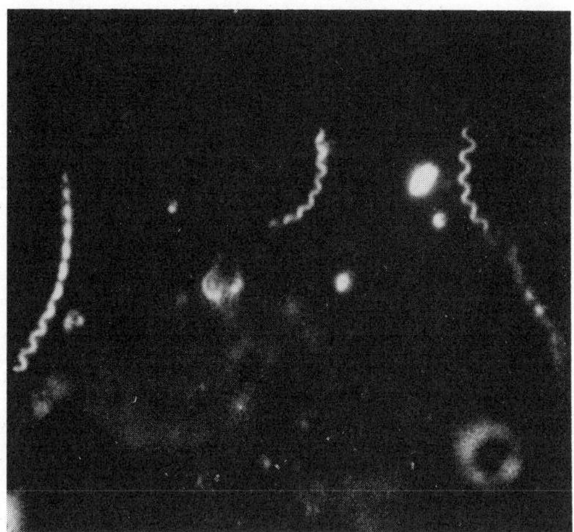

FIG. 1. *Morphology of Treponema pallidum as demonstrated by immunofluorescence. ×1,200. (Courtesy of U. S. G. Kuhn III and P. Cox.)*

in properly obtained specimens from suspect lesions. It is essential that great care be taken in preparing the site to be examined so that saprophytic spirochetes morphologically similar to *T. pallidum*, which may be present on the surface of the lesion, are eliminated. The examiner, wearing rubber gloves, removes any surface crusts or scabs from the lesion, which is then repeatedly cleansed with saline-soaked gauze sponges followed by drying. The surface of the lesion is abraded with a dry sponge until bleeding occurs; blood is removed by gentle sponging until a serum exudate is seen. Application of pressure to the base of the lesion is frequently helpful in obtaining sufficient material for sampling. A clean cover slip (no. 1, 22 by 22 mm) is touched to the surface of the lesion to pick up the exudate and is then inverted onto a microscope slide, care being taken to eliminate air bubbles. For relatively inaccessible lesions of the cervix, vagina, etc., cleansing is done with saline-soaked swabs and exudate is transferred with a sterile bacteriological loop to a slide, over which a cover slip is then placed. If lesions are dry and difficulty is encountered in obtaining exudate even with application of pressure, a drop of sterile physiological saline is applied to the surface of the lesion. Pressure is applied to the base of the lesion and material is then transferred to a cover slip.

Preparations for dark-field microscopy should be sealed. In my laboratory, anhydrous lanolin is liquefied by heating and poured into the barrels of 2.5-ml plastic Luer-lok syringes fitted with 18-gauge needles. The plungers are partially inserted, the syringes are inverted, and air is removed. When cooled to room temperature, lanolin may be expressed from the syringe in a thin ribbon around the edges of the cover slip. This method avoids inadvertently heating the specimen, as may occur when melted paraffin is used. A number of syringes may be prepared and will last several years.

Specimens are examined with a microscope equipped with a dark-field condenser. A drop of oil is applied to the top of the condenser, which is then raised to contact the lower surface of the slide. After initial focusing with the low-power objective and adjustment of the condenser for maximal contrast, the specimen is examined with the high dry objective and then with the oil immersion lens for the presence of spirochetes. Usually, preparations will contain erythrocytes which serve as a reference for estimating the length of observed organisms. *T. pallidum* has an average length one and one-half times the diameter of red cells. Spirals of *T. pallidum* are tightly wound, in contrast to some saprophytic spirochetes. Typical movement is rotation around the axis with a slight forward or backward motion. Marked directional motility or sharp extension or flexion is not seen with *T. pallidum*, but is frequently observed with saprophytic organisms. Observation of many bacteria other than spirochetes in the specimen may be an indication that the site sampled was not properly cleansed before the specimen was taken.

Considerable care must be taken in interpreting specimens taken from the oral cavity, as *T. microdentium*, a saprophyte resembling *T. pallidum*, may be present as part of the normal flora. In problem cases, it may be necessary to resort to regional lymph node aspiration, which should be done by a physician. The presence of typical spirochetes in aspirates is diagnostic of syphilis.

STAINING

In biopsy material or tissue removed at autopsy, spirochetes can be demonstrated in histological sections stained by silver impregnation methods, which add to the width of treponemes and thereby permit observation by conventional microscopy. A modification of the Warthin technique is recommended (2). Regardless of the method employed, it is essential that a known positive control section be stained simultaneously, as the staining methods are somewhat capricious.

T. pallidum can also be demonstrated in smears or frozen sections by immunofluorescence using specific fluorescein-conjugated antisera. In a recent study of the specificity of this procedure, it was found that nonpathogenic treponemes stained equally as well as *T. pallidum* (5). Because of the lack of commercial sources of reagents and the nonspecificity of the staining reactions, this method is not recommended for routine diagnostic purposes.

ANIMAL INOCULATION

T. pallidum and *T. pertenue* infection can be established in mature, male rabbits by intratesticular inoculation of clinical specimens (6). Because of the complexity of the technique and long incubation period, this procedure is rarely used for diagnostic purposes. For use in serological testing or for research purposes, both species may be maintained in the laboratory with retention of virulence by serial intratesticular passage in rabbits. Animals should be housed at a temperature of 20 C and fed antibiotic-free rations. Suspensions of organisms prepared from infected rabbits may be maintained for years with retention of infectivity by adding glycerol to a final concentration of 10 to 15% and storing at −70 C or in liquid nitrogen. Suspensions should be rapidly thawed and immediately inoculated into additional rabbits for recovery of strains.

SEROLOGICAL METHODS

Serological tests for syphilis are covered in chapter 51.

ANTIMICROBIAL SUSCEPTIBILITY

The drug of choice for all treponemal infections is penicillin. Alternate drugs for individuals with penicillin allergy include erythromycin and the tetracyclines (7). With initiation of therapy, a mild Jarisch-Herxheimer reaction may occur; however, this is usually of little significance.

DISCUSSION

Between 1957 and 1972, the reported case rates for primary and secondary syphilis per 100,000 population in the United States more than tripled. The Public Health Service estimates the number of new cases of syphilis during 1972 as 85,000 (1). Thus, despite the availability of effective chemotherapeutic agents, syphilis is not being eradicated, as had been optimistically forecast, but rather is increasing. Experimental data both in humans and in animals indicate that active immunization to *T. pallidum* infection is feasible and may offer a means of controlling syphilis (3). The inability to cultivate the organisms, however, at present rules out vaccine development.

LITERATURE CITED

1. American Social Health Association. 1973. Today's VD control problem, p. 10–11. American Social Health Association, New York.
2. Lillie, R. D. 1965. Histopathologic technic and practical histochemistry, p. 599–602. McGraw-Hill Book Co., Inc., New York.
3. Miller, J. N. 1973. Immunity in experimental syphilis. VI. Successful vaccination of rabbits with *Treponema pallidum*, Nichol's strain, attenuated by γ-irradiation. J. Immunol. **110**:1206–1215.
4. Nelson, R. A., Jr., and M. M. Mayer. 1949. Immobilization of *Treponema pallidum in vitro* by antibody produced in syphilitic infection. J. Exp. Med. **89**:369–396.
5. Ryan, S. F., E. E. Nell, and P. H. Hardy. 1972. A study of the aqueous humor for the presence of spirochetes. Amer. J. Ophthalmol. **73**:250–257.
6. Turner, T. B., P. H. Hardy, and B. Newman. 1969. Infectivity tests in syphilis. Brit. J. Vener. Dis. **45**:183–196.
7. U.S. Public Health Service. 1968. Syphilis: a synopsis. U.S. Public Health Service Publication No. 1660, p. 109–116.

Section IV

ANAEROBIC BACTERIA

Chapter 37
Introduction to Anaerobic Bacteria

LOUIS DS. SMITH

Many clinical microbiologists were long reluctant to make anaerobic procedures part of their laboratory routine because they considered the anaerobes a strange and somewhat exotic group of organisms, difficult to isolate, almost impossible to identify, and productive only of tetanus, gas gangrene, spores, and bad smells. In the past few years, however, the importance of these organisms, especially the nonsporeformers, in human medicine has been generally accepted, and the microbiology laboratories of many hospitals now endeavor to isolate and identify the anaerobes as routinely as they do the facultative and obligately aerobic organisms that they encounter. This development has been stimulated by the clinicians who, as they became acquainted with the infections caused by the anaerobic bacteria, increasingly requested anaerobic culture of specimens from their patients and the identification and determination of antibiotic susceptibility of the organisms that were isolated.

This increased interest in the anaerobic bacteria has resulted in the development of better and more convenient methods for their isolation and identification, and three clinical laboratory manuals have become available describing such methods (1–3). The development of the GasPak jar, the plastic anaerobic chamber, and the roll tube equipment gives the clinical microbiologist a choice of procedures for isolation, and the commercially available anaerobic media spare him the task of preparing special media.

The basic procedures used for the anaerobes differ but little from those which are used for the facultative and aerobic organisms. The media tend to be richer, to contain a higher proportion of peptone and carbohydrate, because anaerobic metabolism is much less efficient than aerobic metabolism in obtaining energy from substrate. Also, longer incubation is required, 2 days generally being used for isolation. If *Actinomyces* strains are expected, 3 days is considered a minimum and 5 days is better.

Although we speak of the anaerobes as though they all had similar requirements for anaerobiosis, this is not the case. Indeed, they form a continuous spectrum, from organisms that are able to grow, though just barely, on the surface of solid media exposed to the air, to organisms that are unable to grow if the atmosphere contains as little as 0.03% oxygen, or if the medium contains even traces of certain oxidized medium constituents. There are two terms that are sometimes applied to the anaerobes that are barely able to grow on the surface of media exposed to the air, but both have been used in such a variety of ways that their meaning is no longer clear, except for the context in which they are used. These are "microaerophile" and "aerotolerant." Microaerophile originally referred to an organism that was an obligate aerobe but which could grow on solid media only if the concentration of oxygen in the atmosphere was appreciably below that normally found. *Brucella abortus* is an example. However, many microbiologists now apply this term to bacteria that are basically anaerobic but (i) also grow well on solid media in an aerobic atmosphere containing 10% CO_2 or (ii) are just able to grow on agar in an aerobic incubator as is the case with *Clostridium histolyticum*. The term aerotolerant was coined to refer to the last-named group of organisms. Unfortunately, this term is also used to refer to anaerobes that, once grown, can be exposed to the air for several hours or longer without being killed.

All of the pathogenic anaerobic bacteria are part of the normal microflora of the body and require special conditions before their pathogenicity can be manifest. The significance of their isolation from a specimen is not a simple matter, for they may be present as important causative agents, as secondary invaders in tissue that has been rendered nonviable by trauma or by other microbes, or simply as contaminants from nearby microflora. That these organisms are part of the normal microflora is no indication that their virulence, once an infection has started, is low. Indeed, the prognosis for a patient with a blood culture positive for *Bacteroides fragilis* is much worse than for a patient with a blood culture positive for *Salmonella typhosa*.

Our knowledge concerning the pathogenicity of the anaerobes for humans is still incomplete. The pathogenic species of the clostridia are well recognized, but we are still in the process of determining the potential pathogenicity of many of the nonsporeforming anaerobes. The great majority of the hundred or so species in the normal human flora are probably without pathogenicity for humans. Others are potential pathogens, even though they may be present during the whole life of most hosts without ever causing overt infection. Among the nonsporeformers that do have pathogenic potentiality are *Actinomyces israelii*, *A. bovis*, *A. naeslundii*, *Bacteroides fragilis* (especially subspecies *fragilis*), *B. melaninogenicus*, *Peptococcus magnus*, *Peptostreptococcus anaerobius*, and *Sphaerophorus* (*Fusobacterium*) *necrophorus*. Also potential pathogens, although probably to a lesser extent, are *Peptococcus prevotii*, *Propionibacterium acnes*, *Eubacterium limosum*, *E. lentum*, *Fusobacterium fusiforme*, and *F. nucleatum*. All, of course, are pathogens of opportunity, and only when they obtain access to tissue with impaired blood supply, or that has been rendered necrotic for whatever reason, can they grow and cause sufficient tissue destruction to bring about a local pathological condition.

The report from the microbiological laboratory to the clinician should not wait upon species identification. The relative numbers of various morphotypes seen in the direct examination of the specimen, as well as the morphological description, should be reported as soon as it has been established by incubation of aerobic, 10% CO_2, and anaerobic subcultures that the isolate is in fact anaerobic and not facultative. The antibiotic susceptibility and species identification can be reported later. Because the anaerobes are part of the normal microflora of the body, and their pathogenicity is often a function of immunosuppressive therapy or implanted prosthetic devices, the assessment of the importance of an anaerobic isolate is often not a simple matter and is usually the function of the clinician. The possibility that the isolate may be a contaminant from the normal microflora must be taken into consideration, as well as the clinical condition of the patient, the therapy, and the source of the culture. Consequently, the microbiologist may be of considerable assistance to the clinician in assessing the importance of the anaerobes that have been isolated.

LITERATURE CITED

1. Dowell, V. R., Jr., and T. M. Hawkins. 1973. Laboratory methods in anaerobic bacteriology. CDC Laboratory Manual. Center for Disease Control, Atlanta, Ga.
2. Holdeman, L. V., and W. E. C. Moore. 1972. Anaerobe laboratory manual. Virginia Polytechnic Institute and State University, Balcksburg.
3. Sutter, V. L., H. R. Attebery, J. E. Rosenblatt, K. Bricknell, and S. M. Finegold. 1972. Anaerobic bacteriology manual. Extension Division, University of California, Los Angeles.

Chapter 38

Isolation of Anaerobic Bacteria

SYDNEY M. FINEGOLD, VERA L. SUTTER, HOWARD R. ATTEBERY, AND JON E. ROSENBLATT

INTRODUCTION

All organs or tissues of the body may be involved in anaerobic infection, and all types of infection seen with aerobic or facultative bacteria (cellulitis, abscess formation, bacteremia, etc.) are also found with anaerobic organisms. Types of infections in which anaerobes are commonly found or are the predominant pathogens include bacteremia, brain abscess, otogenic meningitis or extradural or subdural empyema, chronic otitis media, chronic sinusitis, dental infections, aspiration pneumonia, lung abscess, pulmonary infection secondary to obstructive process, bronchiectasis, thoracic empyema, liver abscess, pylephlebitis, peritonitis, appendicitis, diverticulitis, subphrenic abscess, other intra-abdominal abscess, wound infection following bowel surgery or trauma, puerperal sepsis, post-abortal sepsis, endometritis, tubo-ovarian abscess, other gynecological infections, peri-rectal abscess, gas-forming cellulitis, infected vascular gangrene, and gas gangrene. Anaerobes are also noted for their role in such intoxications as botulism and tetanus.

Clinical hints suggesting possible infection with anaerobes

1. Foul-smelling discharge
2. Location of infection in proximity to a mucosal surface
3. Necrotic tissue, gangrene; pseudo-membrane formation
4. Gas in tissues or discharges
5. Endocarditis with negative routine blood cultures
6. Infection associated with malignancy or other process producing tissue destruction and that associated with impaired circulation
7. Infection related to the use of aminoglycosides (oral, parenteral, or topical)
8. Septic thrombophlebitis
9. Bacteremic picture with jaundice
10. Infection following human or other bites
11. Black discoloration of blood-containing exudates; these exudates may fluoresce red under ultraviolet light (*Bacteroides melaninogenicus* infections)
12. Presence of "sulfur granules" in discharges (actinomycosis)
13. Classical features of gas gangrene
14. Clinical setting suggestive of anaerobic infection (septic abortion, infection following gastrointestinal surgery, etc.)

In the situations listed above, the probability of anaerobic infection is high so that special efforts must be made to obtain proper specimens for anaerobic culture. For example, discharges with a foul or putrid odor essentially always contain anaerobes. On the other hand, feces and gastric contents should not be cultured anaerobically, nor should vaginal discharge, urine, or sputum except when these materials are obtained in special ways as described below. Sputum may be a proper specimen in suspected actinomycosis (chapter 42).

COLLECTION OF SPECIMENS

The preferred technique of collecting most specimens is by aspiration with needle and syringe. In doing so, it is important to protect the specimen as much as possible from contact with air. The plunger should be fully inserted into the barrel at the start and, when the volume is adequate, a drop of specimen should be expelled on an alcohol-cotton pledget. If the site to be sampled will yield very little material, about 1 ml of a sterile pre-reduced solution or broth (see below) is aspirated into the syringe before collection. The sample is then aspirated with this needle and syringe.

Whenever possible, it is desirable to obtain specimens of tissue—rather than just exudate—for anaerobic culture. Tissue specimens may more accurately indicate the bacteriology of the infectious process, and anaerobic bacteria survive more readily in this type of specimen.

Practically all of the anaerobes involved in infections in humans are also found normally on mucous membranes and on other surfaces of the body as indigenous flora. In these areas, they are usually present in such large numbers that even minimal "contamination" of a clinical specimen with normal flora may give misleading results. Specimens obtained from sites that are normally sterile (pleural fluid, blood, spinal fluid, etc.) pose no problem; one must simply take the usual precautions to decontaminate the skin properly before puncturing it to obtain the specimen. Other situations are not so simple, and the following precautions are recommended.

Endometritis. Decontaminate the cervical os before obtaining a specimen for culture; take care to prevent contamination of the swab or other collecting device with normal vaginal flora. The use of a small sterile tube which can be passed through the endocervical canal into the endometrial cavity is desirable. A sterile finger cot can be stretched over this and secured proximally; it is then snipped free by way of the tube lumen after the tube is in place.

Urinary tract infections. Collect urine by percutaneous suprapubic bladder puncture. Voided urine commonly contains anaerobes from the normal urethral flora (7). Because anaerobes are apparently only seldom involved in urinary tract infections, bladder puncture is necessary only in special situations.

Pneumonia, lung abscess, and other pulmonary infection. A more common and more difficult problem is the patient with pulmonary infection. Percutaneous transtracheal needle aspiration (or direct lung puncture) is the most dependable way to obtain a reliable sample for culture since these procedures bypass areas with normal flora. Ordinary sputum specimens must not be used for anaerobic culture because of the large number and variety of anaerobes normally present in the mouth. Even bronchoscopically obtained specimens are not always reliable, although material obtained directly from an involved segmental bronchus through the new fiber optic bronchoscopes may prove to be meaningful.

Abscesses. Liquid pus is always preferable to swabs; therefore, use needle aspiration for a closed abscess.

Sinus tracts or draining wounds. Avoid sampling surface material as it is likely to be "contaminated" by organisms not responsible for the infection. Collection is best done by aspiration by syringe with the use of an intravenous-type plastic catheter placed as deeply as possible through the decontaminated skin opening.

SPECIMEN TRANSPORT

Some anaerobes, such as *Bacteroides fragilis* and *Clostridium perfringens*, are moderately resistant to oxygen contact and can survive for days if only kept moist. However, other anaerobes responsible for clinical infections do not tolerate even very brief exposures to air. Consequently, special transport methods have been designed to insure survival of all anaerobes in clinical material. Obligate aerobes and facultative organisms remain viable in an anaerobic system; therefore, the universal carrier for bacteriological specimens, where anaerobic bacteria as well as other forms are sought, should be an anaerobic container.

Material in a syringe is injected into a tube (Fig. 1) or bottle containing O_2-free gas (2). Suitable containers are also available from commercial sources 1 and 2 (see list at end of this chapter). Dilution of specimens reduces proportionately the chances of full recovery of the microorganisms present and promotes overgrowth of facultative species. Therefore, empty gassed-out collection tubes and bottles should be used for the transport of most specimens. It is important, however, that collection tubes and bottles contain a few drops of aqueous resazurin (0.0003% final concentration), an oxidation-reduction indicator, and that these containers be stored in the dark to preserve the indicator. A pink color, indicating aeration, may develop upon addition of specimens, but it should be only temporary. Cysteine HCl is added to some commercial containers to facilitate reduction. The fluid used to dilute specimens should have a low E_h.

A syringe and needle assembly containing aspirated specimen may be taken directly to the laboratory if the needle is inserted into a sterile rubber stopper (Fig. 2). Use this method only when the specimen is processed promptly (the plastic syringe gradually admits air).

A portable gassing-out device for making a tube anaerobic is useful for tissue scrapings, biopsy specimens, and fluids. Such a device has been described in detail (8). The mini-jar method (3), utilizing a 35-mm film container as an anaerobic jar, is a simple device for transport of tissue specimens. Steel wool immersed in a 5% copper sulfate solution which has previously been acidified to pH 2.0 with H_2SO_4 is the oxygen scavenger. Tissue or other clinical material that can be placed into a 1-dram vial can be placed in the mini-jar for transport (Fig. 3).

The swab method is by far the least desirable for collecting anaerobic specimens. Because of the risk of excessive aeration, it should be used only when aspiration is impossible or extremely difficult. Use two gassed-out (O_2-free CO_2) tubes; one contains a swab; the other contains semisolid Cary and Blair transport medium (chapter 95) and receives the collected specimen. The swab is inserted as rapidly as possible into the second tube while the latter is held in an upright position.

All specimens should be cultured promptly. Specimens should be refrigerated to slow down the growth of facultative species which may be present if the culture cannot be set up within 2 h.

DIRECT EXAMINATION

The direct microscopic examination of clinical material is invaluable. The unique morphology of many of the anaerobes (fusiform bacilli, branching forms, etc.) will often alert the microbiologist or clinician to the possibility of infection with anaerobes, and at the same time is a valuable guide to the selection of special media and procedures. Direct examination also allows one to quantitate roughly the various

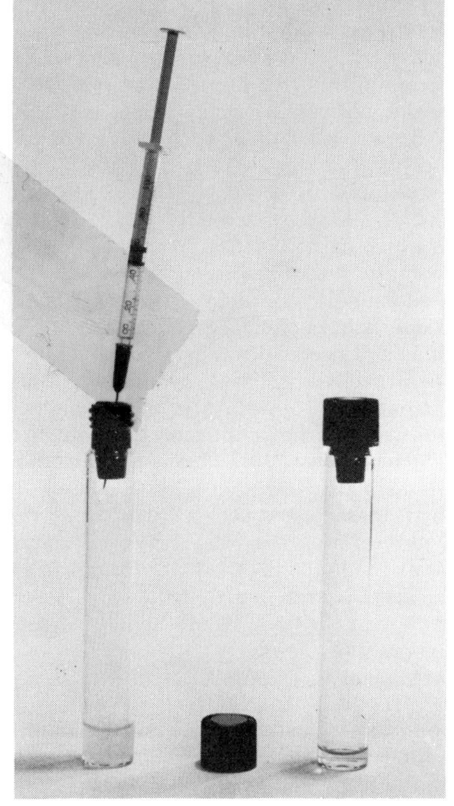

FIG. 1. *Transport tubes for anaerobic specimens. The tubes contain no air, having been flushed out with oxygen-free gas before sterilization. Liquid specimens can easily be injected through the recess in the butyl rubber stopper. Both tubes contain resazurin indicator. The tube on the left has an agar base. The other tube contains a reducing broth.*

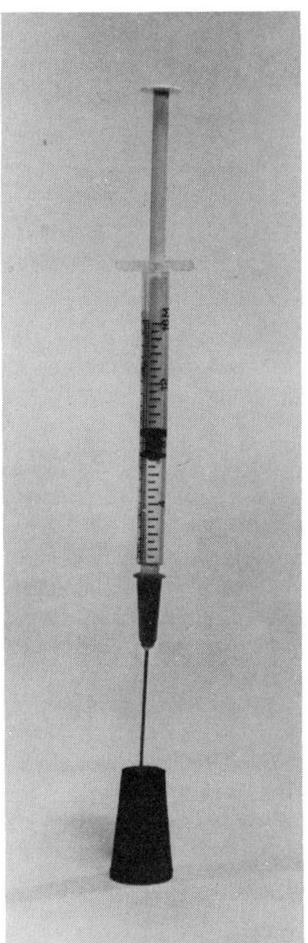

FIG. 2. *A 1-ml syringe is a convenient device for collecting and transporting some specimens for anaerobic bacteriological analysis. See text for details concerning use of syringes.*

types of organisms that are present for use as a check on the adequacy of the techniques employed. One should be able to recover, on culture, in proper relative proportions, all types of organisms seen on direct smear. Since it takes a considerable amount of time to grow anaerobes and to isolate and identify them, the Gram stain may provide important preliminary information to the clinician in the case of fulminant infection.

It is desirable to include both Gram stain and either phase-contrast or dark-field examination. The latter is particularly useful for detection of spirochetes or other motile forms, or spores. Spirochetes may be present in oral, respiratory, and reproductive tract infections, and dark-field examination is the usual method for confirmation of the presence of these organisms. Note the staining, shape, size, and approximate number of the different types of organisms

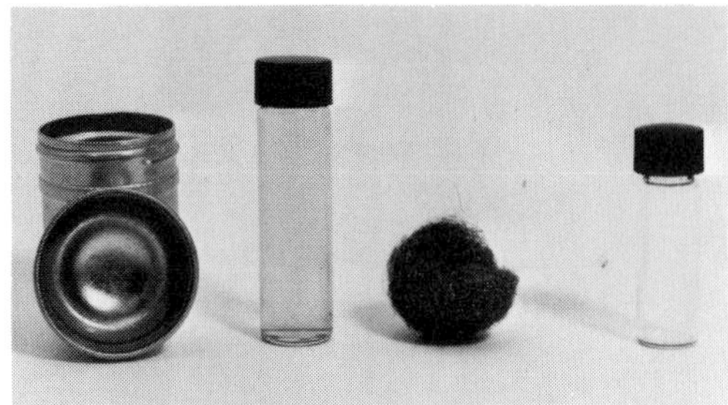

FIG. 3. *Mini-jar anaerobic transporter useful for tissue and other material that can be placed into a 1-dram vial. The vial, with the cap loose, is placed into the jar. Steelwool immersed briefly in an acidified copper-sulfate solution quickly removes oxygen from the container. The lid of the 35-mm film container has a neoprene seal which makes the container gas-tight.*

present, as well as branching or pseudobranching. Also, note the presence of spores and their shape and position in the cell. Do not confuse spores with irregular staining, as is frequently seen in strains of *Bacteroides* and *Fusobacterium*. Because gram-negative anaerobes may stain relatively lightly, examine smears under subdued light. Basic fuchsin counterstain dyes gram-negative anaerobes more deeply than does safranine. For destaining, use 95% alcohol. Some laboratories prefer the Kopeloff modification of the Gram stain procedure because it is thought to reduce the well-known tendency of some anaerobic species to decolorize very readily (10).

Bacteriological hints suggesting possible infection with anaerobes

1. Gram stain of discharge or of culture revealing:
   a. Pale, irregularly staining, pleomorphic, slender gram-negative bacilli (*Bacteroides* or *Fusobacterium*)
   b. Gram-negative rods with tapered ends (possible *F. nucleatum*)
   c. Large, broad, gram-positive bacilli (may appear gram-negative), or smaller bacilli with spores (*Clostridium*)
   d. Thin, branching, or filamentous gram-positive bacilli (*Actinomyces, Arachnia, Bifidobacterium, Eubacterium, Lactobacillus,* or *Propionibacterium*)
   e. Tiny to small gram-negative cocci in pairs or masses (*Veillonella*) or larger gram-negative cocci (*Acidaminococcus*)
2. Failure to grow organisms aerobically or with inadequate anaerobic technique, especially if organisms were seen on Gram stain of original exudate
3. Growth in anaerobic zone of fluid media or of agar deeps
4. Gas, foul odor in specimen or culture
5. Characteristic colonies on agar plates anaerobically
6. Growth on media highly selective for anaerobes

PRIMARY CULTURE

Specimens are inoculated to both solid and liquid media. As is the case with facultative bacteria, greatest dependence is placed upon agar cultures; broth and semisolid media are employed as back-up culture for primary isolation. The composition of these media is generally complex so that the wide nutritional needs of the more fastidious species are supplied. Some additives such as vitamin K_1 for certain strains of *Bacteroides melaninogenicus* (9), for *B. fragilis* (R. Chan et al., unpublished data), and for gram-positive nonsporeformers (R. J. Zabransky, personal communication) may serve a specific purpose. Others, such as yeast extract or autolysate, act as supplements with broader growth-stimulating action. Hemin is also helpful and should be used in primary isolation media which do not contain blood (9).

There are several satisfactory nonselective blood-agar media for primary isolation of anaerobic bacteria from clinical specimens. One good medium is Brucella blood-agar for anaerobes, and the Brucella agar base is available commercially (sources 3 and 5). An equally good solid medium is brain heart infusion supplemented (BHI-S) blood-agar (10). This is also available as commercially prepared plates (source 1). Although these plates become thoroughly oxidized before use, they nevertheless produce almost as good growth of isolates from primary clinical specimens as freshly prepared plates of the same composition (E. H. Spaulding, personal communication).

Laked blood-agar can also be used advantageously as a nonselective medium. *B. melaninogenicus* grows more rapidly and produces brown to black pigment sooner when the blood has been laked (13). It is prepared in the laboratory from either BHI-S blood-agar or Brucella blood-agar for anaerobes (chapter 95). To the melted and cooled medium is added 5% sheep blood which has previously been lysed by alternate freezing and thawing.

Some laboratories like also to inoculate a tube of *nonselective* liquid medium as a back-up for the plate cultures. One medium useful for this purpose is a supplemented thioglycolate medium (13). This is prepared in the laboratory from a commercial dehydrated medium, plus certain additives to provide adequate enrichment for primary culture (See Thioglycolate medium supplemented for anaerobes, chapter 95). Commercially prepared prereduced anaerobically sterilized (PRAS) media such as chopped meat glucose (CMG) broth and BHI-S broth (source 1) are also satisfactory.

Culture in liquid media should never be used as the sole method for isolating anaerobes from clinical specimens. Recovery of anaerobes is generally poorer in liquid media than on agar plates in anaerobic jars (12), and quantitation is not possible.

In many clinical laboratories, liquid "back-up" tubes which have developed turbidity are examined only when there is no growth on the corresponding anaerobic agar plates, or when there has been a jar failure (methylene blue indicator is not colorless after overnight incubation). Alternatively, routine examination of Gram-stained smears from these tubes, whether or not there is growth on the anaerobic plates, may be carried out as shown in Fig. 7. If there are morphological forms different from any seen in the corresponding smears from agar, the tube culture is subcultured as though it were the original specimen. Because this step involves considerable time, effort, and expense, each laboratory must decide whether or not to take it. In this connection, we point out that the same strain may show quite dissimilar appearances when taken from an agar colony and from a broth culture, so that two seemingly different isolates may, after several days of study, turn out to be the same organism.

Some laboratories also inoculate specimens to *selective* media. By inhibition of unwanted varieties, they can facilitate presumptive identification of selected types in the presence of a mixture of facultative and anaerobic species. However, selective media may also be somewhat inhibitory for the target species and should always be used, therefore, in conjunction with nonselective media.

One good selective medium is kanamycin-vancomycin (KV) blood-agar (chapter 95). This is prepared in the laboratory from either Brucella agar or BHI-S agar as the base. KV agar is useful for isolating *Bacteroides* from clinical material; growth of facultative bacteria is greatly inhibited and most gram-positive anaerobes will not grow on this medium. Kanamycin-vancomycin laked blood-agar (KVL) is similar to KV agar except that the concentration of kanamycin is reduced and the blood is laked rather than whole. The presence and presumptive identification of *B. melaninogenicus* can often be made within 48 h after receipt of the specimen, if this medium is included in the initial isolation procedure. See reference 13 for a list of additional selective media which may be prepared in laboratories with special needs and adequate facilities.

Anaerobic collection tubes are not opened during the inoculation of primary cultures. Instead, the screw cap is removed, material is aspirated with a needle and syringe, and two or three drops are placed on the plates and added to tubes.

INCUBATION

The isolation of pure cultures of anaerobic bacteria from clinical specimens requires the use of solid media incubated in an anaerobic environment.

The three principal anaerobic incubation methods available at present are the anaerobic jar method, the roll-tube method, and the anaerobic chamber or glove box procedure. Several studies have shown that recovery of anaerobes from clinical specimens is as good with anaerobic jars as with roll tubes or the chamber, providing proper methods of specimen collection and transport are utilized (6, 12). Certainly, use of the anaerobic jar is simpler, less expensive, less time-consuming, and generally more applicable in the clinical microbiology laboratory than the other more complex and costly methods.

Anaerobic jars

Three different types of anaerobic jars are shown in Fig. 4. The components are a rigid, sturdy jar made of steel (Torbal), polycarbonate (GasPak), or glass (Brewer) and a lid capable of forming an air-tight seal. A wire mesh "cage" attached to the lid contains the "cold" catalyst (palladium coated alumina pellets). Originally, the Brewer jar lid employed a catalyst heated by electrical current. It is desirable to replace these older catalysts with those requiring no heating. Anaerobiosis is established by introducing or producing an oxygen-free, hydrogen-containing gas in the clamped jar. The oxygen remaining in the jar combines, by action of the catalyst, with hydrogen to form water.

The jars can be set up by two different methods. The simplest one uses a commercially available (source 3) packet (GasPak) which is simply placed inside the jar and generates H_2 and CO_2 when 10 ml of water is added to it (4). The lid is then clamped on quickly and the jar is placed in the incubator.

A second method is the evacuation-replacement system (Fig. 5). Here, the air is removed from the jar by drawing a vacuum of 25 inches (625 mm) of Hg and replacing this with N_2 or CO_2. The jar is evacuated and refilled three to five times, the final fill gas being a mixture such as 80% N_2, 10% H_2, and 10% CO_2. Hydrogen must be introduced to activate the palladium catalyst. The final fill gas mixture may be used for all flushes, but the single gases are less expensive (commercial source 6).

An indicator of anaerobiosis should be included in each jar; a convenient type is commercially available (source 3) as a methylene blue-saturated filter-paper strip. Although the E_h at which this becomes reduced (i.e., colorless) is relatively high (+10 mV at pH 7), its use will identify jar failures (usually due to a faulty seal or inactive catalyst). Catalyst becomes inactivated by absorption of excess moisture and of H_2S. Therefore, it *must* be reactivated each time it is used, and this is done by heating to 160 C in a hot air oven for 1.5 to 2 h. Having an extra supply of catalyst "cages" will facilitate their rotation. Reactivated catalysts should be stored in a desiccator until used.

Results with the two-jar systems are comparable and, although the GasPak is very simple to use, the evacuation-replacement system might prove less expensive in the long run. We do not recommend use of jars without catalyst.

A useful adjunct to the use of anaerobic jars has been suggested by Martin (11). Inoculated plates may be placed in a jar covered with an unclamped lid while CO_2 constantly flows through the lid vent from a tank source. The CO_2 is passed over heated copper to remove all traces of O_2. This CO_2 flow protects the inoculated plates from O_2 until enough specimens are accumulated to fill a jar, which is then set up by one of the methods described above.

Roll tubes

The roll tube method includes the use of PRAS media. These are described in detail in the VPI *Manual* (10). Convenient equipment for handling roll tubes is available commercially as the VPI Anaerobic Culture System (source 7). A constant flow of O_2-free gas is required, and either the double mixture of 97% CO_2 and 3% H_2, or a triple mixture of N_2, H_2, and CO_2, is satisfactory (commercial source 6). Traces of O_2 which may be present in tank gases are removed by attaching a Deoxo Gas Purifier assembly (commercial source 8) to the tank. The gas must contain a minimum of 3% H_2 to activate the Deoxo catalyst.

Roll tubes contain PRAS agar as a thin transparent layer. Most clinical laboratories

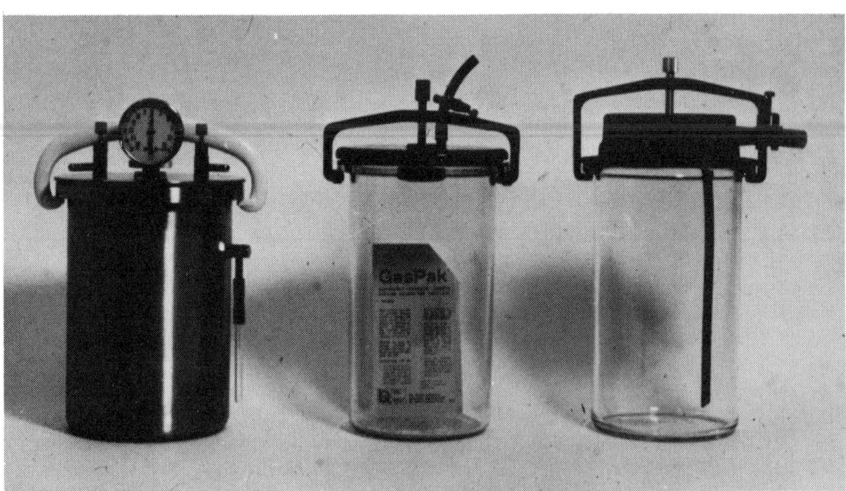

FIG. 4. *Three anaerobic jars in most common use: (left to right) the Torbal, GasPak, and Brewer (modification of McIntosh-Fildes jar) jars. The first two are "cold" catalyst jars and the third can be converted readily for use with this catalyst. All three systems can be used as evacuation-replacement jars and the GasPak jar can, in addition, be used with the commercial envelope that supplies H_2 and CO_2 gas generated by the addition of water to the packet. The Torbal jar is available from commercial source 5 and the GasPak jar from source 3.*

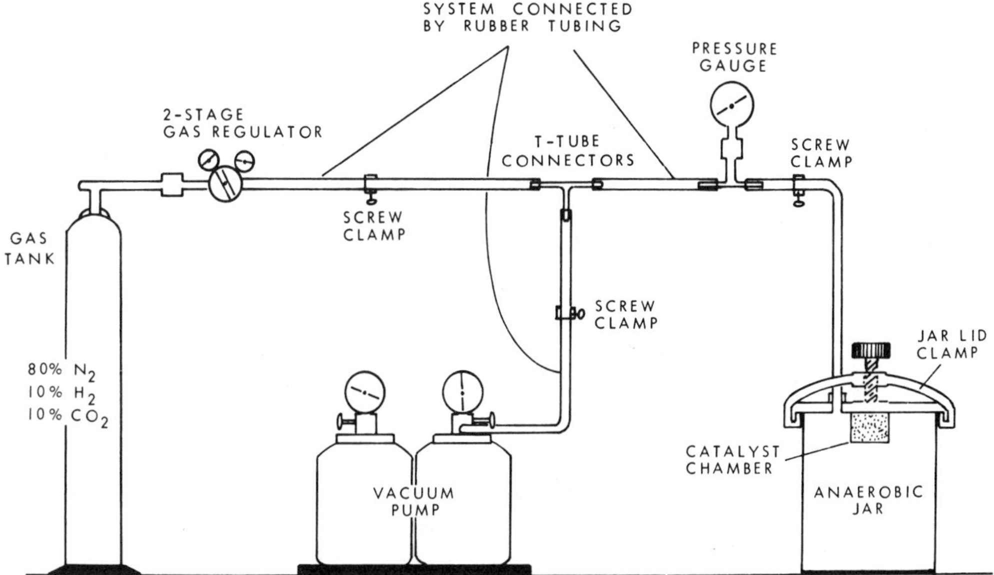

FIG. 5. *Schematic view of apparatus for evacuation-replacement anaerobic jar technique. A mixture of 85% N_2, 10% H_2, and 5% CO_2 is also satisfactory.*

will find it more convenient to use commercially prepared tubes (sources 1 and 2). When received, they are filled with O_2-free gas, and they must remain anaerobic during inoculation. As the stopper is removed, a flamed gassing cannula delivering O_2-free gas is introduced into the tube to maintain reduced conditions (Fig. 6). Roll tubes are inoculated with the aid of a holder-rotator which revolves the tube in a slanted position (Fig. 6C). Two drops of the specimen are deposited on the upper surface and distributed by gently pressing an inoculating loop against the agar surface as the tube is rotated. By gradually inserting the loop to the bottom of the tube and then withdrawing it, a pair of spiral streaks are made. The stopper is replaced rapidly as the cannula is removed. When direct smear examination reveals many bacteria, a second tube should be inoculated with a more dilute inoculum. A simple way to do this is to replace the first tube with a second one and use the same loop as the inoculum.

As in all other types of anaerobic culture work, only stainless-steel or platinum loops should be employed; nichrome wire is unsatisfactory.

Liquid PRAS media are inoculated in a similar manner but with the tubes in upright position.

Anaerobic chamber

Flexible plastic chambers equipped with a metal port or lock are available commercially (source 9). They are extremely useful and highly desirable pieces of equipment for handling large volumes of specimens and particularly for studies of normal flora which contain a wide variety of fastidious species (1). But an anaerobic chamber (glove box) is not needed by the average clinical microbiology laboratory (see reference 13 for a table comparing the tube, jar, and chamber methods).

ISOLATION PROCEDURE

Roll tubes can be examined at frequent intervals and the colonies can be picked as often as desired without disturbing the continuous anaerobic environment. On the other hand, jars containing primary plate cultures should ordinarily not be opened during the first 2 days of incubation so as to avoid the exposure to air that would occur. Examination of plate cultures should be as expeditious as possible. Primary culture plates should be reincubated anaerobically for an additional 5 days or longer and reexamined for the appearance of slow-growing species.

Select the different colony types and subculture each one to aerobic, CO_2, and anaerobic blood-agar plates (BAP) as shown in Fig. 7. Make a Gram stain and note morphology. In some laboratories, as a preliminary step, each colony type is first subcultured to an anaerobic BAP and incubated for 24 h as a check on purity. If the culture appears to be pure, it is safe to use more than one colony (many species produce colonies too small for one to provide adequate inoculum) for subcultures to aerobic and CO_2 plates. The results after overnight incubation demonstrate which of the individual isolates are facultative and which ones are obligate anaerobes. Those types growing on the CO_2 and anaerobic plates, but not on the aerobic plates, are considered microaerophilic. It should be noted, however, that some genera, regarded as obligately anaerobic, contain species, or strains within them, which are capable of some growth on the surface of aerobic agar plates. Fortunately such strains are not encountered frequently in clinical specimens, and their nature can usually be suspected by the scanty growth aerobically compared with the amount of anaerobic growth.

When anaerobic bacteria are not isolated from specimens in which they are actually present, such failure is probably attributable to one or more of the following reasons.

1. Gram stain not prepared directly from clinical specimen. If organisms seen on the smear fail to grow out, this suggests the possible presence of organisms requiring special media or conditions of incubation, or the use of defective techniques.

2. Failure to set up anaerobic cultures promptly from clinical specimens—or to keep these under anaerobic conditions pending culture.

3. Use of fluid medium as the only system for growing anaerobes. Solid media are required to separate the various organisms present in mixed culture. Errors are made at times even when anaerobes have grown in fluid medium. Some workers do not check the broth if growth appears on aerobic plates, assuming that the same organism is growing both. A Gram stain of the broth will often alert one to the additional presence of anaerobes.

4. Failure to use supplements in media. Vitamin K_1 (or similar compounds) is required by some strains of *B. melaninogenicus* and enhances growth of some strains of *B. fragilis* and gram-positive nonsporeformers.

5. Failure to use selective media. Some anaerobes may be overgrown by facultative species and overlooked if selective media are not used.

6. Failure to use a good anaerobic jar. Brewer, Gas Pak, and Torbal jars have been found to perform well.

7. Failure to check jars carefully for leaks after they are set up.

8. Catalysts not in good working order; use

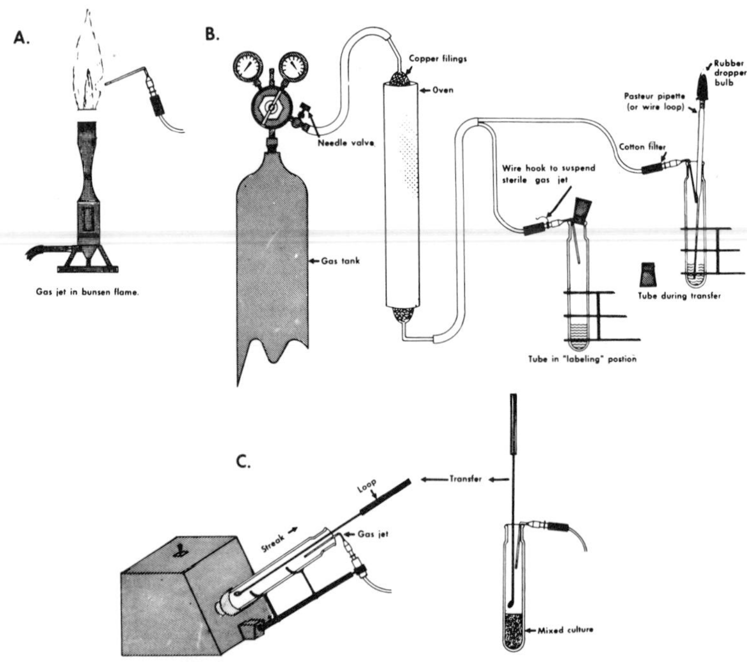

FIG. 6. *Roll-tube technique (PRAS media) for maintaining anaerobiosis. A Deoxo catalyst may be used in place of the oven pictured when gases containing at least 3% hydrogen are used (commercial source 8). (A) Gas cannula flow should visibly indent bunsen flame. (B) Connected gassing-out apparatus. (C) Apparatus for inoculation of streak roll tubes.*

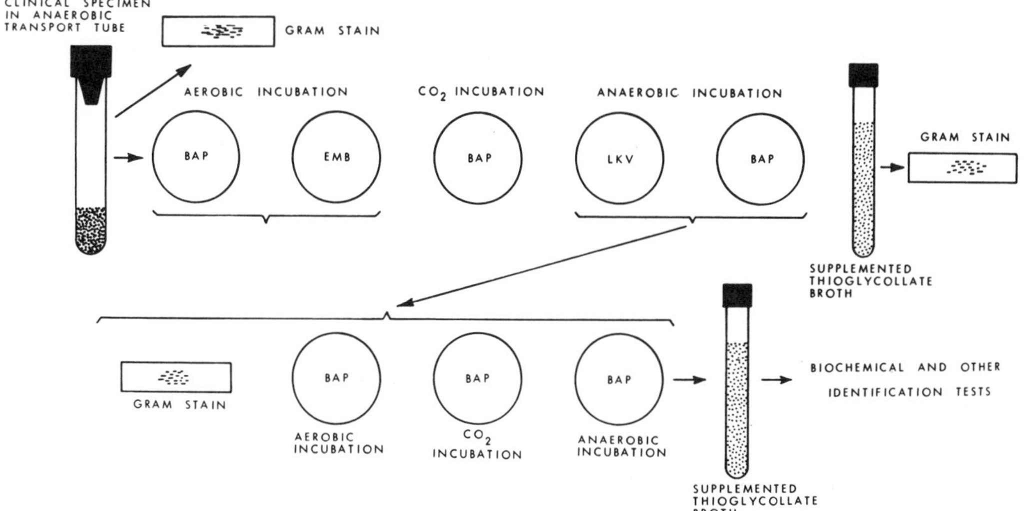

FIG. 7. *Scheme for minimal processing of clinical specimens for anaerobic bacteria (see text for additional media which may be useful). BHI-S or chopped meat may be substituted for thioglycolate broth if desired. Inclusion of a CO_2 plate (10% by volume, or candle jar) in the primary culture set is optional. BAP, blood-agar plate; LKV, kanamycin-vancomycin laked blood-agar.*

freshly regenerated catalysts each time a jar is set up.

9. Using toxic gas in displacement procedure with the Brewer jar; laboratory line gas may contain carbon monoxide.

10. Failure to include CO_2 in atmosphere in jars. Carbon dioxide is desirable for most anaerobes and essential for some.

11. Failure to hold cultures for extended periods. Occasionally, fastidious organisms present in small numbers may require 2 weeks to grow.

At this point the laboratory is able to report the presence or absence of anaerobes or microaerophiles and their morphology and Gram stain reaction. The identification of these isolates is dealt with in the chapters which follow in this section.

PRESERVATION AND SHIPMENT

Laboratories may wish to save cultures or mail them to more specialized laboratories for further study. Cultures of anaerobes may be preserved for prolonged periods either by lyophilization or by freezing at very low temperatures (−65 C) in a suitable colloid medium such as skimmed milk, 10% bovine albumin, fetal calf serum, or defibrinated blood.

Shipment of anaerobic cultures can be accomplished by several means. Lyophilized cultures may be shipped easily. The most practical method is deep stabbing of Brucella agar or brain heart infusion agar with a heavy inoculum of the anaerobe or using an agar shake culture in one of these media. The tube should be filled two-thirds of the way to the top with agar, and the medium should contain a minimal amount of fermentable carbohydrate so that excess acid and gas will not be produced. The tube is incubated until visible growth is present and can then be shipped with the cap tightly sealed and taped. One may ship cultures in liquid media if precautions are taken to avoid tube breakage and spillage.

COMMERCIAL SOURCES

1. Robbins Division of Scott Laboratories, Fiskeville, R.I. 02823.
2. Hyland Laboratories, 3300 Hyland Ave., Costa Mesa, Calif. 92626.
3. BBL Division of Bioquest, Box 243, Cockeysville, Md. 21030.
4. Difco Laboratories, 920 Henry St., Detroit, Mich. 48201.
5. Major laboratory supply houses.
6. Specialty Gas Laboratories of Liquid Carbonic Corp., 670 Essex St., Harrison, N.J. 07029; with branches throughout the U.S.
7. Bellco Glass, Inc., P.O. Box B, Vineland, N.J. 08360.
8. Deoxo Gas Purifier assembly (three parts). Mathewson Gas Products, P.O. Box 85, East Rutherford, N.J. 07073.
9. Coy Manufacturing Co., 1393 Harpst, Ann Arbor, Mich. 48104.

EDITORIAL COMMENT

This chapter contains a number of changes from the original manuscript. These were suggested by the section editor (L.DS.S.) and one of the *Manual* editors (E.H.S.). Thus, the overall procedure described herein represents a synthesis of the experiences in other laboratories as well as in that of the authors. We express our appreciation to them for their cooperative and generous attitude in accepting so many of our suggestions, which in some instances were significant changes from their own methods.

L. DS. Smith
E. H. Spaulding

Supplement to Chapter 38

Susceptibility of Anaerobic Bacteria to Antimicrobial Agents[1]

The susceptibility of anaerobes to various therapeutically useful antibacterial agents is noted in Table S1. Patterns of susceptibility are generally useful, but determination of susceptibility of individual strains may be important for the management of infections, particularly in cases of bacterial endocarditis and other serious infections.

Table S1. *Susceptibility of anaerobes to antimicrobial agents*[a]

Antibiotic	Microaerophilic and anaerobic cocci	*Bacteroides fragilis*	*Bacteroides melaninogenicus*	*Fusobacterium varium*	Other *Fusobacterium* species	*Eubacterium* and actinomyces	*Clostridium perfringens*	Other clostridia
Penicillin G[b]	++++	+	+++	+++[c]	++++	++++	++++[c]	++ to +++
Lincomycin	+++	+ to ++	+++	++	+++	++ to +++	+ to ++	+
Clindamycin	+++	+++	+++	++	+++	+++[c]	+++[c]	++
Metronidazole	++	+++	+++	+++	+++	+ to ++	+++	?+++
Chloramphenicol	+++	+++	+++	+++	+++	+++	+++[c]	+++[c]
Tetracycline[e]	++	+ to ++	+++	++	++ to +++	++	++	++
Erythromycin	++ to +++	+	++	+	+	++ to +++	+	++ to +++[d]
Vancomycin	++ to +++	+	+	+	+	?+++	+++	?+++[c]

[a] ++++, Drug of choice; +++, good activity; ++, moderate activity; +, poor or inconsistent activity. Only drugs which might be useful therapeutically are included; not all of these agents have been used clinically for anaerobic infections and not all are FDA approved.

[b] Other penicillins and cephalosporins may show differences in activity; see text.

[c] A few strains are resistant.

[d] Based on old studies (resistance may have developed subsequently).

[e] Doxycycline and minocycline are more active. Many tetracycline-resistant strains have now been detected.

Three anaerobic species, *Bacteroides fragilis*, *Fusobacterium varium*, and *C. ramosum*, are often resistant to several antimicrobial drugs, and susceptibility tests are very important with isolates of this type. In addition, strains of many other species of *Clostridium* and some of *Eubacterium* are resistant to clindamycin, a drug commonly used and generally very effective in anaerobic infection.

The new penicillins and cephalosporins are often less active (sometimes much less active) than penicillin G; only ampicillin and cephaloridine, among these newer compounds, are comparable to penicillin G in activity. However, drugs such as carbenicillin and cefazolin may be valuable because of the very high blood levels which may be achieved safely. Doxycycline and minocycline are much more active than tetracycline, but there are still strains which exhibit resistance to these. Plate and tube dilution susceptibility tests can be set up in a manner similar to that used for aerobes and then incubated in an anaerobic atmosphere (see Chapter 49). Do not use media containing thioglycolate because thiol compounds inactivate some antibiotics.

[1] Editorial comment. The following supplement was prepared by Sydney M. Finegold and collaborators. Although it is not directly related to the subject matter of this chapter, it is the most appropriate place to insert this useful and authoritative information. (E.H.S.).

LITERATURE CITED

1. Aranki, A., S. A. Syed, E. B. Kenney, and R. Freter. 1969. Isolation of anaerobic bacteria from human gingiva and mouse cecum by means of a simplified glove box procedure. Appl. Microbiol. **17**:568–576.
2. Attebery, H. R., and S. M. Finegold. 1969. Combined screw-cap and rubber-stopper closure for Hungate tubes (pre-reduced anaerobically sterilized roll tubes and liquid media). Appl. Microbiol. **18**:558–561.
3. Attebery, H. R., and S. M. Finegold. 1970. A miniature anaerobic jar for tissue transport or for cultivation of anaerobes. Amer. J. Clin. Pathol. **53**:383–388.

4. Brewer, J. H., and D. L. Allgeier. 1966. Safe self-contained carbon dioxide-hydrogen anaerobic system. Appl. Microbiol. **14:**985–988.
5. Brewer, J. H., D. L. Allgeier, and C. B. McLaughlin. 1966. Improved anaerobic indicator. Appl. Microbiol. **14:**135–136.
6. Dowell, V. R., Jr. 1972. Comparison of techniques for isolation and identification of anaerobic bacteria. Amer. J. Clin. Nutr. **25:**1335–1343.
7. Finegold, S. M., L. G. Miller, S. L. Merrill, and D. J. Posnick. 1965. Significance of anaerobic and capnophilic bacteria isolated from the urinary tract, p. 159–178. *In* E. H. Kass (ed.), Progress in pyelonephritis. F. A. Davis Co., Philadelphia.
8. Fulghum, R. S. 1971. Mobile anaerobe laboratory. Appl. Microbiol. **21:**769–770.
9. Gibbons, R. J., and J. B. Macdonald. 1960. Hemin and vitamin K compounds as required factors for the cultivation of certain strains of *Bacteroides melaninogenicus*. J. Bacteriol. **80:**164–170.
10. Holdeman, L. V., and W. E. C. Moore. 1972. Anaerobic bacteriology manual. Anaerobe Laboratory, Virginia Polytechnic Institute and State University, Blacksburg.
11. Martin, W. J. 1971. Practical method for isolation of anaerobic bacteria in the clinical laboratory. Appl. Microbiol. **22:**1168–1171.
12. Rosenblatt, J. E., A. Fallon, and S. M. Finegold. 1973. Comparison of methods for isolation of anaerobic bacteria from clinical specimens. Appl. Microbiol. **25:**77–85.
13. Sutter, V. L., H. R. Attebery, J. E. Rosenblatt, K. Bricknell, and S. M. Finegold. 1972. Anaerobic bacteriology manual. Extension Division, Univ. of California, Los Angeles.

Chapter 39

Clostridium

LOUIS DS. SMITH AND V. R. DOWELL, JR.

CHARACTERIZATION

The clostridia are spore-forming, anaerobic and aerotolerant bacilli which are widely distributed in terrestrial and marine environments throughout the world. Some reside in the lower intestinal tract of humans and lower animals as part of the normal microbiota. Although more than 300 species of the genus *Clostridium* have been described, fewer than a third of these are now recognized. A much smaller number of species is encountered in clinical specimens. In one study of the occurrence of clostridia in specimens submitted by three clinical laboratories to a reference laboratory, 97% were found to belong to a recognized species, and 90% of these clustered in only 12 species (Table 1).

There have been a few recent changes in the nomenclature of these organisms. Those formerly called *C. capitovale* are now classified as *C. cadaveris; C. butyricum* and *C. beijerinckii* contain strains formerly labeled *C. multifermentans;* and *C. subterminale* includes strains formerly called *C. hastiforme*. The species *C. ramosum*, one of the most frequently encountered clostridia in clinical specimens, includes organisms formerly called *Catenabacterium ramosum*, *Bacteroides terebrans*, and *Bacteroides trichoides*.

Since some aerotolerant clostridia may grow on the surface of a fresh agar medium under aerobic conditions, it is possible to confuse these with certain facultative *Bacillus* species. However, members of the genus *Clostridium* form spores under anaerobic conditions and usually do not produce catalase, whereas *Bacillus* species do not sporulate in an anaerobic environment and usually are catalase-positive. Also, aerotolerant clostridia, e.g., *C. tertium* and *C. histolyticum*, form larger colonies under anaerobic conditions than in air, and the reverse is true for *Bacillus* species.

Although a number of diseases such as botulism, *C. perfringens* foodborne illness, tetanus, gas gangrene (myonecrosis), and cellulitis may involve clostridia from an exogenous source, endogenous infections are much more common. However, special circumstances are required for development of endogenous infections. Common predisposing factors include surgery; an underlying illness such as leukemia, carcinoma, or diabetes mellitus; and prior treatment with immunosuppressants or corticosteroids. Essentially any organ of the body can be invaded by clostridia under the right conditions. Since clostridia are members of the normal intestinal microflora, their presence in a clinical specimen does not necessarily imply association with a pathological condition. Some clostridia, apparently nonpathogenic for humans, can colonize and grow in tissue with impaired blood supply, although they are unable progressively to invade healthy tissue. Moreover, strains of pathogenic species may react in the same way, for their pathogenic properties are manifested only under special circumstances. Therefore, close liaison between the attending physician and the clinical microbiologist is essential for assessing the clinical significance of clostridial isolates and establishing the correct diagnosis.

COLLECTION AND TRANSPORT OF CLINICAL SPECIMENS

Proper selection, collection, and transport of clinical specimens are extremely important for laboratory diagnosis of clostridial infections. Precautions should be taken to exclude surface contaminants from the normal flora when collecting samples. Specimens should be cultured immediately or held in an anaerobic environment until processed. Aspirated materials, blood, and tissue samples are preferred. Several tissue specimens should be taken from the active site of infection when gas gangrene is suspected because the clostridia are often not distributed uniformly in pathological processes. A properly collected (via a speculum) swab specimen from the cervix of the uterus serves in cases of postabortal uterine infection. If it is necessary to hold clinical specimens that may contain clostridia, leave them at room temperature for as short a time as possible. Vegetative cells of some species, such as *C. perfringens*, die rapidly in the cold.

TABLE 1. *Clostridia most frequently encountered in clinical specimens*

Species	Occurrence[a]
C. perfringens	26
C. ramosum	17
C. sporogenes	11
C. bifermentans	7
C. innocuum	6
C. sordellii	6
C. paraputrificum	3
C. subterminale	3
C. cadaveris	3
C. butyricum	3
C. septicum	3
C. tertium	2

[a] Percentage of clostridial isolates.

DIRECT EXAMINATION

Direct microscope examination of clinical materials can provide extremely useful information for the physician's use in the diagnosis and treatment of clostridial infections. Microscopy is especially useful in differentiating clostridial myonecrosis and cellulitis from other bacterial infections. Infection with certain nonsporeforming anaerobes and facultative gram-negative bacilli can resemble these clostridial infections, but the treatment required may be quite different. Radical surgery, such as amputation of a limb, may be required in the treatment of some clostridial infections; therefore, rapid diagnosis is essential.

The usual Gram stain is satisfactory for direct examination of a specimen. Special note should be taken of gram-positive rods with or without spores because sporulation in tissue is not common with the two species most frequently encountered, *C. perfringens* and *C. ramosum*. *C. perfringens* usually appears as large, relatively short, fat, gram-positive rods in tissue smears; the cells of *C. ramosum* are more slender, longer, and often curved. *C. perfringens* may or may not be encapsulated in smears from wounds; capsules usually are present in cervical smears from postabortal *C. perfringens* infections. Gram strains are also usually sufficient for demonstration of spores. Examination with a phase microscope is helpful if the spores are mature or nearly so, but special spore stains offer no advantage. If spores are present, note their shape (spherical or oval) and position (terminal or subterminal to central) in the cells. The best single medium for demonstration of spores is cooked-meat medium made up as an agar slant. Incubate anaerobically at a temperature 5 to 7 degrees below the optimum for growth of the clostridia. For most species, 30 C is satisfactory, but 37 C is better for sporulation of *C. perfringens*.

CULTURE AND ISOLATION

Inoculate plates of blood-agar and egg yolk medium and incubate anaerobically for 2 or 3 days. Examine the blood-agar culture with a stereoscopic microscope, noting particularly the hemolysis pattern, colony structure, and any evidence of swarming or of motile colonies. Examine the egg yolk-agar culture for evidence of lecithinase (phospholipase C) or lipase production. Lecithinase is indicated by a whitish precipitate within the agar, under and around the colony. Lipase activity produces a narrow zone of iridescence most easily seen at the edge of the colonies or at the edge of heavy growth. Good light is essential to see the effects of lipase.

If swarming growth has covered the surface of the agar medium, inoculate another blood-agar plate and incubate anaerobically only overnight. Subculture from colonies as soon as the plates are taken from the anaerobe jar. If swarming is again observed, inoculate a plate of medium made up with 5% agar. When isolated colonies can be picked, subculture to cooked-meat medium, incubate overnight, and use for inoculating differential media.

IDENTIFICATION

Inoculate the media indicated in Table 2 and incubate for 2 to 7 days at 35 to 37 C; 2 days are sufficient if growth is prompt and adequate. Examine Gram stains of the cooked-meat culture to determine the presence, position, and shape of spores. If spores are not found, inoculate a tube of cooked-meat medium, heat at 70 C for 10 min, and incubate. Growth in this heated tube usually indicates the presence of spores, although none may be apparent microscopically.

Determine which of the carbohydrates were fermented by using a pH meter or by adding indicator to the tubes. Determine the metabolic products if at all possible, using a glucose broth culture and a gas chromatograph. Identification of species can be made without the use of a gas chromatograph, but this usually involves more time. The information listed in Table 2 will serve to identify most of the clostridia commonly isolated from clinical specimens.

Toxin tests are necessary for the identification of a few species. *C. sporogenes* cannot be differentiated with certainty from the proteolytic group I strains of *C. botulinum* unless toxin tests are used. Although *C. botulinum* is rarely encountered in clinical material, at least

TABLE 2. *Differential characteristics of commonly encountered clostridia*[a]

Species	Cooked-meat medium		Egg yolk-agar		Growth on aerobic blood-agar	Gelatin hydrolysis	Indole production	Carbohydrate fermentation						Principal fermentation products
	Digestion	Spores	Lec.	Lip.				Glucose	Maltose	Lactose	Sucrose	Salicin	Mannitol	
Toxic, pathogenic for humans:														
C. botulinum[b]														
Group I[c]	+	OS	–	+	–	+	–	+	+	–	–	V	–	A,P,IB,B, IV,V,IC
Group II[c]	–	OS	–	+	–	+	–	+	+	–	–	V	–	A,B
Group III[c]	–	OS	V	+	–	+	–	+	V	–	–	–	–	A,P,B
C. histolyticum	+	OS	–	–	V	+	–	–	–	–	–	–	–	A
C. novyi A[c]	–	OS	+	+	–	+	–	+	+	–	–	–	–	A,P,B,V
C. novyi B[c]	V	OS	+	–	–	+	V	+	+	–	–	–	–	A,P,B,V
C. perfringens	–	OS	+	–	–	+	–	+	+	+	+	V	–	A,B
C. septicum	–	OS	–	–	–	+	–	+	+	+	–	V	–	A,B
C. sordellii	+	OS	+	–	–	+	+	+	+	–	–	–	–	A,F,P,IB, IV,IC
C. tetani	–	RT	–	–	–	+	V	–	–	–	–	–	–	A,P,B
Nontoxic, doubtfully pathogenic for humans:														
C. bifermentans	+	OS	+	–	–	+	+	+	+	–	–	–	–	A,F,P,IB, IV,IC
C. butyricum	–	OS	–	–	–	–	–	+	+	+	+	+	V	A,F,B
C. cadaveris	+	OT	–	–	–	+	–	+	–	–	–	–	–	A,B,IV
C. chauvoei[d]	–	OS	–	–	–	+	–	+	+	+	+	–	–	A,B
C. difficile	–	OS	–	–	–	–	–	+	–	–	–	V	+	A,F,IB,B, IV,V,IC
C. innocuum	–	OT	–	–	–	–	–	+	V	–	V	+	+	A,F,B
C. limosum	+	OS	+	–	–	+	–	–	–	–	–	–	–	A
C. paraputrificum	–	OT	–	–	–	–	–	+	+	+	+	+	–	A,B
C. ramosum	–	R/OT	–	–	–	–	–	+	+	+	+	+	V	A,F
C. sphenoides	–	RS/T	–	–	–	–	+	+	+	V	+	+	+	A
C. sporogenes	+	OS	–	+	–	+	–	+	+	–	–	V	–	A,P,IB,B, IV,V,IC
C. subterminale	+	OS	–	–	–	+	–	–	–	–	–	–	–	A,IB,B,IV
C. tertium	–	OT	–	–	+	–	–	+	+	+	+	+	+	A,B

[a] Key: +, positive reaction; –, negative reaction; V, variable reaction; /, either or; O, oval; R, round; S, subterminal; T, terminal; Lec., lecithinase production; Lip., lipase production. Fermentation products: A, acetic; B, butyric; F, formic; IB, isobutyric; IC, isocaproic; IV, isovaleric; P, propionic; V, valeric.

[b] Group I contains proteolytic strains (A, B, F, G); group II, types C and D; group III, nonproteolytic strains (B, E, F).

[c] Toxin neutralization test required for identification.

[d] Pathogenic for herbivores.

nine cases of type A wound botulism in humans have been reported. A few strains of group III *C. botulinum* produce lecithinase as well as lipase and are difficult to distinguish from type A *C. novyi* except by toxin tests or by the use of *C. novyi* fluorescent-antibody conjugate. To test for toxin, inoculate two tubes of cooked meat-glucose medium, incubate one tube at 37 C overnight and the other at 37 C for 3 days. Test the overnight culture first; if no toxin is found, test the 3-day culture. Centrifuge the culture, remove the liquid, and place 1.2-ml amounts in several tubes. Prepare mixtures using 0.3 ml of appropriate antiserum per tube for the various species suspected. Let stand for 30 min at room temperature or at 37 C and inject 0.5-ml portions intraperitoneally into each of two mice. Observe the mice for 3 days and record deaths that occur. Only specific sera for laboratory testing should be used for toxin identification; therapeutic sera are often unsatisfactory because they may contain antibodies to toxins of species other than those listed on the label. Diagnostic clostridial antisera are available from Burroughs Wellcome Co., Research Triangle Park, Durham, N.C. 27709.

If it is necessary to determine the toxin type of an isolate of *C. perfringens* or *C. botulinum*, it is best to send it to a reference laboratory. *C. perfringens* types other than type A seldom are encountered in clinical specimens from humans. Veterinary clinical microbiology laboratories, however, should be familiar with the technique for determining the toxin type of *C. perfringens* isolates.

PRESUMPTIVE IDENTIFICATION

Presumptive identification of a few species can be accomplished fairly rapidly. Commercially available fluorescent-antibody reagents can be used with confidence for *C. novyi*, *C. septicum*, *C. chauvoei* (found only in infections of herbivores), and *C. sordellii*.

C. perfringens is signaled by colonies on blood-agar plates surrounded by an inner zone of complete hemolysis and an outer zone of discoloration and incomplete hemolysis (with rabbit, human, or sheep blood; zones not so distinct with horse blood) composed of short to intermediate gram-positive rods without spores. Subculture from such a colony to an egg yolk-agar plate, one-half of which has been spread with *C. perfringens* antitoxin, and incubate anaerobically overnight. *C. perfringens* will produce a zone of precipitation around colonies on the control side of the plate and no precipitation, or little, on the side spread with antitoxin. Similar reactions will be given by *C. bifermentans* and *C. paraperfringens*, but these should not cause difficulty. *C. bifermentans* does not form a double zone of hemolysis, sporulates readily, is more proteolytic, and varies from *C. perfringens* in other cultural characteristics. *C. paraperfringens* is so seldom encountered in clinical material that it is not likely to be an appreciable source of error.

It is often difficult to isolate *C. tetani* from a suspected lesion. When this organism is being sought, a freshly poured blood-agar plate should be inoculated lightly. Incubate for 1 day and examine carefully for swarming, which may be in the form of a very thin layer. Transfer cells from the edge of the swarming area to a tube of broth and streak a plate of medium containing 5% agar; incubate and pick an isolated colony.

C. tetani may sometimes be demonstrated in a specimen more readily than it can be isolated. Mix a small amount of material from the lesion in sterile broth and inject 0.1 ml in each of four mice beside the base of the tail. Inject two of the mice with 0.1 ml of tetanus antitoxin. Death, or symptoms of tetanus, in the unprotected but not the protected mice indicates the presence of *C. tetani* in the specimen.

SUSCEPTIBILITY TO ANTIBACTERIAL AGENTS

The clostridia are fairly uniform in their susceptibility to antibacterial agents, most strains being sensitive to penicillin G, chloramphenicol, tetracycline, erythromycin, and most other wide-spectrum antibiotics. There is considerable variation with clindamycin, however, and few strains are susceptible to neomycin and kanamycin at therapeutic levels.

EVALUATION

The isolation of a clostridium from a specimen is without meaning unless it is considered in relation to the patient's clinical condition. Because clostridia are ubiquitous, they are likely to be found in any area that is directly or indirectly contaminated with feces, soil, or dust. Even the toxigenic species are only opportunistic pathogens, and conditions suitable for progressive infection occur only rarely.

This is particularly the case with *C. perfringens*, which is second only to *Bacteroides fragilis* in the frequency with which it is isolated from clinical specimens. Although it may cause gas gangrene, septic abortion, necrotic enteritis, or a host of other pathological conditions, many isolates may have little clinical significance. *C. septicum*, on the other hand, is rarely isolated except from serious, usually fatal clinical conditions, often associated with malignancy. *C.*

novyi is seldom isolated in civilian hospital laboratories. During wartime it has been responsible for gas gangrene as the result of wounds that were contaminated with soil when inflicted. Most *C. novyi* strains encountered in wounds belong to type A; only a few belong to type B. Isolation of either type from a wound should be regarded with concern.

Isolation of a pathogenic strain of *C. sordellii* from a human infection is rare; the great majority of isolates appear to lack toxigenicity. However, this situation is somewhat unclear, for this species is notorious for the rapidity with which cultures can lose pathogenicity in the laboratory.

The isolation of *C. botulinum*, particularly type A, indicates the possibility of wound botulism. Nevertheless, toxigenic strains of *C. botulinum* have been isolated from wounds in the absence of clinical evidence for botulism. In addition to culturing wound samples, the patient's serum should be tested for botulinal toxin when wound botulism is suspected. A similar situation holds for *C. tetani*. Since most people have been immunized with tetanus toxoid, isolation of this organism from a wound may be insignificant clinically. Even in unimmunized persons, it is not uncommon to find this organism in wounds without the patients showing symptoms of tetanus.

C. histolyticum is encountered in less than 1% of wounds of civil life, even when it is searched for. Its presence is without clear significance unless a progressive anaerobic infection of muscle is in progress, and then the prognosis is poor.

LITERATURE CITED

1. Dowell, V. R., Jr., and T. M. Hawkins. 1973. Laboratory methods in anaerobic bacteriology. CDC Laboratory Manual, Publication No. (HSM) 73-8222. Center for Disease Control, Atlanta, Ga.
2. Holdeman, L. V., and W. E. C. Moore. 1972. Anaerobe laboratory manual. Virginia Polytechnic Institute Anaerobe Laboratory, Blacksburg, Va.
3. Merson, M. H., and V. R. Dowell, Jr. 1973. Epidemiologic, clinical, and laboratory aspects of wound botulism. N. Engl. J. Med. **289:**1005–1010.
4. Smith, L. DS., and L. V. Holdeman. 1968. The pathogenic anaerobic bacteria. Charles C Thomas, Publisher, Springfield, Ill.
5. Sutter, V. L., H. R. Attebery, J. E. Rosenblatt, K. S. Bricknell, and S. M. Finegold. 1972. Laboratory methods in anaerobic bacteriology. Department of Continuing Education in Health Sciences, University of California, Los Angeles.
6. Willis, A. T. 1969. Clostridia of wound infection. Butterworths, London.

Chapter 40
Anaerobic Cocci

WILLIAM J. MARTIN

GRAM-POSITIVE COCCI

Characterization

Because of the variability of the biochemical reactions of the anaerobic gram-positive cocci (2), the present classification systems generally are considered to be inadequate.

A recent classification of these bacteria has been developed by the Anaerobe Laboratory, Virginia Polytechnic Institute and State University (7). Gram-positive anaerobic cocci which occur in pairs and chains and require fermentable carbohydrates are classified as members of the genus *Ruminococcus*, of which there is one species, *R. bromii*. Members of the genera *Peptostreptococcus* and *Peptococcus*, on the other hand, do not require fermentable carbohydrates for growth. There presently are seven species in the genus *Peptococcus* and six species in the genus *Peptostreptococcus*. Of the latter, *P. elsdenii* is synonymous with *Megasphaera elsdenii*.

The anaerobic gram-positive cocci are part of the indigenous microflora of the oral cavity, skin, gastrointestinal tract, and genitourinary system (4, 5, 12, 15, 19). These organisms have been described as frequent causative agents in practically every type of human infection (5). Stokes (16) reviewed a 6-year experience with 496 anaerobic organisms and found approximately 200 gram-positive cocci in mixed culture and 100 in pure culture.

Collection of specimens

For a review of collection, transport, and storage of specimens, see chapter 38.

Direct examination

Gram stains should be performed on all specimens, except blood, submitted to the laboratory for anaerobic culture. Gram-positive cocci of the genus *Peptostreptococcus* may be spherical or elongated and occur singly, in pairs, or in chains. However, many of these same characteristics can describe members of the genus *Peptococcus*, the only exception perhaps being that the latter can occur in irregular clumps as well. Obviously, the Gram stain serves only to show the presence of coccus-like organisms in the specimen, and it remains for the subsequent culture procedures to determine whether these organisms are truly anaerobic, microaerophilic, or facultative.

Culture and isolation

With the exception of blood cultures (see chapter 43), all anaerobic specimens should be inoculated onto two 5% sheep blood-agar plates; one plate is incubated anaerobically and the other, under CO_2. In addition, one may find a phenylethyl alcohol-blood-agar plate (chapter 95) and a kanamycin-vancomycin-menadione-blood-agar plate (chapter 95) useful. The former is helpful in suppressing the gram-negative bacteria. The latter suppresses most facultative and anaerobic gram-positive flora and, therefore, is not recommended per se for the isolation of the anaerobic gram-positive cocci. However, because many specimens contain mixtures of both gram-negative and gram-positive anaerobic and facultative bacteria, the inclusion of a kanamycin-vancomycin-menadione plate provides a better perspective of the total flora. In addition, a broth medium (such as Schaedler's broth, supplemented thioglycolate broth, or chopped-meat broth with glucose) should be inoculated. At the Mayo Clinic, we have had good experience with thioglycolate broth (BBL 135-C) enriched with rabbit serum (1 to 2 ml/10 ml of broth).

After 48 to 72 h of anaerobic incubation, all plates and broth tubes should be checked grossly and microscopically for growth. The method described above has worked well in our laboratory (8) and therefore I feel I can recommend it. Readers should consult chapter 38 for additional methods of isolation.

Culture characteristics

On anaerobic blood-agar plates, species of *Peptococcus* or *Peptostreptococcus* appear as small (0.5 to 1 mm) gray to white colonies after 48 to 72 h of incubation. These colonies also may be convex, opaque, shiny, dull, and with entire edges. Occasional strains of both genera may be hemolytic or alpha-hemolytic. Pien et al. (13) reported that approximately half of their *Peptostreptococcus* species had a sharp, pungent odor that was not present with any of the *Peptococcus* species they studied. The remainder of their gram-positive anaerobic cocci had either a fecal or "petroleumlike" odor. This sharp, pungent odor was mentioned by Rogosa (14) as being a distinguishing characteristic for the genus *Peptostreptococcus*.

With pure cultures, growth in thioglycolate broth (BBL 135-C) generally shows small, discrete, compact colonies that grow uniformly throughout the medium. Gas may be produced. This type of growth appears to be characteristic for the majority of the anaerobic gram-positive cocci recovered from clinical material at the Mayo Clinic (unpublished data).

Microscope examination of culture growth

In clinical and bacteriological studies of anaerobic gram-positive cocci by Pien et al. (13), of 85 isolates studied microscopically, 9 (11%) appeared in chains characteristic of the genus *Peptostreptococcus*. The remaining strains appeared in clumps of gram-positive cocci suggestive of the genus *Peptococcus*. Included in this group were 22 organisms that appeared as diplococci and 15 that appeared as tetrads.

Biochemical reactions

The theoretical desirability of definitive speciation of all anaerobic cultures is well recognized. On the other hand, most clinical laboratories (including our own) must contend with practical considerations such as work volume, space, budgetary matters, and clinical requirements, so compromises are made. In this regard, the anaerobic cocci are not routinely speciated in many clinical laboratories. Mainly because the majority of these bacteria are biochemically unreactive (3, 7, 13, 18), the anaerobic gram-positive (and gram-negative) cocci isolated at the Mayo Clinic are routinely identified on the basis of their colonial morphology on anaerobic blood-agar plates, their microscopic morphology with the Gram stain, and, if needed, the catalase test (7). When identification to the species level is needed, three manuals (3, 7, 18) are excellent sources of information. Tables 1 and 2 show the biochemical characteristics and metabolic products identified by gas-liquid chromatography that are helpful in the speciation of the anaerobic gram-positive cocci found in human infections.

Susceptibility to antimicrobial agents

There have been relatively few in vitro studies of the susceptibilities of the anaerobic gram-positive cocci to antibiotics. Hare and associates (6) used the broth dilution technique to test 10 anaerobic cocci and found susceptibility to penicillin, chloramphenicol, and tetracycline with general resistance to streptomycin and polymyxin B. Finegold and associates tested approximately 20 strains of anaerobic cocci, most of which were *Peptostreptococcus*, by the agar dilution technique (S. M. Finegold, P. T. Sugihara, and A. B. Miller, Bacteriol. Proc., p. 96, 1967). Penicillin G and ampicillin were the most active drugs, inhibiting all strains at a concentration of 0.39 μg or less/ml. Cephalothin, oxacillin, erythromycin, lincomycin, and chloramphenicol also showed good activity, but tetracycline gave erratic results. Almost complete resistance was reported to both kanamycin and dihydrostreptomycin. Previously reported (9, 13) in vitro data (Tables 3 and 4) from this laboratory show that *Peptococcus* (145 isolates) and *Peptostreptococcus* (72 isolates) are susceptible to lincomycin, clindamycin, penicillin G, cephalothin, erythromycin, rifampin, and chloramphenicol. A few strains of *Peptococcus* required high concentrations of these antibiotics for inhibition. The susceptibility of *Peptococcus* to tetracycline was erratic. Both gentamicin and kanamycin showed poor activity against the anaerobic gram-positive cocci in vitro.

Evaluation

The majority of the anaerobic gram-positive cocci cultured at the Mayo Clinic (13) were biochemically unreactive, but they could be identified by morphology and to a lesser extent by gas-liquid chromatography (see Table 1 and chapter 39). Most infections caused by anaerobic gram-positive cocci supported the concept that these are opportunistic bacteria which, in cases of decreased local or systemic resistance, can produce clinical infection, especially in areas of normal habitation—the skin, oral cavity, genitourinary tract, and gastrointestinal system. Approximately 50% of the anaerobic cocci were isolated from surgical wound infections related to primarily abdominal or pelvic procedures. Skin infections such as hidradenitis suppurativa and infected epidermoid cysts produced several pure cultures of *Peptococcus*. Approximately 25% of these anaerobic isolates were from ischemic foot or leg ulcers. Only one isolate, a *Peptococcus* strain, was recovered from blood during the study period. In one-

TABLE 1. *Characteristics of members of the genus Peptococcus*[a]

Species	Hemolysis	Catalase	Indole production	Nitrate reduction	Gelatin liquefaction	Fermentation of: Cellobiose	Fructose (levulose)	Glucose	Lactose	Maltose	Sucrose	Esculin hydrolysis	Gas production	Products from peptone-yeast-glucose	Propionate from threonine	Growth stimulation with Tween 80
P. asaccharolyticus	−	−	+	−	−	−	−	−	−	−	−	−	+	Acetic, butyric; sometimes succinic, lactic, formic	−/+	+
P. constellatus	−	−	−	V	−	+	+	+	−	+	+	+	−	Lactic, acetic, formic, succinic	−	−
P. magnus	−	−	−	−	+	−	−	−	−	−	−	−	−	Acetic; sometimes lactic, succinic, formic	−	+
P. morbillorum	Sometimes beta	−	−	−	−	−	−	+	−	+	+	−	+/−	Lactic, acetic, formic	−	+
P. prevotii	Sometimes beta	V	−	−	−	−	−	−	−	−	−	−/+	−/+	Acetic, butyric; sometimes lactic, succinic, propionic, formic	−/+	+
P. variabilis	−	−	−	−	+	−	−	V	−	−	−	−	−/+	Acetic; sometimes lactic, succinic, propionic, butyric	−	+

[a] Adapted from Sutter et al. (18). Symbols: −, negative reaction; +, positive reaction; V, variable reaction.

TABLE 2. *Characteristics of members of the genus Peptostreptococcus*[a]

Species	Hemolysis	Catalase	Indole production	Nitrate reduction	Gelatin liquefaction	Fermentation of						Esculin hydrolysis	Gas production	Products from peptone-yeast-glucose	Propionate from threonine	Growth stimulation with Tween 80
						Cellobiose	Fructose (levulose)	Glucose	Lactose	Maltose	Sucrose					
P. anaerobius	Sometimes beta	–	–	–	–	–	+	+	–	–	–	–	+	Acetic, isovaleric; sometimes isobutyric, isocaproic, butyric, lactic, succinic, propionic, ethanol	+	+
P. intermedius	Sometimes alpha	–	–	–	–	+	+	+	+	+	+	+	+	Lactic; sometimes acetic, succinic, formic	–	+
P. micros	Sometimes beta	–	–	–	–	–	–	–	–	–	–	–	–/+	Acetic; sometimes lactic, succinic, formic	–	+
P. parvulus	–	–	–	–	+	–	–	+	+	–	–	–	+	Lactic, acetic; sometimes propionic, succinic, butyric	–	+
P. productus	Sometimes alpha or beta	–	–	–	–	+	+	+	+	+	+	+	+	Acetic, succinic; sometimes lactic, propionic	–	–

[a] Adapted from Sutter et al. (18). Symbols: –, negative reaction; + positive reaction.

TABLE 3. *In vitro susceptibility of 145 clinical isolates of the genus Peptococcus to 10 antibiotics*[a]

Antibiotic	Cumulative percent susceptible at increasing concentrations (μg/ml)									
	0.1	0.2	0.4	0.8	1.6	3.1	6.2	12.5	25	>25
Penicillin G	48	91	95	96	97	99		100		
Erythromycin	9	10	16	24	58	79	80	86	87	100
Cephalothin	22	38	56	78	88	89	97	98	99	100
Tetracycline	12	15	29	52	56	59	62	74	89	100
Lincomycin	29	45	69	92	95	96			97	100
Clindamycin	62	76	87	94	95	96	97			100
Kanamycin	1				2		4	13	44	100
Chloramphenicol	5	6	8	25	67	97	98		99	100
Gentamicin	2	3		5	7	11	30	62	95	100
Rifampin	47	50	62	76	96	98	99			100

[a] From Pien et al. (13).

TABLE 4. *In vitro susceptibility of 72 clinical isolates of the genus Peptostreptococcus to 10 antibiotics*[a]

Antibiotic	Cumulative percent susceptible at increasing concentrations (μg/ml)									
	0.1	0.2	0.4	0.8	1.6	3.1	6.2	12.5	25	>25
Penicillin G	58	91	97	98	100					
Erythromycin	37	39	46	56	73	88	92	99		100
Cephalothin	40	57	70	78	96		99		100	
Tetracycline	18	26	44	55	65	73	77	83	96	100
Lincomycin	39	58	72	85	96	100				
Clindamycin	81	85	90	98	100					
Kanamycin				1	5	11	12	23	44	100
Chloramphenicol		3	11	37	63	96	100			
Gentamicin	1	2	9	13	18	20	33	58	78	100
Rifampin	68			72	94		96			100

[a] From Pien et al. (13).

fourth of the cases, the anaerobic gram-positive coccus was grown either in pure culture or in the presence of *Corynebacterium* or *Staphylococcus epidermidis*, in one-fifth both anaerobic gram-positive cocci and *S. aureus* were cultured together from wound infections, and in one-fourth there was a mixed culture of anaerobic gram-positive cocci and *Bacteroides*. These observations are important because reports by other authors (10, 11) suggest that the anaerobic gram-positive cocci (especially *Peptostreptococcus*) act in synergism with *Bacteroides* or *S. aureus* to produce necrosis in infection.

In their recent report on anaerobic bacteremia, Wilson et al. (20) described 15 patients with blood cultures positive for anaerobic gram-positive cocci, and 5 of these had clinically significant bacteremia. In these five, *Peptococcus* sp. was isolated from two patients and *Peptostreptococcus* sp. from an additional two patients; the fifth patient had both *Peptococcus* and *Peptostreptococcus* (along with a *Bacteroides* sp.) in the blood. All five patients survived.

GRAM-NEGATIVE COCCI

Characterization

Although the seventh edition of *Bergey's Manual* (2) describes characteristics for six species of *Veillonella*, most of the current literature (3, 7, 18) refers to only two species: *V. alcalescens* and *V. parvula*. On the basis of the nitrate reduction reaction, Dowell and Hawkins (3) included an additional species group (*Veillonella* CDC group 3) consisting of 13 strains, whereas the investigators at the Anaerobe Research Laboratory of Virginia Polytechnic Institute (7) list not only the two species of *Veillonella* (*V. alcalescens* and *V. parvula*) but also the differential characteristics for the gram-negative anaerobic coccus described as *Acidaminococcus fermentans* (the former produce propionic and acetic acids, and the latter produce butyric and acetic acids).

Members of the genus *Veillonella* are small (0.3 to 0.4 μm in diameter), anaerobic, gram-negative cocci. They can occur in pairs, short chains, or masses. Good growth is obtained on most anaerobic culture media. Biochemical activity is considered to be pronounced. Whereas *Peptococcus* and *Peptostreptococcus* can be thought of as the anaerobic counterparts of *Staphylococcus* and *Streptococcus*, *Veillonella* can be considered the anaerobic counterpart of the genus *Neisseria*.

Veillonella is considered to be part of the indigenous microflora of the mouth. Also, these organisms usually are present as normal flora in the upper respiratory tract, intestines, and vagina (5, 19).

TABLE 5. *Characteristics of members of the genus Veillonella*[a]

Characteristic	*V. alcalescens*	*V. parvula*
Hemolysis	−	−
Catalase	+	−
Indole production	−	−
Nitrate reduction	+	+
Gelatin liquefaction	−	−
Fermentation of		
Cellobiose	−	−
Fructose (levulose)	−	−
Glucose	−	−
Lactose	−	−
Maltose	−	−
Sucrose	−	−
Esculin hydrolysis	−	−
Gas production	+	+
Products from peptone-yeast-glucose	Small amounts of acetic and propionic; sometimes lactic	
Propionate from threonine	−/+	−/+
Growth stimulation with Tween 80	−	−

[a] Adapted from Sutter et al. (18). Symbols: −, negative reaction; +, positive reaction.

There is little or no published information describing the clinical significance of the anaerobic gram-negative cocci. Because they are part of the indigenous microflora of the mouth, one would have to implicate these organisms in oral anaerobic infections such as periodontal disease and soft-tissue infections. These bacteria also are implicated in mixed anaerobic infections of the lung and pleural space (19).

Recently, Bartlett and Finegold (1) reported, in their extensive review of anaerobic pleuropulmonary infections, that *Veillonella* was isolated in mixed culture from four of their patients. These authors emphasized the importance of transtracheal aspiration (see chapter 38) for culturing anaerobes from this site because quantitative culture yielded *Bacteroides melaninogenicus*, *B. oralis*, *Fusobacterium* sp., and *Veillonella*, all at $>10^8$/ml.

Collection of specimens

The methods are the same as for gram-positive cocci.

Direct examination

See the information given for gram-positive cocci. Gram stains of specimens submitted to the laboratory for anaerobic culture that show gram-negative cocci in pairs, short chains, or irregular clumps should be interpreted as indicating members of the genus *Veillonella*.

Culture and isolation

Use the methods described for gram-positive cocci.

Culture characteristics

On anaerobic blood-agar plates, colonies of *Veillonella* will be small, translucent, convex, and glistening, with an entire edge, after 48 to 72 h of incubation. They are yellow to white.

TABLE 6. *In vitro susceptibility of 13 clinical isolates of the genus Veillonella to 10 antibiotics*[a]

Antibiotic	Cumulative percent susceptible at increasing concentrations (μg/ml)									
	0.1	0.2	0.4	0.8	1.6	3.1	6.2	12.5	25	>25
Penicillin G	23	77	100							
Erythromycin		8	16		23	31	38	69	77	100
Cephalothin	23	69		84	100					
Tetracycline	23		31	69	76	85			100	
Lincomycin	46	77			92		100			
Clindamycin	100									
Kanamycin	8						23	38	61	100
Chloramphenicol	15		23	46	85	100				
Gentamicin					8		31	46	85	100
Rifampin	23			31	100					

[a] Adapted from Martin et al. (9).

Unlike the anaerobic gram-positive cocci, *Veillonella* will grow on kanamycin-vancomycin-menadione-blood-agar plates. Growth of pure subcultures of *Veillonella* in thioglycolate broth will be of a light, diffuse type with small bubbles of gas usually suspended in the broth.

Microscope examination of culture growth

See direct examination, above.

Biochemical reactions

Tests that are helpful in the speciation of *Veillonella* are shown in Table 5.

Susceptibility to antimicrobial agents

In a recent in vitro study (9), 13 clinical isolates of *Veillonella* were susceptible to penicillin G, cephalothin, lincomycin, tetracycline, clindamycin, chloramphenicol, and rifampin (Table 6). Susceptibility to erythromycin was less than that shown with the anaerobic gram-positive cocci. Poor in vitro activity against the anaerobic gram-negative cocci was noted with gentamicin and kanamycin.

Evaluation

The role of anaerobic gram-negative cocci such as *Veillonella* in infection is unknown. These organisms are occasionally isolated from a wide variety of clinical specimens, usually together with other bacteria (1, 15, 17, 19). Recently, Wilson et al. (20) described the isolation of *Veillonella* from a 71-year-old man with acute myelomonocytic leukemia in whom polymicrobial bacteremia (*Veillonella* sp. and *Peptococcus*) developed.

In another recent study of the role of anaerobes in 226 cases of culture-proved empyema, Sullivan et al. (17) isolated *Veillonella* in mixed culture with other anaerobes from one patient who was defined in their retrospective series as "pulmonary, complicated."

Penicillin G and clindamycin are the drugs of choice.

LITERATURE CITED

1. Bartlett, J. G., and S. M. Finegold. 1972. Anaerobic pleuropulmonary infections. Medicine (Baltimore) **51**:413–450.
2. Breed, R. S., E. G. D. Murray, and N. R. Smith. 1957. Bergey's manual of determinative bacteriology, 7th ed. The Williams & Wilkins Co., Baltimore.
3. Dowell, V. R., Jr., and T. M. Hawkins. 1973. Laboratory methods in anaerobic bacteriology: CDC laboratory manual (Publication [HSM] 73-8222). Center for Disease Control, Atlanta, Ga.
4. Finegold, S. M., L. G. Miller, S. L. Merrill, and D. J. Posnick. 1965. Significance of anaerobic and capnophilic bacteria isolated from the urinary tract, p. 159–178. *In* E. H. Kass (ed.), Progress in pyelonephritis. F. A. Davis Co., Philadelphia.
5. Finegold, S. M., J. E. Rosenblatt, V. L. Sutter, and H. R. Attebery. 1972. Scope monograph on anaerobic infections. The Upjohn Co., Kalamazoo, Mich.
6. Hare, R., P. Wildy, F. S. Billett, and D. N. Twort. 1952. The anaerobic cocci: gas formation, fermentation reactions, sensitivity to antibiotics and sulphonamides; classification. J. Hyg. **50**:295–319.
7. Holdeman, L. V., and W. E. C. Moore. 1972. Anaerobe laboratory manual. Virginia Polytechnic Institute and State University, Blacksburg.
8. Martin, W. J. 1971. Practical method for isolation of anaerobic bacteria in the clinical laboratory. Appl. Microbiol. **22**:1168–1171.
9. Martin, W. J., M. Gardner, and J. A. Washington II. 1972. In vitro antimicrobial susceptibility of anaerobic bacteria isolated from clinical specimens. Antimicrob. Ag. Chemother. **1**:148–158.
10. Meleney, F. L. 1931. Bacterial synergism in disease processes: with a confirmation of the synergistic bacterial etiology of a certain type of progressive gangrene of the abdominal wall. Ann. Surg. **94**:961–981.
11. Mergenhagen, S. E., J. C. Thonard, and H. W. Scherp. 1958. Studies on synergistic infections. I. Experimental infections with anaerobic streptococci. J. Infect. Dis. **103**:33–44.
12. Moore, W. E. C., E. P. Cato, and L. V. Holdeman. 1969. Anaerobic bacteria of the gastrointestinal flora and their occurrence in clinical infections. J. Infect. Dis. **119**:641–649.
13. Pien, F. D., R. L. Thompson, and W. J. Martin. 1972. Clinical and bacteriological studies of anaerobic gram-positive cocci. Mayo Clin. Proc. **47**:251–257.
14. Rogosa, M. 1971. *Peptococcaceae*, a new family to include the gram-positive, anaerobic cocci of the genera *Peptococcus*, *Peptostreptococcus*, and *Ruminococcus*. Int. J. Syst. Bacteriol. **21**:234–237.
15. Smith, L. DS., and L. V. Holdeman. 1968. The pathogenic anaerobic bacteria. Charles C Thomas, Publisher, Springfield, Ill.
16. Stokes, E. J. 1958. Anaerobes in routine diagnostic cultures. Lancet **1**:668–670.
17. Sullivan, K. M., R. D. O'Toole, R. H. Fisher, K. N. Sullivan. 1973. Anaerobic empyema thoracis. Arch. Intern. Med. **131**:521–527.
18. Sutter, V. L., H. R. Attebery, J. E. Rosenblatt, K. S. Bricknell, and S. M. Finegold. 1972. Anaerobic bacteriology manual. Department of Continuing Education in Health Sciences University Extension, and the School of Medicine, U.C.L.A., Los Angeles, Calif.
19. Thomas, C. G. A., and R. Hare. 1954. The classification of anaerobic cocci and their isolation in normal human beings and pathological processes. J. Clin. Pathol. **7**:300–304.
20. Wilson, W. R., W. J. Martin, C. J. Wilkowske, and J. A. Washington II. 1972. Anaerobic bacteremia. Mayo Clin. Proc. **47**:639–646.

Chapter 41

Gram-Negative Nonsporeforming Anaerobic Bacilli

VERA L. SUTTER, HOWARD R. ATTEBERY, AND SYDNEY M. FINEGOLD

The bacteria considered in this chapter are members of the genera *Bacteroides*, *Fusobacterium*, *Butyrivibrio*, *Campylobacter*, *Selenomonas*, and *Leptotrichia*. They are part of the normal flora of humans and animals, and are found in the mouth, upper respiratory tract, intestinal tract, and urogenital tract.

Differentiation of these genera is based on motility, morphology, and identification of metabolic end products by gas-liquid chromatography as shown in Table 1. Further definition of species is based on a battery of biochemical characteristics. However, rapid presumptive identification of those most commonly found (*Bacteroides* and *Fusobacterium*) can often be made on the basis of a few observations such as colonial morphology and fluorescence, cellular morphology and arrangement, a few biochemical characteristics, and susceptibility to certain antibiotics.

After presumptive identification, more definitive identification may be attempted to establish the validity of the presumptive identification. It is often difficult to distinguish between widely divergent taxonomic groups of bacteria on the basis of a few tests. Definitive identification is often helpful in the event of recurrent illness to establish whether a particular infection is a new process or a relapse of a previous condition. Additionally, exact species definition of isolates from various infections is needed to establish which anaerobes are significant in particular types of infections.

BACTEROIDES AND FUSOBACTERIUM

Preliminary tests and observations for rapid, presumptive identification of members of the genera *Bacteroides* and *Fusobacterium*, in addition to colonial and microscopic morphology (Fig. 1–4), are as follows.

From a pure culture on a blood-agar plate:

1. Do a spot indole test by removing a loopful of growth and smearing on filter paper saturated with 1% paradimethyl-aminocinnamaldehyde in 10% (vol/vol) hydrochloric acid. A positive reaction is indicated by the development of a blue color around the growth (4). Negative reactions should be checked by conventional indole tests.
2. Inoculate supplemented thioglycolate medium. Incubate for 4 to 6 h or overnight if necessary. Turbidity should be half that of the No. 1 McFarland standard (2).
   a. Make Gram stain. Test for motility.
   b. Antibiotic disk identification procedure. Swab inoculum from thioglycolate culture evenly over the surface of two blood-agar plates. Place disks of colistin (10 μg), erythromycin (60 μg), kanamycin (1,000 μg), penicillin (2 units), rifampin (15 μg), and vancomycin (5 μg), using three disks per plate. (Erythromycin, kanamycin, and rifampin disks are temporarily available from Bioquest.) Incubate anaerobically for 48 h. Measure and record zones of inhibition.
   c. Lipase reaction and catalase tests. Streak culture to an egg yolk-agar plate and incubate anaerobically up to 1 week. Expose the plate to the air for 30 min or more and perform a catalase test (chapter 96). Observe for lipase production. Lipase production is indicated by a fine white precipitate over the surface of the growth, with a mother-of-pearl iridescence at the edge.
   d. Since further testing may be desirable, hold thioglycolate tube for inoculation of additional differential media.

From results of the above tests, a preliminary group determination can usually be made.

Characteristics of *Bacteroides* species most common in clinical specimens are indicated in Table 2. On initial isolation, *B. corrodens* forms characteristic colonies which corrode and pit the agar (Fig. 5). Young colonies are pinpoint and nondescript, but further incubation (5 days or longer) usually results in this distinctive feature. This species is negative in the reactions of the preliminary tests and is inhibited by all of the antibiotic disks used for identification ex-

TABLE 1. *Differentiation of genera of gram-negative nonsporulating bacilli*

Characteristic	Genus
A. Nonmotile or peritrichous flagella	
1. No butyric acid produced in absence of isobutyric and isovaleric acids	*Bacteroides*
2. Butyric acid produced as major metabolic product	*Fusobacterium*
3. Lactic acid only as a major metabolic product	*Leptotrichia*
B. Motile with polar flagella	
1. Nonfermentative	*Campylobacter*
2. Fermentative, producing butyric acid as major metabolic product	*Butyrivibrio*
C. Motile, with lateral tufts of flagella	*Selenomonas*

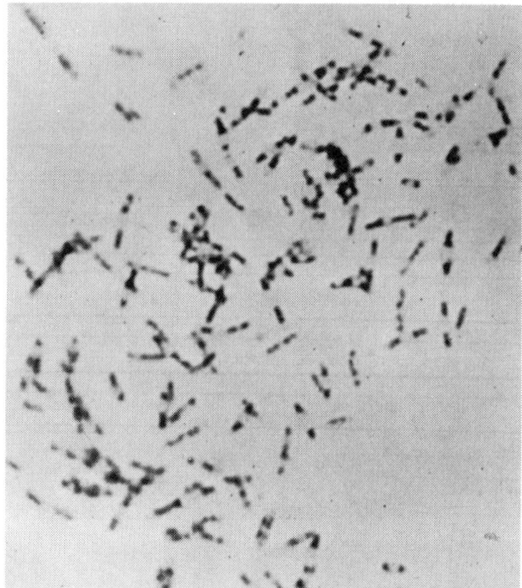

FIG. 1. *Microscopic morphology of Bacteroides fragilis. Note irregularity of staining and moderate pleomorphism.*

cept vancomycin. *Eikenella*, a facultative organism, may pit the agar similarly under anaerobic conditions.

Group definition of *B. fragilis* can be made on the basis of the characteristic reactions shown in Table 2. (A preliminary report indicates that presumptive identification of *B fragilis* can be made with tests for two characteristics: growth on bile and lack of inhibition of growth by disks containing kanamycin, 100 μg (Vargo et al., Abstr. Annu. Meet. Amer. Soc. Microbiol. 1973, p. 84). Further identification into subspecies may be made by utilizing fermentation reactions in a few carbohydrates (1, 3, 4).

B. melaninogenicus and *B. oralis* are similar in their reactions in the preliminary group tests. They may be distinguished by the brick-red fluorescence under ultraviolet light and/or black colony formation exhibited by *B. melaninogenicus* (Fig. 6).

Reactions and characteristics of some of the more common *Fusobacterium* species are given in Table 2. *F. mortiferum* does not produce indole, whereas *F. varium* often does. These two species also may be distinguished by the ability of *F. mortiferum* to hydrolyze esculin, which *F. varium* is unable to do. Other simple tests which have been found useful in characterizing nonsporeforming gram-negative bacilli are those which depend on the ability of some to grow in bile with deoxycholate or in deoxycholate (Table 3).

In addition to tests already mentioned, verification of the presumptive identification should include tests for fermentation of carbohydrates, analysis of metabolic end products from glucose, lactate, and threonine, reduction of nitrate, and hydrolysis of gelatin and starch. Characteristics of the commonly encountered *Bacteroides* and *Fusobacterium* species are shown in Table 3.

Immunoserological methods for the identification of these bacteria are presently not practical, although they are being worked on in a number of laboratories.

Data on susceptibility of *Bacteroides* and

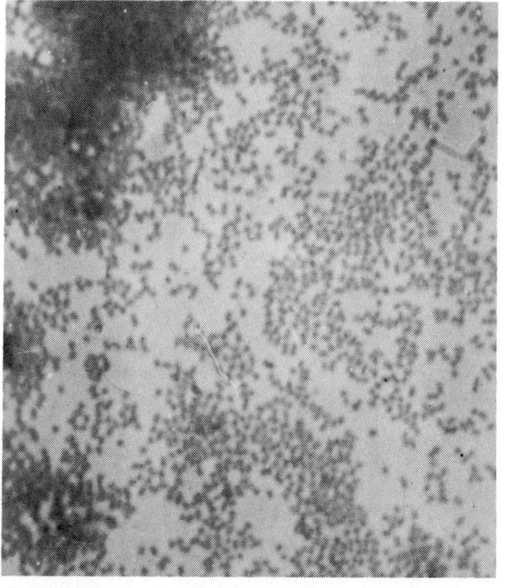

FIG. 2. *Microscopic morphology of Bacteroides melaninogenicus. Organisms are coccobacillary.*

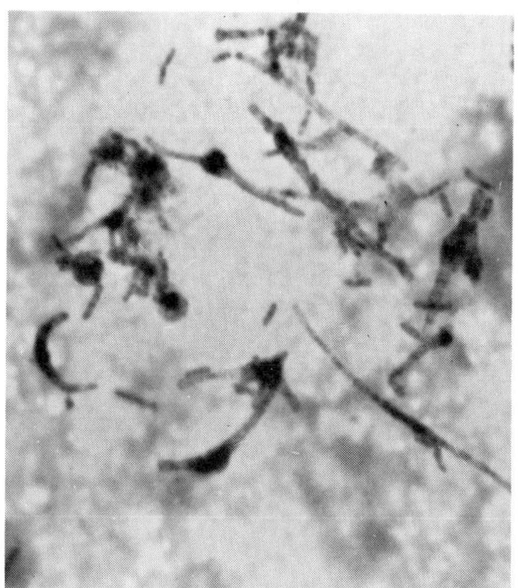

FIG. 3. *Microscopic morphology of Fusobacterium mortiferum. There is marked pleomorphism and irregularity of staining. Note filaments with swellings along their course.*

Fusobacterium species to antibacterial agents are given in Table 4. *B. oralis*, which is of questionable significance clinically, is generally susceptible to most drugs useful against anaerobic infections. Limited data are available on *B. corrodens;* it appears susceptible to penicillin G, tetracycline, chloramphenicol, clindamycin, and metronidazole.

MISCELLANEOUS ANAEROBIC GRAM-NEGATIVE RODS

Leptotrichia buccalis

These organisms are nonmotile rods that have a cell wall structure characteristic of gram-negative bacteria. Young cells, however, stain gram-positive and older cells frequently show gram-positive granules. Gram-variable and gram-positive cells are common. *L. buccalis* has pleomorphic cellular morphology. Broth cultures usually show forms with a filamentous appearance with chains of cells intertwining to give a ropelike appearance (Fig. 7). Filaments up to 200 μm in length can be found. In young cultures, the typical configuration is two cells linked together. The cells frequently have pointed ends and therefore can be confused with fusobacteria. True branching has not been demonstrated, but false branching may occasionally be seen.

Surface colonies of *L. buccalis* on solid media may have a convoluted surface resembling that of the brain (Fig. 8). These organisms require anaerobic to microaerophilic conditions for isolation. Rarely will they grow aerobically even with repeated subculture. Carbon dioxide (10%) stimulates growth. These organisms are catalase-negative. They are saccharolytic, producing lactic acid as the major acid product from fermentation of glucose, fructose, lactose, maltose, mannose, and sucrose. Gas is produced from carbohydrates that are fermented. The organism does not liquefy gelatin or produce indole.

L. buccalis should not be confused with *Bacterionema matruchotii* (*Leptotrichia dentium*), a gram-positive branched rod that grows aerobically, or with *Fusobacterium*, which produces butyric acid as the major acid product from the fermentation of glucose.

The habitat of *L. buccalis* is the oral cavity of humans. *L. buccalis* is not known to be pathogenic but may be mixed with other bacteria in material from infections in or near the oral cavity, and it is occasionally found in clinical material from urogenital areas.

Campylobacter (Vibrio)

These microaerophilic curved rods were first assigned to the genus *Vibrio* but later studies have shown that they differ appreciably from the type species of the genus, *V. cholerae*. The genus *Campylobacter* comprises the gram-negative slender and curved bacteria which are

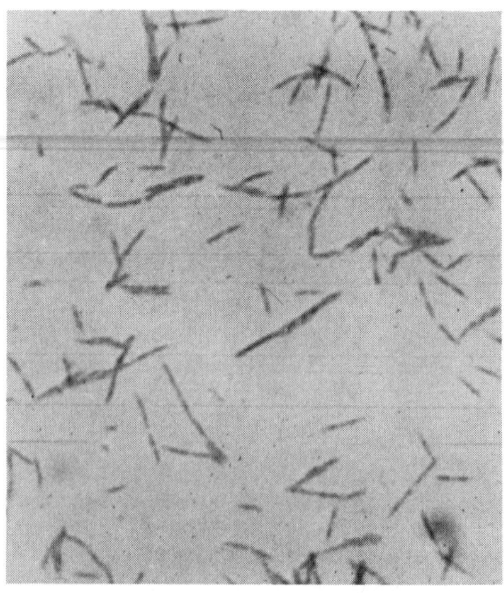

FIG. 4. *Microscopic morphology of Fusobacterium nucleatum. Organisms are thin and delicate with tapered ends. There is little pleomorphism.*

TABLE 2. *Characteristics of some Bacteroides and Fusobacterium species*[a]

Species	Colony morphology on blood-agar	Microscopic morphology	Motility	Indole	Catalase	Lipase	Susceptibility to					
							Colistin, 10 μg	Erythromycin, 60 μg	Kanamycin, 1,000 μg	Penicillin, 2 units	Rifampin, 15 μg	Vancomycin, 5 μg
B. corrodens	Pinpoint with edges spreading and eroding into agar (5 days or more)	Gram-negative bacilli, rounded ends	–	–	–	–	S	S	S	S	S	R
B. fragilis	Convex, white to gray, translucent, glistening	Gram-negative bacilli, rounded ends, may be pleomorphic	–	–/+	–/+	–	R	S	R	R^s	S	R
B. melaninogenicus	Convex, brick-red fluorescence under ultraviolet light (2 days); brown to black pigment (5–7 days)	Gram-negative, often coccobacillary	–	–/+	–	–/+	S/R	S	R	S	S	S/R
B. oralis	Convex, yellowish, translucent, glistening	Gram-negative bacilli, rounded ends	–	–	–	–	S/R	S	R	S	S	R
F. mortiferum and *F. varium*	Flat to convex, opaque center with translucent, irregular edge, "fried egg"	Gram-negative bacilli, highly pleomorphic, with round bodies	–	–/+	–	–	S	R	S	S^r	R	R
F. necrophorum	Convex, umbonate, opaque center with translucent edge	Gram-negative bacilli with rounded to tapered ends, pleomorphic	–	+	–	+	S	S^r	S	S	S	R
F. nucleatum	Convex, glistening with internal iridescent flecking, or raised opaque "bread crumb" colonies	Gram-negative bacilli, slender, with tapered ends	–	+	–	–	S	S^r	S	S	S	R

[a] Reprinted, with minor modifications, from *Progress in Clinical Pathology*, vol. 5, chapter 11, 1973 (Grune and Stratton, New York) with the kind permission of the publishers. Key: +, positive; –, negative; S, susceptible (zones ≧ 10 mm); R, resistant (zones < 10 mm); R^s, usually resistant, occasionally susceptible; S^r, usually susceptible, occasionally resistant.

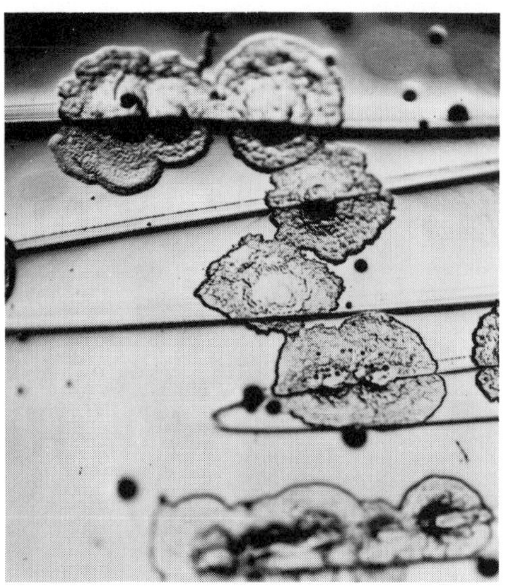

FIG. 5. *Colonies of Bacteroides corrodens, showing etching of agar around colonies.*

motile by means of a single, polar flagellum. All are microaerophilic and do not grow aerobically as surface colonies or under strictly anaerobic conditions. They do not ferment carbohydrates.

Four groups are found in association with humans. *C. fetus fetus*, which is a frequent cause of abortion in sheep and cattle, is sometimes responsible for bacteremia, endocarditis, or enteritis in humans. *C. fetus venerealis intermedius*, whose principal habitat appears to be the genital tract of cattle, occasionally produces human infections. *C. coli*, which is a normal inhabitant of the intestine of swine, poultry, and occasionally of humans, can occasionally be pathogenic for humans, causing bloody diarrhea. *C. sputorum sputorum* has the human mouth as its principal habitat and may occasionally be found in clinical infections. Its pathogenic status is questionable.

For isolation of *Campylobacter*, a Brucella agar plate with 10% defibrinated animal blood, 2 units of bacitracin/ml, and 2 μg of novobiocin/ml is recommended. Brucella broth containing 0.16% agar and tubed in deep tubes is a good liquid medium. Broth tubes can be incubated aerobically if the medium is fresh. Prereduced anaerobically sterilized medium is usually not suitable for growth of the *Campylobacter* species except *C. sputorum*.

Directions for culture and speciation are given in detail elsewhere (1, 5).

Table 5 represents a key for speciation of the genus *Campylobacter*, and chapter 97 contains the media formulations for the needed tests.

Butyrivibrio fibrisolvens.

These organisms are gram-negative slightly curved rods, 0.5 by 2 to 5 μm, with ends usually tapered. The organism is motile by means of a monotrichous flagellum, but motility may be inhibited by some media. Also, preparations for motility must not be exposed to air, even briefly. Cells produce large amounts of butyric acid from the fermentation of fructose, glucose, maltose, cellobiose, sucrose, lactose, xylose, and galactose. Hydrogen gas is produced from fermentations.

B. fibrisolvens is extremely oxygen-sensitive and is isolated by the use of anaerobic chamber techniques or PRAS roll-tube methods. *B. fibrisolvens* has been reported from the intestinal tract of humans (1) and from clinical material. Its role as a pathogen has not been established.

Selenomonas sputigena

This organism occurs commonly in the oral cavity of humans. It is readily identified with suitable stains that show a tuft of flagella on the concave side of the crescent-shaped cell (Fig. 9). *S. sputigena* is saccharolytic, producing lactic acid as the main fermentation product from glucose. It does not reduce nitrate. It has been isolated from clinical material, but is not established as a pathogen. Experimental animals given intraperitoneal or intravenous injections of pure cultures of isolates from the oral cavity of humans only rarely develop a fatal infection.

OCCURRENCE IN CLINICAL MATERIAL AND SIGNIFICANCE

Gram-negative anaerobic bacilli are the most commonly encountered anaerobes in clinical infection; they are found in somewhat more than half of specimens yielding anaerobes. *B.*

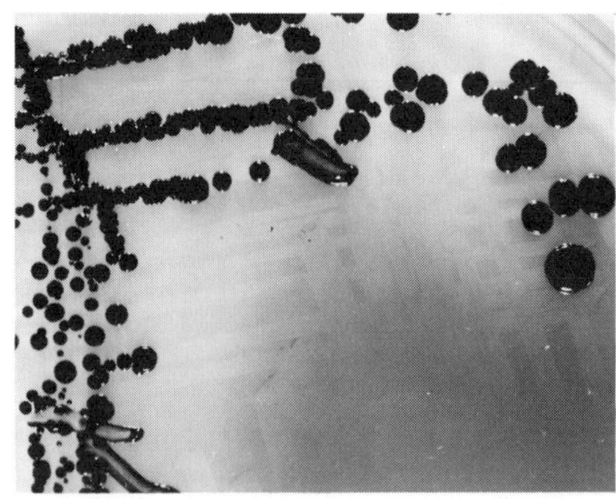

FIG. 6. *Colonies of Bacteroides melaninogenicus. Note black pigmentation.*

TABLE 3. *Definitive characteristics of commonly encountered Bacteroides and Fusobacterium species*[a]

Species	Fermentation of carbohydrates															Hydrolysis of			Effect of		Reduction of nitrate	Production of indole	Conversion of lactate to propionate	Conversion of threonine to propionate	Fatty acids produced[b]
	Amygdalin	Arabinose	Cellobiose	Glucose	Lactose	Levulose	Maltose	Mannitol	Mannose	Melezitose	Raffinose	Rhamnose	Sucrose	Trehalose	Xylose	Esculin	Gelatin	Starch	20% bile + 0.1% deoxycholate	0.1% deoxycholate					
BACTEROIDES																									
corrodens	–	–	–	–	–	–	–	–	–	–	–	–	–	–	–	–	–	–	N	N/S	+	–	–	–	A,L,S
fragilis																									
ss[c] *distasonis*	w^{+}	$+^{-}$	+/–	$+^{w}$	$+^{w}$	$+^{w}$	$+^{w}$	–	$+^{w}$	+/–	$+^{w}$	+/–	$+^{w}$	w^{+}	$+^{w}$	+	$-^{+}$	+/–	S	I	–	–	–	–	A,P,S (IB,IV,L)
ss *fragilis*	w^{+}	–	$-^{w}$	$+^{w}$	w^{+}	$+^{w}$	$+^{w}$	–	$+^{w}$	–	$+^{w}$	–	$+^{w}$	–	$+^{w}$	+	$-^{w}$	+	S	I	–	–	$-^{+}$	–	A,P,S (IB,IV,L)
ss *ovatus*	w^{+}	w^{+}	w^{+}	$+^{w}$	$+^{w}$	$+^{w}$	$+^{w}$	w	$+^{w}$	$-^{w}$	$+^{-}$	+/–	$+^{w}$	+/–	$+^{w}$	+	$-^{w}$	+	S	I	–	+	$-^{+}$	–	A,S (P,IB,IV,L)
ss *thetaiotaomicron*	$+^{w}$	$+^{w}$	$+^{-}$	+	$+^{w}$	$+^{w}$	$+^{w}$	–	$+^{w}$	+/–	$+^{w}$	+/–	$+^{w}$	$+^{-}$	$+^{w}$	+	$-^{w}$	+	S	I	–	+	$-^{+}$	–	A,S (P,IB,IV,L)
ss *vulgatus*	+/–	$+^{-}$	$-^{w}$	$+^{w}$	$+^{w}$	$+^{w}$	$+^{w}$	–	$+^{w}$	–	$+^{w}$	$+^{w}$	$+^{w}$	–	$+^{w}$	$+^{-}$	$-^{+}$	$+^{-}$	S	I	–	–	–	–	A,S (P,IB,IV,L)
melaninogenicus																									
ss *asaccharolyticus*	–	–	–	–	–	–	–	–	–	–	–	–	–	–	–	–	+	–	I	I	$-^{+}$	$+^{-}$	$-^{+}$	–	A,IB,B,IV (P,L,S)
ss *intermedius*	w^{-}	$-^{w}$	–	$+^{w}$	$-^{+}$	+/–	+/–	–	+/–	–	$-^{+}$	–	+/–	$-^{w}$	$-^{w}$	–	+	$+^{-}$	I	I	–	$+^{-}$	$-^{+}$	–	A,IB,IV,S
ss *melaninogenicus*	$+^{-}$	w^{-}	$+^{-}$	+	+	+	+	–	+	–	+	$-^{w}$	+	–	$-^{w}$	$+^{-}$	+	+	I	I	–	–	–	–	L,S (A,IB,IV)
oralis	$+^{w}$	–	$+^{-}$	$+^{w}$	$+^{w}$	$+^{w}$	$+^{-}$	–	$+^{w}$	$-^{w}$	$+^{w}$	$-^{+}$	$+^{w}$	$-^{w}$	$-^{w}$	$+^{-}$	$+^{-}$	+	I	I	–	–	–	–	A,S (IB,IV,L)
FUSOBACTERIUM																									
mortiferum	$-^{w}$	–	w^{-}	$+^{w}$	w^{+}	w^{+}	w^{-}	–	w^{+}	–	+/–	–	+/–	$-^{w}$	$-^{+}$	+	–	$-^{w}$	N	N	–	–	–	+	A,P,B (IV,L,S)
necrophorum	–	–	–	$-^{w}$	–	$-^{w}$	–	–	–	–	–	–	–	–	–	–	+/–	–	I^{N}	I	–	+	+	+	A,P,B (L,S)
nucleatum	–	–	–	$-^{w}$	–	w^{-}	–	–	–	–	–	–	–	–	–	–	$-^{w}$	–	I	I	–	+	–	+	A,P,B,S (L)
varium	–	–	–	w^{+}	–	w	–	–	w	–	–	–	–	–	–	–	$-^{w}$	–	N	N	–	$+^{-}$	–	+	A,B,L (P,S)

[a] Material for this table is taken from references 1 and 4. Key: –, negative reaction or pH above 6.0 in carbohydrate fermentations; w, weak reaction or pH 5.6 to 6.0 in carbohydrate fermentations; +, positive reaction or pH 5.5 or less in carbohydrate fermentations; S, stimulated growth; I, inhibited growth (not necessarily complete inhibition); N, no effect on growth. See reference 1 for additional comments.

[b] Fatty acids: A, acetic; P, propionic; IB, isobutyric; B, butyric; IV, isovaleric; L, lactic; S, succinic; ( ), variable. No quantitation of fatty acids is implied.

[c] Subspecies.

TABLE 4. *Susceptibility of gram-negative anaerobic rods to antimicrobial agents*[a]

Agent	*Bacteroides fragilis*	*B. melaninogenicus*	*Fusobacterium varium*	Other *Fusobacterium* spp.
Penicillin G[b]	+	++++	+++	++++
Lincomycin	+ to ++	+++	++	+++
Clindamycin	+++	+++	++	+++
Metronidazole	+++	+++	++	+++
Chloramphenicol	+++	+++	+++	+++
Tetracycline[c]	+ to ++	+++	++	++ to +++
Erythromycin	+	++	+	+
Vancomycin	+	+	+	+

[a] Only drugs which might be useful therapeutically are included; not all of these agents have been used clinically for anaerobic infections and not all are Food and Drug Administration approved. Symbols: +, poor or inconsistent activity; ++, moderate activity; +++, good activity; ++++, drug of choice.

[b] Other penicillins and cephalosporins may show differences in activity.

[c] Doxycycline and minocycline are more active.

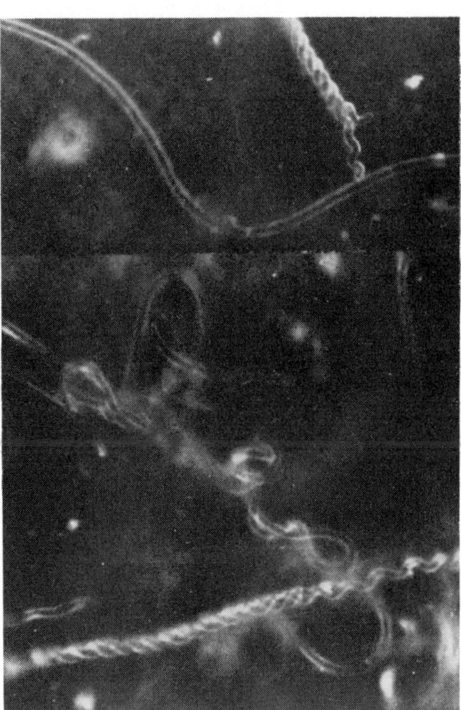

FIG. 7. *Leptotrichia buccalis. Dark-field illumination. "Ropelike" intertwining filaments from a broth culture.*

fragilis is by far the most commonly recovered anaerobe of all types. It is a well-established pathogen and is more resistant to antimicrobial agents than any other anaerobe. To some extent, the frequency with which *B. fragilis* is isolated may relate to the relative ease with

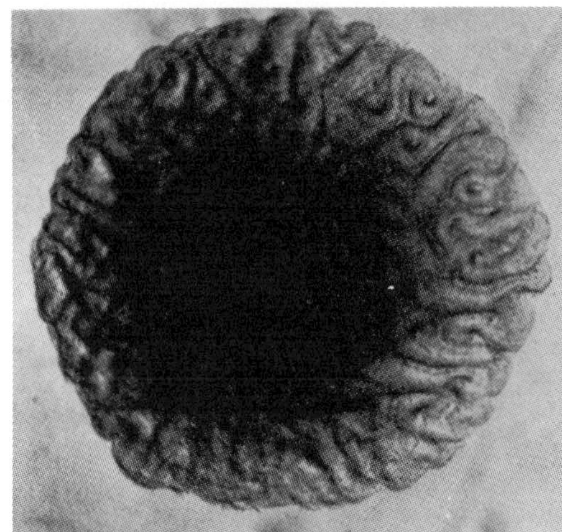

FIG. 8. *Leptotrichia buccalis colony showing irregular surface with convolutions.*

TABLE 5. *Key for speciation of human-associated species of Campylobacter*[a]

Catalase	Growth in 1% glycine	H_2S production[b]	Growth at 25 C	Species
+	+	–	+	*C. fetus fetus*
+	–	–	+	*C. fetus venerealis* biotype *intermedius*
–	Weak	+	–	*C. sputorum sputorum*
+	+	Variable	–	*C. coli*

[a] Characteristics from Veron and Chatelain (5).

[b] Standard medium.

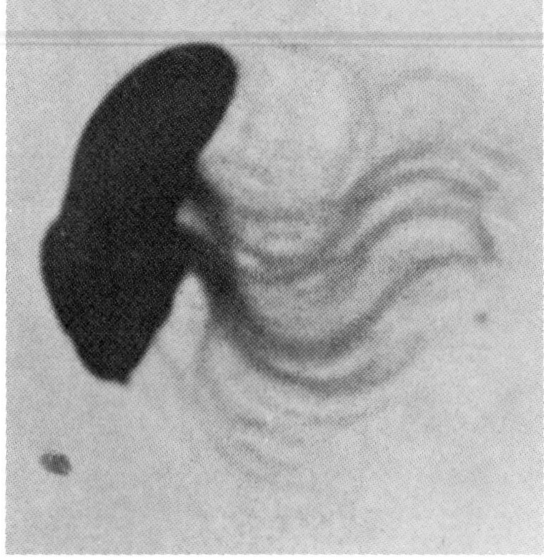

FIG. 9. *Microscopic morphology of Selenomonas. Tufts of flagella on the concave side are characteristic of the genus.*

which it is grown and maintained in culture for identification. Nevertheless, this organism is a dominant member of the normal colonic flora and is involved in infection very often. *B. capillosus* is closely related to *B. fragilis* and may represent a variant of this species. Of the subspecies of *B. fragilis*, subspecies *fragilis* will probably be found to contain most of the pathogenic strains. *B. melaninogenicus*, on the basis of theoretical and experimental data, is probably a key pathogen in mixed anaerobic infections; however, it is difficult to recover and to isolate and is undoubtedly overlooked often. The other two *Bacteroides* species which may be encountered in clinical specimens with some frequency are *B. oralis* and *B. corrodens*. Of the two, *B. corrodens* is probably more pathogenic. *B. oralis* is encountered more often, but is typically found as part of a mixed culture and its pathogenicity is not established.

Next to *B. fragilis*, the gram-negative anaerobic bacillus most commonly recovered from clinical infections is *Fusobacterium nucleatum*. *F. necrophorum*, formerly very commonly encountered, is seen much less frequently since the advent of the antimicrobial era. Other fusobacteria seen with some frequency are *F. mortiferum* and *F. varium*, the latter important because it is relatively resistant to antimicrobials including, at times, penicillin and clindamycin.

Gram-negative anaerobic bacilli of other genera are encountered rarely and are seldom clinically significant, with the exception of *Campylobacter*.

LITERATURE CITED

1. Anaerobe Laboratory. 1972. Outline of clinical methods in anaerobic bacteriology. Virginia Polytechnic Institute, Blacksburg.
2. Bauer, A. W., W. M. M. Kirby, J. C. Sherris, and M. Turck. 1966. Antibiotic susceptibility testing by a single disc method. Amer. J. Clin. Pathol. **45**:493–496.
3. Dowell, V. R., Jr., and T. M. Hawkins. 1973. Laboratory methods in anaerobic bacteriology. CDC Laboratory Manual, Publication No. (HSM) 73-8222. Center for Disease Control, Atlanta, Ga.
4. Sutter, V. L., H. R. Attebery, J. E. Rosenblatt, K. Bricknell, and S. M. Finegold. 1972. Anaerobic bacteriology manual. Extension Division, University of California, Los Angeles.
5. Veron, M., and R. Chatelain. 1973. Taxonomic study of the genus *Campylobacter* Sebald and Veron and designation of the neotype strain for the type species *Campylobacter fetus* (Smith and Taylor) Sebald and Veron. Int. J. Syst. Bacteriol. **23**:122–134.

Chapter 42

Gram-Positive, Nonsporeforming Anaerobic Bacilli

V. R. DOWELL, JR., AND ALEX C. SONNENWIRTH

Gram-positive, nonsporeforming, anaerobic bacilli which may be encountered in clinical specimens include species of *Actinomyces*, *Arachnia*, *Bifidobacterium*, *Eubacterium*, *Lactobacillus*, and *Propionibacterium* (6, 12). Most are obligate anaerobes, but some are capnophiles (microaerophilic) or facultative anaerobes (16). Essentially all are normal inhabitants of the mucous membrane surfaces or the skin of humans (chapter 38). Although a large number of species have been described (5), some are no longer recognized (6, 16), and only a limited number are commonly isolated from properly collected clinical specimens (6).

There have been numerous changes in the taxonomy of this group in recent years. The genera *Catenabacterium*, *Cillobacterium*, and *Ramibacterium* are no longer recognized, some species of the genus *Corynebacterium* are now included in *Propionibacterium*, and species formerly in *Ramibacterium* and *Cillobacterium* are classified in *Eubacterium* (16). A new genus, *Arachnia*, was proposed for the organism formerly described as *Actinomyces propionicus* (18). *Catenabacterium filamentosum*, *Bacteroides terebrans*, and *Bacteroides ramosum* were shown to produce spores, and these are now classified as *Clostridium ramosum* (11).

The organism originally described as *Actinomyces eriksonii* (10) will be listed in the 8th edition of *Bergey's Manual* as Species Incertae Sedis in the family *Actinomycetaceae*. However, on the basis of similarity in end products from glucose fermentation and cell wall analysis, coupled with some evidence of serological cross-reactions, it could be considered a species of *Bifidobacterium* (L. K. Georg, personal communication). The name *Bifidobacterium eriksonii* is now commonly used (6, 12, 24). A list of present and former names of some common species is given in Table 1.

The cellular morphology of actinomyces, arachnia, bifidobacteria, eubacteria, lactobacilli, and propionibacteria, although sometimes distinctive, is usually highly variable and dependent on the culture medium and growth conditions. Microscopically, these bacteria can easily be confused with others such as clostridia, corynebacteria, erysipelothrix, listeria, nocardia, leptotrichia, peptostreptococci, and streptococci. Morphological forms include: (i) small rods, with or without metachromatic staining; (ii) large, plump, evenly stained rods; (iii) club-shaped rods; (iv) rods with bifurcated (bifid) ends; and (v) thin filaments, with or without branching (Table 2). Some show zigzag chains of cells, and "Chinese-letter" configurations are common in others (5).

Differentiation of gram-positive, nonsporeforming bacilli from certain streptococci (e.g., *Streptococcus mutans*) and peptostreptococci (e.g., *Peptostreptococcus productus*; 12) can be difficult. Under certain conditions, especially on agar media, these cocci may form rod-shaped cells which are very similar to bacilli. The tendency of some bifidobacteria, eubacteria, lactobacilli, and propionibacteria to form short coccoid rods resembling cocci can present problems in identification. The failure of certain clostridia (*C. perfringens*, *C. ramosum*) to produce spores readily on ordinary media can also be troublesome. Some nonsporeforming, gram-positive, anaerobic bacilli tend to lose their affinity for crystal violet when stained by the Gram method, and this can lead to incorrect identification of an isolate as a *Bacteroides* or *Fusobacterium* species. Conversely, isolates of *Fusobacterium nucleatum* and *F. necrophorum* are rather frequently submitted to the Center for Disease Control as suspected *Actinomyces*. For these reasons, careful examination of Gram-stained smears of cultures (liquid and agar media) in various stages of growth and a careful search for spores are necessary in the identification of the nonsporeforming, gram-positive, anaerobic bacilli. Use of egg yolk agar can be helpful in differentiating the clostridia from these organisms; none of the nonsporeforming bacilli produces lecithinase and only a few produce lipase on egg yolk

TABLE 1. *Present and former names of some common species of gram-positive, nonsporeforming, anaerobic bacilli*

Present name	Former name(s)
Actinomyces viscosus	*Odontomyces viscosus*
Arachnia propionica	*Actinomyces propionicus*
Bifidobacterium eriksonii	*Actinomyces eriksonii*
Eubacterium alactolyticum	*Ramibacterium alactolyticum*, *Ramibacterium pleuriticum*
Eubacterium lentum	*Corynebacterium diphtheroides*, *Bifidobacterium cornutum*, *Corynebacterium* species CDC group 3 (6)
Propionibacterium acnes	*Corynebacterium acnes*
Propionibacterium granulosum	*Corynebacterium granulosum*

medium. Examination of metabolic products by gas liquid chromatography is the most reliable technique for differentiation of genera (6, 16). The catalase test is helpful in separating *A. propionica* from the propionibacteria (Fig. 1).

Although disease involving gram-positive, nonsporeforming, anaerobic bacilli is not as common as that caused by *Bacteroides fragilis*, *Clostridium perfringens*, and certain other anaerobes, these organisms can cause a variety of human illnesses, either alone or in combination with other bacteria (5). Some of the more important include actinomycosis (cervicofacial, pleuropulmonary, intra-abdominal), brain abscess, endocarditis, liver abscess, lung abscess, osteomyelitis, peridontal disease, and infections following human or animal bites (1, 4, 5, 7, 8; chapter 38). Essentially all are endogenous infections (12, 21, 28; *Anaerobic Bacteria: Role in Disease*, chapters 19 and 34, A. Balows, R. M. DeHaan, V. R. Dowell, Jr., and L. B. Guze (ed.), Charles C Thomas, Publisher, Springfield, Ill., in press) which involve bacteria from the oral cavity, gastrointestinal tract, genitourinary tract, or skin (chapter 38). Factors which can predispose to infection include accidental wounds, tooth extraction or other surgical procedures (especially oral and abdominal surgery), aspiration of material from the oral cavity into the lungs, debilitating disease such as alcoholism, leukemia, carcinoma, or diabetes mellitus, and treatment with immunosuppressant or corticosteroid drugs (1, 8; L. K. Georg, chapter 19 in *Anaerobic Bacteria: Role in Disease*, in press).

A. Produce propionic acid	
1. Catalase usually produced	*Propionibacterium*
2. Catalase not produced	*Arachnia*
B. Propionic acid not produced[a]	
1. Ratio of lactic to acetic acid produced greater than 1:1	
a. Lactic acid only major product	*Lactobacillus*
b. Succinic acid is a major product	*Actinomyces*
2. Ratio of lactic to acetic acid produced less than 1:1	
a. Produce butyric acid plus other acids or no major acids	*Eubacterium* and *Lachnospira*[b]
b. Butyric acid not produced	*Bifidobacterium*

[a] *A. viscosus* produces catalase; the remainder of the organisms under B. are catalase negative.

[b] No isolates of *Lachnospira* from human sources have been reported to date.

FIG. 1. *Differentiation of gram-positive, nonsporeforming, anaerobic bacilli to the genus level.*

COLLECTION AND TRANSPORT OF CLINICAL SPECIMENS

Clinical specimens must be collected so that contamination of the specimens with the normal flora of the mucous membranes and skin is avoided (chapter 38). However, one important exception to the general directions in chapter 38 relates to suspected actinomycosis. In this instance, expectorated sputum is a proper specimen to collect.

Special care must be exercised in the preparation of the skin before venipuncture, lumbar puncture, aspiration of pus from abscesses, thoracentesis, etc., since the skin may contain large numbers of propionibacteria (especially *P. acnes* and *P. granulosum*). The following procedure for preparation of the skin before collecting samples is recommended:

1. Cleanse the area carefully with a soap solution.

2. Remove the soap with 70 to 90% ethyl or isopropyl alcohol.

3. Apply 1% tincture of iodine.

4. Remove with 70 to 90% alcohol. *Do not touch the prepared skin during collection of the specimen.*

DIRECT EXAMINATION

Actinomycosis is usually a chronic disease characterized by suppuration, the formation of draining sinuses, and the presence of granules (so-called "sulfur granules") composed of aggregates of filamentous, branching microorganisms in the exudate. The granules are white or yellowish grains up to 5 mm in diameter and usually rather firm in consistency (9). All suppurative exudates, sputum, and pleural fluid should be inspected for the presence of actinomycotic granules. It is also worthwhile to examine gauze dressings which have been in contact with purulent material from draining lesions for trapped granules in the gauze fibers. However, it should be noted that other bacteria such as *Staphylococcus aureus* can form similar granules, and granules are not always present in actinomycosis.

MICROSCOPE EXAMINATION OF CLINICAL MATERIALS

Microscope examination of unstained as well as stained preparations of clinical materials is useful for presumptive laboratory diagnosis of infections involving gram-positive, nonsporeforming, anaerobic bacilli. If suspect actinomycotic granules are found, place a granule in a drop of water on a glass slide, add a cover slip, press gently, and examine microscopically for the presence of filaments and clubs surrounding the granule. The clubs may or may not be present. Crush suspicious granules by pressing firmly on the cover slip, remove the cover slip, prepare smears, and stain with Gram and acid-fast stains; use an acid-fast stain suitable for *Nocardia asteroides* (9). Examine microscopically for the presence of gram-positive, non-acid-fast filaments or pleomorphic bacilli ("diphtheroids") with or without branching. Examine Gram-stained smears of all clinical specimens, except blood, whether or not granules are observed, and acid-fast-stained smears of materials containing gram-positive filaments or slim rods without spores.

CULTURE AND ISOLATION

Primary isolation

See chapter 38 for a general discussion of primary isolation media and their use. A variety of blood culture media are satisfactory for the gram-positive, nonsporeforming, anaerobic bacilli (12, 17, 24, 27). For all clinical specimens except blood, inoculate at least the following media for isolation of nonsporeforming, anaerobic, gram-positive bacilli:

- one tube of thioglycolate medium (BBL-0135C or equivalent) enriched with sterile serum (0.5 ml per 8 ml of medium) after the medium is heated for 10 min in a boiling-water bath and cooled
- one tube of chopped meat-glucose medium (6) after heating for 10 min in a boiling-water bath or prereduced anaerobically sterilized medium (14)
- two plates of freshly prepared or anaerobically stored blood-agar medium. If a mixture of gram-positive and gram-negative bacilli are observed in direct smears, also inoculate two plates of phenethyl alcohol blood (PEA) agar (6, 9).

Incubate one plate of blood-agar and one plate of the PEA medium in an atmosphere of 6 to 10% CO_2 (candle jar or a CO_2 incubator) and the other plating media in a suitable anaerobic system (6, 12, 14, 19, 24) at 35 to 37 C for a minimum of 2 days and reincubate preferably for 5 days. In some cases it is advisable (particularly when actinomycosis is strongly suspected) to inoculate two sets of primary isolation media with the clinical material and incubate them in separate anaerobic jars. Inspect one set of plates after 2 days of incubation and incubate the others for 5 to 7 days before inspection. Better growth will be obtained if the liquid media are also incubated anaerobically. If screw-capped tubes are used, loosen the caps to allow exchange of gases. Hold liquid cultures at least 2 weeks to detect slow-growing organisms such as *Actinomyces israelii*, *Arachnia propionica*, *Eubacterium alactolyticum*, and *Propionibacterium acnes*. When growth is apparent, prepare and examine Gram-stained smears, and subculture aerobically and anaerobically on plating media as required.

Examination of colonies and subculture

Compare the growth on anaerobically incubated plating media with that obtained on media incubated in CO_2, inspect colonies with a stereoscopic microscope, examine a Gram-stained smear of each colony type, and subculture colonies of gram-positive bacilli to two plates of blood-agar. Incubate one plate anaerobically and the other in CO_2 for 2 to 3 days. Check the purity and aerotolerance (6) of the isolate on blood-agar, and inoculate a tube of enriched thioglycolate broth or chopped meat-glucose medium for use later as a source of inoculum, after incubation, for differential media, or prepare a suspension from colonies in a sugar-free medium and use this for inoculating differential media (6, 23).

PRESUMPTIVE IDENTIFICATION

Some key characteristics which can be used for presumptive identification of the gram-positive, nonsporeforming, anaerobic bacilli include: aerotolerance; microscopic appearance, macroscopic appearance, and rapidity of growth in thioglycolate medium; catalase production; fermentation of glucose; and metabolic products produced in glucose broth (Table 2). To determine these characteristics, inoculate three brain heart infusion agar (BHIA) slants, one tube of enriched thioglycolate broth, and one tube of peptone-yeast extract-glucose (PYG) broth (12). Incubate one BHIA slant in CO_2, one BHIA slant aerobically, and the other media anaerobically until good growth is obtained (usually 24 to 48 h).

After incubation, determine the aerotolerance of the organism by comparing the growth obtained on BHIA aerobically and anaerobically with that in the candle jar. At 30 min (or later) after the BHIA culture is removed from the anaerobic system, add 3% hydrogen peroxide to the slant showing best growth to check for catalase production. Record the degree and appearance of the growth in thioglycolate medium; also prepare and inspect a Gram-stained smear of the growth. Check the pH of the PYG broth culture to determine whether glucose was fermented. Refer to Table 2 and try to make a presumptive identification. If you are reasonably certain that the isolate is a gram-positive, nonsporeforming bacillus and that it is an anaerobic or microaerophilic (rather than an ordinary facultative) species, you may report it in the following manner: "an anaerobic (or microaerophilic) gram-positive nonsporeforming bacillus has been isolated, probably _______(genus)_______(species)"; or "probably a species of ________."

Definitive species identification generally requires the determination by gas chromatography of the volatile and nonvolatile acids produced by the organism in a suitable medium (Table 2), and the use of other biochemical tests (Table 3). If a chromatograph is not available for identification of metabolic products, establish the probable identity of the organism with the conventional tests, and refer the isolate to a reference laboratory for specific identification if it has been isolated more than once from carefully collected specimens of blood, cerebrospinal fluid, bone marrow, pleural fluid, etc., or is the only isolate from wounds.

IMMUNOFLUORESCENCE, FLUORESCENT-ANTIBODY TECHNIQUES

Use of fluorescent-antibody reagents is one of the most promising techniques for rapid, presumptive identification of nonsporeforming,

TABLE 2. *Key differential characteristics of gram-positive, nonsporeforming, anaerobic bacilli commonly isolated from clinical specimens*[a]

Species	Brain heart infusion agar slants		Thioglycolate medium			Peptone-yeast extract-glucose broth							
							Metabolic products detected by gas-liquid chromatography						
	Aerotolerance	Catalase production	Rapidity of growth	Macroscopic appearance	Microscopic appearance	Glucose fermentation	Acetic acid	Propionic acid	Butyric acid	Caproic acid	Lactic acid	Succinic acid
A. israelii	M or An	−	Slow	Granular or diffuse	c,e,g	+	+	−	−	−	+	+
A. naeslundii	F	−	Moderate	Diffuse	a,c,d,e	+	+	−	−	−	+	+
A. odontolyticus	M or An	−	Moderate	Diffuse	a,c,d,e	+	+	−	−	−	+	+
A. viscosus	F	+	Rapid	Diffuse	a,c,d	+	+	−	−	−	+	+
A. propionica	M or An	−	Slow	Granular or diffuse	e,g	+	+	+	−	−	+	+
B. eriksonii	An	−	Rapid	Diffuse	a,c,d	+	+	−	−	−	+	+
E. alactolyticum	An	−	Slow	Diffuse or granular	a,f,e	+	+	−	+	+	−	−
E. lentum	An	−	Moderate	Diffuse	a,e	−	+	−	−	−	+	+
E. limosum	An	−	Rapid	Diffuse	b,c,d	+	+	−	+	−	−	−
P. acnes	An^{F}	$+^{-}$	Slow	Diffuse	a,c,f	+	+	+	−	−	(−)	−
P. granulosum	An^{F}	$+^{-}$	Moderate	Diffuse	a,c,f	+	+	+	−	−	(−)	−

[a] An = obligate anaerobe; F = facultative anaerobe; M = microaerophilic; superscript = occasional reaction or result. Reactions: + = positive; − = negative; (−) = variable. Microscopic appearance: a = small rods with or without metachromatic staining; b = large plump evenly stained rods; c = club-shaped rods; d = rods with bifurcated (bifid) ends; e = thin filaments; f = chinese-letter configurations common; g = branching common.

TABLE 3. *Differential characteristics of gram-positive, nonsporeforming, anaerobic bacilli commonly isolated from clinical specimens*[a]

Species	Motility	Esculin hydrolysis	Gelatin hydrolysis	Nitrate reduction	Indole production	Action on milk	Fermentation of								
							Glucose	Mannitol	Lactose	Sucrose	Maltose	Salicin	Glycerol	Xylose	Arabinose
A. israelii	–	$+^{-}$	–	V	–	(C)	+	V	$+^{-}$	+	+	V	–	$+^{-}$	V
A. naeslundii	–	$+^{-}$	–	$+^{-}$	–	(C)	+	–	$+^{-}$	$+^{-}$	$+^{-}$	V	V	–	$-^{+}$
A. odontolyticus	–	V	–	+	–	(C)	+	–	$+^{-}$	$+^{-}$	+	$+^{-}$	$+^{-}$	V	V
A. viscosus	–	+	–	+	–	NC^{c}	+	–	$+^{-}$	+	+	$+^{-}$	$+^{-}$	–	–
A. propionica	–	$-^{+}$	$-^{+}$	+	–	(C)	+	+	+	+	+	$-^{+}$	$-^{+}$	–	–
B. eriksonii	–	$+^{-}$	–	–	–	(CG)	+	V	+	+	+	+	–	+	+
E. alactolyticum	–	–	–	–	–	NC	+	$+^{-}$	–	–	–	–	–	–	–
E. lentum	–	–	–	V	–	NC	–	–	–	–	–	–	–	–	–
E. limosum	–	V	–	–	–	C(G)	+	$+^{-}$	–	–	–	–	–	–	–
P. acnes	–	–	$+^{-}$	+	$+^{-}$	C(G)	+	V	–	–	–	–	+	–	–
P. granulosum	–	–	V	–	–	(C)	+	–	–	+	+	$-^{+}$	$+^{-}$	–	–

[a] Reactions: +, positive; –, negative; C, coagulated; NC, no coagulation; V, variable reaction; ( ), variable; G, gas; superscript, occasional reaction.

gram-positive bacilli. Fluorescent-antibody conjugates have been used for specific staining of *A. israelii* (serotypes 1 and 2), *A. naeslundii*, *A. odontolyticus*, *A. viscosus*, *A. propionica* (serotypes 1 and 2), *P. acnes* (serotypes 1 and 2), *P. avidum*, *P. granulosum*, and *P. jensenii* in direct smears of clinical materials and in cultures (2–5, 13, 15, 21, 22; L. K. Georg, chapter 19 in *Anaerobic Bacteria: Role in Disease*, in press). The fluorescent-antibody technique is used routinely at the Center for Disease Control as an aid in the identification and serotyping of *Actinomyces*, *Arachnia*, and *Bifidobacterium* cultures (L. K. Georg and J. Brown, personal communication). At present, none of the fluorescent-antibody conjugates mentioned is available commercially.

DEFINITIVE IDENTIFICATION

Other characteristics which are useful for identification include motility, esculin hydrolysis, gelatin hydrolysis, nitrate reduction, indole production, action on milk, and fermentation of glucose, mannitol, lactose, sucrose, maltose, salicin, glycerol, xylose, and arabinose (Table 3). See Holdeman and Moore (12), Dowell and Hawkins (6), Sutter et al. (24), or Georg (9) for detailed descriptions of the media and biochemical tests required. Numerous other species of gram-positive, nonsporeforming, anaerobic bacilli are known to inhabit the oral cavity and gastrointestinal tract but are seldom isolated from properly collected clinical specimens. Unusual isolates from clinical specimens should be referred to a reference laboratory for identification or confirmation of identity.

EVALUATION

Determining the clinical significance of an isolate of one of the gram-positive, nonsporeforming, anaerobic bacilli can be difficult because of the prevalence of these bacteria in the normal flora and their association with other microorganisms in polymicrobic infections. Isolates of propionibacteria from blood, bone marrow, and cerebrospinal fluid cultures can be especially perplexing. Although *P. acnes*, a normal inhabitant of the skin, is frequently a contaminant of blood, bone marrow, and cerebrospinal fluid cultures, isolation of this organism from properly collected specimens can be clinically significant (7, 20; J. M. Felner, chapter 26 in *Anaerobic Bacteria: Role in Disease*, in press).

According to Georg (*Anaerobic Bacteria: Role in Disease*, in press), there are at least five different species of bacteria which can cause actinomycosis. These bacteria, in order of their importance in human disease, are *A. israelii*, *A. propionica*, *A. naeslundii*, *A. viscosus*, and *A. odontolyticus*. All have the ability to induce suppurative lesions and disease that has all the clinico-pathological stigmata of classical actinomycosis. Unfortunately, unless branching filaments are observed, some laboratories report these as "diphtheroids" without attempting identification of isolates.

Despite their prevalence in the normal flora of the oral cavity, gastrointestinal tract, and genitourinary tract, bifidobacteria are seldom isolated from properly collected specimens (6, A. C. Sonnenwirth, chapter 15 in *Anaerobic Bacteria: Role in Disease*, in press). In one series of 3,103 positive blood cultures reported by

Washington (25), only five (0.1%) yielded bifidobacteria; in another series published by Washington (26), only 1 of 847 positive blood cultures contained bifidobacteria. The incidence of eubacteria in blood cultures is also quite low (26–28). Endocarditis due to *Eubacterium ventriosum* has been described, and recently a case of endocarditis involving *Eubacterium aerofaciens* was reported (20).

Establishing the significance of clinical isolates, and the correct diagnosis, requires close cooperation between the attending physician and the microbiologist. The clinician should provide the microbiologist with properly collected clinical specimens and pertinent clinical information pertaining to the patient's condition, and it is the microbiologist's responsibility to employ the best methods available for isolation and accurate identification of the causative agent(s). Otherwise, the patient may undergo unnecessary suffering and unnecessary expenses for hospitalization and treatment.

LITERATURE CITED

1. Bartlett, J. G., and S. M. Finegold. 1972. Anaerobic pleuropulmonary infections. Medicine **51**:413–450.
2. Blank, C. H., and L. K. Georg. 1968. The use of fluorescent antibody for the detection and identification of *Actinomyces* species in clinical material. J. Lab. Clin. Med. **71**:283–293.
3. Brock, D. W., and L. K. Georg. 1969. Determination and analysis of *Actinomyces israelii* serotypes by fluorescent-antibody procedures. J. Bacteriol. **97**:581–588.
4. Brock, D. W., L. K. Georg, J. M. Brown, and M. W. Hicklin. 1973. *Arachnia propionica* as an agent of actinomycosis. Amer. J. Clin. Pathol. **59**:66–77.
5. Dowell, V. R., Jr. 1970. Anaerobic infections, p. 494–543. *In* H. L. Bodily, E. L. Updyke, and J. O. Mason (ed.), Diagnostic procedures for bacterial, mycotic and parasitic infections, 5th ed. American Public Health Association, Inc., New York.
6. Dowell, V. R., Jr., and T. M. Hawkins. 1973. Laboratory methods in anaerobic bacteriology, CDC Laboratory manual. Publication No. (HSM) 73-8222. Center for Disease Control, Atlanta, Ga.
7. Felner, J. M., and V. R. Dowell, Jr. 1970. Anaerobic bacterial endocarditis. N. Engl. J. Med. **283**:1188–1192.
8. Finegold, S. M., J. E. Rosenblatt, V. L. Sutter, and H. R. Attebery. 1972. Scope monograph on anaerobic infections. The Upjohn Co., Kalamazoo, Mich.
9. Georg, L. K. 1970. Diagnostic procedures for the isolation and identification of the etiologic agents of actinomycosis, p. 71–81. *In* Proceedings of International Symposium on Mycoses. Publication No. 205, Pan American Health Organization, Washington, D.C.
10. Georg, L. K., G. W. Robertstad, S. A. Brinkman, and M. D. Hicklin. 1965. A new pathogenic anaerobic *Actinomyces* species. J. Infect. Dis. **115**:88–99.
11. Holdeman, L. V., E. P. Cato, and W. E. C. Moore. 1971. *Clostridium ramosum* (Veillan and Zuber) comb. nov.: emended description and proposed neotype strain. Int. J. Syst. Bacteriol. **21**:35–39.
12. Holdeman, L. V., and W. E. C. Moore (ed.). 1972. Anaerobe laboratory manual. Anaerobe Laboratory, Virginia Polytechnic Institute and State University, Blacksburg.
13. Holmberg, K., and U. Forsum. 1973. Identification of *Actinomyces, Arachnia, Bacterionema, Rothia,* and *Propionibacterium* species by defined immunofluorescence. Appl. Microbiol. **25**:834–843.
14. Killgore, G. E., S. E. Starr, V. E. DelBene, D. N. Whaley, and V. R. Dowell, Jr. 1973. Comparison of three anaerobic systems for isolation of anaerobic bacteria from clinical specimens. Amer. J. Clin. Pathol. **59**:552–559.
15. Lambert, F. W., Jr., J. M. Brown, and L. K. Georg. 1967. Identification of *Actinomyces israelii* and *Actinomyces naeslundii* by fluorescent-antibody and agar-gel diffusion techniques. J. Bacteriol. **94**:1287–1295.
16. Moore, W. E. C., and L. V. Holdeman. 1972. Identification of anaerobic bacteria. Amer. J. Clin. Nutr. **25**:1306–1313.
17. Nastro, L. J., and S. M. Finegold. 1973. Endocarditis due to anaerobic gram-negative bacilli. Amer. J. Med. **54**:482–496.
18. Pine, L., and L. K. Georg. 1969. Reclassification of *Actinomyces propionicus*. Int. J. Syst. Bacteriol. **19**:267–272.
19. Rosenblatt, J. E., A. Fallon, and S. M. Finegold. 1973. Comparison of methods for isolation of anaerobic bacteria from clinical specimens. Appl. Microbiol. **25**:77–85.
20. Sans, M. D., and J. G. Crowder. 1973. Subacute bacterial endocarditis caused by *Eubacterium aerofaciens:* report of a case. Amer. J. Clin. Pathol. **59**:576–580.
21. Slack, J. M., A. Winger, and D. W. Moore. 1961. Serological grouping of *Actinomyces* by means of fluorescent antibodies. J. Bacteriol. **82**:54–65.
22. Slack, J. M., S. Landfried, and M. A. Gerencser. 1971. Identification of *Actinomyces* and related bacteria in dental calculus by the fluorescent antibody technique. J. Dent. Res. **50**:78–82.
23. Starr, S. E., F. S. Thompson, V. R. Dowell, Jr., and A. Balows. 1973. Micromethod system for identification of anaerobic bacteria. Appl. Microbiol. **25**:713–717.
24. Sutter, V. L., H. R. Attebery, J. E. Rosenblatt, K. S. Bricknell, and S. M. Finegold. 1972. Anaerobic bacteriology manual. Department of Continuing Education in Health Sciences, University Extension, and the School of Medicine, Univ. of California, Los Angeles.
25. Washington, J. A. 1971. Comparison of two commercially available media for detection of bacteremia. Appl. Microbiol. **22**:604–607.
26. Washington, J. A. 1972. Evaluation of two commercially available media for detection of bacteremia. Appl. Microbiol. **23**:956–959.
27. Washington, J. A. and W. J. Martin. 1973. Comparison of three blood culture media for recovery of anaerobic bacteria. Appl. Microbiol. **25**:70–71.
28. Wilson, W. R., W. J. Martin, C. J. Wilkowski, and J. A. Washington. 1972. Anaerobic bacteremia. Mayo Clin. Proc. **47**:639–646.

Chapter 43

Anaerobic Blood Cultures

JOHN A. WASHINGTON II

INTRODUCTION

Anaerobic bacteria have been reported to account for between 12 and 27% of positive blood cultures and for 20 to 25% of patients with clinically significant bacteremia (15). Inasmuch as the combination of a penicillin or cephalosporin with an aminoglycoside, commonly used for initial therapy of a bacteremia of unknown etiology, has little activity against *Bacteroides fragilis*, the most frequent cause of anaerobic bacteremia (16), it is important not only to recognize the underlying conditions predisposing to this type of infection but also to isolate and identify the etiological agent as quickly as possible so that appropriate antimicrobial therapy may be administered. Although diseases, and especially malignancies, of the gastrointestinal and genitourinary tracts represent the most common underlying conditions associated with anaerobic bacteremia, gastrointestinal operations or procedures and urogynecological manipulations are common precipitating factors (6). Polymicrobial bacteremia, with other anaerobes or with aerobes or facultative anaerobes, has been found to occur in approximately a quarter of the patients with anaerobic bacteremia (6, 16) and must be taken into consideration in regard to both microbiological diagnosis and therapy.

COLLECTION AND TRANSPORT

Customarily, the blood, collected by venipuncture after proper antisepsis of the skin, is inoculated either directly into liquid media or into a vacuum transport tube containing sodium polyanetholsulfonate (SPS) from which liquid media are inoculated when the specimen has reached the laboratory. There are no published data comparing isolation rates of anaerobic bacteria when these two methods were used concurrently. There are, however, at least two factors which merit careful consideration: (i) it is known that SPS (0.03 to 0.05%) is inhibitory to some strains of anaerobic cocci (2; S. M. Finegold, personal communication), and (ii) most commercially available liquid media under vacuum and with CO_2 have redox potentials (E_h) sufficiently low (-100 to -150 mV) to permit rapid growth of clinically significant anaerobes. With respect to the inhibitory activity of SPS on anaerobic cocci, it should be emphasized that these data were obtained with known inocula of such organisms in simulated cultures. There are no published data documenting the occurrence of this result when blood from patients suspected of having bacteremia was inoculated into liquid media containing 0.03 to 0.05% SPS. In fact, there are limited data, published by Rosner (8, 9), suggesting that the converse may be the case.

One possible means of obviating this theoretical disadvantage of SPS would be to use sodium amylosulfate (SAS, Searle Diagnostic Inc.), a new polyanionic, heat-stable anticoagulant (5) which inactivates antibacterial substances in blood and which does not appear to inhibit anaerobic cocci in simulated blood cultures (4). Further experience with the use of SAS in real blood cultures must be obtained and carefully analyzed before it can be recommended for routine use.

With respect to the second point mentioned above, it would seem advisable to inoculate the blood directly into liquid media with a low E_h as soon as possible after collection to avoid prolonging the lag phase in the growth of any anaerobes which may be present (10). In this connection, it is important to be sure that all air bubbles in the syringe used to collect the blood are eliminated before inoculating the blood into the bottle.

MEDIA

There are various commercially available liquid media which appear to be satisfactory for recovery of anaerobic bacteria. With unvented bottles, each containing 100 ml of liquid medium prepared under vacuum with CO_2, inoculated with blood at a ratio of 1:10 (vol/vol), there were no statistically significant differences between rates or time intervals to detection of anaerobic bacteria in Tryptic Soy (Difco) broth and Thiol (Difco) broth with (1) or without (12) SPS. Similarly, no statistically significant differences in rates or in time intervals to detection of anaerobic bacteria were noted between Trypticase Soy (Becton-Dickinson & Co.) broth and thioglycolate (B-D, 135C) without SPS (13). Finally, no statistically significant differences between rates or times to detection of anaerobic bacteria were noted between Tryptic Soy (Difco) broth and Columbia (Difco) broth with SPS (unpublished data). Rosner's data suggest that SPS in liquid media may enhance recovery of anaerobes from blood (8, 9); however, there are no other published data obtained with clinical material in which the presence or absence of SPS was the only experimental variable in the study.

In recent years, it has been recommended that prereduced, anaerobically sterilized (PRAS) media be used for recovery of anaerobes from clinical material (3). PRAS blood culture media have become available commercially (supplemented prereduced brain heart infusion-yeast extract broth [Robbins Laboratories]; supplemented peptone broth [BBL]); however, there are as yet no data substantiating their superiority over unvented commercially available media under vacuum with CO_2. There were no differences in isolation rates of anaerobic bacteria in one recently published report (14) comparing Tryptic Soy (Difco) broth, thioglycolate medium (Difco), and supplemented brain heart infusion (PRAS) broth (Robbins Laboratories). Studies in this laboratory with a tube containing supplemented peptone broth (B-D) have shown it to be inferior to both Tryptic Soy (Difco) broth and Thiol (Difco) broth for recovery of *Bacteroidaceae* (1).

Sullivan et al. (11) reported an increased recovery of anaerobic bacteria from an osmotically stabilized anaerobic broth with SPS. However, because the liquid media against which this broth was compared were neither osmotically stabilized nor contained SPS, it is not clear which of these two variables was responsible for the enhanced isolation rate of the anaerobes. It is possible that both are beneficial (9); however, in my own experience using samples of blood from patients (unpublished data), Tryptic Soy (Difco) broth with 30% sucrose and no SPS was completely inadequate, when compared with Tryptic Soy broth with SPS and no sucrose, for isolation of anaerobes. Whether or not 30% sucrose is excessive, it is apparent that SPS, or possibly SAS, is an important additive in liquid media used for the isolation of anaerobic bacteria.

Although an automated radiometric system (BACTEC) for detecting bacteremia had a slight advantage over conventional systems, including Tryptic Soy and Thiol broths with SPS, in the time interval to detection of positivity, it detected fewer anaerobes than did the conventional system (7).

It is clear, therefore, at this point that commercially available liquid media under vacuum with CO_2 represent an acceptable means for isolating anaerobic bacteria from blood. It would be reasonable to inoculate two liquid media with equal amounts, on a 10% (vol/vol) basis, of one blood sample and to vent one bottle but not the other. My own practice, however, has been to inoculate two bottles (100 ml each, under vacuum with CO_2) and to vent neither, depending on a routine "blind" subculture of each bottle within the first 24 h after inoculation for recovery of strict aerobes. The rationale for this approach is that initial therapy of presumed septicemia at the Mayo Clinic routinely includes one or more antimicrobial agents active against pseudomonads but not against *B. fragilis*. Emphasis has therefore been placed on rapid and maximal recovery of anaerobes. Obviously, circumstances vary from institution to institution, and practices regarding blood cultures should be adjusted accordingly.

EXAMINATION OF CULTURES

Bottles containing liquid media should be carefully inspected later in the same day they were inoculated and daily thereafter for the presence of turbidity, gas, hemolysis, colonies, or any other evidence of growth. Also, frequent examination of Gram-stained smears of material suspected of containing microorganisms is critically important in the prompt recognition of positive blood cultures. With the types of media already described, it has been our experience that the mean time to detection of positivity of cultures containing *Bacteroidaceae* is approximately 3 days and that approximately 75% of such positive results are detected within 3 days after inoculation of the cultures. Clostridia are detected much more rapidly: two-thirds within 1 day and all within 2 days. Inasmuch as *Bacteroidaceae* may appear pale, irregular, slender, and pleomorphic in Gram-stained smears, their presence in blood cultures can frequently be suspected and tentatively reported as such.

Because anaerobic bacteria generally are rapidly detected in liquid media, the value of a routine "blind" subculture incubated anaerobically is doubtful; however, since anaerobic bacteremias are commonly polymicrobic (16), it is important to subculture samples of any suspected or known positive bottles into media which are incubated both aerobically and anaerobically. It has been my practice, therefore, to subculture known or suspected positive blood cultures into thioglycolate (B-D, 135C) supplemented with sterile rabbit serum, two blood agar plates, and an eosin-methylene blue agar plate or a phenylated alcohol-blood agar plate, depending on the organism's Gram reaction. One blood agar plate is incubated anaerobically and the other is incubated in an atmosphere with 10 to 12% CO_2; the remaining media are incubated aerobically. Care must be taken in examining the anaerobically incubated blood agar plate because (i) facultative anaerobes will grow under these conditions, and (ii) colonies of some anaerobic bacteria may resemble those of some facultative anaerobes.

LITERATURE CITED

1. Hall, M., E. Warren, and J. A. Washington II. 1974. Detection of bacteremia with liquid media containing sodium polyanetholsulfonate. Appl. Microbiol. **27**:187–191.
2. Hoare, E. D. 1939. The suitability of "Liquoid" for use in blood culture media, with particular reference to anaerobic streptococci. J. Pathol. Bacteriol. **48**:573–577.
3. Holdeman, L. V., and W. E. C. Moore. 1972. Anaerobe laboratory manual, p. 2. Virginia Polytechnic Institute and State University, Blacksburg, Va.
4. Kocka, F. E., E. J. Arthur, R. L. Searcy, M. Smith, and B. Grodner. 1973. Clinical evaluation of sodium amylosulfate in human blood cultures. Appl. Microbiol. **26**:421–422.
5. Kocka, F. E., T. Magoc, and R. L. Searcy. 1972. New anticoagulant for combating antibacterial activity of human blood. Proc. Soc. Exp. Biol. Med. **140**:1231–1234.
6. Marcoux, J. A., R. J. Zabransky, J. A. Washington II, W. E. Wellman, and W. J. Martin. 1970. Bacteroides bacteremia. Minn. Med. **53**:1169–1176.
7. Renner, E. D., L. A. Gatheridge, and J. A. Washington II. 1973. Evaluation of radiometric system for detecting bacteremia. Appl. Microbiol. **26**:368–372.
8. Rosner, R. 1968. Effect of various anticoagulants and no anticoagulant on ability to isolate bacteria directly from parallel clinical blood specimens. Amer. J. Clin. Pathol. **49**:216–219.
9. Rosner, R. 1972. A quantitative evaluation of three blood culture systems. Amer. J. Clin. Pathol. **57**:220–227.
10. Smith, L. DS., and L. V. Holdeman. 1968. The pathogenic anaerobic bacteria, p. 8–13. Charles C Thomas, Publisher, Springfield, Ill.
11. Sullivan, N. M., V. L. Sutter, W. T. Carter, H. R. Attebury and S. M. Finegold. 1972. Bacteremia after genitourinary tract manipulation: bacteriological aspects and evaluation of various blood culture systems. Appl. Microbiol. **23**:1101–1106.
12. Washington, J. A., II. 1971. Comparison of two commercially available media for detection of bacteremia. Appl. Microbiol. **22**:604–607.
13. Washington, J. A., II. 1972. Evaluation of two commercially available media for detection of bacteremia. Appl. Microbiol. **23**:956–959.
14. Washington, J. A., II, and W. J. Martin. 1973. Comparison of three blood culture media for recovery of anaerobic bacteria. Appl. Microbiol. **25**:70–71.
15. Washington, J. A., II, W. J. Martin, and P. E. Hermans. 1973. In vitro susceptibility of anaerobic bacteria isolated from blood cultures. *In* Proc. Int. Conf. Anaerobic Bacteria: Bacteriological and Clinical Considerations. Charles C Thomas, Publisher, Springfield, Ill.
16. Wilson, W. R., W. J. Martin, C. J. Wilkowske, and J. A. Washington II. 1972. Anaerobic bacteremia. Mayo Clin. Proc. **47**:639–646.

Section V

LABORATORY TESTS IN CHEMOTHERAPY

Chapter 44
Introduction

JOHN C. SHERRIS

A number of considerations are involved in selecting an appropriate antimicrobic to treat an infection. (The term antimicrobic is used throughout this section to describe both antibiotics and chemotherapeutics.) These include: (i) knowledge of the inherent susceptibility of the infecting organism to appropriate antimicrobics; (ii) clinical pharmacological properties including toxicity, protein binding, distribution, absorption, and excretion; (iii) previous clinical experience of efficacy in treating infections due to the same species; (iv) the nature of the underlying pathological process, its natural history, and its influence on chemotherapy; and (v) the immune status of the host.

Of these factors, the amount of antimicrobic required to inhibit or kill the organism in vitro and the levels of chemotherapeutic attained in body fluids during treatment are subject to direct measurement in the clinical laboratory. The purpose of this section of the *Manual* is to provide detailed descriptions of appropriate procedures for these purposes. The methods described are for use with bacteria other than mycobacteria, which are separately considered in chapter 16.

Influence of technical variation on susceptibility test results

The results of both dilution and diffusion susceptibility tests may be influenced markedly by the reagents and conditions of the tests, and this has been the source of considerable confusion in the past. Inoculum size (especially important), incubation time and temperature, medium constitution and pH, atmosphere, and stability of antibiotic may all influence the end points obtained. In addition, diffusion tests are influenced by the growth rate of the organism and by the type, depth, and concentration of the agar used. For these reasons, special emphasis has been placed on reference procedures and methodological standardization (2, 4, 5, 10–12), because only in this way can adequate reproducibility be obtained in investigative and clinical work.

Selection of susceptibility test methods

The dilution methods described in chapter 45 are derived from those recommended in the report of an International Collaborative Study (2), and the diffusion procedure in chapter 46 is that accepted by the Food and Drug Administration (4, 5) and proposed as a tentative standard by the National Committee on Clinical Laboratory Standards' Subcommittee on Antibiotic Susceptibility Testing (10). These procedures have gained considerable acceptance, and, when performed as directed and shown to be under control with recommended standard strains, they should give good inter- and intralaboratory reproducibility. The methods have been used routinely for a number of years by several of the authors of this section and have been found to be generally satisfactory both as laboratory procedures and as the source of clinically useful information. Deviations from the protocols can lead to significant differences in results, and we recommend that they not be made unless experimentally shown to be more reproducible or more clinically valuable.

There is presently no consensus on the conditions for susceptibility testing of strictly anaerobic organisms, although much work is presently in progress. The considerable differences in growth rates of the different species make it unlikely that a diffusion test with a single set of interpretative standards for all organisms will suffice; however, several different diffusion procedures have been developed for specific purposes, and some appear promising. Meanwhile, the authors of chapter 49 have recommended a dilution test procedure that has proved effective in practice, and we consider that this, or the disk broth method to which they refer, should be employed in the relatively few situations in which susceptibility testing of strictly anaerobic organisms is needed and can yield results in time to influence the clinical outcome.

In each of the susceptibility tests described, the inoculum is derived from several colonies. This is designed to reduce the chance of selecting variants derived from loss-mutations, for example, loss of penicillinase production in staphylococci, or segregants from R-factor resistance markers. It also increases the chance of including representatives of a more resistant organism if more than one strain is represented by colonies that cannot be distinguished morphologically. The final inocula are reasonably heavy, which increases the chance of detecting high-frequency mutations to resistance and also hetero-resistant strains. The media selected show generally good buffering qualities and reproducibility and are of physiological pH.

Interpretation of susceptibility tests: "susceptibility" and "resistance"

The interpretation of a quantitative susceptibility test result has three major components.

1. The relationship of the MIC (minimal inhibitory concentration) or MLC (minimal lethal concentration) for the organism to the concentration in the blood, or in some cases urine or other fluid, obtained with the dosage given. This has proved a clinically useful approach, but is inevitably an incomplete model of the in vivo situation because of the varying degrees of protein binding, the interacting effects of host defense mechanisms, and the arbitrary aspects of the selection of test conditions.

2. The relationship of the susceptibility of the strain under test to that of other members of the same species. This is useful because the selection of resistant mutants or strains with extrachromosomal determinants of resistance has led to the appearance of populations of strains well separated from the "wild" types of some species that were previously uniformly highly susceptible to the antimicrobic. The resulting bimodal distribution of susceptibilities correlates well with clinical responsiveness. Thus, a strain falling in the more resistant population is considered a priori a resistant member of that species.

3. Clinical experience with the treatment of the particular type of infection involved.

An ideal interpretation of susceptibility test results takes account of these factors independently. From a practical point of view, organisms are frequently allocated to predetermined "susceptible," "resistant," and one or more "intermediate" categories, and this approach was considered by the International Collaborative Study to continue to be useful and necessary in the light of presently available technical methods and general understanding of the principles of chemotherapy (2). The three categories recommended for the diffusion test given in chapter 46 have been based on the synthesis of the first two criteria given above. They have been defined (10) as: (i) susceptible (or sensitive), implying that an infection due to the strain tested may be expected to respond to a dosage of antimicrobic recommended for that type of infection and infecting species; (ii) resistant, containing strains not completely inhibited within the usual therapeutic range; and (iii) intermediate, comprising a "buffer zone" which prevents major interpretative discrepancies from small uncontrolled technical factors. The last category also includes strains which may respond to concentrations attainable by unusually high dosage or in areas such as portions of the urinary tract where the antibiotic is concentrated. The clinical extrapolations of these categories are, of course, subject to the considerations given in the first paragraph of this chapter.

This system requires qualification in that it does not consider the blood levels that may be attained with very high dosages of the relatively nontoxic penicillins and cephalosporins, or of the high urine levels of certain antimicrobials. Four-category systems (2, 3) to take account of these factors have been described and may well become more generally used in the future; meanwhile, it is important to recognize the need for an override to the three-category system in special cases.

Indications for susceptibility tests in the clinical laboratory

Tests are indicated for organisms contributing to the infectious process whose susceptibility cannot be predicted from knowledge of their identity. This applies in particular to staphylococci, to gram-negative enteric organisms, and to unusual species playing a pathogenic role. Susceptibility tests will often be set up before species determination, and specific antibiogram patterns may assist correct species allocation. Antibiograms may be determined for epidemiological reasons because the occurrence of a common antibiogram, especially if unusual, often assists the recognition of common-source outbreaks and patterns of cross-infection.

Routine susceptibility tests are not needed when resistance has not been described to the chemotherapeutic of choice, e.g., *Streptococcus pyogenes*, pneumococci, and meningococci to penicillin. Susceptibility testing should be avoided on members of the normal flora in their normal habitat, and on organisms that are known not to be playing a pathogenic role. To make such tests is both wasteful and misleading.

The selection of which antimicrobials to test is considered with each test system (see chapters 45 and 46). Suffice it to say that tests are normally made on only one congener of a "family" of antibiotics when their antimicrobial activity is closely comparable. When they differ as, for example, with benzyl penicillin, ampicillin, and carbenicillin, the different agents need to be tested against species for which they are appropriate.

Special tests and assays

Susceptibility tests make up the bulk of the clinical laboratory tests which are ordered to assist the clinician in his choice of chemotherapeutics. They may need to be supplemented with other procedures in certain complex clinical situations, especially in subacute bacterial endocarditis and in severe infections in the immunologically compromised. In these cases, determination of lethal end points or of the effect of combinations of antimicrobials may need to be measured. Direct tests of the ability of the antimicrobic in the patient's serum to inhibit or kill the infecting organism may also be required to monitor the adequacy of dosage schedules (see chapter 48). So far there has been no general agreement on methods for determining minimal lethal concentrations, studying antimicrobic combinations, or detecting serum inhibition of infecting organisms. The procedures given could serve as a basis for further studies towards methodological standardization of these important tests.

In other situations, it is necessary to determine the amount of antimicrobic present in serum, urine, or other tissue fluids. In clinical practice, this applies particularly to agents such as gentamicin, whose toxic and therapeutic levels for some organisms are very close. Serum assays are thus required to insure that antimicrobic concentrations in the blood are within a safe, but effective, range. This is particularly the case in patients with renal deficit, whose serum levels of antimicrobic may be less predictable. A simple, rapid and accurate method for this procedure is given in chapter 47.

The role of the laboratory in the selection and monitoring of chemotherapy was succinctly expressed by Theodore G. Anderson in the previous edition of this *Manual:* "When selecting an antimicrobial agent for therapy, it is the physician's responsibility to take into consideration the pharmacological characteristics of the several drugs as well as their relative antimicrobial effectiveness. The responsibility of the laboratory is to provide information, through standardized in vitro tests, of the activity of appropriate antimicrobial agents against the organism in question." The methods given in the subsequent chapters constitute accepted approaches among the authors providing this information. Different procedures have been developed by others in a number of countries, and the reader is referred to more detailed reviews for further information and for broader consideration of the theory of the subject (1–3, 6–9, 11).

LITERATURE CITED

1. Balows, A. (ed.). 1974. Current techniques for antibiotic susceptibility testing. Charles C Thomas, Publisher, Springfield, Ill.
2. Ericsson, H. M., and J. C. Sherris. 1971. Antibiotic sensitivity testing. Report of an International Collaborative Study. Acta Pathol. Microbiol. Scand. Sect. B, Suppl. 217.
3. Ericsson, H. M., G. Tunevall, and K. Wickman. 1960. A paper disc method for determination of bacterial sensitivity to antibiotics. Scand. J. Clin. Lab. Invest. **12:**414–422.
4. Federal Register. 1972. Rules and regulations. Antibiotic susceptibility discs. Fed. Regist. **37:**20525–20529.
5. Federal Register 1973. Rules and regulations. Antibiotic susceptibility discs: correction. Fed. Regist. **38:**2576.
6. Garrod, L. P., H. P. Lambert, and F. O'Grady, with a chapter on laboratory methods by P. M. Waterworth. 1973. Antibiotic and chemotherapy, 4th ed. Churchill Livingstone, Edinburgh.
7. Gavan, T. L., E. L. Cheatle, and H. W. McFadden. 1971. Antimicrobial susceptibility testing. Committee on Continuing Education, Council on Microbiology, American Society of Clinical Pathologists. Chicago.
8. Petersdorf, R. G., and J. J. Plorde. 1963. The usefulness of *in vitro* sensitivity tests in antibiotic therapy. Annu. Rev. Med. **14:**41–56.
9. Petersdorf, R. G., and J. C. Sherris. 1965. Methods and significance of *in vitro* testing of bacterial sensitivity to drugs. Amer. J. Med. **39:**766–779.
10. Revised Tentative Standard. 1973. Performance standards for antimicrobial disc susceptibility tests as used in clinical laboratories. National Committee for Clinical Laboratory Standards, Los Angeles.
11. Schoenknecht, F. D., and J. C. Sherris. 1971. New perspectives in antibiotic susceptibility testing, p. 275–292. *In* S. C. Dyke (ed.), Recent advances in clinical pathology. Churchill Livingstone, Edinburgh.
12. World Health Organization. 1961. Standardization of methods for conducting microbic sensitivity tests. Second report of the expert committee on antibiotics. World Health Organ. Tech. Rep. Ser. No. 210, p. 1–24.

Chapter 45
Dilution Test Procedures

JOHN A. WASHINGTON II AND ARTHUR L. BARRY

Dilution tests are used to determine the minimal concentration of an antimicrobial agent required to inhibit or kill a microorganism. Serial dilutions of the antimicrobial agent are inoculated with the organism and incubated. The minimal inhibitory concentration (MIC) is the lowest concentration without apparent growth. The term "broth" (or "tube") and "agar" (or "plate") is added to the term "dilution test," depending on whether the test is performed in liquid or agar media, respectively. Both terms are actually misnomers because it is the antimicrobial agent that is being diluted rather than the broth or agar.

The primary indication for dilution tests is to obtain *quantitative* results of susceptibility tests when this is important or necessary for proper management of antimicrobial therapy. Although qualitative data provided by the disk diffusion test are usually adequate for guiding the therapy of most infections, quantitative data may be needed when drug dosage schedules must be monitored or under conditions in which disk test results are inapplicable, equivocal, or unreliable (15; see chapter 46). These conditions include tests on slow-growing organisms, confirmation of susceptibility (as opposed to resistance) to the polymyxins (B or E), and tests on strains falling into the intermediate category with a potentially toxic antimicrobic if treatment with it is considered. Infections due to microorganisms which are categorized as resistant to the relatively nontoxic penicillins and cephalosporins may occasionally be treated preferentially and safely with massive doses of one of these agents, and certain types of urinary tract infections may respond to ordinary dosages of some antimicrobics, even though the microorganism is intermediate or resistant by the disk test criteria, because of the high levels attained in the urine. In these cases, the precise degree of susceptibility of an organism may influence the choice of antimicrobial, its dosage, and its route of administration. Other indications for dilution testing in liquid media are to determine the bactericidal activity of an antimicrobial agent and synergism or antagonism between antimicrobials against particular microorganisms. These procedures are considered in chapter 48.

Finally, dilution tests have been found to be practical and economical for routine purposes in some large laboratories through the use of micro and semi-automated broth dilution techniques and of agar dilution methods with inoculum replicators.

SOURCES, PREPARATIONS, AND STOCK SOLUTIONS OF ANTIMICROBIAL AGENTS

Standard or reference preparations of antimicrobials should be obtained directly from the manufacturers, from any laboratory supply house which makes available powders specifically for susceptibility tests, or from the U.S. Pharmacopeia Convention, Inc. (12601 Twinbrook Parkway, Rockville, Md. 20852). Clinical preparations should not be used because they are less precisely standardized and because some are esters that develop full activity only after hydrolysis to the active substance in vivo (e.g., chloramphenicol sodium succinate). Containers of powder should bear a label stating activity, expressed in micrograms (μg) or in international units (IU) per milligram, and an expiration date. They should be stored at 5 C in a desiccator, unless received in sealed ampoules.

Powders are weighed on an analytical balance and dissolved to yield the required concentration of active substance per milliliter, as shown in the footnote to Table 1. Although many antimicrobials may be dissolved in distilled water, some require special solvents or pH adjustment for initial solubilization (Table 1). Dilution may subsequently be carried out in distilled water. It is usually not necessary to sterilize stock solutions containing high concentrations of antimicrobials; however, should it be necessary to do so, membrane filtration should be used.

TABLE 1. *Solvents and diluents for stock solutions of antimicrobial agents*[a]

Antimicrobial agent[b]	Solvent	Diluent
Ampicillin	Phosphate buffer, pH 8.0, 0.1 M	Phosphate buffer, pH 6.0, 0.1 M
Carbenicillin	Water	Water
Cephalothin	Phosphate buffer, pH 6.0, 0.1 M	Water
Chloramphenicol	Ethanol	Water
Clindamycin	Water	Water
Cycloserine	Water	Water
Erythromycin	Ethanol	Water
Ethambutol	Water	Water
Flucytosine	Saline, 0.85%	Saline, 0.85%
Gentamicin	Phosphate buffer, pH 8.0, 0.1 M	Water
Isoniazid	Water	Water
Kanamycin	Phosphate buffer, pH 8, 0.1 M	Water
Nalidixic acid	NaOH, 1 N	Water
Nitrofurantoin[c]	Dimethylformamide	Water
Oxacillin	Water	Water
p-Aminosalicylic acid	Water	Water
Penicillin	Water	Water
Polymyxin B	Water	Water
Rifampin	Dimethylsulfoxide	Phosphate buffer, pH 7.0
Streptomycin	Water	Water
Sulfonamides	Hot water + minimal amount of 10% NaOH to dissolve	Water
Tetracycline	Water	Water
Vancomycin	Water	Water

[a] Adapted from reference 27.

[b] The dry weight of the antimicrobial agent must be multiplied by the "activity standard" provided by the manufacturer: e.g., 1 mg = 825 μg of active substance ("activity standard"); therefore, 100 mg = 82,500 μg, and 41.25 ml of solvent must be added to yield a solution with an activity of 2,000 μg/ml.

[c] The sodium salt is water-soluble.

Stock solutions should be stored at −20 C or colder. It should be emphasized that, at −20 C, retention of at least 90% of potency by ampicillin in solution is relatively brief (25). In this instance, preparation of a fresh solution or storage of the solution at −60 or −70 C is necessary. Most stock solutions of antimicrobics remain stable at −60 C for at least 6 months in concentrations of 1,000 μg/ml or greater. Convenient concentrations of stock solutions for most antibiotics are 2,000 or 1,280 μg or IU/ml.

SELECTION OF ANTIMICROBIALS AND CONCENTRATIONS FOR TESTING

For routine dilution procedures, it is generally unnecessary and inadvisable to test more than one representative from a group of related antimicrobials. Similarly, the selection of antimicrobials to be tested should be limited to those that are clinically useful and appropriate for the site of infection. For example, tests with nitrofurantoin and nalidixic acid should be limited to bacteria isolated from the urinary tract. Tests with methenamine mandelate should not be performed because its in vivo activity depends on urinary acidification to a pH of 5.0 or less, and this condition is not reproduced in the ordinary test systems. The selection of antimicrobials for routine testing is also determined by the type of organism isolated and by local preference for particular agents. General guidelines for selection of agents to be tested routinely are shown in Table 2.

For most purposes, a concentration of 128 μg/ml is a satisfactory upper limit for routine testing with any antimicrobic. Important exceptions to this are for carbenicillin, with which inhibition of *Pseudomonas aeruginosa* by concentrations of 100 to 128 μg/ml is considered to signify susceptibility to achievable blood levels, and when results are to be related to urinary concentrations of agents excreted by this route. Under these conditions, higher concentrations will need to be tested. In other cases, such as tests of the macrolides and lincomycins, upper limits of 32 μg/ml are suitable. The lowest

TABLE 2. *General guidelines for selection of antimicrobial agents to be tested routinely against rapidly growing aerobic and facultatively anaerobic bacteria*

Agent	Gram-positive cocci	Gram-negative bacilli	
		Urinary	Other
Ampicillin	×[a]	×	×
Carbenicillin		×	×
Cephalothin	×	×	×
Chloramphenicol	×[b]		×
Clindamycin	×		
Erythromycin	×		
Gentamicin	×[b]	×	×
Kanamycin	×[b]		×
Methicillin[c]	×		
Nalidixic acid		×	
Nitrofurantoin		×	
Penicillin G	×		
Polymyxin B or E			×
Tetracycline	×[b]	×	×
Vancomycin	×[b]		

[a] To be tested against group D streptococci only.

[b] To be tested as secondary agent only.

[c] Oxacillin and nafcillin are acceptable substitutes as representatives of the penicillinase-resistant penicillins.

concentration selected for routine dilution testing will vary according to the antimicrobial agent. In general, however, this concentration should include the upper limit of a high degree of susceptibility, inhibition by which makes in vivo response probable when mild to moderately severe systemic infections are treated with the usual dosage of the antibiotic (Group 1 as defined by The International Collaborative Study [6]). The range of concentrations should include the end point of appropriate standard strains to permit adequate control.

AGAR DILUTION METHOD

This procedure is described first because of its convenience for testing a number of strains simultaneously, its ability to detect microbial heterogeneity or contamination, and its slightly better reproducibility than the broth dilution method (6).

Preparation of antimicrobic dilutions

Dilutions of antimicrobic are prepared at 10 times the concentrations required in the final test. Log_2 dilutions are normally used for determining MICs and may be prepared according to the volumetric schedule shown in Table 3. Dilution schedules should be selected to include a concentration of 1 μg or 1 IU/ml to permit comparison of results from different laboratories and their easy expression as log_2, which facilitates statistical manipulations (6). The dilution method shown in Table 3 is convenient and economical in pipettes because only one need be used for each block of antimicrobic dilutions. It is not subject to the cumulative error inherent in traditional serial dilution methods.

Selection and preparation of medium

For rapidly growing aerobic and facultatively anaerobic bacteria, Mueller-Hinton agar is recommended. Although this medium supports the growth of most bacterial pathogens, supplementation with 5% defibrinated sheep, horse, or other animal blood may be necessary to ensure growth of some more fastidious organisms. Blood supplementation of the Mueller-Hinton agar has little effect on antibiotic susceptibility test end points except in the case of highly protein-bound agents like novobiocin (4, 20). The activity of the sulfonamides and trimethoprim is partly antagonized by components of all bloods except lysed horse blood (7). For routine purposes, supplementation of Mueller-Hinton agar with blood is usually unnecessary; however, defibrinated blood is useful for testing streptococci, and "chocolatized" blood may be used for testing *Haemophilus* and *Neisseria gonorrhoeae* (see below). Unsupplemented Mueller-Hinton agar has been reported as satisfactory for testing of *N. meningitidis* (3).

The appropriate amounts of medium (100-mm plates require 25 ml of agar) are bottled in a screw-capped container and autoclaved; the medium is then allowed to equilibrate in a constant-temperature water bath to 50 C. Addition of the antimicrobic to the agar at higher temperatures may lead to deterioration; its addition to the agar at lower temperatures will preclude adequate mixing. Defibrinated blood may be added to the agar after the

TABLE 3. *System for preparing dilutions for agar dilution method*[a]

Antibiotic solution		+	Sterile water (vol)[b]	=	Intermediate concn (μg or IU/ml)	=	Final concn at 1:10 in agar plates	
Vol[b]	μg or IU/ml						μg or IU/ml	Log_2 concn
6.4	2,000		3.6		1,280		128	7
2	1,280 (from above)		2		640		64	6
1	1,280 (from above)		3		320		32	5
1	1,280 (from above)		7		160		16	4
2	160 (from above)		2		80		8	3
1	160 (from above)		3		40		4	2
1	160 (from above)		7		20		2	1
2	20 (from above)		2		10		1	0
1	20 (from above)		3		5		0.5	−1
1	20 (from above)		7		2.5		0.25	−2

[a] Modified from Ericsson and Sherris (6).
[b] The volume size is determined by number of tests.

antimicrobic has been added and thoroughly mixed.

One volume of each dilution of antimicrobic is added to each 9 volumes of agar. For example, a final concentration in agar of 128 μg/ml is attained by adding 10 ml of the 1,280 μg/ml solution (Table 3) to 90 ml of agar. It is essential to mix the contents of the container thoroughly and to pour the agar into the plates (25 ml per plate) as quickly thereafter as possible to prevent cooling and partial solidification in the container. Although 100-mm round plates may be used, 100-mm square plates with a 13-mm grid embossed on the dish bottom provide a convenient means of identifying the location of each organism. The agar is permitted to solidify in the plates on a level surface. Control plates, with and without defibrinated sheep blood, containing no antimicrobial agent also should be prepared.

Once the agar has solidified, the plates are stored at 4 C. Ryan and co-workers (18) have shown that there is no significant loss of activity of a wide range of antimicrobial agents in agar stored at 4 C in Mylar bags for 1 week. We have confirmed this finding with other antibiotics, including carbenicillin. For routine purposes, antibiotic-containing plates should be used within this period. For reference work, it is desirable to use agar plates that have not been stored for longer than 24 h.

Preparation of inoculum

Portions of four or five discrete colonies representative of the organisms to be tested are inoculated into 4 to 5 ml of a suitable broth medium, such as soybean casein digest (Trypticase soy or Tryptic soy broth), and adjusted to the turbidity of the barium sulfate standard described in chapter 46 and by the methods discussed there. This turbidity is equivalent to approximately 5×10^7 to 9×10^7 colony-forming units (CFU) per ml for *Enterobacteriaceae* and 1×10^8 to 5×10^8 CFU/ml for *Pseudomonas aeruginosa*. A 1:20 dilution is then prepared in saline or Mueller-Hinton broth for inoculation to the antimicrobic-containing plates. Other methods of adjusting the inoculum size of log-phase cultures to approximately this concentration are acceptable. Inoculation of media should be made within 30 min of adjusting the inoculum.

The importance of testing pure cultures at properly standardized concentrations cannot be overemphasized, since mixtures of different types of organisms and the use of improperly standardized inocula confound and confuse results of susceptibility tests (1, 19).

Inoculation of medium

The agar surface of the plates containing the dilutions of antimicrobic and the control plate containing no antimicrobic are spot inoculated (without spreading) with a loop calibrated to deliver 0.001 to 0.002 ml (1 to 2 μliters) or with the inocula-replicating apparatus described by Steers et al. (22). In each case, about 10^4 CFU are delivered to a spot 5 to 8 mm in diameter. The Steers replicator may be purchased with an aluminum head carrying 32 (for 100-mm round petri dishes) or 36 (for 100-mm square dishes) equally spaced inoculating rods (Melrose Machine Shop, Woodlyn, Pa.). Stainless-steel heads are easier to clean and less subject to corrosion. Identical results have been obtained by the loop method and by the replicator (6). If other types of inoculum-replicating apparatus are used, the inoculum should be adjusted so that the equipment delivers the same inoculum and volume to the surface of the plate or yields results identical to those obtained by the methods described above.

When the Steers replicator is used, a portion of the adjusted broth suspension is pipetted to the appropriate well in the seed plate, and then the inocula are picked up and gently transferred onto the agar surface by the replicator to avoid splashing. The plates containing the lowest concentration of antimicrobic should be seeded first, although transfer of significant amounts of antimicrobic back to the wells does not appear to occur. In routine practice, up to six antimicrobics can be tested without changing the replicator head. Control plates should be seeded last to insure that viable organisms were present throughout the procedure. Swarming by *Proteus* is prevented by pressing a glass cylinder (12 by 12 mm Raschig ring; Scientific Glass Apparatus, Bloomfield, N.J.) into the agar surrounding the inoculum spot.

Incubation

Inoculated agar plates are allowed to stand undisturbed until the inoculum spots are completely absorbed and are then incubated at 35 C for 16 to 20 h. Incubation in an atmosphere with CO_2 is not recommended because of the influence of surface pH on various antimicrobial agents (6).

Controls

Staphylococcus aureus ATCC 25923, *Escherichia coli* ATCC 25922, and a strain of *Pseudomonas aeruginosa* are inoculated daily onto each set of agar plates. The means and ranges of MIC values for the *S. aureus* and *E. coli* strains have been determined in arithmetic progression at the Mayo Clinic and are listed in Table 4. It should be emphasized that these data originated from one laboratory and from one lot of Mueller-Hinton agar with the cation content specified in Table 4. Significant deviation (> ±1 twofold dilution) from the nearest $\log_2$ concentration (Table 3) requires careful search for possible errors in the procedure or contamination of the control organism. The agar plates without antimicrobic and with and without added blood are inoculated at the end of the procedure to determine whether each organism was able to grow on agar alone or required blood supplementation.

Although the presence of contamination or a mixture of organisms in one inoculum site on the agar is usually readily detectable on close scrutiny of the control plates, it is recommended that a loopful of the broth culture remaining in each well in the seed plate be streaked onto a properly labeled quadrant of a standard blood-agar plate upon completion of the replicating process. In this manner, detection of mixtures is facilitated and isolated colonies are made available for retesting in pure culture.

TABLE 4. *Means and ranges of minimal inhibitory concentrations with control organisms*[a]

Antimicrobial	Minimal inhibitory concn (μg/ml)			
	Staphylococcus aureus ATCC 25923		*Escherichia coli* ATCC 25922	
	Mean[b]	Range	Mean[b]	Range
Penicillin	0.04	0.04–0.05	—	—
Oxacillin	0.16	0.14–0.19	—	—
Ampicillin	0.06	0.06–0.08	3.4	3.3–3.4
Cephalothin	0.2	0.2–0.3	6.2	0
Erythromycin	0.11	0	—	—
Clindamycin	0.07	0	—	—
Vancomycin	1.2	0	—	—
Tetracycline	0.7	0	1.3	1.2–1.4
Kanamycin	0.9	0	2.3	2.3–2.4
Polymyxin B	—	—	0.5	0.4–0.5
Gentamicin	0.2	0	0.4	0.3–0.5
Chloramphenicol	8.0	0	4.0	0
Carbenicillin	1.0	0.9–1.3	3.7	0
Nalidixic acid	—	—	1.9	1.8–2.0
Nitrofurantoin	18.0	17.0–18.0	10.6	10.0–12.0

[a] Tested on Mueller-Hinton agar (calcium, 50.8 μg/ml; magnesium, 19.3 μg/ml) in arithmetic progression of 0.1 or 0.01 μg/ml.

[b] Means are based on 10 replicate determinations performed at the Mayo Clinic; when all 10 gave same value, range is shown as 0.

Results

The MIC represents the lowest concentration of antimicrobial agent at which complete inhibition occurs; a very fine barely visible haze or a single colony is disregarded.

MACRO BROTH DILUTION METHOD

Media

For testing rapidly growing aerobic and facultatively anaerobic bacteria, Mueller-Hinton broth is recommended; however, fastidious organisms, including some streptococci, may not grow adequately in this medium. In such instances, a casein soy peptone (for example, Trypticase or Tryptic soy) broth or Levinthal medium (21) may be used.

Dilution of antimicrobial agent

The stock solution is diluted to twice the highest final concentration desired. Sterile 13 by 100 mm screw-capped or cotton-plugged test tubes are used. Ordinarily, for a small number of tests, twofold dilutions can be prepared directly in the tubes. To the first tube is added 2 ml of the working solution of antimicrobial agent. To each remaining tube is added 1.0 ml of broth. With a sterile pipette, 1.0 ml is transferred from the first tube to the second tube. After thorough mixing of the contents of the second tube, 1.0 ml is transferred with a separate pipette (for this and each succeeding transfer) to the third tube. This process is continued through the next-to-last tube, from which 1.0 ml is removed and discarded. The last tube receives no antimicrobial agent and serves as a growth control. The final concentrations of antimicrobic in this test are half those of the initial dilution series because of the addition of an equal concentration of inoculum in broth.

A volumetric method or a bulk method of preparation of dilutions similar to that described for the agar dilution procedure may also be used (6).

Inoculum

The inoculum is prepared so as to contain 10^5 to 10^6 CFU/ml. This can be achieved in the case of *Enterobacteriaceae* and staphylococci by making a 1:2,000 dilution of an overnight broth culture. Preferably the inoculum is prepared by adjusting the turbidity of a broth culture incubated for a shorter time to match the turbidity standard (see chapter 46) and then further diluting it 1:200 in broth. To each test tube is added 1.0 ml of the adjusted inoculum. The tubes are incubated at 35 C for 16 to 20 h. Incubation in added CO_2 is not recommended unless essential for growth.

Results

The lowest concentration of antimicrobic resulting in complete inhibition of visible growth represents the MIC; a very faint haziness or a small clump of possible growth is generally disregarded, whereas a large cluster of growth or definite turbidity is considered evidence that the drug has failed to inhibit growth completely at that concentration.

SPECIAL PROBLEMS WITH DILUTION PROCEDURES

Sulfonamides and trimethoprim

The broth dilution method described above is unsuitable for tests with sulfonamides and trimethoprim because susceptible organisms may go through several generations before inhibition, thus obscuring end points. Methods with a lower inoculum and special media have been described for this purpose.

Results with the agar dilution procedure have proved satisfactory, but the end point must be taken as the plate showing sudden sharp (80%) diminution of growth (2, 3). Some growth may be seen up to the highest concentration tested because of delay in inhibition due to carry-over of sulfonamide antagonists in the inoculum. End points are sharper on media containing no thymidine or when 5 to 10% horse blood lysed by freezing and thawing is added (7), but results with unmodified Mueller-Hinton medium obtained in this country have been generally satisfactory (2, 3).

Gentamicin and tobramycin

Susceptibility tests of *Pseudomonas aeruginosa* by broth dilution methods may provide misleadingly low MICs with gentamicin and tobramycin because of the low concentrations of Mg^{2+} and Ca^{2+} in Mueller-Hinton and many other broth media (7, 8). Results with the agar dilution (or diffusion) procedures are more reliable because divalent cations contributed by most agar preparations bring them to concentrations approaching the physiological. There is need for the establishment of performance standards for media for these antibiotics; meanwhile, strains with MICs fourfold or more above the majority of routine isolates and of a representative control strain should be regarded as having increased resistance.

Methicillin

Heteroresistant strains of *Staphylococcus aureus* express their resistance to methicillin, oxacillin, and nafcillin readily with the agar dilution procedure at 35 C, but less rapidly and clearly at temperatures of 37 C or above unless incubated for at least 48 h. Careful control of incubator temperatures at 35 C is thus important (5).

SUSCEPTIBILITY TESTING OF NEISSERIA GONORRHOEAE

Routine susceptibility testing of isolates of *N. gonorrhoeae* is not needed because the penicillin schedule now used in clinical practice in the treatment of gonorrhea is sufficient to attain levels adequate to inhibit the most resistant strains encountered in the U.S. (i.e., MIC of 2 to 4 units/ml). For epidemiological and research purposes, modifications of the agar dilution procedure are needed, including the use of special media, such as GC medium base (Difco; 17, 24), supplemented with the manufacturers' recommended supplements or 5% chocolatized sheep blood. The reader is referred to the method recommended by the Center for Disease Control (24) and to the proposed international reference procedure of Reyn et al. (16).

ROUTINE USE OF DILUTION TESTS

As indicated above, dilution procedures may be used economically for routine purposes when a sufficient number of tests is made. Detailed descriptions for the routine use of the agar dilution procedure with the Steers replicator (22) and with three or four selected concentrations of each antimicrobic have been given elsewhere (26, 27). The antimicrobial concentrations are chosen to correspond to blood levels readily attained with ordinary dosage (oral when applicable) of antimicrobic, levels attained on high systemic dosage, and levels attained in the urinary tract or locally. These correspond to the four-category system described by Ericsson and Sherris (6) in the International Collaborative Study report. Broth dilution methods employing mechanized and semi-automated modifications of the microtitration system have been developed and equipment has been marketed for their use (10–13, 23). Results have been shown to correlate well with those of the macro broth dilution method. The reader is referred to the original literature for descriptions.

INTERPRETATION OF RESULTS OBTAINED FROM DILUTION TESTS

Interpretation for clinical purposes involves the factors discussed in chapter 44. In general, in the treatment of systemic infections the dosage employed should yield a peak concentration in the blood substantially higher than the MIC (14). Factors of three- to fivefold have been suggested, but it must be realized that such recommendations have been made without standardized dilution procedures and on the basis of few well-controlled laboratory-clinical correlative studies. Many uncomplicated urinary tract infections respond to urine levels rather than blood levels sufficient to inhibit the infecting organism, and in such cases account may be taken of the urine levels.

As indicated in chapter 44, interpretation is best made not only on the basis of data correlating blood level and MIC, but also by comparing the susceptibility of the strain under examination with that of others of the same species and by considering clinical experience in therapy with the agent being used. Appendix II of this section summarizes blood level data on different dose schedules for many antibiotics, and Appendix I gives the usual MICs by the agar dilution procedure of susceptible populations from among a number of commonly tested species. Resistant variants or recombinants have substantially higher MICs. For further information on available blood levels and usual MIC data, the reader is referred to the texts by Garrod, Lambert, and O'Grady (7) and by Goodman and Gilman (9).

LITERATURE CITED

1. Barry, A. L., L. J. Joyce, A. P. Adams, and E. J. Benner. 1973. Rapid determination of antimicrobial susceptibility for urgent clinical situations. Amer. J. Clin. Pathol. **59:**693–699.
2. Bauer, A. W., and J. C. Sherris. 1964. The determination of sulfonamide susceptibility of bacteria. Chemotherapia **9:**1–19.
3. Bennett, J. V., H. M. Camp, and T. C. Eickhoff. 1968. Rapid sulfonamide disc sensitivity test for meningococci. Appl. Microbiol. **16:**1056–1060.
4. Brenner, V. C., and J. C. Sherris. 1972. Influence of different media and bloods on the results of diffusion antibiotic susceptibility tests. Antimicrob. Ag. Chemother. **1:**116–122.
5. Drew, W. L., A. L. Barry, R. O'Toole, and J. C. Sherris. 1972. Reliability of the King-Bauer disc diffusion method for detecting methicillin-resistant strains of *Staphylococcus aureus*. Appl. Microbiol. **24:**240–247.
6. Ericsson, H. M., and J. C. Sherris. 1971. Antibiotic sensitivity testing. Report of an International Collaborative Study. Acta Pathol. Microbiol. Scand. Sect. B, Suppl. 217.
7. Garrod, L. P., H. P. Lambert, and F. O'Grady, with a chapter on laboratory methods by P. M. Waterworth. 1973. Antibiotic and chemotherapy, 4th ed. Churchill Livingstone, Edinburgh.
8. Gilbert, D. N., E. Kutscher, P. Ireland, and J. P. Sanford. 1971. Effect of the concentrations of magnesium and calcium on the *in vitro* susceptibility of *Pseudomonas aeruginosa* to gentamicin. J. Infect. Dis. **124:**S37–S45.
9. Goodman, L. S., and A. Gilman. 1970. The pharmacological basis of therapeutics, 4th ed. The Macmillan Co., New York.
10. Goss, W. A., and E. B. Cimijotti. 1968. Evaluation of an automatic diluting device for microbiological applications. Appl. Microbiol., **16:**1414–1416.
11. Harwick, H. J., P. Weiss, and F. R. Fekety, Jr. 1968. Application of microtitration techniques to bacteriostatic and bactericidal antibiotic susceptibility testing. J. Lab. Clin. Med. **72:**511–516.
12. MacLowry, J. D., M. J. Jaqua, and S. T. Selepak. 1970. Detailed methodology and implementation of a semiautomated serial dilution microtechnique for antimicrobial susceptibility testing. Appl. Microbiol. **20:**46–53.
13. Marymont, J. H., Jr., and R. M. Wentz. 1966. Serial dilution antibiotic sensitivity testing with the microtitrator system. Amer. J. Clin. Pathol. **45:**548–551.
14. Petersdorf, R. G., and J. J. Plorde. 1963. The usefulness of *in vitro* sensitivity tests in antibiotic therapy. Annu. Rev. Med. **14:**41–56.
15. Revised Tentative Standard. 1973. Performance standards for antimicrobial disc susceptibility tests, as used in clinical laboratories. National Committee for Clinical Laboratory Standards, Los Angeles.
16. Reyn, A., M. W. Bentzon, J. D. Thayer, and A. E. Wilkinson. 1965. Results of comparative experiments using different methods for determining the sensitivity of *Neisseria gonorrhoeae* to penicillin G. Bull. W.H.O. **32:**477–495.
17. Ronald, A. R., J. Eby, and J. C. Sherris. 1969. Susceptibility of *Neisseria gonorrhoeae* to penicillin and tetracycline. Antimicrob. Ag. Chemother. 1968, p. 431–434.
18. Ryan, K. J., G. M. Needham, C. L. Dunsmoor, and J. C. Sherris. 1970. Stability of antibiotics and chemotherapeutics in agar plates. Appl. Microbiol. **20:**447–451.
19. Shahidi, A., and P. D. Ellner. 1969. Effect of mixed cultures on antibiotic susceptibility testing. Appl. Microbiol. **18:**766–770.
20. Sherris, J. C., A. L. Rashad, and G. A. Lighthart. 1967. Laboratory determination of antibiotic susceptibility to ampicillin and cephalothin. Ann. N.Y. Acad. Sci. **145:**248–265.
21. Sonnenwirth, A. C. 1970. Media, tests, and reagents, p. 1090. *In* S. Frankel, S. Reitman, and A. C. Sonnenwirth (ed.), Gradwohl's clinical laboratory methods and diagnosis: a textbook on laboratory procedures and their interpretation, vol. 2, 7th ed. C. V. Mosby, St. Louis.
22. Steers, E., E. L. Foltz, B. S. Graves, and J. Riden. 1959. An inocula replicating apparatus for routine testing of bacterial susceptibility to antibiotics. Antibiot. Chemother. (Basel) **9:**307–311.
23. Tilton, R. C., L. Lieberman, and E. M. Gerlach. 1973. Microdilution antibiotic susceptibility test; examination of certain variables. Appl. Microbiol. **26:**658–665.
24. U.S. Department of Health, Education, and Welfare. 1963. Gonococcus, procedures for isolation and identification. Publication 499, Public Health Service. U.S. Government Printing Office, Washington, D.C.
25. Warren, E., R. J. Snyder, C. O. Thompson, and J. A. Washington II. 1972. Stability of ampicillin in intrave-

nous solutions. Mayo Clin. Proc. **47**:34–35.
26. Washington, J. A., II. 1971. The agar-dilution method, p. 127–141. *In* T. L. Gavan, H. W. McFadden, Jr., and E. L. Cheatle (ed.), Antimicrobial susceptibility testing. American Society of Clinical Pathologists, Inc., Chicago.
27. Washington, J. A., II. 1974. Laboratory procedures in clinical microbiology. Little, Brown & Co., Boston.

Chapter 46

Susceptibility Testing: Diffusion Test Procedures

JOHN M. MATSEN AND ARTHUR L. BARRY

INTRODUCTION AND PRINCIPLES

In the late 1940's, filter-paper disks impregnated with antimicrobics were first used to measure bacterial susceptibility to penicillin. Disks were often prepared with more than one concentration of penicillin and were then applied to the surface of an agar plate which had been streaked with the test organism. A concentric zone of inhibition resulted, and, within certain limits, its size increased in parallel with the amount of penicillin in the disk. Conversely, when the amount of drug in the disk was held constant, the size of the zone of inhibition could be related directly to the degree of susceptibility of the test organism. This feature led, over the intervening years, to the development of susceptibility testing methods employing single antimicrobic disks of defined content.

The size of the zone of inhibition is also influenced by a number of technical variables other than disk content, and carefully standardized techniques are needed for acceptable intra- and interlaboratory reproducibility. In the United States, the same standardized disk diffusion susceptibility test method, with minor modifications, has been recommended by both the U.S. Food and Drug Administration (FDA) and the Subcommittee on Antimicrobial Susceptibility Testing of the National Committee for Clinical Laboratory Standards (10, 11, 16) and is described in this chapter. Utilization of other techniques or modification of the recommended procedures can be justified only after extensive experimental data have demonstrated that the alternate method is at least as accurate and precise as the recommended method.

When filter-paper disks containing fixed amounts of antimicrobics are applied to the moist agar surface, the antimicrobics diffuse into the surrounding medium, presenting a constantly changing gradient of antimicrobic concentrations at various distances from the edge of the disk. At the same time, the microorganisms are multiplying logarithmically on the agar surface. At a critical time, the position of the zone of inhibition will be determined; i.e., growth will be inhibited in the area where sufficiently high concentrations of drugs have been obtained, but, beyond that, growth will proceed where the concentration of antimicrobic is not great enough. When all of the variables are held constant, the diameter of the zone of inhibition relates approximately linearly to the log minimal inhibitory concentration (MIC) as measured by dilution susceptibility tests for organisms of reasonably comparable growth rates (9, 14). This zone size-MIC relationship is of critical importance in developing interpretive standards for the disk diffusion test. Based on knowledge of the pharmokinetics of each antimicrobic and the behavior of organisms of known clinical responsiveness, it is possible to select MIC breakpoints above which an organism should be considered resistant and below which the organism is classified as susceptible (see chapter 45). Clinical experience over the years has generally proven that these extrapolations predict in vivo response or lack of response reasonably well.

Figure 1 illustrates the type of data that can be collected with different drugs to document the relationship between zone diameters and MICs by use of a standardized method and a fixed disk content. It shows results of tests using the agar dilution procedure described in chapter 44 and the diffusion method described below. Microorganisms are selected whenever possible to provide MICs which are fairly evenly distributed over a relevant range of concentrations and to include representatives of the common species of bacteria for which the antimicrobial agents might be used. At least 100 to 150 strains should be tested by both methods. With most drugs, the distribution of plots indeed is linear and, by using the formula of least squares the line of best fit (regression line), can be calculated mathematically, assuming a straight-line relationship. In calculating a regression line, all MIC values above and below the actual concentrations tested and all disk tests showing no zone of inhibition should be excluded. By convention, zone diameters are usually considered the dependent variable. The results in Fig. 1 are plotted with MICs as the dependent variable because the lines are intended for

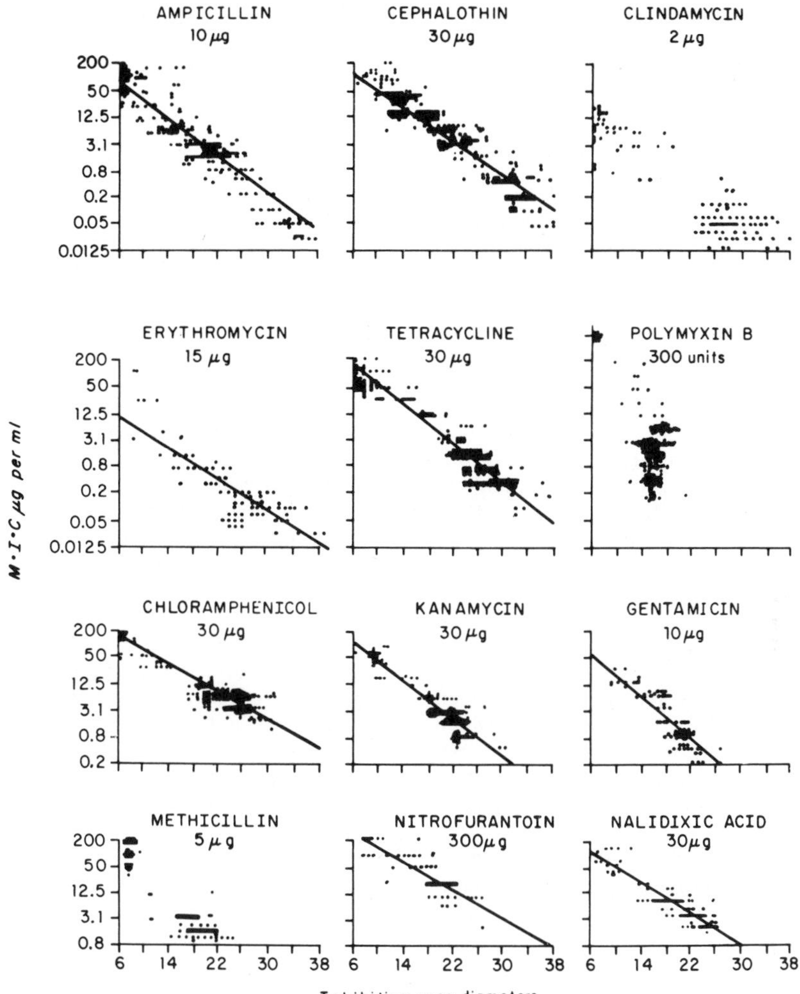

FIG. 1. *Relationship of zone diameter to agar dilution MIC with some commonly used antimicrobics. All except polymyxin and gentamicin show combined data from clinical laboratories of the Universities of Minnesota and Washington. The disk content is shown below each antimicrobic. Polymyxin MICs are in units per milliliter.*

extrapolating ranges of MIC correlates from diffusion test results (14). A regression analysis is valid only when it is possible to obtain a reasonably uniform distribution of points along the entire range of MIC values. Since the MIC values are determined by using doubling dilution steps, whereas the zone diameter is determined with a system which exposes the bacteria to a continual gradient of drug concentrations, the "true" regression line can be depicted more accurately by drawing a second line parallel to the calculated line exactly one-half an MIC below the observed value (9). When the distribution of points does not permit a regression analysis, the relationship of MIC to zone diameter is best expressed as a scattergram (also shown in Fig. 1).

Once a consideration of the pharmokinetics of the antimicrobic has provided MIC values for defining "resistant" and "susceptible" categories, the corresponding zone size breakpoints can be calculated directly from regression lines. Since the actual observed points are found to scatter on either side of the calculated line, it may be necessary to adjust the calculated zone size breakpoints by considering population distributions (chapter 44) in order to avoid major errors in interpretation with those strains giving divergent results. In this way, it is possible to establish for each drug a minimal zone diameter for organisms that are normally considered susceptible and a maximal zone diameter that may be produced by resistant organisms. An intermediate category between these two extremes in zone sizes is thereby created to serve as a "buffer zone" which minimizes the significance of minor variations in zone diameters with those strains which give zones right at the zone size breakpoints, and in addition this intermediate category would include those strains which are truly intermediate in their susceptibility.

INDICATIONS FOR DIFFUSION SUSCEPTIBILITY TESTS

Antimicrobic susceptibility tests should be performed with all microorganisms which are contributing to an infectious process that warrants chemotherapy, providing that the microorganism's susceptibility cannot be predicted from the knowledge of its identity. Thus, susceptibility tests are most often indicated when the causative microorganism has been identified as a species known to be capable of exhibiting resistance to commonly used antimicrobic agents, e.g., *Staphylococcus* sp., the *Enterobacteriaceae*, and *Pseudomonas* sp. Susceptibility tests are rarely necessary when the infection is due to a microorganism that is invariably susceptible to an effective drug; e.g., most pathogenic streptococci and *Neisseria* species are predictably susceptible to one or more highly effective antibiotics. When the nature of the infection is not clear and the specimen contains mixed growth of normal flora in which the microorganisms probably bear little relationship to the infectious process being treated, susceptibility tests are often wasteful or grossly misleading (3).

It is important to understand that the standardized disk diffusion method described below should be used only for rapidly growing organisms for which an end point can be easily determined within an 18- to 24-h period. Beyond that point, diffusion of antimicrobic or its inactivation may give erroneous results. Tests with enterococci can be made by the standardized procedure using blood-supplemented Mueller-Hinton agar. Sometimes it is necessary to test isolates of *Haemophilus influenzae*, and this can be done with chocolatized blood agar. The method has not been standardized for facultative organisms with slower growth rates such as many viridans streptococci. Zone diameters will be larger for equivalent MICs, and susceptibility should be confirmed by dilution tests. Resistance, however, is always significant.

SELECTION OF ANTIMICROBICS FOR ROUTINE DIFFUSION TESTING

In general, routine tests should include only one representative of each group of antimicrobics with closely related in vitro activity. The FDA has recognized specific class disks for testing as noted in Table 2 (10). The agents listed in Table 1 should fulfill the basic requirements for routine diffusion use in most clinical laboratories. Additional antimicrobics should be available for use with special problems of the individual patient or to take account of local preference. Agents other than those used in therapy may be tested to provide epidemiological information and taxonomic data; however, routine reports to physicians should include only those appropriate for therapeutic use to avoid misleading information. Certain antimicrobics may be added to, or removed from, this basic list for educational purposes or for controlling the use of potentially toxic drugs within an institution.

TABLE 1. *Basic sets of antimicrobics suggested for routine disk susceptibility tests in clinical microbiology laboratories*

Staphylococcus aureus	Enterococci	*Enterobacteriaceae*	Pseudomonads
1. Penicillin G	1. Penicillin G	1. Ampicillin	1. Gentamicin
2. Oxacillin or methicillin	2. Ampicillin	2. Cephalothin	2. Carbenicillin
3. Cephalothin	3. Cephalothin	3. Kanamycin	3. Polymyxin B
4. Erythromycin	4. Erythromycin	4. Gentamicin	4. Kanamycin[c]
5. Clindamycin	5. Chloramphenicol[a]	5. Polymyxin B	5. Chloramphenicol[c]
6. Chloramphenicol[a]	6. Tetracycline[a]	6. Tetracycline	6. Tetracycline[c]
7. Tetracycline[a]		7. Chloramphenicol	7. Sulfonamides[b, c]
8. Gentamicin[a]		8. Nitrofurantoin[b]	
9. Kanamycin[a]		9. Nalidixic acid[b]	
		10. Sulfonamides[b]	

[a] Suggested only as secondary drugs.

[b] Only with isolates from urinary tract infections.

[c] Indicated for testing *Pseudomonas* species other than *P. aeruginosa* or for other nonfermentative gram-negative bacilli.

TABLE 2. *Zone diameter interpretive standards and approximate MIC correlates*[a]

Antibiotic	Disk content	Zone diam (nearest whole mm)			Approximate MIC correlates	
		Resistant	Intermediate	Susceptible	Resistant	Susceptible
Ampicillin[b] when testing						
Gram-negative enteric organisms and enterococci	10 μg	≤11	12–13	≥14	≥32 μg/ml	≤8 μg/ml
Staphylococci and penicillin G-susceptible microorganisms	10 μg	≤20	21–28	≥29	≥2 μg/ml Penicillinase[c]	≤0.2 μg/ml
Haemophilus species	10 μg	≤19	—	≥20	—	≤2.0 μg/ml
Carbenicillin[d] when testing						
Proteus species and *Escherichia coli*	50 μg	≤17	18–22	≥23	≥32 μg/ml	≤16 μg/ml
Pseudomonas aeruginosa	50 μg	≤12	13–14	≥15	≥250 μg/ml	≤125 μg/ml
Cephalothin[e, f]	30 μg	≤14	15–17	≥18	≥32 μg/ml	≤10 μg/ml
Chloramphenicol	30 μg	≤12	13–17	≥18	≥25 μg/ml	≤12.5 μg/ml
Clindamycin	2 μg	≤14	15–16	≥17	≥2 μg/ml	≤1 μg/ml
Erythromycin	15 μg	≤13	14–17	≥18	≥8 μg/ml	≤2 μg/ml
Gentamicin	10 μg	≤12	—	≥13	>6 μg/ml	≤6 μg/ml
Kanamycin	30 μg	≤13	14–17	≥18	≥25 μg/ml	≤6 μg/ml
Methicillin[f, g] when testing staphylococci[h]	5 μg	≤9	10–13	≥14	—	≤3 μg/ml
Neomycin	30 μg	≤12	13–16	≥17	—	≤10 μg/ml
Penicillin G[i] when testing						
Staphylococci	10 units	≤20	21–28	≥29	Penicillinase[c]	≤0.1 μg/ml
Other microorganisms[j]	10 units	≤11	12–21[i]	≥22	≥32 μg/ml	≤1.5 μg/ml
Polymyxin B[k]	300 units	≤8	9–11	≥12	≥50 units/ml	—
Streptomycin	10 μg	≤11	12–14	≥15	≥15 μg/ml	≤6 μg/ml
Tetracycline[l]	30 μg	≤14	15–18	≥19	≥12 μg/ml	≤4 μg/ml
Vancomycin	30 μg	≤9	10–11	≥12	—	≤5 μg/ml
Sulfonamides[m]	250 or 300 μg	≤12	13–16	≥17	≥35 mg/100 ml	≤10 mg/100 ml
Sulfonamide-trimethoprim (19:1)[m]	25 μg	≤10	11–15	≥16	≥200 μg/ml	≤35 μg/ml
Nitrofurantoin[m]	300 μg	≤14	15–18	≥19	≥100 μg/ml	≤25 μg/ml
Nalidixic acid[m]	30 μg	≤13	14–18	≥19	≥32 μg/ml	≤12 μg/ml

[a] Interpretations for antibiotics are from those presently recommended by the FDA (10, 11). Those for chemotherapeutics are from the National Committee for Clinical Laboratory Standards tentative recommendation (16) or from the manufacturer in the case of the sulfonamide-trimethoprim combination. Recommendations for bacitracin, cephaloglycin, colistin, lincomycin, novobiocin, and oleandomycin are given in reference 10 or disk package inserts.

[b] Class disk for ampicillin and hetacillin.

[c] Resistant *S. aureus* strains are penicillinase producers.

[d] A carbenicillin change to a 100-μg disk with new interpretative standards is presently under consideration by the FDA. If this occurs, the new standards will be given in package inserts.

[e] Class disk for cephalothin, cephaloridine, cephalexin, and cefazolin.

[f] See section on limitations of method.

[g] Class disk for penicillinase-resistant penicillins in tests with staphylococci.

[h] Authors' addition.

[i] Class disk for penicillin G, phenoxymethyl penicillin, or phenethicillin.

[j] Intermediate category includes some organisms such as enterococci and certain gram-negative bacilli that may cause systemic infections treatable with high dosage of penicillin G, but not of phenoxymethyl penicillin or phenethicillin.

[k] Considered by the authors to apply also to colistin. See also section on limitations of method.

[l] Class disk for tetracyclines.

[m] Use for urinary tract-infecting organisms only.

RECOMMENDED DISK DIFFUSION TECHNIQUES

The disk diffusion test currently recommended by the U.S. FDA (10, 11) and as a tentative standard by the National Committee for Clinical Laboratory Standards is a slight modification of that described by Bauer, Kirby, Sherris, and Turck (4). This method should be followed exactly as outlined if accurate, reproducible results are to be anticipated. Only one alternative method has been adequately studied and shown to give comparable zone sizes, similar precision, and satisfactory correlation with MICs. That is the agar overlay method of Barry, Garcia, and Thrupp (2), which has been recognized formally as an acceptable alternative method for standardizing the inoculum when testing the commonly isolated rapid-growing bacterial pathogens, such as *Staphylococcus aureus*, members of the *Enterobacteriaceae*, and *Pseudomonas aeruginosa* (10).

Agar medium

Both methods have been standardized with Mueller-Hinton agar. The unsupplemented medium supports the growth of most of those microorganisms for which susceptibility tests are most relevant. Other microorganisms may require the addition of 5% defibrinated sheep, horse, or other animal blood. The agar overlay method has not been evaluated for testing those microorganisms which require the addition of defibrinated blood or other supplements to the base medium.

The pH of each batch of Mueller-Hinton agar should be checked at the time the medium is poured for use. The pH should be 7.2 to 7.4 after equilibration at room temperature and may be measured by allowing the agar to solidify around the electrodes of a pH meter, by maceration of the medium in neutral distilled water, or by use of a surface electrode. The freshly prepared and cooled medium is poured into petri plates on a level horizontal surface so as to give a uniform depth of approximately 4 mm; this requires approximately 60 ml of medium in 150-mm plates and approximately 25 ml in 100-mm plates. After the medium has been allowed to cool to room temperature, it should be stored in a refrigerator (2 to 8 C). If the plates are to be stored for more than 5 to 7 days, they should be wrapped in plastic to minimize evaporation. Just before use, the plates should be placed in an incubator (35 C) with lids ajar, until excess surface moisture is lost by evaporation (usually about 10 to 20 min). There should be no droplets of moisture on the surface of the medium or on the petri plate cover. With the agar overlay method of inoculation, the plates must be warmed to room temperature but the surface need not be dried before inoculation.

Storage of antimicrobic disks

Antimicrobic cartridges containing filter-paper disks specifically certified for susceptibility testing are generally supplied in separate containers, each with a desiccant. They should be stored under refrigeration (2 to 8 C) or "frozen" at −14 C or lower until needed. Disks containing drugs which belong to the penicillin or cephalosporin families should always be kept "frozen" to ensure maintenance of their potency (7, 8, 13); however, a small working supply may be held in a refrigerator at 2 to 8 C for as long as 1 week. Unopened containers should be removed from the refrigerator or freezer 1 or 2 h before the disks are to be used and allowed to equilibrate to room temperature before being opened. This is done to minimize the amount of condensation that would occur when warm room air reached the cold containers. If a disk-dispensing apparatus is used, it should be fitted with a tight cover and supplied with an adequate indicating desiccant. Also, it should be allowed to warm to room temperature before being opened. When not in use, the dispensing apparatus should always be kept covered and refrigerated. Only those disks that have not reached the manufacturer's stated expiration date should be used.

Inoculation of test plates

Standard method. An inoculating needle or loop is touched to each of four or five well-isolated colonies of the same morphological type and inoculated into 4 or 5 ml of a suitable broth medium such as soybean casein digest broth. The broth cultures are then allowed to incubate at 35 C until a slightly visible turbidity appears (usually 2 to 5 h). The turbidity of actively growing broth cultures is then adjusted with saline or broth so as to obtain a turbidity visually comparable to that of a turbidity standard prepared by adding 0.5 ml of 0.048 M $BaCl_2$ (1.175%, wt/vol, $BaCl_2 \cdot 2H_2O$) to 99.5 ml of 0.36 N H_2SO_4 (1%, vol/vol). (This is half the density of a McFarland no. 1 standard.) This turbidity standard is agitated on a Vortex mixer immediately prior to use. Unless the standard is contained in heat-sealed glass tubes (20), it should be replaced at least once every 6 months. For proper turbidity adjustment, it is helpful to use a white background and contrasting black line in combination with an adequate light source. The modified Rh-typing view box described by Stemper and Matsen (18) facilitates standardizing cultures. When time does not permit for the development of a turbid broth culture, colonies can be suspended directly into a small volume of saline which is then further diluted until the turbidity matches that of the $BaSO_4$ standard (3). The inoculum suspension should not be allowed to stand longer than 15 to 20 min before the plates are inoculated.

To inoculate the agar medium, a sterile cotton swab on a wooden (not plastic) applicator stick is dipped into the standardized suspension, and excess broth is expressed by pressing and rotating the swab firmly against the inside of the tube above the fluid level. The swab is then streaked evenly in three directions over the entire surface of the agar plate to obtain a uniform inoculum. A final sweep is made of the agar rim with the cotton swab. This plate is then allowed to dry for 3 to 5 min, but no longer than 15 min, before the disks are applied. The inoculum should yield confluent or almost completely confluent growth.

Alternate agar overlay method (2). Four or five isolated colonies of the same morphological type are selected, and a visibly turbid suspension is prepared in 0.5 ml of brain heart infusion broth, in 13 by 100 mm tubes. Changes due to evaporation during storage of this small volume of broth are avoided by transferring it aseptically into sterile tubes on the day it is to be used. The small-volume broth cultures are then allowed to incubate in a 35 to 37 C water bath or heating block for 4 to 8 h. By this time, maximal growth has occurred. A 0.001-ml calibrated loopful of a well-mixed broth culture is transferred to 9.0 ml of a 1.5% aqueous solution of agar which has been melted and cooled to 45 to 50 C. Screw-capped tubes of agar may be held at this temperature before inoculation for up to 8 h in a heating block. After inoculation, the seeded agar is quickly mixed by gentle inversion and spread evenly over the surface of a 150-mm petri plate containing Mueller-Hinton agar (4 mm in depth). This procedure is facilitated by bringing the plates to room temperature before attempting to spread the thin layer of seeded agar. The inoculated plates are allowed to stand for 3 to 5 min undisturbed on a flat and level surface before susceptibility disks are applied.

Test procedure: either method of inoculation

Within 15 min after the plates are inoculated, antimicrobic-impregnated disks are applied to the surface of the inoculated plates either by a mechanical dispenser or by hand with sterile forceps. All disks must be gently pressed down onto the agar with forceps or an inoculating needle to ensure complete contact with the agar surface. The spatial arrangement of the disks should be such that they are no closer than 15 mm from the edges of the plate and far enough apart to prevent overlapping of zones of inhibition. Generally, this limits the number of disks which can be placed on a single plate to 12 or 13 on a 150-mm plate or only 4 or 5 on a 100-mm plate. Within 15 min after the disks are applied, the plates are inverted and placed in an incubator at 35 C. Any longer delay before incubation will allow excess prediffusion of the antimicrobic. Incubation in an environment of increased CO_2 is to be avoided because the CO_2 will alter the surface pH enough to affect the antimicrobial activity of some agents (9).

Reading and interpretation

After 16 to 18 h of incubation, the plates are examined and the diameter of the zones of complete inhibition is measured to the nearest whole millimeter, by use of sliding calipers, a ruler, or a template prepared for this purpose. When unsupplemented medium is used, the measuring device is held on the back of the petri plate, which is illuminated with reflected light. Similar systems using transmitted light may also be used if comparable zone sizes are obtained with quality control strains. Zones on blood-containing media are measured at the agar surface. The end point by all reading systems is complete inhibition of growth as determined visually, ignoring faint growth or tiny colonies which can be detected by very close scrutiny. Large colonies growing within the clear zone of inhibition may represent resistant variants or a mixed inoculum and may require reidentification and retesting. In the case of sulfonamides or sulfonamide-trimethoprim mixtures, the microorganisms may grow through several generations before inhibition occurs. In this instance, slight growth (80% inhibition) is disregarded and the margin of heavy growth is measured (5). The veil of swarming *Proteus* sp. is also disregarded and the margin of heavy growth is measured. In clinically urgent situations, preliminary readings can be obtained often within 5 or 6 h after inoculation, but the plates should always be reincubated and a final report is withheld until a full 16 to 18 h have elapsed.

The zone diameters for individual antimicrobics are translated into prefixed susceptible, intermediate, or resistant categories by referring to an interpretative table. The interpretations for the antibiotics in Table 2 are those presently recommended by the FDA (10, 11). They are supplemented with recommendations from other sources for the chemotherapeutics. Approximate MIC correlates of the breakpoints obtained with the methods described in chapter 45 are also given in the table (16).

Four changes of the zone size recommendations in Table 2 have been proposed in the National Committee for Clinical Laboratory Standards tentative standard (16). They comprise:

(1) Consolidation of the penicillin and ampicillin interpretative criteria. Those given for ampicillin against staphylococci and against *Enterobacteriaceae* and enterococci would apply to both antimicrobics, as would the category "other organisms" listed for penicillin. This change would take account of the high systemic and urine levels that are achieved with doses appropriate for treating gram-negative and enterococcal infections.

(2) A shift in the gentamicin breakpoint for susceptibility to a zone diameter of 15 mm or more, and the establishment of an intermediate category of 13 to 14 mm. This has been proposed because a few strains of *Pseudomonas* have been encountered with zones of 13 and 14 mm and agar dilution MICs as high as 12.5 μg/ml.

(3) A shift in clindamycin breakpoints to 11 mm or less, resistant; and 16 mm or more, susceptible. This would equate to MICs of approximately ≥ 4 and ≤ 2 μg/ml, respectively.

(4) Zone standards for oxacillin and nafcillin 1-μg disks against staphylococci. These have been recommended because the two agents are more stable than methicillin and are equally, or more, effective in detecting resistance to the penicillinase-resistant penicillins. The recommended standards for both are: resistant, 10 mm or less; intermediate, 11 to 12 mm; susceptible, 13 mm or more. It is to be anticipated that some agreed changes in the interpretation chart will result from these proposals and that changes will occur from time to time as further knowledge is gained and new agents become available.

The MIC breakpoints listed in Table 2 are related to blood levels usually expected with frequently used dose schedules or to urine levels in the case of nitrofurantoin or naladixic acid. The breakpoints were tested against the distribution of zone sizes and MICs among a variety of species of known clinical responsiveness or lack of responsiveness to check their appropriateness and were modified where considered necessary for adequate discrimination (4, 16, 17). The resistant and susceptible categories for most drugs were developed to apply to systemic infections and appropriate dosage schedules. In situations where high dosage of nontoxic agents may be given, blood levels may greatly exceed those considered in establishment of the interpretive values. Similarly, concentration of certain antibiotics by the kidney may result in urinary levels many-fold higher than the levels considered in developing breakpoints for systemic infections. In such situations, organisms which are resistant by the disk method might be treated successfully. Extrapolation from data such as that given in Fig. 1 to determine the probable MIC or direct antimicrobic dilution studies should be made before such therapy is considered.

LIMITATIONS OF THE METHOD AND SPECIAL PRECAUTIONS

Slow-growing organisms, obligate anaerobes, and capnophiles should not be tested with the disk diffusion method which has been standardized for testing rapidly growing aerobes or facultative organisms. Special precautions must be taken and special interpretative standards must be used to test *Neisseria meningitidis* against the sulfonamides (6). The method has not been standardized for other tests with *N. meningitidis* or *N. gonorrhoeae*. Dilution methods should be used if susceptibility tests are desired for such microorganisms. Disk diffusion susceptibility testing is not done with either methenamine mandelate or methenamine hippurate as there is no corollary between the in vivo and in vitro conditions (16, 17).

Special problems are posed by hetero-resistant "methicillin-resistant" *S. aureus*. These strains appear to have increased clinical resistance to the penicillins and cephalosporins. They can be detected reliably with methicillin, oxacillin, or nafcillin disks, and at temperatures of 35 C, but often not at 37 C (8, 19). If incubators cannot be controlled at 35 C, separate tests with one of these agents only should be made on segments of Mueller-Hinton agar plates incubated at 30 C. Diffusion tests with these strains often fail to indicate resistance to cloxacillin and cephalothin although dilution tests show it to exist. Thus, strains proved to be resistant to methicillin, oxacillin, or nafcillin should be considered potentially resistant to the whole group of penicillinase-resistant penicillins and cephalosporins, and the clinician should be alerted to this.

Many false reports of methicillin resistance have resulted from deterioration of methicillin disks while refrigerated. Attention to the recommendations given below for disk storage and quality control should avoid this difficulty (7, 8, 13).

As discussed in chapter 45, results of tests for gentamicin susceptibility of *P. aeruginosa* are highly dependent on medium content of magnesium and calcium. Most batches of Mueller-Hinton agar are satisfactory for routine testing and interpretation by the criteria given in Table 2. However, it is important to use a control strain of *P. aeruginosa* to detect errors from this source (12).

The accuracy of this disk test is dependent on adequate diffusion of antimicrobic. The polymyxins (B and E) diffuse very poorly, and, although resistance is significant, it is important to confirm susceptibility by a dilution test if it is proposed to use these agents for systemic therapy (10, 14).

QUALITY CONTROL PROCEDURES

To control the precision and accuracy of disk diffusion tests, the "Seattle strains" of *S. aureus* (ATCC 25923) and *Escherichia coli* (ATCC 25922) have been designated as standard control organisms and should be included with each day's batch of tests (10, 16). A gentamicin- and carbenicillin-susceptible strain of *P. aeruginosa* should also be used. Strain ATCC 27853 is now being recommended by the FDA for this purpose. To avoid variation and contamination, control strains should not be subcultured repeatedly on slants or in broth. They should be maintained lyophilized, frozen at −60C in 15% glycerol broth or 50% inactivated fetal calf serum in broth, or purchased from a laboratory supply house as single-use vials specifically developed for quality control purposes.

Daily tests should be made of the quality control strains and the actual zone of inhibition should be measured to the nearest millimeter and plotted on an easily accessible, easily readable chart (1, 7). Adequate precision and accuracy in this procedure can be determined by standard statistical methods. The maximal and minimal zone diameters that would be expected with the standard *S. aureus* and *E. coli* strains are listed in Table 3. These tolerance limits represent data accumulated from a large number of institutions before acceptance of these control strains, and therefore the limits are rather broad. The table also shows the presently accepted "true" means. Ideally, each laboratory should also establish its own means and standard deviations, which are recalculated every 3 to 6 months. The range represented by the ±2 SD should fall within the tolerance limits listed in Table 3. If the means obtained with all or most antibiotics fall consistently above those listed in Table 3, it is probable that the inoculum is too light. Consistently smaller zones suggest excessive inoculum. Declining zone sizes with one of the penicillins and cephalosporins (especially methicillin) suggest disk deterioration. Divergent results between the aminoglycosides and tetracycline suggest that the pH is incorrect.

Table 3 also lists the maximal standard deviation which could be tolerated on theoretical grounds (16). These values are based on the differences between the minimal zone size for suceptible strains and maximal zone size for resistant strains, and assume that the standard deviations with clinical isolates would be those of the control organisms. If the maximal values are not exceeded, inherent test variables will result in a serious interpretive error no more than once in every 100 tests with strains which give zones just at the interpretative breakpoint. That is to say, the interpretation may vary between resistant and intermediate or between susceptible and intermediate, but very rarely between resistant and susceptible.

If these control limits are exceeded, there is a significant probability that technical errors are sufficient to result in clinically significant misinterpretations with some of the test organisms. The various sources of technical error must be investigated and corrected when the controls indicate unsatisfactory results.

COMMON SOURCES OF ERROR

Though the disk diffusion method is a fairly forgiving procedure, technical errors can compromise accuracy and reliability, and one error may either neutralize or compound the effect of another type of error. Included below is a list of some of the more common sources of error which are encountered in clinical microbiology laboratories.

1. Failure to use Mueller-Hinton agar medium.
2. Improper preparation of Mueller-Hinton agar, especially failure to measure pH at the time of preparation.
3. Use of outdated medium or unsatisfactorily stored plates.
4. Improper storage of disks.
5. Inadequate standardization of broth culture density.
6. Inaccurate preparation or storage of turbidity reference standard.
7. Failure to express surplus fluid from the swab before inoculating plates.
8. Excess delay between culture standardization and plate inoculation.

TABLE 3. *Mean and range of zone diameters (mm) and theoretical maximal standard deviation permissible with standard control organisms*

Antimicrobic (high-content disks)	*E. coli* (ATCC 25922)			*S. aureus* (ATCC 25923)		
	Mean[a]	Zone limits[b]	Max SD[c]	Mean	Zone limits[a]	Max SD[b]
Penicillin G		—	—	31.5	26–37	2.9
Ampicillin	17.5	15–20	1.3	29.5	24–35	2.9
Methicillin		—	—	19.5	17–22	1.6
Cephalothin	20.5	18–23	1.3	31.0	25–37	1.3
Chloramphenicol	24.0	21–27	1.9	22.5	19–26	1.9
Tetracycline	21.5	18–25	1.6	23.5	19–28	1.6
Erythromycin	11.0	8–14	1.6	26.0	22–30	1.6
Clindamycin	—	—	—	26.0	23–29	1.6
Kanamycin	21.0	17–25	1.6	22.5	19–26	1.6
Streptomycin	16.0	12–20	1.3	18.0	14–22	1.3
Gentamicin	22.5	19–26	1.3[d]	23.0	19–27	1.3[d]
Polymyxin B	14.0	12–16	1.3	10.0	7–13	1.3

[a] Means of FDA collaborative study results.

[b] Tolerance limits based on data from FDA collaborative studies (10).

[c] Theoretical maximal standard deviation permissible without altering the interpretation of the test significantly ($P < 0.01$), based on the minimal change in zone size which would be required to alter the interpretation from susceptible to resistant.

[d] Relates to National Committee for Clinical Laboratory Standards tentative recommendation for gentamicin (16).

9. Excess delay in applying disks after inoculation of plates.
10. Excess delay in incubating the plates after application of disks.
11. Incubation deviating from 35 C or use of increased CO_2 atmosphere.
12. Premature reading of test results before the full 16 to 18 h.
13. Failure to measure zone borders carefully.
14. Attempts to test mixed cultures.
15. Application of the procedure to slow growers and to anaerobes.
16. Failure to include quality control strains or to record the results of control tests.
17. Transcription error in recording results of individual tests (15).

INDICATIONS FOR DIRECT SUSCEPTIBILITY TESTING ON CLINICAL MATERIAL

The direct inoculation of susceptibility plates can sometimes provide invaluable preliminary information with urgent clinical infection problems. For example, direct tests may be made on plates seeded with emergency specimens, such as cerebrospinal fluid, other body fluids, or purulent specimens, if direct Gram smears indicate that a large number of bacteria of a single species may be expected to grow. However, routine direct susceptibility tests on clinical material are to be avoided. Mixtures of organisms, common in many specimens, frequently produce inaccurate interpretations (3). Furthermore, it is very difficult to standardize the density of an inoculum from direct clinical material. The use of a purity check plate will be of great assistance in these emergency situations, as will an assessment of the nature of the "lawn" of inoculum on the susceptibility test plate. Results from emergency tests should be reported as preliminary or tentative and should be repeated and confirmed by one of the recommended methods. When directly inoculated test plates are unsatisfactory, valuable preliminary information can be obtained by making preliminary readings of the regular test after 5 to 6 h of incubation at 35 C. When this is done, the plate must be reincubated and a final report is issued after overnight incubation.

LITERATURE CITED

1. Barry, A. L., G. D. Fay, and F. W. Atchison. 1972. Quality control of antimicrobial disc susceptibility testing with a rapid method compared to the standard methods. Antimicrob. Ag. Chemother. **2:**419–422.
2. Barry, A. L., F. Garcia, and L. D. Thrupp. 1970. An improved single-disk method for testing the antibiotic susceptibility of rapidly growing pathogens. Amer. J. Clin. Pathol. **53:**149–158.
3. Barry, A. L., L. J. Joyce, A. P. Adams, and E. J. Benner. 1973. Rapid determination of antimicrobial susceptibility for urgent clinical situations. Amer. J. Clin. Pathol. **59:**693–699.
4. Bauer, A. W., W. M. M. Kirby, J. C. Sherris, and M. Turck. 1966. Antibiotic susceptibility testing by a standardized single disk method. Amer. J. Clin. Pa-

thol. **45:**493–496.

5. Bauer, A. W., and J. C. Sherris. 1964. The determination of sulfonamide susceptibility of bacteria. Chemotherapia **9:**1–19.
6. Bennett, J. V., H. M. Camp, and T. C. Eickhoff. 1968. Rapid sulfonamide disc sensitivity test for meningococci. Appl. Microbiol. **16:**1056–1060.
7. Blazevic, D. J., M. H. Koepcke, and J. M. Matsen. 1972. Quality control testing with the disc antibiotic susceptibility test of Bauer-Kirby-Sherris-Turck. Amer. J. Clin. Pathol. **57:**592–597.
8. Drew, W. L., A. L. Barry, R. O'Toole, and J. C. Sherris. 1972. Reliability of the Kirby-Bauer disc diffusion method for detecting methicillin-resistant strains of *Staphylococcus aureus*. Appl. Microbiol. **24:**240–247.
9. Ericsson, H. M., and J. C. Sherris. 1971. Antibiotic sensitivity testing. Report of an International Collaborative Study. Acta Pathol. Microbiol. Scand. Sect. B, Suppl. 217.
10. Federal Register. 1972. Rules and regulations. Antibiotic susceptibility discs. Fed. Regist. **37:**20525–20529.
11. Federal Register. 1973. Rules and regulations. Antibiotic susceptibility discs—correction. Fed. Regist. **38:**2576.
12. Garrod, L. P., and P. M. Waterworth. 1969. Effect of medium composition on the apparent sensitivity of *Pseudomonas aeruginosa* to gentamicin. J. Clin. Pathol. **22:**534–538.
13. Griffith, L. J., and C. G. Mullins. 1968. Drug resistance as influenced by inactivated sensitivity discs. Appl. Microbiol. **16:**656–658.
14. Matsen, J. M., M. J. H. Koepcke, and P. G. Quie. 1970. Evaluation of the Bauer-Kirby-Sherris-Turck single-disc diffusion method of antibiotic susceptibility testing, p. 445–453. Antimicrob. Ag. Chemother. 1969.
15. Petralli, J., E. Russell, A. Kataoka, and T. C. Merigan. 1970. On-line computer quality control of antibiotic-sensitivity testing. N. Engl. J. Med. **283:**735–738.
16. Revised Tentative Standard. 1973. Performance standards for antimicrobial disc susceptibility tests, as used in clinical laboratories. National Committee for Clinical Laboratory Standards, Los Angeles.
17. Ryan, K. J., F. D. Schoenknecht, and W. M. M. Kirby. 1970. Disc sensitivity testing. Hospital Practice **5:**91–100.
18. Stemper, J. E., and J. M. Matsen. 1970. Device for turbidity standardization of cultures for antibiotic sensitivity testing. Appl. Microbiol. **19:**1015–1016.
19. Thornsberry, C., J. Q. Caruthers, and C. N. Baker. 1973. Effect of temperature on the in vitro susceptibility of *Staphylococcus aureus* to penicillinase-resistant penicillins. Antimicrob. Ag. Chemother. **4:**263–269.
20. Washington, J. A., II, E. Warren, and A. G. Karlson. 1973. Stability of barium sulfate turbidity standards. Appl. Microbiol. **24:**1013.

Chapter 47

Assay of Antimicrobial Agents

L. D. SABATH AND JOHN M. MATSEN

INTRODUCTION

There are six currently used methods for assaying antimicrobial agents in serum, urine, or other biological fluids:

1. agar diffusion
2. turbidimetric
3. inhibition of pH change
4. enzymatic
5. radioimmunoassay
6. chemical

The *agar diffusion* method (2, 4, 6, 7, 13, 14) is currently the most widely used both in industry and in hospitals and is the one that will be described in detail here; it has been used for the assay of virtually all antimicrobial agents in use in medicine. *Enzymatic assays* for aminoglycosides (5, 15) and a *radioimmunoassay* for gentamicin (9; also for kanamycin and tobramycin [J. Lewis, personal communication]) have been developed that are also useful in clinical medicine; they are both more accurate (error <5%) and more specific than the agar diffusion assays, which often have errors of up to 10%. However, the reagents for the enzymatic and radioimmunoassays are not yet commercially available and their requirement for radioactive material and the use of a scintillation counter may limit their implementation. In *enzymatic assays* (5, 15), the antibiotic is the substrate for an enzyme, and the product of the reaction is measured. In the enzymatic assay of gentamicin, a gentamicin adenyl transferase transfers radioactive adenosine monophosphate (from adenosine triphosphate) to gentamicin, and the adenylated gentamicin formed is proportional to the amount of gentamicin in the sample. It is adsorbed onto phosphocellulose paper (because of its net positive charge) for counting, whereas the excess radioactive adenosine triphosphate is not so adsorbed, and not counted. A similar second enzymatic assay (5) utilizes a broader spectrum enzyme that transfers radioactive acetate from acetyl-coenzyme A to most aminoglycoside antibiotics; the acetylated product is adsorbed onto phosphocellulose paper, and the radioactivity is then determined. In the *radioimmunoassay* the complexing of antibody and radioactive antibiotic is inhibited by the nonradioactive antibiotic in the sample for assay.

The *turbidimetric assay* (8) may be performed two different ways:

1. By making serial dilutions of the fluid to be assayed in nutrient broth and seeding the tubes with a 10^{-4} dilution of an overnight culture of the assay organism (e.g., *Staphylococcus aureus* 209P) before incubating, the greatest dilution showing complete inhibition of bacterial growth can be assumed to contain the minimal inhibitory concentration (MIC) for the assay strain, which should be determined with each run. Thus, if the MIC for the assay strain is 0.5 μg/ml, and the greatest dilution of sample showing inhibition is 1:32, the sample contains 16 μg/ml. This procedure carries an inherent error of ± 1 $\log_2$ dilution and is insufficiently precise for most purposes.

2. The more accurate version of the turbidimetric assay requires the construction of a curve (Fig. 1) relating *turbidity* (or optical density) of an assay strain grown at various subinhibitory concentrations of antibiotic to those concentrations. The sample for assay is seeded with the same assay organism and incubated at several dilutions with the plan that one will contain an amount of antibiotic that will provide a turbidity that can be read off the standard curve (i.e., more turbidity than complete inhibition, but less than control growth with no antibiotic). An automated apparatus to perform this assay (Autoturb) is available from Elanco, Indianapolis, Ind.

The *potentiometric assays* (3, 12) are similar to the second version of the turbidimetric assay in that a standard curve is constructed relating the effect of various antibiotic concentrations in inhibiting growth, but the parameter followed is inhibition of change of pH of the medium, rather than change in turbidity.

The *chemical assays*, in general, are not sufficiently sensitive to detect accurately most antibiotics in complex biological fluids at the concentrations (several to less than 1 μg/ml) at which they usually occur; sulfonamides are an exception in being chemically measurable at concentrations used in medicine.

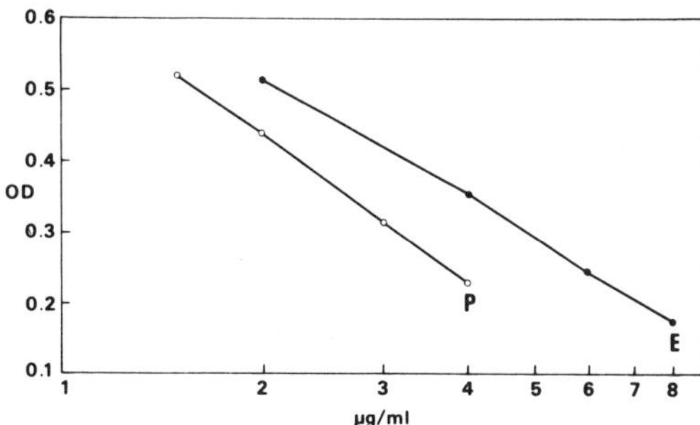

FIG. 1. *Relationship between growth (optical density) and log of antibiotic concentration of penicillin (P) and erythromycin (E) (from reference 7 with permission of the author and publisher).*

DETAILS FOR AN AGAR DIFFUSION ASSAY

The serum concentration of gentamicin, kanamycin, streptomycin, neomycin, tobramycin, or vancomycin can be measured in 2 h with an error of ≤10% with a sample of 0.1 ml by a simple agar diffusion assay (13, 14).

Preparation of assay strain

The assay organism is the spore of *Bacillus subtilis* ATCC 6633 which can be purchased (Difco) as a lyophilized preparation or prepared by seeding the organism on Heart Infusion Agar (Difco) in Roux bottles, incubating at 36 C for 1 week, and then harvesting with the aid of sterile glass beads (0.58 cm in diameter). The spores are heated for 30 min at 65 C both before and after a wash in sterile distilled water, suspended to give about 10^{10} colony-forming units/ml, and stored at 4 C; each preparation can be used for over 6 months.

Preparation and storage of assay plates

The assay plates are prepared by adding 0.1 ml of the *B. subtilis* spore suspension to each 100 ml of molten assay medium (Difco antibiotic assay medium no. 5, or Grove and Randall medium no. 5 [4]) at 48 to 65 C, pouring 5 ml of the uniformly seeded agar into plastic petri dishes (100 mm in diameter, Falcon Plastics), and permitting them to harden on a level bench (check with spirit level) at room temperature. The plates can be used immediately or stored at 4 C in sealed plastic bags for future use; plates stored for less than 2 weeks provide results after 2 h of incubation, and plates stored 2 to 6 weeks require 4 to 5 h of incubation before readings can be made.

Setting up the test

The *assay of a single serum sample* requires two assay plates and sixteen 0.25-inch (0.6-cm) paper disks (Schleicher & Schuell Co., no. 740-E). The disks are placed in four rows of four disks in the inverted lid of one of the assay plates, and 0.02 ml (use Lang-Levy type pipette) of the sample is placed on each of the four disks in the top row. Three standards are used for most clinical assays. Normal human sera (each batch should be checked to be sure it does not contain antibacterial activity before the "standard" amount of antibiotic is added) containing 12, 6, and 1.5 μg/ml are used for the gentamicin serum assay (suggested standards for other assays are as follows: for streptomycin, 25, 12.5, and 3.1 μg/ml; for vancomycin, 40, 20, and 10 μg/ml; for kanamycin, 27, 9, and 3 μg/ml; and for tobramycin and neomycin, 12, 6, and 1.5 μg/ml); 0.02 ml of each standard is placed on each of four paper disks. A reference mark should be made on the bottom of each assay plate, and one paper disk containing the 12-μg standard should be placed on the surface of the seeded agar near the reference mark, about 1 cm from the edge, and pressed firmly in place with metal forceps. In a similar fashion, the 6- and 1.5-μg disks and the disk with the sample for assay are placed on the surface of the agar in the sequence going clockwise. Duplicates for each of these four disks are placed on the agar surface of the same plate so that pairs containing the same fluid are opposite each other. In an identical fashion, the other eight disks are placed to form a ring on the surface of the seeded agar in the second plate, and the two assay plates are placed on a level shelf at 37 C.

Incubation and reading

After about 2 h of incubation (range of 75 to 150 min), zones of inhibition are visible around the disks containing antibiotic (if gentamicin, at ≥0.37 μg/ml). The zone diameters can be measured with a ruler or, for greater accuracy, with a vernier caliper.

Calculation

The results are calculated by forming a standard curve (Fig. 2) on semilog paper relating the concentration of antibiotic in the standard sera (log scale) to the diameter (in millimeters) of the zone of inhibition produced. A separate curve is made for each of the two plates (each point the mean of the duplicate standards), and diameters of the zones around the two sample disks on each plate are averaged before being read off the standard curve for that plate. The final result of the assay is the mean of the values obtained from each plate. Thus, if plate A gave a value of 5.8 μg/ml, and plate B a value of 6.2 μg/ml, the value to be recorded for the sample would be 6.0 μg/ml.

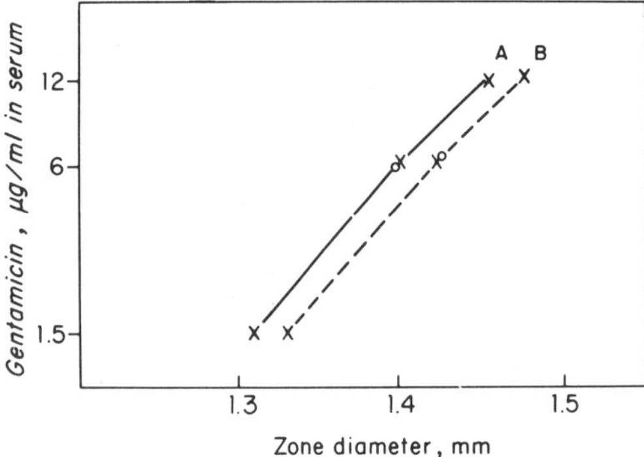

FIG. 2. *Standard curves for gentamicin on plates A and B, relating gentamicin concentration (log scale) to diameter of zone of inhibition. Symbols:* O, *mean diameter of zones for unknown sample;* ×, *mean diameter of standards for plate.*

Assay of samples containing more than one antibiotic

The agar diffusion assay described can conveniently be used to measure gentamicin or other aminoglycosides in the presence of any other penicillin or cephalosporin currently in use in the United States by simply adding 0.02 ml of β-lactamase II-containing fluid (obtainable from Whatman Biochemicals, Maidenhead, Surrey, England) to 0.1 ml of serum for assay a few minutes before loading the disks (in calculating results, allow for dilution of sample by enzyme fluid by increasing "apparent" gentamicin value by 20%). Alternatively, an appropriate β-lactamase II-containing fluid may be prepared by simply growing *B. cereus* 569 (obtainable from the American Type Culture Collection, Rockville, Md.; ATCC 27348) in Difco Brain Heart Infusion broth containing 20 µg of cephalothin per ml, at 37 C for 18 h, and using the supernatant fluid as crude β-lactamase II. Should a non-β-lactamase antibiotic (such as tetracycline or clindamycin) be present, the assay should be performed with an assay organism highly resistant to the antibiotic that is *not* to be measured. Appropriate strains of *Staphylococcus aureus* (1) and of *Klebsiella pneumoniae* (10) have been so used in similar diffusion systems.

Variations of agar diffusion assays

The samples (and standards) for the radial (or horizontal) diffusion method may be held in cylinders (metal, glass, or porcelain; 6, 7) or in wells or holes (2) punched in the agar, as well as on paper disks. The standard metal cylinders hold about 0.2 ml; the punched holes (depending on thickness of agar and size of punch) can conveniently hold as much as 0.3 ml or as little as 0.001 ml. The pH of the medium can be altered to increase or decrease the sensitivity of the system to the antibiotics in the sample.

A linear (or vertical) assay system has been described (7, 11) in which sample and seeded medium are placed in glass tubes, rather than in petri dishes (or larger plates).

LITERATURE CITED

1. Alcid, C. V., and S. J. Seligman. 1973. Simplified assay for gentamicin in the presence of other antibiotics. Antimicrob. Ag. Chemother. **3**:559–561.
2. Bennett, J. V., J. L. Brodie, E. J. Benner, and W. M. M. Kirby. 1966. Simplified, accurate method for antibiotic assay for clinical specimens. Appl. Microbiol. **14**:170–177.
3. Faine, S., and D. C. Knight. 1968. Rapid microbiological assay of antibiotics in blood and other body fluids. Lancet **2**:375–378.
4. Grove, D. C., and W. A. Randall. 1955. Assay methods of antibiotics. Medical Encyclopedia, Inc., New York.
5. Haas, M. J., and J. Davies. 1973. Enzymatic acetylation as a means of determining serum aminoglycoside concentrations. Antimicrob. Ag. Chemother. **4**:497–499.
6. Heatley, N. G. 1944. A method for the assay of penicillin. Biochem. J. **38**:61–65.
7. Heatley, N. G. 1949. The assay of antibiotics, p. 110–199. *In* H. E. Florey, et al. (ed.), Antibiotics, vol. 1. Oxford University Press, London.
8. Kavanagh, F. 1972. Photometric assaying, p. 43–121. *In* F. Kavanagh (ed.), Analytical microbiology, vol. 2. Academic Press Inc., New York.
9. Lewis, J. E., J. C. Nelson, and H. A. Elder. 1972. Radioimmunoassay of an antibiotic: gentamicin. Nature (London) **239**:214–216.
10. Lund, M. E., D. J. Blazevic, and J. M. Matsen. 1973. Rapid gentamicin bioassay using a multiple-antibiotic-resistant strain of *Klebsiella pneumoniae*. Antimicrob. Ag. Chemother. **4**:569–573.
11. Mitchison, D. A., and C. C. Spicer. 1949. A method of estimating streptomycin in serum and other body fluids by diffusion through agar enclosed in glass tubes. J. Gen. Microbiol. **3**:184.
12. Noone, P., J. R. Pattison, and D. Samson. 1971. Simple, rapid method for assay of aminoglycoside antibiotics. Lancet **2**:16–19.
13. Sabath, L. D. 1972. A simple, rapid microassay for nephrotoxic antibiotics. Scope monograph, The Upjohn Co., Kalamazoo, Michigan.
14. Sabath, L. D., J. I. Casey, P. A. Ruch, L. L. Stumpf, and M. Finland. 1971. Rapid microassay of gentamicin, kanamycin, neomycin, streptomycin, and vancomycin in serum or plasma. J. Lab. Clin. Med. **78**:457–463.
15. Smith, D. H., B. Van Otto, and A. L. Smith. 1972. A rapid chemical assay for gentamicin. N. Engl. J. Med. **286**:583–586.

Chapter 48

Special Tests: Bactericidal Activity and Activity of Antimicrobics in Combination

ARTHUR L. BARRY AND L. D. SABATH

Two special procedures that may be useful in regulating antimicrobic therapy are the determination of: (i) the bactericidal activity of antimicrobics against the pathogen from the patient to be treated, and (ii) the effect of antimicrobics in combination.

BACTERICIDAL ACTIVITY

The activity of an antimicrobial agent against a given microorganism is usually expressed quantitatively as the minimal inhibitory concentration or MIC (see chapter 45). At the MIC end point, inhibition of growth is usually reversible, and viable microorganisms can be recovered when the concentration of active drug is reduced to subinhibitory levels, as by dilution. However, with many antimicrobial agents, concentrations slightly greater than the MIC will produce an irreversible inhibition of the growth (a "killing" effect) of most organisms. The following section describes some methods by which such a lethal effect may be measured in the clinical laboratory. No standard techniques have yet been recognized for these procedures, and there are differences of opinion among investigators accustomed to using different methods for doing the same kind of test.

Definition of terms

The broad term "lethal activity" may be used to express a completely irreversible inhibition of microbial growth; more specific terms such as "bactericidal" or "fungicidal" refer to the lethal activity against a particular group of microorganisms. The minimal lethal concentration (MLC) may be defined arbitrarily as the lowest concentration of drug which will produce a minimal number or defined proportion of viable survivors after incubation for a fixed time, under a given set of conditions (5). Alternatively, the lethal activity may be expressed as the rate of killing by a fixed concentration of drug, measured by determining the number of survivors at various time intervals under a given set of laboratory conditions (5).

Indications for determination of lethal activity

In a limited number of clinical situations, chemotherapy should be adjusted to obtain lethal concentrations or some multiple of lethal concentrations at the site of infection, e.g., when host defense mechanisms are unable to function optimally and thus inhibition without "killing" is not likely to effect a permanent cure, as in bacterial endocarditis.

Bactericidal activity in broth

1. The inoculum is prepared for the broth dilution procedure as described in chapter 45. This should contain 10^5 to 10^6 organisms per ml.

2. A viable count is performed on the inoculum. This can be simply done by spreading 0.1 ml of 1:100 and 1:1,000 dilutions of the inoculum evenly over the surfaces of blood-agar plates. After overnight incubation, the colonies are counted and the inoculum is calculated from the plate showing 50 to 200 colonies.

3. A broth dilution test is set up as described in chapter 45, and incubated for 18 to 24 h.

4. The MIC is read, and 0.1 ml is subcultured from tubes showing no growth and spread over at least a quadrant of a blood-agar plate. A separate pipette should be used for each transfer. Alternatively, 0.01 ml delivered by a calibrated loop can be used but with inevitable loss of accuracy in establishing the end point. Carryover of antimicrobic onto the plate is, however, reduced by subculturing the smaller volume.

5. Plates are incubated for 18 to 24 h. Colony counts are performed.

6. The MLC is determined as the lowest concentration which yields no more than a predetermined number of viable cells. We recommend that the MLC be defined as the minimal concentration which will result in

99.9% "kill" after 18 h of incubation of the broth dilution series; i.e., no more than 0.1% of the viable cells in the primary inoculum will be able to survive and grow under the test conditions.

Thus, if the dilution test was shown to have received an inoculum of 10^5 viable cells per ml, a lethal effect would be attributed to those concentrations of drug which contain no more than 100 colony-forming units per ml, i.e., which grow 10 colonies or less from the 0.1 ml subculture, or no more than one colony with a 0.01-ml loop subculture.

In certain experimental situations, it may be desirable to express the lethal activity in terms of rate of killing by fixed concentrations of antimicrobic (concentrations approximating the average blood level during therapy with usual dosage). Tubes are prepared containing 10 ml of broth (Mueller-Hinton is appropriate for enteric organisms and staphylococci) with antimicrobic(s) at the predetermined concentrations. A control tube contains 10 ml of broth. Each is seeded to give about 10^5 organisms per ml in the tube. Growth dynamics are studied during incubation at 37 C. Immediately after inoculation and periodically thereafter, the tubes are mixed, and samples are withdrawn and suitably diluted for colony counts. The total number of survivors should be determined at least after 0, 4, and 24 h; occasionally 48- or 72-h determinations may be indicated. The results may be presented graphically by plotting the total number of viable cells on a logarithmic scale against hours of incubation. By comparing the rate of decline in the number of survivors, it is possible to determine the most rapidly lethal antimicrobic agent under these conditions. An early decrease in the number of survivors may be followed by a marked increase in the number of viable cells. This may be due to the selection of resistant variants or to the partial inactivation of the antimicrobial agent during incubation, or to both. This procedure can be used for study of the effect of antimicrobic combinations (see below).

Certain antimicrobics are markedly bound by serum proteins, and some investigators prefer to test all antimicrobics in normal human serum or in broth with 50% serum added. This presumably mimics the in vivo situation more closely. Since serum itself is a variable product, samples from a large number of healthy individuals should be pooled. It is known that different batches of normal serum may have some bactericidal activity against some strains of bacteria. The activity is complement-dependent and declines during storage (1, 13). In practice, pooled samples of human serum will be stored for various periods of time before being used, and appropriate controls must be incorporated when the addition of human serum to this test system is considered necessary. Pooled serum may be heat-inactivated at 56 C for 30 min.

Serum bactericidal tests

As a guide in the selection of appropriate dosage, it may be necessary to measure the concentration of antimicrobic in the serum of the patient periodically during therapy (see chapter 47). A simple direct method for estimating the bactericidal activity of serum of patients being treated with one or more antimicrobial agents against their own infecting organisms was first described by Schlichter et al. (11, 12) and has been modified many times since then (3). The following represents one such modification.

1. A recent bacterial isolate from the patient is transferred and stored at −20 C or lower in a suitably stabilized broth medium such as broth with 50% inactivated fetal calf serum or with 15% (vol/vol) glycerol, or refrigerated on a nutrient agar slant until needed. Just before the test to be run, the stored culture is subcultured to a nutrient agar plate and, after overnight incubation, growth from four to five colonies is transferred to Mueller-Hinton or other appropriate broth, which then serves as the inoculum after 5 to 6 h of incubation followed by appropriate dilution.

2. Serum samples are collected from the patient before treatment has begun and again 24 h after therapy has been initiated. If intermittent therapy is being given, two samples should be collected: one just before a dose is given (lowest level) and the other when the peak concentration should be expected (usually about 1 h after an intramuscular injection, or immediately after an intravenous infusion). Once separated from the clot, serum samples may be stored at −20 C or lower for several days without loss of antimicrobic activity. In the case of the heat-stable aminoglycosides, the patient's serum can be inactivated at 56 C for 30 min. With the penicillins, this may result in some loss of activity.

3. For each serum sample, twofold dilutions are prepared in 0.5-ml volumes with inactivated normal human pooled serum as diluent, the first tube containing undiluted patient's serum. In this way, each tube contains 0.5 ml of serum although its origin and length of storage before testing are unavoidably different. A control tube containing pretreatment serum is added to exclude inhibition by normal bactericidal mechanisms; this is especially important when

the patient's serum cannot be inactivated by heating.

4. The patient's isolate is then diluted in Mueller-Hinton or other appropriate broth so as to obtain about 2×10^5 viable cells per ml (see chapter 45). Viable counts are made on the inoculum. Each tube is inoculated with 0.5 ml of the suspension. Two controls are always inoculated: one containing 0.5 ml of the pooled serum diluent and the other with 0.5 ml of broth alone. Tubes are incubated overnight.

5. Because of the turbidity inherent in certain serum samples, inhibitory levels are often impossible to determine, and thus subcultures on blood-agar are routinely made from each tube to detect growth and bactericidal end points. These are made as described earlier in this chapter.

6. After appropriate incubation of the subcultures, the maximal dilutions of serum which give 99.9% "kill" are determined. Interpretation may have to be individualized according to the nature and severity of the illness and the toxicity of the drug. In general, dosage is considered to be adequate if a bactericidal activity can be demonstrated in a dilution of 1:8 or 1:16 (6); peak level bactericidal activity of 1:32 or greater is desirable in staphylococcal endocarditis.

EFFECT OF ANTIMICROBICS IN COMBINATION

The clinical advantages of chemotherpay with combinations of two or more antimicrobial agents are clearly documented in the treatment of tuberculosis and the therapy of enterococcal endocarditis (2, 5, 7). Combinations are often used in the treatment of other serious infections in an attempt to exploit the phenomenon of synergism. In tuberculosis, two or three drugs are given together to prevent the selection of resistant variants, which occurs rapidly during single-drug therapy. Enterococcal endocarditis is often treated with benzylpenicillin or ampicillin in combination with one of the aminoglycosides (streptomycin, kanamycin, or gentamicin) because the latter markedly increases the bactericidal activity of the penicillin against strains of enterococci which are not resistant to very high concentrations of the aminoglycosides (8). A combination is considered to be synergistic when the effect observed with the combination is greater than the sum of the effects observed with the two drugs independently. Many other combinations of antimicrobial agents are only additive or indifferent; i.e., the combined effect is equal to the sum of the effects observed with the two drugs tested separately or equal to that of the most active drug in the combination. Some drug combinations are clearly antagonistic; i.e., the combination is less effective than the most active drug in the combination. One of the important reasons for determining the in vitro effect of antibiotic combinations is to avoid antagonism.

The effect of combining antimicrobial agents may be measured in several ways (9, 10), but methods which determine the lethal activity of the combinations are generally preferred. This may be done by adapting one of the two methods outlined above for measuring bactericidal activity to include preselected fixed concentrations of one or both antimicrobics. Further description of this procedure is not needed.

A quantitative detailed method for evaluating the antimicrobial activity of drugs in combination is to test multiple combinations and express the results as an isobologram (10). This is done by serially diluting each drug in large volumes and then combining 0.25-ml samples of each of the two antimicrobics in smaller tubes, arranged in a checkerboard fashion so as to obtain many possible combinations of drug concentrations. For example, 50 sterile tubes could be arranged in 5 files, each 10 tubes long (10 rows). The first file would receive zero drug A (each of the 10 tubes getting 0.25 ml of sterile broth); the second file, drug A at 2 μg/ml (0.25 ml of this into each of the 10 tubes); the third file, drug A at 4 μg/ml; the fourth file, drug A at 8 μg/ml; and the fifth file, drug A at 16 μg/ml. In a similar fashion, zero drug B would be added to row one of each file (each of the five tubes getting 0.25 ml of broth instead); the second row would get drug B at 1 μg/ml (0.25 ml of broth containing 1 μg/ml into each of the 5 tubes in that row); the third row, drug B at 2 μg/ml; the fourth row, 4 μg/ml; the fifth, 8 μg/ml, etc.; and the tenth row would get drug B at 256 μg/ml. Each drug is thus tested separately: drug A in row one and drug B in file one. The tubes are then all inoculated with 0.5 ml of a standardized suspension of the test organism (usually 10^5 organisms per ml). After 16 to 18 h, inhibitory end points are read for each drug alone and for each drug in the presence of the other drug. Subcultures of inhibited tubes to determine the MLCs are made as described above if lethal end points are desired. Isobolograms are plotted as shown in Fig. 1 to determine evidence of synergistic inhibition or killing. (Obviously, the final concentration of drug in each tube is one-fourth what was added, because only 0.25 ml of fluid with each drug was added to each tube that had a final volume of 1 ml; thus, for drug A, the final concentrations in files 1, 2, 3,

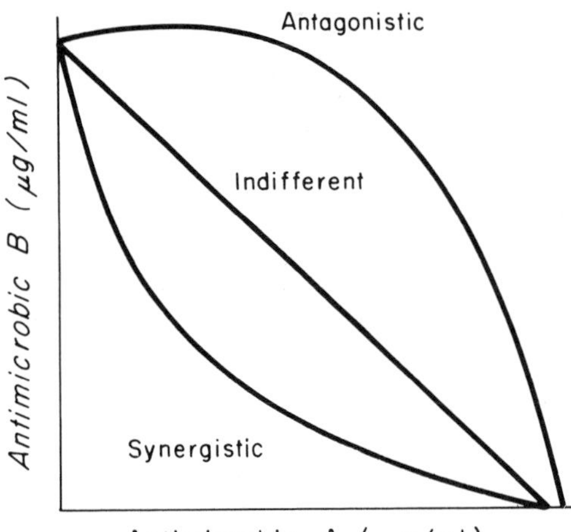

FIG. 1. *Isobologram portraying three possible results when two antimicrobics (A and B) are tested singly and in various combinations; either MIC or MLC end points may be plotted. A straight line joining the values obtained with each drug separately represents an isobol which indicates indifference. Antagonism is indicated by an isobol which bows upward away from the coordinates, and a bowing toward the coordinates indicates synergism.*

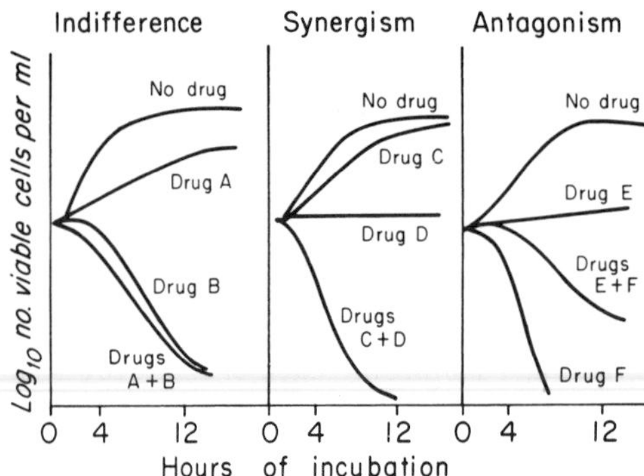

FIG. 2. *Rate of killing with antimicrobial agents singly and in combination. Schematic representation showing three different types of results.*

4, and 5, respectively, were 0, 0.5, 1, 2, and 4 μg/ml. The exact concentrations mentioned would have been appropriate for testing an enterococcus against gentamicin [drug A] and ampicillin or benzylpenicillin [drug B].) Such an approach requires a large number of test tubes and a considerable amount of time. Adaptation to a microdilution technique with mechanization makes it more practical both for large studies or for testing isolates from individual patients.

Another approach to the problem is to document the rate of "killing" by concentrations of the two drugs singly and in combination, as described in the first section of this chapter. The results may then be presented graphically as demonstrated in Fig. 2. The labor involved in multiple colony counts makes both of the above approaches prohibitive for routine use in most clinical laboratories, although Bulger and Nielson (1) have shown that the latter method can be simplified considerably. Sufficiently accurate counts can be obtained by using a 0.001-ml calibrated loop to seed the molten agar for pour plates. With an electronic colony counter and recording device, a large number of colonies can be counted quickly and accurately. In most cases, sufficient information for proper interpretation can be obtained by performing colony counts at the time of the inoculation and again after 4 h of incubation. The tubes should be held and an additional count may be performed after 24 h if the 4-h counts are questionable or unclear.

Finally, bactericidal synergism can be measured by the ingenious cellophane transfer technique of Chabbert. This procedure is well described in Garrod and O'Grady's test (4). It does not provide the quantitative information that can be derived from more laborious tests.

LITERATURE CITED

1. Bulger, R. J., and K. Nielson. 1968. Effect of different media on in vitro studies of antibiotic combinations. Appl. Microbiol. **16**:890–895.
2. Dowling, H. F. 1965. Present status of therapy with combinations of antibiotics. Amer. J. Med. **39**:796–803.
3. Dunlop, S. G. 1965. The serum dilution bactericidal test for antibiotic effectiveness. Amer. J. Med. Technol. **31**:69–76.
4. Garrod, L. P., H. P. Lambert, and F. O'Grady, with a chapter on laboratory methods by P. M. Waterworth. 1973. Antibiotic and chemotherapy, 4th ed. Churchill Livingstone, Edinburgh.
5. Jawetz, E. 1968. Combined antibiotic action: some definitions and correlations between laboratory and clinical results. Antimicrob. Ag. Chemother. 1967, p. 203–209.
6. Klastersky, J., D. Daneau, G. Swings, and D. Weerts. 1974. Antibacterial activity in serum and urine as a therapeutic guide in bacterial infections. J. Infect. Dis. **129**:187–193.
7. McCabe, W. R. 1968. Clinical use of combinations of antimicrobial agents. Antimicrob. Ag. Chemother. 1967, p. 225–233.
8. Moellering, R. C., Jr., C. Wennersten, T. Medrek, and A. N. Weinberg. 1971. Prevalence of high-level resistance to aminoglycosides in clinical isolates of enterococci. Antimicrob. Ag. Chemother. 1970, p. 335–340.
9. Patte, J. C., H. Hirsch, and Y. Chabbert. 1958. Etude des courbes d'effet bacteriostatique des associations d'antibiotiques. Ann. Inst. Pasteur (Paris) **94**:621–635.
10. Sabath, L. D. 1968. Synergy of antibacterial substances

by apparently known mechanisms. Antimicrob. Ag. Chemother. 1967, p. 210–217.

11. Schlichter, J. G., and H. MacLean. 1947. A method of determining the effective therapeutic level in the treatment of subacute bacterial endocarditis with penicillin. Amer. Heart J. **34**:209–211.

12. Schlichter, J. G., H. MacLean, and A. Malzer. 1949. Effective penicillin therapy in subacute bacterial endocarditis and other chronic infections. Amer. J. Med. Sci. **217**:600–608.

13. Traub, W. H. 1969. Assay of the antibiotic activity of serum. Appl. Microbiol. **18**:51–56.

Chapter 49

Susceptibility Testing of Anaerobes

VERA L. SUTTER AND JOHN A. WASHINGTON II

The current increase in interest in clinical anaerobic bacteriology has been stimulated by the more frequent isolation of anaerobes from clinical specimens. Recognition of the role of anaerobic bacteria in infections has brought about a greater demand for information relative to appropriate antimicrobial therapy.

Antimicrobial therapy of anaerobic infections is usually empirically determined since cultivation of clinically significant anaerobic bacteria may be slow (e.g., mean of 3 to 4 days in blood cultures) and since results of susceptibility tests may not be available for an additional 2 to 4 days. In general, there is a high level of predictability of antimicrobial susceptibility of anaerobes which forms the basis of their appropriate initial therapy; however, changing patterns of susceptibility to certain agents have been recognized in recent years. For example, from 50 to 62% of recent isolates of *Bacteroides fragilis* have been reported to be resistant to tetracycline (5, 8, 11, 13). Resistance to tetracycline has also been reported to occur among the anaerobic cocci and *Clostridium* species (5, 7; F. P. Tally, A. Y. Armfield, and S. M. Finegold, Abstr. Annu. Meet. Amer. Soc. Microbiol., 1973, p. 90). Finally, some groups of anaerobes previously thought to be susceptible to penicillin are no longer uniformly susceptible to this agent. It is, therefore, important to tabulate and analyze results of susceptibility tests of anaerobes so that the empirical basis of therapy can reflect any changes in susceptibility patterns. In instances of serious infections involving anaerobic organisms, e.g., endocarditis and brain abscess, or infections requiring prolonged antimicrobial therapy, e.g., pulmonary abscess and osteomyelitis, it is important to determine the antimicrobial susceptibility of individual isolates. It should, however, be emphasized that the "routine" testing of anaerobic or other fastidious organisms is probably seldom indicated and is fraught with problems related to technique and interpretation of results.

There are a number of problems associated with susceptibility testing of anaerobes which are not encountered in the testing of aerobes and facultative bacteria. Anaerobiosis itself appears to decrease the activity of aminoglycoside antibiotics, and the presence of CO_2 in the atmosphere will lower the pH of the medium and affect the activity of many antibiotics. The activity of the aminoglycosides, the macrolides, and the lincomycins is decreased, whereas that of tetracycline, methicillin, and novobiocin is increased. The activity of penicillin, chloramphenicol, bacitracin, polymyxin, and colistin is generally not affected (2, 4, 6, 10). Most studies of these effects have been done with facultative organisms cultivated in an anaerobic or CO_2-containing atmosphere, and their exact definition and significance, as they relate to anaerobes, remain to be determined. In practice, susceptibility tests are generally needed only against penicillin, cephalothin, tetracycline or minocycline, clindamycin, and chloramphenicol. Metronidazole susceptibilities may be indicated if this agent is approved for therapy.

Within the past 2 or 3 years, the International Collaborative Study Group has made recommendations for interim reference dilution methods for aerobic and facultative pathogens (2), and the Food and Drug Administration (FDA) has made recommendations for standardized disk susceptibility testing of these same groups of organisms (3). The FDA recommended using a dilution method for determination of the antimicrobial susceptibility of anaerobes without indicating which of the numerous modifications would be acceptable. There is no general agreement among workers in anaerobic bacteriology with regard to dilution series, choice of medium, age and density of inoculum, or conditions and length of anaerobic incubation. A few studies have been directed toward standardization of a single-disk agar diffusion method and correlating inhibition zone diameters with results of dilution tests (1, 7–11). Correlation appears satisfactory with some drugs, but not with others. Much more work remains to be done before a disk method with inhibition zone diameter standards for interpretation of susceptibility can be recommended.

A broth-disk test has recently been described (12) which may prove to be a reliable method for simple, rapid susceptibility testing of anaerobes. Again, more experience and data need to be gained before this test can be recommended.

In the absence of a national or international standard or reference method for susceptibility testing of anaerobes, a multitude of variations in techniques will be used throughout the country. The individual laboratory should, however, carefully standardize all elements of its procedure so that results are consistent and reproducible from day to day. To provide methods for use until standard or reference methods are recommended, the following dilution procedures are outlined.

BROTH DILUTION TEST

With rapidly growing strains (*Bacteroides fragilis*, most *Clostridium* species) the inoculum is prepared as follows.

1. Portions of three or four colonies or a 3-mm loopful of growth from an overnight culture on blood-agar are inoculated into a tube of modified Thioglycollate medium without indicator (BBL-135C). This medium is enriched with hemin, 5 μg/ml (added prior to sterilization), and $NaHCO_3$, 1 mg/ml, with vitamin K_1, 0.1 μg/ml (added just prior to use). This medium will henceforth be referred to as THCM.
2. After 4 to 6 h of incubation at 35 C, the broth culture is diluted with Brucella broth (Pfizer Co., Inc.) to the density of the barium sulfate standard given in chapter 46 and then is further diluted 1:200 with minimal aeration.

With slower growing strains (anaerobic cocci, *Eubacterium*, and many fusobacteria), colonies are picked from a 2- to 3-day-old blood-agar plate culture, inoculated into THCM, and incubated overnight prior to dilution for the test.

On the day of the test, serial twofold dilutions of antimicrobial agent (see chapter 45 for recommended dilution series) are prepared in Brucella broth, containing either hemin, at a final concentration of 5 μg/ml, or sheep blood, laked by freezing and thawing, at a final concentration of 5%, and vitamin K_1, 0.1 μg/ml. An equal volume of inoculum is added, and the tubes are incubated at 35 C in GasPak (BBL) jars for approximately 48 h. If other systems of anaerobic incubation are used, the CO_2 content of the atmosphere should be 7 to 10%. An inoculated broth containing no antimicrobial agent is included as a growth control for each strain tested, and a tube of uninoculated broth is also included with each day's tests. Slight turbidity often develops in broth during incubation without actual growth. This latter tube is included to aid in distinguishing between this type of turbidity and growth. The minimal inhibitory concentration (MIC) is the lowest concentration of drug with no visible growth.

Bactericidal end points can be determined as described in chapter 48.

AGAR DILUTION TEST

The inoculum is prepared in the same manner as that used in the broth dilution test, except that it is diluted to match the turbidity of a No. 1 McFarland standard. The standard is prepared by adding 1.0 ml of 0.048 M $BaCl_2$ (1.175%, wt/vol, $BaCl_2 \cdot 2H_2O$) to 99.0 ml of 0.36 N H_2SO_4 (1%, vol/vol). Note that this is double the density of the standard described for the diffusion procedure in chapter 46.

On the day of the test, dilutions of stock antibiotic solutions are prepared as described in chapter 45 and then incorporated into 5% laked or whole defibrinated sheep blood-agar plates (Brucella agar base, or brain heart infusion agar base with vitamin K_1, 10 μg/ml).

The plates are spot-inoculated with a 0.001-ml calibrated loop or a Steers replicator (see chapter 45), allowed to dry, and incubated at 35 C in GasPak (BBL) jars for approximately 48 h. Two plates each of the blood-agar medium are inoculated before and after the series of antibiotic-containing plates. One set is incubated with the tests in the GasPak jars to serve as growth controls, and one set is incubated in air to determine whether aerobic contamination has occurred. The MIC of each strain is the lowest concentration of drug yielding no growth, one to two discrete colonies, or a fine, barely visible haze.

LITERATURE CITED

1. Bodner, S. J., M. G. Koenig, L. L. Treanor, and J. S. Goodman. 1972. Antibiotic susceptibility testing of *Bacteroides*. Antimicrob. Ag. Chemother. **2**:57–60.
2. Ericsson, H. M., and J. C. Sherris. 1971. Antibiotic sensitivity testing. Report of an International Collaborative Study. Acta Pathol. Microbiol. Scand. Sect. B, Suppl. 217.
3. Federal Register 1972. Rules and regulations. Antibiotic susceptibility discs. Fed. Regist. **37**:20525–20529.
4. Ingham, H. R., J. B. Selkon, A. C. Codd, and J. H. Hale. 1970. The effect of carbon dioxide on the sensitivity of *Bacteroides fragilis* to certain antibiotics *in vitro*. J. Clin. Pathol. **23**:254–258.
5. Martin, W. J., M. Gardner, and J. A. Washington II. 1972. In vitro antimicrobial susceptibility of anaerobic bacteria isolated from clinical specimens. Antimicrob. Ag. Chemother. **1**:148–158.
6. Rosenblatt, J. E., and F. Schoenknecht. 1972. Effect of several components of anaerobic incubation on antibiotic susceptibility test results. Antimicrob. Ag. Chemother. **1**:433–440.
7. Sapico, F. L., Y.-Y. Kwok, V. L. Sutter, and S. M. Finegold. 1972. Standardized antimicrobial disc susceptibility testing of anaerobic bacteria: in vitro susceptibility of *Clostridium perfringens* to nine antibiotics. Antimicrob. Ag. Chemother. **2**:320–326.

8. Sutter, V. L., Y.-Y. Kwok, and S. M. Finegold. 1972. Standardized antimicrobial disc susceptibility testing of anaerobic bacteria. I. Susceptibility of *Bacteroides fragilis* to tetracycline. Appl. Microbiol. **23**:268–275.
9. Sutter, V. L., Y.-Y. Kwok, and S. M. Finegold. 1973. Susceptibility of *Bacteroides fragilis* to six antibiotics determined by standardized antimicrobial disc susceptibility testing. Antimicrob. Ag. Chemother. **3**:188–193.
10. Thornton, G. F., and J. A. Cramer. 1971. Antibiotic susceptibility of *Bacteroides* species. Antimicrob. Ag. Chemother. 1970, p. 509–513.
11. Wilkins T. D., L. V. Holdeman, I. J. Abramson, W. E. C. Moore. 1972. Standardized single-disc method for antibiotic susceptibility testing of anaerobic bacteria. Antimicrob. Ag. Chemother. **1**:451–459.
12. Wilkins, T. D., and T. Thiel. 1973. Modified broth-disk method for testing the antibiotic susceptibility of anaerobic bacteria. Antimicrob. Ag. Chemother. **3**:350–356.
13. Zabransky, R. J., J. A. Johnston, and K. J. Hauser. 1973. Bacteriostatic and bactericidal activities of various antibiotics against *Bacteroides fragilis*. Antimicrob. Ag. Chemother. **3**:152–156.

Chapter 50
Future Needs

JOHN C. SHERRIS

During the past decade, there has been considerable progress towards the selection and acceptance of standardized procedures for susceptibility tests and of the strains needed to control them. Technical approaches have varied in different countries, but generally the emphasis has been on standardizing diffusion testing procedures (5–9, 11, 15). Paradoxically, less progress has been made towards agreement on dilution test methods despite the fact that the minimal inhibitory concentration (which is method-dependent) has been generally regarded as the ultimate arbiter of in vitro results. The dilution methods described in chapter 44 conform to those recommended as potential reference procedures by the International Collaborative Study (5), have been quite widely used in published reports, and are the nearest approach to a standard that we now have. There remains, however, need for wider acceptance of reference procedures so that results reported from different laboratories may be related to one another. There is particular need to develop agreed reference and routine procedures for anaerobic organisms (see chapter 49).

Some problems remain to be resolved with the susceptibility testing methods described in this section. An improved testing medium of expanded growth range is needed with content or production details sufficiently defined to insure reproducibility of the products of different manufacturers (4, 13). Meanwhile, performance standards for Mueller-Hinton medium are required to improve reproducibility with all commonly tested organisms and antimicrobics (4). Some significant discrepancies have been reported, particularly with *Pseudomonas* and the gentamicin group of antimicrobics (10, 12; L. B. Reller et al., in preparation).

As discussed in chapter 44, there continues to be a need for the use of agreed qualitative categorizations of susceptibility with the diffusion test. The boundaries of these categories inevitably involve some subjective best judgment decisions, and a mechanism is required for periodic review and updating to take account of new information and changing dose schedules. Improved mechanisms for developing and disseminating interpretative recommendations for new antimicrobics are needed so that they are available to laboratories when the agents are first introduced. As suggested in the report of the International Collaborative Study (5), such recommendations should come from a broad-based group of experts working with one or more reference laboratories, and the basis for their recommendations and decisions should be reported. This could be achieved in the United States by coordinating the activities of the Food and Drug Administration, the National Committee for Clinical Laboratory Standards, and the Center for Disease Control in this field.

Because the results of all susceptibility tests are method-dependent, increasing importance has been placed on quality control and external proficiency testing. A quality control strain of *Pseudomonas aeruginosa* is now being added to the two, *Staphylococcus aureus* and *Escherichia coli*, presently recommended by the Food and Drug Administration for use in the United States. Accepted limits of variation should be narrowed for present quality control strains because those now used were developed before many laboratories had experience with the recommended diffusion test. External proficiency testing is particularly valuable to enable laboratories to insure that their results are under control, and should become a feature of the work of all laboratories undertaking susceptibility tests. Its effectiveness depends on the complete characterization of the antimicrobic response of the test strains by two or more reference laboratories. Computer techniques greatly facilitate quality control, proficiency testing, and statistical approaches towards interpretative breakpoints (16, 17). Within the individual laboratory, they may be used to detect improbable reports of antibiograms on the basis of previous experience (17). This approach will be used increasingly in the future.

Susceptibility tests and assays are essentially titration procedures involving a number of steps which are subject to automation and mechanization. These include inoculum standardization and application, the preparation of dilutions or diffusion gradients of antimicrobics, and end point readout. Mechanized inoculum replication and microtitration dilution systems (see references in chapter 45) are well established, and procedures for the other steps are becoming available or are under development. Fully integrated systems are technically feasible and could improve the accuracy and reproducibility of orthodox procedures by reducing technical error and subjectivity. More sophisticated approaches towards automation are being explored to determine test results in less than 4 h after inoculation. They depend on changes in light scattering from organisms (1) (J. McKie et al., Proc. Symp. Rapid Methods and Automation in Microbiology, Stockholm, 1973, in press) or developing colonies (3), particle counts (14), changes in electrical impedance during growth (P. Cady, Proc. Symp. Rapid Methods and Automation in Microbiology, Stockholm, 1973, in press), and on microcalorimetric measurements (2). These and other methods were described at the symposium on Rapid Methods and Automation in Microbiology in Stockholm in 1973, and will shortly be published (Techniques in Pure and Applied Microbiology Series, John Wiley & Sons, Inc., New York). Complete correlation with the results of orthodox procedures may be difficult to achieve because some organisms respond to subinhibitory concentrations with a prolonged lag phase or detectable morphological changes, so that early readings may indicate degrees of susceptibility greater than those measured after overnight incubation (P. G. Dennis et al., Abstr. Annu. Meet. Amer. Soc. Microbiol., 1973, p. 87). This could pose problems of interpretation by traditional concepts; however, there is evidence that better correlation may be obtained by increasing the inoculum to be used with early reading methods (J. C. Sherris and F. D. Schoenknecht, unpublished data). It seems highly probable that one or more automated early reading systems will prove satisfactory in practice and be approved for use in clinical laboratories.

Methodological agreement is needed on techniques for determining bactericidal end points, for measurements of the effects of combinations, and for Schlichter-type tests. In the absence of agreed methods or reference procedures, results from different laboratories cannot be compared with confidence, and an adequate base of experience has not been developed for fully satisfactory interpretation of the results. For all of these procedures, the kinetics of microbial killing by antimicrobics make it essential that statistical end points be accepted, such as those recommended in chapter 48.

In summary, we may reasonably look forward to improved performance of media and of procedures for orthodox susceptibility tests, to improvements in selecting and disseminating interpretative recommendations, and to improved quality control. Beyond that, rapid fully or semi-automated procedures for susceptibility testing are likely to come into use and should result in better reproducibility through elimination of many sources of technical error. There is a need for reference or agreed procedures for determining lethal end points, interactions of combinations, and bactericidal activities of serum so that their interpretations can be refined through cumulative experience. These developments should increase the usefulness of laboratory procedures in the selection and monitoring of chemotherapy.

LITERATURE CITED

1. Berkman, R. M., P. J. Wyatt, and D. T. Phillips. 1970. Rapid detection of penicillin sensitivity in *Staphylococcus aureus*. Nature (London) **228**:458–460.
2. Binford, J. S., L. F. Binford, and P. Adler. 1973. A semi-automated microcalorimetric method of antibiotic sensitivity testing. Amer. J. Clin. Pathol. **59**:86–94.
3. Bowman, R. L., P. Blume, and G. G. Vurek. 1967. Capillary-tube scanner for mechanized microbiology. Science **158**:78–83.
4. Brenner, V. C., and J. C. Sherris. 1972. Influence of different media and bloods on the results of diffusion antibiotic susceptibility tests. Antimicrob. Ag. Chemother. **1**:116–122.
5. Ericsson, H. M., and J. C. Sherris. 1971. Antibiotic sensitivity testing. Report of an International Collaborative Study. Acta Pathol. Microbiol. Scand. Sect. B, Suppl. 217.
6. Ericsson, H. M., G. Tunevall, and K. Wickman. 1960. A paper disc method for determination of bacterial sensitivity to antibiotics. Scandinav. J. Clin. Lab. Invest. **12**:414–422.
7. Federal Register 1972. Rules and regulations. Antibiotic susceptibility discs. Fed. Reg. **37**:20525–20529.
8. Federal Register 1973. Rules and regulations. Antibiotic susceptibility discs—correction. Fed. Reg. **38**:2576.
9. Garrod, L. P., H. P. Lambert, and F. O'Grady, with a chapter on laboratory methods by P. M. Waterworth. 1973. Antibiotic and chemotherapy, 4th ed. Churchill Livingstone, Edinburgh.
10. Garrod, L. P., and P. M. Waterworth. 1969. Effect of medium composition on the apparent sensitivity of *Pseudomonas aeruginosa* to gentamicin. J. Clin. Pathol. **22**:534–538.
11. Garrod, L. P., and P. M. Waterworth. 1971. A study of antibiotic sensitivity testing with proposals for simple uniform methods. J. Clin. Pathol. **24**:779.
12. Gilbert, D. N., E. Kutscher, P. Ireland, and J. P. Sanford. 1971. Effect of the concentrations of magnesium and calcium on the *in vitro* susceptibility of *Pseudomonas aeruginosa* to gentamicin. J. Infec. Dis. **124**:S37–S45.
13. Hoeprich, P. D., A. L. Barry, and G. D. Fay. 1971. Synthetic medium for susceptibility testing. Antimicrob. Ag. Chemother. 1970, p. 494–497.
14. Isenberg, H. D., A. Reichler, and D. Wiseman. 1971. Prototype of a fully automated device for determina-

tion of bacterial antibiotic susceptibility in the clinical laboratory. Appl. Microbiol. **22:**980–986.

15. Kanazawa, Y. 1966. Single disc method for minimum inhibitory concentration (MIC) determination. J. Antibiot. (Tokyo) Ser. A **19:**175–189.
16. O'Brien, T. F., R. L. Kent, and A. A. Medeiros. 1969. Computer-generated plots of results of antimicrobial-susceptibility tests. J. Amer. Med. Ass. **210:**84–92.
17. Petralli, J., E. Russell, A. Kataoka, and T. C. Merigan. 1970. On-line computer quality control of antibiotic-sensitivity testing. N. Engl. J. Med. **283:**735–738.

APPENDIX I

Approximate MIC (μg/ml)[a] Expected with the More Susceptible Strains Among Some Common Bacterial Pathogens (Excluding Resistant Variants and Recombinants)[b]

Organisms	Erythromycin	Clindamycin	Nafcillin	Benzyl penicillin	Ampicillin	Carbenicillin	Cephalothin	Tetracycline	Chloramphenicol	Polymyxin B (units/ml)	Streptomycin	Kanamycin	Gentamicin	Nitrofurantoin	Nalidixic acid
S. aureus															
Penicillinase negative	0.25	0.06	0.5	0.06	0.12	1.0	0.8	0.5	8.0	>128	4.0	2.0	0.5	16	>128
Streptococcus sp.															
α- or nonhemolytic	0.01	0.01	0.12	0.12	0.12	2.0	0.25	0.5	2.0		8.0	64	4.0		
Enterococci	0.40	16	16	4.0	2.0	64	16	1.0	8.0	>128	128	64	8.0	32	>128
Escherichia	128	>128	>128	64	4.0	4.0	8.0	8.0	8.0	4.0	4.0	4.0	1.0	16	4.0
Klebsiella	>128	>128	>128	>128	64	>128	4.0	4.0	4.0	4.0	4.0	4.0	0.5	128	8.0
Enterobacter	>128	>128	>128	>128	>128	4.0	>128	4.0	8.0	8.0	4.0	4.0	1.0	64	4.0
Serratia	>128	>128	>128	>128	128	>128	>128	>128	16	>128	4.0		1.0	256	
Proteus															
P. mirabilis	>128	>128	>128	8.0	2.0	2.0	4.0	64	16	>128	8.0	4.0	1.0	128	8.0
Other species	>128	>128	>128	>128	32	2.0	>128	64	8.0	>128	4.0	2.0	0.5	64	8.0
P. aeruginosa	>128	>128	>128	>128	>128	64	>128	64	>128	16	64	128	2.0	>256	>256
H. influenzae	4.0	4.0	>128	0.5	0.5	0.5	16	1.0	1.0		4.0	2.0	0.5		
B. fragilis	2.0	0.5	>128	16	16	32	64	1.0	8.0	>128	>128	>128	>128		>128

[a] The values listed represent an estimate of the modal MIC when a fairly large series of strains are tested; in most cases, the MIC for a normal member of the population can be expected to fall within two dilutions above or below the mode. In different studies, the mode may differ between strains because of differences in methodology. The above data were based largely upon broth and agar dilution studies (A. L. Barry, unpublished data) supplemented with data collected from a large variety of published works in which similar methods were used.

[b] Prepared by Arthur L. Barry.

APPENDIX II

Peak Serum Concentrations Frequently Obtained With Some Antimicrobial Agents[a]

Antimicrobial agent	Serum concn (μg/ml)
Penicillins[b]	
Depot (benzathine penicillin G)	0.01–0.06
Depot (procaine penicillin G)	0.1–18
Oral	3–20[c]
Intramuscular or intravenous	2–200[c]
Cephalothin	15–150
Cephaloridine	14–28
Cefazolin	38–118
Cephalexin	5–35
Tetracycline	
Oral	1–5
Intravenous	5–30
Doxycycline	1–6
Minocycline	0.7–4.5
Clindamycin	5–26
Lincomycin	2–20
Erythromycin	2–10
Gentamicin	1–8
Kanamycin	10–25
Streptomycin	10–25
Chloramphenicol	3–12
Vancomycin	20–50
Polymyxin B	2–8
Colistin	6
Sulfonamides	100–150
Isoniazid	2–3
Rifampin	10
Ethambutol	5–10
Metronidazol	4–10
Amphotericin B	0.2–2
5-fluorocytosine	20–100

[a] Prepared by L. D. Sabath.

[b] Penicillins include benzylpenicillin, phenoxymethylpenicillin, ampicillin, amoxicillin, carbenicillin, methicillin, oxacillin, cloxacillin, dicloxacillin, and nafcillin.

[c] Wide ranges represent the effect of different doses, routes of administration and/or preparations.

Section VI

IMMUNOSEROLOGICAL TESTS

Chapter 51

Tests for Syphilis

RONALD M. WOOD[1]

Infection with *Treponema pallidum*, the etiological agent of syphilis, produces in the host antibodies of two known types: (i) nontreponemal antibodies or reagin, which react with lipid antigens, and (ii) treponemal antibodies, which react with *T. pallidum* and closely related strains.

REAGIN TESTS

Serological testing in the management of syphilis traditionally has been based on the detection of reagin by use of antigens prepared from normal tissues, most commonly beef heart. An example of a reliable, inexpensive, and easily performed reagin test is the Venereal Disease Research Laboratory (VDRL) slide technique which can be used qualitatively and quantitatively for detecting reagin in serum and cerebrospinal fluid. The procedure is given below.

In the original rapid plasma reagin (RPR) test (23), the basic VDRL antigen modified by the incorporation of choline chloride permits the testing of plasma without preliminary heating. An extension of this principle is seen in the plasmacrit (PCT) test (1), unheated serum reagin (USR) test (20, 22), RPR (teardrop) card test (21), RPR (circle) card test (19), and automated reagin (AR) test (15, 28). These are especially useful in surveys and under field conditions. Suitable commercial products are available for these tests.

VDRL slide test with serum (8, 9, 26)

Principle. In this test, a buffered saline suspension of cardiolipin-lecithin-cholesterol antigen is mixed with patient's serum, agitated on a mechanical rotator, and examined microscopically for degrees of flocculation. If any reactivity is obtained in the undiluted serum, the test is repeated on serum dilutions to determine the relative amount of reagin present.

[1] This chapter was prepared by the staff of the Microbial Diseases Laboratory of the California State Department of Health.

Equipment.

1. Rotating machine, adjustable to 180 rpm, circumscribing a circle 1.9 cm in diameter on a horizontal plane.
2. Hypodermic needles, without bevels: 18, 19 or 20, and 23 gauge.

Glassware.

1. Slides or plates with paraffin or ceramic rings approximately 14 mm in diameter. Glass slides with concavities or glass rings are not satisfactory for this test.
2. Syringe, Luer-type, 1- or 2-ml, or observation tube with rubber bulb.
3. Bottles, 30-ml, round, flat-bottomed, glass-stoppered, narrow mouth.

Reagents. Serologically standardized antigen and buffered saline are commercially available from several manufacturers.

1. VDRL antigen is an alcoholic solution containing 0.03% cardiolipin, 0.9% cholesterol, and sufficient purified lecithin (usually 0.21 ± 0.01%) to produce a standard reactivity. Each lot of antigen has been serologically standardized. Store antigen at room temperature in sealed ampoules or in screw-capped (vinylite liners) brown bottles. If precipitate forms, discard antigen.
2. VDRL buffered saline containing 1.0% sodium chloride, pH 6.0 ± 0.1: formaldehyde, neutral, reagent grade, 0.5 ml; secondary sodium phosphate (Na_2HPO_4), 0.037 g; primary potassium phosphate (KH_2PO_4), 0.170 g; sodium chloride (A.C.S.), 10.0 g; distilled water, 1,000.0 ml. Check pH of solution and store in screw-capped or glass-stoppered bottles.
3. Saline, 0.9%.

Controls. To control serological procedures adequately and to maintain a standard level of reactivity from day to day, the following control sera are recommended: titered reactive serum (TR), tested quantitatively; weakly reactive serum (W), tested qualitatively; nonreactive serum (N), tested qualitatively. Each antigen suspension should be checked quantitatively with the TR and qualitatively with the W and N controls before acceptance for test purposes. A log of control results as well as reagent lot numbers is recommended as an aid in locating and corrrecting test difficulties. Sterile preserved control sera are available from commercial sources, or controls may be prepared as follows.

Prepare controls by collecting two pools of serum (one of reactive serum and one of nonreactive serum) from routine syphilis serology specimens. Sterilize pools by filtration and, if desired, add sodium azide (final concentration, 1:1,000). Prepare controls of desired reactivity by combining reactive and nonreactive serum and mixing well. Establish the pattern of reactivity for each control by testing several times in duplicate with a reference serum of known reactivity. Distribute in portions sufficient for each day's testing and store at −20 C or at 4 C. Serum stored in this way will maintain its reactivity for several months.

Preparation of antigen suspension. The temperature of buffered saline and antigen should be in the range of 73 to 85 F (23 to 29 C) at the time the antigen suspension is prepared.

1. Pipette 0.4 ml of buffered saline to the bottom of a 30-ml, round, glass-stoppered bottle. Be sure the saline completely covers bottom in a thin layer.

2. Add 0.5 ml of antigen (from the lower half of a 1.0-ml pipette graduated to the tip) directly onto the saline while continuously but gently rotating the bottle on a flat surface. Add antigen drop by drop, rapidly, allowing 6 s for each 0.5 ml of antigen. The pipette tip should remain in the upper third of bottle, and rotation should not be vigorous enough to splash saline onto pipette. The proper speed of rotation is obtained when the center of the bottle circumscribes a 5-cm diameter circle approximately three times per second.

3. Blow last drop of antigen from pipette without touching pipette to saline.

4. Continue rotation of bottle for 10 s.

5. Add 4.1 ml of buffered saline from a 5-ml pipette.

6. Place top on bottle and shake bottom to top and back approximately 30 times in 10 s.

7. Antigen suspension then is ready for preliminary testing (see below) before use. Suspension may be used for a period of 1 day.

8. Double this amount of antigen suspension may be prepared at one time by using doubled quantities of antigen and saline. Use a 10-ml pipette for delivering the 8.2-ml volume of saline. If larger quantities of antigen suspension are required, prepare two or more batches. Test each batch of antigen suspension and pool those showing proper reactivity with control sera. Test the pool with control sera.

9. Mix antigen suspension gently each time it is used. Do not force back and forth through the syringe and needle since this procedure may cause loss of reactivity.

Testing accuracy of delivery needles. The proportion of antigen suspension to serum is important in all flocculation tests. An improper ratio of antigen suspension to serum may lead to inaccurate results. Needles used for dispensing antigen suspensions for slide tests should be checked to determine the size of the drop *each time* tests are performed. Check needles for correct delivery as follows.

Fill 1-ml pipette graduated in 0.01 ml with *reagent to be dispensed* and attach needle to be calibrated. Hold pipette *vertically* and count number of drops in 0.5 ml. The amount delivered should check within ±1 drop per 0.5 ml of reagent (Table 1). Although the above-specified needles are usually satisfactory, they must be calibrated and checked frequently. The reagent drop size rather than the needle gauge is the important factor. Needles must be checked with the reagent to be used and adjusted so that the proper number of drops is obtained.

Preliminary testing of antigen suspension. Check each antigen suspension against control sera before it is used for each day's test. The suspension should give expected results with titered reactive, weakly reactive, and nonreactive control sera. The antigen control (suspension in saline) should be smooth in appearance, with antigen particles well dispersed.

Do not use antigen suspension which does not meet control pattern.

Preparation of patient's serum. Heat serum, obtained from centrifuged, clotted blood, in a water bath at 56 C for 30 min. Allow to cool to room temperature before testing. Recentrifuge any serum showing particulate debris. Sera to be tested more than 4 h after the original heating period should be reheated at 56 C for 10 min.

Procedure for VDRL slide qualitative test.

TABLE 1. *Calibration of needles*

Reagent	No. of drops/ml	Needle gauge
VDRL qualitative antigen suspension	60 ± 2	18
VDRL quantitative antigen suspension	75 ± 2	19 or 20
VDRL sensitized antigen suspension	100 ± 2	21 or 22
Saline (0.9%)	100 ± 2	23

For uniform results, temperature of room where VDRL slide tests are performed should be in the range of 23 to 29 C.

1. Pipette 0.05 ml of heated serum into one ring of a paraffin-ringed or ceramic-ringed slide.

2. Add one drop (0.017 ml) of antigen suspension onto each serum with a calibrated 18-gauge needle.

3. Rotate slides for 4 min. Mechanical rotators that circumscribe a 1.9-cm diameter circle should be set at 180 rpm.

4. Read test microscopically immediately after rotation with low-power objective, at 100× magnification using as much light as possible. Report results as follows: medium and large clumps, reactive (R); small clumps, weakly reactive (W); no clumps or very slight roughness, nonreactive (N).

Zonal reactions occasionally occur in serological tests. In such cases, a strongly reactive serum may show a weak or atypical reaction in undiluted serum. A completely negative reaction due to a prozone in very strongly reactive sera is extremely rare. Test quantitatively any serum suspected of giving a prozone reaction.

Procedure for VDRL slide quantitative test. Retest quantitatively to an end point titer all sera that show any reactivity in the qualitative VDRL slide test. Test dilutions of the serum as follows: 1:1 (undiluted), 1:2, 1:4, 1:8, 1:16, and 1:32.

1. Place sera for quantitation in the front row of a rack with a tube containing 0.7 ml of 0.9% saline directly behind each serum.

2. Prepare a 1:8 dilution of each serum by adding 0.1 ml of the serum to 0.7 ml of the 0.9% saline using a 0.2-ml pipette graduated in 0.01 ml.

3. Mix thoroughly and allow the pipette to stand in the dilution tube until all dilutions are prepared.

4. Using this pipette, transfer 0.04, 0.02, and 0.01 ml of the 1:8 serum dilution into the fourth, fifth, and sixth paraffin rings, respectively.

5. With the same pipette, transfer 0.04, 0.02, and 0.01 ml of the undiluted serum into the first, second, and third paraffin rings, respectively.

6. With a calibrated 23-gauge needle, add two drops (0.01 ml/drop) of 0.9% saline to the serum in the second and fifth rings and add three drops of 0.9% saline (delivered in the same manner) to the serum in the third and sixth rings.

7. Rotate slides gently by hand for about 15 s to mix the serum-saline dilution.

8. Add one drop (0.013 ml) of antigen suspension to each ring with a calibrated 19-gauge needle.

9. Complete tests in the manner described for the VDRL slide qualitative test with serum.

10. Report results in terms of the highest serum dilution that produces a reactive (not weakly reactive) result. If all serum dilutions tested produce reactive results, prepare a 1:64 dilution of that serum by adding 0.1 ml of the 1:8 serum dilution to 0.7 ml of saline. Mix and test this 1:64 dilution in three amounts (as was done for the 1:8 serum dilution) to give 1:64, 1:128, and 1:256 dilutions.

Interpretation of results. A reactive or weakly reactive test result indicates the presence of reagin, which almost invariably is formed in treponemal infection, but which may be produced by a variety of other conditions (17, 24). Medical practice considers a reactive result in the presence of clinical symptoms as confirmatory evidence of syphilitic infection. However, in the absence of clinical findings, test reactivity can represent any of the following: (i) latent syphilis; (ii) a biological false-positive reaction, either temporary or chronic; or (iii) a technical or clinical error. The simplest step open to the physician is to request VDRL testing on a repeat specimen. The titer on the second specimen can then be compared with that of the first: a drop to nonreactive suggests a prior technical problem or a temporary biological false-positive condition in the patient; a rise in titer suggests the likelihood of syphilis; a stable titer remains inconclusive, requiring further medical follow-up as well as serological testing for treponemal antibodies.

Pitfalls and sources of error. It is important for physicians and laboratory workers to be familiar with those conditions other than syphilis which can cause reagin reactivity. Acute or chronic infections such as malaria, leprosy, infectious mononucleosis, and upper respiratory diseases, as well as collagen and immunological diseases such as rheumatoid arthritis and lupus erythematosus (13, 17, 24), can produce false-positive reagin tests. Other less well-known physiological conditions contributing to this problem include: tissue regeneration, pregnancy, heroin addiction, and the use of certain drugs for hypertension (13, 17, 24). Reliable test results require strict attention to details of technique including proper identification of specimens, accurate measurement, temperature control, correct timing, and use of principles of quality control. Additional information on test interpretation, biological false-positive reactions, and sources of error can be found in many publications (13, 17, 24).

VDRL slide test with spinal fluid (7, 26)

Equipment.

1. Rotating machine (refer to VDRL test with serum).
2. Hypodermic needle, without bevel: 21 or 22 gauge.

Glassware. Agglutination slides, 2.25 by 3 inches (5.7 by 7.6 cm), with 12 concavities, each measuring 16 mm in diameter and 1.75 mm in depth.

Reagents (refer to VDRL test with serum).

1. VDRL antigen.
2. VDRL buffered saline.
3. Saline, 0.9%.
4. Saline, 10.0%.

Controls. Although this test is performed with spinal fluids, it is more convenient to prepare controls from a high-titered reactive serum.

1. Select serum with a VDRL slide test titer of 1:80 or greater.
2. Prepare additional dilutions of serum with 0.9% saline, selecting those that produce reactive, minimally reactive, and nonreactive results in the VDRL slide spinal fluid test.
3. Dispense quantities of control sera sufficient for one testing period into properly labeled tubes and stopper tightly with paraffin-coated corks. Store in a freezer.
4. For daily use, remove one tube of reactive serum, thaw and mix thoroughly, and prepare the proper dilutions in 0.9% saline. Control sera are tested without preliminary heating in the slide test.

Preparation of sensitized antigen suspension.

1. Prepare antigen suspension as described for the VDRL slide test.
2. Add one part of 10% saline to one part of VDRL slide test suspension.
3. Mix well and allow to stand at least 5 min, but not more than 2 h, before use.

VDRL slide qualitative test with spinal fluid.

1. Pipette 0.05 ml of control serum diluted to produce reactive (R), minimally reactive (R_m), and nonreactive (N) results into each of three concavities of an agglutination slide.
2. Pipette 0.05 ml of spinal fluid into one concavity of the slide.
3. Add one drop (0.01 ml) of sensitized antigen suspension to each control and spinal fluid with a calibrated 21- or 22-gauge needle.
4. Rotate slides for 8 min on a mechanical rotator at 180 rpm.
5. Immediately after rotation, read tests microscopically at 100× magnification and report the results as follows: definite clumping, reactive (R); no clumping or very slight roughness, nonreactive (N).

VDRL slide quantitative test with spinal fluid. Quantitative tests are performed on all spinal fluids found to be reactive in the qualitative test.

1. Prepare spinal fluid dilutions as follows. Pipette 0.2 ml of 0.9% saline into each of five or more tubes. Add 0.2 ml of unheated spinal fluid to tube 1, mix well, and transfer 0.2 ml to tube 2. Continue mixing and transferring 0.2 ml from one tube to the next until the last tube is reached. The respective dilutions are 1:2, 1:4, 1:8, 1:16, 1:32, etc.
2. Test each spinal fluid dilution and undiluted spinal fluid as described for the VDRL slide qualitative test with spinal fluid.
3. Report results in terms of the greatest spinal fluid dilution that produces a reactive result.

TREPONEMAL TESTS

Tests for syphilis employing treponemal antigens are of most value in testing sera from patients presenting diagnostic problems. Such individuals most frequently have reactive reagin tests in the absence of clinical or historical evidence of syphilis, but may have nonreactive reagin tests and clinical signs of late syphilis. A reactive treponemal test is considered good evidence of past or present syphilitic infection, providing that other treponematoses can be ruled out.

The *Treponema pallidum* immobilization (TPI) test determines the presence of immobilizing antibodies in the serum of patients with syphilis or other treponematoses (18). The test antigen is the virulent Nichols strain of *T. pallidum* freshly harvested from rabbit testicular syphilomas. Motile treponemes suspended in Nelson's medium are exposed to patient's serum and active guinea pig complement during overnight incubation at 37 C in an atmosphere of 95% nitrogen and 5% carbon dioxide. These organisms are observed by dark-field microscopy for loss of motility as compared with organisms in serum controls treated in a similar fashion but exposed to inactivated complement (18).

The TPI test has undergone extensive clinical and laboratory evaluation and has been accepted as the treponemal test of reference. Because of its specificity, it is most useful in evaluating diagnostic problem cases. Like other treponemal tests, the TPI test remains reactive over long periods of time, it is not useful in assessing therapy, and it does not distinguish between the treponematoses. The TPI test is insensitive in early syphilis. It is the test of choice for spinal fluids, especially for detecting neuro-syphilis when reagin tests give nonreactive or equivocal results (13, 17).

Fluorescent treponemal antibody absorption test (26, 27, 29)

Following the development of the TPI test, many other procedures were devised to overcome the complexities of the TPI test and make reliable treponemal testing available to most medical laboratories. Although some of these procedures (TPCF, RPCF) were widely used, they were found to lack sensitivity and reproducibility (13, 24). The most promising and useful technique to date is an indirect fluorescence procedure originally described by Deacon et al. in 1957 (5). The fluorescent treponemal antibody absorption (FTA-ABS) test, an improved procedure utilizing absorption of sera with Reiter sorbent was first published by the VDRL in 1968 (27).

Because of problems experienced in some laboratories with apparent loss of treponemes from acetone-fixed slides in the FTA-ABS test, Wood and his associates (29) developed an alternate method of fixation employing methanol. Fresh methanol-fixed slides give reactions in the FTA-ABS test comparable to those obtained with acetone. Methanol-fixed slides may give slightly lower plus readings on some sera than does acetone, but this does not appear to affect the reportable reactivity.

The FTA-ABS test employing either acetone or methanol-fixed slides (26) is described below. The procedure is well standardized, and commercial reagents are available from several manufacturers.

Principle. In the FTA-ABS test, nonviable *T. pallidum* (Nichols strain) cells are allowed to react with patient's serum which has been treated to remove substances reacting nonspecifically with *T. pallidum* (6, 10). Specific antitreponemal antibodies present in the serum combine with the treponemal antigens and are detected by the addition of antihuman globulin labeled with fluorescein isothiocyanate.

Equipment.

1. Incubator, adjustable, 35 to 37 C.
2. Dark-field fluorescence microscope assembly.
3. Bibulous paper.
4. Slide board or holder.
5. Moist chamber. Any convenient cover for slides may be made into a moist chamber by placing wet paper inside cover.
6. Loop, bacteriological, standard 2-mm, 26-gauge, platinum.
7. Small dropper bottle.
8. Polyethylene bottle with faucet, 5-gallon size.

Glassware.

1. Microscope slides, 1 by 3 inches (2.5 by 7.6 cm), frosted end, approximately 1 mm thick with two etched circles 10 mm in diameter. (Pre-etched slides are available commercially.) Slides should be cleaned by soaking in 70% alcohol for 1 h and wiping dry, or by washing in detergent, rinsing well, and wiping dry.
2. Cover slips, no. 1, 22 by 50 mm or 22 by 22 mm. Cover slips should be cleaned by soaking in 70% alcohol for 1 h and wiping dry.
3. Disposable capillary pipettes, 5.75 inches (14.6 cm) in length.
4. Dish, staining, with removable glass tray. Inside dimensions: 3⅝ by 2¾ by 2½ inches in height (9.2 by 7.0 by 6.4 cm). Coplin staining jars may be used when few slides are involved.
5. Glass rods, approximately 100 by 4 mm, both ends fire polished.

Reagents. All reagents for the FTA-ABS test are available commercially.

1. Antigen for this test is *T. pallidum* Nichols strain. Lyophilized antigen suspensions are reconstituted according to the manufacturers' directions. A satisfactory reconstituted antigen suspension should contain a minimum of 7 to 10 organisms per high dry field (for methanol-fixed slides) or a minimum of 30 organisms per high dry field (for acetone-fixed slides). The suspension should be free from extraneous material such as tissue fragments, fibrin, etc. Antigen suspensions stored in a refrigerator may be used for 2 weeks if the antigen does not become badly clumped or contaminated and if satisfactory results are obtained with control sera.
2. Reiter sorbent is a standardized extract of nonpathogenic Reiter treponemes. Sorbent stored at 6 to 10 C can be used indefinitely if it does not become contaminated and if satisfactory results are obtained with controls.
3. Fluorescein-labeled antihuman globulin. Store rehydrated conjugate in convenient quantities (0.3 ml or more) at −20 C or lower. High-titered antihuman globulin can be reconstituted to volume and diluted 1:10 in sterile phosphate-buffered saline (containing Merthiolate in a concentration of 1:5,000) or sterile phosphate-buffered saline containing 2% Tween 80 before freezing. When thawed for use, do not refreeze but store undiluted at 6 to 10 C for not more than 1 week.

4. Phosphate-buffered saline. Formula per liter: NaCl, 7.65 g; Na_2HPO_4, 0.724 g; KH_2PO_4, 0.21 g. The pH reading should be 7.2 ± 0.1. If change in pH is noted or if solution is contaminated by molds or bacteria, discard and prepare a fresh solution. Store in a large polyethylene bottle.

5. Tween 80. To prepare a solution of 2% Tween 80 in phosphate-buffered saline, heat the two reagents in a water bath at 56 C for 15 to 30 min. To 98 ml of buffered saline, add 2 ml of Tween 80, measuring from the bottom of a pipette, and rinse out the pipette. The pH reading should be 7.0 to 7.2. This solution keeps well at refrigerator temperature but should be discarded when found to contain precipitate. Prepare a fresh solution with each fresh preparation of phosphate-buffered saline.

6. Mounting medium. To prepare the mounting medium, add 1 part buffered saline (pH 7.2 ± 0.1) plus 9 parts of glycerol (reagent grade).

7. Absolute methanol. A.C.S. reagent grade. To prepare 10% solution of methanol, add 1 part absolute methyl alcohol to 9 parts of distilled water. Prepare fresh solution on day of use. Do not use solution for more than one fixation period or more than 20 slides per 200 ml. Slides fixed with methanol should be used on the day of preparation.

8. Acetone. A.C.S. reagent grade. Not more than 60 slides should be fixed with 200 ml of acetone. Acetone-fixed smears may be used on the day of preparation or may be stored at −20 C or below. Fixed, frozen smears are usable indefinitely, provided that satisfactory results are obtained with the controls. Do not thaw and refreeze antigen smears.

9. Oil, immersion, low fluorescence, nondrying.

Preliminary testing of antigen suspension. Mix antigen suspension well according to the manufacturers' directions to insure an even distribution of treponemes. Determine by darkfield examination that treponemes are adequately dispersed before making smears for the FTA test.

Compare a new lot of antigen, or an antigen of unknown quality, with an antigen of known reactivity using control sera and individual sera of graded reactivity before incorporating into the routine test procedure. A satisfactory antigen preparation should give comparable results with control sera and individual sera. It should not stain nonspecifically with a diluted conjugate of known quality.

Preliminary testing of Reiter sorbent. Compare a new lot of sorbent with a sorbent of known activity using control sera and individual sera of graded reactivity before use in routine test procedures. A satisfactory sorbent should give comparable results with control sera and individual sera. It should not cause nonspecific staining of antigen with a diluted conjugate of known quality.

Preliminary testing of fluorescein-labeled antihuman globulin conjugate.

1. Determine the titer of each new lot of fluorescein-labeled conjugate before use in routine testing.

2. Prepare serial twofold dilutions of the new conjugate in phosphate-buffered saline containing 2% Tween 80 to include two to three dilutions greater than the manufacturer's titer.

3. Test each conjugate dilution with the reactive (4+) control serum diluted 1:5 in phosphate-buffered saline in accordance with the FTA-ABS technique.

4. Test each conjugate dilution with antigen as a check on nonspecific staining (antigen smear treated with 0.03 ml of buffered saline in place of serum).

5. A reference conjugate is tested at its previously determined dilution with the reactive (4+) control serum, the minimally reactive (1+) control serum, and the nonspecific staining control for the purpose of controlling reagents and test conditions.

6. Read the control slides to insure reagents are working properly and test conditions are satisfactory. Then examine the slides with the new conjugate, starting with the lowest dilution of conjugate. Record readings in pluses.

7. The end point of the titration is the highest dilution giving maximal (4+) fluorescence. The working titer of the new conjugate is one doubling dilution below the end point.

8. The new conjugate should not stain nonspecifically at three doubling dilutions below the working titer of the conjugate.

9. Using the reference conjugate at its working dilution and the new conjugate at the titer determined by the titration, test the following sera in parallel: (i) Control sera, unabsorbed and absorbed; (ii) 10 sera of graded reactivity, absorbed. Results obtained with both conjugates should be comparable.

Controls. The following controls must be included in each test run.

1. Reactive control serum (syphilitic human serum). Reactive control serum should show 4+ fluorescence in unabsorbed test and may show slightly reduced fluorescence in absorbed test. (i) Unabsorbed: using a 0.2-ml pipette, measuring from the bottom, add 0.05 ml of reactive control serum to a tube containing 0.2 ml of buffered saline. Mix at least eight times with the same pipette. (ii) Absorbed: using another 0.2-ml pipette, measuring from the bottom, add

0.05 ml of reactive control serum to a tube containing 0.2 ml of Reiter sorbent. Mix at least eight times with the same pipette.

2. Minimally reactive control serum (syphilitic human serum). The minimally reactive control serum should show 1+ fluorescence. Control serum showing 2+ to 3+ fluorescence in the unabsorbed test and 1+ fluorescence in the absorbed test may be used. (i) Unabsorbed: same as for the reactive control. (ii) Absorbed: same as for the reactive control.

A dilution of the reactive control serum, showing 1+ fluorescence, may also be used. (i) Unabsorbed: dilute the reactive control serum in phosphate-buffered saline to the predetermined titer showing 1+ fluorescence.

3. Nonspecific control serum (a nonsyphilitic human serum known to demonstrate nonspecific reactivity to *T. pallidum*, Nichols strain (at a 1:5 or higher dilution). (i) Unabsorbed: same as for reactive control. (ii) Absorbed: same as for reactive control.

4. Control of nonspecific staining by conjugate. (i) Unabsorbed: 0.03 ml of buffered saline in place of serum. (ii) Absorbed: 0.03 ml of Reiter sorbent in place of serum.

Preparation of sera. Heat the test and control sera in a water bath at 56 C for 30 min. Previously heated sera should be reheated for 10 min at 56 C on the day of testing.

Procedure for fluorescent treponemal antibody absorption test with serum.

1. Prepare antigen smears on day of test by spreading 0.005 ml or one loopful of *T. pallidum* antigen from a standard 2-mm, 26-gauge platinum wire loop within each circle on grease-free slides. Allow to air-dry.

2. Immerse in or cover slides with freshly prepared 10% methanol for 20 s. Remove slides and blot dry with bibulous paper. If acetone fixation is preferred, fix smears in acetone for 10 min and allow to air-dry thoroughly.

3. Arrange 12 by 75 mm test tubes in suitable racks so that there is one tube for each serum to be tested. Add tubes for dilutions of control sera prepared as described under Controls.

4. For each serum to be tested, pipette 0.2 ml of standardized Reiter sorbent into a test tube. Using a 0.2-ml pipette, measuring from the bottom of the pipette, add 0.05 ml of the test serum into each tube. Mix at least eight times with same pipette. Test should be performed within 30 min after dilutions are made. If it is necessary to test specimen after this period, make a new serum dilution.

5. Cover the *T. pallidum* smears with 0.03 ml of the serum-sorbent mixture to be tested. Include controls as described above.

6. Place slides in a moist chamber to prevent evaporation of serum.

7. Place moist chamber containing the slides in an incubator at 35 to 37 C for 30 min.

8. Rinse slides with running buffered saline for approximately 5 s. Soak in two changes of buffered saline for a total of 10 min. (At the end of 5 min of the soaking period, rinse the slides by dipping them in and out of buffered saline 10 times.) Follow with a brief rinse of running distilled water to remove salt crystals.

9. Blot slides with bibulous paper to remove all water drops.

10. On the day of use, dilute fluorescein-labeled antihuman globulin to its working titer in phosphate-buffered saline containing 2% Tween 80.

11. Place approximately 0.03 ml of diluted fluorescein conjugate on each smear. Spread conjugate with a glass rod in a circular pattern so that smears are completely covered. A disposable pipette, calibrated needle, or dropper may be used for dispensing conjugate.

12. Repeat steps 6, 7, 8, and 9.

13. Place a small drop of mounting medium on each smear, apply a cover slip, and place slides in a covered slide holder.

14. Slides should be examined immediately or may be stored in a darkened room for several hours before reading. Exposure to light will cause fading of fluorescence and make readings, particularly those in the moderately fluorescent (2+) zone, difficult to read.

15. Smears are studied microscopically, by use of ultraviolet light and a high-power dry objective. The total magnification should approximate 400×. A combination of BG 12 (primary) filter and Zeiss 50/- (II/0) or OG 1 (secondary) filter has been found to be satisfactory for routine use.

16. Nonreactive smears should be checked by switching from ultraviolet to white light to verify the presence of treponemes.

17. Using the minimally reactive (1+) control slide as the reading standard, record the intensity of fluorescence of the treponemes according to the chart given in Table 2.

Control pattern illustration.

Reactive control serum:

1:5 in buffered saline	R 4+
1:5 in sorbent	R 3–4+

Minimally reactive control serum:

1:5 in buffered saline	R 2–3+
1:5 in sorbent	MR 1+

or

Minimally reactive control serum:	
Predetermined dilution in buffered saline of the reactive control serum	MR 1+
Nonspecific control serum:	
1:5 in buffered saline	R 2+
1:5 in sorbent	N
Control for nonspecific staining by conjugate:	
Buffered saline	N
Sorbent	N

Interpretation. Reactive: confirms presence of treponemal antibodies, but does not indicate stage or activity of infection.

Nonreactive: no treponemal antibodies detected. If early infection suspected, repeat serological testing may be helpful.

Borderline: results are inconclusive and cannot be interpreted. May indicate a very low level of treponemal antibody, or may be due to nonspecific factors. Further follow-up and repeat serological testing may be helpful.

The FTA-ABS test is most often used to determine whether a reactive reagin test is due to latent syphilis or to some condition other than syphilis. It may also be used on patients with nonreactive reagin tests but with clinical evidence of syphilis (24). It is more sensitive than the TPI test in all stages of syphilis, especially in the very early and very late stages. Once the FTA-ABS test becomes reactive, it tends to remain so for long periods of time, regardless of therapy. Extensive evaluation by several investigators (6, 25, 29) indicated good agreement between the FTA-ABS and TPI tests in patients presenting diagnostic problems. Although the specificity of the FTA-ABS test is considered to be extremely good, the possibility of false-positive reactions in some patient groups should be considered. False-positive reactions have been reported in patients with diseases associated with increased or abnormal globulins (2, 16), in patients with lupus erythematosus and antinuclear antibodies (11, 14), and during pregnancy (3, 4). The majority of these reactions are in the borderline to minimally reactive range.

Pitfalls and sources of error. The FTA-ABS test does not distinguish between syphilis and other treponematoses such as pinta, yaws, and bejel. It is not useful in measuring the effectiveness of therapy. The technical procedure, although simple and reliable in the hands of well-trained laboratory workers, involves subjective readings of degrees of fluorescence and requires careful standardization and checking of reagents and controls.

TABLE 2. *Fluorescence intensity of treponemes*

Reading	Intensity of fluorescence	Report
4+	Very strong	Reactive (R)
3+	Strong	Reactive (R)
2+	Moderate	Reactive (R)
1+	Equivalent to minimally reactive (1+) control	Reactive (R)[a]
<1+	Weak but definite, less than minimally reactive (1+) control	Borderline (B)[a]
– to ±	None to barely visible	Nonreactive (N)

[a] Retest all specimens with intensity of fluorescence of 1+ or less. When a specimen initially read as 1+ is retested and is subsequently read as 1+ or greater, the test is reported as "Reactive." All other results on retest are reported as "Borderline." It is not necessary to retest nonfluorescent (Nonreactive) specimens.

Detection of Treponema pallidum by the fluorescent-antibody dark-field technique (12)

Principle. The diagnosis of infectious syphilis can be made by the demonstration of *T. pallidum* from external lesions or from the aspirate of regional lymph nodes. The organisms may be demonstrated by conventional dark-field or by fluorescent-antibody dark-field (FADF) techniques. In either method, it is essential that specimens be taken for examination prior to the beginning of therapy.

In the conventional dark-field method, *T. pallidum* is differentiated from other treponemes by its characteristic morphology and motility. In the FADF method, *T. pallidum* is differentiated from other treponemes by the use of specific absorbed conjugates. The FADF test has not been extensively evaluated because of the unavailability of commercial reagents. The use of the FADF test has been limited to those laboratories preparing their own conjugates.

Collection of material. Material should be collected by the physician, who should attempt to obtain tissue serum from the deeper layers of the lesion, avoiding if possible red blood cells and tissue debris.

Remove any crust or scab from the surface of the lesion. Clean with a gauze sponge moistened with water or saline only. Do not use antiseptics or detergents. Abrade lesion with sponge, needle, or suitable instrument to provoke slight bleeding. When the lesion is oozing, blot successively with gauze until relatively clear serum appears. Press glass slide against the oozing lesion until an adequate amount of serum adheres to the slide. Material should be confined within a small area of the slide, approximately 10 mm in diameter. Air-dry slide, label, and insert in container provided for transportation to the laboratory, together with the appropriate laboratory request form.

Treat lesions of the body cavities in a similar manner to those of the surfaces. Obtain serum with a fine pipette and express onto the surface of the slide, using a wire loop if necessary. Remove vaginal, cervical, or anal discharges by the usual preliminary cleansing.

In the event that a regional node is to be aspirated, prepare for aseptic skin puncture. Perform local infiltration of an anesthetic solution down to the surface of the node, if necessary. With the node stabilized by external pressure, puncture with a large-gauge needle on a syringe holding approximately 0.5 ml of sterile normal saline. Inject saline and move the needle tip about within the substances of the node. Apply suction until the needle tip is withdrawn from the node capsule. Release plunger traction and withdraw needle through the skin. Prepare slides from aspirated material in needle shaft, in the manner described above.

Scarify or incise suspected secondary skin lesions to produce bleeding and treat serum as above.

Examination of slides by the FADF technique. Equipment and glassware are the same as described above for the FTA-ABS procedure.

Reagents.

1. FTA-ABS antigen, *T. pallidum*, Nichols strain, for use as a positive control.

2. Fluorescein-labeled anti-*T. pallidum* conjugate, prepared by labeling the globulin fraction of high-titered syphilitic serum of human origin with fluorescein isothiocyanate. Conjugate must be absorbed with Reiter treponemes to remove antibodies reacting with spirochetes other than *T. pallidum* and titrated to determine the optimal dilution for use (12). Store stock conjugate in a refrigerator in the dark.

3. Other reagents: phosphate-buffered saline, Tween 80, mounting fluid, and immersion oil are as described above for the FTA-ABS procedure.

Procedure.

1. Heat-fix the smears to be tested by flaming smears three times over a Bunsen burner. After fixation, smears can be stored at 4 to 6 C for several days before examination. Be sure to allow the smears to come to room temperature before proceeding with the staining procedure.

2. Mark off an area of the smear approximately 10 mm in diameter to be stained.

3. Dilute conjugate according to previously determined titer with equal parts of 2% Tween 80 in phosphate-buffered saline and sterile normal rabbit serum.

4. Apply the diluted conjugate to test and control smears.

5. Incubate slides in a moist chamber at 35 to 37 C for 30 min.

6. Rinse slides under running phosphate-buffered saline (pH 7.2) and soak in buffered saline for 10 min with a change of saline at the end of 5 min.

7. Rinse the slides briefly under running distilled water. Blot smears dry with bibulous paper. Place a small amount of phosphate-buffered glycerol (pH 7.2) on each smear and apply a cover slip.

8. Examine smears using ultraviolet light and high-power dry objective with total magnification of approximately 400 to 450×. A combination of BG 12 (primary) filter and Zeiss 50/- (II/0) or OG 1 (secondary) filter has been found satisfactory. Examine smears for spirochetes with morphology characteristic of *T. pallidum* which show fluorescence of 2+ or greater.

9. Report presence or absence of spirochetes resembling *T. pallidum*, as seen by the FADF technique.

Interpretation of results. The presence in suspicious lesions of spirochetes detected by FADF examination is presumptive evidence of syphilitic infection. Recent studies (12, 30) indicate that this procedure is as accurate as the traditional examination by dark-field microscopy and does not depend on the presence of motile treponemes of typical morphology. The test is applicable to specimens sent through the mails.

Pitfalls and sources of error. A reliable FADF test is dependent on thorough examination of microscopic smears so that even small numbers of treponemes will be detected. A high-titered conjugate, adequately absorbed to eliminate cross-reactions with saprophytic spirochetes, is essential.

LITERATURE CITED

1. Andujar, J. J., and E. E. Mazurek. 1959. The plasmacrit

(PCT) test on capillary blood. Amer. J. Clin. Pathol. **31**:197–204.
2. Bradford, L. L., D. L. Tuffanelli, J. Puffer, M. L. Bissett, H. L. Bodily, and R. M. Wood. 1967. Fluorescent treponemal absorption and *Treponema pallidum* immobilization tests in syphilitic patients and biologic false positive reactions. Amer. J. Clin. Pathol. **47**:525–532.
3. Buchanan, C. S., and J. R. Haserick. 1970. FTA-ABS test in pregnancy: a probable false positive reaction. Arch. Dermatol. **102**:322–325.
4. Cohen, P., G. Stout, and N. Ende. 1969. Serologic reactivity in consecutive patients admitted to a general hospital: a comparison of the FTA-ABS, VDRL, and automated reagin tests. Arch. Intern. Med. **124**:364–367.
5. Deacon, W. E., V. H. Falcone, and A. Harris. 1957. A fluorescent test for treponemal antibodies. Proc. Soc. Exp. Biol. Med. **96**:477–480.
6. Deacon, W. E., J. B. Lucas, and E. V. Price. 1966. Fluorescent treponemal antibody absorption (FTA-ABS) test for syphilis. J. Amer. Med. Ass. **198**:624–628.
7. Duncan, W. P., H. N. Bossak, and A. Harris. 1961. VDRL slide spinal fluid test. Amer. J. Clin. Pathol. **35**:93–95.
8. Harris, A., A. A. Rosenberg, and E. R. Del Vecchio. 1948. The VDRL slide flocculation test for syphilis. II. A supplementary report. J. Vener. Dis. Inform. **29**:72–75.
9. Harris, A., A. A. Rosenberg, and L. M. Riedel. 1946. A microflocculation test for syphilis using cardiolipin antigen. Preliminary report. J. Vener. Dis. Inform. **27**:169–174.
10. Hunter, E. F., W. E. Deacon, and P. E. Meyer. 1964. An improved test for syphilis—the absorption procedure (FTA-ABS). Pub. Health Rep. **79**:410–412.
11. Jokinen, E. J., A. Lassus, and E. Linder. 1969. Fluorescent treponemal antibody (FTA) reaction in sera with antinuclear factors. Ann. Clin. Res. **1**:77–80.
12. Jue, R., J. Puffer, R. Wood, G. Schochet, W. Smartt, and W. Ketterer. 1967. A comparison of fluorescent and conventional darkfield methods for the detection of *Treponema pallidum* in syphilitic lesions. Amer. J. Clin. Pathol. **47**:809–811.
13. King, A. 1964. Recent advances in venereology. Little, Brown and Co., Boston.
14. Kraus, S. J., J. R. Haserick, and M. A. Lantz. 1970. Fluorescent treponemal antibody-absorption test reactions in lupus erythematosus: atypical beading pattern and probable false-positive reactions. N. Engl. J. Med. **282**:1287–1290.
15. McGrew, B. E., M. J. F. Du Cros, G. W. Stout, and V. H. Falcone. 1968. Automation of a flocculation test for syphilis. Amer. J. Clin. Pathol. **50**:52–59.
16. Mackey, D. M., E. V. Price, J. M. Knox, and A. Scotti. 1969. Specificity of the FTA-ABS test for syphilis: an evaluation. J. Amer. Med. Ass. **207**:1683–1685.
17. Miller, S. E. 1966. The laboratory diagnosis of venereal infections, p. 757–790. *In* S. E. Miller (ed.), A textbook of clinical pathology, 7th ed. The Williams & Wilkins Co., Baltimore.
18. Nelson, R. A., Jr., and M. M. Mayer. 1949. Immobilization of *Treponema pallidum* in vitro by antibody produced in syphilitic infection. J. Exp. Med. **89**:369–393.
19. Portnoy, J. 1963. Modifications of the rapid plasma reagin (RPR) card test for syphilis for use in large scale testing. Amer. J. Clin. Pathol. **40**:473–479.
20. Portnoy, J., H. N. Bossak, V. H. Falcone, and A. Harris. 1961. Rapid reagin test with unheated serum and new improved antigen suspension. Pub. Health Rep. **76**:933–935.
21. Portnoy, J., J. H. Brewer, and A. Harris. 1962. Rapid plasma reagin card test for syphilis and other treponematoses. Pub. Health Rep. **77**:645–652.
22. Portnoy, J., and W. Garson. 1960. New and improved antigen suspension for rapid reagin test for syphilis. Pub. Health Rep. **75**:985–988.
23. Portnoy, J., W. Garson, and C. A. Smith. 1957. Rapid plasma reagin test for syphilis. Pub. Health Rep. **72**:761–766.
24. Sparling, P. F. 1971. Medical progress. Diagnosis and treatment of syphilis. N. Engl. J. Med. **284**:642–653.
25. Tuffanelli, D. L., K. D. Wuepper, L. L. Bradford, and R. M. Wood. 1967. Fluorescent treponemal-antibody absorption tests: studies of false-positive reactions to tests for syphilis. N. Engl. J. Med. **276**:258–262.
26. U.S. Department of Health, Education, and Welfare, National Communicable Disease Center, Venereal Disease Branch. 1969. Manual of tests for syphilis. U.S. Government Printing Office, Washington, D.C.
27. Veneral Disease Research Laboratory. 1968. Technique for the fluorescent treponemal antibody-absorption (FTA-ABS) test. Health Lab. Sci. **5**:23–30.
28. Venereal Disease Research Laboratory, Venereal Disease Program, National Communicable Disease Center. 15 January 1970. Provisional technic for the automated reagin (AR) test. Center for Disease Control, Atlanta.
29. Wood, R. M., Y. Inouye, W. Argonza, L. Bradford, R. Jue, Y. Jeong, J. Puffer, and H. L. Bodily. 1967. Comparison of the fluorescent treponemal antibody absorption and *Treponema pallidum* immobilization tests on serums from 1182 diagnostic problem cases. Amer. J. Clin. Pathol. **47**:521–524.
30. Yobs, A. R., L. Brown, and E. F. Hunter. 1964. Fluorescent antibody technique in early syphilis. Arch. Pathol. **77**:220–225.

Chapter 52
Immunoserological Tests Other Than Syphilis

WALLIS L. JONES

A. AGGLUTINATIONS, FEBRILE

Febrile agglutination tests have frequently been used in the diagnosis of certain febrile diseases. They should not be substituted for intensive attempts to isolate etiological agents and may represent a retrospective opportunity to implicate a particular disease if the more important cultural attempts have failed.

The agglutination reaction usually becomes positive during the second week after typhoid fever infection. These reactions are quantitatively determined by using either a micro dilution test system or the tube test.

To interpret any febrile agglutination test, paired acute and covalescent phase sera should be collected 1 to 2 weeks apart. A fourfold or greater increase in titer is usually considered significant. It must be kept in mind that cross-reactions do occur, and diagnosis should not be based on serological results only. The patient's immunization history must also be considered.

Typhoid carriers may have elevated Vi agglutinins in their sera, which may be demonstrated by a hemagglutination procedure (1, 17). The validity of this approach for detection of carriers has been challenged (3). Sera of patients with typhoid fever may or may not show titers against the Vi antigen.

When serological tests are performed to demonstrate antibodies against *Brucella* antigen, care should be taken to use a standard antigen preparation such as that prepared by the National Animal Disease Laboratory (NADL), Ames, Iowa, or an equivalent preparation from a commercial source. The NADL antigen is prepared in accordance with World Health Organization recommendations and is standardized against an International Reference Serum. Antigen should be diluted with phenolized saline (0.85% NaCl with 0.5% phenol) and should be prepared fresh each day. Problems occasionally arise with these tests. They include prozone reactions which usually appear in lower dilutions. Typical agglutination appears in the higher dilutions. "Blocking" antibodies, another problem, also are usually found only in lower dilutions and are diluted out. Some workers report instances when the standard tube test gave low or negative titers but other tests gave titers of significant levels. Tests which have been used in these cases include the Coombs and centrifugation methods (15). Heat inactivation and 2-mercaptoethanol treatment have been used to detect immunoglobulin G antibody. These tests may also be helpful in cases where nonspecific agglutination is suspected. Cross-reactions may be seen with tularemia and cholera antigens.

With tularemia sera, a significant titer may be observed during the second week of illness, and titers usually reach a maximum level between the fourth and sixth week after onset. Titers begin to drop after 1 year, but with a tube agglutination test results may be positive for several years.

Other febrile agglutination tests employing Proteus OX19, OXK, and OX2 that imply rickettsial infection have been used, but are being replaced in many laboratories by more specific complement fixation tests.

Quality control measures are important in attempts to standardize tests. Each new lot of antigen should be checked for proper reactivity with a control or reference serum of known titer.

Time and temperature of incubation, two frequently found variables, should be standardized. The Center for Disease Control recommends 37 C for *Brucella* over a period of 24 h and 37 C for tularemia over an 18-h period.

End point reporting is another variable frequently found. It is recommended that the last tube with a 2+ (50% agglutination) reaction be used as the end point.

Sera should not be mixed so vigorously that foaming results, since this will denature some antibodies. Serum should be removed from the clot as soon as possible and put into a clean, sterile tube. Hemolyzed serum should not be used because it may give false positive reactions.

Reference controls or preparations should be run with each set of test specimens, and, if possible, high titer, low titer, and negative reactions should be included.

B. ANTINUCLEAR ANTIBODY

Sera from patients with systemic lupus erythematosus have antibodies that react in various serological tests. These include latex particle tests, indirect fluorescent antibody tests, and radioimmunoassays. Several commercial sources have "kits" available to perform these tests.

The indirect fluorescent antibody test is a very sensitivie procedure in which various tissue preparations or even blood smears are used. These preparations are reacted with the patient's serum, washed, and then reacted with a fluorescent conjugate of anti-human globulin. Patterns of nuclear fluorescence in the smears are then observed (2).

In the radioimmunoassay, an intrinsic label is used in the deoxyribonucleic acid antigen. This procedure is more specific for systemic lupus erythematosus than the other tests mentioned.

C. ANTISTREPTOLYSIN "O" MICTROTITRATION TESTS

Antistreptolysin "O", antideoxyribonuclease, and antihyaluronidase procedures are defined in detail by the commercial suppliers of the respective tests (10). (Refer to part J of this chapter for references.)

D. DIPHTHERIA AND TETANUS ANTITOXIN LEVELS

Two tests that are frequently used to evaluate a patient's immune response to antigenic stimulation are tetanus and diphtheria antitoxin levels. At this time the most frequent tests are hemagglutination procedures (16).

Reagents

1. Prepare a 2.5-ml sheep red blood cell suspension in phosphate-buffered saline (PBS), pH 7.2.
2. Prepare tannic acid stock. For each milligram of this stock add 1 ml of pH 7.2 PBS to yield a final dilution of 1:1,000.
3. Working tannic acid solution is prepared by diluting the 1:20 stock 1:1,000 to obtain a 1:20,000 dilution.
4. Mix equal volumes of 2.5% cells and 1:20,000 tannic acid together in a centrifuge tube.
5. Incubate in a 37 C water bath for 20 min.
6. Centrifuge for 5 min at the speed used for washing cells, remove the supernatant, suspend the cells in 2 to 3 volumes of PBS, pH 7.2, and centrifuge again for 5 min.
7. Remove the supernatant and resuspend the cells to a 2.5% suspension by adding the proper amount of physiological saline to return the cells to their original volume.

Sensitization of cells

1. Make the optimal dilution of antigen in PBS, pH 6.4. (The optimal dilution is determined in a block titration which is described below.)
2. Into a 15-ml graduated centrifuge tube, pipette the following materials: 1 volume of 2.5% tanned cells (0.5 ml), 1 volume of toxoid dilution (0.5 ml), 4 volumes of PBS, pH 6.4 (2.0 ml). Into another 15-ml graduated centrifuge tube, pipette the following materials: 1 volume of 2.5 tanned cells (0.5 ml), 5 volumes of PBS, pH 6.4 (2.5 ml).
3. Incubate the two tubes for 15 min at room temperature.
4. Centrifuge the tubes for 5 min at the speed used for washing cells; remove supernatant.
5. Suspend the cells in two to three times their volume with 1% rabbit serum diluent.
6. Recentrifuge, remove supernatants, and resuspend the packed cells in two times the original volume of tanned cells; use the 1% normal rabbit serum diluent. This will give a 1.25% concentration of tanned sensitized cells, and a 1.25% concentration of tanned, nonsensitized cells.
7. The cells are now ready for use in the test.

Procedure

1. a. Set up two rows of tubes for each serum—10 tubes to each row.
   b. Make a starting dilution of the unknown sera and known positive sera for each antigen. Inactivate at 56 C for 30 min.
   c. Add 1 ml of the starting dilution of each serum to the first tube in each row.
2. Add 0.5 ml of 1% rabbit serum to all other tubes in each row.
3. Add 0.5 ml of a 1% normal rabbit serum to each of the two tubes labeled cell controls for sensitized and nonsensitized cells.
4. Make doubling dilutions of serum in 0.5-ml amounts. Discard 0.5 ml from the last tube in each row.
5. Into the first row of tubes for each serum and the diluent cell control tube, add 0.1 ml of tanned sensitized cells. Into the second row of tubes for each serum and diluent control tube, add 0.1 ml of tanned, nonsensitized cells.
6. Shake all tubes thoroughly.
7. Incubate at room temperature for 3 to 4 h.
8. Read and record.

Antigen block titration

1. Prepare tanned cells as described in steps 1a and b of Procedure.

2. Prepare twofold master dilutions of the toxoid which will cover the expected titer. Dilutions of toxoid from 1:4 to 1:128 are usually sufficient.
3. Prepare sensitized cells with these dilutions of toxoid as described in step 1c of Procedure.
4. Prepare serial dilutions of standard antitoxin which will cover the expected titer. Make twofold dilutions starting with a 1:20 dilution of the appropriate standard antitoxin.
5. Set up a rack with the proper tubes to cover the block titration plus tubes for the diluent controls and for the nonsensitized tanned cells.
6. Add 0.5 ml of serum dilutions to proper tubes.
7. Add 0.5 ml of rabbit serum diluent to diluent-cell control tubes.
8. Add 0.1 ml of sensitized cells to proper tubes and 0.1 ml of nonsensitized cells to the proper tubes.
9. Incubate at room temperature for 3 to 4 h.
10. The optimal dilution is that dilution of sensitized cells which agglutinates with the highest dilution of the standard antitoxin. Control tubes must show no agglutination. A level of 0.01 antitoxin units/ml is considered to be a protective level for both tetanus and diphtheria antitoxin levels.

E. IMMUNOGLOBULIN DETERMINATIONS

Immunoglobulins are presently being quantitated most often by use of radial immunodiffusion plates (12). These are prepared by mixing class-specific immunoglobulin antisera with agar and pouring the mixture into a suitable container. Wells are punched into the agar, and the test serum is placed in them. After a period of incubation, the diameter of the precipitin ring is measured and then related to a standard curve of known immunoglobulin levels. Numerous commercial kits for this procedure are available.

In performing this test it is important not to overfill or underfill the wells and to avoid bubbles. Standard reference curves should be run simultaneously with the test specimen.

These tests are a valuable aid in the diagnosis of such conditions as Walderstroms macroglobulinemia, agammaglobulinemia, certain myelomas, dysgammaglobulinemia, certain liver diseases, hyperimmunization, and a wide variety of infections.

F. INFECTIOUS MONONUCLEOSIS: LABORATORY METHODS FOR DIAGNOSIS

The etiology of infectious mononucleosis as yet is unconfirmed, and until it is confirmed there cannot be an ideal serological test.

Two currently popular procedures are the Davidsohn differential (6, 7) and the ox cell hemolysis (13) tests.

Commercial companies have developed rapid slide tests based on various immunological principles. Since the protocols for the various kits differ, the directions supplied by the manufacturer must be strictly adhered to in performing these tests.

Ox Cell Hemolysis Test

Reagents

1. Veronal-buffered saline.
2. Veronal-buffered water.
3. Ox erythrocyte suspension, 2%.
4. Complement, lyophilized.

Controls

1. Positive sera 1:40 or greater.
2. Negative sera.
3. Ox cell control.
4. Complement-ox cell control

Procedure

1. Make a 1:10 dilution of each test and control sera and incubate at 56 C for 30 min.
2. Place ten 12 × 75 mm test tubes in a test tube rack for each serum specimen, and one tube each for the ox cell control and the complement ox cell control.
3. Add 0.5 ml of VBD to the second through the tenth tube in each row. Pipette 1 ml of VBD into the ox cell control tube and 0.5 ml of VBD into the complement ox cell control tube.
4. Add 0.5 ml of the 1:10 dilution of inactivated serum to the first and second tubes of the appropriate row. Beginning with the second tube (1:20 dilutions), mix and transfer 0.5 ml to the third tube. Continue making twofold dilutions through the tenth tube, discarding the last 0.5 ml from the tenth tube.
5. Prepare a 50% hemolytic end point standard by adding the following to a 12 by 75 mm test tube.
   a. 0.25 ml of a 2% ox cell suspension.
   b. 1.0 ml of buffered water.
   c. An 0.25-ml dilution (1:15) of complement.

6. Add 0.5 ml of a 2% ox cell suspension to each tube.
7. Add 0.5 ml of a 1:15 dilution of complement to each tube except the ox cell control tube.
8. Shake the tubes to mix the contents.
9. Incubate tubes in a 37 C waterbath for 30 min.
10. Centrifuge tubes at 150 × *g* for 2 min.
11. Read and record results.

(Note: The 50% hemolytic end point is usually read by visual inspection of the tubes. The tube which most nearly matches the 50% hemolysin standard is considered the end point.)

Interpretation

An end-point dilution of 1:40 or greater is usually considered serological evidence of infectious mononucleosis.

G. LEPTOSPIROSIS SEROLOGY

A diagnosis of leptospirosis should be considered for patients with febrile illness of unknown origin. Clinical manifestations which suggest aseptic meningitis or nonparalytic poliomyelitis-like infections frequently are caused by leptospiral infections.

A variety of tests have been developed for the serodiagnosis of leptospirosis. The most widely used test has been the microscopic agglutination procedure (8) in which live antigen is used. This test is still considered the reference procedure for evaluating other tests.

A modified semi micromethod and improved microtechnique (5) have proved to be beneficial to smaller clinical laboratories. The improved microtechnique is performed as follows.

Equipment

1. Disposal plastic microdilutions plates with flat-bottom wells (Microtest II, Falcon Plastics, Oxnard, Calif., and Linbro Chemical Co., New Haven, Conn.).
2. Disposable microtiter pipettes equipped with an 0.05-ml dropper tip (Linbro Chemical Company, New Haven, Conn.).
3. Multimicrodiluter handle equipped with 0.05-ml microdiluters (Cooke Engineering Co., Alexandria, Va.).
4. Plate covers (Microtest II, Falcon Plastics, Oxnard, Calif., and Linbro Chemical Co., New Haven, Conn.).

Before use, plastic fibers or dust particles should be blown from the flat-bottom wells with a jet of clear air. The microdilution plates may be used repeatedly if they are washed immediately after each use with a sodium hypochlorite solution, rinsed in distilled water, and dried.

Procedure

1. Place one drop (0.05 ml) of PBS in each well in the plate except for the wells in the first row.
2. Add two drops (0.10 ml) of a 1:25 serum dilution to the first row of wells.

With the 0.05-ml microdiluter, the dilutions in the first row are mixed by twirling the diluters 10 to 15 times. Diluters are transferred to the next row and mixed. Mixing with the diluters is repeated for the desired number of dilutions.

Antigens are 4- to 7-day-old cultures of leptospira grown in polysorbate (EMJH) medium (Difco Laboratories, Detroit, Mich.). The antigen concentration is adjusted to 100 to 200 organisms per high-power field (×450), which is equivalent to a McFarland no. 0.5.

A separate 0.05-ml dropper is used for each antigen. One drop of antigen is added to each serum dilution. Each antigen is added to each serum dilution. Each antigen is added in a separate column. The plates are gently shaken to mix contents, covered, and incubated at room temperature (25 to 30 C) for 2 h.

Reading of tests

The plates are placed on the stage of a dark-field microscope equipped with a long-working-distance, 10× objective (no. 599-003, E. Leitz, Inc., Rockleigh, N.J.), and the wells are examined for agglutination. The end point is the highest dilution in which at least 50% of the leptospires are agglutinated.

Indirect hemagglutination test

Recently an indirect hemagglutination test has been reported that detects antibody as early as 4 days after onset of illness (C. R. Sulzer and W. L. Jones, submitted for publication). This test has been developed to replace the Galton rapid macroscopic slide test as a presumptive test for detecting antibodies in the diagnosis of leptospirosis. The rapid slide test was frequently positive with convalescent sera and negative with sera taken during the early stages of the disease. The indirect hemagglutination test is positive during the early stages of the disease and becomes negative a few weeks later. Since the indirect hemagglutination test is a presumptive test, positive results by this test should be confirmed by the regular microscopic agglutination test.

Reagents

Reagents include stock sensitized human "O" negative cells concentrated 10 times, stock nonsensitized human "O" negative cells concentrated 10 times, and positive *Leptospira andamana* control rabbit serum.

Kent buffer

A. Stock solution: NaCl, 75.0 g; NaCl (1 N), 180.0 ml; Triethanolamine (2,2[1],2[11]nitrilotriethanol), 28.0 ml; 4.15 M $MgCl_2 \cdot 6H_2O$, 1.2 ml; 1.25 M $CaCl_2 \cdot 2H_2O$, 1.2 ml. (Measure the triethanolamine carefully. Special care should be taken to assure complete transfer of triethanolamine from the graduate.) Dissolve the NaCl in 700 ml of distilled water in a 1-liter volumetric flask. Add the indicated volumes of the other components in the order given, and adjust the volume to 1,000 ml with distilled water.

B. Working solution. Dilute stock solution 1:10 with distilled water containing either 0.1% fetal calf serum or 0.1% bovine serum albumin. Adjust to pH 7.3 to 7.4. Make fresh each week.

Equipment

1. Microtiter diluters, 0.05 ml.
2. Microtiter pipettes, 0.025 and 0.05 ml.
3. Microtiter plates, U bottom.
4. 37 C and 60 C water bath.
5. Microtest plate shaker, vertical vibrator.

Procedure

1. Dilute test serum 1:25 with Kent buffer.
2. Inactivate at 60 C for 1 h with occasional shaking.
3. Place 0.05 ml of each serum into two microtiter wells (one for test and one for the heterophil control).
4. Add 0.025 ml of a 1:10 dilution of sensitized cells in working Kent buffer to each test well with a 0.025-ml microtiter dropper.
5. Add 0.025 ml of a 1:10 dilution of nonsensitized cells in working Kent buffer to each heterophil control well with a 0.025-ml microtiter dropper.
6. Prepare the following control wells.
   a. Buffer controls: (i) Kent buffer + sensitized cells; (ii) Kent buffer + nonsensitized cells.
   b. Positive control serum diluted 1:25 with Kent buffer.
   c. Negative control serum diluted 1:25 with Kent buffer.
7. Mix contents on a vibrator.
8. Incubate for 6 h or overnight at room temperature.
9. Read and record results.

Interpretation

The results are interpreted as follows: 4+, compact granular agglutination; 3+, smooth mat on bottom of well with folded edges; 2+, smooth mat on bottom of well, edges somewhat ragged; 1+, small ring on bottom of well; negative, discrete button in center of well bottom. If the heterophil and cell controls are negative, a 2+ agglutination or greater is considered to be a positive test, and the test should be repeated by titrating serum samples.

H. LISTERIA SEROLOGY

Listeriosis in humans has been reported with increasing frequency (4). The serological confirmation of suspected human listeriosis (10) can be a valuable aid if both acute and convalescent sera are tested.

Preparation of antigen

Cultures of *Listeria monocytogenes* strains and *Staphylococcus aureus* are incubated for 24 h at 37 C in tryptose broth and then transferred to tryptose agar and incubated for 48 h. Cells are harvested with normal saline and then steamed at 100 C for 1 h. The cells are washed in Sorensen phosphate-buffered saline, pH 7.3, and resuspended in a concentrated state. This concentrated suspension is treated with 0.1% trypsin by adding one part 1% trypsin to nine parts of concentrated cells. The cells are trypsinized for 15 min at 37 C, and then washed twice in saline and adjusted to a concentration that gives about a 50% optical transmission reading when diluted 1:20. Antigens are preserved with Merthiolate at a final concentration of 1:10,000.

Procedure

Twofold serial dilutions of sera are prepared in normal saline of 0.25-ml volumes. An equal volume of 1:20 diluted antigen is added. The tubes are incubated at 50 C for 2 h and then at 4 C for 24 h. Tests are read against a black background with a fluorescent lamp for viewing. The titer is recorded as the highest dilution having a 2+ or greater agglutination.

Two listeria antigens (1a, 1b, or 2) and (4a, 4b, 4c, 4d, or 4e) are used along with a *Staphylococcus aureus* antigen prepared in the same manner. If cross-reaction appears with *S. aureus*, the sera should be absorbed with *S. aureus* antigen and the test should be repeated. A fourfold greater rise in titer of the convalescent specimen is indicative of listeriosis.

I. RHEUMATOID FACTOR

The presence of rheumatoid factor in a serum is one of several criteria for the diagnosis of rheumatoid arthritis. A number of serological tests have been developed including the use of globulin-sensitized human or sheep cells, globulin-coated bentonite particles, and globulin-coated latex particles. The latex agglutination test of Singer and Plotz (14, 18) or modifications of this procedure are probably the tests most widely used in clinical laboratories at this time for diagnosis of rheumatoid arthritis. The reagents for these procedures are usually combined by commercial companies into some form of kit. Several variables are found in the methods and material of these kits; they include different species as globulin source for coating the latex particles, size of particles, incubation time and temperature, antigen concentration, and the dilution of antigen. One procedure for standardizing the method of reporting results of these tests with commercial latex reagents (W. L. Jones and G. L. Wiggins, Amer. J. Clin. Pathol., in press) is to convert titer results into units per milliliter. This is done by running a reference preparation at the same time and using the following formula to convert to units: units/ml of test serum = (units/ml of reference × titer of test serum)/titer of reference. Although reporting in units does not correct for all problems found with these reagents, it helps to normalize varying titers to a common denominator and should help the physician interpret results.

J. STREPTOCOCCAL SEROLOGY

Serological tests used as laboratory aids in the detection of group A (some C and G) streptococcal infection are the popular *antistreptolysin O test* and the less known *antideoxyribonuclease B* and *antihyaluronidase tests.* A commercial product, "Streptozyme," which is a test in which multiple streptococcal antigens adsorbed on red blood cells are used, is available but should be used for screening purposes only (10).

A positive test indicating a recent streptococcal infection is generally considered to be one in which there is a two-dilution-step rise in titer between acute and convalescent serum specimens or a specimen with titers above the normal levels for these tests (9).

Reagents for these tests are available from commercial sources. Manufacturer's directions for each product should be followed explicitly. The dilution of serum, however, may be adjusted to meet various recommendations of proficiency testing groups.

LITERATURE CITED

1. Ayres, J. C., and R. F. Feemster, 1950. Serologic tests in the diagnosis of infectious diseases. N. Engl. J. Med. **243**:996–1002; 1034–1043.
2. Beck, J. S. 1961. Variations in the morphological patterns of "autoimmune" nuclear fluorescense. Lancet **1**:1203–1205.
3. Bokkenheuser, V., P. Suit, and N. Richardson. 1954. A challenge to the validity of the Vi test for the detection of chronic typhoid carriers. Amer. J. Pub. Health **54**:1507–1513.
4. Busch, L. A. 1971. Human listeriosis in the United States 1967–1969. J. Infect. Dis. **123**:328–332.
5. Cole, J. R., C. R. Sulzer, and A. R. Pursell. 1973. Improved microtechnique for the leptospiral microscopic agglutination test. Appl. Microbiol. **25**:976–980.
6. Davidsohn, I. 1937. Serologic diagnosis of infectious mononucleosis. J. Amer. Med. Ass. **108**:289–295.
7. Davidsohn, I., K. Stern, and C. Kashiwagi. 1951. The differential test. Amer. J. Clin. Pathol. **21**:1101–1113.
8. Gochenour, W. S., C. A. Gleiser, and N. K. Ward. 1958. Laboratory diagnosis of leptospirosis. Ann. N. Y. Acad. Sci. **70**:421–426.
9. Klein, G. C., C. N. Baker, and W. L. Jones. 1971. "Upper limits of normal" antistreptolysin O and antideoxyribonuclease B titers. Appl. Microbiol. **21**:999–1001.
10. Klein, G. C. and W. L. Jones. 1971. Comparison of the streptozyme test with the antistreptolysin O, antideoxyribonuclease B, and antihyaluranidase test. Appl. Microbiol. **21**:257–259.
11. Larsen, S. A., and W. L. Jones. 1972. Evaluation and standardization of an agglutination test for human listeriosis. Appl. Microbiol. **24**:101–107.
12. Mancini, G., A. O. Carbonara, and J. F. Heremans. 1965. Immunochemical quantitation of antigens by single radial immunodiffusion. Immunochemistry **2**:235–254.
13. Mikkelsen, W., C. J. Tupper, and J. Murray. 1958. The ox cell hemolysin test as a diagnostic procedure in infectious mononucleosis. J. Lab. Clin. Med. **52**:648–652.
14. Plotz, C. M., and J. M. Singer. 1956. The latex fixation test II. Results in rheumatoid arthritis. Amer. J. Med. **21**:893–896.
15. Schubert, J. H., and J. F. Colvin. 1964. Non-specificity of the *Brucella* antibody blocking reaction. Health Lab. Sci. **1**:309–315.
16. Schubert, J. H., and R. G. Cornell. 1958. Determination of diphtheria and tetanus antitoxin by hemagglutination test in comparison with tests in vivo. J. Lab. Clin. Med. **52**:737–743.
17. Schubert, J. H., P. R. Edwards, and C. H. Ramsey. 1959. Detection of typhoid carriers by agglutination tests. J. Bacteriol **77**:648–654.
18. Singer, J. M., and C. M. Plotz. 1956. The latex fixation test. I. Application to the serologic diagnosis of rheumatoid arthritis. Amer. J. Med. **21**:888–892.

Section VII

FUNGI

Chapter 53
Introduction to Clinical Mycology

B. H. COOPER

Quite often a clinical laboratory worker who has been trained primarily in bacteriology will be left confused by his initial encounter with the fungi because of their unfamiliar names and the different procedures which must be utilized for their isolation and identification. With careful study, however, the person with an adequate background in the principles and techniques of bacteriology will soon put aside this momentary confusion to realize that fungi are, in many respects, more easily dealt with than bacteria. To begin with, most fungi have distinct morphological properties in the form of characteristic spores that can be observed with a microscope using only high-power (400×) magnification. Fungi grow more slowly than bacteria, and a certain amount of patience is required for their study; however, identification based on their gross colonial characteristics and microscopic morphology is somewhat less difficult than is the identification of bacterial species. Proper collection and handling of clinical specimens for the isolation of fungal pathogens require some special considerations, and these will be discussed in some detail in this and subsequent chapters.

Fungi are ubiquitous, eukaryotic microorganisms, and the majority of species survive quite successfully in nature as saprophytes on nonliving organic materials. Relatively few of the thousands of known species of fungi are capable of causing human diseases. Most of those species which do infect humans are limited by their own nutritional requirements and by host-defense mechanisms to invasion of the superficial skin and subcutaneous tissues. The species that are capable of invading the deeper tissues to cause serious life-threatening infections are, fortunately, quite few in number. Systemic fungus infections are acquired by accidental inhalation of spores carried about on wind currents, or by traumatic inoculation from contaminated soil or plant materials, and are unusual in most hospitals except in certain geographic areas where a specific disease may affect almost 100% of the total population with varying degrees of severity. In the majority of hospitals, patients having systemic mycoses are still seen relatively infrequently, and most clinical laboratories are only prepared to deal with the most frequently isolated species of fungi. A recent survey (3) revealed that a majority of clinical laboratories were inadequately prepared to handle mycology specimens, and the overall level of training in mycology has been a matter of concern to a number of professional mycologists. Even specimens of superficial tissues infected with dermatophytes are not always properly handled, although these are the most frequently encountered of all mycology specimens.

Two seemingly unrelated factors, the mobility of modern human populations and the widespread therapeutic use of drugs that alter immune defenses make it imperative for the personnel of every sizeable modern clinical laboratory to be well trained in techniques for isolation and identification of pathogenic fungi. The availability of rapid transportation by jet aircraft makes it possible for a person to acquire a particular fungus disease in an area where it is highly endemic but then not manifest symptoms until some time after returning to his home where the disease may be unusual or unexpected. Unless physicians and laboratory personnel have a high level of suspicion for the disease in question, the correct diagnosis can be missed altogether or unnecessarily delayed, much to the disadvantage of the patient. Drugs that alter a patient's immune defenses predispose that patient to infection by a number of fungi that are ordinarily considered to be harmless saprophytes. Patients with diabetes mellitus, severe burns, leukemias, and other debilitating diseases are similarly susceptible to serious systemic infections with fungi that are not ordinarily considered to be human pathogens. In a clinical setting involving a compromised host, any fungus capable of growth at 37 C should be considered a potential pathogen. Repeated isolation of the same fungus in significantly large numbers from the same kind of specimen or demonstration of tissue invasion by direct microscope examination of biopsy specimens may be necessary to document pathogenicity of the fungus isolated. Concurrent use of serological tests to demonstrate a specific rising titer often helps to clarify the diagnosis in clinical settings of this type.

COLLECTION AND HANDLING OF SPECIMENS

Once a fungus has been isolated in pure culture, an identification can usually be made by reasonably well-trained microbiologists. It is imperative, however, that certain essential steps in collecting and handling specimens be taken before pathogenic fungi can successfully be isolated, particularly from specimens naturally contaminated with rapidly growing bacteria and nonpathogenic fungi. A brief scheme for processing specimens for direct microscopic examination and for isolation of the major human pathogens is presented in Fig. 1. The procedures summarized in the figure are dealt with in greater detail in subsequent chapters.

Prompt handling of freshly collected clinical specimens and addition of antibiotics to contaminated specimens are two steps that can be taken to improve the chances for isolating human pathogenic fungi. The selection of media for plating specimens suspected of containing fungi should be given careful consideration, and, since no one medium is adequate for isolating all species of fungi, it is important to plate each specimen on a battery of media including selective, enriched, and relatively simple mycological culture media. It is also helpful to incubate cultures both at 37 C and at room temperature of 25 to 30 C. It should be kept in mind that pre-prepared commercial media may not be satisfactory, so that individual laboratories will have to prepare their own or perhaps modify dehydrated media that are commercially available at the present time.

One of the common failings of clinical laboratories is that they do not hold cultures long enough to permit development of the slower-growing pathogens. Cultures must be kept at least 2 weeks and preferably up to 4 weeks or longer. With such a long incubation time, precautions to prevent dehydration of culture media—such as keeping a pan filled with water in the bottom of the incubator or partially sealing (do not create anaerobic conditions) petri dishes with masking tape—must be taken. The use of media in screw-capped tubes or bottles offers advantages of safety and lessens the problem of dehydration, but the caps of such containers must be kept partially loosened to provide proper growth conditions. Another common failing is to discard cultures when a known pathogen such as *Candida albicans*, which is also a member of the normal flora of the mouth, throat, intestinal tract, and vagina, has been isolated without waiting for more significant pathogens to develop. Cultures should be held for a full 4 weeks even though one or more pathogens may have already been isolated.

IDENTIFICATION OF FUNGI

Identification of fungi is accomplished rather simply by noting the development of their colonies, and their gross and microscopic morphology. The surface texture, color, and growth rate of fungal colonies, along with the pigmentation of the reverse side of the colony, are important identifying characteristics. For specific identification, it is necessary to induce a fungus to display its characteristic spores; although this may require the use of special media or growth conditions, it is not ordinarily a difficult procedure. Biochemical tests are also useful, especially for the identification of yeasts, but the emphasis should be placed on morphological characteristics for correct identification of species.

Fungi can easily be differentiated into two types based on the macroscopic appearance of their colonies. Those that produce opaque, creamy, or pasty colonies are called yeasts, and those that produce cottony, woolly, fluffy, or powdery aerial growths above the culture medium are referred to as molds. A third group can be demonstrated to develop as yeasts when cultivated at 37 C and as molds when they are grown at 25 to 30 C. This environmentally controlled interconversion of morphological phases is called dimorphism. Most systemic human pathogens as well as other species of fungi exhibit dimorphism, and it is essential that conversion from one phase to the other be accomplished for exact identification of those species. Upon microscopic examination the yeasts will be observed to be small, unicellular microorganisms that produce daughter cells from the parent cell by budding. The molds are multicellular microorganisms whose cells are joined together to make up long, tubelike filaments called hyphae. As some hyphae elongate, they form cross walls or septa behind the growing hyphal tip. Other hyphae which do not form cross walls are said to be coenocytic. As hyphae multiply, they become intertwined to form a mycelium or mold colony. That portion of the mycelium which penetrates into the

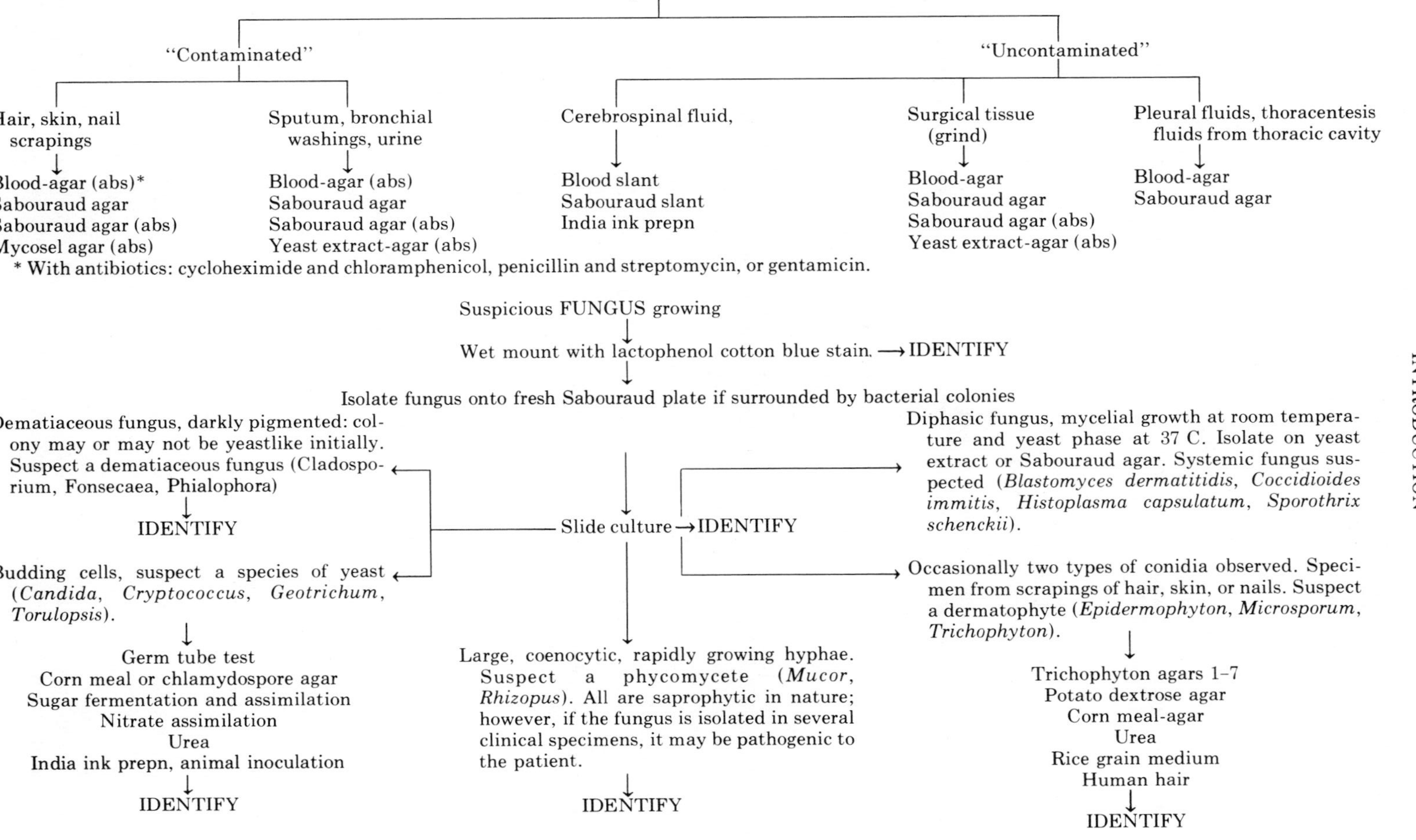

FIG. 1. *Flow chart illustrating procedures for laboratory isolation and identification of fungi from clinical specimens. (From an original chart by Norman L. Goodman and Howard W. Larsh. Used with permission.)*

substrate from which it absorbs nutrients is called the submerged mycelium. The portion of the mold colony that grows above the substratum in an erect fashion is called the aerial mycelium.

Microorganisms classified as actinomycetes resemble true fungi in many respects; they cause diseases which resemble fungus diseases, and they will be encountered in many of the same clinical specimens as fungi. The actinomycetes, however, have distinctive cellular and molecular properties which make them different from fungi so that they are properly classified as gram-positive filamentous bacteria. For these reasons they have not been included in the chapters dealing with higher fungi.

In addition to their gross macroscopic properties, fungi are quite distinctive at the cellular and molecular level. First of all, they possess an organized nucleus surrounded by a nuclear membrane, i.e., they are eukaryotic microorganisms. Unlike bacteria, the fungi grow slowly and their cell walls are composed of polysaccharide polymers such as glucan, mannan, cellulose, and chitin. The teichoic and muramic acids found in bacterial cell walls are not present in the cell walls of fungi. Finally, the true fungi or *Eumycotina* reproduce both sexually and asexually. Sexual reproduction occurs by the fusion of specialized cells called gametes, and the end result of their fusion is the development of a conspicuous fruiting body in which spores are produced following meiosis. The growth state induced by sexual recombination is referred to as the perfect state and provides the basis for classification of fungi as *Phycomycetes*, *Ascomycetes*, or *Basidiomycetes*. A fourth form class, the *Deuteromycetes* or Fungi Imperfecti, was created to accommodate those species for which the perfect state is unrecognized.

Asexual reproduction occurs by the formation of vegetative spores of one type or another. Observation of the size, shape, color, and arrangement of vegetative spores under a microscope is the single most important criterion for laboratory identification of fungi. Vegetative spores produced directly from the body or thallus of the fungus without involvement of specialized spore-bearing structures are called thallospores. Arthrospores, formed by fragmentation of hyphae into individual cells, blastospores, formed by budding as in the yeasts, and chlamydospores, which are thick-walled, resting spores, are the important kinds of thallospores. Vegetative spores formed on specialized hyphal branches called conidiophores are named conidia, and there are as many different kinds of conidia as there are species of fungi. Conidia are named microconidia if they are small and unicellular and macroconidia if they are larger and multicellular.

Conidia and other spores can be demonstrated by removing a small piece of spore-bearing mycelium from a mold colony with a dissecting needle and then gently teasing the mycelium apart in a drop of lactophenol cotton blue (LPCB). The size, shape, and color of spores can readily be observed by this technique, but, because the spores are usually knocked apart by this procedure, demonstration of the characteristic arrangement of spores requires that a special microculture called a slide culture be made. For this a small block of agar is placed on a sterile microscope slide supported on a bent glass rod in a sterile petri dish. The agar block is inoculated on all four sides with the fungus to be studied, and a sterile cover slip is placed over the block of agar. Water is added to the petri dish to prevent dehydration, and the culture is incubated at 25 to 30 C. The slide can be removed from the chamber from time to time and the fungus can be observed with a microscope as it develops in situ. When the fungus is fully developed, a permanent mount can be made by removing the cover slip from the agar and placing it face downward in a drop of LPCB. The edges of the cover slip are then sealed with nail polish or another mounting medium, creating a permanent mount of the fungus. Much the same thing can be accomplished by coating a cover slip with mounting resin and then pressing it down onto a fungus colony with the sticky side down. The cover slip is next removed and mounted in a drop of LPCB as described above, creating a permanent mount. Scotch tape can be used for the same purpose, but caution should be used when any systemic pathogen is examined with this technique.

The identifying characteristics of the major human pathogens are described in the following chapters. As anyone who is experienced in mycology is well aware, typically sporulating human pathogens are less of a problem to identify than are the numerous fungal contaminants that grow luxuriantly on laboratory culture media. Some of the more confusing contaminants are described in the following chapters. However, it is not within the scope of this *Manual* to provide detailed descriptions of all of the fungi that contaminate laboratory cultures. Barnett's *Illustrated Genera of Imperfect Fungi*

(1) and *The Genera of Hyphomycetes from Soil*, by Barron (2), can be recommended as useful guides to the identification of most laboratory contaminants.

MAINTENANCE OF STOCK CULTURES

It is desirable to maintain stock cultures of typical strains of pathogenic fungi for reference and teaching purposes. Stock cultures may be maintained on Sabouraud agar at room temperature if they are transferred at least every 6 weeks. Cultures stored in a refrigerator at 4 C can be maintained 3 to 4 months without transferring. Agar slant cultures covered with sterile mineral oil can be maintained without transferring for up to 12 months. Stock cultures can also be stored in a freezer at −20 C on agar slants for longer periods of time; lyophilized cultures can be preserved for several years without losing their typical characteristics.

SEROLOGICAL TECHNIQUES

Mycoserological techniques are covered in a separate chapter because of the importance attached to development of an accurate understanding of these procedures. Serological testing with fungal antigens presents two major difficulties: (i) the lack of commercial availability of sensitive and specific antigens for all fungus diseases, and (ii) the broad cross-reactivity of antigens, which makes interpretation of test results more complex than might be desired. The complexities of mycoserology derive not from the kinds of tests that are employed, but from the crudeness and complexity of the antigens that must be used in the tests.

Individual clinical laboratories that want to provide serological tests to assist in diagnosis of fungus diseases must often be prepared to manufacture their own antigens. Such antigens need to be carefully standardized by using known positive reference antisera that can be obtained from the Center for Disease Control in the United States and from other reference laboratories. As the demand for mycoserological tests increases, it is hoped that commercial production of high-quality antigens will become a reality. As new test materials become available, it is essential that trained personnel be on hand in hospital, private, and state and local public health laboratories to evaluate their efficacy. The information presented in a subsequent chapter of this *Manual* should be of great value to persons seeking current information on serological tests for fungus diseases.

CONCLUSION

The methods described in the following chapters represent the most up-to-date procedures available at the time of publication. If the recommended procedures are followed, a reasonably well-trained microbiologist should be able to isolate and identify human pathogenic fungi from clinical specimens without much difficulty. New chapters dealing with the fungi that cause keratomycosis and aspergillosis have been added to this edition in recognition of the importance that these two diseases have assumed in recent years. A third new chapter dealing with testing of susceptibility to antifungal drugs has also been added because of the necessity for making information of this nature available to clinical laboratories that assist physicians in managing the therapy of fungus diseases. Other chapters have been updated to take into account development of new techniques and the availability of more accurate information in medical mycology.

A few selected references that are not directly cited in the text have been listed under References for Further Study to aid those who desire more training in mycology. The Center for Disease Control in Atlanta, Ga., and a number of universities in the United States conduct training programs in medical mycology on a regular basis. The *ASM News* and the Newsletter of the Medical Mycological Society of the Americas can be consulted for current announcements concerning these programs. The Center for Disease Control has made available at nominal cost a set of medical mycology teaching slides, which can be obtained from Color Film Laboratories, Inc., Mamaroneck, N.Y.

In the opinion of this writer the quality of the mycology chapters in this edition of the *Manual* has been upgraded appreciably by following a system of peer review. Libero Ajello, C. W. Emmons, Morris A. Gordon, and George S. Kobayashi generously contributed their time as reviewers, and we wish to express our appreciation to them for their valuable contributions.

LITERATURE CITED

1. Barnett, H. L. 1960. Illustrated genera of imperfect fungi, 2nd ed. Burgess Publishing Co., Minneapolis.
2. Barron, G. L. 1968. The genera of hyphomycetes from soil. The Williams & Wilkins Co., Baltimore.
3. Bump, C. M. 1973. A survey of procedures used in clinical mycology laboratories. Amer. J. Med. Technol. **39**:40–51.

REFERENCES FOR FURTHER STUDY

Ajello, L., L. K. Georg, W. Kaplan, and L. Kaufman. 1963. Laboratory manual for medical mycology. Public Health Service Publication No. 994, U.S. Government Printing Office, Washington, D.C.

Alexopoulous, C. J. 1962. Introductory mycology, 2nd ed. John Wiley & Sons, Inc., New York.

Beneke, E. S., and A. L. Rogers. 1971. Medical mycology manual, 3rd ed. Burgess Publishing Co., Minneapolis.

Conant, N. F., D. T. Smith, R. D. Baker, and J. L. Callaway. 1971. Manual of clinical mycology, 3rd ed. W. B. Saunders Co., Philadelphia.

Cooper, B. H. 1972. The superficial and subcutaneous mycotic agents. *In* R. Clark (ed.), Topics in clinical microbiology. The Williams & Wilkins Co., Baltimore (24 lessons on compact tape cassettes with accompanying explanatory manual).

Cooper, B. H. 1972. Identification of yeast-like fungi. *In* R. Clark (ed.), Topics in clinical microbiology. The Williams & Wilkins Co., Baltimore.

Cooper, B. H. 1972. Isolation and identification of the systemic mycotic agents. *In* R. Clark (ed.), Topics in clinical microbiology. The Williams & Wilkins Co., Baltimore.

Emmons, C. W., C. H. Binford, and J. P. Utz. 1970. Medical mycology, 2nd ed. Lea and Febiger, Philadelphia.

Hazen, E. L., M. A. Gordon, and E. C. Reed. 1970. Laboratory identification of pathogenic fungi simplified, 3rd ed. Charles C Thomas, Publisher, Springfield, Ill.

Jones, J. W., H. W. McFadden, C. A. McWhorter, and N. G. Miller. 1967. Atlas of medical mycology. American Society of Clinical Pathologists, Chicago (Kodachrome slides and accompanying descriptive manual).

Koneman, E. W., and S. E. Fann. 1971. Practical laboratory mycology. Medcom Press, New York (Kodachrome slides and accompanying descriptive manual).

Krickel, J. H., and L. D. Haley. 1970. An audio-tutorial kit for training in basic medical mycology. Proc. Int. Symp. Mycoses, p. 225–227. Scientific Publication No. 205. Pan American Health Organization, Washington, D.C.

Moss, E. S., and A. L. McQuown. 1969. Atlas of medical mycology, 3rd ed. The Williams & Wilkins Co., Baltimore.

Chapter 54

Dermatophytes and the Agents of Superficial Mycoses

LIBERO AJELLO AND ARVIND A. PADHYE

The laboratory diagnosis of suspected cutaneous mycotic infections requires that two basic procedures be carried out to determine whether or not a given disease is mycotic in nature: (i) direct examination of clinical material with a microscope, and (ii) isolation and subsequent identification of the fungi recovered. Both of these procedures will be described in detail in the presentations that follow of the various superficial and cutaneous mycoses.

SUPERFICIAL MYCOSES

All mycotic diseases that affect only the cornified layers of the epidermis and the superfollicular portion of the hair are classified as superficial mycoses. The stratum corneum is not attacked in these diseases. In addition, the nails are not known to be infected by the agents of the superficial mycoses. Four diseases are classified in this category: black piedra, white piedra, tinea nigra, and tinea versicolor.

Black piedra

Black piedra is a fungus infection of scalp hair but rarely of the axillary and pubic hair of humans. Many genera and species of lower primates and other mammals are also susceptible to this disease (8).

In black piedra, hair filaments above the follicular orifice are overgrown by the mycelium of the dematiaceous ascomycete *Piedraia hortae*. The dark-walled mycelium spreads over and around the hair shaft and forms a cemented mat of hyphae. Nodules eventually are formed from this mycelium that may attain a diameter of 0.1 cm and a thickness of 100 μm (Fig. 1). At maturity, asci and ascospores develop in their interior. The nodules are hard and gritty, hence the Spanish name of "piedra" (i.e., stone) for this disease.

Black piedra primarily occurs in the tropical areas of the world. Cases have been recorded in Africa, Asia, and Latin America. The etiological agent, *P. hortae*, is not known to be transmitted from person to person or from infected animals to humans. Presumably this mold occurs as a saprophyte in nature, but it has not as yet been isolated from a nonliving source.

Direct examination. Portions of hairs with nodules from suspected cases of black piedra are examined in wet mounts of 10% KOH. After the preparation has been gently heated, microscope examination of the edges of the nodules will reveal the presence of septate, dematiaceous mycelium (4 to 8 μm in diameter) on the surface of the hair filament. The nodules themselves are composed of cemented mycelium that forms a pseudoparenchymatous tissue. Mature nodules, when crushed, reveal the presence of oval asci (44 to 50 μm by 24 to 30 μm). At maturity they contain eight aseptate, curved, spindle-shaped ascospores that bear a filament at each pole. The ascospores range from 35 to 55 μm in length and from 5 to 8 μm in width.

P. hortae usually invades the hair shaft under the cuticle where its mycelium proliferates. It then breaks out and begins to grow around the hair shaft. In other instances, the fungus invades the hair shaft and causes extensive damage through destruction of the cortex and medulla.

Isolation and culture identification. Sabouraud agar is recommended for isolation of *P. hortae*. Media with cycloheximide cannot be used since *P. hortae* is inhibited by that antibiotic. Antibacterial antibiotics such as chloramphenicol are useful, however, to reduce bacterial contamination. Growth is slow but it is stimulated by thiamine (0.01 mg/ml). Colonies are dark to dark brown and heaped. They are glabrous or covered with a fine downy mycelium. On Sabouraud agar and most other media, the fungus generally fails to produce asci and ascospores. The hyphae are dematiaceous and of variable diameter.

White piedra

White piedra is an uncommon disease encountered in both tropical and temperate regions of the world. The disease is characterized by the development of soft, yellowish or pale

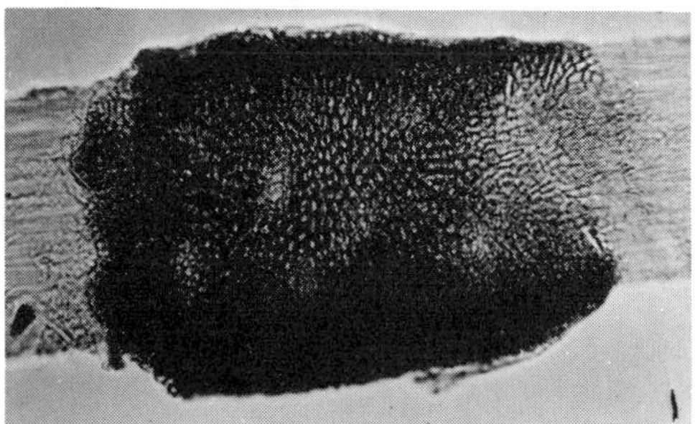

FIG. 1. *Nodule of black piedra.* ×*200.*

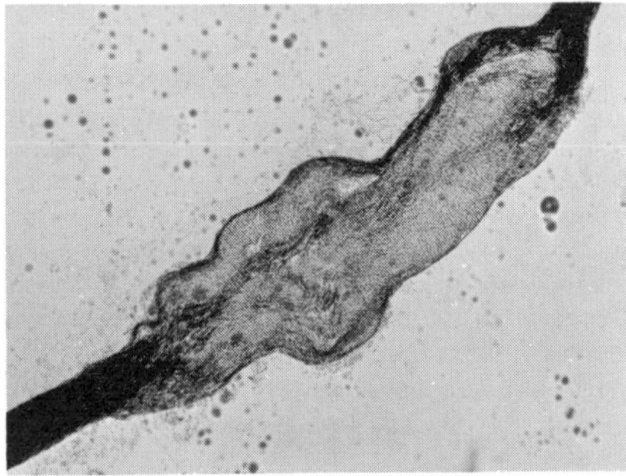

FIG. 2. *Nodule of white piedra.* ×*100.*

brown accretions around the shaft of hairs in the axillary, facial, genital and scalp regions of the body (Fig. 2). Humans and lower animals are infected.

The fungus responsible for this disease is properly identified as *Trichosporon beigelii.* It is frequently, but erroneously, referred to as *T. cutaneum* in various publications (9).

The accretions are made up of hyaline hyphae that tend to form arthrospores. The mycelium of *T. beigelii* frequently invades the cortex of hair filaments with resultant damage to the hair.

Direct examination. In mounts of 10% KOH, the nodules of white piedra are readily crushed by covering them with a cover slip and applying light pressure. Hyaline mycelium and arthrospores will be found in the preparation. The width of these mycelia ranges from 2 to 4 μm, and a cementlike material binds them together.

In some instances, the interior of the hair is found to have been destroyed by the activity of the fungus. In the early stages of hair invasion, pilar swelling will be present, caused by the proliferation of mycelium under the cuticle or within the hair shaft.

Isolation and culture identification. *T. beigelii* is readily isolated on Sabouraud agar that contains chloramphenicol or other bacterial growth inhibitors. Cycloheximide cannot be used since it inhibits the growth of *T. beigelii.* This fungus grows rapidly and in a few days produces a cream-colored yeastlike colony. Microscopically the growth will be composed of hyaline mycelium that produces blastospores and that fragments into arthrospores. Some blastospores arise directly from the mycelium whereas others develop in chains and clusters.

Eight species of *Trichosporon* are accepted as valid members of this genus (9). Their differentiation and identification is based on specific biochemical reactions. *T. beigelii* is distinguished from all other members of the genus by its inability to ferment sugars and its ability to assimilate certain compounds (chapter 56).

Biochemical characteristics. *T. beigelii* assimilates dextrose, lactose, and xylose. The following carbon compounds are assimilated by some isolates and not by others: cellobiose, erythritol, galactose, inositol, maltose, melibiose, melizitose, raffinose, rhamnose, sucrose, and trehalose. Among nitrogenous compounds, potassium nitrate and sodium nitrite are not assimilated.

Tinea nigra

Tinea nigra is a disease manifested by the development of blackish-brown macular patches on the smooth skin of the body. Most lesions develop on the palm of a hand, and hence the infection is sometimes referred to as tinea nigra palmaris. The agent of tinea nigra is a black yeast belonging to the family *Dematiaceae,* Fungi Imperfecti. For that reason, it is described in chapter 59 and will not be covered here.

Tinea versicolor

Tinea versicolor or pityriasis versicolor is a cosmopolitan disease of the smooth skin of the body. It generally manifests itself by the development of fine, slightly raised scaly patches on the neck and torso. The infection spreads and the patches of infection enlarge and merge with adjacent ones. The infected sites on white-skinned subjects tend to be brownish and lighter than normal skin in the dark races. After exposure to sunlight, infected skin fails to tan as deeply as normal skin. A rare form of tinea versicolor involves the hair follicles. In such infections, involvement tends to be localized and the lesions become elevated.

Most infected areas when irradiated with a

Wood's lamp in a dark room fluoresce with a dull reddish to orange color.

A growing number of medical mycologists contend that the lipophilic yeast *Pityrosporum orbiculare* is the etiological agent of tinea versicolor (6). On the basis of priority, however, this fungus is validly named *P. furfur*, and the old name, *Malassezia furfur*, for the etiological agent of tinea versicolor becomes a synonym of *P. furfur*.

Direct examination. As mentioned above, the use of a Wood's lamp in a dark room is extremely useful in detecting areas of infection by *P. furfur* and their distribution.

For microscopic confirmation of infection, the suspected site should be cleaned with 70% alcohol and scraped with a sterile scalpel. The scales so collected are then mounted in a drop of lactophenol cotton blue or Loeffler's methylene blue, covered with a cover slip, and examined under a microscope.

Alternatively, infected scales can be stripped from a suspected site by applying a piece of transparent vinyl tape to the area and lifting it off. The tape, with gummed surface down, is placed on a drop of lactophenol cotton blue on a slide. The preparation is then examined under a microscope for the presence of hyphal elements 2.5 to 4 μm in diameter and of variable length along with unicellular oval or round cells 3 to 7 μm in diameter (Fig. 3).

Isolation and culture identification. Although cultivation of the fungus is not required to establish a diagnosis of pityriasis, at times isolation may be necessary or desired.

In such cases, an oil-enriched isolation medium must be used. Sabouraud agar overlaid with olive oil or Sabouraud agar with cycloheximide with an olive oil overlay are recommended. The inoculated tubes should be incubated at 37 C and maintained at an angle to keep the agar surface covered with oil.

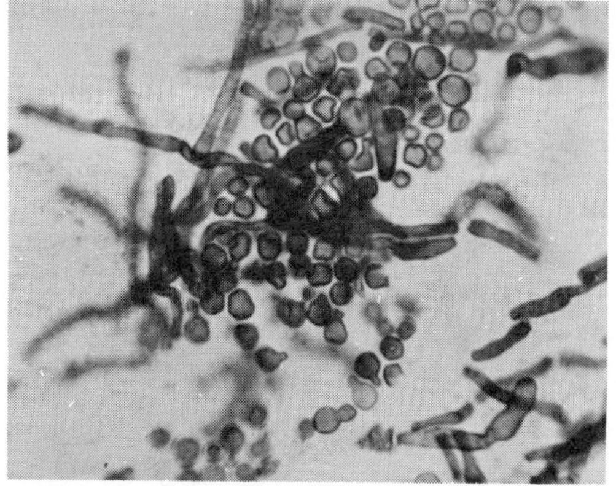

FIG. 3. *Tinea versicolor. Skin scraping. Periodic acid-Schiff stain.* ×*1,200.*

Growth is slow. At first it is cream colored, glossy, and raised. With age the colony becomes dull, dry, and beige colored. The colony will be found to be composed of globose to ellipsoidal, hyaline cells ranging from 3 to 7 μm in diameter. Successive budding takes place at a given locus on a mother cell.

Mycelium is not produced in culture; however, germ tubes are extruded by some cells, and these resemble short mycelial filaments.

Although some investigators doubt whether *P. furfur* differs from *P. ovale*, others hold them to be distinct species. The differentiation is based on two points. (i) There is a difference in the shape of the cells; they are ellipsoidal in *P. ovale* and globose in *P. furfur*. (ii) The growth of *P. ovale* on Littman's oxgall agar is long-lived, but the growth of *P. furfur* subcultures on that medium is short-lived.

CUTANEOUS MYCOSES (RINGWORM)

The cutaneous mycoses are infections of the epidermal tissues of humans and animals caused by a group of specialized fungi, the dermatophytes. Unlike the agents of the superficial mycoses, these penetrate and parasitize all of the fully keratinized tissues of the body (skin, hair, and nails) and produce infections that give rise to mild to severe symptoms. The dermatophytes are unable, in general, to invade the subcutaneous or deeper tissues of the body, probably because of inhibitory factors in serum and body fluids (4, 10).

Characterization of the dermatophytes

The dermatophytes are mycelial fungi that until recently were classified as *Deuteromycetes* (Fungi Imperfecti). Some species are now known to reproduce sexually producing ascospores. These species are classified in the family *Gymnoascaceae* of the class *Ascomycetes*. All of the dermatophytes possess keratinolytic abilities that enable them to parasitize skin, hair, and nails, causing diseases known as the dermatomycoses, ringworm, or tineas. The majority of the dermatophytes have a worldwide distribution; however, some species are limited geographically.

The dermatophytes have marked host preference. Some are animal parasites, others almost exclusively infect humans, and others are essentially soil organisms that only rarely infect humans and animals. As a result, the dermatophytes are classified, more or less arbitrarily, into three separate groups: the anthropophilic, the zoophilic, and the geophilic (1).

Diagnosis of ringworm

Dermatophyte infections of the skin produce reactions that vary from mild erythema and scaling to severe vesicular, heavily crusted, suppurative or rarely granulomatous lesions. The infections may be asymptomatic or extremely itchy and painful. Ringworm-infected nails are thickened, discolored, and deformed. The distal ends are raised from the nail bed. Usually there is no inflammation of the paronychial tissues and no pain. Infections of the bearded areas of the face and neck in adults (male) are frequently suppurative and painful, and resemble bacterial infections. Scalp infections are manifested by scattered loss of hair, or by discrete, usually circular lesions with loss of hair, erythema, scaling, vesiculation, and suppuration. In some cases, raised fluctuant, suppurative lesions known as kerions occur. Favus is another type of clinical manifestation characterized by cup-shaped crusts, "scutulae," which may form heavy confluent masses on the scalp or smooth skin. This type of lesion is usually incited by *Trichophyton schoenleinii*. Depending upon the site involved, dermatophyte infections are clinically classified as *tinea pedis* (athlete's foot), *tinea cruris* (jock itch), *tinea capitis*, etc. (5).

Examination of patients

Suspected ringworm of the scalp. Patients are examined first under normal lighting conditions for loss of hair, presence of broken-off hairs, or skin lesions. The patient is then examined in a darkened room with a Wood's lamp. In certain types of ringworm, infected hairs fluoresce a bright yellow-green under such conditions. Even minimal infections, where only a few hairs are infected, can be detected by use of a Wood's lamp. Fluorescence is not observed in early infections or in some cases during treatment. False fluorescence may result from the presence of certain oils or medications on the hair. When hairs are plucked and the roots are examined under the lamp, true fluorescence can be determined.

Suspected ringworm of the skin. The Wood's lamp is also useful in differentiating dermatophyte infection from erythrasma (a bacterial infection of the skin) caused by *Corynebacterium tenuis*. Ringworm lesions do not fluoresce whereas the lesions of erythrasma, which are clinically similar to ringworm, glow with an orange to coral-red fluorescence.

Suspected ringworm of the nails (onychomycosis, tinea unguium). Nail lesions suspected of being mycotic in origin must be differentiated from a variety of other diseases that resemble onychomycosis (viz., psoriasis, lichen planus, etc.). This is readily done by directly examining nail scrapings and clippings in 10% KOH. The detection of mycelial elements in the nail cells virtually establishes the mycotic nature of the condition. The etiological agent involved is established through cultures of the nail material.

Collection of specimens

The following equipment is needed: a disinfectant for cleansing the skin, sterile scalpels, epilating forceps, nail clippers or scissors, and clean paper envelopes. Disposable combs or brushes have been recommended for the collection of specimens from the scalp or from animal bodies (11). The scales from the active borders of the lesions should be scraped with a scalpel. Hair from the scalp is plucked out with forceps. Infected hairs can be easily pulled out but normal hairs are harder to remove. In the case of infected nails, friable material is removed from under the edge of the nail or clipped from the distal border.

Specimens should be enclosed in paper packets or envelopes and should not be enclosed in rubber stoppered tubes. In closed tubes the specimens become moist, and contaminating bacteria and saprophytic fungi may overgrow any pathogenic fungus present.

Direct examination

Fragments of hair, skin scrapings, or nail clippings are placed in a drop of 10% KOH on a slide, and a cover slip is added. The slide is gently heated over a flame for a few seconds; then it is examined under a microscope. Reheating may sometimes be necessary to clear the specimen.

Infected skin and nail scrapings show hyaline, septate, branched hyphae and arthrospores in chains (Fig. 4). Infected hairs show hyphae in the interior of the hair shaft during early stages of invasion. Arthrospores formed by the fragmentation of the hyphae may be evident later inside the hair shaft (endothrix infections; Fig. 5). In ectothrix infections, the arthrospores are observed outside the hair shaft surrounding it in the form of a sheath (Fig. 6). The manner of hair invasion varies with the dermatophyte species involved. In general, there are three

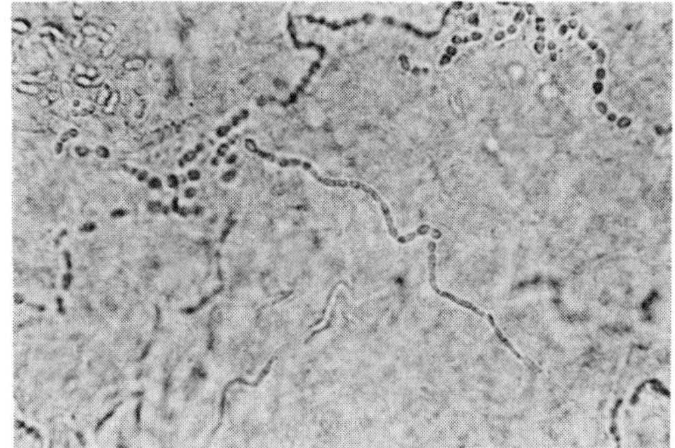

FIG. 4. *Dermatophyte mycelium in skin scraping. KOH mount.* ×*475.*

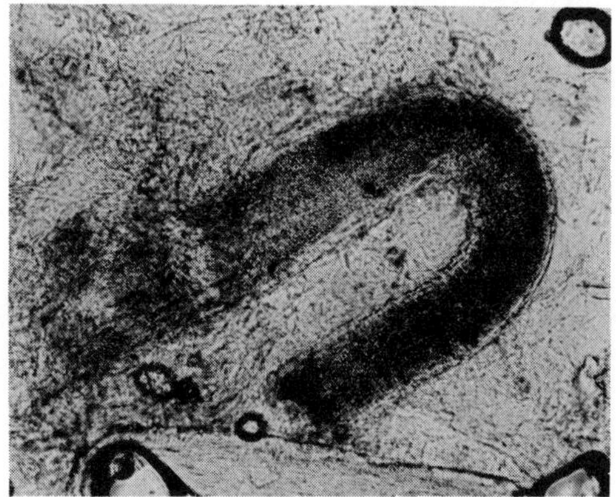

FIG. 5. *Endothrix type of hair invasion caused by Trichophyton tonsurans. Hair stub filled with arthrospores.* ×*100.*

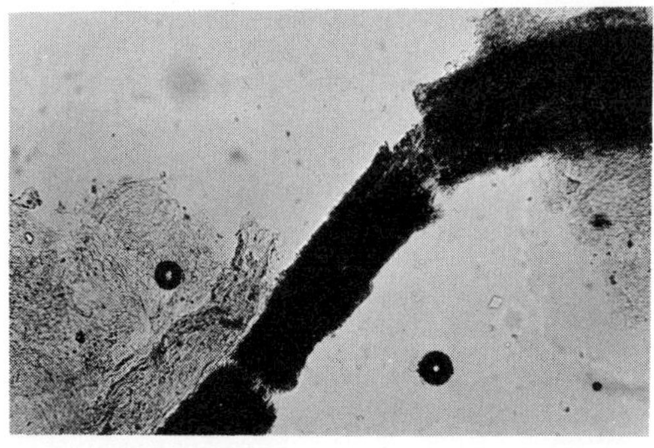

FIG. 6. *Ectothrix type of hair invasion caused by Microsporum audouinii. Note sheath of small arthrospores surrounding the hair shaft.* ×*100.*

types of hair parasitism: ectothrix, endothrix, and favic. The terms ectothrix and endothrix refer to the location of the arthrospores in relationship to the hair. In favic hair invasion. the interior of the hair is filled with long hyphal filaments, with few if any arthrospores present (Fig. 7).

When septate, branched hyaline hyphae with only a few chains of arthrospores are observed in direct examination of KOH mounts of the skin and nail scrapings, the diagnosis of ringworm infection is confirmed. But the causative agents involved cannot be determined in this manner. The etiological agent can only be identified through the isolation and study of cultures. It should also be remembered that KOH-negative specimens may yield positive cultures. In the direct examination of the hair, the following key may be used as an aid to the preliminary diagnosis of ringworm.

Key to Direct Examination of Hair

Wood's lamp

(1) Bright yellow-green fluorescence of hair shafts: *Microsporum audouinii, M. canis; M. distortum, M. ferrugineum*; rarely *T. schoenleinii.*

(2) No fluorescence: all the other dermatophyte species.

KOH mounts

(1) *Ectothrix hairs*

  (a) Spores 2 to 3 μm is diameter in mosaic, forming a sheath around the hair: *M. audouinii, M. canis, M. distortum, M. ferrugineum* (Fig. 6).

  (b) Spores 3 to 5 μm forming a sheath, or in isolated chains on the surface of hairs: *T. mentagrophytes.*

  (c) Spores 5 to 8 μm forming a sheath, or in isolated chains on the surface of hair: *T. equinum*; rarely *T. rubrum.*

  (d) Spores 5 to 8 μm in chains, or in irregu-

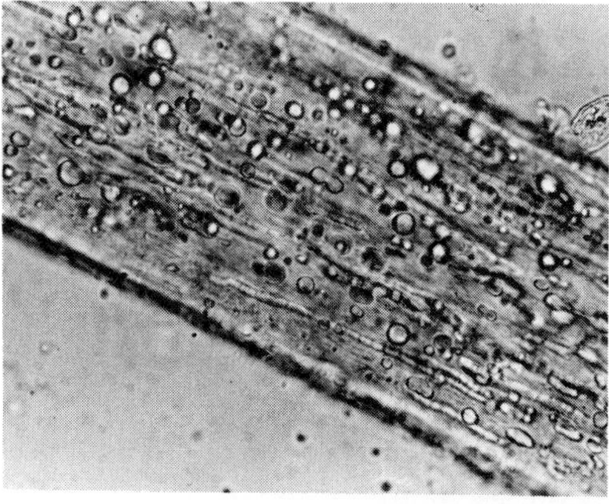

FIG. 7. *Favic-type hair invasion caused by Trichophyton schoenleinii. Note mycelial filaments and air spaces in the hair shaft.* ×*522.*

lar masses on the hair surface: *M. fulvum*, *M. gypseum*, *M. nanum*.

(e) Spores 8 to 10 μm forming a sheath, or in isolated chains on surface of hair: *T. verrucosum*.

(2) *Endothrix hairs*

Short hair stubs, thick and usually twisted, filled with chains of large spores 4 to 8 μm: *T. soudanense*, *T. tonsurans*, *T. violaceum*, *T. yaoundii* (Fig. 5).

(3) *Favic hairs*

Hairs invaded throughout their length by hyphal elements. Empty areas (tunnels) where hyphae have degenerated and fat droplets are commonly seen inside the hair: *T. schoenleinii* (Fig. 7).

Culture examination

Sabouraud agar, pH 5.6, is the most commonly used medium for the isolation of dermatophytes from clinical material. A modification with less dextrose (2%) and a pH between 6.8 and 7.0 is preferable, especially when antibiotics are added to inhibit bacteria and saprophytic fungi as in cycloheximide medium (see chapter 95). This is available commercially as Mycosel Agar or Mycobiotic Agar. The use of the antibiotic gentamicin has been recommended for specimens heavily contaminated with bacteria (14).

Nail clippings may be ground in a mortar before being inoculated onto media. Animal hairs that are heavily contaminated with bacteria and saprophytic fungi may be teased apart and soaked in an aqueous solution of antibiotics (chloramphenicol and cycloheximide in amounts used in the selective medium) before being inoculated onto selective agar media. Specimens should be pressed gently into the agar surface.

The cultures are incubated at room temperature (25 to 30 C) and examined every 4 to 6 days. When colonies appear, they should be transferred to fresh medium to avoid contamination by possible associated bacteria or saprophytic fungi. Clinical material from individuals who may have contracted their infection from cattle should be incubated at 37 C, since *T. verrucosum*, the common cause of cattle ringworm, develops more rapidly at this temperature. Cultures should be held for 4 weeks before being considered negative. The chance of isolating the etiological agent is increased if four to six tubes of media are inoculated with the clinical specimens.

Morphological study of cultures

The identification of the dermatophyte species is based on both their gross colony characteristics and their microscopic morphology. The colony characteristics described are based on growth on Sabouraud agar with or without antibiotics. When the colony characteristics are considered, rate of growth, texture, topography of the colony, color of the colony, and production of pigment on the reverse of the colony should be studied. Microscope examination should be made of the colony by preparing teased, wet mount preparations in lactophenol cotton blue, which is usually adequate to demonstrate the characteristic structures. Slide cultures, Pablum cereal agar, and special sporulation media, such as potato dextrose agar, often must be used to identify some isolates.

Nutritional tests

In many instances, characteristic spores are not produced or are produced infrequently. In such cases, nutritional tests are of utmost importance. Basal media are casein (vitamin-free) agar, to which various vitamin solutions are added, and ammonium nitrate agar, to which amino acids are added. Basal media without additives serve as controls. Inocula may be taken from cultures grown on the usual isolation media. It is important, however, to take only a fragment (about the size of the head of a pin) to avoid carrying over an excess of the media (7). Nutritional media for dermatophytes may be obtained commercially in desiccated form (Fig. 8).

In vitro hair perforation test

The test is most useful in the differentiation of *T. rubrum* and *T. mentagrophytes* (3). Hair filaments exposed to *T. mentagrophytes* are radially penetrated by organized groups of hy-

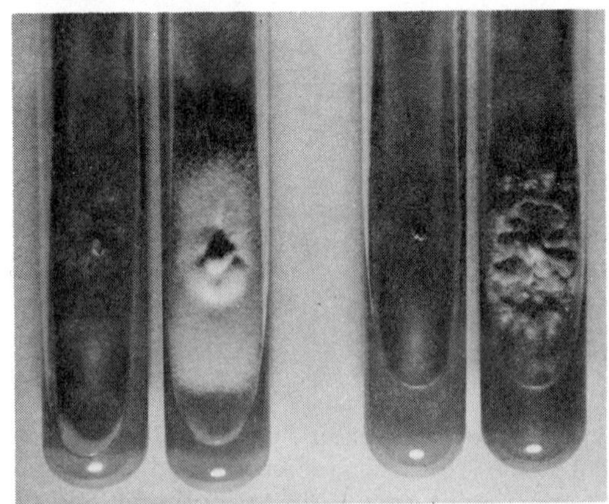

FIG. 8. *Dermatophyte nutritional test. Two isolates of T. tonsurans on media with and without thiamine. Note growth stimulation by thiamine.*

phae that form wedge-shaped perforations. *T. rubrum* grows on the hair and gradually erodes it, but does not form perforations.

Short strands of human hair are placed in petri dishes and sterilized at 120 C for 10 min. A 25-ml amount of sterile distilled water and two or three drops of 10% sterilized yeast extract are added; then the strands of hair are inoculated with several small fragments of the test fungi that have been grown on Sabouraud agar. The strands are incubated at room temperature and examined at regular intervals over a period of 4 weeks. Hair fragments overgrown with mycelium are removed with sterile forceps and examined in wet mounts of lactophenol cotton blue. Gently heating the slide aids in the detection of perforations (Fig. 9).

Generic and species descriptions

The majority of dermatophyte species produce two types of asexual aleuriospores (conidia) when grown in artificial culture: small unicellular microconidia and large, septate, thin- or thick-walled macroconidia. On the basis of the presence or absence of these spores, the dermatophytes are divided into three genera: *Epidermophyton*, *Microsporum*, and *Trichophyton*. The perfect states of the *Microsporum* species that are known to reproduce sexually belong to the genus *Nannizzia* and those of the *Trichophyton* sp., to the genus *Arthroderma* (2, 12). The distinguishing features of the three genera are as follows.

Epidermophyton. Macroconidia smooth, large, fusiform to obovate, multiseptate, borne in groups of two or three. Size 20 to 40 μm by 6 to 8 μm with two to four cells. Microconidia not produced.

The genus *Epidermophyton* is monotypic and is based on only one species—*E. floccosum*.

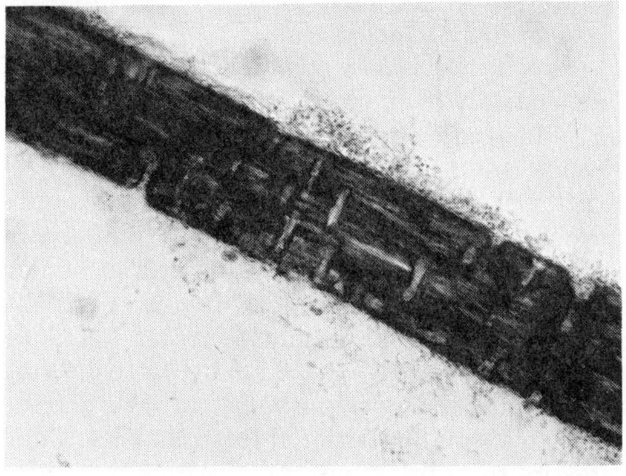

FIG. 9. *Positive in vitro hair perforation test. Note perforations caused by Trichophyton mentagrophytes. ×250.*

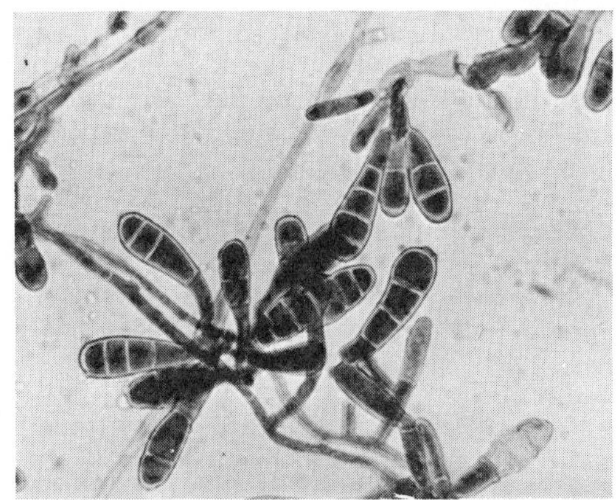

FIG. 10. *Clusters of smooth macroconidia of Epidermophyton floccosum. ×522.*

Microsporum. Macroconidia echinulate, multiseptate, variable in shape (fusiform to obovate), thin- or thick-walled. Borne singly on hyphae 5 to 100 μm by 3 to 8 μm with 2 to 15 cells. Macroconidia may be numerous or rare. Microconidia pyriform to obovate.

Fourteen species are classified under the genus *Microsporum*. Type species—*M. audouinii*.

Trichophyton. Macroconidia smooth-walled, thin- or thick-walled, and range from clavate to fusiform in shape. Borne singly or in clusters. Microconidia spherical, pyriform or clavate, borne singly or in grapelike bunches.

The genus *Trichophyton* has 20 valid species. Type species—*T. tonsurans*.

Characteristics of the common dermatophyte species

The dermatophyte species listed below (in alphabetical sequence) represent species that are commonly isolated from human ringworm lesions in the United States. For other species, refer to Rebell and Taplin (13).

Epidermophyton floccosum. Perfect state: unknown.

Gross colony characteristics. Growth slow. White and fluffy at first, becoming velvety and powdery, greenish yellow to tan. Surface flat or radially folded. Reverse tan. Tufts of white sterile growth (pleomorphic) are common.

Microscopic characteristics. Macroconidia numerous in young colony. At first aseptate and fingerlike in groups of two or three, becoming widely clavate, two- to three-celled with roundish distal ends and with smooth walls (Fig. 10). Microconidia absent. Spiral hyphae extremely rare. Chlamydospores numerous in old cultures.

Physiological and pathological characteris-

tics. No special nutritional requirements. Common agent of ringworm of the skin, particularly of the feet, groin (tinea cruris), and nails of humans. Does not invade hairs. Rarely reported from animals. Anthropophilic.

Microsporum audouinii (M. langeronii, M. rivalierii). Perfect state: unknown.

Gross colony characteristics. Colony slow-growing, flat with short aerial hyphae. Surface gray, cream to tan. Reverse salmon pink to reddish brown.

Microscopic characteristics. Hyphae usually sterile with occasional chlamydospores. Microconidia usually rare, except on enriched media. Clavate, small, borne laterally or terminally on short pedicels or sessile. Macroconidia usually absent, but small number produced by rare isolates; when present, large, irregularly spindle-shaped, thick-walled with a smooth or echinulate surface. Abortive or bizarre-shaped macroconidia more commonly seen.

Physiological and pathological characteristics. Grows poorly on rice-grain medium (see chapter 95). Common agent of epidemic tinea capitis in young children. Invades skin and hair, very rarely nails. Very rarely infects adults or animals. Anthropophilic.

Microsporum canis (M. felineum, M. equinum, M. lanosum). Perfect state: unknown.

Gross colony characteristics. Fast-growing, white, fluffy at first, becoming silky with bright-yellow pigment showing through the periphery. After 2 to 4 weeks, aerial mycelium is dense, cottony, and tan, sometimes in irregular tufts or concentric rings. Reverse at first bright yellow, becoming buff orange-brown. Rare strains show no pigment on reverse.

Microscopic characteristics. Microconidia clavate, small, usually less numerous than the macroconidia. Macroconidia usually numerous, large, fusiform, 35 to 110 μm by 12 to 25 μm with up to 14 septa. Thick-walled (up to 4 μm) and with verruculose walls (Fig. 11). Isolates from equine ringworm (considered by some mycologists to be a distinct species, *M. equinum;* treated as synonymous or as a variety of *M. canis* by others) show few macroconidia. Those produced are elliptical to broadly fusiform, echinulate, 18 to 60 μm by 5 to 15 μm with up to eight septa and walls up to 3.5 μm thick. Typical large macroconidia similar to those of *M. canis* are also produced by these strains and hence their retention in *M. canis*.

Physiological and pathological characteristics. No special nutritional requirements. Grows very well and sporulates abundantly on rice-grain medium. Common agent of ringworm in cats and dogs. Most infections in humans are acquired from infected animals rather than from infected humans. Zoophilic.

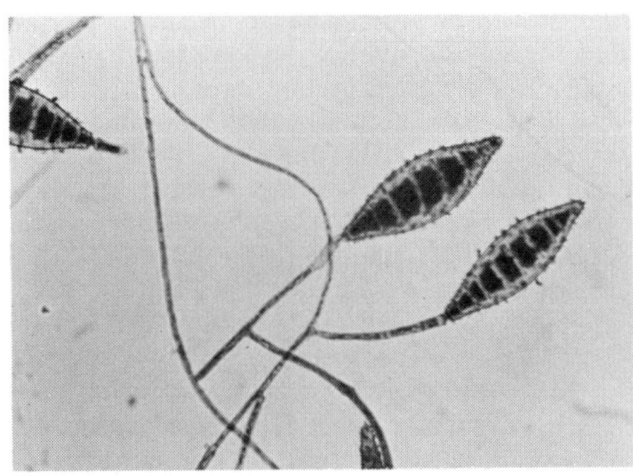

FIG. 11. *Echinulate macroconidia of Microsporum canis. ×522.*

Microsporum gypseum. Perfect states: *Nannizzia gypsea, N. incurvata.*

M. gypseum is a complex of species. Before 1963, *M. fulvum* was also considered to be conspecific with *M. gypseum*. The discovery of the perfect states of the *M. gypseum* complex conclusively proved that *M. fulvum*, though morphologically similar to *M. gypseum*, is a distinct species. The conidial states of *Nannizzia incurvata* and *N. gypsea* are referable to *M. gypseum*, and that of *N. fulva* is referable to *M. fulvum*. Minor but consistent differences in colonial and micromorphology exist among the three perfect states that are evident only to a well-trained eye. The conclusive identification and differentiation of *M. gypseum* and *M. fulvum* is best achieved by mating the conidial isolates with the tester strains of *N. fulva, N. gypsea*, and *N. incurvata*.

Gross colony characteristics. Growth rapid, flat, coarsely or finely granular, with an irregularly fringed border, buff to rosy buff with reverse rosy buff to cinnamon.

Microscopic characteristics. Macroconidia numerous, ellipsoid to fusiform, 25 to 60 μm by 8.5 to 15 μm with up to five septa, and moderately thick-walled (up to 1.2 μm; Fig. 12). Microconidia few in number, clavate, sessile or on short pedicels, 1.7 to 3.3 μm by 3.3 to 8.4 μm.

Physiological and pathological characteristics. No special nutritional requirements. Common in soil. Infection rare in humans; more common in animals, particularly dogs and horses. Geophilic.

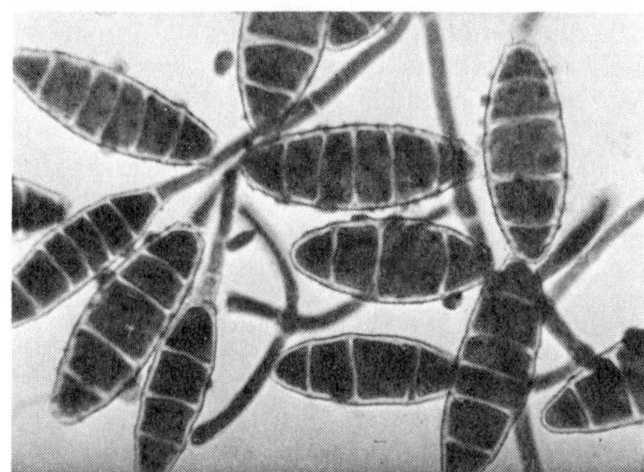

FIG. 12. *Echinulate, elliptical macroconidia of Microsporum gypseum complex.* ×522.

Microsporum fulvum. Perfect state: *Nannizzia fulva.*

Gross colony characteristics. Growth rapid, dense, downy to granular, pale buff to rosy buff, usually with white cottony periphery. Reverse rosy buff to amber.

Microscopic characteristics. Macroconidia numerous, predominantly cylindrical, slightly tapering towards each end and with a rounded apex, or clavate, occasionally ellipsoid to fusiform, 25 to 58 μm by 7.5 to 12 μm with up to five (rarely seven) septa, and with verruculose walls. Microconidia clavate, 1.7 to 3.3 μm by 3.3 to 8.3 μm, unicellular, sessile or on short pedicels, borne on both sides of hyphae.

Physiological and pathological characteristics. No special nutritional requirements. Common in soil. Infection rare in humans. Geophilic.

Microsporum nanum. Perfect state: *Nannizzia obtusa.*

Gross colony characteristics. Growth rapid, flat, powdery to fluffy, cream to buff to cinnamon colored. Reverse orange-tan becoming brownish red. (Colony very similar to that of *M. gypseum.*)

Microscopic characteristics. Macroconidia numerous, small, ovate to elliptical with one to two cells (rarely up to four-celled), echinulate (Fig. 13). Microconidia few, clavate to pyriform, sessile on hyphae.

Physiological and pathological characteristics. No special nutritional requirements. Grows well and sporulates on rice-grain medium. Geophilic. Common agent of ringworm in pigs. Rarely infects humans.

Microsporum persicolor. Perfect state: *Nannizzia persicolor.*

Gross colony characteristics. Growth moderately rapid, downy velvety, or rarely powdery, white at first becoming peach, light buff colored. Reverse reddish brown. On Pablum cereal agar (see chapter 95), the majority of the isolates turn peach to rose-violet colored or even deep vinaceous red.

Microscopic characteristics. Microconidia numerous, pyriform to spherical, borne along the sides of hyphae or in grapelike bunches. Macroconidia produced by the majority of freshly isolated strains, evident after 20 to 24 days of incubation at 25 C. Macroconidia clavate, thin-walled, and finely echinulate (Fig. 14). The echinulations on the outer walls are evident under oil immersion and become more pronounced when grown on sterile soil baited with hair. Tightly wound and loose spirals are numerous in fresh isolates.

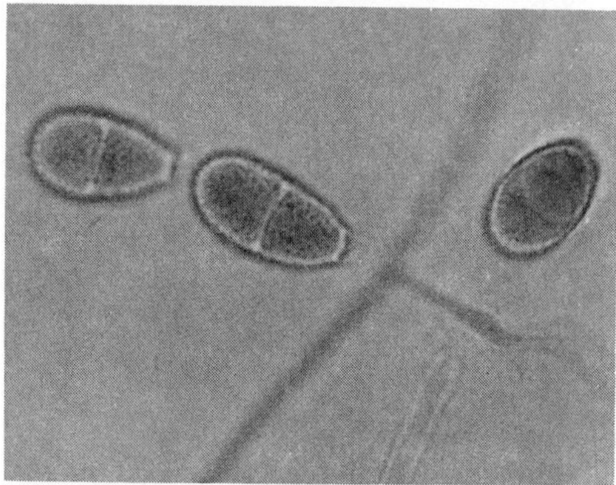

FIG. 13. *Two-celled, echinulate macroconidia of Microsporum nanum.* ×1,000.

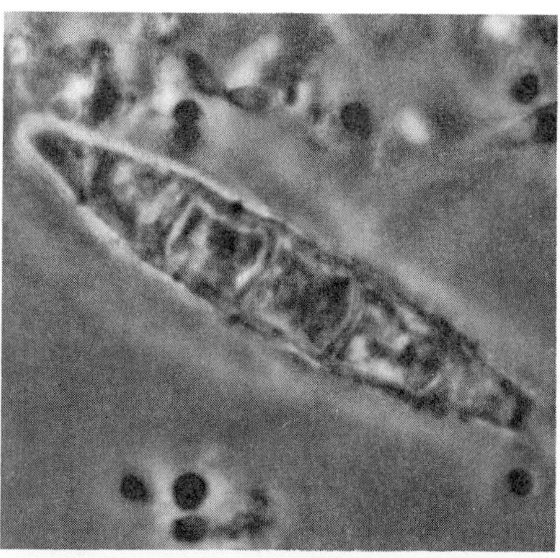

FIG. 14. *Echinulate, clavate macroconidium of Microsporum persicolor.* ×1,650.

Physiological and pathological characteristics. No special nutritional requirements. *M. persicolor* is a frequent, but mild, pathogen of small wild rodents, particularly bank voles and field voles. It infrequently infects humans. Geophilic.

Until recently, *M. persicolor* was believed to be endemic only in western European countries. Recent studies show that it has a wide geographic distribution. It occurs as an infrequent pathogen of man in the United States, Canada, Africa, and Australia. *M. persicolor* closely resembles *T. mentagrophytes* except for its echinulate macroconidia. It can be differentiated from *T. mentagrophytes* by growing it on Pablum cereal agar on which the majority of *M. persicolor* isolates develop characteristic peach- to rose-violet-colored colonies. *T. mentagrophytes* shows no such change on Pablum cereal agar.

Trichophyton equinum. Perfect state: unknown.

Gross colony characteristics. Growth rapid and at first white and fluffy with bright yellow pigment in peripheral growth. Surface velvety, folded, and cream to tan in older colonies. Reverse bright yellow at first, turning pinkish to deep red-brown.

Microscopic characteristics. Microconidia numerous, thin, pyriform, occasionally globose, sessile or on short pedicels and borne along the sides of the hyphae. Macroconidia very rare. When produced, they are cylindrical with thin smooth walls.

Physiological and pathological characteristics. Most isolates have a complete requirement for nicotinic acid. Recently, isolates not dependent on nicotinic acid have been described from New Zealand and Australia as *T. equinum* var. *autotrophicum*. Common cause of ringworm in horses. Zoophilic. Occasionally infects humans and other animals.

Trichophyton mentagrophytes (T. asteroides, T. granulosum, T. gypseum, T. interdigitale, T. quinckeanum). Perfect state: *Arthroderma benhamiae.*

Gross colony characteristics. Growth rapid, flat with powdery to granular surface (var. *mentagrophytes*), flat with downy to fluffy surface (var. *interdigitale*), or heaped and irregularly folded with downy to velvety surface (var. *quinckeanum*). Surface usually white to tan, or pale yellowish. Reverse usually pale yellowish or rose-brown, occasionally pink to red or orange-red (nodular variety).

Microscopic characteristics. Microconidia numerous, small, spherical or clavate, borne singly along the sides of hyphae, sessile or on short pedicels or in grapelike bunches. Macroconidia usually rare, but abundant in some isolates, two- to five-celled, clavate, thick and smooth-walled. Spirally coiled hyphae and nodular bodies numerous in some isolates (Fig. 15).

Physiological and pathological characteristics. Common agent of all types of ringworm in humans and animals, especially rodents. Anthropophyilic (var. *interdigitale*); zoophilic (var. *mentagrophytes*).

Trichophyton rubrum (T. purpureum). Perfect state: unknown.

Gross colony characteristics. Growth slow, flat or heaped at the center with a white, fluffy surface turning pink-tan with wine red reverse (downy type), or surface powdery suede with radial furrows, creamy white, pink, with reverse dark red-tan to wine red (granular type). Some strains (dysgonic type) are slow-growing, deeply pigmented purple with wooly or granular texture and with submerged, feathery peripheral growth. Some downy forms are characterized by the production of diffusible (melanoid type) pigment on reverse. Some strains (African type) are powdery with compactly-heaped folded center, buff-pink surface, and red-tan on reverse. Occasionally some African strains produce a diffusible red pigment. The hyperpigmented type produce a violet to red-violet velvety surface with radial furrows with wine-red color on reverse. The pigment in older colonies may diffuse into the medium. Isolates of the rodhainii type are slow-growing, glabrous, acuminate, folded, deep purple with a white fringe and white granular center.

Microscopic characteristics. Microconidia

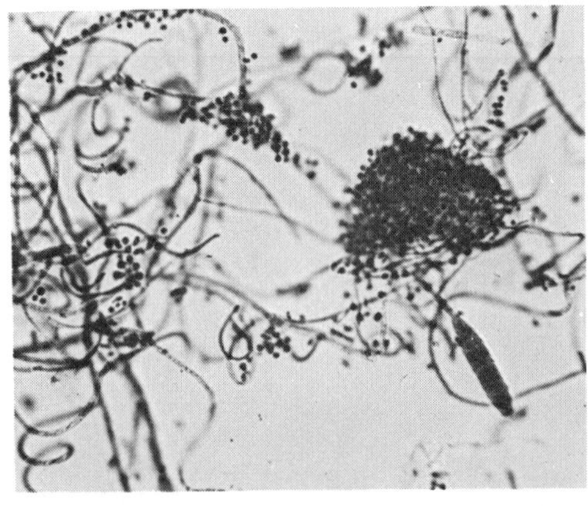

FIG. 15. *Micro- and macroconidia of Trichophyton mentagrophytes.* ×522.

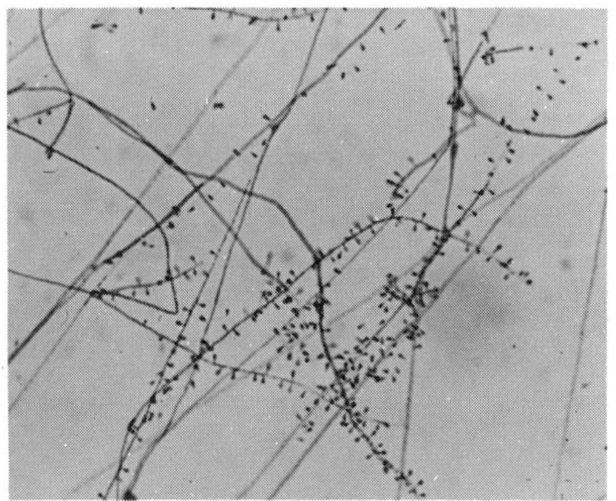

FIG. 16. *Microconidia of Trichophyton rubrum. ×522.*

thin, clavate, borne laterally on undifferentiated hyphae or on short stalks (Fig. 16). Macroconidia typically long, narrow, cylindric with rounded apices three- to eight-celled with thin smooth walls (Fig. 17). The production of microconidia and macroconidia varies greatly in different types of colonies. In the downy type, microconidia are moderate in number, and there are no macroconidia. In the granular type, both microconidia and macroconidia are produced in comparatively large numbers. In the dysgonic type, microconidia are produced in varying numbers, and macroconidia are occasionally observed. In the African type, macroconidia are more numerous than microconidia. In hyperpigmented colonies, macroconidia are occasionally produced. On the other hand, both microconidia and macroconidia are numerous in older colonies of the rodhainii type. In the dysgonic African, melanoid, hyperpigmented, and rodhainii types, many chlamydospores are frequently seen (15).

Physiological and pathological characteristics. No special nutritional requirements. Common agent of ringworm of the skin and nails. Rarely invades hair. Occasional parasite of animals. Anthropophilic.

Trichophyton schoenleinii. Perfect state: unknown.

Gross colony characteristics. Growth slow, irregularly heaped and folded. Surface usually glabrous or waxy and cream to yellowish tan. Old colonies become tough and leathery and may develop white powdery or downy surface on some areas of the colony. Occasionally some isolates grow largely submerged in the agar.

Microscopic characteristics. Mycelium highly irregular in diameter. Coarser hyphae become knobby and irregularly branched at ends (favic chandeliers; Fig. 18). Chlamydospores usually numerous. Microconidia rare. Macroconidia absent.

Physiological and pathological characteristics. No special nutritional requirements. Does not have a complete requirement for thiamine, but growth of some isolates is stimulated by thiamine. Growth not stimulated at 37 C. Common cause of favus, a clinical form of ringworm characterized by heavy cup-shaped crusts (scutulae) and hair invaded throughout its length by hyphae which do not fragment into arthrospores. Also infects skin and nails. Anthropophilic.

Trichophyton tonsurans (T. acuminatum, T. crateriforme, T. sulfureum). Perfect state: unknown.

Gross colony characteristics. Growth slow, flat at first with finely powdery surface, later

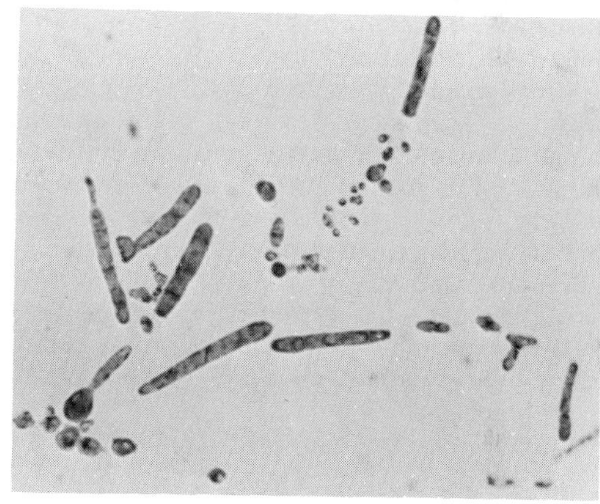

FIG. 17. *Smooth, elongated macroconidia of Trichophyton rubrum. ×522.*

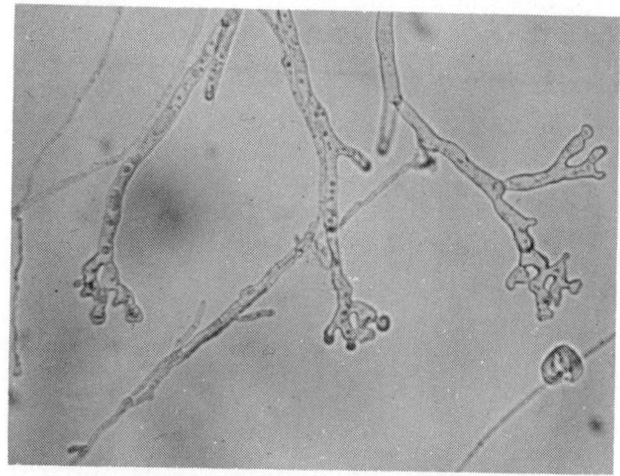

FIG. 18. *Favic chandeliers of Trichophyton schoenleinii. ×522.*

becoming highly heaped, folded with a velvety surface. Center may be acuminate or depressed or entire surface may be irregularly folded (cerebriform). Surface usually cream to tan, rarely rose or bright yellow (var. *sulfureum*). Reverse yellowish to mahogany red (Fig. 19).

Microscopic characteristics. Microconidia numerous, delicate, elongate when young, larger and irregular in size and shape in older colonies (Fig. 20). Macroconidia rare in many isolates; when produced, cylindric to clavate, slightly curved at the tips, two- to three-celled or sometimes five- to seven-celled.

Physiological and pathological characteristics. Grows poorly on vitamin-free media. Growth greatly stimulated by thiamine. Common cause of epidemic tinea capitis in both children and adults. Causes large-spored endothrix infections. Also commonly infects skin and nails. Infection rare in animals. Anthropophilic.

Trichophyton verrucosum (T. album, T. discoides, T. faviforme, T. ochraceum). Perfect state: unknown.

Gross colony characteristics. Growth very slow. At first small, heaped, glabrous, and tough leathery. May become disk-shaped (var. *discoides*) or highly heaped and folded (var. *album*). Most isolates grayish-white, few yellowish-tan (var. *ochraceum*). Old colonies may develop white powdery to downy aerial growth.

Microscopic characteristics. On Sabouraud agar at room temperature, growth thin consisting of hyphae with many chlamydospores. At 37 C, chlamydospores become numerous, often in chains. On thiamine-enriched media, mycelium is more regular in form, and microconidia may be numerous. Microconidia small, thin, borne along the sides of the hyphae. Macroconidia extremely rare, three- to five-celled, variable in shape, thin and smooth walled.

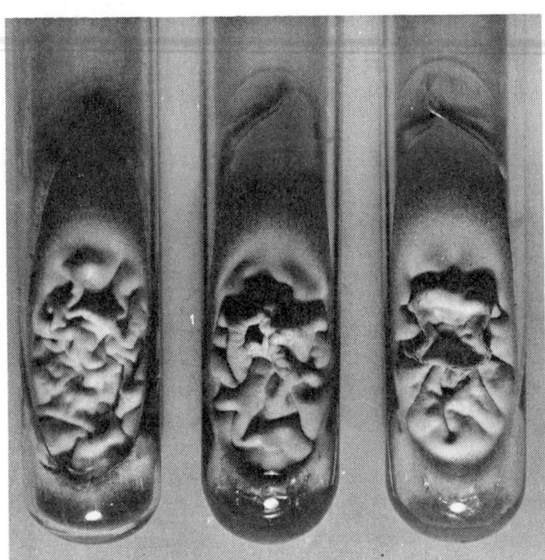

FIG. 19. *Colony variation in Trichophyton tonsurans.*

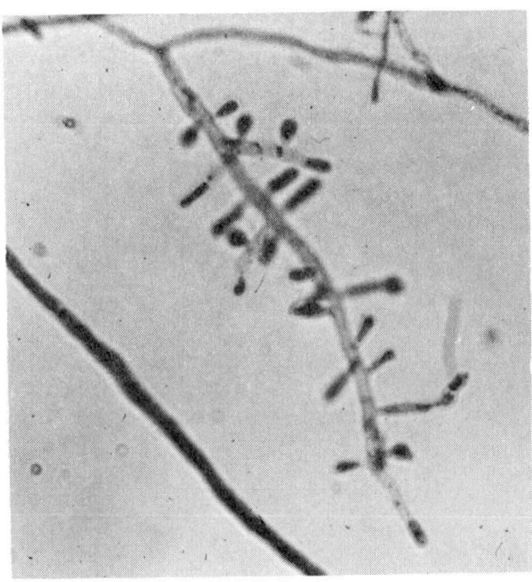

FIG. 20. *Microconidia of Trichophyton tonsurans. ×1,070.*

Physiological and pathological characteristics. No growth on vitamin-free media. Some strains require thiamine, others require a combination of thiamine and inositol. Growth more rapid at 37 C than at room temperature. Common agent of ringworm in cattle. Occasionally infects humans and other animals. Zoophilic.

Trichophyton violaceum (T. glabrum). Perfect state: unknown.

Gross colony characteristics. Growth very slow, heaped or finely folded with a glabrous or waxy surface. At first cream-colored, becoming pinkish then lavender to deep purple. Old cultures may develop color-free sectors with downy grayish aerial hyphae. A few strains lack pigment when first isolated (var. *glabrum*).

Microscopic characteristics. Mycelium thin and usually sterile. Occasionally chlamydospores may be found. Microconidia very rare; macroconidia absent on most media. In some isolates, spores are produced in old cultures when grown on thiamine-enriched media.

Physiological and pathological characteristics. Grows poorly on vitamin-free media. Growth greatly stimulated by thiamine. Cause of tinea capitis in both children and adults. Also infects skin and nails. Infection very rare in animals. Anthropophilic.

LITERATURE CITED

1. Ajello, L. 1962. Present day concepts of the dermatophytes. Mycopathol. Mycol. Appl. **17**:315–324.
2. Ajello, L. 1968. A taxonomic review of the dermatophytes and related species. Sabouraudia **6**:147–159.
3. Ajello, L., and L. K. Georg. 1957. *In vitro* cultures for differentiating between atypical isolates of *Trichophyton mentagrophytes* and *Trichophyton rubrum*. Mycopathol. Mycol. Appl. **8**:3–17.
4. Blank, H., S. Sabami, C. Boyd, and J. Roth, Jr. 1959. The pathogenesis of superficial fungous infections in cultured human skin. Arch. Dermatol. **79**:524–535.
5. Conant, N. F., D. T. Smith, R. D. Baker, and J. L. Callaway. 1971. Manual of clinical mycology, 3rd ed., p. 548–586. W. B. Saunders Co., Philadelphia.
6. Emmons, C. W., C. H. Binford, and J. P. Utz. 1970. Medical mycology. 2nd ed. Lea & Febiger, Philadelphia.
7. Georg, L. K., and L. B. Camp. 1957. Routine nutritional tests for the identification of dermatophytes. J. Bacteriol. **74**:113–121.
8. Kaplan, W. 1959. The occurrence of black piedra in primate pelts. Trop. Geogr. Med. **11**:115–126.
9. Lodder, J. 1970. The yeasts. North-Holland Publishing Co., Amsterdam.
10. Lorincz, A. L., J. O. Priestly, and P. J. Jacob. 1958. Evidence for humoral mechanism which prevents growth of dermatophytes. J. Invest. Dermatol. **31**:15–17.
11. Mackenzie, D. W. R. 1963. "Hairbrush diagnosis" in detection and eradication of nonfluorescent scalp ringworm. Brit. Med. J. **2**:263–265.
12. Padhye, A. A., and J. W. Carmichael. 1971. The genus *Arthroderma* Berkeley. Can. J. Bot. **49**:1525–1540.
13. Rebell, G., and D. Taplin. 1970. Dermatophytes, their recognition and identification. University of Miami Press, Coral Gables, Fla.
14. Taplin, D. 1965. The use of gentamycin in mycology. J. Invest. Dermatol. **45**:549–550.
15. Young, C. N. 1972. Range of variation among isolates of *Trichophyton rubrum*. Sabouraudia **10**:164–170.

Chapter 55

Fungi of Keratomycosis

GERBERT C. REBELL AND RICHARD K. FORSTER

After synonyms are taken into account, reported causes of keratomycosis (mycotic ulcers of the cornea) comprise some 80 species in 35 genera of the Eumycota, most of which occur in nature as common saprobes and plant pathogens, and only a few of which are known as causes of nonocular mycoses (8, 11, 15). Identification usually requires assistance from mycologists with specialized knowledge of groups of fungi outside the field of medical mycology. The task is somewhat simplified, however, by the fact that only a relatively few species and genera account for the majority of corneal ulcers. Beginning with the most frequent, the common causes of keratomycosis are *Fusarium solani*, *Candida albicans*, *Aspergillus fumigatus*, *Curvularia spp.* and other dematiaceous hyphomycetes, *Acremonium spp.* and related genera, *Aspergillus flavus* and other species of *Aspergillus* and *Penicillum*, *Fusarium episphaeria* and other species of *Fusarium* and *Cylindrocarpon*, *Volutella spp.*, *Allescheria boydii*, and *Lasiodiplodia theobromae*. Corneal infections resembling keratomycosis are also caused by *Actinomycetales*, principally *Nocardia asteroides* and *Mycobacterium fortuitum*. With the single exception of ocular infections caused by *C. albicans*, keratomycosis is exogenous in origin, and is encountered in apparently healthy persons, usually originating from outdoor material, particularly vegetable matter, which appears to introduce the fungus into the cornea. Both incidence and prevailing etiological agents vary geographically. In Miami, Fla., 10 cases per year is the usual incidence.

Prompt institution of antifungal therapy and avoidance of the therapeutic use of corticosteroids are important to the clinical outcome of keratomycosis and depend on early diagnosis. The most serious consequence of keratomycosis is penetration of the fungus deeper into the tissues of the eye and perforation of the globe, with ensuing endophthalmitis. Other ocular mycoses include canaliculitis and dacryocystitis, orbital cellulitis, endophthalmitis following surgery or trauma, and the extension of cutaneous and systemic mycotic diseases to the eye.

The first step in diagnosis of keratomycosis requires an alert ophthalmologist, who must correctly evaluate the ulcer clinically and then obtain adequate scrapings from the lesion for direct examination and culture. Characteristics of the lesions of mycotic corneal infection are an elevated ulcer with an infiltrate having hyphate margins, satellite lesions, and occasionally a hypopyon (Fig. 1). Frequently there is an "immune" infiltrate halo, and there may be moderate to severe conjunctival reaction and discomfort.

COLLECTION OF SPECIMENS

The two procedures required to confirm keratomycosis are (i) direct observation of fungal hyphal elements in scrapings from the cornea and (ii) isolation of the fungus in culture by inoculating the scrapings on culture media. Slides and culture media are usually inoculated by the ophthalmologist directly from the patient. Scraping of the corneal lesion with a platinum spatula must be vigorous enough to obtain material for direct microscope examination and culture, and should be performed under biomicroscopy. Corneal fragments are scraped from the base and margins of the ulcer. A swab culture is not adequate for laboratory diagnosis.

DIRECT EXAMINATION

The most useful method for the direct examination of corneal scrapings is the Giemsa-stained slide. For this procedure, corneal scrapings are smeared on a slide, and the slide is fixed in methanol and stained in diluted Giemsa solution for 1 h. At the same time, a Gram stain and KOH wet mount should also be examined. KOH preparations are not very reliable and can be omitted when material obtained by scraping is limited. The KOH preparation tends to clear slightly in the course of a few minutes or longer and should be examined at intervals during this clearing process. The characteristic appearance of positive slides by Giemsa and KOH methods is shown in Fig. 2.

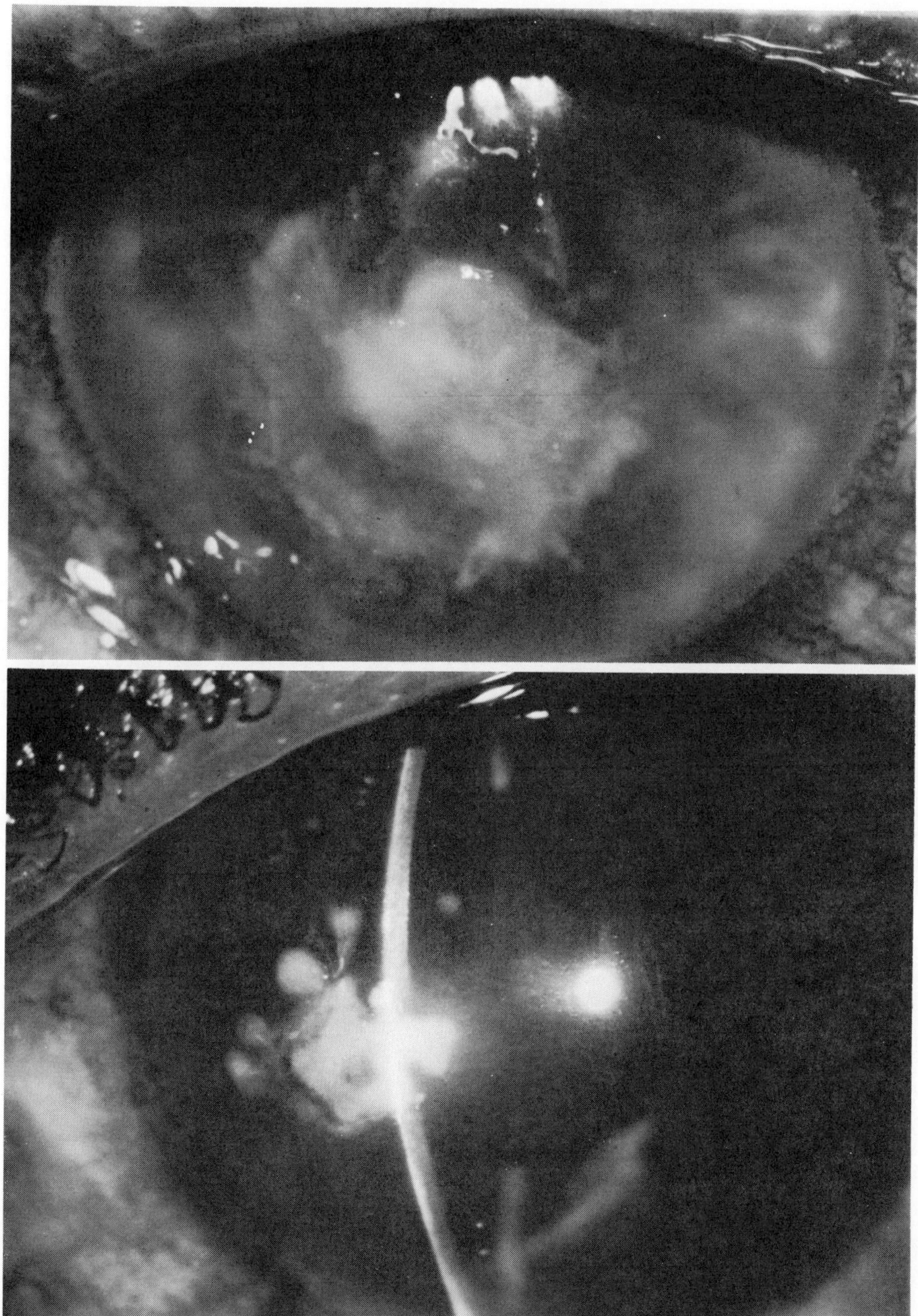

FIG. 1. *Keratomycosis.* (*A*) *Typical ulcer showing shaggy, hyphate margins* (*F. solani*). (*B*) *Ulcer with satellite lesions* (*F. solani*).

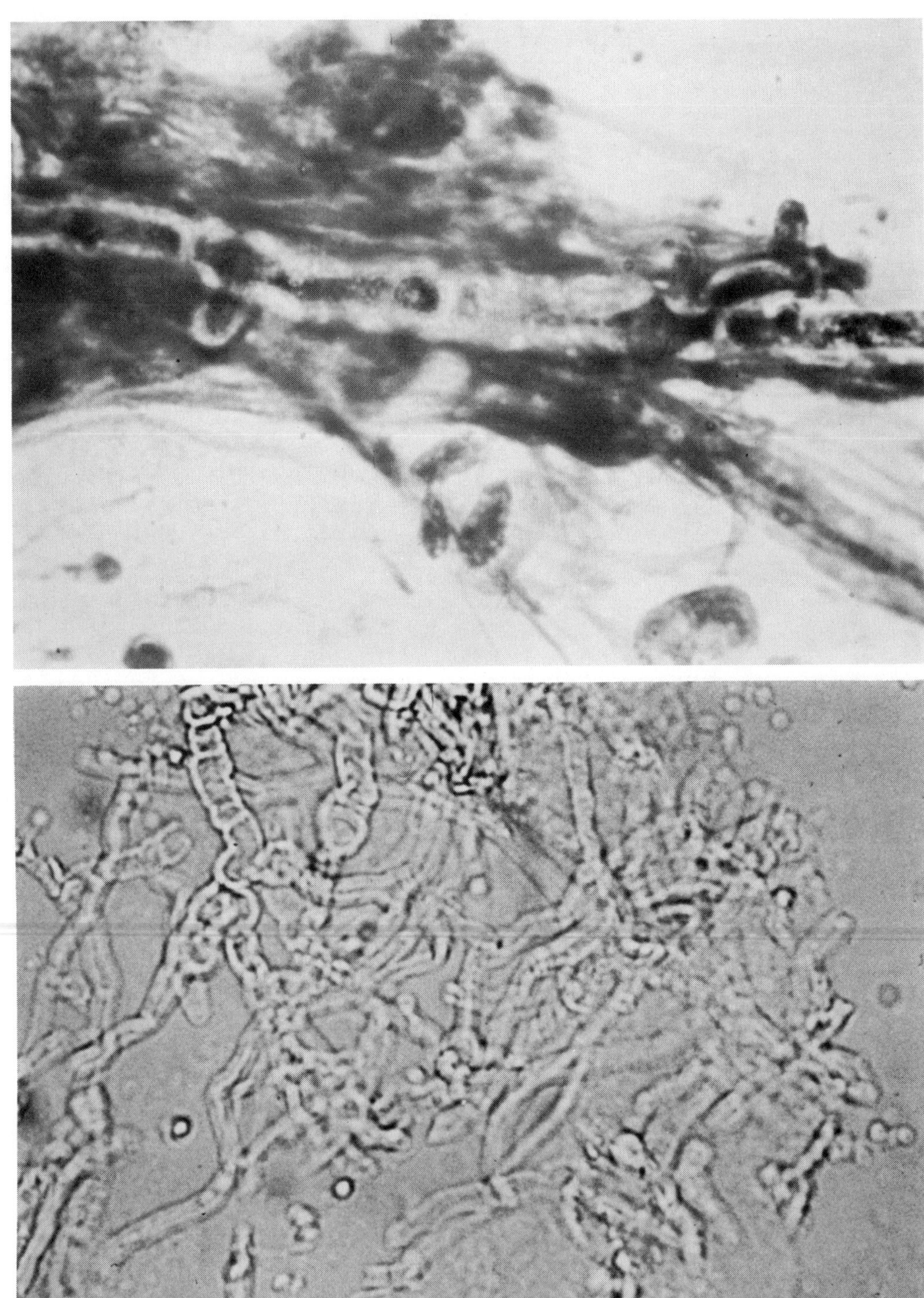

FIG. 2. *Direct examination of corneal scrapings. (A) Giemsa stain (C. senegalensis). (B) KOH preparation (F. solani).*

CULTURE

The culture media used routinely are blood-agar plates (casein soy peptone agar base), incubated both at room temperature and at 37 C, and Sabouraud agar plates, incubated at room temperature. If tubed medium is used, multiple tubes should be inoculated. The Sabouraud agar should contain an antibacterial antibiotic (50 μg of either gentamicin or chloramphenicol per ml). Cycloheximide should not be present in isolation media used for keratomycosis. Usually bacteria are sparse in fungal ulcers, and growth of the fungus without bacteria is obtained on blood-agar incubated at room temperature. A 250-ml flask containing 50 ml of brain heart infusion broth with gentamicin or chloramphenicol has occasionally proven to be an alternate safeguard method for isolating fungi which did not appear on solid media (21). The flask is incubated at room temperature (27 C), preferably on a rotary shaker. Studies in our laboratory have shown that gentamicin in liquid media is somewhat inhibitory for *Fusarium solani*.

The common etiological fungi of keratomycosis appear on solid media 24 to 48 h after inoculation. However, plates should be incubated for at least 1 week before they are discarded as negative for growth. Every effort should be made to reduce contamination by airborne fungi. Primary isolation plates should be incubated in dust-free areas, away from other fungus cultures, and should be removed from these areas as soon as growth is detected to prevent contamination of subsequent cultures. The best assurance against mistaking airborne contaminants for positive outgrowths from mycotic keratitis is the technique by which the plates are inoculated. This technique consists of marking the scrapings into the agar with a platinum spatula in a series of "C"-shaped cuts (Fig. 3). The "C" cuts localize the sites of implantation of the corneal scrapings on the

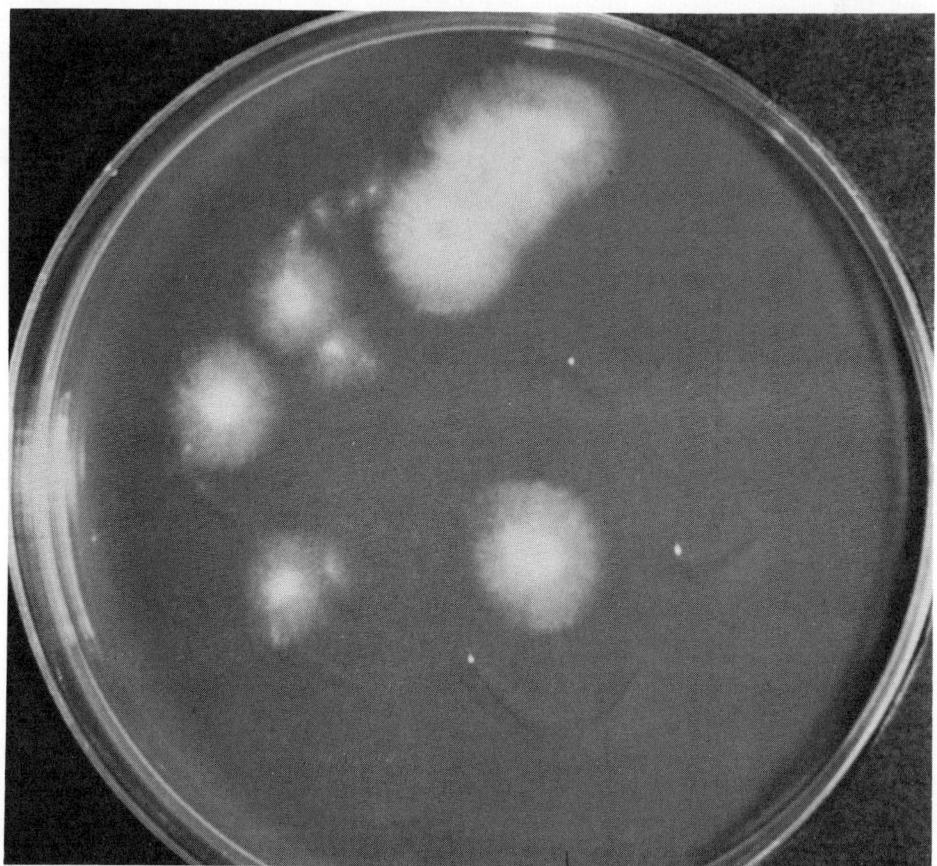

FIG. 3. *Primary inoculation plate showing outgrowth from "C" cuts (F. solani).*

agar media and provide a crude graded dilution of the specimen. Fungal outgrowths from the "C" cuts are therefore significant. Outgrowths away from the "C" cuts may be discarded as contaminants.

Once the fungus outgrowth has appeared, it should be subcultured promptly to fresh media for isolation in pure culture, identification, and preservation as a stock culture before mutation occurs. If the facilities exist for lyophilization or storage at −70 C, reserve cultures, consisting of conidia suspended in skim milk, may be so maintained to prevent mutation.

Potato dextrose agar, cornmeal-agar, Czapek agar, and other special media may be required for sporulation and identification of isolates. However, a scotch tape mount made directly from the primary outgrowth will usually confirm the isolation of *F. solani*, *A. fumigatus*, *A. boydii*, etc., within 48 h (Fig. 4). For making this mount, a flag of no. 800 acetate-back tape (3M Co.) is fastened to a wooden applicator stick, and the sticky surface of the tape is touched to the surface of the fungus outgrowth. The tape is then pressed sticky side down on a slide with a drop of lactophenol cotton blue stain and examined under a microscope.

IDENTIFICATION OF AGENTS

It is obviously impossible to provide a complete guide to the identification of fungi from keratomycosis. What will be attempted here are brief notes on the most frequent causative agents, and recommendations concerning publications and sources of help for the identification of known or potential agents of keratomycosis.

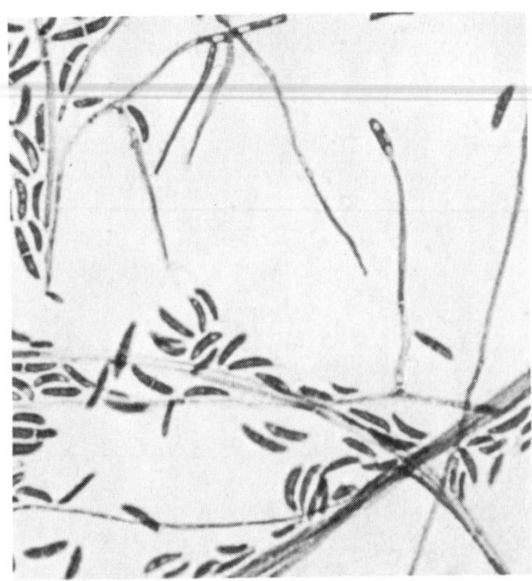

FIG. 4. *Tape mount from primary outgrowth made 30 h after inoculating scrapings from the cornea, showing characteristic microconidia and phialids of F. solani.*

Books which may be adopted as standards for identifications and nomenclature are listed in the Literature Cited and mentioned below. For overall identification and nomenclature of genera, we recommend von Arx (3), backed up by the taxonomic reviews published as volume 4 of *The Fungi* edited by Ainsworth (1). In addition to these books, the publications by Barron (5) and Barnett and Hunter (4) provide additional help, illustrations, and bibliographies useful in identification of species.

We strongly recommend that all fungi isolated from keratomycosis lesions be sent to an appropriate mycological laboratory or authority to confirm identification. Authors of the manuals cited below are obvious first sources of help. Subcultures should be made promptly and mailed before they mutate. Cultures in screw-top tubes should be mailed with the caps slightly loosened to provide aeration. Subcultures should also be sent to a repository for maintenance as stock cultures for future reference. A culture repository for ocular mycoses has been established at the Bascom Palmer Eye Institute, University of Miami School of Medicine, P.O. Box 875, Biscayne Annex, Miami, Fla. 33152.

Fusarium and Cylindrocarpon

A recent manual for identification of *Fusarium* species (6) and a separate paper on *Cylindrocarpon* (7) by Booth may be used for species identification. The simple nine-species system devised for *Fusarium* by Snyder and Hansen (20) has also been satisfactory for identifying isolates from keratomycosis. The Fusarium Research Center, Pennsylvania State University, University Park, Pa. 16802, provides an identification service based principally on the Snyder-Hansen taxonomy.

F. solani is the most important cause of keratomycosis. Curiously, it was not reported until recently (2, 13, 14, 16). Less commonly isolated are *F. episphaeria* and *F. moniliforme*. Reports of *F. oxysporum* and other species from keratomycosis are questionable, however, as apparent or possible misidentifications of *F. solani*. There is one valid report of *C. tonkinense* (17).

Acremonium (Cephalosporium) and related genera

The genus *Cephalosporium*, along with other nondematiaceous fungi which produce small conidia from simple phialides, has recently been revised by Gams (12), providing a much needed reference with a key in English for species identification. Three genera, *Acremonium*, *Cephalosporium*, and *Paecilomyces*, have been combined by Gams under the single name *Acremonium*.

Although reports of *Cephalosporium* isolations are prominent in the ophthalmological literature, there is a dearth of information on which to base a discussion of *Cephalosporium* species isolated from proven cases of keratitis. Some reports are probably based on misidentification of microconidia of *F. solani*. Others are referable to *Verticillium*. Only *A. potroni* and *A. kiliense* have been specifically identified, each from a single instance of ocular infection.

In *Volutella*, conidia resembling those of *Acremonium* are produced from discrete sporodochia in association with awl-like setae. *Volutella* has been reported to cause endophthalmitis and keratitis. Two isolates from keratitis lesions have been identified as *V. cinerescens*.

Aspergillus and Penicillium

Identification of species is based on standard books by Raper and Fennel (18) and Raper and Thom (19; see also chapter 61). *A. fumigatus* is a major cause of exogenous keratomycosis, second only to *F. solani* in incidence. *A. flavus* is the next most common *Aspergillus* to be involved in ocular infections. There are three reports of isolation of *P. lilacinum* from keratomycosis and endophthalmitis.

Curvularia and other dematiaceous hyphomycetes

Fungi with brown-pigmented conidia or hyphae, and hence blackish colonies, may be conveniently categorized as dematiaceous. The first volume of a continuing taxonomic review of dematiaceous hyphomycetes by Ellis is available as a major reference for species identification (9). *Phialophora gougerotti* (17) and *P. verrucosa* (21), which have been isolated from keratomycosis, are described in chapter 59. In addition to the dematiaceous hyphomycetes, many fungi in the orders *Sphaeropsidales* and *Melanconiales* are brown-pigmented and appear in cultures as dematiaceous fungi; see *Lasiodiplodia* (17).

Dematiaceous hyphomycetes account for approximately 10% of mycotic ulcers. *Curvularia* species are the most frequent dematiaceous causative agents. In our experience, *C. senegalensis* and *C. verruculosa* are the most commonly isolated species. Some published reports of *C. geniculata* and *C. lunata* are in fact also referable to these species; however, the occurrence of *C. lunata* in keratomycosis has been verified (Fig. 5).

Candida albicans

C. albicans is responsible for corneal ulcers and other ocular infections in patients whose resistance has been compromised by trauma, surgery, medication, disease, and age. The fungus can usually be tentatively identified from direct microscope examination of corneal scrapings by the presence of pseudomycelium and budding yeast cells (Fig. 6). See chapter 56 for laboratory identification of *C. albicans*.

C. parapsilosis, which has been reported as a cause of keratomycosis, is frequently isolated from normal skin and conjunctiva, as well as from mascara, etc. Budding cells of *Malassezia* (*Pityrosporon*) may be present in slides from the conjunctiva and lids, but are without significance in keratomycosis.

Fusarium solani (Mart.-Sacc.) Snyder & Hansen, 1941

Colony off-white to buff, frequently with patches of purple-brown or cyan-blue pigment, and umber-colored sporodochia. Undersurface yellow, colorless, or purple-brown. Single-celled and double-celled microconidia usually abundant in young cultures, and produced on slender, relatively unbranched phialides (Fig. 4). Macroconidia are produced separately, either diffusely or in slimy masses in sporodochia, and are relatively untapered, banana-shaped, with blunt, hooked ends, usually having a foot cell, and a relatively straight short side (Fig. 7). Both micro- and macroconidia have rather thick walls when compared with other species of *Fusarium*. Rough-walled chlamydospores are present in older cultures. Keratitis isolates have consistently been capable of moderate growth at 37 C, usually with a characteristic colony appearance on brain heart infusion agar.

Fusarium episphaeria (Tode) Snyder & Hansen, 1945

Colony typically slow-growing and virtually devoid of aerial hyphae, presenting instead a shiny, yellow to deep orange, mucilagenous surface. Macroconidia curved, pointed, and usually without a prominent foot cell. Separate phialides with microconidia not present. Chlamydospores may be present. *F. episphaeria* as defined by Snyder and Hansen is treated by Booth as two species: *F. dimerum* Pensig-Saccardo, 1882, characterized in part by short macroconidia, and *F. merismoides* Corda, 1838, characterized in part by longer, slender macroconidia. The question of whether orange *F.*

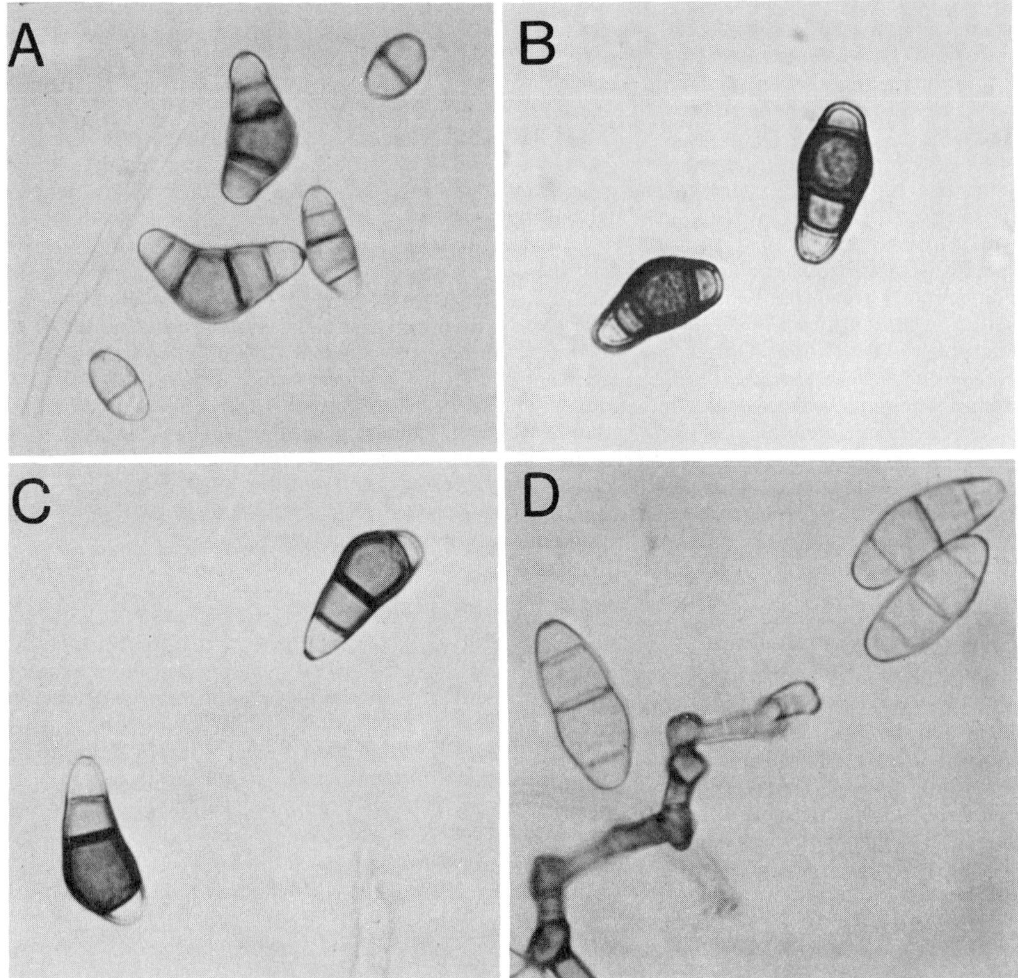

FIG. 5. *Conidia of Curvularia species isolated from keratomycosis. (A) C. senegalensis. (B) C. verruculosa. (C) C. lunata. (D) C. pallescens. Conidia of C. senegalensis and C. geniculata typically have four septa; those of C. verruculosa, C. lunata, and C. pallescens, three septa. Conidia of C. senegalensis average 24 μm in length, those of C. geniculata average 30 μm. Conidia of C. pallescens are uniformly pale; those of C. verruculosa are slightly roughened.*

episphaeria isolates from ocular infections are taxonomically or physiologically homogenous is not settled.

Fusarium moniliforme Sheldon, 1904

Colony white and rather loosely fluffy, frequently with dark violet undercolor and blue-black sclerotia. Typically, microconidia are produced in chains, although *Cephalosporium*-like clusters of microconidia held in a droplet of moisture also occur, as in other species of *Fusarium*. If present, macroconidia are slender. Chlamydospores are absent.

Aspergillus fumigatus Fresenius, 1863

This fungus is well described in medical texts (10; see also chapter 61). Colonies are flat and blue-green, changing to gray-black with age. Conidial heads form compact columns, as seen under lower-power magnification. Vesicles are tapered basally and are fertile over the upper half only. Sterigmata are arranged in a single series and curved toward the vesicle.

Growth typically is excellent at 40 C. As in other tissues, *Aspergillus* hyphae in the cornea, as seen in histological sections, exhibit dichotomously forked branching.

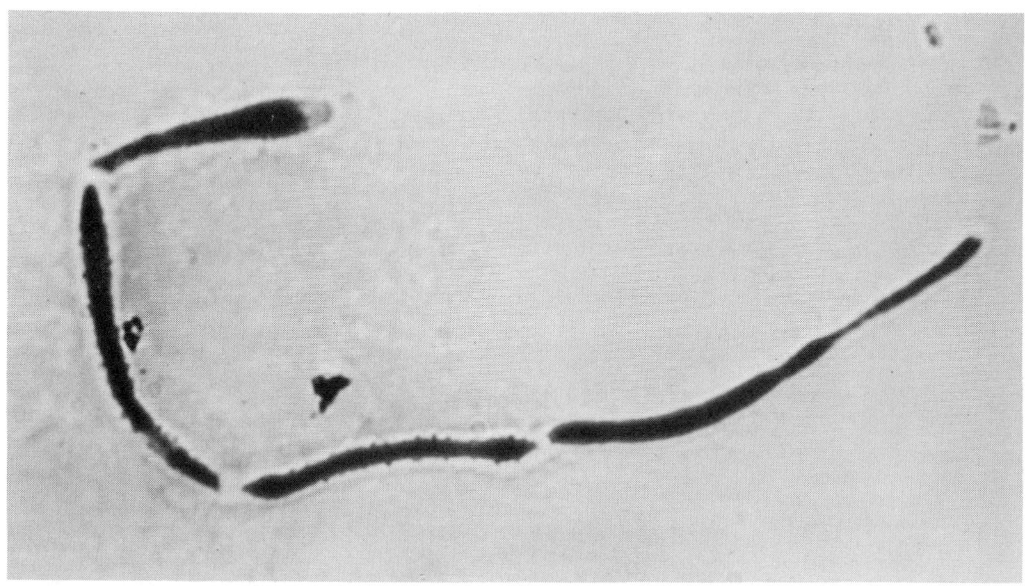

FIG. 6. *Direct scrapings of corneal ulcers caused by C. albicans showing pseudohyphae (Gram stain).*

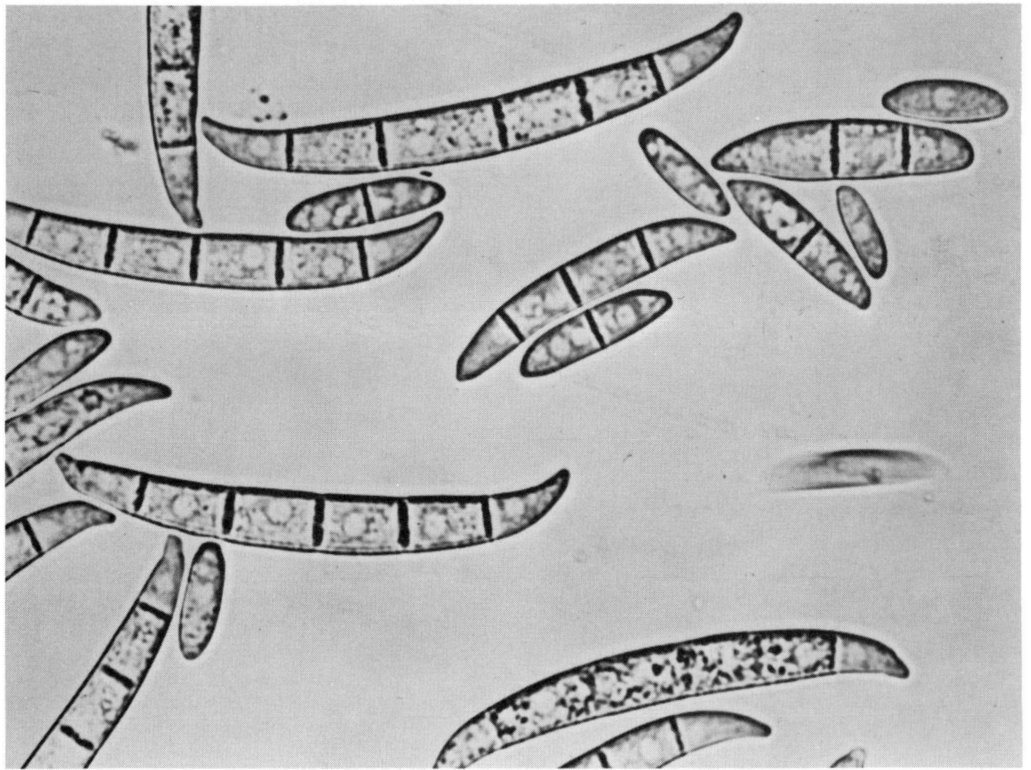

FIG. 7. *Macroconidia and microconidia of F. solani.*

Aspergillus flavus Link, 1809

Colony typically yellow to yellow-green, usually with a dense, deep pile of conidiophores. In the related species *A. oryzae*, the colony turns brown with age. Conidial heads usually appear in shaggy columns or they are globose. Conidiophores frequently vary in size; some small, sparse, and with clavate vesicles. Sterigmata usually in part biserate and distributed over the entire bulbous surface of the vesicle.

LITERATURE CITED

1. Ainsworth, G. C., F. K. Sparrow, and A. S. Sussman (ed.). 1973. The fungi, an advanced treatise., vol. 4A. Academic Press Inc., New York.
2. Arrechea, A. de, R. C. Zapater, E. Storero, and V. H. Guevara. 1971. Queratomicosis por Fusarium solani. Arch. Oftalmol. Hisp.-Amer. **46:**123–127.
3. Arx, J. A. von. 1970. The genera of fungi sporulating in pure culture. Verlag von J. Cramer, Germany.
4. Barnett, H. I., and B. B. Hunter. 1972. Illustrated genera of imperfect fungi, 3rd ed. Burgess Publishing Co., Minneapolis, Minn.
5. Barron, G. L. 1968. The genera of hyphomycetes from soil. The Williams & Wilkins Co., Baltimore (Krieger Publishing Co., Hunting, N.Y., 1971).
6. Booth, C. 1971. The genus Fusarium. Commonwealth Mycological Institute, Kew, Surrey, England.
7. Booth, C. 1966. The genus Cylindrocarpon. Mycology Paper No. 104, Commonwealth Mycological Institute, Kew, Surrey, England.
8. De Voe, A. G., and M. Silva-Hutner. 1972. Fungal infections of the eye, p. 208–240. *In* D. Locatcher-Khorazo and B. C. Siegel (ed.), Microbiology of the eye. C. V. Mosby, St. Louis, Mo.
9. Ellis, M. B. 1971. Dematiaceous hyphomycetes. Commonwealth Mycological Institute, Kew, Surrey, England.
10. Emmons, C. W., C. H. Binford, and J. P. Utz. 1970. Medical mycology, 2nd ed. Lea & Febiger, Philadelphia.
11. Francois, J., and M. Rysselaera. 1968. Oculomycoses (Engl. Transl.). Charles C Thomas, Publisher, Springfield, Ill.
12. Gams, W. 1971. Cephalosporium-artige Schimmelpiltze (Hyphomycetes). Gustav Fischer, Jena.
13. Halde, C., and M. Okumoto. 1966. Ocular mycoses: a study of 82 cases. Proc. 20th Int. Congr. Ophthalmol., Munich **2:**705–712.
14. Jones, B. R., D. B. Jones, S. M. Lim, et al. 1970. Corneal ulcer and intra-ocular infection due to a *Fusarium solani*. Trans. Ophthalmol. Soc. U.K. **84:**757–779.
15. Jones, B. R., A. B. Richards, and G. Morgan. 1969. Direct fungal infection of the eye in Britain. Trans. Ophthalmol. Soc. U.K. **84:**727–741.
16. Jones, D. B., R. Sexton, and G. Rebell. 1970. Mycotic keratitis in South Florida: a review of thirty-nine cases. Trans. Ophthalmol. Soc. U.K. **84:**781–797.
17. Laverde, C. L., L. H. Moncada, A. Restrepo, and C. L. Vera. 1973. Mycotic keratitis: 5 cases caused by unusual fungi. Sabouraudia **11:**119–123.
18. Raper, K. B., and D. I. Fennel. 1965. The genus Aspergillus. The Williams & Wilkins Co., Baltimore.
19. Raper, K. B., and C. Thom. 1968. Manual of the Penicillia. The Williams & Wilkins Co., Hafner Publishing Co., New York.
20. Toussoun, T. A., and P. E. Nelson. 1968. A pictorial guide to the identification of *Fusarium* species according to the taxonomic system of Snyder and Hansen. The Pennsylvania State University Press, University Park.
21. Wilson, L. A., R. R. Sexton, and D. Ahearn. 1966. Keratochromomycosis. Arch. Ophthalmol. **76:**811–816.

Chapter 56
Medically Important Yeasts

MARGARITA SILVA-HUTNER AND B. H. COOPER

GROUP CHARACTERIZATION

Summary of distinguishing characteristics

The yeasts are fungi which are predominantly unicellular when actively growing (logarithmic phase) under normal conditions of temperature, aeration, pressure, and humidity. Their colonies are therefore glabrous, with a moist, creamy or membranous texture, and lack the aerial hyphae that impart a fluffy or velvety texture to the colonies of filamentous fungi (molds). It is true that many yeasts can form filaments as either true or pseudohyphae, but these are produced under reduced O_2 conditions such as exist in the submerged portions of solid culture media, an atmosphere of 5 to 10% CO_2, or the tissues of a parasitized host.

The normal vegetative cells of yeasts are round or oval, 2.5 to 6 μm in diameter, and reproduce asexually by budding, bud-fission, or fission. Buds (blastospores) can remain attached to the mother cell and in turn continue to bud, thus producing branching clusters of blastospores. Individual blastospores still adhering to their neighbors in a chain can elongate to produce filaments called pseudohyphae. True septate hyphae result from germination of "transitional cells" (rounded or flattened blastospores, or chlamydospores).

The taxonomic affinities of yeasts with one another and with other fungi are becoming clearer as a result of more detailed knowledge of their life cycles and cytology, and of their antigenic and chemical composition.

According to their method of sexual reproduction, yeasts can be divided into three main groups, *Ascomycetes* (*Saccharomyces*, *Endomycopsis*, *Pichia*, and *Nematospora*), *Heterobasidiomycetes* (*Leucosporidium* and *Syringospora*), and *Deuteromycetes* or Fungi Imperfecti (*Candida*, *Cryptococcus*, *Rhodotorula*, *Torulopsis*, and *Trichosporon*) (19).

Clinical significance

Yeast infections are among the commonest fungal infections affecting humans; their incidence has greatly increased since the advent of broad-spectrum antibiotics, corticosteroids, and antitumor agents. Their severity ranges from benign and transient through more severe, chronic, and recalcitrant. Although intertriginous cutaneous and mucocutaneous localizations are the most common, dissemination can occur to produce systemic infections which are sometimes fatal. Yeast fungaemia occurs frequently in patients with indwelling catheters, and can result in endocarditis or pyelonephritis in recipients of organ transplants, artificial heart valves, or other prosthetic devices (25). Endopthalmic candidiasis resulting in loss of an eye has occurred in several such patients (20).

Yeast endocarditis is also frequent in drug addicts who inject themselves intravenously using nonsterile syringes or needles.

Yeasts exist in nature in a wide variety of organic substrates, including fruits, vegetables, and home-made fermented beverages. *Candida albicans*, the most frequent pathogen, is a normal inhabitant of the gastrointestinal tract of humans, various surveys showing an incidence of 20 to 40% in asymptomatic individuals. Another yeast, *Rhodotorula glutinis*, is a common inhabitant, in the tropics, of moist skin; its role as a pathogen is questionable, except for transient *Rhodotorula* fungaemia.

Because of the frequent association of yeasts with the internal and external environment of humans, their incidence in clinical specimens is rather high. For example, yeast colonies grew out in cultures from 1,606 out of 7,336 clinical specimens received at the mycology laboratory of the Columbia-Presbyterian Medical Center (CPMC) during the 12 months immediately preceding this writing. Whereas the number of positive yeast cultures amounted to 69% of all positive fungal isolations (2,325), it is estimated that less than 10% of the patients examined actually had systemic yeast infections.

For these reasons, collaboration between physician and laboratory is essential in assessing the possible etiological role of a yeast growing out in a clinical culture. Besides clinical and laboratory evaluation of the patient, critical mycological studies must include direct microscopic examination of fresh specimens and serological tests for specific antigens and antibodies as well as cultural isolation of significant yeasts.

COLLECTION, TRANSPORT, AND STORAGE OF SPECIMENS

Clinical specimens to be examined for the presence of yeasts of etiological significance can be collected in the same way as bacteriological specimens (see chapter 6), bearing in mind certain precautions and exceptions. A minimum of 5 ml of cerebrospinal fluid is essential for adequate sampling when culturing for *Cryptococcus* (17).

Commercial "Transport Media" should be avoided until their effects on yeasts have been evaluated.

Whenever possible, specimens for yeasts should be examined and cultured at the patient's bedside, or a portion of the specimen should be fixed as a dry smear or preserved in 10% Formalin to permit microscopic evaluation of the amount and morphology of the yeast at the moment of collection. For bedside cultures, Sabouraud agar slants in screw-capped tubes or bottles should be available at the locations where patients are examined. Other culture media will be described later.

DIRECT EXAMINATION

The identification of yeasts in a clinical specimen begins with the direct microscopic examination of stained or unstained samples of the specimen. Such examination does not permit exact species identification but does provide early clues which aid the physician in making a presumptive diagnosis and which aid the laboratory technologist in deciding which cultural and biochemical tests to utilize for further study. The mere presence of yeasts in properly collected specimens of body fluids which are normally sterile is immediately significant; however, the significance of yeasts in naturally contaminated specimens such as sputum, feces, and urine depends upon other considerations. The important clues to be gained from direct microscopy include: (i) the presence or absence of encapsulated yeasts (Fig. 1), (ii)

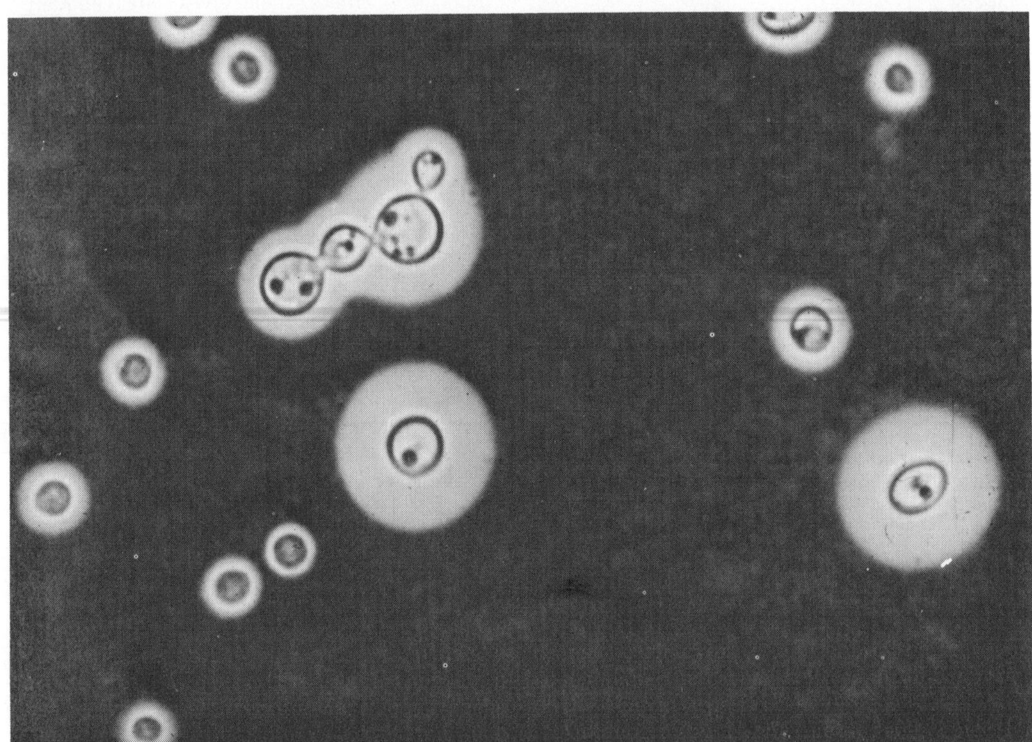

FIG. 1. *Cryptococcus neoformans. Nigrosin-stained wet preparation of sediment from centrifuged cerebrospinal fluid. Note encapsulated cells, some with wide capsules which probably originated in vivo; narrow capsules are probably on daughter cells "budded out" in vitro.*

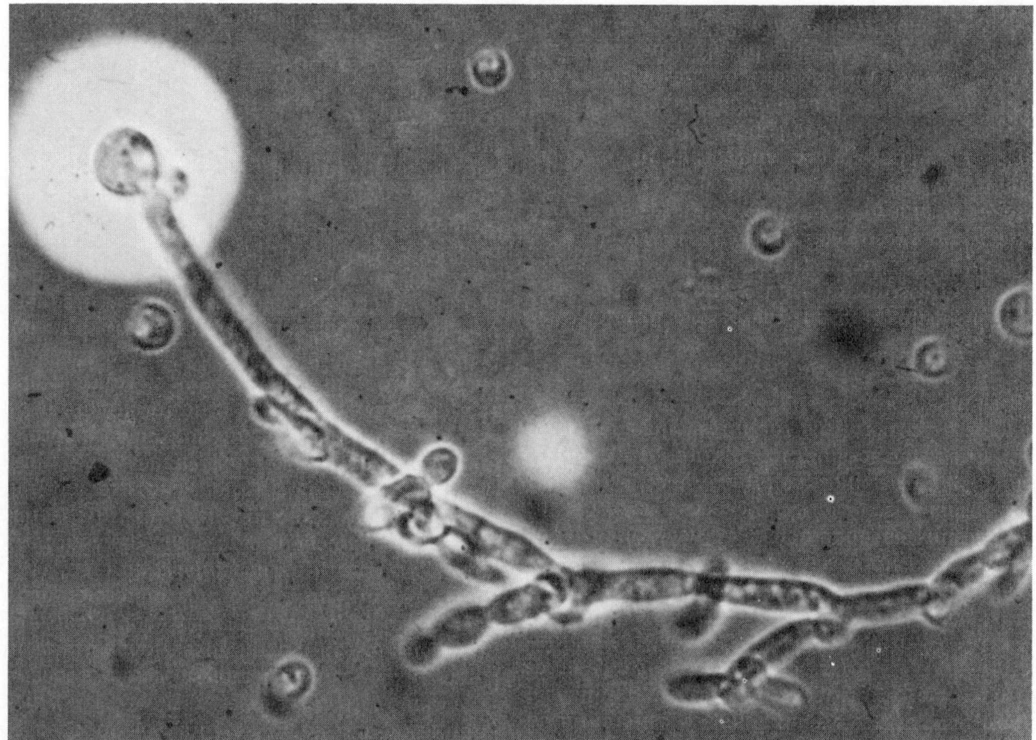

FIG. 2. *Cryptococcus neoformans. Unusual strain which produced pseudohyphae. Nigrosin-stained wet preparation of sediment from centrifuged cerebrospinal fluid.* ×*1,200.*

the presence or absence of pseudohyphae (Fig. 2), (iii) the presence or absence of true hyphae and arthrospores (Fig. 3), (iv) the size and shape of the yeast, and (v) the number of buds and the nature of their attachment to the mother cell.

To facilitate handling, specimens received by the laboratory should be sorted into groups according to type of material submitted.

Smears or scrapings

Smears or scrapings on glass slides can be examined by adding a drop of saline solution or of 10% NaOH. The latter should be used with fecal smears or with thick exudates or skin scrapings. Stains are seldom necessary, but yeasts can be detected in smears stained by the Gram, Ziehl-Neelsen, Giemsa, periodic acid-Schiff, or Gomori methenamine silver methods.

Cerebrospinal fluid, thoracentesis, or urine specimens

Specimens should be centrifuged or passed through a membrane filter to concentrate the sediment and increase the probability of finding yeasts. If urinary sediment is too heavy, dilute accordingly. Direct examination of a drop of sediment or of a piece of the membrane filter (cut and handled aseptically) can then be carried out. India ink or nigrosin may be added by capillarity under the cover slip as a negative "capsule stain" to reveal *Cryptococcus*, if present. Besides wet preparations, dry smears can be stained as described above.

Sputum or other mucous secretions

Flood the sputum cup with saline to reduce the viscosity of the mucus and enable particles or granules to float. These usually represent bits of tissue or cell accumulations which contain the fungi and should be selected for direct examination and culture. Alternatively, the specimen may be concentrated as described in chapter 57 before being examined microscopically and cultured.

Biopsy or autopsy tissue

Slice with sterile scalpel and examine all surfaces in search of ulcerations or granulomatous areas which usually contain the fungi. Eliminate residual tissue for reason given above.

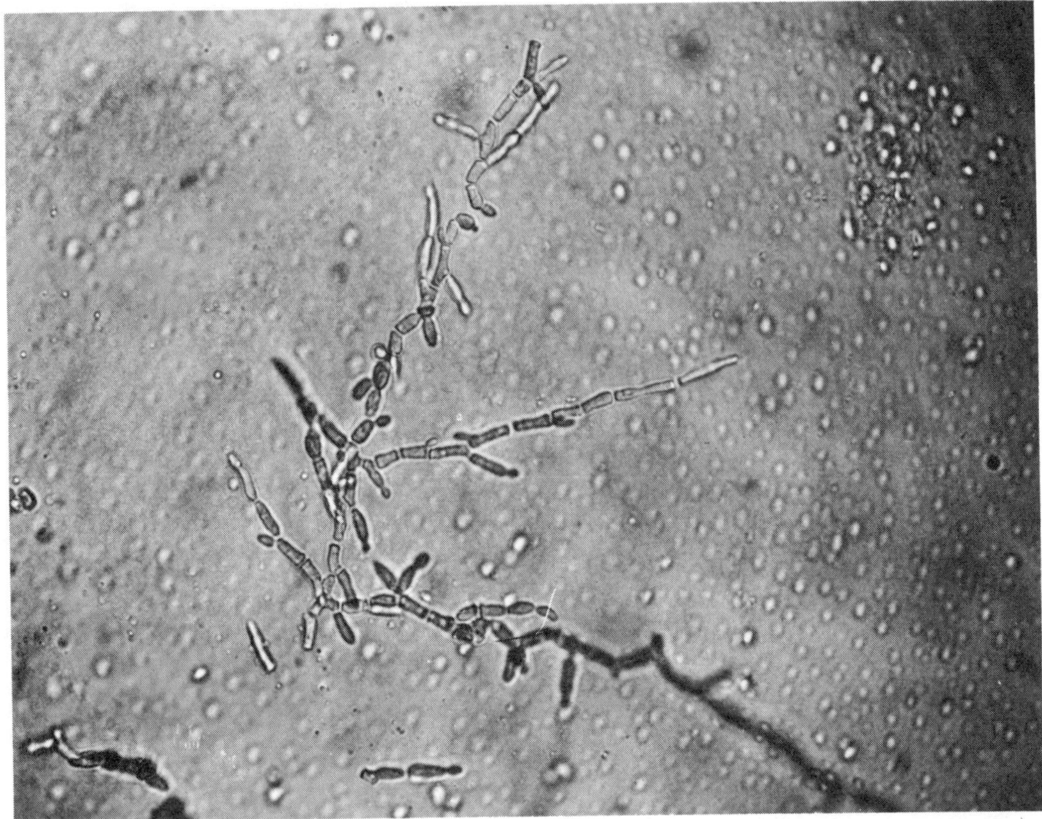

FIG. 3. *Trichosporon beigelii in fresh unstained preparation of sputum. ×600. Note arthrospores and blastospores characteristic of genus Trichosporon.*

Because of the possible occurrence of yeasts and yeastlike fungi as part of the transient or resident flora of the body and because they may proliferate rapidly in vitro, direct microscopic examination of clinical specimens must be done soon after collection. All specimens should be delivered to the diagnostic laboratory as soon as possible, even within minutes of collection.

CULTURE AND ISOLATION

The procedures for preparing specimens for primary culture of yeasts have been described in preceding sections of this chapter, and in chapters 53 and 57.

Media of choice

The routine isolation medium for yeasts is Sabouraud agar, without antibiotics. This can be used as slants or agar plates depending on the specimen. Supplementary media (not to be used at the *exclusion* of Sabouraud because they inhibit certain yeasts) are media with antibiotics. Especially useful among these is the same Sabouraud base plus chloramphenicol and cycloheximide (chapter 95) and Littman oxgall agar with streptomycin and gentian violet. Oxgall restricts colony diameter in fast-growing mold contaminants, which can overgrow the plate and prevent or mask growth of yeast colonies. It should be noted that cycloheximide inhibits *Cryptococcus* and several other yeasts (Table 1). Agar plates should be employed with sputum, soil, or other heavily contaminated specimens since this enables one to "touch spot" several points on the surface of the agar to attain spatial separation necessary for dilution or elimination of possible contaminants.

For primary isolation of yeasts from peripheral blood, a fungal blood culture vessel has been designed and used by the senior author for several years at the CPMC. This consists of a biphasic combination of a 1-cm layer of agar in a rectangular bottle overlaid with a 1-cm layer of Sabouraud broth. The advantage of such a bottle is that the broth dilutes any antibodies or other inhibitors in the blood (13) while stimulating yeast multiplication in the liquid phase. The agar layer permits the development of discrete yeast colonies which can be detected sometimes sooner than broth turbidity (often obscured by blood cells).

In addition to these media, a variety of agar media which contain salts of metals such as bismuth and molybdenum or which contain a tetrazolium dye are commercially available and provide early clues for the identification of yeast colonies based on color reactions. Such media are especially useful for detecting individual colonies in a mixed population of more than one yeast. An excellent differential medium for isolating *C. neoformans* can be prepared by adding to Littman oxgall agar an extract of seeds from the Indian thistle plant, *Guizotia abyssinica* (a seed common to birdseed mixtures) (6). *C. neoformans* characteristically produces brown colonies on this medium in 1 week when incubated at 25 C, a property not shown by other yeasts, including other *Cryptococcus* species. The medium was adapted from the original descriptions by Staib (31) and by Shields and Ajello (30), and all three media have come to be known by the common name "birdseed agar." The chemical responsible for pigment production has recently been identified (33), and the color reaction has been shown to be catalyzed by a phenol oxidase (29).

No matter which medium is employed, most human pathogenic yeasts will form pasty, opaque colonies at both 37 C and at ambient room temperature. For early presumptive identification of yeasts producing pseudohyphae, specimens positive on direct microscopic examination can be cut directly into corn meal agar as well as plated onto other isolation media.

IDENTIFICATION

Recommended procedures

The methods used for identifying yeast species are schematized in Fig. 4, and the cultural and biochemical characteristics of the most frequently encountered species in clinical specimens are summarized in Table 1. The initial steps include: (i) making a wet mount and stained smears for microscopic observation; (ii) making an India ink preparation; (iii) doing a germ tube test; and (iv) inoculating Wolin-Bevis or cornmeal agar for detecting pseudohyphae and chlamydospores (1, 3, 8, 11). At the same time that these tests are being done, each distinct colony type should be restreaked on bacteriological media such as brain heart infusion agar with or without 10% blood and incubated at 37 C, as well as on Sabouraud agar and incubated at 25 C, to ensure that pure cultures are obtained for further biochemical testing.

Cultural characteristics

Most yeasts grow well on the common mycological and bacteriological media, producing visible colonies within 48 to 72 h. Most pathogens grow readily at both 25 and 37 C. Although many pathogenic yeasts grow best at 37 C, most saprophytic yeasts encountered in clinical specimens fail to grow at 37 C. The ability to grow at this temperature is an important characteristic for differentiating species. Some species are inhibited by cycloheximide or chloramphenicol. In certain species, sporulation may be enhanced by the use of special media. The growth and temperature requirements for the several genera and the indications for using special media are summarized at the end of this section.

Pellicle formation on broth. When yeasts are cultivated in tubes of liquid media such as Sabouraud broth or malt extract broth, their growth takes the form of (i) a sediment in the bottom of the tube, (ii) a ring around the circumference of the broth surface, (iii) a film on the surface, or (iv) a surface pellicle. These growth characteristics depend largely on the oxygen requirements of the yeast. In the past, emphasis was placed on the ability to form a surface pellicle on liquid media as an important taxonomic property, but more recent evidence has demonstrated this to be a variable characteristic (15) and it is no longer stressed as much as it once was. However, the appearance of the growth of a yeast in liquid media can be used as one clue to identification of species. Pellicle-forming yeasts often isolated from clinical specimens include *C. tropicalis*, *C. krusei*, and especially *Trichosporon* species.

Microscope examination of culture growth

Wet preparations of primary cultures in distilled water, India ink, nigrosin, or lactophenol cotton blue, or dried smears stained by the Gram or Ziehl-Neelsen method, provide clues for microscopic morphology, presence or absence of capsules, presence or absence of ascospores, and purity of cultures. For further morphological study, special media are necessary. Incubation of yeast cells in blood serum or egg white at 37 C for 1 to 4 h permits observation of germ tube production (*C. albicans*). Subculture by cut-streaking cornmeal infusion agar or Wolin-Bevis (39) agar plates followed by incu-

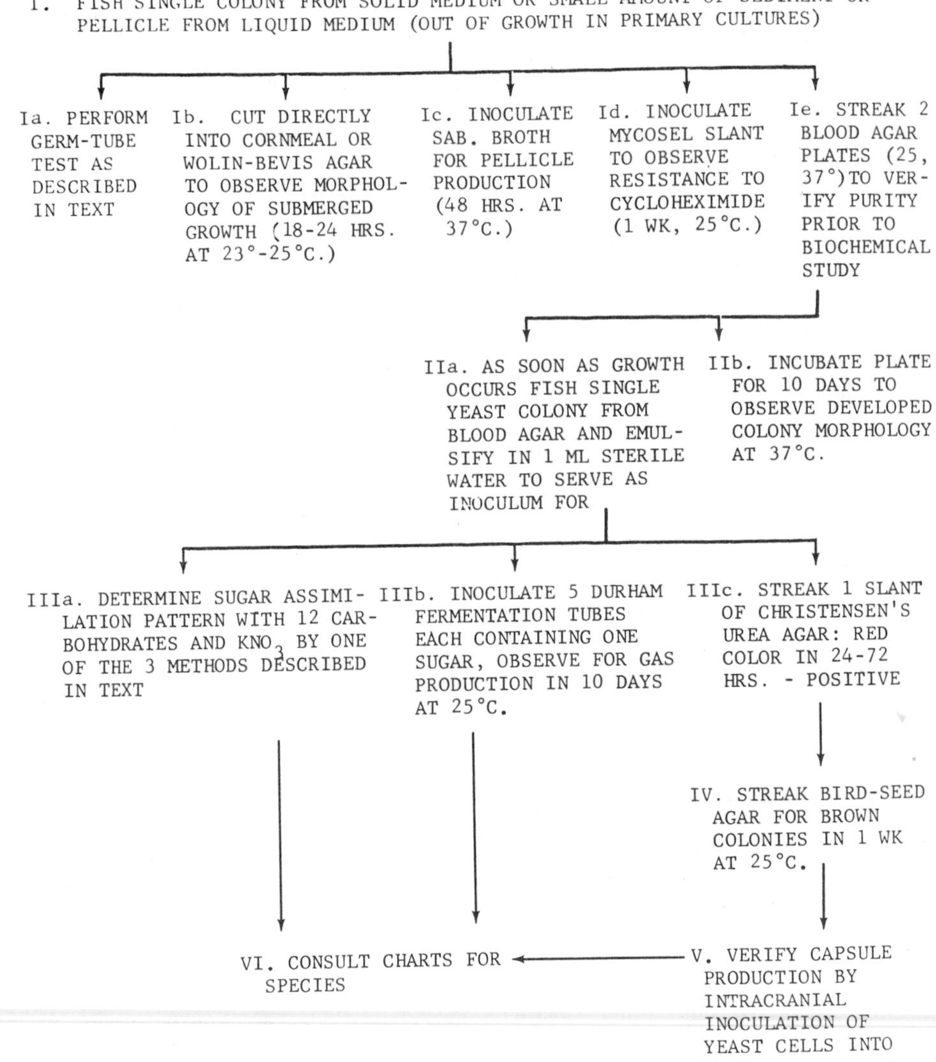

FIG. 4. *Schema for a step-by-step procedure that can be followed in the isolation and identification of yeasts from primary cultures of clinical specimens.*

bation at 23 to 25 C for 18 to 48 h permits detection of pseudomycelium, true mycelium, and/or chlamydospores (see Table 1). Special sporulation media (chapter 95) may be necessary to detect ascospore production whose presence and characteristic morphology are essential to identification of ascosporogenous genera found in clinical specimens such as *Saccharomyces*, *Pichia*, *Endomycopsis*, and *Nematospora*.

Many of these procedures can be carried out directly with primary cultures prior to purification, and even with the original specimen.

Germ tube test. One of the most valuable tests for rapid, presumptive identification of *C. albicans* is the germ tube test. In this test, one only needs to make a dilute suspension of a yeast colony in 0.5 to 1.0 ml of serum, accomplished by touching the tip of a sterile Pasteur pipette to a yeast colony and then gently emulsifying the cells which adhere to the pipette in the serum. The mixture is then incubated at 37 C for 2 to 4 h after which a drop of the mixture is examined microscopically for germ tubes, which can be seen in Fig. 5. As a convenience, the pipette can be left in the

TABLE 1. *Cultural and biochemical characteristics of yeasts frequently isolated from clinical specimens*

Species	Growth at 37 C	Pellicle, broth	Pseudo/true hyphae	Chlamydospores	Germ tubes	Capsule, India ink	Assimilations												Fermentations					Urease activity	KNO_3 utilization	Brown colonies on birdseed agar	Cycloheximide resistance
							Glucose	Maltose	Sucrose	Lactose	Galactose	Melibiose	Cellobiose	Inositol	Xylose	Raffinose	Trehalose	Dulcitol	Glucose	Maltose	Sucrose	Lactose	Galactose				
Candida albicans	+	−	+	+	+	−	+	+	+	−	+	−	−	−	+	−	+	−	F	F	−*	−	F	−	−	−	+
C. stellatoidea	+	−	+	+	+	−	+	+	−	−	+	−	−	−	+	−	+*	−	F	F	−	−	−	−	−	−	+
C. tropicalis	+	+	+	+[b]	−	−	+	+	+	−	+	−	+*	−	+	−	+	−	F	F	F	−	F	−	−	−	−
C. parapsilosis	+	−	+	−	−	−	+	+	+	−	+	−	−	−	+	−	+	−	F	−	−	−	F*	−	−	−	−
C. krusei	+	+	+	−	−	−	+	−	−	−	−	−	−	−	−	−	−	−	F	−	−	−	−	+*	−	−	−
C. pseudotropicalis	+	−	+	−	−	−	+	−	+	+	+	−	+	−	+*	+	−	−	F	−	F	F	F	−	−	−	+
C. guillermondii	+	−	+	−	−	−	+	+	+	−	+	+	+	−	+	+	+	+	F	−	F	−	F	−	−	−	+
C. rugosa	−	−	+	−	−	−	+	−	−	−	−	+	−	−	+	−	−	−	−	−	−	−	−	−	−	−	−
Cryptococcus neoformans	+	−	*R*	−	−	+	+	+	+	−	+	−	+	+	+	+*	+	+	−	−	−	−	−	+	−	+	−
C. albidus var. *albidus*	−*	−	+*	−	−	+	+	+	+	+*	−*	−*	+	+	+	+	+*	+	−	−	−	−	−	+	+	−	−
C. albidus var. *diffluens*	+	−	−	−	−	+	+	+	+	−	−*	+*	+	+	+	+	+	+*	−	−	−	−	−	+	+	−	−
C. luteolus	−	−	−	−	−	−	+	+	+	−	+	+	+	+	+	−*	+	+*	−	−	−	−	−	+	−	−	−
C. laurentii	+	−	−	−	−	+	+	+	+	+	+	+*	+	+	+	+*	+	+	−	−	−	−	−	+	−	−	−
C. uniguttulatus	−	−	−	−	−	+	+	+	+	−	−*	−	−*	+	+	+*	+*	−	−	−	−	−	−	+	−	−	−
C. terreus	+	−	−	−	−	+	+	+*	−*	−*	+*	−	+	+	+	−	+	+*	−	−	−	−	−	+	+	−	−
C. gastricus	−	−	−	−	−	+	+	+	−*	−	+	−	+	+	+	−	+	−	−	−	−	−	−	+	−	−	−
Rhodotorula glutinis	−	−	−	−	−	−	+	+	+	−	+*	−	+	−	+	+	+	−	−	−	−	−	−	+	+	−	−
R. rubra (mucilaginosa)	+*	−	−	−	−	−	+	+	+	−	+*	−	+*	−	+	+	+	−	−	−	−	−	−	+	−	−	+*
Saccharomyces cerevisiae	+	−	+*	−	−	−	+	+	+	−	+	−	−	−	−	+	+*	−	F	F	F	−	F	−	−	−	−
Torulopsis glabrata	+	−	−	−	−	−	+	−	−	−	−	−	−	−	−	−	+	−	F	−	−	−	−	−	−	−	−
T. pintolopesii	+[c]	−	−	−	−	−	+	−	−	−	−	−	−	−	−	−	−	−	F	−	−	−	−	−	−	−	−
Trichosporon beigelii	+*	+	+	−	−	−	+	+*	+*	+	+	+*	+	+*	+	+*	+*	+*	−	−	−	−	−	+*	−	−	+
T. capitatum	+	+	+	−	−	−	+	−	−	−	+	−	−	−	−	−	−	−	−	−	−	−	−	−	−	−	+
T. pullulans	+	+	+	−	−	−	+	+	+	+	+	+*	+	+*	+	+*	+	−	−	−	−	−	−	+	+	−	+
T. penicillatum	+	+	+	−	−	−	+	−	−	−	+	−	−	−	+	−	−	−	−	−	−	−	−	−	−	−	+
T. inkin	+	+	+	−	−	−	+	+	+	+	+	−	+	+	+	−	+	−	−	−	−	−	−	−	−	−	−
Geotrichum candidum	−	+	+	−	−	−	+	−	−	−	+	−	−	−	+	−	−	−	−	−	−	−	−	−	−	−	−

[a] Asterisks indicate strain variation; R, rare. Under Assimilations, plus signs indicate growth greater than the control; under Fermentations, F indicates that sugar is fermented (i.e., gas is produced).

[b] Occasional strains of *C. tropicalis* produce tear drop-shaped chlamydospores.

[c] *T. pintolopesii* is a thermophilic yeast capable of growth at 40 to 42 C.

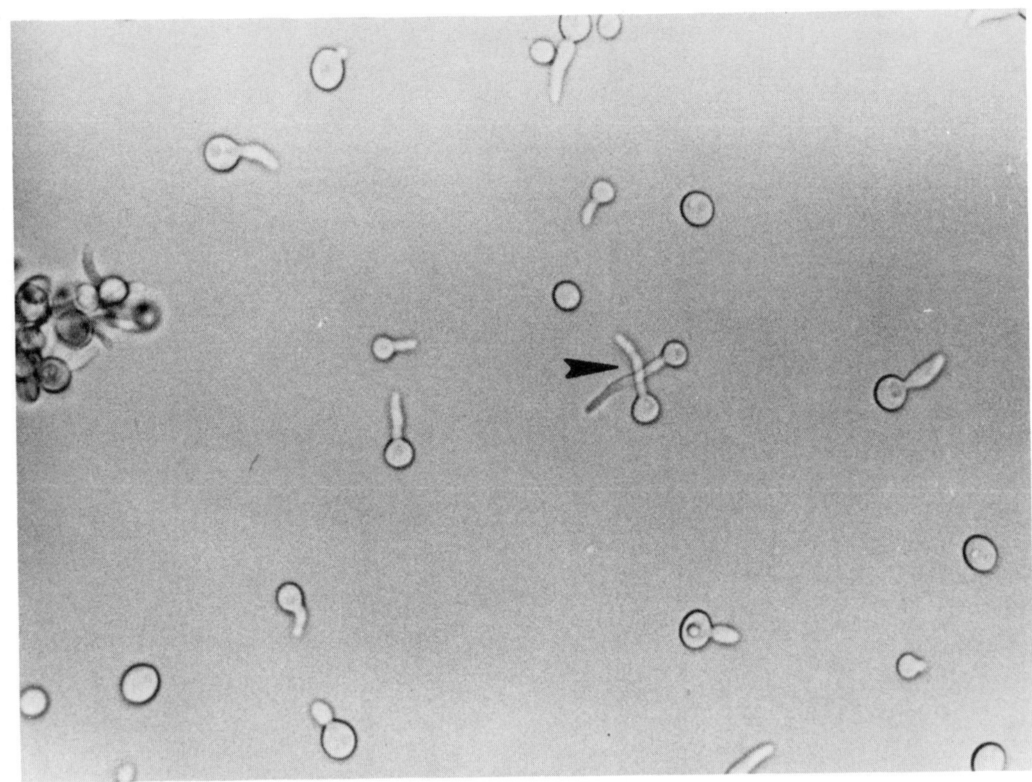

FIG. 5. *Candida albicans. Germ tubes (arrow) formed after incubation in serum for 2 h at 37 C. ×1,500.*

serum during the incubation period and used to transfer a drop of the serum to a slide for microscopic examination. When incubated in this fashion, individual yeast cells of *C. albicans* and/or *C. stellatoidea* produce short lateral hyphal filaments called germ tubes which are not produced by other *Candida* species. *C. stellatoidea* and *C. albicans* are easily differentiated by a sucrose assimilation test. *C. albicans* assimilates sucrose; *C. stellatoidea* does not. Human and bovine serum, including fetal calf serum which is commercially available, bovine serum albumin, or ovalbumin, can be used with success in this procedure, and a recent report (14) described the use of peptone for the germ tube test. Known strains of *C. albicans* and *C. tropicalis* should be included as positive and negative controls, respectively.

Chlamydospores. Another standard technique for identifying yeasts is to test for production of chlamydospores. A variety of media are available for this test including chlamydospore agar, Wolin-Bevis (39) agar, cornmeal Tween 80 agar, and rice Tween 80 agar. The choice of medium is based largely on individual preference. The technique described here utilizes Wolin-Bevis or cornmeal Tween 80 agar. Spherical chlamydospores are produced by *C. albicans* and to a lesser extent by *C. stellatoidea*, when inoculated into these nutritionally poor media. *C. tropicalis* occasionally produces distinct oval- to teardrop-shaped chlamydospores. Chlamydospores of the type formed by *C. albicans* are shown in Fig. 6. In addition, all species of *Candida* will form pseudohyphae, and species of *Trichosporon* will form true hyphae and arthrospores on this type of medium.

For the test, cut the yeast colony or original specimen in two or three parallel lines 1 cm apart on the agar. Incubate at room temperature (23 to 25 C) for 18 to 48 h, by which time most strains of *C. albicans* and *C. stellatoidea* will have formed typical chlamydospores. This technique is also useful for demonstrating giant pseudohyphae of *C. parapsilosis*. The experienced eye can also recognize the typical morphological patterns of other *Candida* species (3). Confirmation by biochemical reactions is recommended.

Biochemical reactions

Before any biochemical reactions are measured, it is *essential* to purify yeast cultures as described above. This should be done even if contamination is not immediately apparent, since a hidden contaminant can significantly alter the results.

Biochemical reactions useful in yeast identification include (i) assimilation of carbohydrates (currently 12 sugars are used with clinical isolates), (ii) assimilation of KNO_3, (iii) fermentation reactions (i.e., gas production using five sugars), (iv) urease production, (v) ability to produce brown colonies on birdseed agar, and (vi) resistance to cycloheximide. Other biological characteristics tested are (i) ability to grow at 37 C, (ii) ability to form a pellicle on broth, and (iii) animal pathogenicity (1, 3, 8, 9, 11).

Besides the above routine tests, mention should be made of certain other characteristics currently employed by research investigators as taxonomic criteria for yeasts. Some of these may eventually be adapted for use in clinical laboratories. They include (i) analysis of cell wall components by gas chromatography, nuclear magnetic resonance spectra, and methylation techniques, (ii) determination of the percentage of guanine plus cytosine in the deoxyribonucleic acid (DNA) of a given strain, (iii) amino acid sequencing of cytochrome *c* or other protein components, (iv) somatic cell hybridization or DNA hybridization techniques, and (v) determination of temperature for growth, and of other nutritional imbalances.

Following the flow sheet for identification procedures (Fig. 4), a description is given of the methods we recommend as routine procedures. Alternate methods are also listed.

Urease. Urea is split by yeasts having urease, including all species of *Cryptococcus* and *Rhodotorula*, and some species of *Trichosporon* (26). Occasional strains of *Candida krusei* are urease-positive. The test is performed by transferring with a sterile loop a portion of a yeast colony to a slant of Christensen urea agar. The slant is incubated at 25 to 30 C and examined daily for 4 days. Change in the amber color of the medium to pink or red denotes a positive reaction due to alkalinization of the phenolphthalein indicator in the medium.

Carbohydrate assimilation tests. Tests to

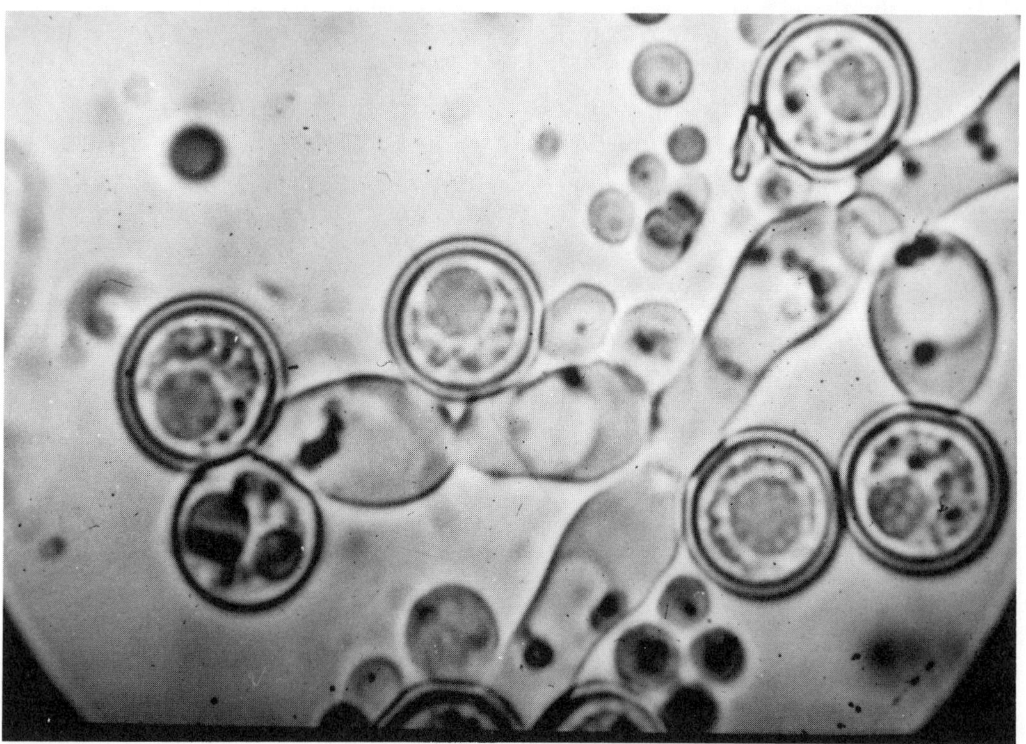

FIG. 6. *Candida albicans. Submerged mycelium with spherical clusters of blastospores and double-walled spherical chlamydospores on corn meal agar.* ×*1,500.*

determine the ability of a yeast to utilize a carbohydrate as sole source of carbon in a chemically defined medium have long been a major tool of yeast taxonomists (38), but such tests are avoided by many technologists who regard them as being difficult to set up and interpret.

In actual fact, assimilation tests provide a definitive biochemical basis and shorten the time required for speciating yeasts. A brief review of these methods is presented in the following paragraphs.

(*1*) *Auxanography*. Modifications of Beijerinck's auxanographic technique (4) for determining assimilation patterns are widely used. In this method, small amounts of dry carbohydrates are placed on a heavily inoculated synthetic agar medium. Growth occurs in the area where an assimilated compound was placed. No growth denotes lack of those enzymes necessary for utilization of the test carbohydrate; the pattern of carbohydrates supporting growth is called an auxanogram. Although mutations involving enzymes essential to carbohydrate utilization are well known for yeasts, the auxanogram is an adequately dependable characteristic for identification of each species when used in conjunction with other tests. Modification of Beijerinck's method currently in use include: (i) streaking the surface, rather than seeding the agar plate; (ii) using filter paper disks impregnated with the carbohydrates; (iii) placing drops of carbohydrate solutions on the agar; and (iv) placing the carbon sources in wells cut out of the agar in a petri dish.

Auxanography is the method of choice for assimilation tests at CPMC. For inoculation, each of two agar plates containing basal medium (Wickerham yeast nitrogen base, Difco) is streaked thoroughly and completely with a cotton swab containing a heavy inoculum of the test organism so as to obtain confluent growth over the entire plate. Immediately after streaking, 6 of the 12 carbohydrate disks, separated by equal distances, are placed on each plate. For maximal separation, the disks are placed at the extreme circumference of the agar surface against the vertical wall of the petri dish. Plates are incubated at room temperature (25 C) and read for growth around the carbohydrate disks occurring between 72 h and 7 days (Fig. 7).

(*2*) *Wickerham broth technique*. This technique as originally recommended by Wickerham (36, 38) uses the same chemically defined medium as above, but in liquid form. The broth tubes containing individual sugars (or carbohydrate disks as employed at CPMC) is inoculated either with a "starved" suspension of the yeast grown for 48 h in the basal medium without a carbon source or with a drop from a dilute suspension of a yeast colony in distilled water. Twelve tubes, each containing one of the sugars listed in Table 1, are inoculated for each isolate, the tubes are incubated at room temperature

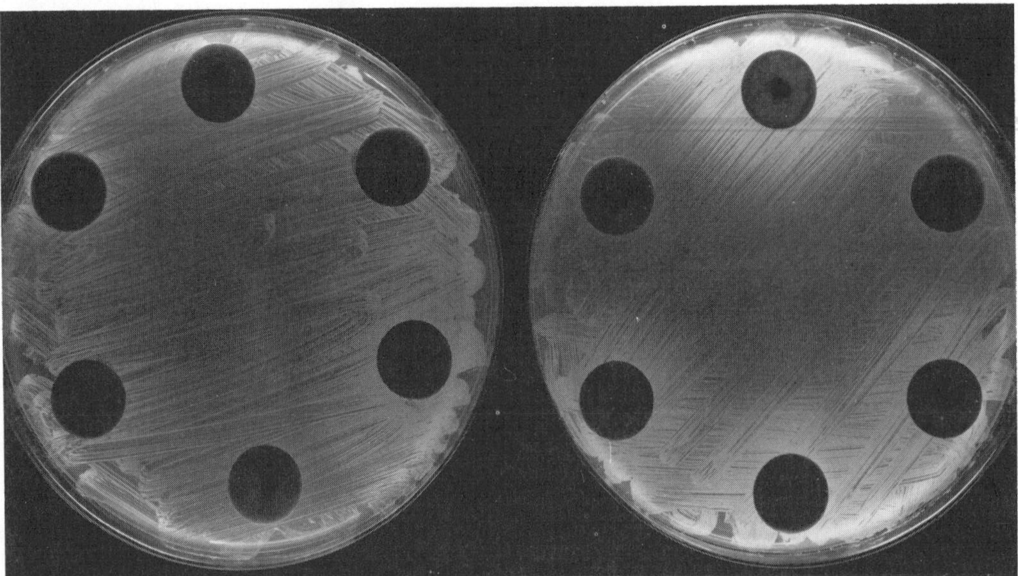

FIG. 7. *Candida pseudotropicalis. Auxanographic plates showing growth around disks of glucose, sucrose, lactose, galactose, cellobiose, xylose, and raffinose. One-half actual size.*

(25 C) and growth is evaluated turbidimetrically. When a carbon source is assimilated, the growth clouds the medium so that black lines or letters will not show through. Ahearn et al. (2) recommend shaking the tubes during incubation.

(3) *Assimilation agar slant technique.* A recent modification of the Wickerham broth method which involves neutralizing the medium to pH 7.0, adding a pH indicator (bromocresol purple), and solidifying the individual carbohydrates in yeast nitrogen base in agar slants has been used with success at Temple University Hospital (E. D. Adams and B. H. Cooper, Amer. J. Med. Tech., in press). The exact procedure for preparation of this medium is given in chapter 95. For inoculation, a dilute suspension of the yeast to be tested is prepared by suspending a single colony in 9 ml of sterile distilled water. This suspension is then inoculated in 0.1-ml volumes onto each assimilation slant, incubated at 25 C, and observed for growth. Assimilations are considered positive when abundant growth appears on a test medium with negligible or no growth on the control slant; results may be reported in 72 h, but slants should be held for 14 days to allow for delayed reactions. Assimilations are considered negative where there is no significant difference between the carbohydrate medium and the control medium. As growth occurs, acid production changes the indicator from purple to yellow (Fig. 8).

Nitrate assimilation. Tests of ability of a yeast to utilize nitrate as sole nitrogen source can be carried out by any one of these same procedures except that Wickerham yeast carbon base is used as the basal medium, and potassium nitrate (final concentration 0.078 g/100 ml) and peptone (1%) are used as the test nitrogen sources. The peptone serves as a positive growth control.

Fermentation reactions. Carbohydrate fermentation tests are familiar, useful tests for identifying yeasts. However, these tests are more subject to variation and are less dependable than carbohydrate assimilation tests. The only reliable evidence for carbohydrate fermentation by yeasts is production of gas; therefore, Durham tube inserts should be employed for gas detection. The basal medium employed includes peptone, yeast extract, and bromocresol purple indicator; the pH is adjusted to 7.0. The carbohydrates routinely employed are glucose, maltose, sucrose, lactose, and galactose. For inoculation, the same suspension used in inoculating assimilation tests in liquid media may be employed. Readings are made after incubation at 25 C for 10 to 14 days. All fermented carbohydrates will also be assimilated; however, certain carbohydrates will be assimilated, but not fermented.

Serological methods

Fluorescent-antibody techniques with specific conjugates are extremely useful in those instances where cultures have failed and yet yeasts are observed in histological sections, body fluids, or exudates (chapters 4 and 62). These techniques, along with agar gel precipitins, slide or tube agglutination, or immunoelectrophoresis, are also useful in specific differentiation of yeasts provided suitably absorbed, species-specific antisera are employed (34).

Differentiation from related species

Since yeasts, as already stated, are a heterogeneous conglomerate of various fungal taxa, this chapter by necessity points out differences among yeast genera and species. It is important, however, to mention also certain other organisms encountered in clinical specimens that produce colonies resembling yeasts on the same isolation media. For the most part these microorganisms must be identified by methods other than those used for yeasts. The following are examples of such microorganisms.

Geotrichum. This is a filamentous fungus whose initial growth may be glabrous and creamy to pasty, but becomes velvety with aging on repeated subculture. Microscopically, *Geotrichum* produces true hyphae and arthrospores, but neither pseudohyphae nor blastospores, thus differing morphologically from the yeast genus *Trichosporon*. Further differentiation can be obtained by physiological and biochemical tests (24). Fluffy strains of *Geotrichum* superficially resemble the systemic pathogen *Coccidioides immitis* and must be differentiated from it.

Prototheca. This colorless alga which is also encountered in clinical specimens (and may be a pathogen) produces colonies resembling those of *Cryptococcus* on Sabouraud agar. It differs in having no capsule, a less refringent cell wall, and in producing characteristic endospores by internal segmentation into eight (or more) compartments (7). *Prototheca* species can also be differentiated by staining with specific immunofluorescent conjugates (34).

Ustilago. This basidiomycetous genus is another filamentous fungus which can occasionally grow out of sputum specimens and produce yeastlike colonies. At first unicellular, it soon produces short hyphae with clamp connections,

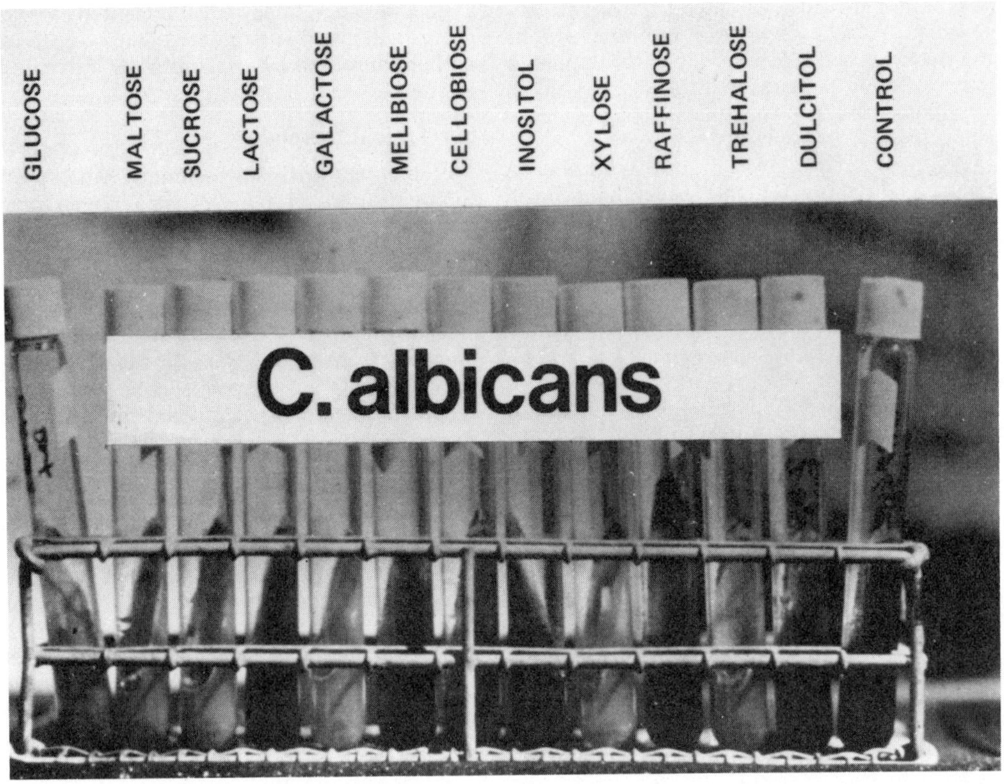

FIG. 8. *Candida albicans. Assimilation test using modified Wickerham medium in agar slants. Growth and acid production on slants of glucose, maltose, sucrose, galactose, xylose, and trehalose. One-half actual size.*

and its colonies become finely powdery or velvety. Even at the unicellular stage, the elongated cells characteristic of this genus differentiate it from yeasts.

Animal inoculation

Techniques for isolating *C. neoformans* and other pathogenic yeasts from contaminated specimens by animal inoculation are discussed in chapter 57. Demonstration of pathogenicity as an aid to differentiation of *C. neoformans* from other cryptococci can be accomplished by intracranial inoculation of 0.05 ml of a saline suspension containing a 0.2% concentration of yeast cells (1:500 by volume of packed cells) into each of two 20- to 30-g white mice. Alternatively, 0.5 to 1 ml of the yeast cell suspension can be injected intravenously or intraperitoneally into mice. The majority of strains of *C. neoformans* are lethal for mice when injected intracranially within 4 to 5 days, and microscopic examination of brain tissue from infected mice clearly demonstrates encapsulated yeast cells.

Pathogenicity of *C. albicans* can be demonstrated by injecting 0.2 to 0.8 ml of a 1% suspension of packed cells into the marginal ear vein of a 1- to 2-kg rabbit, or of a similar volume of an 0.2% suspension into the tail vein of a 20- to 30-g mouse. Death of the animal usually occurs within 1 week, and at autopsy miliary abscesses in the kidneys and sometimes in the spleen and liver will be observed. Pathogenicity of *C. albicans* can also be demonstrated by chick embryo inoculation (22).

CHARACTERISTICS OF INDIVIDUAL MEDICALLY IMPORTANT YEAST GENERA

Genus Candida

A heterogeneous genus presently classified within the family *Cryptococcacea*, Fungi Imperfecti (*Deuteromycetes*). *Candida* species are frequently present as members of the normal flora of the mouth, throat, large intestine, vagina, and skin, and are often present as contaminants in exudates or other specimens taken from these areas. In patients whose immune defenses have been compromised by disease or by the secondary effects of drugs used to treat their diseases, these normal flora organisms may invade the deeper tissues to produce severe, life-threatening infections. *C. albicans*, the principal pathogenic species, causes mild to severe or chronic superficial infections of skin, nails, and mucous membranes in individuals with normal immune defenses, as well as serious systemic infections in debilitated patients. *C. parapsilosis*, *C. tropicalis*, and *C. guillermondii* have become important causes of endocarditis of patients with indwelling intravenous catheters, patients undergoing cardiovascular surgery, and drug addicts.

Cultural characteristics. Budding cells (blastospores) round, oval, or oblong, 2.5 by 3 to 14 μm, single or in clusters or chains. Abundant pseudohyphae usually produced on nutritionally poor media, along with secondary blastospores in species-characteristic patterns. Production of germ tubes (Fig. 5) and spherical chlamydospores (Fig. 6) by *C. albicans* and *C. stellatoidea* are useful identifying characteristics. Ascospores have been reported in certain species which subsequently have been assigned to perfect genera. For example, ascospore-forming strains of *C. guillermondii* have been assigned to the genus *Pichia* (37).

Growth is aerobic. Tiny colonies may be visible as early as 24 to 36 h and attain a size of 1.5 to 2 mm in 5 or 7 days on Sabouraud agar. Colonies are usually stark white in color, but may become cream-colored or tan with age. They are glabrous, creamy, or membranous, and may have a fringe of submerged hyphae. Optimal growth temperature is 25 to 37 C.

Biochemical characteristics (Table 1). Carbohydrates are utilized in oxidative (assimilation) or fermentative patterns, or both, that are helpful in differentiating species. Urease is negative except for occasional strains of *C. krusei*. KNO_3 is not utilized by frequently encountered clinical isolates.

Animal pathogenicity. *C. albicans* is lethal to mice and rabbits when injected intravenously, causing miliary abscesses in the kidneys and other organs. Other *Candida* species may also produce lesions (12), but they are seldom lethal for experimental animals that have not been pretreated with corticosteroids or other immunosuppressive drugs (16).

Genus Cryptococcus

Formerly classified in the same family as the genus *Candida* and, like *Candida*, now believed to be a heterogeneous genus. Its only recognized pathogenic species, *Cryptococcus neoformans*, and probably also *C. albidus*, are believed to be in the heterobasidiomycete genus *Leucosporidium* (27). Infections by *C. neoformans* are exogenous, this yeast living naturally on soil contaminated with bird droppings, particularly from pigeons and other seed-eating birds. Meningitis is the most frequently recognized type of cryptococcal infection, followed by localized abscesses or granulomas (cryptococcoma or toruloma) in the lungs, brain, lymph nodes, skin, or bones. Diffuse pulmonary infection is perhaps the most common type of cryptococcal infection, though often asymptomatic and unrecognized. The respiratory tract is believed to be the portal of entry for most, if not all, cryptococcal infections.

Blastospores are chiefly spherical in shape and exhibit a wide range of diameters (from 5 to 30 μm). A polysaccharide capsule (Fig. 1) is a constant feature, although it is much more prominent in infected tissues or when suspended in immune sera than in cultures (10). The capsule can be demonstrated in wet preparations by negative staining with India ink or nigrosin or by mounting the cells in a drop of normal serum with a drop of 1% acetic acid, or it can be demonstrated in immune serum. The capsule also is revealed by mucin stains such as mucicarmine or alcian blue. This feature permits the specific identification of *C. neoformans* in histopathological sections since other yeasts which invade human tissues are not revealed by these dyes.

Colony morphology often is mucoid, becoming dull and progressively drier with age. Colonies on Sabouraud agar initially are pale buff in color, changing from tan to brown as they age. This genus does not ordinarily form mycelium or ascospores, though occasional isolates have been encountered which produce pseudomycelium (28) (Fig. 2) and structures suggestive of endospores (5). Hyphae-forming strains of *C. neoformans* which produce clamp connections have been observed (27), suggesting an affinity with *Leucosporidium*.

Growth. Aerobic. Grows well on ordinary bacteriological and mycological media, attaining colony diameters of 1 to 3 mm in less than 1 week; inhibited by cycloheximide. Bacteria, serum factors, or tissue inhibitors in clinical specimens may delay appearance of colonies by as much as 2 to 4 weeks. Optimal temperature varies with the species (see Table 1).

Biochemical characteristics. Metabolism is

strictly oxidative; the assimilation of certain sugars and of KNO_3 is useful in differentiation of species (Table 1). The utilization of inositol (23) and the usual absence of carotenoid pigments distinguish this genus from *Rhodotorula;* both genera have capsules, produce starchlike compounds, and are urease-positive. *C. neoformans* can be differentiated from other *Cryptococcus* species by (i) ability to grow at 37 C, (ii) production of brown colonies on birdseed agar, (iii) characteristic assimilation pattern, (iv) pathogenicity for experimental animals, and (v) ability to utilize creatinine as its sole carbon source (9, 32).

Animal pathogenicity. *C. neoformans*, but not other species of *Cryptococcus*, is lethal for mice by invasion of the brain, which is reached by direct intracranial inoculation or by neurotropic extension from the intravenous or intraperitoneal routes.

Genus Pichia

This genus contains the perfect form of *Candida guilliermondii* and belongs to the subfamily *Saccharomycetoideae* of the family *Saccharomycetaceae* of the *Ascomycetes*. Of many strains of *C. guilliermondii* tested, only a few have been found to produce ascospores (37), which are hat-shaped and occur in numbers ranging from one to four per ascus. The growth characteristics, biochemical reactions, and other laboratory reactions of the perfect form should be the same as those of the imperfect species which are listed in Table 1.

Genus Pityrosporum

Members of the *Cryptococcaceae*, responsible for blepharitis, dacryocystitis, and ocular invasion. Associated with dandruff and seborrhea and probable cause of tinea versicolor. May be identical with *Malassezia*, but *Pityrosporum* has priority (see chapter 54). Isolated from clinical specimens of above lesions and also from comedones and from oily areas of the skin and scalp of various mammals.

Bottle-shaped small budding cells 1 to 2 by 2 to 4 μm, reproducing by a process known as bud fission in which the bud detaches from the mother cell by a septum. Short hyphae were reported by Panja in vitro (21) but are more generally observed in tinea versicolor scales. No ascospores.

Growth. Aerobic, on media containing lipids or fatty acids. Grows well at 37 C, forming colonies that are creamy and punctiform when young; later membranous and confluent.

Biochemical characteristics. No fermentative ability. Requires lipids or specific fatty acids, such as myristic, palmitic, and oleic acids, for growth.

Genus Rhodotorula

This genus (family *Cryptococcaceae*, subfamily *Rhodotoruloideae*) may be reduced to synonymy with the genus *Cryptococcus*, which it resembles in rate of growth, colony topography, cell size and shape, occasional rudimentary pseudomycelium, presence of a capsule, ability to split urea, and lack of fermentative ability. Its lack of pathogenicity, different serotype, and conspicuous carotenoid pigment have maintained *Rhodotorula* as a distinct genus (23). *Cryptococcus*, further, can use inositol, invade human and animal tissues, and cause death (*C. neoformans*). *Rhodotorula* is a normal symbiont of humid skin (due to climate or to patient's abnormal physiology); *R. rubra* (*mucilaginosa*) and *R. glutinis* have caused transient blood stream invasion (fungaemia) but not actual infection of host tissues. A frequent source of this problem is the contamination of rubber or plastic tubing left in place during prolonged intravenous therapy. *Rhodotorula* spp. are also cultured readily from shower curtains, bath tub-wall junctions, and the rubber tips and handles of tooth brushes if not properly aerated.

Genus Saccharomyces

Member of family *Saccharomycetaceae* (ascosporogenous). *S. cerevisiae* responsible for occasional cases of thrush and vulvovaginitis; also reported from urine specimens in diabetics.

Oval to spherical cells, 3 by 5 μm. Can exist as budding cells in either haploid or diploid conditions (following fusion). May form short chains and elongate as pseudohyphae. Ascospores, one to four in number, in either tetrahedral or linear arrangement (Fig. 9), gram-negative (vegetative cells are gram-positive). An excellent sporulation medium is the potassium acetate-yeast extract-glucose medium (ascospore medium) of McClary (18) modified from Adams (chapter 95).

Occasional production of rudimentary pseudomycelium; this genus is the perfect state of *Candida robusta*, a nonpathogen.

Growth. Rapid growth on most media, both aerobically and anaerobically; optimal temperature, 25 to 37 C.

Biochemical reactions. Fermentative and assimilative action on sugars in pattern that is useful for identification (Table 1). *S. cerevisiae*

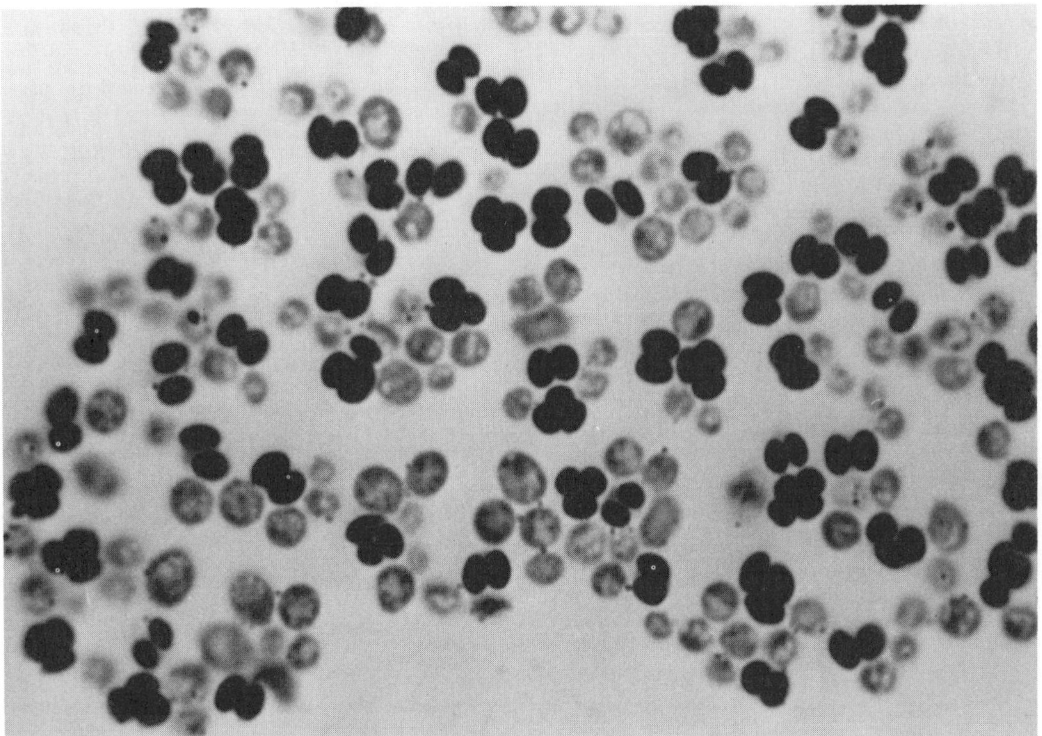

FIG. 9. *Saccharomyces cerevisiae. Ascospores (darkly stained cells) from culture grown on acetate medium of McClary (18). Stained with Kinyoun acid-fast stain. Approximately* ×*2,000.*

does not assimilate KNO_3, split urea, or grow on creatine.

Serological examination. A slide agglutination method (35) is used in identifying species with specific antisera.

Genus Torulopsis

Family *Cryptococcaceae*, a symbiont of man frequently found in abundant numbers in urine specimens (*T. glabrata*) without invasion of genitourinary tissues; occasionally reported as lung invader; *T. pintolopesii* is a commensal in the intestine of mice.

Cells oval to spherical, small, 1 to 2 by 2 to 4 μm; no capsule; no hyphae or pseudohyphae; no ascospores.

Growth. Aerobic. Rapid on ordinary media. *T. pintolopesii*, a thermophilic species, does not grow below 30 C. No pellicle in liquid media.

Biochemical reactions. Fermentative and assimilative action on sugars. *T. glabrata*, the most frequent clinical isolate, assimilates glucose and trehalose only, and does not split urea or assimilate KNO_3.

Animal pathogenicity. *T. glabrata* will form small granulomas when injected intraperitoneally into mice or rats and produces an intracellular pattern resembling that of *Histoplasma capsulatum*, from which it should be differentiated by cultures.

Genus Trichosporon

Members of the subfamily *Trichosporoideae*, family *Cryptococcaceae*. *T. beigelii* (*cutaneum*) causes superficial nodules on distal portion of hair (white piedra) and occasional opportunistic invasion of the mucous membranes or skin. *T. capitatum* invades rabbit kidneys, causing death a few days after intravenous injection. Pulmonary invasion in humans has been reported.

Well-developed hyphae and pseudohyphae, reproducing also by blastospores and arthrospores; no chlamydospores or ascospores reported. *T. capitatum* produces arthrospores in verticillate pattern suggesting "capitate" arrangement.

Growth. Aerobic. Grows in all of the usual culture media except those containing cycloheximide. Smooth shiny colonies, 3 to 6 mm, within

1 week; later become membranous, dry, and cerebriform. Optimal temperature, 25 to 30 C; some species grow equally well at 37 C.

Biochemical characteristics. Mostly oxidative but in occasional species also fermentative. Heavy surface pellicle formed. Assimilation of KNO_3 generally absent, but present in *T. pullulans*; urease-positive species are *T. beigelii* and *T. pullulans* (15).

Trichosporon can be distinguished from *Geotrichum* by its production of blastospores as well as arthrospores, by its ability to grow rapidly at 37 C, and by its assimilation of a greater number of the usual sugars (see Table 1).

Animal pathogenicity. *T. capitatum* is lethal to rabbits by intravenous inoculation. Produces miliary abscesses in the kidneys resembling those produced by *Candida albicans*.

LITERATURE CITED

1. Ahearn, D. G. 1969. Systematics of yeasts of medical interest. Proc. Int. Symp. Mycoses Sci. Publ. Pan-Amer. Health Organ. **205:**64–70.
2. Ahearn, D. G., F. J. Roth, Jr., J. W. Fell, and S. P. Myers. 1960. Use of shaken cultures in the assimilation test for yeast identification. J. Bacteriol. **79:**369–371.
3. Ajello, L., L. K. Georg, W. Kaplan, and L. Kaufman. 1963. Laboratory manual for medical mycology. U.S. Department of Health, Education, and Welfare, Public Health Service, Atlanta, Ga.
4. Beijernick, M. W. 1889. L'auxanographie ou la méthode de l'hydro diffusion dans la gélatine appliquee aux recherches microbiologiques. Arch. Néer. Sci. Exactes Natur. **23:**367–373.
5. Benham, R. W. 1955. *Cryptococcus neoformans:* "an ascomycete." Proc. Soc. Exp. Biol. Med. **89:**243–245.
6. Botard, R. W., and D. C. Kelley. 1968. Modified Littman oxgall agar to isolate *Cryptococcus neoformans*. Appl. Microbiol. **16:**689–690.
7. Davies, R. R. 1972. Protothecosis and opportunistic fungal infections. Trans. St. John's Hosp. Dermatol. Soc. **58:**38–42.
8. Dolan, C. T. 1971. A practical approach to identification of yeast-like organisms. Amer. J. Clin. Pathol. **55:**580–590.
9. Dolan, C. T., and M. R. Woodward. 1971. Identification of *Cryptococcus* species in the diagnostic laboratory. Amer. J. Clin. Pathol. **55:**591–595.
10. Farhi, F., G. S. Bulmer, and J. R. Tacker. 1970. *Cryptococcus neoformans*. IV. The not-so-encapsulated yeast. Infect. Immunity **1:**526–531.
11. Haley, L. D. 1971. Identification of yeasts in clinical microbiology laboratories. Amer. J. Med. Technol. **37:**125–131.
12. Hurley, R. 1966. Pathogenicity of the genus *Candida*, p. 13–25. *In* W. I. Winner and R. Hurley (ed.), Symposium on *Candida* infections. E. & S. Livingstone, Ltd., London.
13. Isenberg, H. D., and J. I. Burkman. 1962. Microbial diagnostics. Ann. N.Y. Acad. Sci. **98:**647–669.
14. Joshi, K. R., J. B. Gavin, and D. A. Bremmer. 1973. The formation of germ tubes by *Candida albicans* in various peptone media. Sabouraudia **11:**259–262.
15. Lodder, J. (ed.) 1970. The yeasts. North-Holland Publishing Co., Amsterdam.
16. Louria, D. B., N. Fallon, and H. G. Browne. 1960. The influence of cortisone on experimental fungus infections in mice. J. Clin. Invest. **39:**1435–1449.
17. Louria, D. B., N. Feder, W. Mitchell, and C. W. Emmons. 1959. Influence of fungus strain and lapse of time in experimental histoplasmosis and of volume of inoculum in cryptococcosis upon recovery of the fungi. J. Lab. Clin. Med. **53:**311–317.
18. McClary, D. O., W. L. Nulty, and G. R. Miller. 1959. Effect of potassium versus sodium in the sporulation of *Saccharomyces*. J. Bacteriol. **78:**362–368.
19. Medical Research Council. 1967. Nomenclature of fungi pathogenic to man and animals, p. 7. Her Majesty's Stationery Office, London.
20. Myers, B. R., T. W. Lieberman, and A. P. Ferry. 1973. *Candida* endophthalmitis complicating candidemia. Ann. Intern. Med. **79:**647–653.
21. Panja, G. 1946. A new medium for enhancement of growth of the *Malassezia*. Indian Med. Gaz. **81:**171.
22. Patridge, B. M., M. A. Athar, and H. I. Winner. 1971. Chick embryo inoculation as a pathogenicity test for *Candida* species. J. Clin. Pathol. **24:**645–648.
23. Phaff, H. J., and J. W. Fell. 1970. *Cryptococcus* Kützing emend. Phaff et Spencer, p. 1078–1145. *In* J. Lodder (ed.), The yeasts. North-Holland Publishing Co., Amsterdam.
24. Saëz, H. 1964. Action de la temperature sur le developpement in vitro de quelques especes de "*Geotrichium*". Rev. Pathol. Comp. N.S. (Ann. 64) **1:**229–301.
25. Seelig, M. S. 1966. Mechanisms by which antibiotics increase the incidence and severity of candidiasis and alter the immunological defenses. Bacteriol. Rev. **30:**442–459.
26. Seeliger, H. P. R. 1956. Use of a urease test for the screening and identification of cryptococci. J. Bacteriol. **72:**127–131.
27. Shadomy, H. J. 1970. Clamp connections in two strains of *Cryptococcus neoformans*, p. 67–72. *In* Recent trends in yeast research, vol. 1, Spectrum: Monograph Series in the Arts and Sciences. Georgia State University, Atlanta.
28. Shadomy, H. J., and J. P. Utz. 1966. Preliminary studies on a hypha-forming mutant of *Cryptococcus neoformans*. Mycologia **58:**383–390.
29. Shaw, C. E., and L. Kapica. 1972. Production of diagnostic pigment by phenoloxidase activity of *Cryptococcus neoformans*. Appl. Microbiol. **24:**824–830.
30. Shields, A. B., and L. Ajello. 1966. Medium for selective isolation of *Cryptococcus neoformans*. Science **151:**208–209.
31. Staib, F. 1962. *Cryptococcus neoformans* and *Guizotia abyssinica* (syn. *G. oleifera* D.C.) (Farbreaktion für *C. neoformans*.) Z. Hyg. Infektionskr. Med. Mikrobiol. Immunol. Virol. **148:**466–475.
32. Staib, F. 1963. Zur Kreatinin-Kreatin-Assimilation in der Hefepilzdiagnostik. Zentralbl. Bakteriol. Parasitenk. Infektionskr. Hyg. Abt. Orig. **191:**429–432.
33. Strachan, A. A., R. J. Yu, and F. Blank. 1971. Pigment production of *Cryptococcus neoformans* grown with extracts of *Guizotia abyssinica*. Appl. Microbiol. **22:**478–479.
34. Sudman, M. S., and W. Kaplan. 1973. Identification of the *Prototheca* species by immunofluorescence. Appl. Microbiol. **25:**981–990.
35. Tsuchiya, T., Y. Fukazawa, S. Kawakita, M. Imai, and T. Shinoda. 1965. Serological classification of the genus *Saccharomyces* (III). Jap. J. Microbiol. **9:**149–159.
36. Wickerham, L. J. 1951. Taxonomy of yeasts. U.S. Dept. Agr. Tech. Bull. 1029.

37. Wickerham, L. J. 1966. Validation of the species *Pichia guilliermondii*. J. Bacteriol. **92:**1269.

38. Wickerham, L. J., and K. A. Burton. 1958. Carbon assimilation tests for the classification of yeasts. J. Bacteriol. **56:**363–371.

39. Wolin, H. L., M. L. Bevis, and N. Laurora. 1962. An improved synthetic medium for the rapid production of chlamydospores by *Candida albicans*. Sabouraudia **2:**96–99.

Chapter 57

Fungi of Systemic Mycoses

HOWARD W. LARSH AND NORMAN L. GOODMAN

CHARACTERISTICS OF MICROORGANISMS

The fungi classically referred to as the etiological agents of the systemic mycoses include *Blastomyces dermatitidis*, *Coccidioides immitis*, *Cryptococcus neoformans*, *Histoplasma capsulatum*, *Histoplasma duboisii*, *Paracoccidioides brasiliensis*, and *Sporothrix schenckii*. These fungi, with the exception of *C. neoformans*, are diphasic; i.e., they grow as complex mycelial elements in their "natural" state or on media at 25 C, and they assume a yeast or "tissue" form in human or animal tissue or on complex media at 37 C. These fungi primarily cause pulmonary infections but may progress systemically to affect any or all organs of the body and may include cutaneous and subcutaneous manifestations.

The epidemiology of the systemic mycoses is quite complex. Soil is generally considered to be the natural habitat of these organisms; however, this is questionable in the case of *B. dermatitidis*. Infection occurs by inhalation of the fungal spores, which, with the exception of *C. immitis* and *C. neoformans*, presumably convert to the yeast state shortly after inhalation and continue to multiply in the host, eliciting various stages of disease, depending on factors such as size of the inoculum, susceptibility of the host, etc.

The geographic distribution of the fungi causing systemic disease is also quite variable. *H. capsulatum* and *B. dermatitidis* have been isolated from widely divergent geographic areas, even though the areas of high incidence of disease are somewhat limited. *H. capsulatum* has been isolated from various areas throughout the world, but the isolation of *B. dermatitidis* is more limited. *C. immitis*, on the other hand, is known to occur only in the arid and semi-arid regions of North, Central, and South America. *P. brasiliensis* is found in most countries of South America, in Mexico, and in several of the republics of Central America. Thus far, isolation of *H. duboisii* has been restricted to the continent of Africa.

As mentioned earlier, all of the above species, except *C. neoformans*, produce mycelia when grown under natural conditions at ambient temperatures; the hyphae forming the mycelial mat are septate and vary considerably in size and morphology with environmental conditions. Asexual spores are produced by all species; however, the tuberculate spore of *H. capsulatum* is the only one that is distinctive for the individual species.

Taxonomically, the systemic fungi are placed in the class *Deuteromycetes*, division Mycota, with *H. capsulatum* and *B. dermatitidis* having perfect stages in the class *Ascomycetes*. The perfect stage of *H. capsulatum* is designated *Emmonsiella capsulata* (8) and of *B. dermatitidis*, *Ajellomyces dermatitidis* (10).

COLLECTION, TRANSPORT, AND STORAGE OF SPECIMENS

The correct laboratory diagnosis of a systemic mycosis is dependent not only upon the mycological expertise of the laboratorian but also upon the quality of the specimen provided for laboratory analysis. The proper collection, transmission, and processing of specimens, as well as prompt inoculation on appropriate mycological media, are essential factors which govern the success of mycological analysis for pathogenic fungi. Since collection and transmission of specimens are not usually the primary responsibility of the laboratorian, it is imperative that those responsible for these duties be thoroughly informed of the correct procedures for obtaining the appropriate specimen at the proper time and then immediately delivering the specimen to the laboratory for prompt processing.

Since the classical systemic mycoses are primarily respiratory in origin, the major clinical specimens to be examined and cultured are respiratory secretions, i.e., sputum, bronchial lavage, and transtracheal aspirate, or tissue taken at biopsy. These diseases, however, are not limited to the respiratory tract and often become disseminated, affecting one or more internal organs of the body, with frequent cutaneous manifestations. One must then be prepared to examine fluids, exudates, or tissue from any organ, orifice, or system of the body, including urine, spinal fluid, pleural fluid, pericardial fluid, or exudate from subcutaneous or cutaneous lesions.

The specimen most frequently received for the laboratory diagnosis of systemic mycoses is sputum. Because of the probability of contamination by transient fungi, the collection of expectorated sputum samples from patients with pulmonary mycotic infections presents a serious problem. If successful isolation of the etiological agent is to be attained, proper procedures must be followed to eliminate excessive contamination by endogenous or saprophytic microorganisms present in the upper respiratory system. Failure to isolate pathogenic fungi from the sputum of patients with suspected mycotic infections has resulted in severe criticism of the collecting methods, and this has caused clinical mycologists to advocate abandonment of tests based on expectorated sputum. More complicated and sophisticated procedures for obtaining lung secretions have been suggested; these include bronchoscopy, transtracheal aspiration, and even transthoracic needle specimens. There is little doubt that specimens obtained by these methods are less likely to be contaminated than expectorated sputum. Nevertheless, such methods cannot be used routinely in an institution where large numbers of patients with chest diseases are observed daily. Catheterized sputum specimens are certainly welcomed by the laboratory mycologist.

On the other hand, it has been shown that carefully collected sputum is useful in the isolation of pathogenic fungi that cause systemic diseases. Diagnostic mycological procedures begin not in the laboratory but in the clinic where the specimens originate, and the first step in collecting expectorated sputum depends upon the individual charged with obtaining it. It is absolutely essential to instruct the patient on the part he must play. A useful specimen can be obtained only from a highly cooperative patient, and the instructions given him often must be repeated. It is desirable to gain the confidence of the patient as well as his cooperation, and this can best be done by explaining the rationale for obtaining satisfactory specimens.

Intensive oral hygiene is one of the prime prerequisites for obtaining a quality sputum specimen. The patient's teeth must be brushed thoroughly, or his dentures removed, and the mouth cleansed by extensive use of a mouth wash. Only a specimen from deep in the lungs should be obtained; nasopharyngeal secretions, saliva, and other superficial oral specimens should not be collected.

The specimen should be collected in a sterile container with a wide mouth to permit deposit of the sputum without undue difficulty. A sterile 4-oz (120-ml) wide-mouth glass jar with a Bakelite screw cap is a good specimen container. These are not placed in the patient's room until the morning the specimen is to be obtained. Experience has proved that if the sterile jar is accessible to the patient, it is likely to be contaminated prior to use. The first specimen expectorated in the morning is usually the best, and the amount collected need not exceed 10 to 15 ml. Casual observation of the specimen usually gives sufficient evidence as to its source; for this reason the volume, consistency, and color are recorded. The clinician may request a 12- to 72-h collection of sputum for other reasons, but not for isolation of the disease-producing fungi.

There are times when it is necessary to obtain nebulized specimens by using mucolytic agents. After aerosolization, an increased volume of liquefied secretions may occur and may be mistaken for saliva. In view of this, it is imperative that the specimen be labeled correctly to assure that it is processed and not discarded as an inadequate sample. Nebulized "sputum" obtained from patients not producing adequate expectorated material may be the only source of the pathogenic fungus.

Swabs are of limited use in the isolation of systemic fungi, except in disseminated cases with cutaneous abscesses. When possible, exudate, or pus, should be aspirated; however, if swabs must be used, collect as much specimen as possible. After the specimen is collected, the swab should be placed into a sealed, sterile tube and taken immediately to the laboratory before drying occurs.

Tissue collected for culture should be collected under aseptic conditions, placed into a sterile screw-capped container, sealed tightly, and taken immediately to the laboratory for processing. Specimens in Formalin are not suitable for isolating fungi. Care should be taken to prevent drying and contamination.

Transport

Clinical specimens should be examined and cultured as soon as possible after collection. The systemic fungi will survive in most clinical specimens for several hours; however, the presence of rapidly growing bacteria and fungi may overgrow and mask the presence of the slower-growing systemic fungi. Sputum may be transported in glass or heavy-plastic screw-capped containers. Care must be taken to secure caps to prevent leakage. Antibiotics may be added to the specimen to prevent heavy bacterial growth. Penicillin (20 units/ml) and streptomycin (40 units/ml) or chloramphenicol (0.05 mg/ml) are generally recommended. Note: Penicillin should not be added to specimens to be examined for *Nocardia* sp. or *Actinomyces* sp. Bronchial washes, aspirates, and urine may be transported under the same conditions as sputum. Swabs should be transported in containers that will prevent drying. Specimens to be transported by mail should be collected and mailed so that the specimen will arrive in the laboratory during working hours, not on weekends or holidays. Tissue transported to the laboratory for culture should be placed in a small amount of sterile physiological saline and kept cool (not frozen) in transit. Antibiotics, in the above amounts, can be used in the saline if the tissue is possibly contaminated.

Storage

Clinical specimens should not be stored prior to primary culture unless absolutely necessary. If storage is necessary prior to culture or desirable after primary culture for reference purposes, use the procedures outlined above for transport and store the specimen at 4 C.

At this point, it should be made clear that all diagnostic mycological work should be carried out in a *biological* hood. All plating of specimens and examination of plated or tubed cultures or specimens should be done inside the hood. Aerosols and spores from the organisms are infective and if inhaled may cause severe disease.

DIRECT EXAMINATION

Direct microscopic examination of the clinical specimens often saves considerable time in the diagnosis of a systemic fungal disease. Observations can be made on stained or unstained preparations of specimens taken directly from the patient. Sputum and exudate lend themselves especially well to direct examination for fungi.

The consistency of the specimen determines what procedure is necessary prior to microscopy. If the specimen is viscid or opaque, it is imperative that some type of partial digestion, homogenization, or mixing be instituted. There are several satisfactory digestants; however, if the specimen is to be cultured, digestion can be successfully accomplished with *N*-acetyl-cysteine, dithiothreitol, or enzyme preparations. Any of these agents will liquefy the specimen rapidly and produce a preparation that can be readily observed microscopically, while preserving the viability of any fungi present for culture.

Specimens can be examined without prior digestion, but it is usually best to mix a sample with 10% sodium hydroxide on a glass slide. The slide preparation should be warmed gently to expel air bubbles and to clear the specimen. Most systemic fungi can be recognized in these preparations without specific staining; the procedure is rapid and permits a tentative identification in only a few minutes. Nevertheless, many investigators find greater success or more rapid differentiation of the organisms by using selective staining. One frequently used procedure involves the addition of equal parts of 20% NaOH and Parker's Superchrome Ink to sputum specimens. This selective stain readily permits identification of the larger fungi such as species of *Aspergillus*, *Blastomyces*, *Coccidioides*, *Cryptococcus*, and *Mucor*. However, dried and heat-fixed smears stained by the Giemsa, Gram, or Wright stains should be used for the detection of *Histoplasma capsulatum* and other small yeasts.

Direct microscopy of unconcentrated sputum may not reveal the presence of pathogenic fungi. Many fruitless hours can be spent screening such smears, whereas cultures from the same specimen may be positive. In addition, unequivocal identification may be impossible because diagnostic stages of the fungus may not occur in preparations containing few infectious units.

Digestion and concentration of the sputum specimen increase the probability of finding pathogenic fungi in smear preparations. Furthermore, the sputum sediment may be embedded and sectioned by standard histological techniques. Paraffin sections stained with either hematoxylin-eosin or methenamine silver frequently reveal pathogenic fungi which cannot be observed in unstained smears.

Cytological studies for the detection of tumor cells have opened up an area of great value to the medical mycologist. Sputum smears stained by the Papanicolaou method are excellent for the rapid detection of pathogenic fungi; fungus cells have been observed in smears of untreated material and in centrifuged sediments by this technique. Yeast cells in pulmonary infections caused by *H. capsulatum*, *B. dermatitidis*, and *C. neoformans* can be differentiated by this stain. It is an efficient procedure because routine cytological techniques permit more direct and rapid diagnosis than the time-consuming culture method.

Staining with fluorescent-antibody techniques, although not infallible, can be an excellent adjunct for the detection of pathogenic fungi in clinical specimens. When absorption techniques are used, the procedure may be specific for a particular fungal agent, and in many instances a tentative diagnosis can be made from fluorescent-antibody reactions several days prior to cultural confirmation. In highly contaminated specimens, fluorescent staining may be the only laboratory evidence supporting the clinical diagnosis.

In observing wet or stained preparations of clinical specimens, good microscopic technique should be observed, to prevent morphological aberrations. The use of phase microscopy in observing wet preparations of clinical specimens is helpful.

In wet or stained preparations, *B. dermatitidis* appears as large yeast cells (8 to 15 μm in diameter) that are uniformly spherical with thick, refractile walls (Fig. 7). A single bud is attached to the mother cell by a wide (4 to 5 μm) septum.

C. immitis appears as a mixture of immature and mature spherules. These are nonbudding, spherical, thin-walled structures (30 to 60 μm in diameter) that are filled with numerous endospores (2 to 5 μm) at maturity.

H. capsulatum occurs as a single-budding, ovate yeast (1 to 5 μm). Oil immersion is usually required for viewing. It should be noted that other fungi may be morphologically similar to *H. capsulatum*.

Direct examination of specimens containing *P. brasiliensis* reveals fungal cells varying in size from 19 to 25 μm in diameter. The cells are spherical to ovate or elliptical, with occasional chaining of three or four cells. Budding occurs, with the cell producing one or more buds simultaneously, each bud being attached to the parent cell by a narrow neck.

CULTURE AND ISOLATION

Processing of specimens

Processing of specimens should be delayed no longer than 2 h, and immediate processing is preferable. Long periods between collection and culturing encourages significant increases in the number of rapidly growing organisms. At room temperature, reproduction of contaminating organisms may lead to excessive overgrowth by these species on various isolation media, preventing the successful isolation of pathogenic fungi.

For mycological studies, it is preferable not to digest sputum specimens because some procedures that are used may destroy the mycotic agents. This is particularly true if the concentration of the digestant and the length of exposure to it are not critically controlled. If the sputum is too viscid, sterile L-cysteine saline can be added to assist in dilution; the process can be hastened by use of a mechanical shaker. Specimens satisfactory for quantification are obtained by shaking at 275 strokes per min for 30 min.

Antibiotics can be added to the specimens, provided that a control sample is retained for study. Specimens highly contaminated with rapidly growing organisms seldom yield pathogenic fungi unless they, or the inoculated media, contain antibiotics. Of these, cycloheximide, chloramphenicol, penicillin, and streptomycin have been most frequently used. However, precautions must be taken, as indiscriminate use of antibiotics will lead to failure in isolating certain pathogenic fungi: *C. neoformans* is extremely sensitive to cycloheximide, as are isolates of *Allescheria boydii*, *Aspergillus*, and *Phycomycetes*, and many isolates of *H. capsulatum* are inhibited by high dosages of chloramphenicol. In addition, *Actinomyces* or species of *Nocardia* are susceptible to penicillin and some broad-spectrum antibiotics.

In carefully controlled investigations, digestion of sputum by sodium hydroxide and specific enzymes did not appreciably reduce the pathogenic fungi in the specimens. It was evident, however, that long exposures to these agents reduced the total number of viable organisms, as is also true when *Mycobacterium tuberculosis* is subjected to excessive periods of digestion, but sputum specimens protected either by an efficient buffer or by neutralization after digestion will frequently permit the isolation of pathogenic fungi.

Digestion of sputum specimens with either *N*-acetyl-L-cysteine or dithiotreitol has proved useful for isolation of pathogenic fungi. The specimens may be rapidly liquefied, neutralized, and concentrated without any apparent effect on the pathogenic organisms. Best results are obtained when the concentration of sodium hydroxide in the digestion procedure is minimal (2 to 4%) and the pH does not exceed 8.0.

Culturing of specimens

Specimens that have been carefully collected and processed should be inoculated on artificial culture media as soon as feasible, for reasons previously discussed. Procedures for plating specimens on suitable media are outlined in

Fig. 1. The primary isolation medium used by most medical mycologists is modified Sabouraud agar. However, use of this medium to obtain isolates of pathogens from sputum specimens frequently results in complete overgrowth by bacteria and saprophytic molds. Nevertheless, knowledge that certain antibiotics have a marked effect of the growth of specific pathogens makes it mandatory that plain Sabouraud or some other type of plain, artificial culture medium such as brain-heart infusion agar, with or without blood, be included in the battery of isolation media used. Although Sabouraud medium has its limitations, it is adequate if contaminating organisms can be controlled.

Another factor which discourages the use of plain Sabouraud agar is that it will not support the growth of certain pathogens from expectorated sputum specimens. This is especially true of *H. capsulatum*. However, when the pathogen has first been isolated and is then transferred to this medium, excellent growth occurs.

Selective isolation media have proved very effective in the isolation of pathogens from primary clinical specimens. These include modified Sabouraud agar and either brain-heart infusion agar or blood-agar base with specific antibiotics. The latter two media usually include 8 to 10% defibrinated human, sheep, or rabbit blood and antibiotics which either inhibit or retard the growth of contaminating organisms. As stated earlier, the commonly used antibiotics are chloramphenicol, cycloheximide, penicillin, and streptomycin. Commercial mycological media contain chloramphenicol and cycloheximide, but they cannot be considered ideal because they may completely or partially inhibit various species of pathogenic fungi. The yeast phase of some isolates of *H. capsulatum* is sensitive to chloramphenicol, and, for this reason, it is preferable to use penicillin, streptomycin, and cycloheximide in the selective isolation medium. The concentration of penicillin and streptomycin does not seem to be critical. The usual amounts added are 20 units of penicillin, 40 units of streptomycin, and 0.5 mg of cycloheximide per ml of specimen. No inhibition was apparent when 200,000 units of penicillin, 400,000 units of streptomycin, and 1.5 mg of cycloheximide per ml of specimen were used for sputum containing *H. capsulatum*. However, penicillin and streptomycin are heat-labile, and they must be added aseptically to the cooled agar prior to plating. In our laboratory, the use of the antibiotic gentamicin in the medium has proved effective in controlling the growth of

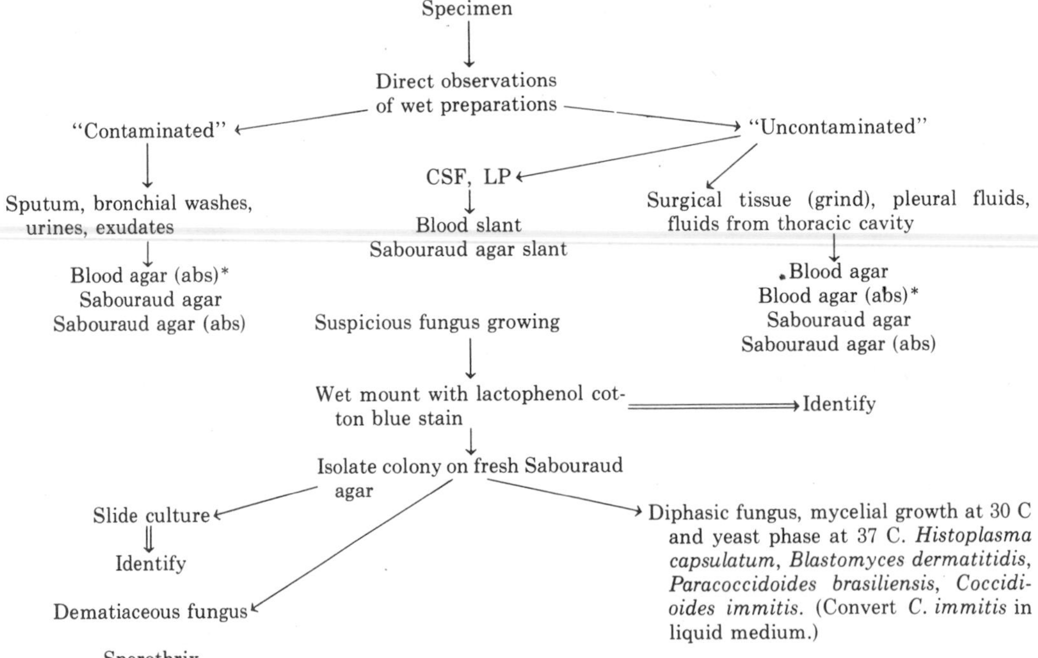

* With antibiotics: cycloheximide and chloramphenicol, penicillin and streptomycin, or gentamicin.

FIG. 1. *Procedures used for identifying systemic fungi in the clinical laboratory.*

gram-negative bacteria. In particular, species of *Proteus* and *Pseudomonas* are effectively controlled by incorporating 50 μg of gentamicin per ml of blood-agar.

Modified Sabouraud antibiotic agar has proved successful for the isolation of most pathogenic fungi. *H. capsulatum* has frequently been recovered from clinical specimens, especially sputum, on brain-heart-blood-agar or a blood-agar containing antibiotics when there was no recovery on Sabouraud agar, either with or without antibiotics.

These antibiotic-containing media should be incubated at 25 to 30 C, since many pathogens are inhibited by cycloheximide at 37 C. *C. immitis* is an exception to this rule, for it has been recovered from clinical specimens much more rapidly at 37 C on blood-agar containing penicillin and streptomycin. Growth of the mycelial phase of this fungus occurs within 3 to 5 days at 37 C. At this time, there is usually a distinct metallic sheen on the medium, and the diagnostic arthrospores appear. The plates must be sealed with masking tape to prevent rapid dehydration and to provide environmental conditions conducive for growth of the fungus.

There are other selective and differential media available to the laboratory medical mycologist, but these are required only in a limited number of cases.

ANIMAL INOCULATION

Animal inoculation has proved valuable in isolating pathogenic fungi from contaminated clinical specimens. Unfortunately, however, there is no experimental animal that is universally susceptible to fungi pathogenic to man. The white Swiss mouse has been most frequently used, but this species is only slightly susceptible to many of these pathogens. Rats, hamsters, rabbits, and guinea pigs have also been of value for establishing the pathogenicity of various fungi.

Specific routes of inoculation are followed when pure cultures are studied, but the intraperitoneal route is the one of choice when contaminated specimens are used.

The rationale for animal inoculation with sputum is much different from that for establishing the pathology or observing the tissue phases of pure cultures. Specimens contaminated with bacteria and saprophytic fungi usually overgrow culture plates and mask or prevent the growth of pathogens. Treatment of highly contaminated specimens with antibiotics or other chemicals to inhibit or retard saprophytic fungi and bacteria on artificial media has proved difficult. When these in vitro procedures fail, the last resort is animal inoculation. Injection with untreated specimens often results in fulminating bacteremia and death of animals within 48 h, which is not sufficient time for the pathogenic fungus, if present, to establish disease. Histological studies have shown that pathological reactions do occur in those animals that survive for at least 2 weeks. Earlier attempts to isolate pathogens from such animals usually fail, since only contaminating fungi may be recovered from them for at least the first 2 weeks. Therefore, it has been found that the inoculation of treated specimens into experimental animals is the most successful means of isolating pathogens from highly contaminated material. Even with this procedure, however, the rate of isolation is still relatively low. Most of the broad-spectrum antibiotics are satisfactory for the treatment of sputum, but some strains of white mice are highly susceptible to streptomycin. Not only should the specimen be treated prior to inoculation but also the animals may require antibiotics *ad libitum* or by intraperitoneal inoculation for several days after receiving the contaminated material. Animal inoculation has proved useful for all mycoses but may be necessary for the isolation of *B. dermatitidis*, *C. immitis*, *C. neoformans*, and *H. capsulatum*.

If a small number of pathogenic microorganisms are present in the inoculum, the animals may not develop a lethal infection. Also, there are variants of the systemic fungi that react differently in inoculated animals. Earlier studies reported that experimental animals died within a few days from infections with *C. immitis* and *C. neoformans*. However, it is a common occurrence, especially in the self-limiting chronic pulmonary disease caused by many of the systemic fungi, that animals inoculated with cultures of the causative organisms fail to die in 4 to 5 days. In recent investigations of self-limiting pulmonary cryptococcosis, animals inoculated with large doses of *C. neoformans*, either intracerebrally or intraperitoneally, lived from 15 to 28 days. It is for this reason that certain clinicians place more emphasis on morphological and physiological findings for identification of *C. neoformans* than on animal inoculation. Actually, laboratory mycologists must recognize that variations occur and that animals, like culture plates, must be observed for longer periods. In all experimental studies, large numbers of animals should receive the inoculum so that some can be sacrificed at specific intervals for isolation attempts before spontaneous death. Since there is variation in the host-parasite reaction, it is common to sacrifice and autopsy inoculated mice at 2 and 4 weeks. The organs most frequently removed for culture are the liver and spleen, from which pieces are clipped and placed on various media. This procedure may prove successful; however, many investigations have shown that infected tissues may not yield the pathogen on artificial culture media. These failures may be due to changes in the pH of the tissue, which rapidly destroy the pathogenic phase, or the pathogen may be localized within the tissue and not come in contact with the medium. Grinding or homogenization of organs under aseptic conditions, followed by dilution with 0.85% sterile L-cysteine-saline, is a more satisfactory technique. Plating of approximately 1 ml of the tissue homogenate onto each of three isolation media is the preferred procedure. The inoculated plates should be incubated at 30 C and observed for at least 30 days.

It has been shown that highly pigmented inbred mice are more susceptible to many of the pathogenic fungi than are white Swiss mice. These strains can be used advantageously in isolation, pathological, and immunological studies.

IDENTIFICATION

The laboratory identification of the fungi which cause systemic mycoses is primarily dependent upon recognition of morphological characteristics exhibited in all phases of growth, i.e., mycelial, yeast, and tissue phases. In the case of dimorphic fungi, the organisms should be converted from one phase to another to assure that both phases do indeed exist and thus strengthen the laboratory diagnosis. A confirmed report should never go to the physician without first proving dimorphism in the fungus isolated.

As all students of medical mycology know, there is considerable variation in the fungi causing systemic disease, not only because of genetic changes but also due to environmental factors within the host, on the laboratory media, and in the methods of incubation within the laboratory. To avoid the confusion created by this variation, the laboratorian must become familiar with the fungi as they occur in the laboratory by carefully studying stock cultures and keeping up with the current literature in the field.

There are many procedures for identifying systemic fungi, and certainly each laboratory must adjust its procedures to fit practical considerations; however, certain basic procedures have been developed and proved successful.

In isolating and identifying the systemic fungi, it is convenient and simple to isolate the mycelial phase of the diphasic fungus. This is accomplished by incubating the primary isolation plates at 25 to 30 C, for at least 4 weeks. Frequent examination of the plates will allow the early observation of colony growth and thus a better chance to examine an isolated colony.

In the early stages of colony growth, prepare a lactophenol cotton blue wet mount of the mycelial growth and examine it microscopically for the characteristic mycelium and spores.

At the same time, transfer another small piece of the isolated colony to a plate of modified Sabouraud agar and incubate it at 25 to 30 C. This culture will serve to demonstrate characteristic colony morphology and microscopic characteristics.

Also, at this time, transfer yet another small piece of the isolated colony to a tube of fresh blood-agar, or brain-heart infusion agar. Place the inoculum firmly onto the medium and smear over a small area. Incubate this medium at 37 C, and after 48 h observe daily for conversion to the yeast phase. If conversion does not occur in 4 to 5 days, transfer this culture to another fresh tube of conversion medium and repeat the process. If *C. immitis* is suspected, conversion to the spherule form may be accomplished in special liquid media instead of blood-agar or brain-heart infusion agar. However, the dimorphic nature of *C. immitis* is best demonstrated by inoculating the fungus into animals such as mice or guinea pigs.

When a pure culture has been obtained on the isolation medium, the fungus can be identified by its gross colony morphology and microscopic characteristics. Again, one must keep in mind that there are variants of all microorganisms.

Histoplasma capsulatum

On Sabouraud agar incubated at room temperature, the fungus grows slowly, producing white, cottony, aerial mycelium that turns buff to brown with age. Microscopy reveals round to pyriform, smooth or echinulate microconidia (2.5 to 3 μm in diameter) which may be sessile on the sides of hyphae or attached to short lateral conidiophores. Later, the "so-called" characteristic and diagnostic large, round, or pyriform tuberculate macroconidia (7.5 μm in diameter) appear in the culture (Fig. 2). Similar cultural and microscopic findings occur on blood-agar. These results are contrary to those usually reported when an enriched blood-agar medium is used to culture sputum at room temperature. Investigators must be cognizant that macroconidia may be absent or have

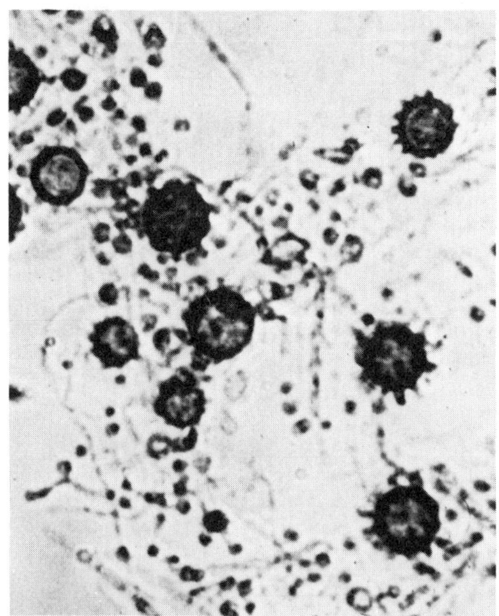

FIG. 2. *Microscopic appearance of a wet preparation of Histoplasma capsulatum mycelial phase from Sabouraud agar incubated at 30 C. Lactophenol cotton blue stain. ×540.*

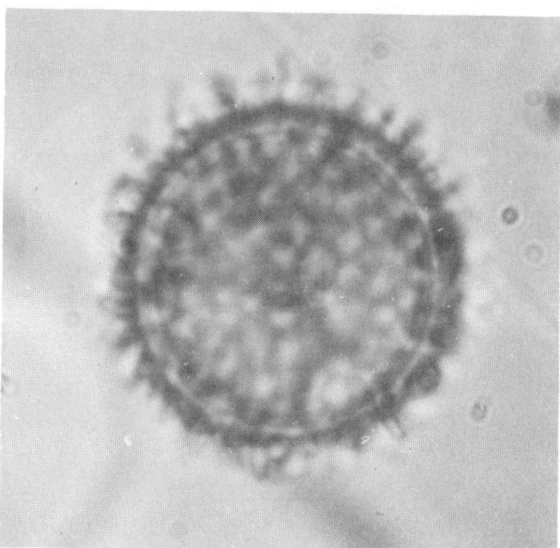

FIG. 3. *Tuberculated conidium of Sepedonium species. ×1,000.*

only smooth walls when the isolate is from a patient with chronic histoplasmosis. In addition, there are several variants of this fungus, and the mycelial growth is not always typically white and cottonlike, with aerial hyphae. Also, one must be aware of the saprophytic fungus *Sepedonium*, which has a tuberculated spore similar to *H. capsulatum* (Fig. 3). These can be differentiated, however, by the conversion of *H. capsulatum* to its yeast form.

The yeast (parasitic) form of *H. capsulatum* may be grown on blood-agar or other enriched media at 37 C as a typical oval, budding yeast 2 to 3 by 4 to 5 μm in size. The cell reproduces by budding at the small end of the cell, and the pore between the bud and parent cell remains small (Fig. 4).

In tissue sections or smears, the fungal cell is seen to be intracellular in macrophages, giant cells, or polymorphonuclear leukocytes. The yeast may show typical budding, with the cells having the same dimensions given above (Fig. 5). *H. capsulatum* can be stained in tissue by many techniques, with the methenamine-silver technique giving the highest contrast between fungal cell and host cell.

Blastomyces dermatitidis

The mycelial form of *B. dermatitidis*, when growing on Sabouraud agar at room temperature (25 to 30 C), is a white mold. Seven to 10 days are required to produce a mature colony,

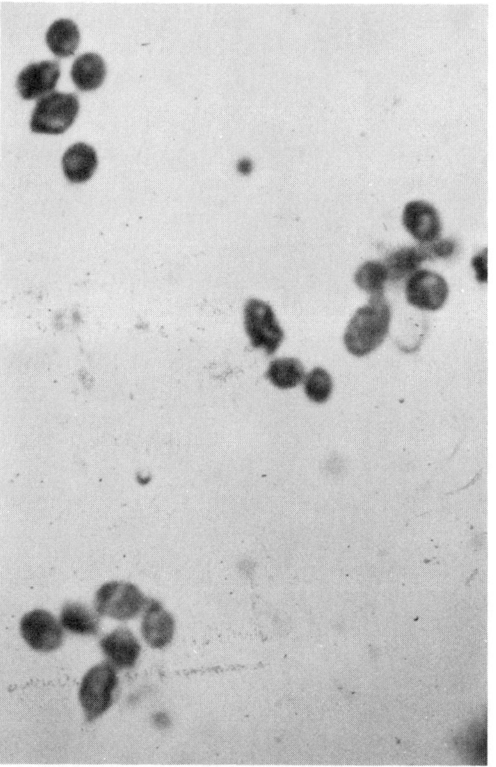

FIG. 4. *Wet preparation of Histoplasma capsulatum yeast form from blood-agar incubated at 37 C. Lactophenol cotton blue stain. ×900.*

which may continue growing to fill the petri plate or agar slant. Occasional isolates may be encountered that grow more slowly and sporulate poorly. Also, isolates may be found that become brown or produce a dark pigment in the medium.

Conidia that are borne on slender, lateral conidiophores, or terminally on hyphal branches, are smooth-walled, spherical to oval, and vary in size from 2 to 10 μm (Fig. 6). In its early stage, the mycelial form of *B. dermatitidis* may resemble very closely and be confused with isolates of *Monosporium apiospermum*. In most typical isolates, *B. dermatitidis* becomes tan to brown with age, whereas *M. apiospermum* turns gray.

The yeast form of *B. dermatitidis* can be grown at 37 C on enriched media such as blood-agar. The organisms are uniformly spherical with thick, refractile walls and are 8 to 15 μm in diameter. The single bud is characteristically attached to the mother cell by a wide septum 4 to 5 μm wide, which is a diagnostic character (Fig. 7). In a young bud, the wall is much thinner than in the mother cell, and the attachment may be as wide as the bud; the wall gains refractivity with age and is sometimes termed a double-contoured wall. Single budding distin-

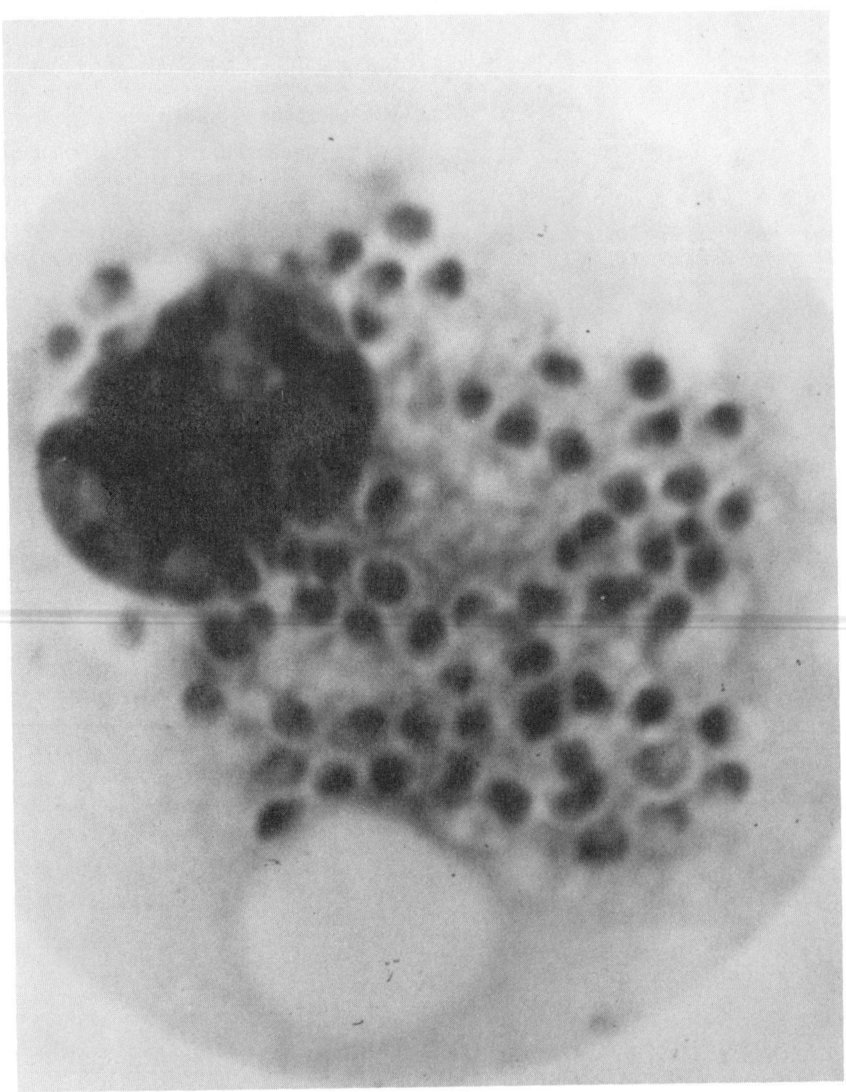

FIG. 5. *Histoplasma capsulatum in tissue. Hematoxylin and eosin stain. ×900.*

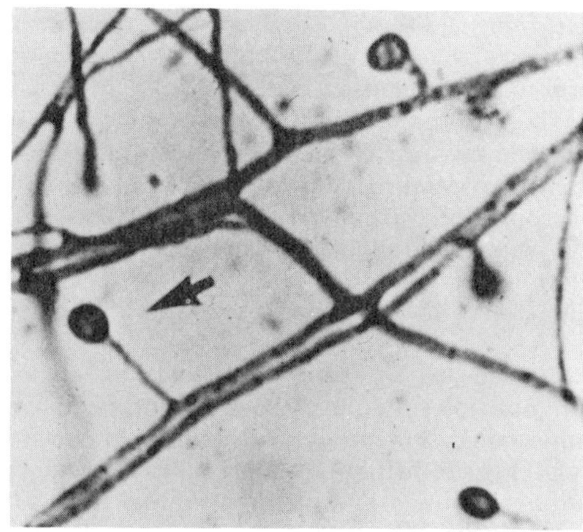

FIG. 6. *Wet preparation of mycelial phase Blastomyces dermatitidis grown on Sabouraud agar. Lactophenol cotton blue stain.* ×590. (*Photomicrograph courtesy of L. Ajello.*)

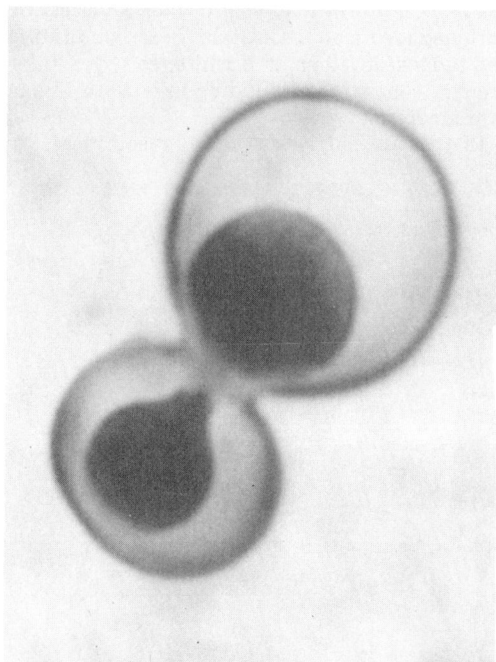

FIG. 7. *Wet preparation of Blastomyces dermatitidis yeast form. Lactophenol cotton blue stain.* ×900.

guishes *B. dermatitidis* from its South American counterpart, *P. brasiliensis*, whose pathogenic phase is a multiple-budding yeast.

B. dermatitidis reproduces in tissue by budding, the bud being characterized by its large size, the attachment to the parent cell by a wide septum, and the presence of a thick refractile wall (Fig. 8).

Coccidiodes immitis

C. immitis grows rapidly on Sabouraud agar, the mycelium covering the plate or slant within a few days. The young culture is floccose, and with age the color darkens, some isolates producing a brown or yellow pigment. A darkening of the peptone-containing medium is common.

Spores first appear on the side branches of the hyphae. The septation of the hyphae produces arthrospores that exhibit alternation of arthrospores with empty spaces. The arthrospores are barrel-shaped, 2 to 4 by 3 to 6 μm, and are dispersed by the fragmentation of the walls of the empty spaces between spores. With age, the entire hyphal mass of the culture may form arthrospores (Fig. 9).

In cultures on artificial media incubated at room temperature *C. immitis* must be differentiated from other fungi such as species of *Arthroderma* and *Geotrichum*. All of these fungi produce arthrospores by hyphal fragmentation, and casual microscopic observation may result in misidentification. Careful and thorough studies of the type of growth on Sabouraud agar and of lactophenol cotton blue preparations are of value in reaching a correct laboratory diagnosis. Nevertheless, if there is any doubt, definitive diagnosis can be made by intraperitoneal inoculation of mice or intratesticular inoculation of guinea pigs with the culture and

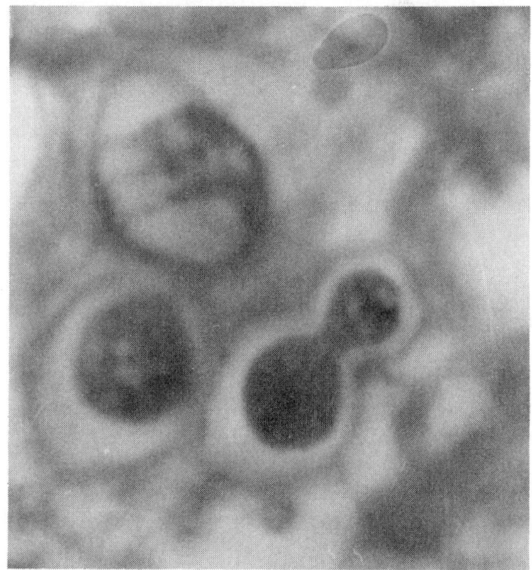

FIG. 8. *Blastomyces dermatitidis in tissue. Hematoxylin and eosin stain.* ×720.

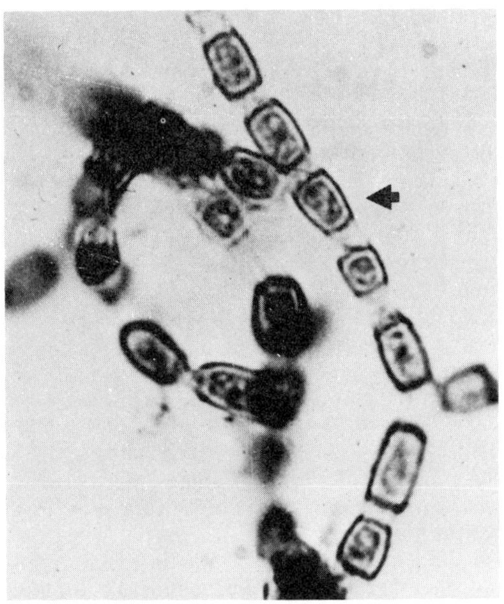

FIG. 9. *Wet preparation of Coccidioides immitis grown on Sabouraud agar at 30 C. Lactophenol cotton blue stain. ×620.*

subsequent examination of the tissue for the characteristic spherules of *C. immitis*.

C. immitis appears in tissue as a nonbudding, spherical, thick-walled structure 30 to 60 μm in diameter, which may be filled with numerous small (2 to 5 μm in diameter) endospores. The fungus reproduces by means of these endospores, which are released by rupture of the spherule cell wall. These infectious units increase in size and develop into large spherules. In direct examination of tissue, it is possible to observe only immature forms of *C. immitis*, which do not contain endospores. This stage is easily confused with nonbudding yeasts, especially *B. dermatitidis* and *C. neoformans*, because of variation in the size of spherules. In view of this, several microscopic preparations of the tissue may be required, and each must be examined for the characteristic, endospore-filled, mature spherules (Fig. 10–11).

Paracoccidioides brasiliensis

P. brasiliensis is slow growing compared with the other systemic fungi. On Sabouraud agar, at 25 to 30 C, the fungus develops as a heaped, glabrous or wrinkled colony with a short, white aerial mycelium which often turns brown with age. Microscopically, chlamydospores and a few sessile, oval-to-round conidia may occur. These conidia, when present, are indistinguishable from those of *B. dermatitidis*; thus, it is necessary to convert the culture to the yeast form for identification.

When *P. brasiliensis* is grown at 37 C on enriched medium, it grows slowly and develops smooth to cerebriform, yeastlike colonies. Microscopically, the culture is composed of single- and multiple-budding yeasts. The multiple-budding cells are thick-walled, 10 to 25 μm in diameter, with buds from 1 to 10 μm in diameter.

In tissue, *P. brasiliensis* appears as single- and multiple-budding yeasts with the above dimensions; however, care should be taken to look for the multiple-budding cells, as the singly budding cells are indistinguishable from *B. dermatitidis* (Fig. 12–13).

Histoplasma duboisii

The mycelial form of *H. duboisii*, grown at 25 to 30 C, is indistinguishable from *H. capsulatum*.

The yeast form may be grown on a variety of enriched media at 37 C. Under these conditions, the fungus develops as a white, soft, yeastlike growth, consisting of budding cells 10 to 15 μm in diameter.

In tissue, *H. duboisii* resembles *B.*

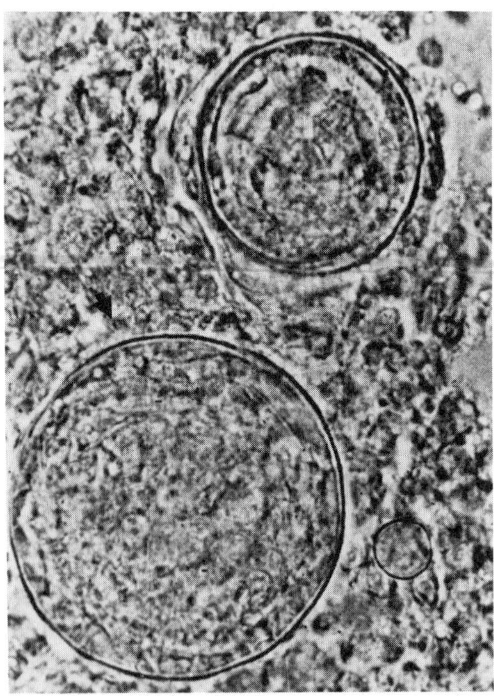

FIG. 10. *Spherules of coccidioides immitis seen in an unstained wet preparation of sputum. ×265.*

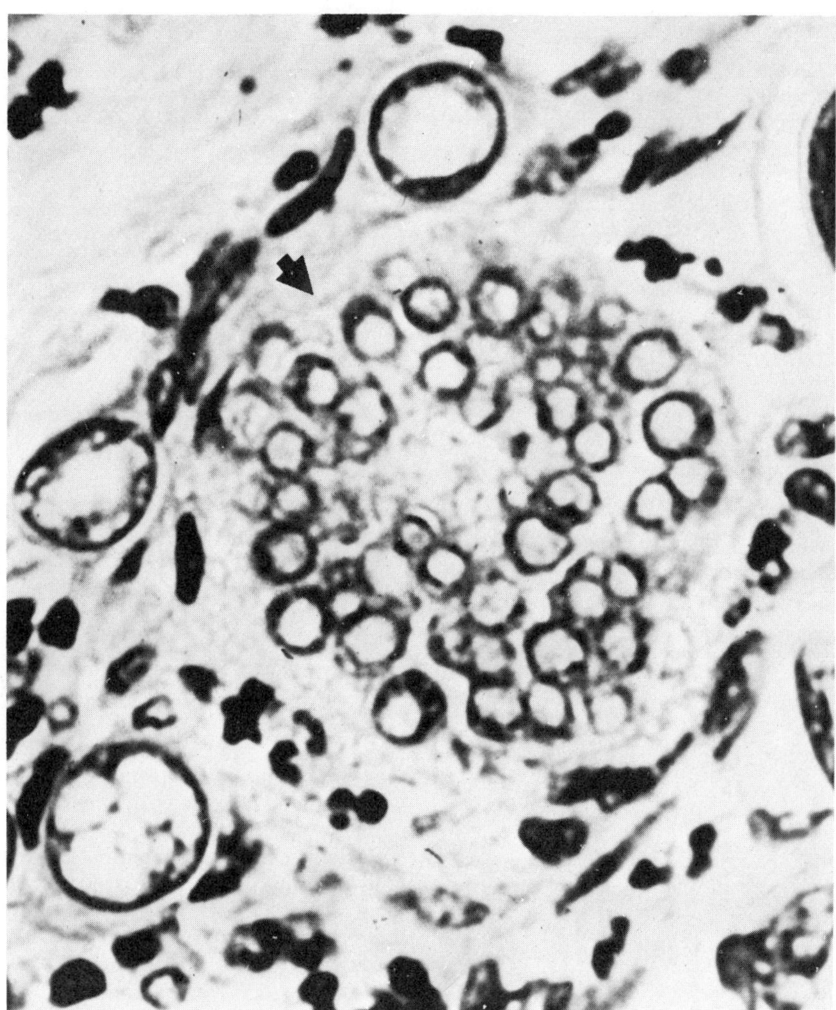

FIG. 11. *Spherule of Coccidioides immitis in tissue. Hematoxylin and eosin stain. ×900.*

dermatitidis in size, shape, and thick-walled appearance. The cells are approximately 10 μm in diameter with numerous budding forms that stain well with most histological dyes (Fig. 14).

Sporothrix schenckii

S. schenckii is a diphasic fungus that can be grown under the same conditions outlined for the previous systemic fungi. For complete identification procedures, refer to the chapter on the dematiaceous fungi (chapter 59).

Cryptococcus neoformans

C. neoformans is a spherical, thick-walled, single-budding yeast (5 to 20 μm in diameter) surrounded by a wide, refractile, gelatinous capsule that may be encountered in the same specimens as other systemic pathogens. In sputum, and particularly in tissue, the type of budding permits rapid laboratory identification. The bud is attached to the mother cell by a relatively small slender neck giving it a "pinched-off" appearance that resembles a tear drop. The organism is urease-positive, but other yeasts are known to produce this enzyme. Growth at 37 C, assimilation pattern, and pathogenicity to mice are criteria which separate this species from other cryptococci. For detailed procedures for isolation and identification of *C. neoformans*, see the chapter on yeasts (chapter 56).

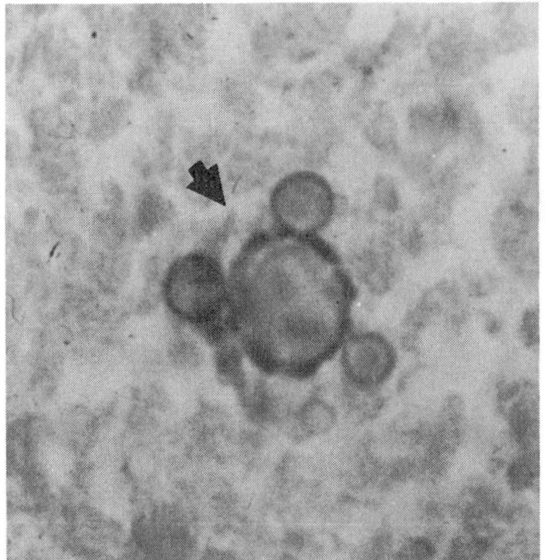

FIG. 12. *Yeast form of Paracoccidioides brasiliensis. Methenamine silver stain.* ×*900.*

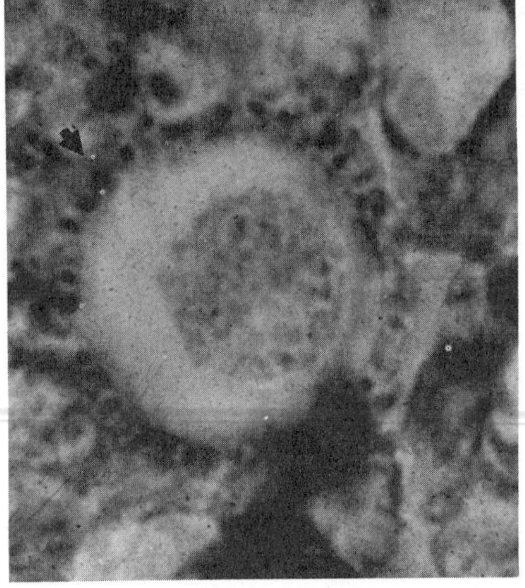

FIG. 13. *Paracoccidioides brasiliensis in tissue. Note multiple budding yeast "Mariner's wheel." Hematoxylin and eosin stain.* ×*600.*

DISCUSSION

With the increasing incidence and awareness of chronic pulmonary disease and use of immunosuppressive agents, the diagnostic medical mycologist must be acutely aware of the possible pathogenic role of fungi isolated in the laboratory. The appearance of one or two colonies of a fungus on the primary plate should not be considered of no consequence, or "a contaminant."

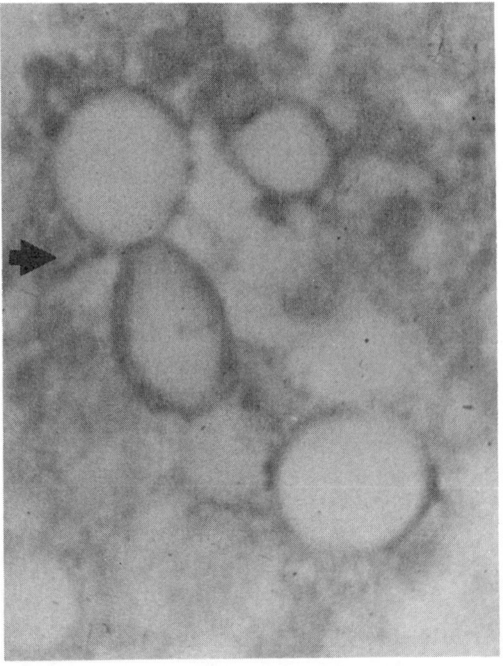

FIG. 14. *Histoplasma duboisii in tissue. Hematoxylin and eosin stain.* ×*1,000.*

Patient, consistent examination of all fungal growth from plates incubated for sufficiently long periods of time will result in more efficient and increased laboratory diagnosis of the mycoses.

LITERATURE CITED

1. Ajello, L. (ed.). 1967. Coccidioidomycosis. University of Arizona Press, Tucson.
2. Ajello, L., E. W. Chick, and M. L. Furcolow. (ed.). 1971. Histoplasmosis. Proc. 2nd Nat. Conf. Charles C Thomas, Publisher, Springfield, Ill.
3. Carbonell, L. M., and J. Rodriguez. 1965. Transformation of mycelial and yeast forms of *Paracoccidioides brasiliensis* in cultures and in experimental inoculations. J. Bacteriol. **90:**504–510.
4. Conant, N. F., D. T. Smith, R. D. Baker, and J. L. Callaway. 1971. Manual of clinical mycology, 3rd ed. W. B. Saunders Co., Philadelphia.
5. Emmons, C. W. 1942. Isolation of Coccidioides from soil and rodents. Pub. Health Rep. **57:**109–111.
6. Emmons, C. W., C. H. Binford, and J. P. Utz. 1970. Medical mycology, 2nd ed. Lea and Febiger, Philadelphia.
7. Fiese, M. J. 1958. Coccidioidomycosis. Charles C Thomas, Publisher, Springfield, Ill.
8. Kwon-Chung, K. J. 1973. Studies on *Emmonsiella capsulata*. I. Hetero-thallism and development of the ascocarp. Mycologia **65:**109–121.

9. Larsh, H. W. 1970. Isolation and identification media for systemic fungi. Proc. Int. Symp. Mycoses. Pan-Amer. Health Organ. Sci. Publ. No. 205.
10. McDonough, E. S., and A. L. Lewis. 1968. The ascigerous stage of *Blastomyces dermatitidis*. Mycologia **60:**76–83.
11. Symposium. 1972. Paracoccidioidomycosis. Proc. 1st Pan-Amer. Symp., Medellin, Colombia. Pan-Amer. Health Organ. Sci. Publ. No. 254.

Chapter 58

Fungi of Maduromycosis

JOHN D. SCHNEIDAU, JR.

CHARACTERIZATION

Maduromycosis is a chronic, suppurative infection caused by various species of the higher fungi (Eumycophyta). The lesions are characterized by the presence of multiple, draining sinus tracts that exude pus containing granules of varying size and color. Most lesions occur on the extremities, but lesions may occasionally be located on other parts of the body. Direct examination and culture of the granules are the most important procedures in the laboratory diagnosis, as the fungal agents are usually confined to the granules and are only rarely present as isolated filaments or spores in the pus. Direct examination is also important in differentiating maduromycosis from actinomycotic mycetoma (see chapter 17) since the lesions are indistinguishable clinically and in both infections granules are present in the pus.

DESCRIPTION OF AGENTS

The agents of maduromycosis are all species of filamentous fungi that produce broad, septate, branched hyphae both in culture and in granules in the lesions. The diameter of hyphae in the granules varies somewhat depending on the species but usually averages 4 to 5 μm. In some granules the terminal portions of the hyphae near the periphery of the granule and within it are greatly expanded and may attain diameters of 30 to 40 μm.

The species of fungi most frequently isolated from cases of maduromycosis are *Madurella grisea*, *Madurella mycetomi*, and *Monosporium apiospermum* (*Allescheria boydii*). *M. apiospermum*, a species that produces white granules, is the agent most frequently isolated from cases reported from the United States. *M. grisea*, *M. mycetomi*, and a fourth agent, *Phialophora jeanselmei*, all produce brown to black granules in the lesions and have been reported from the United States only rarely (6). The following additional species also cause maduromycosis: *Leptosphaeria senegalensis*, *Pyrenochaeta romeroi*, *Neotestudina rosatii*, and several species of *Cephalosporium*. *L. senegalensis* is prevalent in African countries, especially Senegal and Mauritania. *P. romeroi*, *N. rosatii*, and the *Cephalosporium* species must be considered of relatively minor importance until more information regarding their prevalence and distribution becomes available. Many other species of fungi have been described as possible etiological agents of maduromycosis, but convincing proof of their pathogenic role is lacking.

All of the fungi that cause maduromycosis grow readily on Sabouraud agar at room temperature. A few species can be identified by means of the conidial structures that they produce in culture. Others are ascomycetes and produce cleistothecia and asci. Some species may fail to produce any type of sporulation at all so that identification based solely on cultural features can be quite difficult.

COLLECTION AND EXAMINATION OF GRANULES

Pus from the lesions should be carefully examined for the presence of granules. Brown or black granules are readily seen, but white to cream-colored granules may be difficult to find, especially if they are quite small, since they may easily be confused with other particulate material in the pus. If the pus is thick and opaque, it should first be diluted with saline and then a small amount should be placed in a petri dish and spread out evenly over the surface of the dish in a thin layer. Granules should be searched for by holding the plate over a fluorescent light, or by examining the plate under low magnification on the stage of a stereoscopic microscope. Granules appear as discrete, opaque, rounded to oval bodies with a somewhat lobulated, smooth, shiny surface. Granules can be fished out with a Pasteur pipette, or with a forceps if they are large enough, and placed on a slide for microscopy. At least one granule should be smeared out in a thin film between two slides, and the smear should be heat-fixed and then gram-stained. A second granule should be placed on a slide in 20% potassium hydroxide and lightly crushed between slide and cover glass. At this stage of the laboratory procedure, it is important to differentiate between granules produced by the higher fungi and those produced by actinomycetes, and this differentiation can readily be accomplished by examination of the gram-stained smear and KOH wet mount of the granules. The broad, septate hyphae of the higher fungi are easily seen in the KOH wet mount, whereas on the gram-stained smear they may be more difficult to recognize. Although higher fungi are considered to be gram-positive, not all hyphae in a granule stain well with this stain, and hyphal walls do not stain. If they adhere to the slide at all, hyphae in granules also containing pus cells and debris are often unrecognizable as such because of the distortion caused by heat fixation and subsequent dehydration. On the other hand, the actinomycetes, because of their small size, are not visible in the KOH wet mount, but in the gram-stained smear appear as delicate, branched, gram-positive filaments with a diameter of 1 nm or less. Lactophenol cotton blue mounts of the crushed granules may also be used to demonstrate the filaments of the higher fungi (Fig. 1). In addition, crushed granules are sometimes stained with special fungal stains such as the periodic acid-Schiff stain or the Gomori methenamine-silver stain, but these stains are used only rarely and are often unsatisfactory because of the thickness of the smear, or because the small friable particles of the smeared granule often become detached from the slide during the staining procedure. In both cases, when no granules can be found, wet mounts of the pus, both with and without KOH, should be examined directly for hyphal fragments.

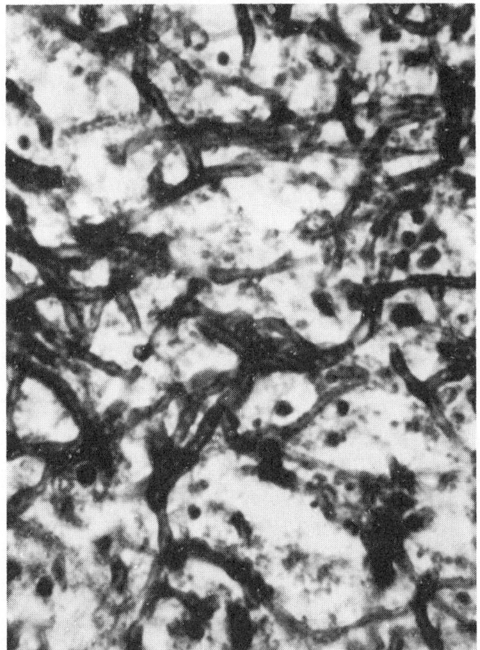

FIG. 1. *Monosporium apiospermum in smear of crushed granule. Wet mount in lactophenol cotton blue.* ×*550.*

In addition to the microscope examination, the granules should be examined grossly for size, color, and consistency, since such characteristics may give clues to the specific identity of the etiological agent (Table 1).

CULTURAL PROCEDURES

Granules obtained from pus should be washed by repeated centrifugation in sterile physiological saline to eliminate as much surface contamination as possible. The washed granules should then be emulsified in 1 ml of saline by gentle grinding in either a mortar and pestle or a tissue grinder. The saline suspension should then be serially streaked on plates of Sabouraud agar containing 100 μg of chloramphenicol per ml. Plates of Littman oxgall agar (Difco) should be similarly inoculated because many of the fungi that cause maduromycosis grow well on this medium, whereas the growth of saprophytic contaminating fungi is restricted. Plates should be incubated at 25 to 30 C and examined for growth at intervals for at least 3 weeks. When no granules can be found, the pus should be streaked for isolation on the media described above, but the likelihood of obtaining positive cultures is greatly reduced. Media containing cycloheximide, which are routinely used in other mycotic infections have limited usefulness for the isolation of the agents of maduromycosis because many of the species involved will not grow on these media.

IDENTIFICATION OF SPECIES

The species can be divided into the following three groups on the basis either of the ease with which they may be identified or of their prevalence or rarity as agents of maduromycosis.

Group I: Monosporium apiospermum (Allescheria boydii), Cephalosporium species, and Phialophora jeanselmei

The organisms in group I exhibit distinctive microscopic and macroscopic characteristics that make cultural identification relatively easy. *M. apiospermum* is the most common causative agent of maduromycosis in the United States and is prevalent worldwide. Both *M. apiospermum* and *Cephalosporium* species

TABLE 1. *Gross characteristics of the granules*

Species	Color	Consistency	Size range (mm)[a]
Monosporium apiospermum (*Allescheria boydii*)	White to cream	Soft	0.5–3
Cephalosporium species	White	Soft	1–3
Neotestudina rosatii	Buff to light brown	Soft	0.3–1
Phialophora jeanselmei	Brownish yellow to dark brown	Soft to firm	0.5–2
Madurella mycetomi	Dark brown to black	Hard	0.5–5
Madurella grisea	Black	Firm to hard	0.5–3
Leptosphaeria senegalensis	Black	Hard	0.5–3
Pyrenochaeta romeroi	Black	Hard	0.5–2

[a] The size range given here refers to the size of the granules as usually seen in tissue sections. In exudate from the lesions, the granules tend to be smaller than those seen in sections from deeper parts of the lesion, and the minimal size may be considerably less than that indicated in the table.

produce white to yellowish granules in the lesions, but the microscopic structure of these granules is not distinctive enough to allow specific identification. The granules of *P. jeanselmei* are brown to black, and stained sections present a characteristic appearance that permits a specific identification by an experienced histopathologist.

M. apiospermum. Colonies develop rapidly on Sabouraud agar and reach maturity in 8 to 9 days, at which time numerous conidia are present. The color of the aerial mycelium may vary from white to some shade of gray, but most primary isolates are mouse gray in color and become white only after several transplants. The reverse of the colony is dark gray. Conidia vary somewhat in size, but most are approximately 6 by 9 μm with a fairly thick double contoured wall containing a yellowish to tan pigment. Most conidia are produced singly at the tips of the conidiophores, but they may occasionally occur in clusters of two and three, and some may be laterally attached (Fig. 2). The perfect stage of *M. apiospermum* is the ascomycete *Allescheria boydii*, and in some cultures cleistothecia may be produced. These appear as dark brown spherical bodies embedded in the mycelium and measuring 150 to 200 μm at maturity. They are seen only in old cultures (4 to 6 weeks) and are not essential for identification.

Cephalosporium species. Members of the genus *Cephalosporium* produce conidial structures in culture that readily permit generic identification. Conidia arise successively from the tips of short, slender conidiophores, and are held together in a ball by a secretion of slime (Fig. 3). The conidia may be round, oval, elongate, or slightly curved, depending upon the species. The sparse aerial growth is usually white to cream, but may be tan, peach, or salmon in color. Coremia are produced by some species. *C. falciforme*, *C. granulomatis*, *C. infestans*, *C. madurae*, and *C. recifei* have been implicated as causative agents of maduromycosis. Of these, *C. falciforme* and *C. recifei* are known to be pathogenic, whereas the pathogenic role of the other species is dubious (1). There are many other species within the genus, and a number of these may occur as saprophytes on the skin or in open lesions, so that the

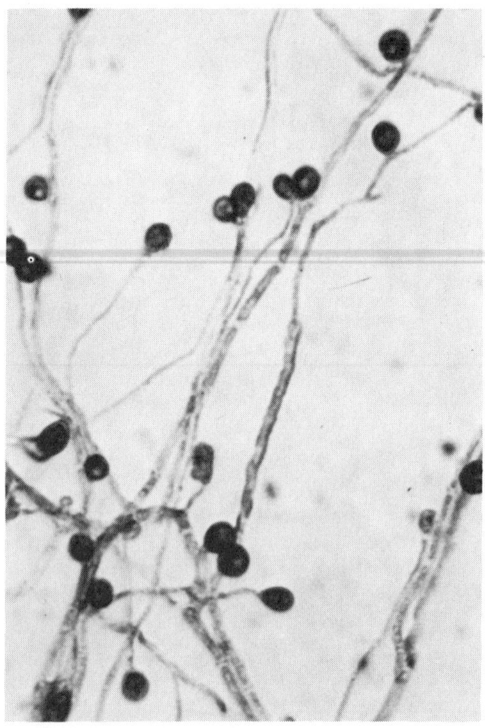

FIG. 2. *Conidia and conidiophores of Monosporium apiospermum. ×800.*

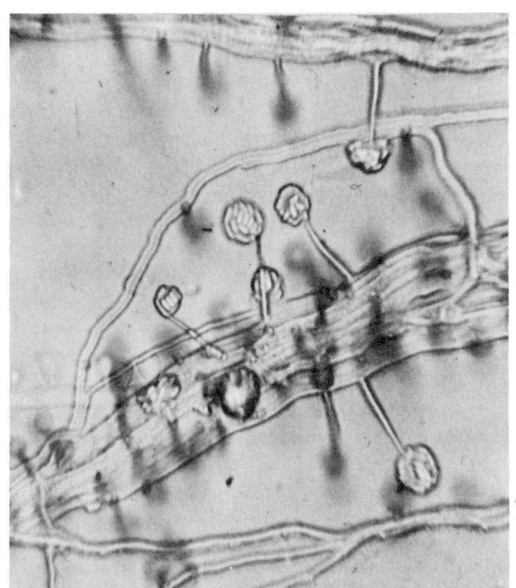

FIG. 3. *Conidia and conidiophores typical of Cephalosporium sp.*

isolation of a *Cephalosporium* species from a lesion is not proof of its pathogenic role. The same species must be repeatedly isolated in large numbers from the washed, crushed granules before it can be considered to be the causative agent of the lesion. The identification of species of *Cephalosporium* is quite difficult because of the minor differences that separate the large number of species. Isolates suspected of being pathogenic should be forwarded to a specialist for identification.

P. jeanselmei. The species *P. jeanselmei* produces hyphae with a dark, smokey pigment in the walls, and is dimorphic in culture. The very early growth is smooth, moist, and shiny black, and consists almost entirely of budding yeast cells with darkly pigmented walls, but after 3 to 4 days hyphae begin to form and the yeasty growth is then rapidly overgrown with a greenish-gray to black mycelium. Phialids are produced, but they lack the collarette usually seen in other species of *Phialophora* and are thus difficult to recognize as true phialids. They appear as slender, short hyphae, sometimes branched, with clusters of conidia at the tips. There is a superficial resemblance to the *Cephalosporium* type of sporulation, except that the conidia are loosely aggregated around the tips of the phialid and are not embedded in mucus. Conidia are also produced directly on the sides of the hyphae from minute apiculi (Fig. 4).

Group II: Madurella grisea and Madurella mycetoma

The two species in group II present similar problems in identification since only rarely can they be readily and unequivocally identified on the basis of cultural characteristics alone. Both species are quite variable in culture, with overlapping characteristics, so that one may sometimes be mistaken for the other. Some of the features that they possess in common include the color and gross aspect of the colony, production of a diffusible pigment in the medium, the formation of numerous chlamydospores, and the lack of spore production on Sabouraud agar. The species differ in their optimal growth tem-

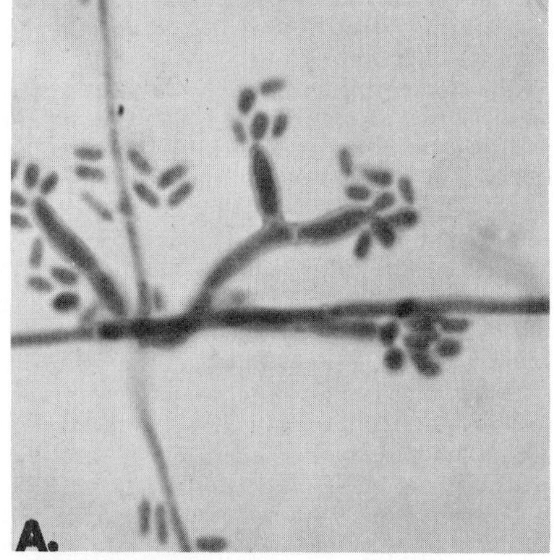

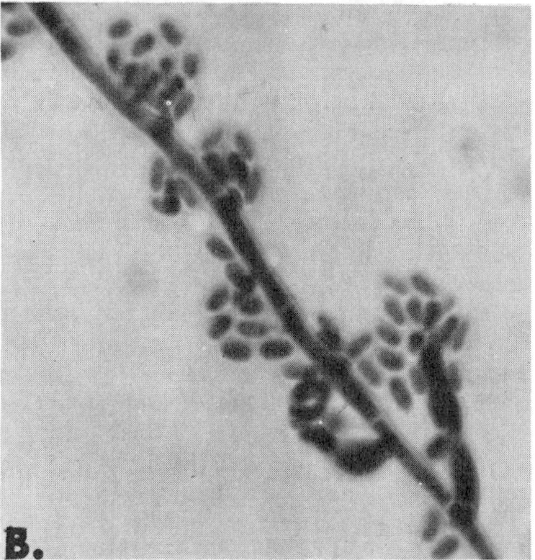

FIG. 4. *Sporulation in Phialophora jeanselmei. (A) Phialids. (B) Conidia arising laterally from the hypha. (From N. F. Conant et al., Manual of clinical mycology, 3rd ed. W. B. Saunders Co.)*

peratures, their sugar assimilations, the production of phialids by some strains of *M. mycetoma* on cornmeal-agar, and in the formation of sclerotia in old cultures of *M. grisea*. However, the two species produce granules in tissues that differ markedly in their microscopic structure in stained sections, with distinctive features that permit specific identification by an experienced histopathologist. For this reason, an exchange of information between the pathologist and the clinical microbiologist is valuable and may often be necessary for final identification of the cultures. Numerous isolates of both *M. mycetomi* and *M. grisea* that currently exist in stock culture collections were originally identified because the colonial features of the cultures were compatible with the pathologist's identification based on the appearance of granules in tissue sections.

A brief description of each species is given below. For a more detailed description and discussion of these fungi, the publications of Mackinnon (7) and Segretain (11) should be consulted.

M. mycetomi. Most rapid growth occurs at 35 C, with visible growth present in 3 days. The growth is compact, leathery, and wrinkled or folded, usually brownish in color with a powdery or velvety surface nap which may be white at first but which rapidly becomes yellow-brown or deep brown. In old cultures (6 to 8 weeks), some strains produce small (0.5 to 1 mm), hard, oval to spherical black bodies (sclerotia). On Sabouraud agar spores are not usually produced; however, on cornmeal-agar some strains produce phialids and phialospores which resemble the type of sporulation seen in cultures of *Phialophora jeanselmei* (Fig. 4a). The diffusible pigment, when present, is yellowish-brown.

M. grisea. Grows most rapidly at 25 to 30 C, with visible growth present in 4 to 5 days. A compact, leathery, cerebriform growth develops which becomes covered with abundant dark gray to black-brown aerial hyphae. Reverse of the colony is black. Diffusible pigment, when present, is red-brown. No conidia are produced on Sabouraud agar or on corn meal-agar. Physiologically, *M. grisea* differs from *M. mycetomi* in that the latter assimilates lactose but not sucrose, whereas the reverse is the case for *M. grisea*. Pycnidia have been reported in a few strains.

Group III: Leptosphaeria senegalensis, Pyrenochaeta romeroi, and Neotestudina rosatii

The three species in group III have not been implicated as agents of maduromycosis in the United States. *L. senegalensis* is prevalent in Africa and appears to be restricted almost entirely to that continent. Infections due to *P. romeroi* and *N. rosatii* are quite rare; only three to four cases have been reported in the world literature. Colonies of *L. senegalensis* and *P. romeroi* are dark grayish-brown to black with a black reverse, whereas those of *N. rosatii* are tan to brown, with a deep brownish-black reverse. Both *L. senegalensis* and *N. rosatii* are ascomycetes and produce deep brown to black ascocarps in culture. The ascospores of *L. senegalensis* are multicellular with six to eight cells, whereas those of *N. rosatii* are two-celled. *P. romeroi* is a member of the order *Sphaeropsidales*, which is characterized by the production of pycnidia that are usually black in color, are ostiolate, and contain numerous conidia. A number of species belonging to this order may occur in clinical materials as contaminants. Specific identification based on the micoscopic morphology of the ascocarps or pycnidia is difficult and in most instances will require the services of a specialist in the taxonomy of these fungi. Complete descriptions of the above three species may be found in the publications of Baylet et al. (2), Segretain et al. (12, 13), and Borelli (3). For additional general information regarding maduromycosis, consult the texts of Conant et al. (4) and Emmons et al. (5), and the publications of Mariat (9) and Vanbreuseghem (14, 15).

SEROLOGY

Studies by Murray and Mahgoub (8, 10) on the diagnosis of maduromycosis by gel diffusion techniques offer promise that serological methods may eventually provide a relatively rapid and accurate means of specific diagnosis. However, such procedures are still in an experimental stage, and they are not currently adaptable for routine use in the diagnostic laboratory.

LITERATURE CITED

1. Avram, A. 1964. Étude clinique et mycologique concernant le premier cas Europeen de mycétome déterminé par *Cephalosporium sp.* Mycopathol. Mycol. Appl. **24**:177–194.
2. Baylet, J., R. Camain, and G. Segretain. 1959. Identification des agents des maduromycosis due Sénégal et la Mauritanie. Bull. Soc. Pathol. Exot. **52**:448–477.
3. Borelli, D. 1959. *Pyrenochaeta romeroi, n. sp.* Rev. Dermatol. Venezolana **1**:1–3.
4. Conant, N. F., D. T. Smith, R. D. Baker, and J. L. Callaway. 1971. Manual of clinical mycology, 3rd ed., p. 458–481. W. B. Saunders, Co., Philadelphia.
5. Emmons, C. W., C. H. Binford, and J. P. Utz. 1970. Medical mycology, 2nd ed., p. 389–418. Lea & Febiger, Philadelphia.
6. Green, W. O., and T. E. Adams. 1964. Mycetoma in the United States. Amer. J. Clin. Pathol. **42**:75–91.

7. Mackinnon, J. E. 1954. A contribution to the study of the causal organisms of maduromycosis. Trans. Roy. Soc. Trop. Med. Hyg. **48:**470–480.
8. Mahgoub, E. S. 1964. The value of gel-diffusion in the diagnosis of mycetoma. Trans. Roy. Soc. Trop. Med. Hyg. **58:**560–563.
9. Mariat, F. 1963. Sur la distribution géographique et la repartition des agents de mycétomes. Bull. Soc. Pathol. Exot. **56:**35–351.
10. Murray, I. G., and E. S. Mahgoub. 1968. Further studies on the diagnosis of mycetoma by double diffusion in agar. Sabouraudia **6:**106–110.
11. Segretain, G. 1957. Diagnostic biologique des maduromycoses. Pathol. Biol. **33:**951–955.
12. Segretain, G., J. Baylet, H. Darasse, and R. Camain. 1959. *Leptosphaeria senegalensis, n. sp.* agent de mycetomes a gran noirs. C. R. Acad. Sci. **248:**3730–3732.
13. Segretain, G., and P. Destombes. 1961. Description d'un nouvelle agent de maduromycose. *Neotestudina rosatii,* n. gen. n. sp. isole en Afrique. C. R. Acad. Sci. **253:**2577–2579.
14. Vanbreuseghem, R. 1967. The early diagnosis of mycetoma. Dermatol. Int. **6:**123–140.
15. Vanbreuseghem, R. 1967. Early diagnosis, treatment, and epidemiology of mycetoma. Rev. Med. Vet. Mycol. **6:**49–60.

Chapter 59

Dematiaceous Fungi

HARRY S. NIELSEN, JR.

DESCRIPTION OF AGENTS

The dematiaceous fungi comprise the darkly pigmented molds which sporulate from simple or branched conidiophores produced singly on the vegetative hyphae. It should be emphasized, however, that not all fungi developing a smoky appearance in culture are classified in the family *Dematiaceae*. The etiological agent of sporotrichosis, which is considered in this chapter, is not a member of this taxonomic group, but is included because many strains are deeply pigmented.

Agent of Sporotrichosis

Sporothrix schenckii Hektoen and Perkins, 1900 is the causative agent of sporotrichosis. Synonymy: *Sporotrichum* sp. Smith, 1898; *Sporotrichum beurmanni* Matruchot and Ramond, 1905; *Sporotrichum schenckii* Matruchot, 1910. The binomium *Sporothrix schenckii*, as opposed to the more familiar name *Sporotrichum schenckii*, is adopted on the basis of priority and of morphological disagreement between this fungus and *S. aureum*, the type species of the genus *Sporotrichum* (11). *Ceratocystis stenoceras* has been suggested as the possible sexual stage of *S. schenckii* (40–42). Comparative studies of certain polysaccharides of *S. schenckii* and *Ceratocystis* species indicate that some similarities exist between the rhamnomannans of *S. schenckii* and *C. stenoceras* (60).

Sporotrichosis is primarily a granulomatous disease of the skin, subcutaneous tissue, and lymphoid tissue, usually involving body extremities. Less frequently, infection may be extracutaneous, with localized or disseminated lesions of the musculoskeletal, pulmonary, genitourinary, ocular, and central nervous systems (37, 64). Although the usual subcutaneous form of the infection with node involvement is highly suggestive of the mycosis, the disease may be confused with tularemia, anthrax, glanders, and the cutaneous forms of tuberculosis and other mycoses. In addition to its observation in humans, naturally acquired infection has been reported in several animals, including horses and cows (2).

The disease is worldwide in distribution and occurs most often in persons exposed to soil and vegetation. The etiological agent has been isolated repeatedly from saprophytic sources (30, 39, 59) and is known to infect humans after abrasion or minor wounds (23, 26). Growth of the fungus on lagging timber in South African gold mines resulted in a single epidemic involving over 2,500 human cases (59).

Examination of clinical material. Unlike the etiological agents of other mycoses (blastomycosis, cryptococcosis, and coccidioidomycosis), *S. schenckii* is not readily demonstrated by the microscopic examination of fresh preparations of serosanguineous exudates, pus, or cellular debris from lesions. Unless these materials or tissues are stained with Gomori methenamine-silver stain or periodic acid-Schiff stain, microscopic preparations are of little value in the diagnosis of the disease (22).

Histopathology. In tissue, *S. schenckii* appears as an elongate or oval budding yeast (Fig. 1). It rarely occurs as hyphae (38) or as an asteroid body (36), and the fusiform cells, which are frequently described as being cigar-shaped, are most characteristic of experimental infection in laboratory animals (Fig. 2). The fungus is not usually seen in sections stained with hematoxylin and eosin, but can be adequately demonstrated with the Gomori methenamine-silver stain, the Gridley stain, or with the diastase modification of the periodic acid-Schiff stain (22).

Cultural examination. The use of culture media containing antibiotics is recommended if specimens are obtained from lesions which are secondarily infected with bacteria or contaminated with the spores of saprophytic fungi. The yeast form of the fungus is readily cultured on brain heart infusion agar containing 5% whole blood, or on Francis' glucose-cystine-blood-agar (10). The culture should be incubated at 35 to 37 C and examined within 3 to 5 days for small, glistening, cream-colored colonies. Yeast cells are nonencapsulated, 2 by 3 to 2 by 6 μm in size,

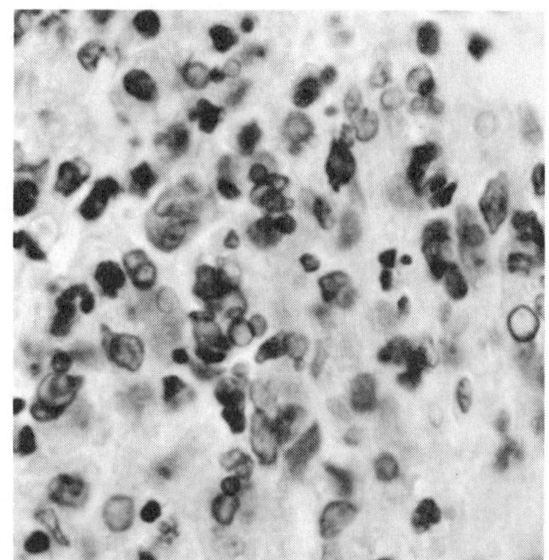

FIG. 1. *Spherical budding yeast of Sporothrix schenckii in tissue. Periodic acid-Schiff stain. ×922.*

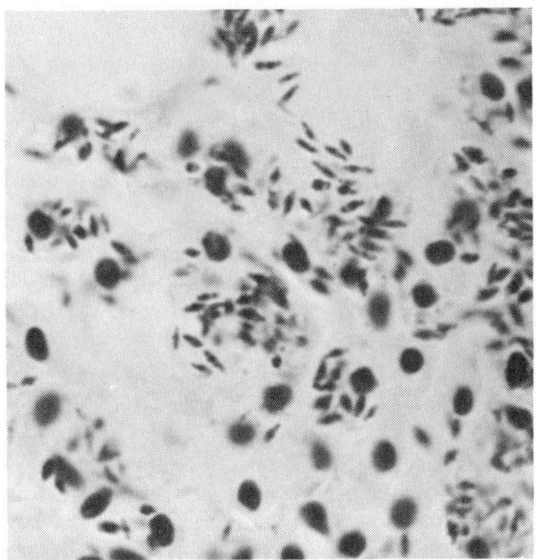

FIG. 2. *Fusiform-shaped yeast of Sporothrix schenckii in peritoneal exudate from mouse. Gram stain. ×922.*

and frequently exhibit a tadpole appearance because of the elongate nature of some buds (Fig. 3).

The hyphal form of *S. schenckii* can be isolated at room temperature on conventional media such as Sabouraud glucose agar. The colony is slow-growing, napform or leathery, and changes from white or cream-colored to nearly black with age. Microscopically, the fungus consists of delicate hyphae (1 to 2 μm in diameter) from which simple conidiophores are borne usually at a 45° to 90° angle from the supporting hyphal cell. Sporulation occurs from several apicular sites, resulting in a loose cluster of pyriform spores at the tip of the conidiophore (Fig. 4). As the culture matures, the conidia develop basipetally and eventually on the hypha itself.

Biochemical properties. Biochemical properties are of no value in the identification of this species. The fungus is known to have an absolute requirement for thiamine (17); however, this characteristic has not been used diagnostically.

Immunological properties. Delayed hyper-

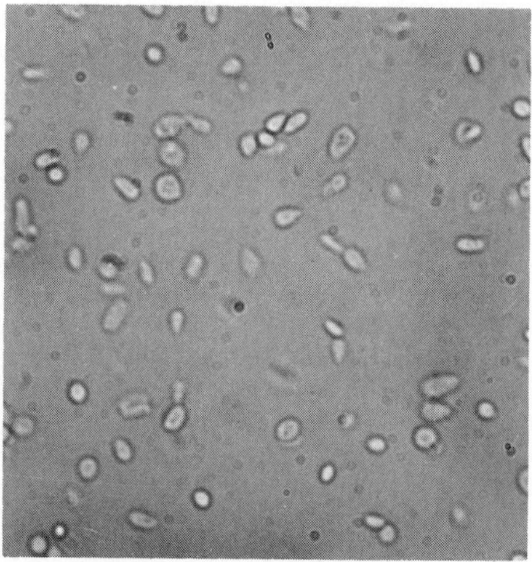

FIG. 3. *Yeast of Sporothrix schenckii from 37 C culture. Brain heart infusion-blood agar. ×922.*

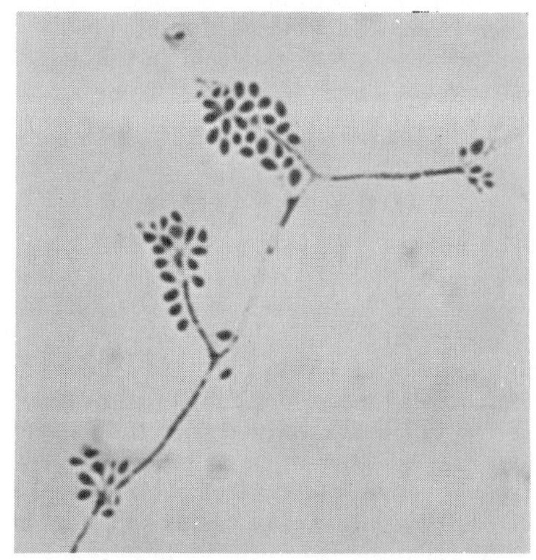

FIG. 4. *Mycelial form of Sporothrix schenckii illustrating delicate hyphae and conidiophores bearing spores at the tips and sides. Sabouraud glucose agar. Room temperature. ×922.*

sensitivity to *S. schenckii* can be demonstrated in persons with active or past infection by use of a 1:2,500 (vol/vol) suspension of heat- or Merthiolate-killed yeast or conidia. Soluble antigens prepared from extracts of the yeast cell or culture broth are usually less reliable as skin test agents, although antigen-containing cell wall material appears to be as good as whole yeast in eliciting a skin response (47).

Serum of individuals suspected of having sporotrichosis should be tested for agglutinins, in which a titer of 1:40 or greater is considered suggestive of the mycosis. The test is performed with whole yeast antigen (1:2,500, vol/vol) and is read after 1 h of incubation at 37 C followed by a second incubation at 4 C for 12 to 18 h and centrifugation for 5 min at 2,500 rpm, in that order. Precipitins are usually less reliable than are agglutinins but, nevertheless, can be demonstrated by immunodiffusion in agar gel in approximately 75% of culturally confirmed cases. In this test, the broth filtrate of the yeast form of the fungus is a suitable antigen at a concentration of 0.5 to 1.0 mg/ml. Complement fixation with yeast antigen has been employed (50), but this test is usually less satisfactory than either agglutination or precipitation procedures. In addition to the above techniques, immunofluorescence has been successfully used in demonstrating the fungus in smears of lesion exudate and tissue (33).

Animal pathogenicity. With the possible exception of some soil isolates of *S. schenckii*, the fungus is virulent for mice (30, 51). Peritonitis, orchitis, and bone and visceral involvement usually occur after intraperitoneal inoculation of either yeast or hyphal elements. Rats and hamsters are also susceptible, but guinea pigs are resistant to progressive disease with this agent.

FAMILY DEMATIACEAE

The medically important fungi belonging to the *Dematiaceae* are differentiated in the following key. (*Phialophora jeanselmei* has been purposely omitted from this key because of its consideration in chapter 58. This species is closely related morphologically to *P. gougerotii*. The two fungi differ primarily in the nature of their in vivo growth forms. *P. gougerotii* is characterized by budding elements and hyphae, whereas *P. jeanselmei* occurs as spherical and hyphal cells aggregated in the form of a granule.)

Key to the Medically Important Fungi Belonging to the Family Dematiaceae

I. Colony initially yeastlike, becoming hyphal with age.
   A. Yeast septate, fusiform or bizarre in shape ...... *Cladosporium werneckii*.
   B. Yeast aseptate or rarely septate, ellipsoid to round.
      1. Sporogenous, peglike sterigmata present on hyphae but more or less inconspicuous; conidiophores regularly consisting of several cells that frequently resemble a short lateral branch; good growth at 37 C ...... *Phialophora dermatitidis*.
      2. Sporogenous, peglike sterigmata usually conspicuously dark and elevated; conidiophores usually tubular, easily distinguished from cells of the hyphae; little or no growth at 37 C ..... *P. gougerotti*.
      3. Sporogenous, peglike sterigmata relatively uncommon; conidiophores dark, rigid, and spinelike; little or no growth at 37 C ...... *P. spinifera*.

II. Colony typically that of a mold during early and late stages of growth.
   A. Conidia produced predominantly from semiendogenous loci.
      1. Phialids flask-shaped, extensions cuplike ...... *P. verrucosa*.
      2. Phialids long and tubular, extensions nearly flat or saucer shaped ...... *P. richardsiae*.
   B. Conidia produced from exogenous and endogenous loci; sporeheads primarily of a reduced *Cladosporium* type, sometimes accompanied by conidiophores of the *Acrotheca* and *Phialophora* types.
      1. Spores ellipsoid to elongate ...... *F. pedrosoi*.
      2. Spores compressed, ovoid to round ...... *F. compactum*.
   C. Conidia produced entirely from exogenous loci; conidiophores of the *Cladosporium* type.
      1. Proteolytic ...... saprophytic *Cladosporium* species.
      2. Nonproteolytic.
         a. Colonies moderately slow-growing; temperature maximum 42 to 43 C; conidia to 11 μm; neurotropic ...... *C. trichoides*.
         b. Colonies slow-growing; temperature maximum 35 to 36 C; conidia 1.5 to 7.5 μm; not neurotropic ...... *C. carrionii*.

Agents of Chromoblastomycosis

Chromoblastomycosis is caused by five different dematiaceous fungi belonging to the genera *Phialophora*, *Cladosporium*, and *Fonsecaea*. Two species, *P. verrucosa* and *C. carrionii*, are essentially monosporulating. *P. dermatitidis* sporulates by abstriction and by semiendogenous development, and *F. pedrosoi* and *F. compactum* produce conidia according to methods described below for *Phialophora*, *Cladosporium*, and *Acrotheca*. Sporulation in the genus *Phialophora* occurs by the successive production of conidia from a single semiendogenous locus (Fig. 5). Sporulation in *Cladosporium* involves budding from one or more loci, resulting in branching chains of conidia (Fig. 6), and that observed in *Acrotheca* is characterized by budding from a terminal locus and from multiple lateral loci, resulting in aggregates of

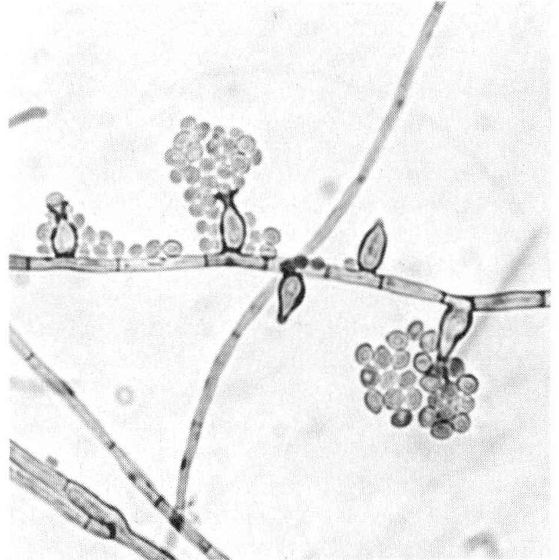

FIG. 5. *Flask-shaped conidiophores of Phialophora verrucosa illustrating flaring tips surrounded by clusters of semiendogenously produced spores. Corn meal-agar.* ×*678.*

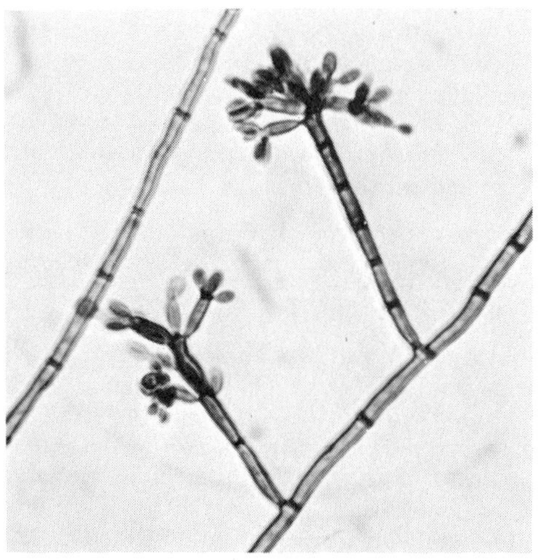

FIG. 6. *"Cladosporium"-type conidiophores of Fonsecaea pedrosoi. Corn meal-agar.* ×*678.*

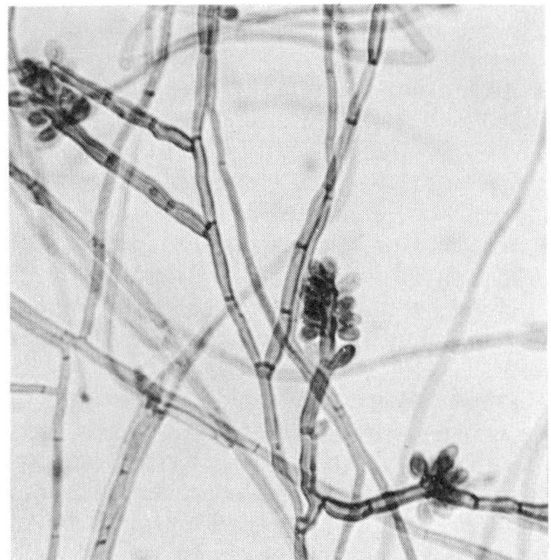

FIG. 7. *"Acrotheca"-type conidiophores of Fonsecaea pedrosoi. Corn meal-agar.* ×*678.*

spores surrounding the distal end of the conidiophore (Fig. 7).

These agents are believed to be closely related despite their separation into three different taxa. This system of classification is employed because it avoids amending the descriptions of definitive taxonomic groups. The publications of Conant et al. (14), Emmons et al. (20), Carrion (12), and Trejos (61) should be consulted for general discussions concerning the nomenclature of this group of pathogens. Of the five fungi involved, *F. pedrosoi* is isolated most frequently from the disease. *C. trichoides*, a common cause of cerebral abscess, has been isolated from a case simulating chromoblastomycosis (20), although this agent is not usually associated with this mycosis.

Chromoblastomycosis is a chronic, granulomatous infection, usually localized and limited to the skin and subcutaneous tissues. Lesions first appear as nodular processes, but become verrucous, ulcerated, or crusted as the disease evolves. Rarely, cutaneous chromoblastomycosis may develop into a generalized infection (25, 32). Immature lesions must be distinguished from the cutaneous forms of other mycoses, particularly blastomycosis, as well as tuberculosis, leishmaniasis, syphilis, and yaws.

The disease is seen most frequently in tropical and subtropical climates (12), but it also occurs in temperate regions of the world (31, 44). Adult males whose occupation brings them in contact with soil and wood are chiefly affected. The saprophytic existence of the fungi causing chromoblastomycosis has been reviewed by Ridley (52), Ahearn and Kaplan (1), and Gezuele et al. (27). A detailed treatise on chromoblastomycosis has been published by Al-Doory (3).

Examination of clinical material. Crusts or exudative materials from lesions should be placed in 10% KOH, gently heated, and examined for ovoid, deeply pigmented, sclerotia-like bodies. These elements are 4 to 12 μm in diameter and are either unicellular or septate through one or more planes of division (Fig. 8). Branching hyphae may be observed in superficial scales, but this growth form is relatively rare.

Histopathology. The epidermis of infected areas is usually irregularly thickened and shows pronounced hyperkeratosis. Keratolytic microabscesses containing the spherical, sometimes septate forms, either within giant cells or extracellular, are usually circumscribed by fibrotic tissue. Because of the natural yellowish-brown pigmentation of the fungus, it can be adequately demonstrated with routine stains such as hematoxylin and eosin. It is impossible to distinguish among the five etiological agents of chromoblastomycosis on the basis of their in vivo morphology.

Cultural examination. Each of the five fungi associated with chromoblastomycosis can be isolated by streaking slants of Sabouraud antibiotic medium with crusts or other material from lesions. Cultures should be incubated at room temperature and retained for at least 3 weeks before being discarded as negative. Species identification is based primarily on micromorphology, and is best accomplished from slide culture preparations. The following descriptions summarize the most salient characteristics of these fungi (see also Table 1).

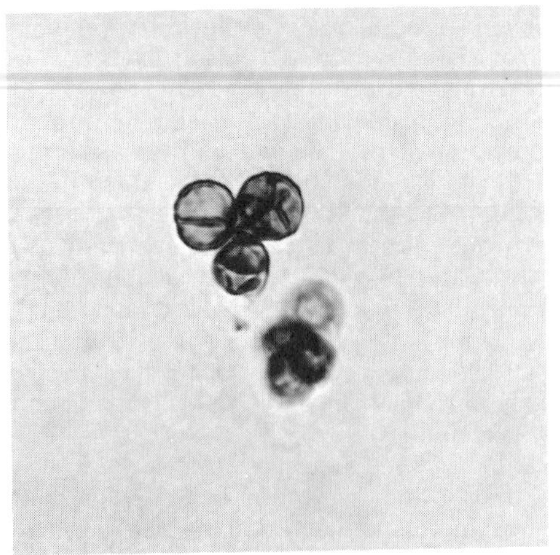

FIG. 8. *Pigmented bodies which characterize the tissue morphology of the fungi of chromoblastomycosis. In pus from a lesion, unstained.* ×678.

Phialophora verrucosa Thaxter in Medlar 1915. Synonymy: *Cadophora americana* Nannfeldt, 1927; *Phialophora macrospora* Moore and Almeida, 1936; *Fonsecaea pedrosoi* var. *phialophorica* Carrion, 1940.

Colonies of this fungus are slow-growing, dark olive-gray in color, and have a velvety or nap-form surface. Vegetative growth is most pronounced on Sabouraud glucose agar; however, sporulation is increased on a sparse medium, such as corn meal-agar. Conidia, 1 by 3 to 2 by 4 μm in size, develop semiendogenously from flask-shaped phialids which are borne singly or in groups on terminal or lateral aspects of the hyphae (Fig. 5). A small number of strains are said to sporulate from conidiophores of the *Cladosporium* and *Acrotheca* types (20).

Phialophora dermatitidis (Kano 1937) Emmons 1965. Synonymy: *Hormiscium dermatitidis* Kano, 1937; *Fonsecaea dermatitidis* Carrion, 1950; *Hormodendrum dermatitidis* Conant, 1953.

Young colonies of this fungus are moist and glistening, olive to black, and consist of aseptate budding yeast (Fig. 9). As the culture matures, feathery strands of submerged or tightly oppressed hyphae radiate outwardly from the margin of the colony, or appear as sectors, and eventually give rise to olive-gray aerial filaments. Microscopic preparations of this growth form reveal septate hyphae from which conidia are borne successively from peg-like sterigmata and from the tips and sides of poorly differentiated conidiophores (Fig. 10). This appendage is multicellular and frequently resembles a short lateral branch. Extensions which constitute the *Phialophora* cup are usually inconspicuous unless confined to short cup-shaped phialids. In contrast to previously reported observations (13), neither true *Cladosporium* nor *Acrotheca* methods of sporulation are present in this species.

Fonsecaea pedrosoi (Brumpt, 1922) Negroni, 1936. Synonymy: *Hormodendrum pedrosoi* Brumpt, 1922; *Acrotheca pedrosoi* da Fonseca and Leao, 1923; *Hormodendrum algeriensis* Montpellier and Catanei, 1927; *Trichosporium pedrosianum* Ota, 1928; *Trichosporium pedrosoi* Langeron, 1929; *Hormodendron rossicum* Meriin, 1930; *Gomphinaria pedrosoi* Dodge, 1935; *Botrytoides monomorpha* Moore and Almeida, 1936; *Hormodendroides pedrosoi* Moore and Almeida, 1936;

TABLE 1. *Salient characteristics of the medically important fungi belonging to the family Dematiaceae*[a]

Fungus	Primary mycosis	Tissue morphology	Dermatotropic	Neurotropic	Cultural characteristics				Growth at 37 C
					Generalized disease	Yeast form	Hyphal form	Sporulation	
Fonsecaea pedrosoi	Chromoblastomycosis	Spherical, septate cells	+	±	±	−	+	Conidia produced from dentrically branched conidiophores; less commonly from irregular club-shaped conidiophores and from semiendogenously sporulating phialids.	+
F. compactum	Chromoblastomycosis	Spherical, septate cells	+	−	−	−	+	Similar to above, sporeheads more reduced, spores oval and flattened as opposed to elongate.	+
Cladosporium carrionii	Chromoblastomycosis	Spherical, septate cells	+	−	−	−	+	Long flexuous branching chains of conidia.	±
Phialophora verrucosa	Chromoblastomycosis	Spherical, septate cells	+	−	−	−	+	Semiendogenous formation of conidia from flask-shaped phialids.	+
P. dermatitidis	Chromablastomycosis	Spherical cells; yeastlike forms; hyphae	+	+	+	+	+	Abstriction at the tips and sides of simple, hyphalike appendages; semiendogenously from cuplike phialids; successively from peglike sterigmata.	+
P. gougerotii	Subcutaneous abscess (cyst)	Spherical cells; yeastlike forms; hyphae	+	−	−	+	+	Abstriction at the tips and sides of simple or branched tubular conidiophores; semiendogenously from the above structure; successively from peglike sterigmata.	±
P. richardsiae	Subcutaneous abscess (cyst)	Hyphae	+	−	−	−	+	Semiendogenously from tubular conidiophores with expanded, or saucer-shaped apices.	+
P. spinifera	Granuloma	Spherical budding cells	+	−	−	+	+	Abstriction at the tips and sides of simple or branching spinelike conidiophores; semiendogenously from urn-shaped phialids.	±
C. trichoides	Brain abscess	Spherical cells; hyphae	−	+	−	−	+	Long flexuous branching chains of conidia.	±
C. werneckii	Tinea nigra	Branching hyphae; bacillary elements	+	−	−	+	+	Abstriction from poorly developed conidiophores; successively from peglike sterigmata of hyphae; chains of spores rarely produced.	−

[a] *Phialophora jeanselmei* is not included in this table because of its consideration in chapter 58.

Phialoconidiophora guggenheimia Moore and Almeida, 1936; *Hormodendrum japonicum* Takahaski, 1937; *Phialophora pedrosoi* Emmons in Binford et al., 1944.

This fungus is slow-growing, olivaceous to black, and produces a colony that is smooth, heaped, or irregular. As mentioned for *P. verrucosa*, sporulation is most pronounced on a sparse medium. Conidiophores of a reduced *Cladosporium* type (Fig. 6) intermixed with those characterizing *Acrotheca* (Fig. 7) and *Phialophora* (Fig. 5), in that order, constitute the micromorphology of this species. Since the fungus is extremely polymorphic, it should be recognized that variation from this pattern is not unusual. Some strains appear to produce only *Cladosporium*-type appendages, which necessitates their careful distinction from the saprophytic cladosporia. Conidia produced from *Cladosporium* heads are 1.5 by 3 to 3 by 6 μm in size, and exhibit distinctly darkened ends (disjunctors). The characteristic "shield"-shaped cell is formed from spores or terminal cells of a conidiophore which have two fertile loci.

Fonsecaea compactum Carrion, 1940. Synonymy: *Hormodendrum compactum* Carrion, 1935; *Phialoconidiophora compactum* Moore and Almeida, 1936; *Phialophora compactum* Emmons in Binford et al., 1944.

This fungus is slow-growing, producing a heaped colony that is usually brittle in texture, but otherwise indistinguishable from *F. pe-*

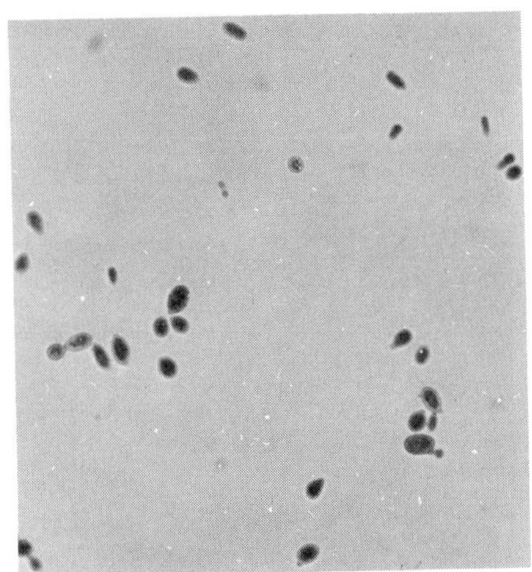

FIG. 9. *Aseptate yeast of Phialophora dermatitidis from a young colony. Corn meal-agar. ×678.*

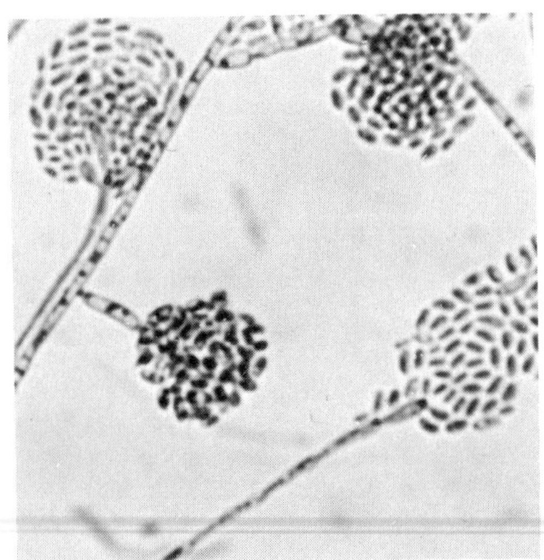

FIG. 10. *Hyphal form of Phialophora dermatitidis showing fertile sterigmata of the hyphae and a conidiophore surrounded by spores. Corn meal-agar. ×678.*

drosoi. With age, tufts of brownish aerial hyphae appear out of the napform surface of the mold. Conidiophores are similar to those of *F. pedrosoi* except for the compact nature of the sporeheads. In contrast to the elliptical conidia of *F. pedrosoi*, the spores of this species are ovoid, ranging in size from 1.5 by 2 to 2 by 3 μm. The fungus is seen infrequently as an etiological agent of chromoblastomycosis, and may represent a morphological variant of *F. pedrosoi*.

Cladosporium carrionii Trejos 1954. Synonymy: *Fonsecaea pedrosoi* var. *cladosporium* Simson, 1946; *Fonsecaea cladosporium* Powell, 1952.

This fungus is slow-growing with a dark olive-black colony which may be smooth or irregular. The margin is usually well defined, with a halo of darker submerged hyphae. Conidia are 1.5 by 2 to 3.0 by 7.5 μm in size and are produced entirely from *Cladosporium*-type conidiophores. Spore chains are long and flexuous and resemble those of saprophytic species. It has been isolated from cases of chromoblastomycosis occurring only in South Africa, Venezuela, and Australia.

Biochemical properties. The etiological agents of chromoblastomycosis do not hydrolyze starch, coagulate milk, or liquefy gelatin, Loffler's medium, or other substrates containing protein. These properties afford a useful means of distinguishing this group of fungi from saprophytic species of *Cladosporium* that are proteolytic (24).

Serological properties. Both complement-fixing antibodies and precipitins have been demonstrated in the sera of persons with chromoblastomycosis (9, 44). Antigens employed in these tests were obtained by extracting mechanically disrupted fungus cells with diluent, followed by centrifugation or filtration to remove particulate matter. The fluorescent-antibody procedure has been applied to the intergeneric study of these fungi (28), but it has not been used diagnostically.

Animal pathogenicity. Animal inoculation is of little value in the diagnosis of chromoblastomycosis or in the identification of the etiological agents. Experimental studies have shown that *F. pedrosoi* produces granulomatous lesions in the lungs and kidneys of mice when inoculated intraperitoneally (35). *F. pedrosoi*, *F. compactum*, and *P. verrucosa* have been isolated from cerebral lesions in mice after intraperitoneal and or intracranial exposure (18, 21), and *F. pedrosoi* is pathogenic for guinea pigs and rats when inoculated intratesticularly (5).

Agents of Chromomycotic Infection Involving the Brain and Subcutaneous Tissue

Infections of the brain and subcutaneous tissue are caused by several different species of fungi belonging to the genera *Phialophora* and *Cladosporium*. Cerebral involvement may occur as a complication of generalized disease (25, 57), or as an independent mycosis (7). The latter is believed to result from inhalation of the etiological agent, followed by metastasis from a primary pulmonary lesion. In contrast, infection of the subcutaneous tissue occurs after trauma. The lesions are usually small, single, and asymptomatic. They are seen most frequently on body extremities (6, 19, 43, 65) and may be diagnosed as subcutaneous abscesses, cysts, or ganglion or foreign body granulomas (34, 49). The agents are best described according to the lesions which they produce.

Brain abscess

Cladosporium trichoides Emmons in Binford et al., 1952, is the most commonly reported dematiaceous agent of cerebral infection in the United States, South America, Europe, India, and Africa (7, 15, 18, 53). The term "cladosporiosis" is used by some investigators to refer to brain abscess caused by *C. trichoides* (7). In Asia, *P. dermatitidis* has been isolated from disseminated disease including the brain (57, 62), and a report of *F. pedrosoi* from this organ (25) necessitates the addition of this species to the list of possible etiological agents.

Direct examination. Purulent material from the center of the abscess or fibrous tissue from the surrounding area should be mounted directly or in 10% KOH and examined microscopically for yellowish-brown to olive branching hyphae or single cells (Fig. 11). These growth forms may be accompanied by short chains of spherical bodies or bizarre forms which reproduce by budding or, less commonly, by septal formation.

Histopathology. Histological sections of brain show a predominance of pigmented hyphae free in the granulomatous wall of the abscess or within giant cells of the foreign body type. These elements are in marked contrast to

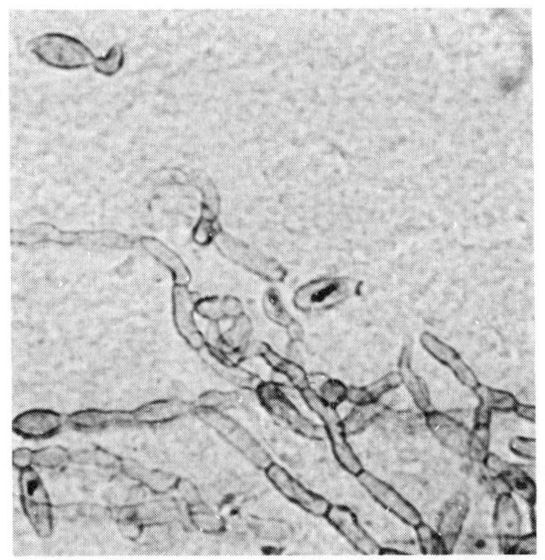

FIG. 11. *Hyphae and single-celled elements of Cladosporium trichoides in pus. Unstained. ×678.*

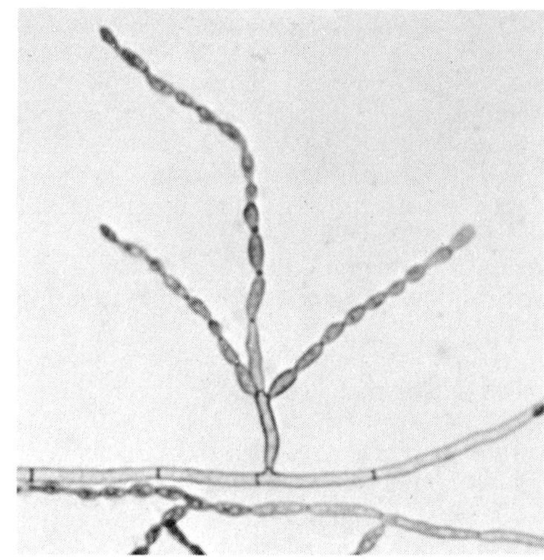

FIG. 12. *Conidiophore of Cladosporium trichoides supporting long flexuous chains of conidia. Corn meal-agar. ×678.*

the spherical septate bodies found in the cutaneous lesions of chromoblastomycosis.

Cultural examination. *C. trichoides*, as well as the other agents mentioned, can be isolated on Sabouraud glucose agar containing antibiotics at either 25 or 37 C. In culture, this species is characterized by a spreading olive-gray to brown colony and long flexuous chains of spores that are borne on sparsely branched conidiophores (Fig. 12). Among the pathogenic cladosporia, the fungus is most similar to *C. carrionii*. It differs from the latter in that it has larger conidia (4 to 11 μm in contrast to 2.5 to 7.5 μm), is capable of growing at a higher temperature (42 to 43 C as opposed to 35 to 36 C), and is neurotropic (61). Borelli (8) believes *C. trichoides* to be the same as *C. bantianum*, although there is some question as to the synonymy of the two fungi. The spores of *C. bantianum* are larger than those of *C. trichoides* and are borne in unbranched chains (19, 20).

P. dermatitidis and *F. pedrosoi* are identified by the characteristics described under chromoblastomycosis.

Biochemical properties. Failure to hydrolyze starch, liquefy gelatin, or coagulate milk readily distinguishes *C. trichoides* from saprophytic species of *Cladosporium*. *Phialophora dermatitidis* is nonproteolytic, but the property is of limited value in the identification of this species because similar nonpathogenic fungi, such as *Pullularia pullulans*, also fail to hydrolyze proteinaceous substrates.

Immunological properties. The value of immunological procedures in diagnosis of cerebral infections of dematiaceous origin is unknown. However, it is possible that serological techniques might be used diagnostically, as *C. trichoides* can be differentiated from morphologically similar fungi by immunofluorescence (4), and antigenic differences are known to exist between *P. dermatitidis* and other yeastlike forms (48).

Animal pathogenicity. *C. trichoides, P. dermatitidis,* and *F. pedrosoi* can be isolated from the brains of mice after intraperitoneal and intravenous inoculation (18, 21, 57). A dosage of 300,000 spores of *C. trichoides*, given intravenously, has been reported to be lethal for this laboratory animal (20). Multiple lesions of the brain also have been observed in rabbits inoculated with *C. trichoides*.

Subcutaneous abscesses, cysts, and granulomas

Phialophora gougerotii is the most important cause of these mycoses. The fungus was originally isolated from a subcutaneous abscess by Beurmann and Gougerot in 1907 (6) and described by Matruchot (45) in 1910. It has been reported from similar cases in separate parts of the world since that time (16, 29, 43, 65). In addition to this fungus, two other species of *Phialophora* have been isolated from humans on single occasions. Schwartz and Emmons (56) identified *P. richardsiae* from a lesion of the finger, and *P. spinifera*, a newly described species, has been reported from a granuloma of the nose (49).

Direct examination. Pus from an abscess or infected tissue should be examined directly by placing the specimen on a glass slide and overlaying with a cover slip. When necessary, clearing of the preparation can be accomplished with 10% KOH. The specimen is examined microscopically for yellowish-brown hyphae or spherical cells which occur individually or in moniliform chains.

Histopathology. Lesions are usually well encapsulated and consist of dense connective tissue lined by a layer of granulomatous inflammatory tissue. The etiological agents may be found within giant cells, free among fibroblasts and epitheloid cells, or in necrotic debris. The fungi appear as yellow- to brown-pigmented elements in the forms of single yeastlike cells, short moniliform chains, or true hyphae, or in a combination of these forms (Fig. 13). Reproduction of spherical cells occurs by budding or, rarely, by the formation of septae as seen in chromoblastomycosis.

Cultural examination. Clinical material should be streaked on Sabouraud glucose agar with antibiotics and incubated at room temperature. *P. gougerotii* and *P. spinifera* are initially yeastlike, but become hyphal with age. The colony of *P. richardsiae* is typically that of a mold throughout all stages of growth. Species identification is based on microscopic morphology and is best accomplished from slide culture preparations with the use of corn meal-agar. The following descriptions summarize the salient characteristics of these fungi.

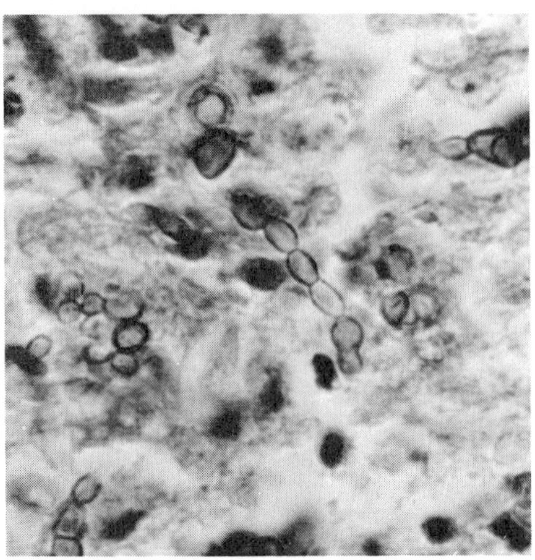

FIG. 13. *Yeast cells and "moniliform" hyphae of Phialophora gougerotii in the wall of a subcutaneous abscess. Hematoxylin and eosin. ×828.*

Phialophora gougerotii (Matruchot, 1910) Borelli 1955. Synonymy: *Sporotrichum gougerotii* Matruchot, 1910; *Dematium gougerotii* Grigoraki, 1924; *Pullularia gougerotii* Langeron, 1945; *Cladosporium gougerotii* Carrion and Silva, 1955.

This species begins as an olive to black, yeastlike colony which eventually is overgrown with olive-gray aerial hyphae. Microscopically, the fungus is characterized by numerous clusters or bouquets of blastospores which are produced from dark, elevated sterigmata (Fig. 14). True conidiophores (Fig. 15) are borne at 45° to 90° angles from the hyphae and usually consist of one or two cells. The appendage terminates with a slight flaring extension, a tubular process, or an attenuated, somewhat irregular tip. Conidia are elongate to ellipsoid and range in size from 2 by 3 to 2.5 by 4 μm.

This species is closely related to *P. jeanselmei*, an etiological agent of mycetoma. The two fungi differ primarily in their in vivo growth forms and in the extent of sporulation from peglike sterigmata of the hyphae. Conidiophores of *P. gougerotii* are reported to be more flexuous than those of *P. jeanselmei* (19); however, this property is an extremely variable one and is difficult to demonstrate in many strains.

Phialophora richardsiae (Nannfeldt) Conant, 1937. Synonymy: *Cadophora richardsiae* Nannfeldt, 1934; *Cadophora brunnescens* Davidson, 1935.

In culture, this species appears as a flat, umbonate, dull-brown colony consisting of short, wooly, aerial hyphae. Spores are borne from well-defined, tubular conidiophores that may be undifferentiated at first, but which show an expanded, saucer-shaped tip at maturity. Conidia are spherical, 2.3 to 3.2 μm, or elongate, 1.5 to 4.8 μm, and usually do not remain aggregated at the orifice of the phialid.

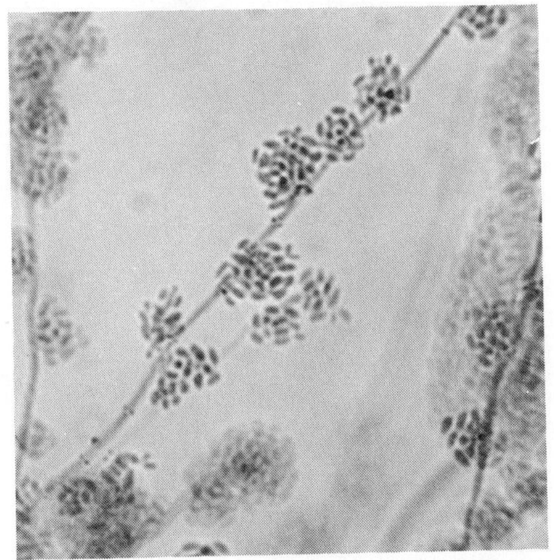

FIG. 14. *Hyphal form of Phialophora gougerotii illustrating "bouquets" of spores produced from fertile sterigmata. Corn meal-agar.* ×678.

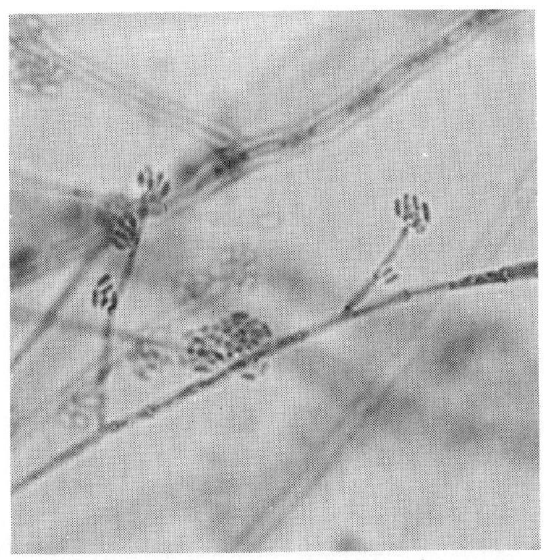

FIG. 15. *Hyphal form of Phialophora gougerotii showing a conidiophore with fertile sites at the tip and side of the appendage. Corn meal-agar.* ×678.

Phialophora spinifera Nielsen and Conant, 1968.

In culture, this species is slow-growing, olive to black, and remains yeastlike almost indefinitely on Sabouraud glucose agar. Microscopic preparations of aerial filaments from corn meal-agar reveal numerous, deeply pigmented conidiophores. These structures have a definite spine-like appearance and terminate with either a smooth or irregularly extended tip.

Spores are produced successively from a single, sometimes extending, site, and remain clustered at the apex or accumulate along the side of the conidiophore. The conida are unicellular, spherical to ellipsoid, and 1 by 1.5 to 2.5 by 3.5 μm in size. Short flask-shaped phialids with distinct apical cups also occur in corn meal-agar cultures.

Biochemical properties. It is reported that *P. gougerotii* slowly hydrolyzes hypoxanthine, whereas *P. richardsiae* does not affect this substrate (19). Similar data are not available for *P. spinifera*.

Immunological properties have not been used in the diagnosis of these mycoses, and the virulence of these fungi for laboratory animals is unknown.

Agent of Tinea Nigra

Cladosporium werneckii Parreiras Horta, 1921, is the causative agent of tinea nigra (tinea nigra palmaris). Synonymy: *Dematium werneckii* Dodge, 1935; *Aureobasidium mansonii* Cooke, 1962. Attempts have been made to adopt *Cladosporium mansonii* as the proper binomium for the etiological agent of this mycosis; however, the name was originally associated with pityriasis versicolor, and therefore must be considered a nomen dubium.

Tinea nigra is a superficial infection characterized by dark macular patches on the palms or palmar aspects of the wrist and fingers. In rare instances, other areas of the body can be involved (14). The lesions are of varied sizes, are round to irregular in shape, and resemble a silver nitrate stain. Clinically, they must be differentiated from junctional nevi, contact dermatitis, lesions of syphilis, pinta and yaws, and the pigmentation of Addison's disease (58).

The mycosis is seen in both tropical and temperate climates (46, 63) and is believed to occur after introduction of the fungus into abraded skin. At the present time, the disease

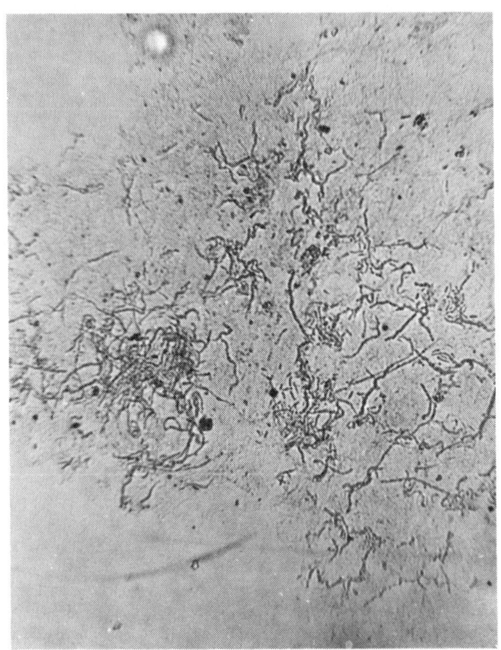

FIG. 16. *Septate branching hyphae of Cladosporium werneckii in scales of infected skin. KOH. ×150. (Courtesy of A. L. Carrion.)*

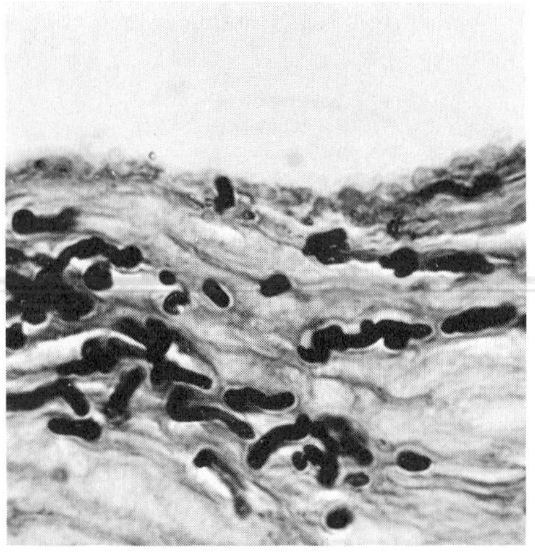

FIG. 17. *Transverse section of skin showing hyphal elements of Cladosporium werneckii. Periodic acid-Schiff stain. ×678.*

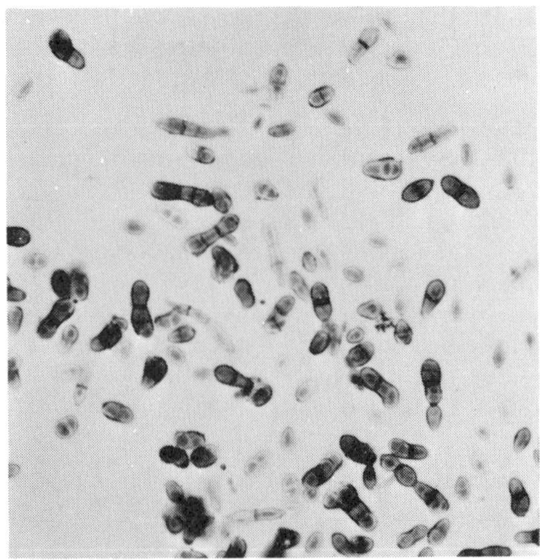

FIG. 18. *Septate yeast cells of Cladosporium werneckii from a young colony. Corn meal-agar. ×678.*

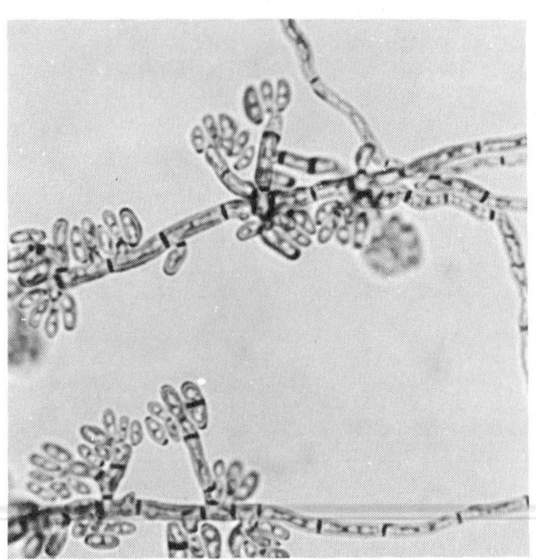

FIG. 19. *Hyphae of Cladosporium werneckii illustrating spore formation from stipular protuberances and conidiophores. Corn meal-agar. ×678.*

has no established race or occupational boundaries, although the incidence of infection appears to be highest in young females. Experimental tinea nigra of humans has been demonstrated by autoinoculation (54).

Examination of clinical material. Epidermal scales from a discolored area of the skin should be placed in a drop of 10% KOH, gently heated, and examined microscopically. The fungus can be seen as a mixture of dark, olivaceous, septate, branching hyphae, and occasionally as budding cells (Fig. 16).

Histopathology. Sections of biopsied tissue show a normal dermis with a thickened corneal layer. The fungus is confined to the epidermis and exists as short segments of hyphae and bacillary elements (Fig. 17).

Cultural examination. *C. werneckii* is readily isolated by placing epidermal scrapings from a lesion on Sabouraud glucose agar containing antibiotics. The culture should be incubated at room temperature and examined after 3 to 4 days for a moist, deeply pigmented yeastlike colony. Microscopically, the fungus consists of fusiform, sometimes bizarre, conspicuously septate budding cells (Fig. 18). With age, this growth form gives rise to olive-gray to black hyphae. Sporulation from aerial filaments occurs from short stipular protruberances and from poorly differentiated conidiophores (Fig. 19).

Biochemical properties. The fungus assimilates a variety of monosaccharides, disaccharides, and some polysaccharides. It is the only human pathogenic yeastlike dematiaceous fungus that utilizes lactose.

Serological properties. Serological procedures are of no value in the diagnosis of tinea nigra. It is doubtful that persons with the mycosis have antibodies to the fungus. Antigenic studies employing rabbit antiserum and the techniques of agglutination, antibody absorption, and immunodiffusion indicate that the species consists of a single serological group (48).

Animal pathogenicity. Macular lesions similar to those observed in humans have been experimentally induced in guinea pigs 5 to 7 weeks after cutaneous inoculation (55).

LITERATURE CITED

1. Ahearn, D. G., and W. Kaplan. 1969. Occurrence of *Sporotrichum schenckii* on a cold-stored meat product. Amer. J. Epidemiol. **89**:116–124.
2. Ainsworth, G. C., and P. K. C. Austwick. 1959. Fungal diseases of animals. Commonw. Bur. Anim. Health Rev. Ser. No. 6.
3. Al-Doory, Y. 1972. Chromomycosis. Mountain Press Publishing Co., Missoula, Mont.
4. Al-Doory, Y., and M. A. Gordon. 1963. Application of fluorescent-antibody procedures to the study of pathogenic dematiaceous fungi. I. Differentiation of *Cladosporium carrionii* and *Cladosporium bantianum*. J. Bacteriol. **86**:332–338.
5. Azulay, R. D. 1945. Experimental studies on chromoblastomycosis. J. Invest. Dermatol. **6**:281–292.
6. Beurmann, L., and H. Gougerot. 1907. Associations morbides dans les sporotrichosis. Bull. Mem. Soc. Med. Hosp. Paris, Ser. 3 **24**:591–596.
7. Binford, C. H., R. K. Thompson, M. E. Gorham, and C. W. Emmons. 1952. Mycotic brain abscess due to *Cladosporium trichoides*, a new species. Amer. J. Clin. Pathol. **22**:535–542.
8. Borelli, D. 1960. Torula bantiana, agent di un granuloma cerebrale. Riv. Anat. Patol. Oncol. **17**:617–622.
9. Buckley, H. R., and I. G. Murray. 1966. Precipitating antibodies in chromomycosis. Sabouraudia **5**:78–80.
10. Campbell, C. C. 1945. Use of Francis' glucose cystine blood agar in the isolation and cultivation of Sporotrichum schenckii. J. Bacteriol. **50**:233.
11. Carmichael, J. W. 1962. *Chrysosporium* and some other aleuriosporic hyphomycetes. Can. J. Bot. **40**:1137–1174.
12. Carrion, A. L. 1950. Chromoblastomycosis. Ann. N. Y. Acad. Sci. **50**:1255–1282.
13. Carrion, A. L. 1950. Yeastlike dematiaceous fungi infecting the human skin. Arch. Dermatol. Syphilol. **61**:996–1009.
14. Conant, N. F., D. T. Smith, R. D. Baker and J. L. Callaway. 1971. Manual of clinical mycology, p. 267–278. W. B. Saunders Co., Philadelphia.
15. Desai, S. C., M. L. Bhatikar, and R. S. Mehta. 1966. Cerebral chromoblastomycosis due to *Cladosporium trichoides* (Bantianum). Part II. Neurology India **14**:6–18.
16. Di Salvo, A. F., and W. H. Chew. 1968. Phialophora gougerotii: an opportunistic fungus in a patient treated with steroids. Sabouraudia **6**:241–245.
17. Drouhet, E., and F. Mariat. 1950. La pyrimidine. Facteurs de croissance pour les *Sporotrichum*. Ann. Inst. Pasteur (Paris) **79**:306–313.
18. Duque, O. 1961. Meningo-encephalitis and brain abscess caused by *Cladosporium* and *Fonsecaea*. Review of the literature, report of two cases, and experimental studies. Amer. J. Clin. Pathol. **36**:505–517.
19. Emmons, C. W. 1966. Pathogenic dematiaceous fungi. Jap. J. Med. Mycol. **7**:233–245.
20. Emmons, C. W., C. H. Binford, and J. P. Utz. 1963. Medical mycology, p. 282–291. Lea & Febiger, Philadelphia.
21. Felger, C. E., and L. Friedman. 1962. Experimental cerebral chromoblastomycosis. J. Infect. Dis. **111**:1–7.
22. Fetter, B. F. 1961. Human cutaneous sporotrichosis due to *Sporotrichum schenckii*. Technique for demonstration of organisms in tissues. Arch. Pathol. **71**:416–419.
23. Foerster, H. R. 1929. Sporotrichosis. An occupational dermatosis. J. Amer. Med. Ass. **87**:1605–1609.
24. Fuentes, C. A., and Z. E. Bosch. 1960. Biochemical differentiation of the etiological agents of chromoblastomycosis from nonpathogenic *Cladosporium* species. J. Invest. Dermatol. **34**:419–421.
25. Fukushiro, R., S. Kagawa, S. Nishiyama, and H. Takahashi. 1957. Un cas de chromoblastomycose cutanee avec metastase cerebrale mortelle. Presse Med. **65**:2142–2143.
26. Gastineau, F. M., L. W. Spolyar, and E. Hagnes. 1941. Sporotrichosis: report of six cases among florists. J. Amer. Med. Ass. **117**:1074–1077.
27. Gezuele, E., J. E. Mackinnon, and J. A. Conti-Diaz. 1972. The frequent isolation of *Phialophora verrucosa* and *Phialophora pedrosoi* from natural sources. Sabouraudia **10**:266–273.
28. Gordon, M. A., and Y. Al-Doory, 1965. Application of fluorescent-antibody procedures to the study of pathogenic dematiaceaous fungi. II. Serological relationships of the genus *Fonsecaea*. J. Bacteriol. **89**:551–556.
29. Gougerot, H., and J. Duche. 1939. Epidermite due au *Sporotrichum gougerotii*. Bull. Soc. Fr. Dermatol. Syphiligr. **46**:1455.
30. Howard, D. H., and G. F. Orr. 1963. Comparison of strains of *Sporotrichum schenckii* isolated from nature. J. Bacteriol. **85**:816–821.
31. Howles, J. K., C. B. Kennedy, W. H. Garvin, J. W. Brueck, and G. T. Buddingh. 1954. Chromoblastomycosis. Report of nine cases from a single area in Louisiana. Arch. Dermatol. Syphilol. **69**:83–90.
32. Iwata, K., and T. Wada. 1957. Mycological studies on the strains isolated from a case of chromoblastomycosis with a metastasis in the central nervous system. Jap. J. Microbiol. **1**:355–360.
33. Kaplan, W., and A. Gonzalez Ochoa. 1963. Application of the fluorescent antibody technique to the rapid diagnosis of sporotrichosis. J. Lab. Clin. Med. **62**:835–841.
34. Kempson, R. A., and W. H. Sternberg. 1963. Chronic subcutaneous abscesses caused by pigmented fungi. A lesion distinguishable from cutaneous chromoblastomycosis. Amer. J. Clin. Pathol. **39**:598–606.
35. Levy, B., and B. Black-Schaffer, 1945. Studies in experimental systemic mycosis. I. Systemic chromomycosis

(chromoblastomycosis) in mice: Preliminary study. Amer. J. Trop. Med. **25:**117–127.

36. Lurie, H. I. 1963. Histopathology of sporotrichosis. Notes on the nature of the asteroid body. Arch. Pathol. **75:**421–437.
37. Lurie, H. I. 1963. Five unusual cases of sporotrichosis from South Africa showing lesions in muscles, bones, and viscera. Brit. J. Surg. **50:**585–591.
38. Maberry, J. D., J. F. Mullins, and O. Stone. 1966. Sporotrichosis with demonstration of hyphae in human tissue. Arch. Dermatol. **93:**65–67.
39. Mackinnon, J. E., I. A. Conti-Diaz, E. Gezuele, E. Civila, and S. da Luz. 1969. Isolation of *Sporothrix schenckii* from nature and considerations on its pathogenicity and ecology. Sabouraudia **7:**38–45.
40. Mariat, F. 1971. Adaptation de *Ceratocystis* à la vie parasitaire chez l'animal. Etude de l'aquisition d'un pouvoir pathogène comparable à celui de *Sporothrix schenckii*. Sabouraudia **9:**191–205.
41. Mariat, F., and E. Diez. 1971. Nature des spores endogènes de *Sporothrix schenckii* Hektoen et Perkins. Remarques à propos de l'éventuelle sexuée de ce champignon. C.R. Acad. Sci. Paris **272:**1075–1077.
42. Mariat, F., and E. Diez. 1971. Adaptation de *Ceratocystis stenoceras* (Robak) C. Moreau à la vie parasitaire chez l'animal. Etude de la souche sauvage et des mutants pathogènes. Comparaison avec Sporothrix schenckii Hektoen et Perkins. Rev. Mycol. **36:**3–24.
43. Mariat, F., G. Segretain, P. Destombes, and H. Darasse. 1967. Kyste sous-cultane mycosique (phaeo-sporotrichosis) á *Phialophora gougerotii* (Matruchot 1910) Borelli, 1955, observe au Senegal. Sabouraudia **5:**209–219.
44. Martin, D. S., R. D. Baker, and N. F. Conant. 1936. A case of verrucous dermatitis caused by *Hormodendrum pedrosoi* (chromoblastomycosis) in North Carolina. Amer. J. Trop. Med. **16:**593–619.
45. Matruchot, L. 1910. Sur un nouveau groupe de champignons pathogènes, agents des sporotrichoses. C. R. Acad. Sci. Paris **150:**543–545.
46. Neves, J. A., and O. G. Costa. 1947. Tinea nigra. Arch. Dermatol. Syphilol. **55:**67–84.
47. Nielsen, H. S., Jr. 1968. Biologic properties of skin test antigens of yeast form of *Sporotrichum schenckii*. J. Infect. Dis. **118:**173–180.
48. Nielsen, H. S., Jr., and N. F. Conant. 1967. Practical evaluation of antigenic relationships of yeastlike dematiaceous fungi. Sabouraudia **5:**283–294.
49. Nielsen, H. S., Jr., and N. F. Conant. 1968. A new human pathogenic *Phialophora*. Sabouraudia **6:**228–231.
50. Norden, A. 1951. Sporotrichosis. Clinical and laboratory features and serological study in experimental animals and humans. Acta Pathol. Microbiol. Scand. Suppl. **89:**49–81.
51. Okudaira, M., E. Tsubura, and J. Schwarz. 1961. A histopathological study of experimental murine sporotrichosis. Mycopathol. Mycol. Appl. **14:**284–296.
52. Ridley, M. F. 1961. The saprophytic occurrence of fungi causing chromoblastomycosis. Recent advances in botany. Toronto University Press, Toronto.
53. Riley, O., Jr., and S. H. Mann. 1960. Brain abscess caused by *Cladosporium trichoides*. Amer. J. Clin. Pathol. **33:**525–532.
54. Ritchie, E. B., and T. E. Taylor. 1964. A study of tinea nigra palmaris: report of a case and inoculation experiments. Arch. Dermatol. **89:**601–603.
55. Sartory, A., R. Sartory, B. Rietmann, and J. Meyer. 1930. Contribution a l'étude d'une epidermomycose bresilienne palmaire noire, provoqué par un cladosporium noveau. C.R. Soc. Biol. **104:**878–881.
56. Schwartz, I. S., and C. W. Emmons. 1968. Subcutaneous cystic gramulama caused by a fungus of wood pulp (*Phialophora richardsiae*). Amer. J. Clin. Pathol. **49:**500–505.
57. Shimazono, Y., I. Kiminori, H. Torii, R. Otsuka, and T. Fukushiro. 1963. Brain abcess due to *Hormodendrum dermatitidis* (Kano) Conant 1953. Report of a case and review of the literature. Folia Psychiat. Neurol. Jap. **17:**80–96.
58. Smith, J. G., Jr., W. M. Sams, and F. J. Roth, Jr. 1958. Tinea nigra palmaris: a disorder easily confused with junctional nevus of the palm. J. Amer. Med. Ass. **167:**312.
59. Symposium. 1947. Sporotrichosis infection in mines of the Witwaterstrand. Proc. Transvaal Mine Med. Officers' Assoc. Transvaal Chamber of Mines, Johannesburg.
60. Travassos, L. R., P. A. J. Gorin, and K. O. Lloyd. 1973. Comparison of the rhamnomannans from the human pathogen *Sporothrix schenckii* with those from the ceratocystic species. Infect. Immunity **8:**685–693.
61. Trejos, A. 1954. *Cladosporium carrionii* n. sp. and the problem of cladosporia isolated from chromoblastomycosis. Rev. Biol. Trop. **2:**75–112.
62. Tsai, C. Y., Y. C. Lu, L.-T. Wang, T. L. Hsu, and J.-L. Sung. 1966. Systemic chromoblastomycosis due to *Hormodendrum dermatitidis* (Kano) Conant. Report of the first case in Taiwan. Amer. J. Clin. Pathol. **46:**103–114.
63. Van Velsor, H., and H. Singletary, 1964. Tinea nigra palmaris. A report of 15 cases from coastal North Carolina. Arch. Dermatol. **90:**59–61.
64. Wilson, D. E., J. J. Mann, J. E. Bennett, and J. P. Utz. 1967. Clinical features of extracutaneous sporotrichosis. Medicine **46:**265–279.
65. Young, J. M., and E. Ulrich. 1953. Sporotrichosis produced by *Sporotrichum gougerotii*. Report of a case and review of the literature. Arch. Dermatol. Syphilol. **67:**44–52.

Chapter 60
Fungi of Phycomycosis

DONALD L. GREER

CHARACTERIZATION OF ZYGOMYCETES

The phycomycetes are a heterogeneous group of lower fungi now classified into six classes (1). All species of phycomycetes known to be pathogenic for humans are members of the class *Zygomycetes*. (Other classes of these fungi are primarily aquatic forms not known to be pathogenic for humans.) Two orders in this class, *Mucorales* (bread molds) and *Entomophthorales* (insect fungi), contain all the five genera presently recognized as the principal pathogens of humans: *Mucor, Rhizopus, Absidia, Entomophthora*, and *Basidiobolus*. On two occasions, unidentified species, probably of the genus *Mortierella*, have been isolated from humans, and *Hyphomyces destruens* has been reported from horses and mules (8). The zygomycetes are responsible for diseases of humans and animals commonly known as phycomycoses, and the term zygomycoses has been used to refer to infections by fungi of this class. The term mucormycosis is reserved for infections by genera of the order *Mucorales*, and the term entomophthoromycosis is used for infections by genera of the order *Entomophthorales*.

These diseases occur as acute necrotic infections of rhinocerebral, pulmonary, abdominal, and cutaneous tissues (mucormycosis, rhinophycomycosis) or as chronic granulomatous infections of subcutaneous tissues (entomophthoromycosis, subcutaneous phycomycosis, rhino-entomophthoromycosis). The disease process produced by genera of each order is distinct, clinically and histologically; therefore, the correct diagnosis of the mycoses usually can be made in tissues without cultural confirmation.

Class Zygomycetes

Terrestrial fungi with well-developed, broad, usually nonseptate hyphae. Sexual spores (zygospores) are nonmotile. All grow rapidly on routine laboratory media, but most are sensitive to cycloheximide. Temperature range is from 25 to 55 C with an optimal temperature of 28 to 30 C. All of the pathogenic species grow at 37 C. All are saprophytic in nature and occur worldwide. No serological or biochemical classification is available. The Zygomycetes are identified primarily upon the basis of their morphological characteristics (1).

Order Mucorales

Rapidly growing ubiquitous fungi which form loose, gray, wooly colonies filling a petri plate in 2 to 5 days with aseptate mycelium. Asexual spores (sporangiospores) are borne in a closed sac (sporangium) supported on a slender stalk (sporangiophore). Sporulation appears as black pinpoints scattered throughout the mycelial mass of the colony.

Species of the *Mucorales* are opportunistic fungi; i.e., they have a low ability to produce disease and usually can cause disease only in immunologically defective, metabolically unbalanced, or chronically debilitated individuals (12). Diabetes mellitus is the disease most commonly associated with mucormycosis. In over 50% of the individuals, the diabetes is uncontrolled and acidosis is present. In other predisposing conditions, acidosis also appears to be the most common characteristic (13).

The incidence of mucormycosis infections is increasing. Patients with severe burns, children with acute leukemia, and patients treated with cytotoxic or immunodepressive drugs and corticosteroids are prime victims (2).

Since species of *Mucorales* are considered common laboratory contaminants, the significance of isolating the fungi from pathological material depends upon the source of the specimen and the symptoms of the patient. Observation by direct examination of either broad aseptate hyphal fragments (Fig. 1) in sterile body fluids or invading hyphae in tissue scrapings or biopsy materials has etiological significance, and may mean more to the clinician than the isolation of the fungus. Repeated isolation of the same species of phycomycete from contaminated sources, e.g., nose, throat, sputum, etc., may be of some diagnostic value, especially if associated with signs of clinical infection in a debilitated person.

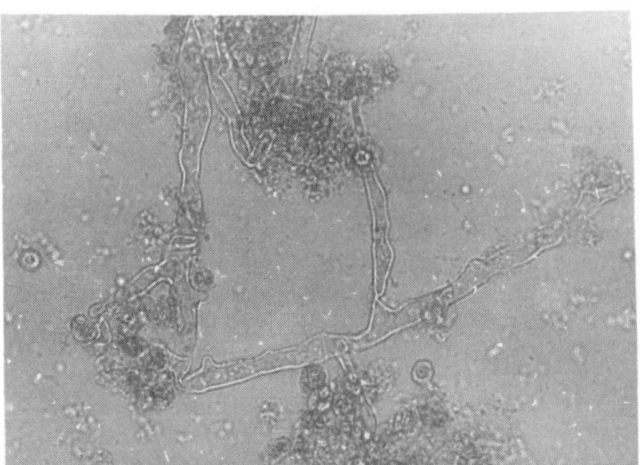

FIG. 1. *Mucor sp. Aseptate hyphae in unstained wet mount of sputum. ×400 (Photomicrograph courtesy of B. H. Cooper).*

Order Entomophthorales

Ubiquitous fungi forming flat, waxy colonies, which may develop a white fuzz on the surface. The hyphae are septate. Asexual spores are conidia or uninucleate sporangia which are forcibly expelled from the conidiophore at maturity.

There are no reports of laboratory contamination by the two pathogenic genera, *Basidiobolus* and *Entomophthora*. Isolation of either of these fungi from clinical material warrants attention. As yet, predisposing factors for infections caused by these species are not known (18).

Entomophthoromycosis in humans caused by *Basidiobolus* and *Entomophthora* has not been reported from the United States, although *Entomophthora coronata* has been isolated from horses from several southern states (8). A recent case of human entomophthoromycosis diagnosed by histopathology was reported from a child in the United States (9), but unfortunately the fungus was not cultured. Entomophthorales infections have been reported primarily from the tropical countries of Central Africa and Southeast Asia (14). Only a few cases are known from South America.

COLLECTION, TRANSPORT, AND STORAGE OF SPECIMENS

Care must be taken to obtain an adequate sample. Light scrapings or swabs, such as used for bacteriological methods, are usually unsatisfactory. Sufficient materials for all laboratory examinations may be obtained by aspiration of abscesses, irrigation, and scraping of mucosal membranes and multiple biopsies.

Rhinocerebral infections are acute and often fatal; clinical materials received for examination and culture are frequently tissues from autopsy. Antemortum specimens from central nervous system (CNS) infections usually include exudates from the sinuses, scrapings from nasal or oral mucosa, or cerebrospinal fluid (4). Other specimens from pulmonary or abdominal infections may include sputum, bronchial washings, or stools. Biopsy material should be obtained whenever possible; in burned patients, the biopsy should be taken at the growing edge of the lesion (5).

The primary responsibility in diagnosing mucormycosis lies with the physician. An alert doctor will make a rapid clinical diagnosis, notify the mycology laboratory, and send the material immediately to the laboratory. A responsible laboratory must rapidly examine the clinical specimens received and report any findings to the physician. The examination of clinical material by a direct KOH preparation can provide the physician with a diagnosis sufficient to begin treatment. Frequently, there is not enough time to culture the specimen and identify the fungal agent.

Clinical specimens should be transported immediately to the laboratory for examination because of (i) the need for rapid information and (ii) the fragility of the fungal elements. If overnight storage is necessary, the specimen should be placed in a Stuart's bacteriological transport medium and stored at room temperature. Zygomycetes do not survive long at refrigerator temperature.

DIRECT EXAMINATION

A direct wet mount preparation should be made on all clinical specimens. Necrotic or purulent material may contain only dead or degenerated hyphal elements which, though visible on direct examination of the material, may not grow on culture. A direct examination showing hyphal invasion of viable tissue gives a rapid diagnosis of a phycomycetous infection and verification of later cultural findings. The absence of fungal elements, however, does not necessarily rule out the diagnosis.

Examine a portion of the necrotic tissue or purulent material by mixing the specimen with several drops of 20% aqueous potassium hydroxide on a slide. Add a cover slip, warm the preparation slightly to enhance the clearing action of the KOH, and observe under a microscope. Clear body fluids, e.g., cerebrospinal fluid may be centrifuged and the sediment examined directly on a slide with a few drops of KOH.

Study the wet mount preparations under a

microscope for broad, aseptate hyphal fragments (Fig. 1). In tissue, abundant, irregularly branching hyphal elements are seen.

CULTURE AND ISOLATION

No special nutritive media or environmental requirements are necessary for culturing the zygomycetes. Sabouraud agar is an adequate isolation medium. However, isolations have been improved by adding sterilized bread to the agar (19). Antibacterial antibiotics may be added to the medium, but cycloheximide (Actidione) should not be used as most phycomycetes are sensitive to this antibiotic. Therefore, media such as Mycosel or Mycobiotic agar, which contain cycloheximide and are commonly used for the isolation of pathogenic fungi, cannot be used.

In mucormycosis, the most common tissue reaction is necrosis; therefore, specimens received for culture are often heavily contaminated with bacteria. To prevent overgrowth of bacteria, such specimens as purulent exudates, mucosal scrapings, necrotic biopsies, and sputum should be streaked onto petri plates of Sabouraud agar containing antibacterial antibiotics. (Gentamicin and polymyxin B are two useful broad-spectrum antibiotics.) Do not be afraid to use a large inoculum; the number of viable fungal elements in the clinical specimens is usually small. Streak the materials over the plate, using most, if not all, of the specimen. Laboratory cultures are incubated in duplicate under aerobic conditions at both 25 and 37 C.

Growth of species of *Mucorales* is observed in 2 to 5 days. Observe the cultures early for colonies growing within the area of the inoculum. The fungus grows rapidly, filling the petri plate with an abundance of grayish-white aerial mycelium. The mycelia are tenacious and have the consistency of "steel-wool" when an attempt is made to remove some for microscopy.

Entomophthorales infections are chronic, and virtually all are diagnosed from tissue biopsy. The tissue should be minced aseptically into pieces of 1 to 2 mm, as the fungi are difficult to isolate when the specimen is ground or macerated too vigorously.

Inoculate the tissue fragments onto petri plates of Sabouraud agar containing only antibacterial antibiotics, and incubate the cultures at 25 to 30 C. Temperatures of 37 C or higher are not recommended for primary isolation.

The fungus grows in 3 to 4 days as a thin, flat, waxy colony at the site of inoculation, and the growth adheres to the surface of the agar. The colony appears gray to pale yellow and may develop radial furrows and a short, white, velvetlike "bloom" composed of conidia. The conidia are forcibly expelled and adhere to the top of the petri plate, giving the plate a "ground-glass" appearance.

CULTURAL AND MICROSCOPIC CHARACTERISTICS

The specific identification of the zygomycete isolated from clinical material rests upon the morphology of the fungus. Identification is made by preparing a lactophenol cotton blue wet mount of a small portion of the colony and observing the morphology of the characteristic fungal structures as described below.

No special biochemical reactions or nutritional requirements are known to aid in the identification of the pathogenic species of zygomycetes. Growth temperature requirements may be used to identify some species, particularly *Rhizopus*, since the "pathogenic" species often grow better than the "saprophytic" ones at 37 C.

Identification of genera: Rhizopus species (R. arrhizus, R. oryzae, R. nigricans)

Rapidly growing colony with voluminous white to gray aerial mycelium (Fig. 2). Mycelium tenacious, coarse, and wooly. Hyphae are nonseptate and colorless. Sporangiophores are long, unbranched, and clustered at nodes oppo-

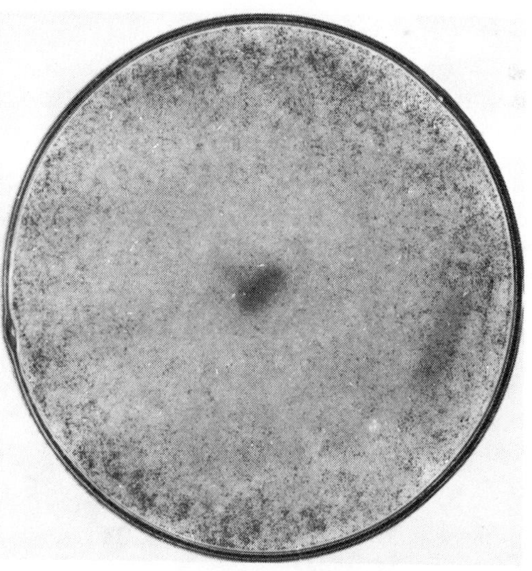

FIG. 2. *Colonial morphology of Rhizopus sp. grown on Sabouraud agar at room temperature for 4 days. Note voluminous aerial mycelium and production of sporangia (black dots).*

site holdfasts (rhizoids) which form along a horizontal runner (stolon). Sporangia are dark-walled, spherical, and filled with round hyaline spores. A columella is present (Fig. 3).

Absidia species (A. corymbifera)

Colonial morphology and rate of growth are similar to *Rhizopus*. Microscopically, rhizoids are present but the sporangiophores arise *between* the nodes of the stolon instead of opposite the nodes as in *Rhizopus*. Sporangia are pear-shaped, filled with round to oval spores, and contain a columella (Fig. 4).

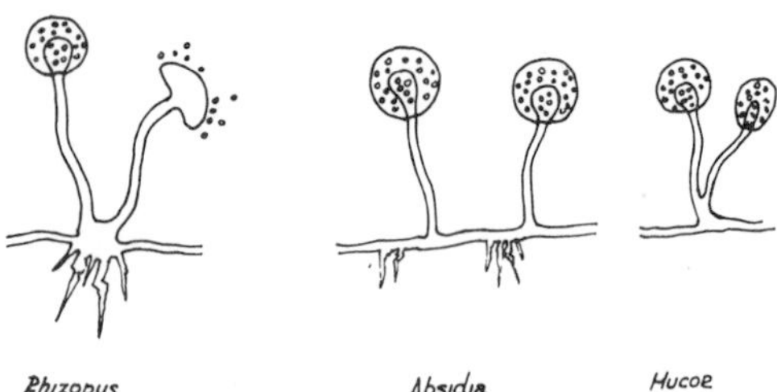

FIG. 4. *Diagrammatic representation of morphological distinction between the genera Rhizopus, Absidia, and Mucor.*

Mucor species (M. pusillus, M. ramosissimus)

Colony is rapidly growing, forming a cottony surface which fills the culture plate in 5 to 7 days. Aerial mycelium is white, later becoming gray to brown. Grossly the colony resembles that of *Rhizopus*.

Microscopically, no rhizoids are present. Sporangiophores arise from hyphae. Sporangia are spherical and have a columella (Fig. 5). Considerable variation occurs among the different species of *Mucor*.

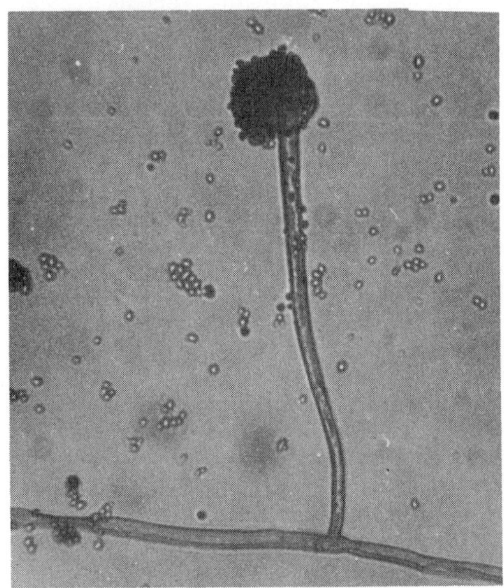

FIG. 5. *Mucor sp. Aseptate hypha forming single or branched sporangiophores. No rhizoids are present. Sporangium contains a columella. ×400.*

Mortierella species (unidentified)

Colony is flat and gray or yellowish in color. Usually few sporangia and little mycelium are produced.

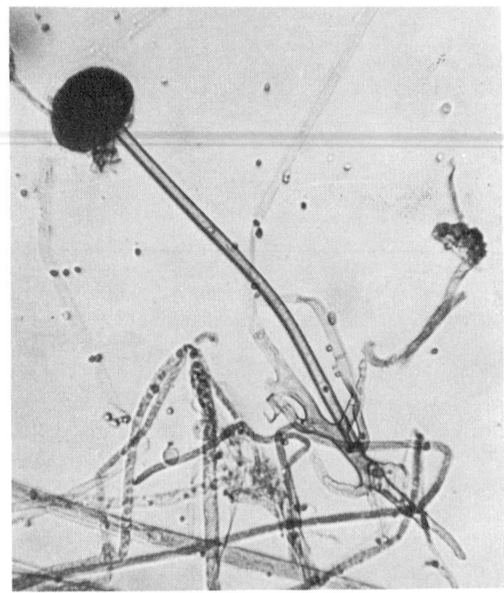

FIG. 3. *Rhizopus sp. Aseptate hyphae with rhizoids at the base of sporangiophores. Sporangium is black, spherical, and contains a columella. ×400.*

Microscopically, both sporangia and conidia ("stylospores") are present. Sporangia have no columella and are borne on a sporangiophore which tapers to a hairlike tip. Conidia are round, unicellular, and spiny, and are borne singly at the tip of an attenuated conidiophore.

Basidiobolus species (B. haptosporus, synonym B. meristosporus)

The fungus grows rapidly as a flat, waxy, gray to pale yellow colony which becomes covered with numerous conidia (uninucleate sporangia) and short, white aerial mycelia (Fig. 6).

Microscopically, the hyphae are divided by septa into short elements called hyphal bodies. Large numbers of chlamydospores and zygospores are usually formed beginning in the center of the colony. Zygospores are the identifying

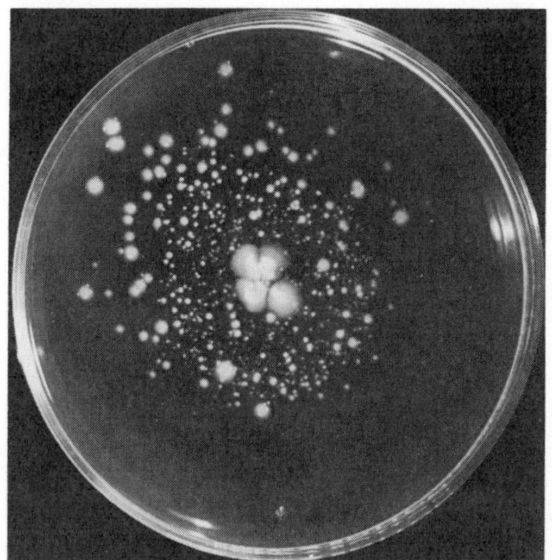

FIG. 6. *Colonial morphology of Basidiobolus sp. grown on Sabouraud agar at room temperature for 5 days. Note numerous satellite secondary colonies.*

feature and appear as round thick-walled smooth structures having two protuberances or beaks on their surface (Fig. 7). The beaks are not part of the wall of the zygospore. Numerous globose uninucleate sporangia are borne singly on short club-shaped sporangiophores arising directly from the hyphae. The sporangium and a fragment of the sporangiophore ("basidium") are forcibly ejected at maturity and collect on the glass surface of the culture container (Fig. 8).

Temperature tolerance, zygospore wall morphology, and production of odor have been used as criteria to distinguish between strains of *Basidiobolus* isolated from humans and those isolated from nature (10). However, a recent review (6) shows variations in temperature requirements among strains isolated from the same patient as well as variation in zygospore wall morphology. Apparently, as seen in another study, these criteria, although helpful, are not absolute for identification of species of *Basidiobolus* (11).

Entomophthora species (E. coronata)

Fungus develops as a flat, gray colony similar to *Basidiobolus*, but sporulation is usually heavier (Fig. 9).

Microscopically, the hyphae are sparingly septate and produce many chlamydospores. Zygospores, if present, are not obvious. Numerous globose true conidia are borne singly on short slender conidiophores. These are forcibly expelled at maturity without an attached hyphal fragment (Fig. 10). The conidia differ from those of *Basidiobolus* by having a prominent papilla and producing multiple secondary co-

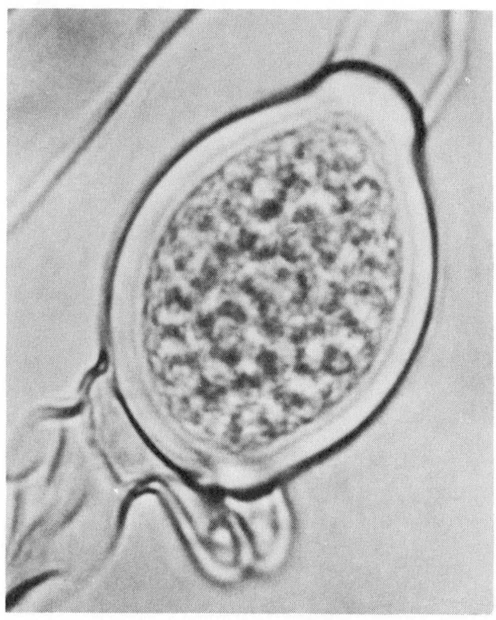

FIG. 7. *Basidiobolus sp. Smooth-walled intercalary zygospore showing remnants of copulatory tubes ("beaks"). ×400.*

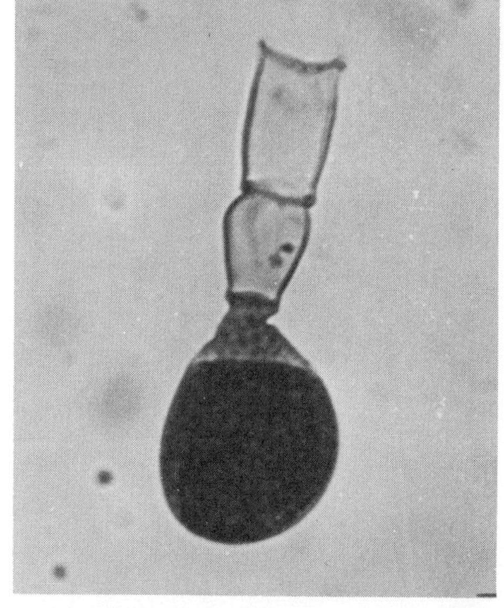

FIG. 8. *Basidiobolus sp. Smooth, globose uninucleate sporangium which has been forcibly expelled from the sporangiophore. A fragment of the sporangiophore (basidium) is attached. ×400.*

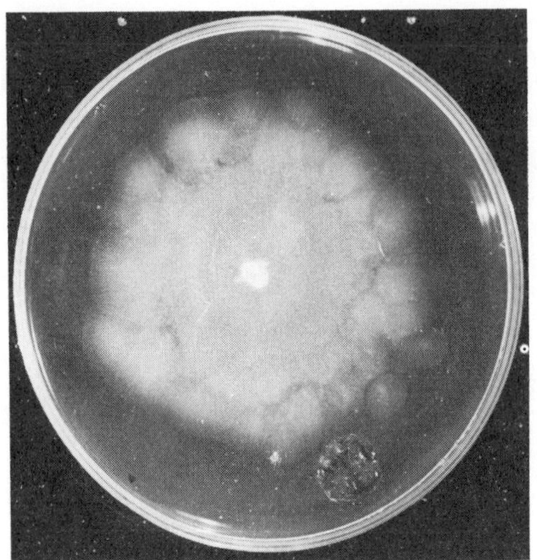

FIG. 9. *Colonial morphology of Entomophthora coronata grown on Sabouraud agar at room temperature for 5 days. Note presence of short aerial mycelia, "bloom," and "ground glass" appearance.*

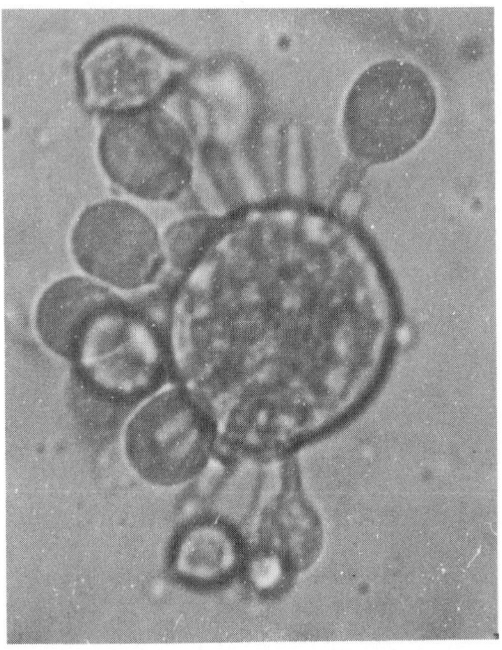

FIG. 11. *Entomophthora coronata. Production of secondary globose conidia by multiple replication showing a "corona" effect. ×400.*

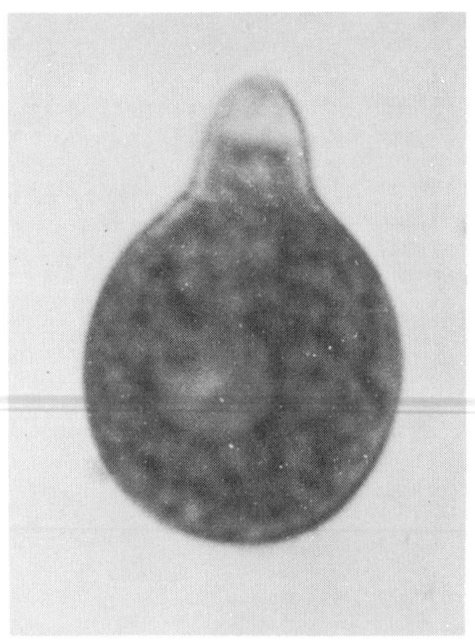

FIG. 10. *Entomophthora coronata. Globose smooth conidium showing prominent papilla. The true conidium has been forcibly expelled without hyphal attachment. ×400.*

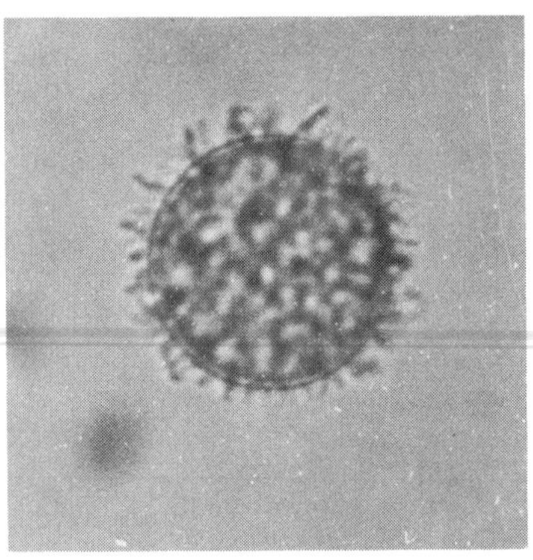

FIG. 12. *Entomophthora coronata. Degenerating globose conidium showing fine hairlike projections over the surface.*

nidia in the form of a "corona" from which the species derives its name (Fig. 11). Under unfavorable conditions, the conidia may develop short hairlike filaments over their surface (Fig. 12).

SEROLOGICAL METHODS

No satisfactory serological methods have been developed for the diagnosis of phycomycetous infection. Skin test material obtained from the zygomycetes is not specific enough to be of diagnostic value.

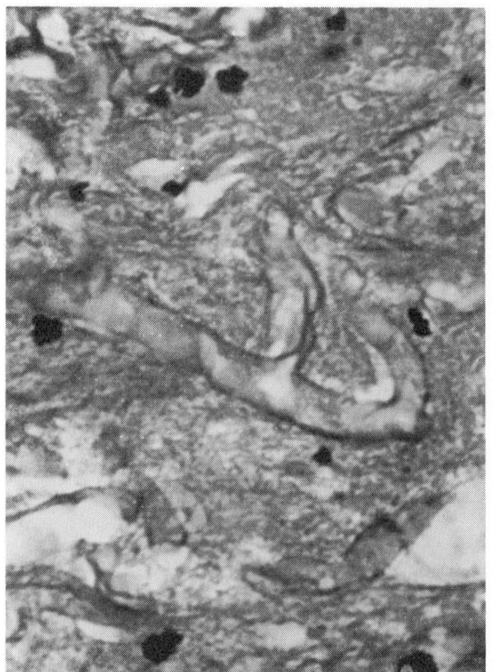

FIG. 13. *Mucormycosis. Tissue section (hematoxylin and eosin) showing broad, aseptate hyphae. Tissue reaction is one of necrosis.* ×*400.*

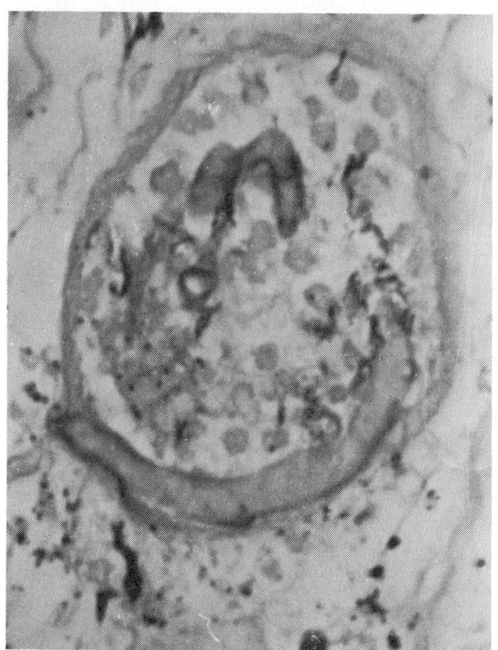

FIG. 14. *Mucormycosis. Tissue section (hematoxylin and eosin) showing invasion of blood vessel by broad, aseptate hyphae.* ×*400.*

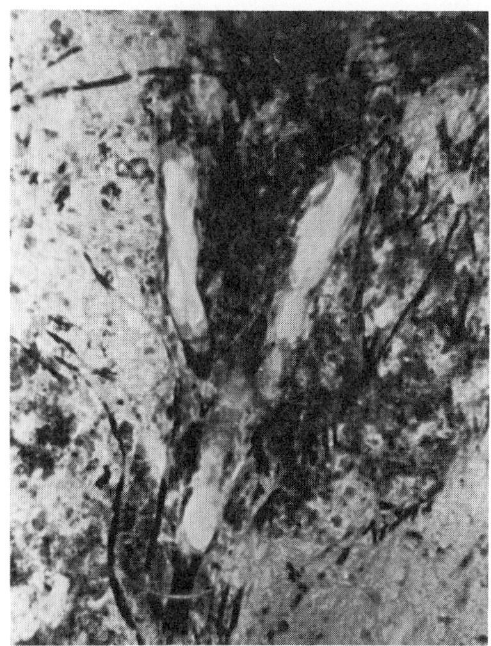

FIG. 15. *Entomophthoromycosis. Tissue section (hematoxylin and eosin) showing hyphal fragment surrounded by typical eosinophilic necrotic debris.* ×*400.*

ANIMAL PATHOGENICITY

Zygomycetous infections in animals are usually possible after alteration of the host defenses. Experimental mucormycosis has been successful in alloxan-treated rabbits (17). Attempts to produce entomophthoromycosis in animals with species of *Basidiobolus* and *Entomophthora* have been unsuccessful (10).

HISTOLOGICAL IDENTIFICATION

Since zygomycoses are frequently diagnosed from biopsy sections, it is important for the laboratory technician to be aware of their morphology in tissue. Special histological stains for these infections are seldom necessary, as the hyphae in tissue sections are easily observed with hematoxylin and eosin (3). Special stains for fungi such as Gridley or Grocott may be used, if necessary.

The typical tissue reaction of *Mucorales* infection is distinctly different from the tissue reaction caused by the *Entomophthorales*. Usually a diagnosis of a zygomycetous infection more compatible to one group of fungi than the other can be made by histopathological methods (15). Species identification, however, cannot be made in tissue sections.

Mucorales infections in tissue are characterized by the presence of abundant broad, branched, usually aseptate hyphae 15 to 20 μm in diameter and often 200 μm in length. Crossfolds of the hyphal walls may resemble septa (Fig. 13).

The tissue reaction is usually acute, revealing extensive necrosis and edema with diffuse infiltrations of polymorphonuclear leukocytes. The fungus has a strong predilection to invade blood vessels, resulting in thrombosis and tissue necrosis (4; Fig. 14).

The genus *Mortierella* produces a chronic eosinophilic tissue reaction similar to the *Entomophthorales* genera *Basidiobolus* and *Entomophthora*.

Entomophthorales infections in tissue are characterized by sparse, degenerating, thin-walled, broad hyphae surrounded by an eosinophilic necrotic precipitate similar to the Hoeppli phenomenon (3). The tissue reaction is one of an intense, chronic inflammatory process of a granulomatous type (Fig. 15). Fragments of hyphae may be seen in disseminated microabscesses composed of eosinophils, neutrophils, and foreign body giant cells (Fig. 16). The hyphal fragments stain poorly by any stain (16). Infections by *Basidiobolus* and *Entomophthora* are indistinguishable in tissue sections.

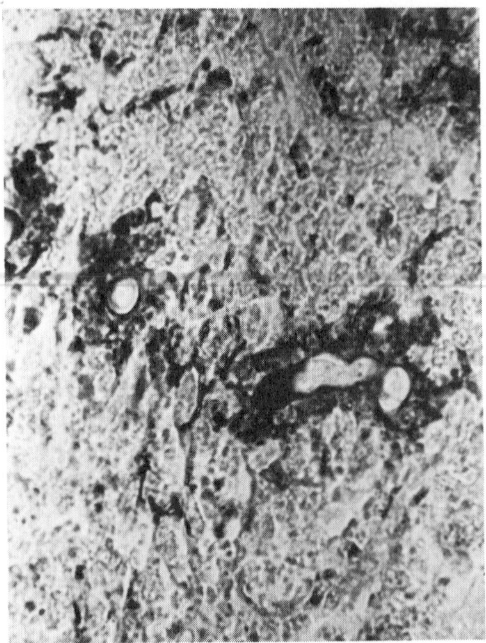

FIG. 16. *Entomophthoromycosis. Tissue section (hematoxylin and eosin) showing transverse section of hyphal fragments. Tissue reaction is chronic and granulomatous, with foreign body giant cells and microabscesses. ×400.*

Rhizopus and *Mucor* must be differentiated in tissue sections from species of *Aspergillus* and *Candida*. The hyphae of *Aspergillus* and *Candida* do not take the hematoxylin and eosin stain as readily as the Zygomycetes, and usually special histological stains are needed to observe them. The hyphae of Aspergillus have numerous septa, are narrow (5 μm), and have straight even parallel walls. Usually in tissue a large number of prominent hyphae branching at an acute angle are seen growing in a radiating pattern (7). *Candida* species produce both true septate hyphae and club-shaped pseudomycelia in tissue. Often, the tissue section shows a mixture of yeast cells and hyphal elements. The hyphae are narrow (4 μm wide).

EVALUATION

Antemortum diagnosis of mucormycosis depends upon rapid and intensive collaboration between the laboratory and physician. Because of the acute nature of the disease, often there is no time for culture confirmation of the diagnosis. Therefore, a report of broad, aseptate branching hyphae from purulent nasal exudates or such hyphal invasion from biopsies of necrotic tissue is pathognomonic for mucormycosis. Less urgent but equally important, the finding of hyphal fragments surrounded by an eosinophilic debris in a biopsy of chronic granulomatous tissue confirms diagnosis of entomophthoromycosis. When possible, the etiological agent should be isolated in culture so that the species of the fungus involved can be identified.

LITERATURE CITED

1. Alexopoulos, C. J. 1962. Introductory mycology, 2nd ed. John Wiley & Sons, Inc., New York.
2. Baker, R. D. 1970. The phycomycoses. Ann. N.Y. Acad. Sci. **174:**592–605.
3. Baker, R. D. 1971. Human infection with fungi actinomycetes and algae. Springer-Verlag, New York.
4. Bauer, H., L. Ajello, E. Adams, and D. U. Hernandez. 1955. Cerebral mucormycosis: pathogenesis of the disease: description of fungus, *Rhizopus oryzae*, isolated from fatal case. Amer. J. Med. **18:**822–831.
5. Bruck, H. M., G. Nash, F. D. Foley, and B. A. Pruitt. 1971. Opportunistic fungal infection of the burn wound with Phycomycetes and Aspergillus. A clinical-pathologic review. Arch. Surg. **102:**476–482.
6. Clark, B. M. 1968. The epidemiology of phycomycosis. Systemic Mycoses, Ciba Found. Symp., p. 179–205.
7. Conant, N. F., D. Smith, R. D. Baker, and J. E. Callaway. 1971. Manual of clinical mycology, 3rd. ed. W. B. Saunders, Philadelphia.
8. Emmons, C. W., C. H. Binford, and J. P. Utz. 1970.

Medical mycology, 2nd. ed. Lea and Febiger, Philadelphia.

9. Gilbert, E. F., G. H. Khoury, and R. S. Pore. 1970. Histopathological identification of entomophthoraphycomycosis. Deep mycotic infection in an infant. Arch. Pathol. **90**:583–587.
10. Greer, D. L., and L. Friedman. 1966. Studies on the genus *Basidiobolus* with reclassification of the species pathogenic for man. Sabouraudia **4**:231–241.
11. Hutchison, J. A., D. S. King, and M. A. Nickerson. 1972. Studies on temperature requirements, odor production and zygospore wall undulation of the genus *Basidiobolus*. Mycologia **64**(3):467–474.
12. Hutter, R. V. P. 1959. Phycomycetous infection (mucormycosis) in cancer patients. Cancer **12**:330–350.
13. Landau, J. W., and V. D. Newcomer. 1962. Acute cerebral phycomycosis (mucormycosis). J. Pediat. **61**:363–385.
14. Lie, K. J., and N. T. Eng. 1962. Phycomycosis in tropical countries. Med. J. Malaya **16**:206–213.
15. Martinson, F. D. 1963. Rhinophycomycosis. J. Laryngol. Otol. **77**:691–705.
16. Martinson, F. D., and B. M. Clark. 1967. Rhinophycomycosis entomophthorae in Nigeria. Amer. J. Trop. Med. Hyg. **16**:40–47.
17. Reinhardt, D. J., W. Kaplan, and L. Ajello. 1970. Experimental cerebral zygomycosis in alloxan-diabetic rabbits. I. Relationship of temperature tolerance of selected zygomycetes to pathogenicity. Infect. Immunity **2**:404–425.
18. Symmers, W. St. C. 1962. Histopathologic aspects of the pathogenesis of some opportunistic fungal infections as exemplified in the pathology of aspergillosis and the phycomycosis. Lab. Invest. **11**:1073–1090.
19. Watson, K. C., P. B. Neame, and C. B. Durban. 1960. In vitro activity of Amphotericin B on strains of mucoraceae pathogenic to man. J. Lab. Clin. Med. **56**:251–257.

Chapter 61

Medically Important *Aspergillus* Species

PETER K. C. AUSTWICK

CHARACTERIZATION OF THE ASPERGILLI

The aspergilli are filamentous saprophytic molds of which at least eight species are known to be primary pathogens of humans and animals or to occur as secondary invaders of damaged tissues. The distinguishing generic character is the swollen apex of the conidiophore (the vesicle) bearing peglike sterigmata over its surface, each of which produces a chain of conidia (phialospores). The septate branching hyphae may undergo extensive morphological changes in living tissues, but the yeast-mycelial dimorphism seen in other pathogenic fungi is absent. A wide range of cultural characteristics is produced, and the structure of the sporing head and the color of the colony are of great importance in identification. Optimal temperatures for growth range from 15 to 50 C.

The genus belongs to the *Deuteromycotina* (*Deuteromycetes*, Fungi Imperfecti), class *Hyphomycetes*, but those species with sexual reproduction are placed in the genera *Eurotium*, *Emericella*, and *Sartorya* of the *Ascomycotina* (*Ascomycetes*), class *Plectomycetes*, and are characterized by closed ascocarps (cleistothecia) with eight-spored asci.

Many common antigens exist between the different species of *Aspergillus* and other filamentous fungi, but certain polysaccharide and protein components appear specific.

CLINICAL SIGNIFICANCE

The aspergilli show a wide range of pathogenic activity in humans and animals which goes far beyond the generally accepted meaning of "aspergillosis" when it is restricted to pulmonary infection (1). Estimates of the incidence of the disease are not reliable except when applied to a predisposing debilitating disease such as leukemia in which up to 5% of patients may become infected (15).

Almost every body organ has been reported affected, and three basic disease types have been observed:

Infection—invasion of living tissue by hyphae (infectious aspergillosis, including pulmonary aspergilloma).

Allergy—sensitization through exposure to fungal antigens by inhalation, ingestion, or contact with spores, mycelium, or metabolites.

Toxicosis—poisoning from the ingestion of toxic metabolites.

Because each type of disease can be associated with several *Aspergillus* spp., the problem of the clinical significance of each species is complicated. *A. fumigatus* is involved in about 90% of infections and in the first two types of allergy listed below, whereas *A. clavatus* is a proven cause of allergic alveolitis (17) and *A. flavus* is the most notorious and widely studied of toxin-producing fungi which can also be carcinogenic (9). Diagnosis of infection rests on the observation of the fungus in the tissues, supported by cultural identification. Allergy may be diagnosed by immunoserological methods for the demonstration of hypersensitivity and antibody formation. Toxicosis has rarely been proven in humans, and its diagnosis rests on the histopathology of the affected tissues and the identification of the mycotoxin in the food.

Pulmonary infection

Three types of infection are caused by *A. fumigatus*, *A. flavus*, *A. niger*, *A. nidulans*, and *A. terreus*, with rare cases associated with *A. carneus* and *A. restrictus*.

Primary invasive aspergillosis. A few cases of primary invasive aspergillosis have been recorded in young children. It is also known in debilitated patients and those undergoing immunosuppressive therapy. A feature is the frequent presence of miliary lesions up to 5 mm in diameter arising from inhaled spores.

Pulmonary aspergilloma. A chronic infection generally arising secondarily in an old tubercular cavity or bronchial dilatation. The single lesion can be up to 30 mm in diameter, showing a characteristic crescentic apical air space on X ray and consisting of a firm, caseated mass composed of necrotic tissue and tightly branched radiating hyphae (a "fungus ball"; Fig. 1).

Bronchopulmonary invasive aspergillosis. With the formation of small colonies of *A.*

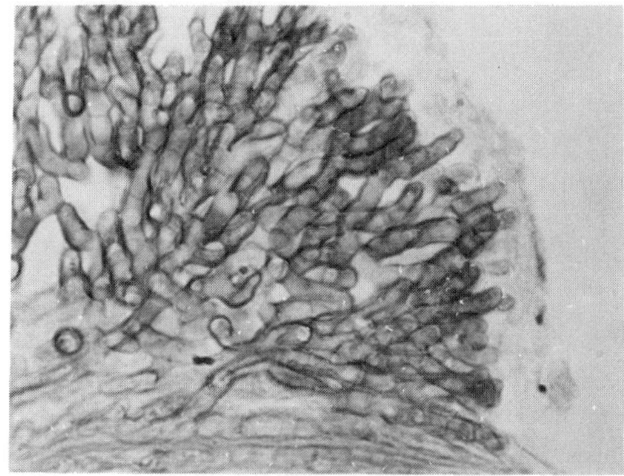

FIG. 1. *Aspergillus fumigatus. Actinomycetoid hyphae at margin of human pulmonary aspergilloma. Stained hematoxylin and eosin.* ×365.

fumigatus in bronchial luminal plugs followed by invasion of the underlying epithelium.

Pulmonary allergy

Asthma and rhinitis. From the inhalation of *Aspergillus* spores by atopic subjects with type I hypersensitivity (6).

Bronchopulmonary allergy. From the inhalation of spores and their germination in the sputum plugs of atopic subjects with both type I and type III sensitivity (6).

Allergic alveolitis (farmer's lung). Primarily from the inhalation of large numbers of the spores of thermophilic actinomycetes from moldy hay, etc., by both atopic and nonatopic persons. Occasionally *Aspergillus* spores have acted as the type III sensitizing antigens (6).

Nasal and orbital infections

A. fumigatus occurs infrequently in nasal sinuses and may form colonies on the epithelium in the turbinate and ethmoid regions. *A. flavus* causes orbital granuloma, and several species are known to cause keratomycosis and other eye infections, mostly arising from trauma (8; see also chapter 55).

Ear infection

Most fungal infections of the ears are caused by aspergilli and frequently involve the growth of the fungus on wax and epidermal squamae with penetration to the underlying epidermis which becomes inflamed. Postoperative aural cavities are especially affected (15).

Cardiovascular and visceral infection

Aspergilli are rarely reported from individual viscera, but following generalization of infection they may be observed in many organs. Both the widespread use of immunosuppressive drugs in the treatment of cancer, especially leukemia, and recent developments in heart surgery and kidney transplantation have led to more secondary infections by these fungi, emphasizing the need for better techniques in diagnosis, especially the monitoring use of serological tests.

Skin infection

Keratinized tissues are not generally suitable substrates for aspergilli, but some species, especially *A. terreus*, invade nails, causing onychomycosis. Subcutaneous abscesses have also been found containing hyphae of this species.

Genital system

Infection of the reproductive organs is uncommon in humans, and few cases of uterine infection are reported.

Natural occurrence

The aspergilli are ubiquitous fungi, and all species at some time have been isolated from dead plant and animal substrates or from soil or air. Pathogenic species, especially *A. fumigatus*, are more often present in spontaneously heated substrates, e.g., moldy hay, grain, and composting plant debris. Habitats of aspergilli in houses are damp and warm areas, and especially badly stored foodstuffs.

COLLECTION, TRANSPORT, AND STORAGE OF SPECIMENS

Methods of collection

The ease of collecting suitable diagnostic material from patients with suspected aspergillosis depends on the site and type of the lesion, but the main emphasis must be on the avoidance of contamination from extraneous *Aspergillus* spores possibly of the same species as that present in the lesion (3). The only certain method of verifying the causal significance of an isolate is the tedious process of dissecting out individual hyphae and directly observing their continued growth in the isolation medium. This method is generally outside normal laboratory practice, but there must always be an element of risk in assigning a causal role to an isolate obtained otherwise. Difficulties may also arise when the lesion is healing and the hyphae in the specimen are already dead.

Aspergillotic lesions are often substantial enough to be removed whole or have pieces cut off them, which should then be placed in a sterile screw-topped bottle. Swabs are difficult to examine directly, but the sediment from centrifuged washings can be used for direct examination and culture. Skin scrapings and nail clippings should be collected dry, together with the scalpel blade used for sampling. Sputum may be collected in the standard way and should be processed rapidly (see chapter 57).

Transport and storage

Most specimens retain their fungal content in little-changed condition over a period of several days if kept at 5 C, but secondary growth and bacterial decomposition will eventually occur. Addition of antibacterial antibiotics to specimens will help preservation, but delay in examination provides chances for invasion by saprophytic aspergilli. Frozen material stored at −20 C is satisfactory for subsequent direct examination, but hyphae do not generally survive this treatment.

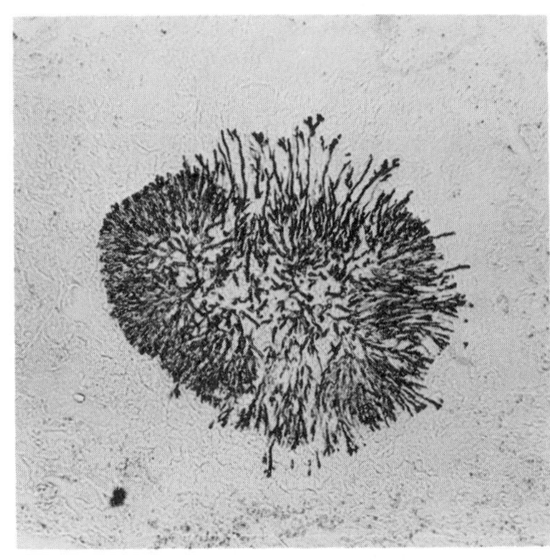

FIG. 2. *Aspergillus fumigatus. Per acute pulmonary lesion in lamb. Stained Gomori-Grocott.* ×161.

DIRECT EXAMINATION

Clinical material

Lesions. Small portions of the specimen ca. 1 mm in diameter should be dissected off under a ×30 stereomicroscope, and each should be mounted in a drop of 20% potassium hydroxide solution. Dissection of this fragment into smaller pieces is helpful, and a no. 1 cover slip should then be placed over the specimen followed by slow gentle warming until the tissue softens. Slight pressure will generally crush the material. Despite this treatment, caseated tissues frequently do not soften sufficiently, and the presence of fat may obscure hyphae completely or allow only short fragments to be seen protruding from dense masses of tissue. The pepsin digest described below is particularly useful in these cases. The fungal structures seen in these preparations will depend upon the type of disease, the material itself, its source, and the stage of infection.

Chronic lesions, including pulmonary aspergillomas, have hyphae 2.5 μm in diameter, showing extensive pseudo-dichotomous branching of the "actinomycetoid" type (Fig. 1 and 2). The tips of these hyphae are usually refractile because of the living cytoplasmic contents, whereas the less well-branched hyphae behind may appear empty. Septa are usually present at regular intervals without constriction of the parallel-walled hyphae. Occasional lack of septa, especially at the margins of lesions, may cause confusion with phycomycete hyphae. Lesions may be found with conidiophores on their surfaces (Fig. 3), especially in the ears and the nasal cavity in humans. In acute lesions caused by *A. fumigatus*, the central part of the nodule may have swollen hyphae present, possibly representing germinated conidia (Fig. 4). These cells may appear empty, are up to 30 μm in diameter, and often occur in groups. In some

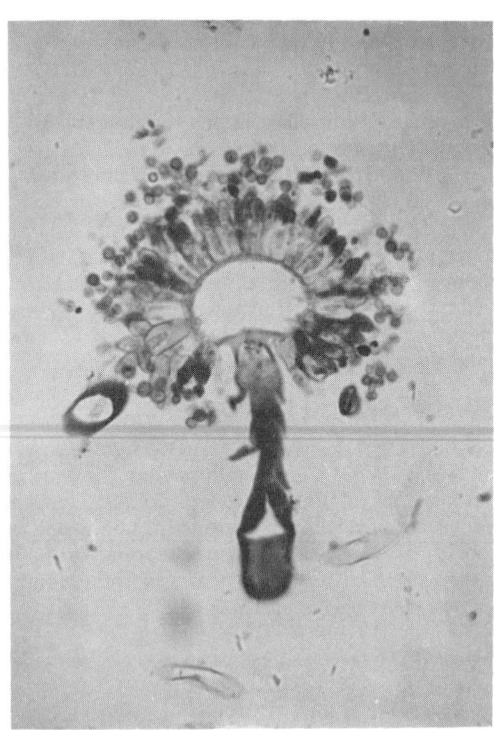

FIG. 3. *Aspergillus flavus. Conidiophore in human lung cavity lesion. Stained Gomori-Grocott.* ×475.

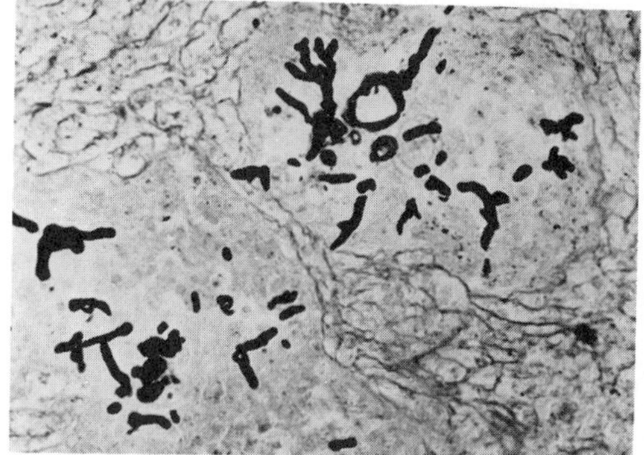

FIG. 4. *Aspergillus fumigatus. Swollen hyphae in infiltrated alveoli of lamb. Stained Gomori-Grocott.* ×365.

animal tissues, they have been found up to 100 μm across, but always with hyphae radiating from them, distinguishing them from the spherules of other pathogenic fungi, e.g., *Coccidioides immitis*.

Sputum. Sputum has to be examined on a more extensive scale than other material and may require digestion in potassium or sodium hydroxide followed by centrifugation before characteristic hyphae and spores can be found. Bronchial plugs may have to be cut into smaller pieces before this is carried out (see Pepsin digestion).

Earwax. Solubilization in warm 20% potassium hydroxide will clear earwax, but emulsification can be carried out by incubating small pieces in 1% Teepol or Tween 80 at just under 100 C for 1 h.

Special methods

Biopsy specimens. Minute portions of tissue such as biopsy specimens, from which cultural confirmation is required, should be dissected under aseptic conditions in a sterile mountant, e.g., saline containing antibacterial antibiotics. The same material can thus be examined microscopically and later plated out.

Pepsin digestion. A most useful method for dealing with samples from chronic lesions which consist of caseated and fibrous material is the pepsin digestion used extensively in parasitology. The pepsin solution is prepared by dissolving 6 g of pepsin in 600 ml of water and then adding 10 ml of concentrated hydrochloric acid. The solution should be stored at 5 C. A portion of the lesion is placed in an excess of this solution and incubated at 37 C for 24 to 48 h. A quick shake of the tube at the end of digestion generally causes the fragment to disintegrate so that the sediment can then be directly mounted or spun down before clearing in potassium hydroxide. Staining of this deposit in ink can be very effective.

Ink staining of slide mounts. Mounting of fresh or Formalin-fixed specimens directly in a solution of equal parts 40% potassium hydroxide and Parker Blue-Black Quink, or drawing the ink beneath the cover slip after mounting in potassium hydroxide, is the best method of staining *Aspergillus* hyphae in wet mounts (2). Although some staining occurs quickly, deeper staining and differentiation will occur if the preparation is kept in a damp chamber overnight. Hyphal walls stain well, but rapidly growing hyphal tips may remain unstained. This method is most useful in differentiating hyphae from collagen fibers and elongated cells, whose chief distinguishing features are their tapering and twisted, flattened aspects. Sometimes capillaries and nerve fibers may simulate branching hyphae in unstained preparations.

CULTURE AND ISOLATION

Recommended procedure for primary culture

Culture media. Isolation must be carried out on media containing one of the following antibacterial antibiotic supplements or its equivalent: 20 units of penicillin plus 40 units of streptomycin per ml, 0.05 mg of chloramphenicol (Chloromycetin, Parke, Davis & Co.) per ml, or 0.05 mg of chlortetracycline (Aureomycin, Lederle Laboratories) per ml. Plates or tubes may be used, depending on the risk of isolating the more dangerous respiratory pathogens, e.g., *Histoplasma capsulatum* (18). The classical isolation medium used is Sabouraud agar (= glucose peptone), on which most aspergilli grow luxuriantly but not characteristically. Two percent malt extract agar is the most useful isolation medium, but other media such as brain-heart infusion agar are also used. Certain members of the *A. glaucus* series and *A. restrictus* grow well only when competition is reduced by the use of media with high osmotic pressures, e.g., malt-salt, or Czapek-Dox agar containing 20% sucrose. Incubation should be at both 25 and 37 C, and cultures must be retained for up to 3 weeks. On no account should cycloheximide (Actidione) be incorporated into the medium since this is inhibitory.

Preparation of material. Material from caseated lesions and other firm tissue should be washed in several changes of sterile water, preferably containing an antibacterial antibiotic, and then blotted on sterile filter paper. Small pieces about 1 to 2 mm in diameter should be cut from the same part of the material used for the microscope examination and plated out with four or five pieces to a plate or one or two to a tube.

With large aspergillomas, it is possible to sear the outside of the specimen and dissect out the inoculum aseptically.

In cases where doubt exists as to the significance of an *Aspergillus* isolate, it may be necessary to take further material and dissect out individual hyphae or hyphal groups under ×30 magnification of a stereo microscope by use of very fine needles. After being washed in several drops of sterile water containing an antibacterial antibiotic on a sterile slide, these hyphae can be transferred to the surface of agar, observed under the microscope, and their positions marked. The culture should be examined frequently from 6 h onwards to ascertain the origin of any colonies.

Sputum, pus, and urine may be plated directly by streaking or dilution, or they may be treated with a surface-active agent (e.g., 1% Tween 80) and antibacterial antibiotics, homogenized, and centrifuged before streaking or dilution-plating the sediment. Whenever possible, the hyphae observed directly should be plated out. *Aspergillus* hyphae do not survive the normal sodium hydroxide digestion used for bacteriological examination of sputum.

Blood and cerebrospinal fluid are preferably centrifuged and the sediment is dilution-plated. This method may also be used for bone marrow and ulcer scrapings. In all cases, very close observation of the origin of any colonies is required.

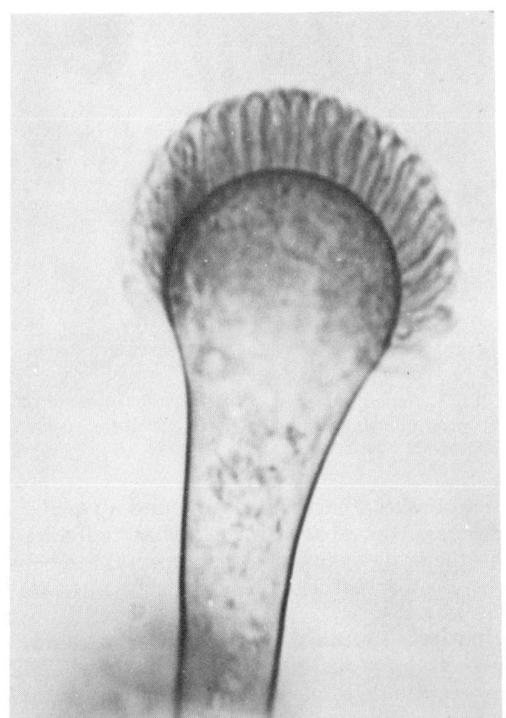

FIG. 5. *Aspergillus fumigatus. Conidiophore from culture showing single row of sterigmata. Stained Parker ink.* ×1170.

IDENTIFICATION

Recommended procedure

If conidiophores have formed in the tissues, it is sometimes possible to identify *A. fumigatus* directly, but other species require isolation. With practice, identification can often be made from the isolation plate (Fig. 5), and the diagnostic characters of the commoner pathogenic species are described in Table 1 from Czapek-Dox agar. Reference must be made to the monograph by Raper and Fennell on *The Genus Aspergillus* (16), in which detailed keys to all the groups and species are given. The data necessary for the identification of an unknown isolate include: colony texture, color, and rate of growth; conidiophore morphology including the numbers of rows of sterigmata; conidial characters of columnar or radiate arrangement, size, shape, and ornamentation of the wall; and characters of cleistothecia and ascospores if present.

Occasionally atypical aspergilli are isolated from chronic lesions. The most common variant is a white, fluffy form of *A. fumigatus* which produces very few conidiophores. Cases of dual infection of *A. fumigatus* with either *Mucor pusillus* or *Allescheria boydii* have been reported.

Cultural characteristics

Cultural characteristics of the *Aspergillus* species are given in Table 1.

Microscope examination of cultures

Colonies should be examined under a low-power microscope for the type of fruiting head. Considerable care is required in the preparation of microscopical mounts to avoid inhalation of conidia, and it is advisable to open culture tubes and plates only in a microbiological safety cabinet. Small portions of growth from the margins and from the centers of mature colonies should be removed, mounted on a slide in a drop of lactophenol (with or without cotton blue), and crushed gently under a cover slip.

Other procedures

Biochemical reactions have not yet been used to differentiate the species of aspergilli, and serological methods have little application in the identification of cultures but can be used, e.g., by fluorescent-antibody staining, to attempt the identification of hyphae observed in lesions. Animal or tissue culture inoculations are not used.

IMMUNOSEROLOGICAL DIAGNOSIS

Preferred procedures

Fungi elicit a wide range of immune reactions because of the volume and chemical complexity of their hyphae, other cells, and spores (11), and immunoserological methods play an important part in the diagnosis of diseases associated with *Aspergillus* spp., especially in pulmonary infection and allergy. Five types of aspergillotic disease are listed in Table 2 under their respective antibody responses (4, 10, 14, 19). Details of antigen preparation are given by Pepys and Longbottom (14) (see also chapter 62).

The skin prick test is important in screening atopic patients with asthma, and the 4- to 6-h late (Arthus) type reaction after an intracutaneous test provides confirmatory diagnosis of allergic bronchopulmonary aspergillosis. In these latter patients the serological tests are

TABLE 1. *Key to Aspergillus species grown on Czapek-Dox medium*[a]

Key	Species	Colony color		Max conidiophore length	Max vesicle diam. (μm)	No. of rows of sterigmata	Conidia (μm)	Ascospore color
		Surface	Reverse (none to:)					
1. Conidial heads yellow, or blue- or gray-green 2.								
Conidial heads in other shades 8.								
2. Conidial heads and vesicles clavate	*A. clavatus*	Pale blue- or gray-green	Brown	2–3 mm 10 mm+	50 180	1	3.5–4.5 × 2.4–3.0	—
Conidial heads columnar 3.								
Conidial heads radiate 5.								
3. Vesicles flask-shaped, sterigmata strictly 1 rowed	*A. fumigatus*	Dark blue-green	Brown	300 μm	30	1	2.5–3.5	—
Vesicles elliptical to globose sterigmata 1–2 rowed 4.								
4. Sterigmata strictly 1 rowed	*A. restrictus*	Green to dark olive-gray	Dark green	150 μm	12	1	4.5–5.5 × 3.0–3.5	—
Sterigmata 1–2 rowed, without Hülle cells[b] 5.								
Sterigmata strictly 2 rowed, with Hülle cells	*A. nidulans*	Dark cress green	Purplish red	130 μm	10	2	3.0–3.5	Red
5. Cleistothecia present 6.	*A. glaucus* group							
Cleistothecia absent 7.								
6. Ascospores rough	*A. amstelodami*	Olive-green[c]	Yellow	350 μm	25	1	4.5–5.0 × 3.5–4.0	Colorless
Ascospores smooth, ridges absent	*A. repens*	Dull green[c]	Maroon	1 mm	40	1	5.0–6.0	Colorless
Ascospores smooth, ridges thin, flexuous	*A. chevalieri*	Gray-green[c]	Maroon	850 μm	35	1	4.5–5.5	Colorless
7. Sterigmata 1–2 rowed	*A. flavus*	Yellow to dark green	Red-brown	2 mm	65	1–2	3.5–4.5	—
Sterigmata 2 rowed	*A. versicolor*	Yellow to blue-green	Wine red	500 μm	16	2	2.0–3.0	—
8. Conidial heads brown to black	*A. niger*	Brown to black	Yellow	6 mm	100	2	5.5–8.0	
Conidial heads pale cinnamon to orange-brown	*A. terreus*	Cinnamon-brown	Brown	250 μm	16	2	1.8–2.4	—
Conidial heads white to cream 9.								—
9. Conidial heads radiate	*A. candidus*	White to cream	Pale pink or yellow	1 mm	40+	2	2.5–3.5	—
Conidial heads columnar	*A. carneus*	White to vinaceous	Brown	1 mm	9	2	2.4–2.8	—

[a] *A. glaucus* series and *A. restrictus* grown on 20% sucrose.
[b] See reference 17 for a description of Hülle cells.
[c] To yellow or orange according to density of cleistothecia.

TABLE 2. *Immunological findings in aspergillosis*

Clinical status	Skin reactivity		Serological precipitins IgG	Type of allergy[a]
	Immediate IgE	Late (Arthus) IgG		
Asthma, rhinitis	+	−	−	I
Allergic aspergillosis	+	+	+weak (60–90%)	I + III
Allergic alveolitis	−	+	+[b]	III
Aspergilloma	±[c]	±[c]	+strong[b] (95%)	I? + III?
Invasive	NK[d]	NK	+[b]	NK

[a] See reference 6.
[b] Specific to the species of *Aspergillus* isolated.
[c] No skin test in majority, but if type I then type III may also develop.
[d] NK, Not known.

weak, with 60% positivity, but with concentration of sera this value may be raised to 90%. This reaction may be compared with that of patients with pulmonary aspergilloma in which the serological precipitin test is virtually diagnostic. Surgical or natural removal (by expectoration) of a pulmonary aspergilloma is followed by a rapid loss of precipitins. In these tests it is also important to exclude nonspecific C-reactive protein/C-substance reactions by the use of citrate in gel diffusions.

SUSCEPTIBILITY TO ANTIMICROBIAL AGENTS

The in vitro susceptibility of *A. fumigatus* to antifungal agents is given in chapter 63, but, because of variation of both individual patient and of fungal species and strain, the in vivo performance of a drug may not always correspond to that given. Therapeutic procedures should be based on both previous experiences with the drug in other cases (5, 7) and on the circumstances of the case, e.g., the existence of an underlying debilitating disease (12).

LITERATURE CITED

1. Austwick, P. K. C. 1965. Pathogenicity, p. 82–126. *In* K. B. Raper and D. I. Fennell (ed.), The genus *Aspergillus*. The Williams & Wilkins Co., Baltimore.
2. Balogh, N. 1964. Diagnostik Pilzkrankheiten bei Tieren mit modifizierte Parker Blue-Black Superchrome Tintensärbung. Deut. Tieraerztl. Wochenschr. **71**:327–330.
3. Buckley, R., C. K. Campbell, and J. C. Thompson. 1969. Techniques for the isolation of pathogenic fungi, p. 113–126. *In* D. A. Shapton and G. W. Gould (ed.), Isolation methods for microbiologists, part 1. Academic Press Inc., London.
4. Coleman, R. M., and L. Kaufman. 1972. Use of the immunodiffusion test in the serodiagnosis of aspergillosis. Appl. Microbiol. **23**:301–308.
5. Conant, N. F., D. T. Smith, R. D. Baker, and J. L. Callaway. 1971. Manual of clinical mycology. W. B. Saunders, Philadelphia.
6. Coombs, R. R. A., and P. G. H. Gell. 1968. Classification of allergic reactions responsible for clinical hypersensitivity and disease, p. 575–596. *In* P. G. H. Gell and R. R. A. Coombs (ed.), Clinical aspects of immunology, 2nd ed. Blackwell, Oxford.
7. Emmons, C. W., C. H. Binford, and J. P. Utz. 1970. Medical mycology, 2nd ed. Lea & Febiger, Philadelphia.
8. Gingrich, W. D. 1962. Keratomycosis. J. Amer. Med. Ass. **179**:602–608.
9. Goldblatt, L. A. (ed.). 1969. Aflatoxin, scientific background, control and implications. Academic Press Inc., New York.
10. Hipp, S. S., D. S. Berns, V. Tompkins, and H. Buckley. 1970. Latex slide agglutination test for Aspergillus antibodies. Sabouraudia **8**:237–241.
11. Longbottom, J. L., I. G. Murray, and J. Pepys. 1968. Diagnosis of fungal diseases, p. 71–111. *In* P. G. H. Gell and R. R. A. Coombs (ed.), Clinical aspects of immunology, 2nd ed. Blackwell, Oxford.
12. Meyer, R. D., L. S. Young, D. Armstrong, and B. Yu. 1973. Aspergillus complicating neoplastic disease. Amer. J. Med. **54**:6–15.
13. Peña, C. E. 1971. Aspergillosis, p. 762–831. *In* R. D. Baker (ed.), The pathologic anatomy of mycoses. Human infection with fungi, actinomycetes and algae. Springer Verlag, Berlin.
14. Pepys, J., and J. L. Longbottom. 1973. Immunological methods in mycology, p. 381. *In* D. M. Weir (ed.), Handbook of experimental immunology. Blackwell, Oxford.
15. Powell, D. E. B., M. P. English, and E. H. L. Duncan. 1962. Clinical, bacteriological and mycological findings in post-operative ear cavities. J. Laryngol. **76**:12–21.
16. Raper, K. B., and D. L. Fennell. 1965. The genus *Aspergillus*. The Williams & Wilkins Co., Baltimore.
17. Riddle, H. F. V., S. Channell, W. Blyth, D. M. Weir, M. Lloyd, W. M. G. Amos, and I. W. B. Grant. 1968. Allergic alveolitis in a maltworker. Thorax **23**:271–280.
18. Shapton, D. A., and R. G. Board (ed.). 1972. Safety in microbiology. Society of Applied Bacteriologists Technical Series No. 6. Academic Press Inc., London.
19. Walter, J. E., and R. D. Jones. 1968. Serologic tests in diagnosis of aspergillosis. Dis. Chest **53**:729–735.

Chapter 62
Serodiagnosis of Fungal Diseases

LEO KAUFMAN

INTRODUCTION

Meticulous consideration of symptoms and epidemiological circumstances may result in an accurate clinical diagnosis of a mycotic disease; however, such diagnoses should be confirmed by standard cultural and histological laboratory procedures. Unfortunately, the diagnosis of a mycotic infection cannot always be proven by culture or histology, despite repeated efforts to isolate a fungus from patients or to demonstrate its presence in biopsy and autopsy material. In such situations, immunological procedures can be used to provide rapid and presumptive evidence of infection. Such evidence often provides the first clue to the existence of a fungus infection. Positive serological results can yield information on the effects of chemotherapy, and, in many cases, lead to increased efforts for the isolation and identification of the etiological agent.

A positive serological reaction, particularly at a high titer, even though on a single specimen can be diagnostically significant. Many of the diagnostic antigens used in medical mycology are crude mixtures of multiple antigenic factors, some of which are shared by fungi of different genera and between fungi and other microorganisms. When cross-reactions are encountered, a prudent diagnosis rests upon (i) results of serological tests performed with a battery of antigens (including those representing antigenically related species), (ii) examination of serial serum specimens for titer changes, and (iii) information as to the acquisition of hypersensitivity. Some individuals suffering with a systemic mycosis are immunologically unresponsive. Others may not demonstrate antibody levels against a fungus because of immunosuppressant medication or because there is not enough time to build up antibody levels before the serum is taken. Consequently, one must always bear in mind that negative immunological results do not exclude a diagnosis of mycotic infection.

DETECTION OF HYPERSENSITIVITY

Most patients affected with coccidioidomycosis and histoplasmosis develop a hypersensitive state that is readily and reliably demonstrated by coccidioidin and histoplasmin skin tests. The hypersensitive state has been demonstrated in individuals suffering from blastomycosis, candidiasis, and cryptococcosis, but not with sufficient frequency or specificity to warrant widespread use of these skin test antigens.

The skin test is administered by intradermally injecting 0.1 ml of an appropriate dilution of antigen into the volar surface of the forearm. In sensitized persons, an area of induration and erythema develops at the injection site. The coccidioidin test should be read at 24 to 36 h for maximal reaction and the histoplasmin test at 48 to 72 h. The largest diameter of induration, not erythema, is recorded. An induration 5 mm or more in diameter is considered a positive reaction.

The skin test is most useful in defining endemic areas for a disease. It has limited value as a diagnostic tool, since it does not distinguish between a past or present infection. In general, a positive reaction is of diagnostic value only if a negative reaction had been obtained prior to the onset of clinical symptoms. Except in infants, a positive reaction with no past history has little diagnostic value. A negative reaction is of greater significance because it shows definite absence of the disease, except in cases in which the patient is in the very early stages of infection, is in the terminal stages, or suffers from a defective cellular immune system, at which times the test becomes negative.

In certain diseases, especially coccidioidomycosis, the skin test is relied upon by physicians in assessing the prognosis of the disease. A reversion to the negative state indicates a state of anergy and a poor prognosis. In a healthy person, a positive coccidioidin skin test implies resistance to infection. It is not known whether a positive histoplasmin skin test in a healthy subject implies such a state.

Because of the sharing of common antigens among fungi, it is suggested that skin tests with several antigens such as coccidioidin and histoplasmin be performed simultaneously. Interpretation is thus facilitated in instances when only one antigen is positive or possibly when one elicits a larger area of induration than the other.

The magnitude of the reaction, however, does not necessarily indicate the homologous reaction. Proper interpretation of tests with multiple antigens must be balanced with the clinical picture and other laboratory data.

COLLECTION, PRESERVATION, AND SHIPMENT OF SPECIMENS

Specimens for serological tests must be taken aseptically, and 10 ml of blood should be drawn. After the blood has clotted and the serum has separated, the serum is removed aseptically and preserved by adding Merthiolate to make a final concentration of 1:10,000.

It is convenient to maintain a 1% stock solution of Merthiolate in the laboratory. This is prepared by dissolving 1.4 g of sodium borate in distilled water, adding 1.0 g of Merthiolate, and adjusting to a final volume of 100 ml with distilled water. Use 0.1 ml of the stock solution per 10 ml of serum or other clinical specimen. Specimens so treated do not require refrigeration during shipment.

Spinal fluid specimens should be aseptically taken when meningeal involvement is suspected. No preservative should be added if the material will be cultured before serological examination, but preservative may be added if no attempt will be made to culture the specimen. It is preferable that the specimen be frozen if it is to be shipped to a laboratory for testing. This will curtail bacterial growth should contamination occur during transit.

All specimens should be enclosed in heavy-walled tubes secured with a tight-fitting cork or soft-rubber stopper. The stoppers should be held in place with adhesive tape or sealed with paraffin. It is desirable to ship specimens by airmail or air express to assure prompt arrival.

DETECTION OF CIRCULATING ANTIBODIES AND ANTIGENS

Antibody responses are useful indices in determining the diagnosis and the prognosis of a mycosis. Dependable diagnoses can frequently be made from a single serological test. However, low titers or cross-reactions in the complement fixation (CF) test are difficult to interpret. In such cases, serum specimens taken 3 weeks apart should be studied. Ideally, to establish a diagnosis and to monitor the course of an infection properly, sera should be taken early in the course of illness, at its height, during convalescence, and several weeks after recovery. Fourfold or greater rises in titer are usually acceptable diagnostic signs of disease, although cross-reactions with heterologous antigens may appear early in illness and cause confusion. Usually, cross-reacting antibody titers remain stable or move at a lower rate than the homologous titer as the disease progresses. False serodiagnoses may be avoided through the use of reference sera in immunodiffusion (ID) tests.

Aspergillosis

Many workers have shown the ID test to be an effective and specific method for establishing a diagnosis of aspergillosis (12, 14, 65, 79). The maximal number of aspergillosis cases may be detected by the concurrent use of *Aspergillus fumigatus*, *A. flavus*, and *A. niger* precipitinogens (44). Uniform and reproducible antigens that do not react with C-reactive protein are prepared from acetone-precipitated culture filtrates of 5-week-old Sabouraud broth cultures grown at 31 C. The carbohydrate content of the 8×-concentrated antigens is determined by the anthrone test and adjusted to 1,000 μg/ml. Only sera that demonstrate a line or lines of identity with a reference serum from a proven human case of aspergillosis should be considered positive. The presence of one or more precipitins in a patient's serum is considered to be indicative of allergic aspergillosis, an aspergilloma, or infection due to an *Aspergillus* species. Precipitins can be found in over 90% of fungus ball cases and 50% of the cases of allergic bronchopulmonary aspergillosis. One or two precipitins could occur with any clinical form of aspergillosis; however, the demonstration of three or more precipitins is indicative of aspergilloma or invasive aspergillosis. Although Young and Bennett (92) found serology of no value in patients with invasive aspergillosis, others have reported the ID test to be helpful in diagnosing systemic aspergillosis (12, 26, 60).

The ID test when used with reference sera is entirely specific. Although aberrant lines may occur with sera from individuals with aspergillosis, a specific diagnosis cannot be achieved in the absence of lines of identity with reference bands, since sera from patients with candidiasis and histoplasmosis may contain precipitins reactive with *Aspergillus* antigens. A decrease in the number of precipitin lines or in the titer reflects recovery.

CF tests for aspergillosis have been developed and found useful for detecting active or very recent infection (64, 90). A decline or disappearance of CF titer appears to be associated with recovery from infection. The CF test is less specific than the ID test.

Blastomycosis

Sensitive ID tests for blastomycosis have been developed, but they lack specificity (1, 7). Recently, a modified and specific ID test for blastomycosis was evaluated at the Center for Disease Control (51). The test permitted the serodiagnosis of approximately 80% of 113 proven cases of blastomycosis. Two diagnostically important precipitins, designated A and B, were frequently recognized in sera of patients with blastomycosis. The routine use of reference sera containing the A and B precipitins in ID tests permits the specific diagnosis of blastomycosis without the need for parallel tests with coccidioidin and histoplasmin.

Macro- and micro-CF tests (85), in which an optimal dilution of a suspension of ground-yeast-form antigen of *Blastomyces dermatitidis* (24) is used, are used widely in the diagnosis of blastomycosis. Titers of 1:8 or greater with the *B. dermatitidis* antigen are considered positive. When reactions occur solely with the *B. dermatitidis* antigen, one is inclined to suspect blastomycosis. This antigen, however, frequently reacts in low titers with sera from patients who show no evidence of blastomycosis and also with sera from persons with confirmed coccidioidomycosis and histoplasmosis. With such sera, a serological diagnosis should be based upon the reactions of several serum specimens taken 3 to 4 weeks apart to observe titer movement. High titers or rising titers indicate that the patient probably has blastomycosis. The testing of serial serum specimens to establish a diagnosis is unnecessary if precipitins are demonstrated in the blastomycosis ID test. Unfortunately, less than 50% of the sera from persons with proven blastomycosis react in the CF test. Thus, a negative reaction has little value and does not exclude the presence of active blastomycosis. Although the CF test for blastomycosis may have limited diagnostic value, it frequently is of prognostic value in the study of culturally proven cases.

Candidiasis

Agglutination, latex agglutination (LA), and ID tests are valuable in the diagnosis of systemic candidiasis (68, 80–84). In contrast, the serodiagnosis of candidiasis by CF tests has proven to be of little value because of positive responses by healthy subjects or by individuals with superficial candidiasis and without systemic involvement (84). Hollister-Stier (HS) 1:10 extracts of *C. albicans* (Hollister-Stier Laboratories, Spokane, Wash.) and homogenate or cytoplasmic sonic extracts of *C. albicans* are most satisfactory as antigens in these tests (81, 84). Stickle et al. (81) encountered cross-reactions with *Torulopsis glabrata* antisera. The LA test has a greater sensitivity than the ID test, but reactions have also been noted in some patients with cryptococcosis and tuberculosis. Rising titers of either precipitins or agglutinins are believed to be reliable indicators of the presence of visceral candidiasis. The precipitin titer represents the highest dilution of serum producing a band after reaction with antigen. Although a decline in the number of precipitins or the precipitin titer may prove useful as an index of recovery, it does not invariably accompany or indicate disease regression after successful treatment. The LA test has prognostic value, and quantitative tests on sera taken at biweekly intervals are of value in monitoring the progress of infection before and after therapy.

Coccidioidomycosis

The CF and tube precipitin tests are invaluable aids in the diagnosis and prognosis of coccidioidomycosis (77). Both test systems incorporate the soluble antigen coccidioidin, a pool of culture filtrates derived from multiple strains of *Coccidioides immitis*. The tests may be applied to sera, cerebrospinal fluid (CSF), plasma, and pleural and joint fluids. The microadaptation of the CF test for coccidioidomycosis gives results comparable to those of the macrotest (49).

Coccidioidin is prepared by a variety of procedures, the most widely known of which employs filtrates from cultures grown in a modified Bureau of Animal Industry tuberculin medium (78). The preparation of coccidioidin in this medium usually requires incubation for 8 weeks or more at room temperature. Coccidioidins are also prepared in Trypticase-yeast extract-dextrose broth inoculated with a single strain of *C. immitis* and incubated for 8 weeks at 28 C (24). Antigens can be prepared within 1 week by the toluene lysis technique of Pappagianis et al. (63).

Heating coccidioidin at 60 C for 30 min destroys the antigen responsible for the CF activity but has no effect on the precipitinogens (32, 63). The two tests measure at least two different antigen-antibody systems. The tube precipitin test is most effective in detecting early primary infection or patients undergoing an exacerbation of existing disease. It is diagnostic but not prognostic in nature. Precipitins are rarely detected 6 months after infection. The CF test becomes positive later than the precipitin test, and it is most effective in determining disseminated disease. The CF titer tends to parallel the severity of the infection (77); titers rise as the disease progresses and decline as the patient improves.

Any tube precipitin or CF titer with coccidioidin should be considered presumptive evidence for *C. immitis* infection. CF reactions, i.e., titers of 1:2 and 1:4, have been found to be indicative of early, residual, or meningeal coccidioidomycosis (77). However, sera demonstrating such titers have also been obtained from patients not known to have coccidioidomycosis. It is thus apparent that when low titers are obtained a diagnosis of coccidioidomycosis must be based on subsequent serological tests and preferably on clinical and mycological studies. Generally, CF titers greater than 1:16 are indicative of disseminating disease. Negative serology does not exclude a diagnosis of coccidioidomycosis.

For those laboratories not in a position to perform the tube precipitin or CF tests, screening tests that yield results comparable to the aforementioned procedures have been developed.

One, the latex particle agglutination test (Hyland Laboratories, Los Angeles, Calif.), uses latex particles sensitized with coccidioidin heated at 60 C for 30 min. Although considered to give results comparable to the tube precipitin test, the latex particle agglutination test is more sensitive than the tube precipitin test and yields a higher percentage of positive results with sera from persons with proven coccidioidomycosis. Results can be obtained in 4 min (33).

The second screening procedure is an ID test (31) which gives results that correlate with those obtained with the CF test. The antigen consists of a heat-labile toluene extract of mycelium. Evaluation studies have shown that the combination of the latex particle and ID tests enables detection of more than 90% of cases (33). It is recommended that sera positive by either of these techniques be analyzed with the standard CF and tube precipitin tests to clarify their clinical significance.

The coccidioidin skin test is considered a valuable screen for serological testing. Conversion from negative to positive is pathognomonic and is the earliest immunological response to infection. Smith and his co-workers (77) never observed positive serological results in patients with primary coccidioidomycosis infection without impending or concomitant dissemination in the absence of a positive skin test. Unlike the serological reactions sometimes noted after administration of the histoplasmin skin test (10, 53), coccidioidin skin testing does not produce a homologous humoral antibody response (89).

Cryptococcosis

Conventional methodology for the diagnosis of cryptococcosis is time-consuming and in many cases inadequate. Until recently, individuals suffering from cryptococcosis were considered to be essentially immunologically inert. Previous immunological tests had only limited successful applications (9, 41), and even then interpretation of results was difficult. Recent work on serological procedures for cryptococcosis has resulted in the development of diagnostically and prognostically useful tests. These procedures are an indirect fluorescent-antibody (IFA) technique (86–88), a charcoal particle agglutination test (22), an agglutination test for cryptococcal antibodies (23), and a latex slide agglutination test for cryptococcal antigen (5).

Although the IFA test is not entirely specific, it is a valuable and sensitive tool for the serological diagnosis of cryptococcosis. This is particularly evident in those cases of cryptococcosis that are negative for *C. neoformans* agglutinins and antigens. This test is performed as follows. Heat-killed *C. neoformans* cells representing serotypes A and R (86) are heat-fixed to a slide and covered with a 1:20 dilution of the heat-inactivated serum specimen. After incubation, the preparation is washed and air-dried, and then is treated with anti-human globulin conjugated to fluorescein isothiocyanate. A positive reaction is indicated by staining of the cells to an intensity of 2+ or greater.

Gordon and Vedder (23) used the conventional agglutination test for detection of cryptococcal antibodies and found it to be specific. Agglutinins were detected in the early stages of central nervous system infection and in infections with no central nervous system involvement.

Formalin-killed whole yeast cells heated at 56 C for 30 min are used in the agglutination test. The cells are adjusted to a concentration of 15 million cells/ml, and 0.5-ml volumes of serial twofold dilutions of serum or spinal fluid are mixed with equal volumes of antigens. The mixtures are shaken for 2 min, incubated at 37 C for 2 h, and then refrigerated at 4 C for 72 h, during which time readings are taken at 24-h intervals.

The charcoal particle test (22) is more sensitive than the whole cell agglutination test for detection of antibody to *C. neoformans*, but it is not as specific. There is evidence that low titers obtained with the charcoal procedure may not always indicate cryptococcal infection. The test uses specially prepared charcoal particles sensitized at room temperature with cryptococcal capsular polysaccharide antigen.

The latex slide agglutination test (5) has been successfully used for the specific detection of cryptococcal antigen in sera and CSF from humans with proven cryptococcosis. The height of the titer appears to be correlated with the severity of the disease. Under certain conditions, antigen tests may be negative in a patient who gives positive cultures. However, in such situations antibodies may be demonstrable. A decline in antigen reactivity or the appearance of agglutinins, with an associated favorable clinical response to chemotherapy, suggests that the tests have prognostic as well as diagnostic value.

False-positive reactions are rare and occur only with some sera from patients with severe rheumatoid arthritis. This presents no problem, however, when all LA-positive sera are routinely evaluated for rheumatoid factor. If this factor is absent, the cryptococcal LA reaction is considered specific.

The latex test basically involves the reaction between latex particles sensitized with anti-*C. neoformans* globulin and the patient's body fluids suspected of containing cryptococcal antigen. Sera and CSF are routinely heated at 56 C for 30 min, whereas urine is heated in a boiling-water bath for 10 min. Amounts of 0.04 ml of the heat-inactivated specimen, in serial dilutions, are allowed to react with 0.02-ml amounts of the latex-globulin suspension on a slide. The slide contents are mixed and agitated for 10 min at 150 rpm, and agglutination is read on a scale of negative to 4+. Reactions less than 2+ are considered negative, but suggest the desirability of follow-up study.

Recently, a cryptococcal antigen LA kit in which a modified procedure is used was developed by Industrial Biological Laboratories, Inc., (Rockville, Md.).

Kaufman and Blumer (47) observed that maximal serological diagnosis of cryptococcosis is accomplished through the concurrent use of three tests: the LA test for cryptococcal antigen and the IFA and tube agglutination tests for *C. neoformans* antibodies.

Of the three tests, the LA test is the most useful for detecting cryptococcal meningitis. Of 39 patients recently studied with culturally proven meningeal cryptococcosis, 36 (92%) had spinal fluid positive by the LA test (18).

Contrary to established thought, *C. neoformans* does stimulate antibody production in humans. Both cryptococcal antibody and antigen tests should be used, since there appears to be an inverse relationship between the two.

Histoplasmosis

Serological evidence is often the prime factor responsible for a definitive diagnosis of histoplasmosis. Such evidence is obtainable through CF, ID, and LA tests, used either alone or in some combination. Of these procedures, the most widely used is the CF test. Properly performed, either as a tube or a microtitration procedure (49), it can yield information of diagnostic and prognostic value. Unfortunately, CF tests are complex and expensive, and should be performed only by highly trained technicians.

Two antigens are used in the Center for Disease Control Laboratory Branch Complement Fixation (LBCF) test (85). One is a suspension of Merthiolate-treated intact yeast-form cells of *H. capsulatum* (73), and the other is a soluble mycelial filtrate antigen, histoplasmin, harvested after growth of the fungus for approximately 6 months in Smith's Aspargine Medium (24). The optimal dilution for use of each antigen is determined by a block titration in which one or more known positive human sera are used.

Use of only one of the two antigens fails to provide adequate diagnostic coverage, because sera from patients with culturally confirmed histoplasmosis may react to only one of the antigens (27, 52). Interpretation of test results can be difficult, because it is not uncommon for these antigens to be cross-reactive or to be nonspecific. In such instances, titers usually range between 1:8 and 1:16, and are mainly noted with the yeast-form antigen. However, many sera from culturally proven cases of histoplasmosis demonstrate titers of only 1:8. Consequently, titers of 1:8 and 1:16 with either antigen are generally considered only presumptive evidence of histoplasmosis. Titers of 1:32 or greater are highly suggestive of *H. capsulatum* infection and are of more diagnostic significance than lower titers; however, they cannot be relied upon as the sole means of diagnosis. Titer movement is often of great assistance in making a diagnosis of histoplasmosis. Fourfold changes in titer in either direction are significant indicators of disease progression or regression. Occasionally in some patients positive titers are obtained that slowly decline over a prolonged period of time after the patient has been cured. Reactions with heterologous antigens may complicate interpretation of results when only a single serum specimen has been tested. For example, in some situations, the first serological response noted in an individual suffering from histoplasmosis may be obtained only with the *B. dermatitidis* antigen. Some patients suffering from histoplasmosis respond to all of the antigens (*H. capsulatum*, *B. dermatitidis*, and *C. immitis*), to only some of them, or to none. It should be emphasized, however, that a lack of immunological response does not exclude histoplasmosis, particularly when only a single specimen has been tested and when the clinical picture strongly suggests pulmonary mycotic disease. In disseminated or terminal histoplasmosis, a state of anergy frequently exists, and immunological responses are negative. The CF test is more frequently positive with sera from chronic active pulmonary histoplasmosis than with sera from primary acute pulmonary histoplasmosis (2, 28).

The yeast-form antigen has the greatest sensitivity (42). It is recommended that the CF test with the yeast-form antigen be used in the diagnostic laboratory (52), and where possible it should be supplemented with either the ID or counterelectrophoresis test with histoplasmin (20, 54). There is a greater than 90% agreement between results obtained in the CF test with histoplasmin and those obtained by ID and counterelectrophoresis. The latter tests are very useful for examining anticomplementary sera, and, because of their greater specificity, they allow a more accurate diagnosis with sera which cross-react in CF tests.

The histoplasmosis counterelectrophoresis test procedure (54) is basically performed as follows: 10 ml of an equal mixture of 0.85% agarose and 0.85% Ionagar No. 2, dissolved in 0.01 M Veronal buffer, pH 7.2, is applied to a 3.25 by 4 inch (8.2 by 10.2 cm) projector slide cover glass, and 5-mm wells are cut into the agar. Each antigen well is 3 mm from each of two serum wells. Sera are placed in the anodic wells of each pair and histoplasmin is placed in the cathodic wells. A control serum containing H and M antibodies is placed in the well adjacent to the serum to be tested. Electrophoresis is performed at room temperature with 0.05 M Veronal buffer, pH 7.2, in each chamber. A constant current of 25 mA is applied across the narrow dimension of the slide for 90 min. After electrophoresis, the slides are removed and read.

The ID test is a useful screening procedure or adjunct in the serological diagnosis of histoplasmosis. The results usually obtained are qualitative in nature. The test was first applied to the diagnosis of histoplasmosis in 1958 by Heiner (25). He was able to demonstrate six precipitin bands when concentrated histoplasmin antigen interacted with serum from patients having histoplasmosis. Two of these bands had diagnostic value. One, designated "h," was uninfluenced by skin testing and was consistently found in the serum of patients with active histoplasmosis. The second, designated "m," was found in acute and chronic histoplasmosis and also appeared after skin testing of sensitized normal individuals with histoplasmin. Although the "h" band is usually associated with the "m" band, the "m" band frequently occurs alone. The "m" band has been considered presumptive evidence of infection with *H. capsulatum* (74). Finding only "m" antibodies in sera may be attributed to active or inactive disease or to skin testing (6, 91).

Proper interpretation of the ID reaction requires that the laboratory workers be cognizant of whether the patient whose serum is being analyzed was recently skin-tested. In the absence of a recent histoplasmin skin test, detection of an "m" band may serve as an early indicator of disease, since this band appears before the "h" factor and disappears more slowly. The demonstration of both the "m" and "h" bands is highly suggestive of active histoplasmosis, regardless of other serological results.

Busey and Hinton's (6) micro-ID test is recommended. In this procedure, 6.5 ml of agar is pipetted into a petri dish and allowed to harden. Then 3.5 ml of hot agar is overlaid, and a 0.125-inch (3 mm) Plexiglas matrix with a 17-7 well pattern (L. L. Pellet Co., Dallas, Tex.) is immediately placed in the liquid agar to eliminate bubbles. Excess agar is removed from the wells down to the first layer with a spatula. Reference serum is placed in the top and bottom wells of each system, and unknown sera are placed in the lateral wells. Histoplasmin is added to the center wells, and the reactants are incubated in a moist chamber for 24 h at 25 C. After incubation, the matrix is removed and agar is overlaid with distilled water and examined for lines of identity with reference sera.

Another useful test is the LA test. Commercially prepared antigen, in the form of histoplasmin-sensitized latex particles, is available. When the test is performed, serial twofold dilutions of sera ranging from 1:4 to 1:512 are prepared in tubes, and optimally diluted antigen is added. The tubes are shaken, incubated for 2 h in a water bath at 37 C, and refrigerated overnight. The centrifuged reactants are then examined for strong agglutination (2, 28).

The test yields results in 24 h and may even be used with anticomplementary sera. Although the test may be negative with sera from persons with chronic histoplasmosis, it is considered an excellent aid in the diagnosis of acute histoplasmosis (2). However, because of the transitory nature of these agglutinins, the latex test cannot be considered a replacement for the CF test, especially with the intact yeast-form antigens (28).

Hill and Campbell (28) considered a latex agglutinin titer of 1:16 or greater to be significant, whereas Bennett (2) considered titers of 1:32 or greater strong evidence for active or very recent disease. A positive LA test should be confirmed by a CF test.

Recent investigations indicate that levels of CF antibodies, precipitins, and agglutinins to *H. capsulatum* antigens may be significantly increased in histoplasmin-sensitized individuals after a single histoplasmin skin test (3, 10, 58, 61). This provocation of antibody makes subsequent changes in CF titers uninterpretable. For this reason, patients with suspected active histoplasmosis should not be skin-tested. A comprehensive study by Kaufman et al. (53) confirmed the antibody-inducing action of the skin test. For the most part, these antibody responses were detected in serum specimens drawn 15 days after skin testing. Although it is preferable that blood be drawn for serological studies prior to skin testing, it is apparent that the patient can be bled within 2 or 3 days after the skin test without antibody induction. Furthermore, one must bear in mind that it is the serum reaction with the histoplasmin antigen which is affected, although effects on the yeast titer have also been reported (58). A single histoplasmin skin test produced no serological response in nonsensitized individuals.

The fluorescent-antibody (FA) inhibition test has been shown to be a simple and effective means for the rapid detection of antibody against whole yeast cells of *H. capsulatum*. However, the test is ineffectual for the detection of antibody to histoplasmin (52). The FA inhibition and agar-gel precipitin tests (48) may help provide rapid diagnosis in cases where sera are anticomplementary.

Paracoccidioidomycosis

CF and ID tests are useful in diagnosing paracoccidioidomycosis and in following the response to treatment (16, 70, 71). LBCF tests with pooled filtrate antigens of the yeast form of *Paracoccidioides brasiliensis* indicate that the paracoccidioidomycosis CF test, like other fungus CF tests, is subject to cross-reactions. These cross-reactions, however, are infrequent and occur mainly at the 1:8 level. The ID tests with the same antigen (70) used with reference sera are entirely specific (43). An initial serodiagnosis of paracoccidioidomycosis can be obtained in over 95% of the cases by the concomitant use of the ID and CF tests (71, 72).

Sporotrichosis

Serological tests can be used in establishing a diagnosis of sporotrichosis. These tests are especially helpful in the diagnosis of the extracutaneous or systemic form of sporotrichosis, where distinct clinical features are lacking. Two tests, the tube agglutination (TA) and LA tests, are reliable and sensitive. Comparable sensitivity is not obtained in CF and ID tests with *Sporothrix schenckii* antigens. The slide LA test is preferred because it is highly sensitive and specific. It is easy to perform and provides results in minutes (8). The slide LA test is performed by adding 0.04 ml of inactivated (56 C, 30 min) serum to 0.02 ml of latex particles sensitized with culture filtrate antigens from the yeast form of *S. schenckii*. The reactants are mixed by rotating the reactants at 150 rpm for 5 min. Sera demonstrating 2+ agglutination or greater at dilutions of 1:4 or more are considered positive in the LA test.

The TA test is performed essentially as reported by Norden (62) except that 0.85% NaCl containing Merthiolate (1:10,000) is used as the diluent and the initial dilution of serum is 1:8.

IN VITRO AND IN VIVO IDENTIFICATION OF FUNGI BY FLUORESCENT-ANTIBODY TECHNIQUES

FA procedures provide mycologists with a valuable adjunct to conventional diagnostic tests. In addition to enabling the rapid gathering of presumptive diagnostic data, they also permit the rapid screening of clinical material designated for isolation and cultural studies. Above all, with fungus cultures these procedures permit rapid identification which by ordinary procedures might take 2 weeks or longer. The technique may be applied to viable and nonviable fungi in culture as well as to clinical materials or tissue sections.

It is my experience that a combination of a 5113 Corning glass primary filter, 3 mm in thickness, and a Wratten 2A secondary filter, 2 mm in thickness, is satisfactory for use with the fungi. Some workers use a BG-12 3-mm-thick primary filter with the secondary filter. Recent studies indicate that an American Optical interference exciter filter used in combination with a Schott GG-9 ocular filter gives excellent results with FA-stained fungi (68). The following information pertains to those FA procedures that have been developed to a practical level.

Actinomyces species and related organisms

Immunofluorescence procedures readily permit the detection and identification of the principal etiological agents of actinomycosis in man. FA reagents have been produced for the specific staining of the serotypes of *A. israelii*, *A. naeslundii*, and *Arachnia* (*Actinomyces*) *propionica* either in smears of tissue and exudates or in culture (4, 17, 55).

Blastomyces dermatitidis

Specific FA preparations for *B. dermatitidis* have been developed (38) by adsorbing rabbit antiyeast-form *B. dermatitidis* labeled antiglobulins with yeast-form cells of *H. capsulatum* and *Geotrichum candidum*. These yeast-form-specific conjugates enable the rapid and accurate detection of *B. dermatitidis* in culture and in clinical materials. FA techniques still cannot be used to identify the mycelial form of this fungus.

Candida species

Numerous studies have been performed on the application of the FA technique to the detection and identification of *C. albicans* and other *Candida* species. All revealed that the *Candida* species are closely related antigenically. Attempts to isolate species-specific FA preparations useful for the definitive identification of *C. albicans* in clinical materials and cultures have failed. To date, no single specific reagent is available for use in the clinical laboratory. Some workers have reported the successful use of a combination of reagents to identify *Candida* cultures (19, 21, 37). In spite of the lack of species-specific FA reagents, some reagents which demonstrate broad intrageneric cross-staining qualities can be used for screening clinical specimens for the presence of *Candida* sp. (34).

Coccidioides immitis

FA reagents specific for the tissue form of *C. immitis* have been developed (35). Such conjugates have been produced from antisera of rabbits infected with viable *C. immitis* cultures. These reagents generally stain the walls of endospores and the contents of spherules. Cross-staining of heterologous fungal antigens by these conjugates is eliminated by dilution or adsorption with yeast-form cells of *H. capsulatum*. Alternatively, specific conjugates can be prepared from antisera of rabbits immunized with suspensions of Formalin-killed arthrospores of *C. immitis*. Cross-staining can be eliminated by adsorption with yeast-form cells of *H. capsulatum*.

The specific conjugates are used for the detection of *C. immitis* in a variety of specimens from human and animal cases of coccidioidomycosis. They can be used in the diagnostic laboratory for the rapid and specific demonstration of the tissue form of *C. immitis* in clinical materials from laboratory animals injected with *C. immitis* cultures.

Cryptococcus neoformans

Eveland et al. (15) successfully used unadsorbed *C. neoformans* conjugates to study the distribution of *C. neoformans* and its polysaccharide products in Formalin-fixed tissue. Similarly, Marshall et al. (59) stained histopathological sections from human cases of cryptococcosis with Mayer's mucicarmine stain and FA preparations. They observed that the conjugate, although nonspecific for *C. neoformans*, stained the yeast cells more intensely and rapidly than did mucicarmine. An effective and practical diagnostic FA reagent of higher specificity is produced by the adsorption of *C. neoformans* conjugate with cells of *C. diffluens* and *Candida krusei* (66).

Histoplasma capsulatum

A specific FA reagent for *H. capsulatum* is produced by adsorbing conjugated homologous antiglobulins with cells of *B. dermatitidis* (50). This conjugate is used to identify yeast-form cells of *H. capsulatum* in culture and in impression smears made from tissues from humans with histoplasmosis and from experimentally infected mice. Several workers have investigated the applicability of FA reagents to the rapid detection of *H. capsulatum* in human clinical specimens (11, 57). The direct FA procedure has been recommended as a rapid screening procedure for *H. capsulatum* and for staining of sputum smears as an adjunct to conventional cultural criteria.

Investigations have demonstrated the existence of five *H. capsulatum* serotypes (45). Of these serotypes, only one, the 1:4 type, consistently failed to react with the available FA reagent. Recent studies indicate this serotype to be closely related to *H. capsulatum* var. *duboisii* and *B. dermatitidis*. A diagnostically useful polyvalent reagent has been developed (46) for detection and identification of *H. capsulatum* regardless of serotype. Adsorption of labeled antibodies produced against the most complete *H. capsulatum* serotype (1:2:3:4) with cells of *C. albicans* yielded a reagent that intensely stained only *H. capsulatum*, *H. capsulatum* var. *duboisii*, and *B. dermatitidis*. Despite its cross-staining, the *C. albicans*-adsorbed reagent can be used diagnostically. This is accomplished through the use of the *B. dermatitidis*-specific FA reagent in conjunction with the polyvalent conjugate. Both of these FA reagents stain isolates of *B. dermatitidis*, whereas only the polyvalent conjugate stains *H. capsulatum*. *H. capsulatum* and *H. capsulatum* var. *duboisii* cannot, thus far, be differentiated from each other by use of FA reagents.

Paracoccidioides brasiliensis

FA reagents for the diagnosis of paracoccidioidomycosis have been developed (76). Tissue-form specific reagents are produced from antisera of rabbits immunized with suspensions of Formalin-killed yeast-form cells of *P. brasiliensis*. Cross-reactions are eliminated by multiple adsorptions with selected heterologous organisms. These reagents are used in the direct FA procedure for the demonstration of *P. brasiliensis* cells in smears of clinical materials. These conjugates are especially useful in clinical materials in which *P. brasiliensis* cells are few and when morphologically typical cells are not present.

Sporothrix schenckii

Good quality reagents for the detection of the tissue form of *S. schenckii* both in clinical materials and in culture have been developed (36). Such reagents are produced from antiserum obtained by immunizing rabbits with suspensions of whole, Formalin-killed yeast cells of *S. schenckii*. Cross-reactions are readily eliminated by dilution without compromising staining qualities. Although, as a rule, few *S. schenckii* cells are found in lesion exudates, they are usually readily observed with the FA tests. In a few cases, particularly after therapy has been initiated, diligent search of a number of fields may be required before the fungi are found.

Comments on the application of fluorescent-antibody reagents to clinical materials

The FA technique is most effective for detecting fungus antigens in cultures, pus, exudates, blood, tissue impression smears, and spinal fluid specimens. It is, however, more difficult to use with sputum and tissue sections. Not only does one have to cope with tissue elements that autofluoresce, but for some reason the staining capacity of the conjugate is impaired in sputa and tissue sections. This impairment may be due to lack of surface interaction between antigen and antibody, as shown by the fact that enzymatic and chemical digestion of sputum specimens enables more effective staining of fungus elements (57, 69, 75). Such treatment may also be applied to tissue sections (39). In those instances when the FA procedure has been successfully applied to tissue sections, it has been noted that fungus elements are stained more intensely in sections cut to a thickness of 4 μm than they are in thicker preparations (40). It is also suggested that glass slides 1 mm or less in thickness be used.

Direct FA staining permits the rapid detection of fungi in paraffin sections of Formalin-fixed tissue. In addition, one can also identify fungi in tissue sections which were previously stained with hematoxylin and eosin, the Brown and Brenn, and the Giemsa stains. The conjugates, however, will not stain fungi in tissues that have been stained previously by the Gomori methenamine-silver nitrate, the periodic acid-Schiff, or the Gridley procedure (39).

Prolonged storage of Formalin-fixed tissues, either wet or in paraffin blocks, does not appear to have adverse effects on the antigens of fungi contained therein. Therefore the FA procedure may also be used in making a retrospective immunohistological diagnosis. It is also interesting to note that, although fluorescein-labeled *H. capsulatum* antiglobulins regularly stain *H. capsulatum* in sections of fixed tissue with active histoplasmosis, they do not regularly stain *H. capsulatum* in healed calcified lesions (29).

LITERATURE CITED

1. Abernathy, R. S., and D. C. Heiner. 1961. Precipitation reactions in agar in North American blastomycosis. J. Lab. Clin. Med. **57**:604–611.
2. Bennett, D. E. 1966. The histoplasmin latex agglutination test. Clinical evaluation and a review of the literature. Amer. J. Med. Sci. **251**:175–183.
3. Bennett, D. E. 1966. Laboratory diagnosis of histoplasmosis: a review. S. Med. J. **59**:922–926.
4. Blank, C. F., and L. K. Georg. 1968. The use of fluorescent antibody methods for the detection and identification of *Actinomyces* species in clinical material. J. Lab. Clin. Med. **71**:283–293.
5. Bloomfield, N., M. A. Gordon, and D. F. Elmendorf, Jr. 1961. Detection of *Cryptococcus neoformans* antigen in body fluids by latex particle agglutination. Proc. Soc. Exp. Biol. Med. **114**:64–67.
6. Busey, J. F., and P. F. Hinton. 1965. Precipitins in histoplasmosis. Amer. Rev. Resp. Dis. **92**:637–639.
7. Busey, J. F., and P. F. Hinton. 1967. Precipitins in blastomycosis. Amer. Rev. Resp. Dis. **95**:112–113.
8. Blumer, S. O., L. Kaufman, W. Kaplan, D. W. McLaughlin, and D. E. Kraft. 1973. Comparative evaluation of

five serological methods for the diagnosis of sporotrichosis. Appl. Microbiol. **26**:4–8.
9. Campbell, C. C. 1967. Serology in the respiratory mycoses. Sabouraudia **5**:240–259.
10. Campbell, C. C., and G. B. Hill. 1964. Further studies on the development of complement-fixing antibodies and precipitins in healthy histoplasmin sensitive persons following a single histoplasmin skin test. Amer. Rev. Resp. Dis. **90**:927–934.
11. Carski, T. R., G. C. Cozad, and H. W. Larsh. 1962. Detection of *Histoplasma capsulatum* in sputum by means of fluorescent antibody staining. Amer. J. Clin. Pathol. **37**:465–469.
12. Coleman, R. M., and L. Kaufman. 1972. Use of the immunodiffusion test in the serodiagnosis of aspergillosis. Appl. Microbiol. **23**:301–309.
13. Drouhet, E., G. Segretain, G. Pesle, and L. Bidet. 1963. Etude des precipitins seriques en milieu gelose pour le diagnostic des aspergilloses bronchopulmonaires. Ann. Inst. Pasteur Paris **105**:597–604.
14. English, M. P., and A. H. Henderson. 1967. Significance and interpretation of laboratory tests in pulmonary aspergillosis. J. Clin. Pathol. **20**:832–834.
15. Eveland, W. C., J. D. Marshall, A. M. Silverstein, F. B. Johnson, L. Iverson, and D. J. Winslow. 1957. Specific immunochemical staining of *Cryptococcus neoformans* and its polysaccharide in tissue. Amer. J. Pathol. **33**:616–617.
16. Fava Netto, C. 1965. The immunology of South-American blastomycosis. Mycopathologia **26**:349–358.
17. Gerencser, M. A., and J. M. Slack. 1967. Isolation and characterization of *Actinomyces propionicus*. J. Bacteriol. **94**:109–115.
18. Goodman, J. S., L. Kaufman, and M. G. Koenig. 1971. Diagnosis of cryptococcal meningitis. Value of immunologic detection of cryptococcal antigen. N. Engl. J. Med. **285**:434–436.
19. Gordon, M. A. 1962. Differentiation and classification of yeasts by the Coons fluorescent antibody technique, p. 207–219. *In* G. Dalldorf (ed.), Fungi and fungous diseases. Charles C Thomas, Publisher, Springfield. Ill.
20. Gordon, M. A., R. E. Almy, C. H. Greene, and J. W. Fenton. 1971. Diagnostic mycoserology by immunoelectroosmophoresis: a general, rapid, and sensitive microtechnic. Amer. J. Clin. Pathol. **56**:471–474.
21. Gordon, M. A., J. C. Elliott, and T. W. Hawkins. 1967. Identification of *Candida albicans*, other *Candida* species and *Torulopsis glabrata* by means of immunofluorescence. Sabouraudia **5**:323–329.
22. Gordon, M. A., and E. Lapa. 1971. Charcoal particle agglutination test for detection of antibody to *Cryptococcus neoformans:* a preliminary report. J. Lab. Clin. Pathol. **56**:354–359.
23. Gordon, M. A., and D. K. Vedder. 1966. Serologic tests in diagnosis and prognosis of cryptococcosis. J. Amer. Med. Ass. **197**:961–967.
24. Harrell, W. K., H. Ashworth, L. E. Britt, J. R. George, S. B. Gray, J. H. Green, H. Gross, and J. E. Johnson. 1970. Procedural manual for production of bacterial, fungal, and parasitic reagents. Biological Reagents Section, Center for Disease Control, Atlanta, Ga.
25. Heiner, D. C. 1958. Diagnosis of histoplasmosis using precipitin reactions in agar gel. Pediatrics **22**:616–627.
26. Henderson, A. H., M. P. English, and G. Stewart-Smith. 1967. Fungal infections. Lancet **1**:502.
27. Hill, G. B., and C. C. Campbell. 1956. A further evaluation of histoplasmin and yeast phase antigens of *Histoplasma capsulatum* in the complement fixation test. J. Lab. Clin. Med. **48**:255–263.
28. Hill, G. B., and C. C. Campbell. 1962. Commercially available histoplasmin sensitized latex particles in an agglutination test for histoplasmosis. Mycopathol. Mycol. Appl. **18**:169–176.
29. Hotchi, M., J. Schwarz, and W. Kaplan. 1972. Limitations of fluorescent antibody staining of *Histoplasma capsulatum* in tissue sections. Sabouraudia **10**:157–163.
30. Huppert, M., and J. W. Bailey. 1963. Immunodiffusion as a screening test for coccidioidomycosis serology. Sabouraudia **2**:284–291.
31. Huppert, M., and J. W. Bailey. 1965. The use of immunodiffusion tests in coccidioidomycosis. Amer. J. Clin. Pathol. **44**:364–368.
32. Huppert, M., and J. W. Bailey. 1965. The use of immunodiffusion tests in coccidioidomycosis. Amer. J. Clin. Pathol. **44**:369–373.
33. Huppert, M., E. T. Peterson, S. H. Sun, P. Chitjian, and W. Derrevere. 1968. Evaluation of a latex particle agglutination test for coccidioidomycosis. Amer. J. Clin. Pathol. **49**:96–102.
34. Kaplan, W. 1973. Direct fluorescent antibody tests for the diagnosis of mycotic diseases. Ann. Clin. Lab. Sci. **3**:25–29.
35. Kaplan, W., and M. K. Clifford. 1964. Production of fluorescent antibody reagents specific for the tissue form of *Coccidioides immitis*. Amer. Rev. Resp. Dis. **89**:651–658.
36. Kaplan, W., and M. S. Ivens. 1960. Fluorescent antibody staining of *Sporotrichum schenckii* in cultures and clinical materials. J. Invest. Dermatol. **35**:151–159.
37. Kaplan, W., and L. Kaufman. 1961. The application of fluorescent antibody techniques to medical mycology—a review. Sabouraudia **1**:137–144.
38. Kaplan, W., and L. Kaufman. 1963. Specific fluorescent antiglobulins for the detection and identification of *Blastomyces dermatitidis* yeast-phase cells. Mycopathol. Mycol. Appl. **19**:173–180.
39. Kaplan, W., and D. E. Kraft. 1969. Demonstration of pathogenic fungi in formalin-fixed tissues by immunofluorescence. Amer. J. Clin. Pathol. **52**:420–437.
40. Kaufman, L. 1965. The application of fluorescent antibody techniques for the detection and identification of mycotic disease agents. Mycopathol. Mycol. Appl. **26**:257–263.
41. Kaufman, L. 1966. Serology of systemic fungus diseases. Pub. Health Rep. **81**:177–185.
42. Kaufman, L. 1970. Serology: its value in the diagnosis of coccidioidomycosis, cryptococcosis, and histoplasmosis. Proc. Int. Symp. Mycoses. Sci. Publ. Pan-Amer. Health Organ. No. 205, p. 96–100.
43. Kaufman, L. 1972. Evaluation of serological tests for paracoccidioidomycosis: preliminary report. Proc. Pan. Amer. Symp. Paracoccidioidomycosis. Sci. Publ. Pan-Amer. Health Organ. No. 254, p. 221–223.
44. Kaufman, L. 1973. Value of immunodiffusion tests in the diagnosis of systemic mycotic diseases. Ann. Clin. Lab. Sci. **3**:141–146.
45. Kaufman, L., and S. Blumer. 1966. Occurrence of serotypes among *Histoplasma capsulatum* strains. J. Bacteriol. **91**:1434–1439.
46. Kaufman, L., and S. Blumer. 1968. Development and use of a polyvalent conjugate to differentiate *Histoplasma capsulatum* and *Histoplasma duboisii* from other pathogens. J. Bacteriol. **95**:1243–1246.
47. Kaufman, L., and S. Blumer. 1968. Value and interpretation of serological tests for the diagnosis of cryptococcosis. Appl. Microbiol. **16**:1907–1912.
48. Kaufman, L., B. Brandt, and D. McLaughlin. 1964. Evaluation of the fluorescent antibody and agar gel

precipitin tests for detecting *Histoplasma* antibodies in anticomplementary sera. Amer. J. Hyg. **79**:181–185.

49. Kaufman, L., E. C. Hall, M. J. Clark, and D. McLaughlin. 1970. Comparison of macrocomplement and microcomplement fixation techniques used in fungus serology. Appl. Microbiol. **20**:579–582.
50. Kaufman, L., and W. Kaplan. 1961. Preparation of a fluorescent antibody specific for the yeast phase of *Histoplasma capsulatum*. J. Bacteriol. **82**:729–735.
51. Kaufman, L., D. W. McLaughlin, M. J. Clark, and S. Blumer. 1973. Specific immunodiffusion test for blastomycosis. Appl. Microbiol. **26**:244–247.
52. Kaufman, L., J. H. Schubert, and W. Kaplan. 1962. Fluorescent antibody inhibition test for histoplasmosis. J. Lab. Clin. Med. **58**:1033–1038.
53. Kaufman, L., R. T. Terry, J. H. Schubert, and D. McLaughlin. 1967. Effects of a single histoplasmin skin test on the serological diagnosis of histoplasmosis. J. Bacteriol. **94**:798–803.
54. Kleger, B., and L. Kaufman. 1973. Detection and identification of diagnostic *Histoplasma capsulatum* precipitates by counterelectrophoresis. Appl. Microbiol. **26**:231–238.
55. Lambert, F. W., J. M. Brown, and L. K. Georg. 1967. Identification of *Actinomyces israelii* and *Actinomyces naeslundii* by fluorescent-antibody and agar-gel diffusion techniques. J. Bacteriol. **94**:1287–1295.
56. Longbottom, J. L., and J. Pepys. 1964. Pulmonary aspergillosis: diagnostic and immunological significances of antigens and C-substance in *Aspergillus fumigatus*. J. Pathol. Bacteriol. **88**:141–151.
57. Lynch, H. J., and K. L. Plexico. 1962. A rapid method for screening sputums for *Histoplasma capsulatum* employing the fluorescent-antibody technic. N. Engl. J. Med. **28**:811–814.
58. McDearman, S. C., and J. M. Young. 1960. The development of positive serologic tests with *Histoplasma capsulatum* antigens following single histoplasmin skin tests. Amer. J. Clin. Pathol. **34**:434–438.
59. Marshall, J. D., L. Iverson, W. C. Eveland, and A. Kase. 1961. Application and limitations of the fluorescent antibody stain in the specific diagnosis of cryptococcosis. Lab. Invest. **10**:719–728.
60. Murray, I. G., 1966. Aspergillosis. Lancet **1**:1373.
61. Nicholas, W. M., J. A. Wier, L. R. Kuhn, C. C. Campbell, L. B. Nolte, and G. B. Hill. 1961. Serologic effects of histoplasmin skin testing. Amer. Rev. Resp. Dis. **83**:276–279.
62. Norden, A. 1951. Sporotrichosis: clinical and laboratory features and a serologic study in experimental animals and humans. Acta Pathol. Microbiol. Scand. (Suppl.) **89**:1–119.
63. Pappagianis, D., C. E. Smith, G. S. Kobayshi, and M. T. Saito. 1961. Studies of antigens from young mycelia of *Coccidioides immitis*. J. Infect. Dis. **108**:35–44.
64. Parker, J. D., G. A. Sarosi, I. L. Doto, and F. E. Tosh. 1970. Pulmonary aspergillosis in the South Central United States. Amer. Rev. Resp. Dis. **101**:551–557.
65. Pepys, J. 1969. Hypersensitivity diseases of lungs due to fungi and organic dusts. Monogr. Allergy **4**:21.
66. Pepys, J., R. W. Riddell, K. M. Citron, Y. M. Clayton, and E. I. Short. 1959. Clinical and immunological significance of *Aspergillus fumigatus* in the sputum. Amer. Rev. Resp. Dis. **80**:167–180.
67. Pidcoe, V., and L. Kaufman. 1968. Fluorescent-antibody reagent for the identification of *Cryptococcus neoformans*. Appl. Microbiol. **16**:271–275.
68. Preisler, H. D., H. F. Hasenclever, A. A. Levitan, and E. S. Henderson. 1969. Serologic diagnosis of disseminated candidiasis in patients with acute leukemia. Ann. Intern. Med. **70**:19–30.
69. Reep, B. R., and W. Kaplan. 1972. The use of n-acetyl-1-cysteine and dithiothreitol to process sputa for mycological and fluorescent antibody examinations. Health Lab. Sci. **9**:118–124.
70. Restrepo, M. A., 1966. La prueba de immunodiffusion en el diagnostic de la paracoccidioidomycosis. Sabouraudia **4**:223–230.
71. Restrepo, M. A. 1967. Comportamiento immunologico de zo pacientes con paracoccidioidomycosis. Antioquia Med. **17**:219–230.
72. Restrepo, M. A., and L. H. Moncada F. 1970. Serologic procedures in the diagnosis of paracoccidioidomycosis. Proc. Int. Symp. Mycoses. Sci. Publ. Pan-Amer. Health Organ. No. 205, p. 101–110.
73. Schubert, J. H., and L. Ajello. 1957. Variation in complement fixation antigenicity of different yeast phase strains of *Histoplasma capsulatum*. J. Lab. Clin. Med. **50**:304–307.
74. Schubert, J. H., H. L. Lynch, and L. Ajello. 1961. Evaluation of the agar-plate precipitin test for histoplasmin. Amer. Rev. Resp. Dis. **84**:845–849.
75. Shamiyeh, B., and E. L. Shipe. 1964. Chlorox digestion of sputum for detection of *Histoplasma capsulatum* yeast cells by fluorescent antibody techniques. Pub. Health Lab. **22**:198–199.
76. Silva, M. E., and W. Kaplan. 1965. Specific fluorescein-labeled antiglobulin for the yeast form of *Paracoccidioides brasiliensis*. Amer. J. Trop. Med. Hyg. **14**:290–294.
77. Smith, C. E., M. T. Saito, R. R. Beard, R. McF. Kepp, R. W. Clark, and B. U. Eddie. 1950. Serological tests in the diagnosis and prognosis coccidioidomycosis. Amer. J. Hyg. **52**:1–21.
78. Smith, C. E., E. G. Whiting, E. E. Baker, H. G. Rosenberger, R. R. Beard, and M. T. Saito. 1948. The use of coccidioidin. Amer. Rev. Tuberc. **57**:330–360.
79. Stallybrass, F. C. 1963. The precipitin test in human systemic aspergillosis. Mycopathol. Mycol. Appl. **21**:272–278.
80. Stallybrass, F. C. 1964. *Candida* precipitins. J. Pathol. Bacteriol. **87**:89–97.
81. Stickle, D., L. Kaufman, S. O. Blumer, and D. McLaughlin. 1972. Comparison of a newly developed latex agglutination test and an immunodiffusion test in the diagnosis of systemic candidiasis. Appl. Microbiol. **23**:490–499.
82. Taschdjian, C. L., G. B. Dobkin, L. Caroline, and P. J. Kozinn. 1964. Immune studies relating to candidiasis. Paper II. Sabouraudia **3**:129–139.
83. Taschdjian, C. L., P. J. Kozinn, and L. Caroline. 1964. Immune studies in candidiasis. Paper III. Sabouraudia **3**:312–320.
84. Taschdjian, C. L., P. J. Kozinn, A. Okas, L. Caroline, and M. A. Halle. 1967. Serodiagnosis of systemic candidiasis. **117**:180–187.
85. U.S. Public Health Service. 1965. Standardized diagnostic complement fixation method and adaption to micro test. U.S. Pub. Health Serv. Publ. No. 1228.
86. Vogel, R. A. 1966. The indirect fluorescent antibody test for the detection of antibody in human cryptococcal disease. J. Infect. Dis. **116**:575–580.
87. Vogel, R. A., and J. F. Padula. 1958. Indirect staining reaction with fluorescent antibody for detection of antibodies to pathogenic fungi. Proc. Soc. Exp. Biol. Med. **98**:135–139.
88. Vogel, R. A., T. F. Sellers, and P. Woodward. 1961. Fluorescent antibody techniques applied to the study

of human cryptococcosis. J. Amer. Med. Ass. **178**:921–923.

89. Wallraff, E. B., R. M. Van Liew, and S. Waite. 1967. Skin reactivity and serological response to coccidioidin skin tests. J. Invest. Dermatol. **48**:553–559.
90. Walter, J. E., and K. D. Jones. 1968. Serologic tests in diagnosis of aspergillosis. Dis. Chest **53**:729–735.
91. Wiggins, G. L., and J. H. Schubert. 1965. Relationship of histoplasmin agar-gel bands and complement-fixation titers in histoplasmosis. J. Bacteriol. **89**:589–596.
92. Young, R. C., and J. E. Bennett. 1971. Invasive aspergillosis—absence of detectable antibody response. Amer. Rev. Resp. Dis. **104**:710–716.

Chapter 63

Susceptibility Testing of Antifungal Agents

SMITH SHADOMY AND ANA ESPINEL-INGROFF

Susceptibility testing with antifungal antimicrobials is basically the same as with antibacterial agents. With both, the purpose of such testing is to define those minimal amounts of drug which will either inhibit the growth of a microorganism or destroy it in vitro. Although experimental design is similar in testing with both types of antimicrobials, there are certain differences which make testing with antifungal compounds somewhat more difficult. Of primary importance among these differences are, first, the basic properties of the compounds to be tested and, second, the growth characteristics of some of the organisms involved.

Three chemotherapeutic agents are now available in the United States for treatment of serious or systemic mycotic infections in man: amphotericin B, nystatin, and 5-fluorocytosine (5-FC). The first of these agents, amphotericin B, is a polyene compound and is used primarily for the treatment of life-threatening fungal infections including blastomycosis, disseminated coccidioidomycosis, disseminated and chronic cavitary histoplasmosis, cryptococcosis, and various forms of candidosis or other opportunistic fungal infections (8). It is administered most commonly by intravenous infusion, although other routes such as intrathecal infusion, topical application, and bladder infusion may be employed.

Nystatin, also a polyene compound, is used primarily in the treatment of nonsystemic *Candida* infections (8). As such, it is administered only orally or topically. Oral administration, as used in the treatment of intestinal candidosis, does not lead to significant serum levels of the drug since absorption of nystatin from the gastrointestinal tract of man is minimal in most instances (2).

The chemical properties of both amphotericin B and nystatin present certain problems relative to in vitro susceptibility testing. Both are light-sensitive and subject to thermal decay upon incubation. Both are water-insoluble and unstable in the presence of acid. Accordingly, certain requirements exist for the preparation of solutions of these drugs for testing as well as for the conditions under which they are tested.

5-FC is a water-soluble, stable, oral antifungal compound employed primarily in the treatment of systemic infections caused by pathogenic or opportunistic yeasts (6). It acts as a competitive antimetabolite for uracil in the synthesis of yeast ribonucleic acid (3) and can be antagonized in vitro by a variety of purine and pyrimidine bases and nucleosides (5). Because of this, the antifungal activity of 5-FC can be measured only in synthetic media.

In vitro testing with 5-FC is more critical clinically than testing with the polyene compounds because of the repeated demonstration of the development of resistant strains of yeasts after exposure to the drug (4). Two metabolic sites appear to be responsible for this resistance (5): the first, the enzyme cytosine permease, is responsible for the uptake of 5-FC, and the second, the enzyme cytosine deaminase, is responsible for deamination of 5-FC to 5-fluorouracil, which then competes with uracil in the synthesis of ribonucleic acid. Fortunately, similar resistance to the polyenes does not occur commonly in vivo, although it can be induced in vitro.

When one is testing with antibacterial agents, in vitro test conditions are simplified by the fact that most bacterial isolates will produce visible growth in broth or on agar within 18 to 24 h, and also by the fact that only one phase of growth is involved. Unfortunately, such is not the case when testing with antifungal compounds, particularly with amphotericin B.

Testing with antifungal compounds is also complicated by selection of conditions for incubation. Although this need not be a problem with rapidly growing yeasts, it is of importance with the slower growing filamentous and dimorphic fungi. The lack of thermal stability of amphotericin B and nystatin is of major concern in this regard. Thus, when testing with polyenes against filamentous or dimorphic organisms, it may be necessary to select a lower temperature such as 30 C and to test with the hyphal phase, rather than testing with the yeast phase at 37 C, to avoid excessive drug inactivation.

The methods available for testing with antifungal compounds are limited. The most suitable ones include broth and semisolid agar dilution procedures. Testing with the agar dilution method is not practical in the clinical laboratory. Representative data for amphotericin B and 5-FC obtained with the broth and semisolid agar dilution procedures to be described here are presented in Table 1.

Diffusion disks are not available in this country for in vitro testing with any of the three agents, although studies are underway to per-

TABLE 1. *Inhibitory and fungicidal activity of amphotericin B and 5-fluorocytosine against pathogenic fungi*[a]

Organism	Amphotericin B[b]			5-Fluorocytosine[b]		
	MIC (μg/ml)	MFC (μg/ml)	Resistance	MIC (μg/ml)	MFC (μg/ml)	Resistance
Pathogenic yeasts						
Cryptococcus neoformans	0.05–0.78 (0.39)	0.10–12.5 (1.3)	Resistance rare	0.10–50 (8.7)	0.39–>100 (22.3)	Resistance uncommon in pretreatment isolates (<3.0%) but common in isolates from inadequately treated patients
Candida albicans	0.20–0.78 (0.54)	0.39–0.78 (0.88)	Resistance rare	0.05–12.5 (0.95)	0.10–>100 (9.8)	Resistance common (ca. 40%), induced resistance rare
Candida parapsilosis	0.39–0.78 (0.52)	0.78–3.13 (2.3)	Resistance not known	0.20–3.13 (1.1)	Generally >100	Resistance common (ca. 50%), induced resistance rare
Candida tropicalis	0.20–1.56	0.39–6.25	Resistance not known	0.10–50 (5.6)	0.20–50 (18.3)	Resistance common (27%)
Torulopsis glabrata	0.10–0.39	0.20–0.78	Resistance not known	0.20–1.56	0.39–1.56	Resistance uncommon (<10%)
Trichosporon sp.	0.78–3.13	1.56–3.13	Resistance not known	25–100	>100	Resistance not known
Geotrichum sp.	0.39–1.56	0.78–3.13	Resistance not known	1.56–12.5	25–>100	Resistance not known
Filamentous fungi[c]						
Allescheria boydii	6.25–>100	>100	Susceptible but not at clinically significant concentrations	Resistant		
Aspergillus fumigatus	0.39–1.56 (1.0)	12.5–25 (7.2)	Resistance rare but MICs in excess of achievable serum levels common	0.20–1.56 (1.9)	>100	Resistance common (ca. 25%)
Aspergillus sp.	0.05–8.0 (1.4)	6.25–>100 (12.6)	Resistance rare	0.20–1.56 (0.8)	>100	Resistance common
Blastomyces dermatitidis	0.05–0.20 (0.18)	0.10–0.39 (0.25)	Resistance not known	Resistant		

TABLE 1.—*Continued*

Organism	Amphotericin B[b]			5-Fluorocytosine[b]		
	MIC (μg/ml)	MFC (μg/ml)	Resistance	MIC (μg/ml)	MFC (μg/ml)	Resistance
Cladosporium trichoides	3.13->100	3.13->100		3.13–12.5	12.5->100	
Coccidioides immitis	0.20–0.78	0.78–1.56	Resistance not known	Resistant		
Histoplasma capsulatum	0.05–0.10 (0.08)	0.05–0.20 (0.1)	Resistance not known	Resistant		
Mucor and *Rhizoous* sp.	0.78–1.56	1.56->100				
Phialophora and *Fonsecaea* sp.	0.05–0.10 (0.08)	6.25->100		Resistant		
Sporothrix schenckii	1.56–12.5	3.13->100		Resistant		

[a] Based on available clinical and research data collected at the Medical College of Virginia, Virginia Commonwealth University, Richmond.

[b] The expected ranges of minimal inhibitory and minimal fungicidal concentrations are shown; averages for more than 10 isolates tested are given in parentheses. Information on frequency of resistance is noted when sufficient data permit.

[c] Dimorphic organisms were generally tested in the mycelial phase.

mit application of the diffusion disk method to susceptibility testing with 5-FC.

BROTH DILUTION METHOD

The broth dilution method provides a quantitative in vitro assessment of the minimal inhibitory concentration (MIC) of a given antifungal agent for a specific microorganism. In addition, the test may be extended to provide an in vitro assessment of the minimal fungicidal concentration (MFC) of the compound. This procedure is employed primarily when testing yeasts or yeast-like organisms but can be adapted to testing with filamentous fungi.

Media

Selection of medium depends upon the drug being tested. Yeast nitrogen base (YNB, Difco) supplemented with glucose and asparagine is used in tests with 5-FC. This is most conveniently prepared as a 10× concentrate, sterilized by filtration, and stored at 4 C. A 1× solution is prepared by making a 1:10 dilution of the 10× concentrate in sterile distilled water. Tests with amphotericin B or nystatin are performed in Antibiotic Medium 20 (M-20, Difco). YNB is not suitable for testing with polyenes because of the low pH (<5.0) which develops as a result of fermentation or assimilation of glucose.

Drug solutions

A 10,000 μg/ml solution of standard 5-FC powder (Hoffmann-La Roche, Inc.) is prepared in distilled water and sterilized by filtration. This solution may be used indefinitely if uncontaminated and stored at −30 C. When testing with amphotericin B or nystatin (E. R. Squibb & Sons, Inc.), sufficient standard is weighed to prepare a 5,000 μg/ml solution. The actual amount to be weighed must be adjusted according to the biological activity of the specific standard. If standard amphotericin B is not available, Fungizone (amphotericin B for injection, E. R. Squibb & Sons, Inc.) may be substituted. A preparation of nystatin designed for use in viral tissue culture media is available and may be used if standard material is not available (Mycostatin suspension, 10,000 units/ml, Grand Island Biological Co.). Both amphotericin B and nystatin may be solubilized in dimethylsulfoxide (DMSO) or dimethylformamide. Solutions of these compounds must be protected from light and should be allowed to stand for 30 min before use to permit autosterilization. The 5,000 μg/ml solution may be used for 1 week if stored in the dark at 4 C.

Preparation of inocula

Inocula are prepared from 24- to 48-h-old cultures grown either on Sabouraud agar or in

YNB. Sabouraud broth cultures should not be used in tests with 5-FC because of possible antagonism. Suspensions are prepared in sterile saline and adjusted to a transmission of 95% measured at 530 nm (Bausch & Lomb Spectronic 20 colorimeter). An alternative method of preparing inocula employs the "Wickerham card technique." In this procedure, the suspension to be adjusted is diluted into a tube of sterile saline which is then placed against a white card bearing several sharply ruled lines. The desired end point is reached when there is obvious turbidity but the lines still are sharply defined when viewed through the suspension. A similar suspension also should be prepared for a control organism. Such controls may be selected from previously tested organisms but more appropriately would be selected from such organisms as *Saccharomyces cerevisiae* ATCC 9763, *S. cerevisiae* ATCC 2601, or *Candida tropicalis* ATCC 13803.

Drug dilutions and performance of the test

The following procedure gives sufficient material to test (in duplicate) one isolate and the appropriate control organism. Using either 1× YNB or M-20 as required, prepare 10 ml of a 100 μg/ml solution of the drug to be tested. In tests with 5-FC, a 1:100 dilution of the 10,000 μg/ml solution in 1× YNB is required; in tests with amphotericin B or nystatin, a 1:50 dilution of the 5,000 μg/ml solution in M-20 is required.

For the test, place 12 sterile, disposable tubes (16 by 125 mm) in a rack and add 5.0 ml of the appropriate broth medium to tubes 2 through 12. Add 5.0 ml of the 100 μg/ml solution of drug in broth to tubes 1 and 2. Mix the contents of tube 2 and then serially dilute the drug, using 5.0-ml volumes and fresh pipettes for each dilution, through the remaining 10 tubes, discarding 5 ml from the last tube. This will give a dilution serial ranging in concentration from 100 to 0.05 μg/ml. Transfer 1.0 ml from each dilution to each of four 12 by 75 mm sterile, disposable tubes. The remaining 1.0-ml volumes in the large tubes may be kept as controls for contamination of the serial dilution. Add 1 ml of drug-free broth to each of four additional sterile 12 by 75 mm tubes for use as growth controls.

A volumetric dilution system may be used to prepare the serial dilutions of drug. In this procedure, specified volumes of standard drug previously diluted into sterile broth are added to specified volumes of broth. Details of such a procedure are presented in Table 2.

Inoculate two tubes of each concentration of drug with 0.05 ml of a standardized suspension

TABLE 2. *Volumetric system for preparing serial dilutions of drugs in broth*

Volumes and concn of drug in broth[a]		To be added to indicated volumes of broth[a]	Final concn (μg/ml)
Volumes	Concn (μg/ml)		
4	100	—	100
2	100	2	50
1	100	3	25
1	100	7	12.5
2	12.5	2	6.25
1	12.5	3	3.13
1	12.5	7	1.56
2	1.56	2	0.78
1	1.56	3	0.39
0.5	1.56	3.5	0.20
0.25	1.56	3.75	0.10

[a] Either M-20 when testing with nystatin or amphotericin B or YNB when testing with 5-FC.

of the test organisms. Also inoculate two tubes of drug-free media for the growth controls. Incubate at 30 C for 48 h or until growth is visible in the growth control tubes. Tests with 5-FC should not be read in less than 48 h. Investigations both by us and by others have shown the time of incubation to be highly critical in susceptibility testing with 5-FC and *Candida* species (7) or *Cryptococcus neoformans* (1). Tests with nystatin and amphotericin B should be read as early as possible.

After incubation, the tubes are examined and the MIC is recorded. The MIC is defined as the lowest concentration of drug which inhibits visible growth. The MFC is determined by subculturing approximately 0.01 ml from each negative tube and from the growth control tubes onto Sabouraud agar with subsequent incubation at 30 C for 48 h or until growth of the subculture from the growth control tubes is apparent. The MFC is defined as the lowest concentration of drug from which subcultures were negative or which yielded fewer than three colonies.

Expected results

Most isolates of susceptible yeasts will be inhibited by 12.5 μg or less of 5-FC per ml and killed by 25 μg or less per ml (Table 1). Isolates of *C. neoformans* with intermediate susceptibilities (MIC of 25 or 50 μg/ml) as well as totally resistant isolates (MIC > 1,000 μg/ml) can be recovered from inadequately treated patients during treatment. Amphotericin B is both inhibitory and fungicidal for most yeasts at a concentration of 0.39 μg or less/ml (Table 1). An MIC of 1.56 μg/ml for amphotericin B suggests probable clinical resistance, as this exceeds concentrations routinely achievable in serum and cerebrospinal fluid. Nystatin is inhibitory and fungicidal for most isolates of *Candida* at concentrations of 3.13 μg or less/ml. However, prolonged incubation or incubation at 37 C may result in erroneously high MIC values because of thermal inactivation of the drug.

SEMISOLID AGAR DILUTION METHOD

The semisolid agar dilution method is applicable primarily for testing the susceptibility of filamentous fungi to amphotericin B and may be of value in testing isolates of *Aspergillus* species for susceptibility to 5-FC. It is not applicable to tests with nystatin. It can provide data regarding both minimal inhibitory and minimal fungicidal concentrations.

Media

Two media are required for testing with amphotericin B: an enriched brain heart infusion broth (BHIB, Difco) and modified SABHI agar medium (Difco). Tests with 5-FC require the 10× concentrate of supplemented YNB and sterile 0.5% agar.

Drug solutions

The stock solutions of 5-FC and amphotericin B used in the broth dilution procedure are also used in the semisolid agar dilution procedure.

Preparation of inocula

Sabouraud agar slants of mature sporulating fungi are washed with sterile saline containing 0.05% Tween 80. The resulting suspension of conidia and hyphae is then adjusted to a transmission of 85 to 90% as measured at 530 nm (Bausch & Lomb Spectronic 20 colorimeter). If desired, inocula can be prepared in Sabouraud broth rather than in saline and incubated overnight prior to use. This provides a suspension of germinated spores and vegetative cells rather than resting spores. Approximately 3.0 ml of inoculum is required for each test.

Susceptibility testing with amphotericin B

The following procedure provides sufficient material for testing one isolate and the appropriate control organism, in duplicate.

For the test, dilute 1.0 ml of the 10,000 μg/ml stock solution in 1.0 ml of DMSO; dilute the resulting 5,000 μg/ml solution 1:25 in modified BHIB to provide a solution containing 200 μg/ml. Place 12 sterile 16 by 125 mm disposable test tubes in a rack; add 5.0 ml of modified BHIB to tubes 2 through 12. Add 5.0 ml of the 200 μg/ml solution of amphotericin B in broth to tubes 1 and 2. Thoroughly mix tube 2, and then serially dilute the drug, using fresh pipettes and 5.0-ml volumes, through the remaining 10 tubes, discarding 5 ml from tube 12. This gives a dilution serial ranging in concentration from 200 to 0.10 μg/ml. In sequence, starting with the first dilution, add 5.0 ml of cool, melted modified SABHI agar to each drug dilution, mix, and immediately dispense in 2.0-ml volumes in sterile test tubes. Do not hold any dilution of drug at 50 C longer than is required to dispense the medium. Allow the tubes to cool in a vertical position. Final drug concentrations will range from 100 to 0.05 μg/ml. For the growth control tubes, mix 5.0 ml each of the two media and dispense in 2.0-ml volumes.

A volumetric dilution procedure may also be used in the semisolid agar dilution method. In this procedure, 10-fold higher concentrations of drug are first prepared in sterile water with subsequent dilution into melted, semisolid media. The diluted preparations of drug are then dispensed as above. Details for this procedure are given in Table 3.

After the tubes have hardened, they should be inoculated by dropping approximately 0.05 ml of the spore or mycelial suspension on the surface of the semisolid medium. Two tubes are inoculated at each concentration and are incubated at 30 C for 48 h or until the growth control tubes are positive.

Interpretation of results may be difficult, as several different end points may be observed. With isolates of *Blastomyces dermatitidis* and

TABLE 3. *Volumetric system for preparing serial dilutions of drugs in semisolid agar*

Volumes and concn of drug in sterile water		To be added to indicated volumes of sterile water	Intermediate concn (μg/ml)[a]
Volumes	Concn (μg/ml)		
4	1,000	—	1,000
2	1,000	2	500
1	1,000	3	250
1	1,000	7	125
2	125	2	62.5
1	125	3	31.3
1	125	7	15.6
2	15.6	2	7.8
1	15.6	3	3.9
0.5	15.6	3.5	2.0
0.25	15.6	3.75	1.0

[a] Final concentrations will be reduced 10-fold when intermediate concentrations are diluted 1:10 in semisolid media.

Histoplasma capsulatum, clear-cut end points showing "no growth" will be obtained at concentrations of 0.20 μg or less/ml (Table 1). In contrast, isolates of *Aspergillus* or *Penicillium* species may show several end points with total inhibition of growth at higher concentrations and inhibition of sporulation only at lower concentrations. The MIC is defined as the lowest concentration which inhibits growth. Minimal fungicidal concentrations may be determined in the same manner as described for the broth dilution procedure.

Susceptibility testing with 5-fluorocytosine

A solution containing 1,000 μg of 5-FC/ml is prepared in 10× YNB. Place 12 sterile 16 by 125 mm disposable tubes in a rack. Add 0.5 ml of 10× YNB to tubes 2 through 12. Add 0.5 ml of the 1,000 μg/ml solution of 5-FC in 10× YNB to tubes 1 and 2. Mix the contents of tube 2 and then serially dilute the drug, using 0.5-ml volumes and fresh pipettes, through the remaining 10 tubes, discarding 0.5 ml from the last tube. Individually add 4.5 ml of the melted 0.5% agar to each dilution of drug, mix, and dispense in 1.5- to 1.7-ml volumes in sterile, disposable tubes. This step dilutes each drug concentration 1:10, giving a final concentration range of 100 to 0.05 μg/ml.

Inoculate each set of tubes, in duplicate, as directed above, and incubate at 30 C for 48 h or until the growth controls are positive.

Isolates of *Aspergillus* sp. or *A. fumigatus* will show a wide range of inhibitory end points, but most isolates should be inhibited at 50 μg or less/ml. As with amphotericin B, end points for both inhibition of growth and of sporulation may be observed.

Control organisms can be selected from previously tested organisms. However, the recommended controls include *S. cerevisiae* ATCC 9763 for tests with either amphotericin B or 5-FC and *Paecilomyces variotii* MSCC 5605 (Mycology Stock Culture Collection, National Institutes of Health) for tests in semisolid agar with amphotericin B.

LITERATURE CITED

1. Block, E. R., A. E. Jennings, and J. E. Bennett. 1973. Variables influencing susceptibility testing of *Cryptococcus neoformans* to 5-fluorocytosine. Antimicrob. Ag. Chemother. **4**:392–395.
2. Hildick-Smith, G., H. Blank, and I. Sarkany. 1964. Fungus diseases and their treatment, p. 378–381. Little, Brown and Co., Boston.
3. Jund, R., and F. Lacroute. 1970. Genetic and physiological aspects of resistance to 5-fluoropyrimidines in *Saccharomyces cerevisiae*. J. Bacteriol. **102**:607–615.
4. Normark, S., and J. Schönebeck. 1972. In vitro studies of 5-fluorocytosine resistance in *Candida albicans* and *Torulopsis glabrata*. Antimicrob. Ag. Chemother. **2**:114–121.
5. Polak, A., and H. J. Scholer. 1973. Fungistatic activity, uptake and incorporation of 5-fluorocytosine in *Candida albicans* as influenced by pyrimidines and purines. I. Reversal experiments. Pathol. Microbiol. **39**:148–159.
6. Shadomy, S. 1972. What's new in antifungal chemotherapy. Clin. Med. **79**:14–18.
7. Shadomy, S., C. B. Kirchoff, and A. E. Ingroff. 1973. In vitro activity of 5-fluorocytosine against *Candida* and *Torulopsis* species. Antimicrob. Ag. Chemother. **3**:9–14.
8. Weinstein, L. 1970. Antibiotics. IV. Miscellaneous antimicrobial, antifungal and antiviral agents, p. 1299–1302. *In* L.S. Goodman and A. Gilman (ed), The pharmacological basis of therapeutics, 4th ed. The MacMillan Co., New York.

Section VIII

PARASITES

Chapter 64
Clinical Parasitology: Introduction and General Methods

J. CLYDE SWARTZWELDER

GENERAL INFORMATION

For the many parasitic infections which involve the intestine or blood stream, two basic necessities to achieve correct diagnosis are (i) preparation of suitable smears of stools or blood and (ii) making a systematic and adequate search, with optimal illumination, for finding and identification of the diagnostic stages of the parasites. The appropriate procedures for preparing suitable smears are described in the following respective chapters on identification of parasites and in texts (1).

Immunological procedures play a major role in or contribute significantly to the diagnosis of many parasitic infections. Examples are toxoplasmosis, trichinosis, echinococcosis, filariasis, visceral larva migrans, cysticercosis, schistosomiasis, Chagas' disease, amebiasis, malaria, and other systemic parasitoses.

MISDIAGNOSES AND MISSED DIAGNOSES

From the standpoint of morphology, major problems in the diagnosis of parasitic infections include missed diagnoses and misdiagnoses (false diagnoses). Errors in the laboratory diagnosis of amebiasis, for example, are due to : (i) failure, because of poor technique or inadequate search, to detect the organism; (ii) confusion of various nonparasitic objects in the stool or in sigmoidoscopic aspirate with *Entamoeba histolytica*; and (iii) confusion of other intestinal protozoa with this pathogen. Erroneous laboratory findings, in turn, lead to incorrect clinical diagnoses.

INFLUENCE OF ILLUMINATION ON DIAGNOSIS

Proper illumination is essential for satisfactory stool examination. Too much light will render amoebas invisible, whereas insufficient light will fail to make clear the morphological details. Inadequate attention is usually given to the adjustment of illumination. *Failure to maintain optimal illumination is one of the major causes for difficulty in the detection and identification of protozoa.*

The following details may appear elementary, but they influence greatly the correct diagnosis of amebiasis. They represent the difference between finding or missing parasites, especially protozoa.

A satisfactory method of controlling the intensity of light during examination of stools is by means of elevating and lowering the substage condenser. Meanwhile, the diaphragm on the substage apparatus is kept wide open or adjusted to individual preference. One hand is kept on the substage condenser control knob constantly. The other hand is used to control both the mechanical stage and the fine adjustment focusing knob. *The substage condenser should be raised and lowered frequently during microscopic work* to assure that the optimal illumination is being obtained. It should be adjusted with each change of magnification and when any object in a fecal smear is studied. This will accentuate morphological details, permit study of objects under various intensities of illumination, and provide optimal illumination of each object and with each magnification.

The entire area of the two smears (saline and iodine) on the fecal slide should be examined systematically with a 10× objective. Obviously, a mechanical stage is an absolute necessity. First, examine the saline smear completely; then examine the entire iodine-stained smear. The 43× objective is employed to study objects suggestive of parasites. It is profitable even for experienced personnel to examine a part of each smear with the higher magnification. This reduces the chances of overlooking small organisms. *Furthermore, a careful, methodical, and diligent search, not merely a glance, is required to complete a satisfactory stool examination* (1).

ERRORS IN IDENTIFICATION

Confusion of various nonparasitic objects in stools, sigmoidoscopic aspirates, blood films, and tissue sections leads to misdiagnoses. Ex-

TABLE 1. *Location in the body of some parasites of man*

Name	Stage	Location
		BLOOD
Plasmodium vivax *Plasmodium malariae* *Plasmodium falciparum*	Trophozoites, schizonts, and gametocytes	In red blood cells
Trypanosoma gambiense *Trypanosoma rhodesiense* *Trypanosoma cruzi*	Trypaniform	Free in blood
Leishmania donovani	Leishmaniform	Occasionally present in leukocytes and monocytes
Wuchereria bancrofti *Brugia malayi* *Loa loa* *Mansonella ozzardi* *Dipetalonema perstans*	Microfilariae	Free in blood
Schistosoma japonicum	Adults	Attached to walls of mesenteric and intrahepatic portal blood vessels
Schistosoma haematobium	Adults	Attached to walls of vesical, pelvic, and portal blood vessels
Schistosoma mansoni	Adults	Attached to walls of intrahepatic portal and mesenteric blood vessels
		LUNGS
Entamoeba histolytica	Trophozoites	In wall of abscess
Ascaris lumbricoides	Larvae	In tissue
Toxocara canis	Larvae	In tissue
Strongyloides stercoralis	Eggs, larvae, adults	Occasionally in alveoli and bronchial epithelium
Dirofilaria spp.	Adult	In blood vessels and in "coin lesions"
Echinococcus granulosus	Hydatid cyst	In tissue
Paragonimous westermani	Adults	In tissue
Schistosoma japonicum *Schistosoma mansoni*	Eggs	In tissue
		BRAIN
Plasmodium falciparum	Trophozoites Schizonts Pigment	In red blood cells; red blood cells parasitized by *P. falciparum* adhere to endothelial lining of blood vessels (marginal distribution)
Trypanosoma gambiense	Trypaniform	In tissue and blood
Trypanosoma rhodesiense	Trypaniform	In tissue and blood
Trypanosoma cruzi	Leishmaniform	In neuroglia cells
Toxoplasma gondii	Multiplicative and pseudocyst forms	In cells and interstitial fluid
Entamoeba histolytica	Trophozoites	At margin of abscess
Naegleria and *Hartmannella* spp.	Trophozoites	In tissue
Toxocara canis	Larvae	In tissue
Taenia solium	Cysticercus	In tissue
Echinococcus granulosus	Hydatid cyst	In tissue
Schistosoma japonicum *Schistosoma mansoni*	Eggs	Occasionally present in tissue
		MUSCLE
Trypanosoma cruzi	Leishmaniform	Intracellular (cardiac muscle)
Toxoplasma gondii	Multiplicative stage and pseudocyst	Intracellular (cardiac and skeletal muscle)
Trichinella spiralis	Larvae	In skeletal muscle
Taenia solium	Cysticercus	In skeletal and cardiac muscle

TABLE 1.—*Continued*

Name	Stage	Location
		LIVER
Plasmodium vivax *Plasmodium malariae* *Plasmodium falciparum*	(1) Pigment; (2) exoerythrocytic stages (rarely seen)	(1) Küpffer cells; (2) parenchymal cells
Trypanosoma cruzi	Leishmaniform	Küpffer cells
Leishmania donovani	Leishmaniform	Küpffer cells
Entamoeba histolytica	Trophozoites	Wall of abscess
Toxocara canis	Larvae	In tissue
Echinococcus granulosus	Hydatid cyst, unilocular	In tissue
Echinococcus multilocularis	Hydatid cyst, alveolar	In tissue
Schistosoma japonicum *Schistosoma mansoni* *Schistosoma haematobium*	Eggs	In tissue
Fasciola hepatica	Adults	Bile ducts and in tissue
Clonorchis sinensis	Adults	Bile ducts
		SPLEEN
Plasmodium vivax *Plasmodium malariae* *Plasmodium falciparum*	Pigment	Reticuloendothelial cells
Trypanosoma cruzi	Leishmaniform	Reticuloendothelial cells
Leishmania donovani	Leishmaniform	Reticuloendothelial cells
Toxoplasma gondii	Multiplicative forms	Intracellular
Schistosoma japonicum *Schistosoma mansoni* *Schistosoma haematobium*	Eggs	In tissue
		SMALL INTESTINE
Giardia lamblia	Trophozoites	Trophozoites attached to and in mucosa
Strongyloides stercoralis	Parasitic adult females, embryonated eggs, and rhabditiform larvae	Imbedded in mucosa (not below muscularis mucosae) and in mucus adherent to mucosa
Ascaris lumbricoides	Adults	Free in lumen
Necator americanus	Adults	Attached to mucosa
Ancylostoma duodenale	Adults	Attached to mucosa
Trichinella spiralis	Adults	Imbedded in mucosa and mucus adherent to mucosa (for about 2 months after inoculation)
Taenia solium	Adults	Free in lumen; scolex attached
Taenia saginata	Adults	Free in lumen; scolex attached
Hymenolepis nana	Adults	Free in lumen; scolex attached
Hymenolepis diminuta	Adults	Free in lumen; scolex attached
Dipylidium caninum	Adults	Free in lumen; scolex attached
Diphyllobothrium latum	Adults	Free in lumen; scolex attached
Fasciolopsis buski	Adults	Attached to mucosa
		LARGE INTESTINE
Entamoeba histolytica	Trophozoites and cysts	Trophozoites in ulcers; cysts free in lumen
Dientamoeba fragilis	Trophozoites	Free in lumen; possibly in tissue
Trichomonas hominis	Trophozoites	Free in lumen
Balantidium coli	Trophozoites	In ulcers and free in lumen
Trichuris trichiura	Adults	Anterior end imbedded in mucosa; posterior end in lumen
Enterobius vermicularis	Adults	Free in lumen (occasionally in wall of intestine)
Schistosoma japonicum *Schistosoma mansoni*	Eggs and adults	Eggs in wall; adults in submucosal blood vessels

TABLE 1.—*Continued*

Name	Stage	Location
		EYE
Toxoplasma gondii	Multiplicative and pseudocyst forms	Intracellular
Toxocara canis	Larvae	In tissue
Loa loa	Larvae; adults	Migrate under conjunctiva of orbit
Onchocerca volvulus	Microfilariae	In tissue and fluid
Taenia solium	Cysticercus	In vitreous and anterior chamber
		LYMPH NODES
Trypanosoma gambiense	Trypaniform	In fluid
Trypanosoma rhodesiense	Trypaniform	In fluid
Trypanosoma cruzi	Leishmaniform	Intracellular
Wuchereria bancrofti	Adults	In vessels and tissue of lymph node
Brugia malayi	Adults	In vessels and tissue of lymph node
		GENITOURINARY SYSTEM
Entamoeba histolytica	Trophozoites	In tissue (vagina, cervix, penis)
Trichomonas vaginalis	Trophozoites	On surface of vaginal mucosa; in prostatic and seminal fluid of male; in urine of male and female
Enterobius vermicularis	Adults and eggs	Free in vagina (occasionally in tissue of female genital tract)
Schistosoma haematobium	Eggs	In urine and semen
		SKIN
Entamoeba histolytica	Trophozoites	In wall of ulcer
Leishmania brasiliensis	Leishmaniform	In reticuloendothelial cells of skin and mucous membranes
Leishmania tropica	Leishmaniform	In reticuloendothelial cells which infiltrate corium
Loa loa	Adults	Migrate in subcutaneous tissue
Onchocerca volvulus	Adults and microfilariae	Adults in nodule; microfilariae in nodule and free in adjacent skin
Dipetalonema streptocerca	Microfilariae	Adults in subcutaneous tissue
Dirofilaria spp.	Adults	In subcutaneous tissue
Dracunculus medinensis	Adults	In cutaneous lesion
Ancylostoma braziliense	Larvae	In serpiginous tunnels in stratum germinativum
Strongyloides spp. (*S. stercoralis*, *S. myopotami*)	Filariform larvae	In superficial layers
Gnathostoma spinigerum	Immature forms	In deep burrow, boils, and abscesses
Spirometra mansonoides	Sparganum (larva)	In subcutaneous tissues; also found in the breast, joints, muscle, spermatic cord, and elsewhere in the body
Schistosoma spp. (birds and rodents)	Cercariae	In papular lesions of skin
Sarcoptes scabiei	Adults, larvae, eggs	In stratum corneum
Eutrombicula alfreddugesi	Larvae	In superficial layers
Demodex folliculorum	Adults	In follicles and sebaceous glands of nose and forehead
Dermacentor andersoni, *Dermacentor variablis*, *Ambylomma americanum*	Larvae, nymphs, or adults	"Head" imbedded in skin
Tunga penetrans	Adult females	In superficial layers
Dermatobia spp. and other fly larvae	Larvae (myiasis)	In superficial layers; in skin and subcutaneous tissues

cellent illustrations of artifacts are included in *The Color Atlas of Intestinal Parasites* by F. M. Spencer and L. S. Monroe (2). Confusing artifacts include: macrophages, leukocytes, tissue cells, and yeast confused with amoebas; plant cells and plant spines resembling helminth eggs and larvae; spores similar in appearance to helminth eggs in stools; septate fungi, contaminants of blood films, which resemble microfilariae (e.g., *Helicosporium lumbricoides*); eggs and larvae of plant nematodes (e.g., *Meloidogne javanica*) and of free-living nematodes (e.g., *Rhabditis* spp.); fibrin strands with the appearance of trypanosomes; seeds in appendices resembling helminths; and a variety of other pseudoparasites.

One should require that objects observed in fecal smears or sigmoidoscopic aspirate meet the accepted morphological criteria for *E. histolytica* and other parasites instead of adapting the criteria of the parasite to meet the characteristics of the object in question. Otherwise, cells or artifacts present in fecal or other specimens may be mistaken for this amoeba or other parasites. One must not allow his enthusiasm for a diagnosis of amebiasis to lead to an erroneous diagnosis.

A few examples of the confusion and errors in clinical and laboratory diagnosis of parasitic diseases are noted below. The misdiagnosis of ulcerative colitis as intestinal amebiasis perhaps is the most frequent error. Recognition of an amoebic liver abscess has been obscured by a tentative diagnosis of hepatoma. A search for brucellosis, without considering the possibility of a malarial etiology, has delayed correct diagnosis of falciparum malaria. Sophisticated hematological studies, including bone-marrow puncture, could have been obviated by stool examination in a case of severe hookworm disease. An "epidemic of malaria," due to misdiagnosis of platelets superimposed on red blood corpuscles as plasmodia, immobilized an aircraft carrier. It is also a common error to fail to search for more than a single etiology. A case of amoebic liver abscess appeared to fail to respond to antiamoebic therapy until a concurrent malarial infection was discovered.

COINCIDENTAL OCCURRENCE OF PARASITOSIS WITH OTHER DISEASES

In population groups, depending upon the geographic area, prevalence of amebiasis may range from less than 1% to more than 50%. Asymptomatic or mild clinical infections with *E. histolytica* may be present and coincidental to other diseases in the same patient. Thus, amebiasis may occur in persons with carcinoma, ulcerative colitis, shigellosis, colonic dysfunction of psychosomatic origin, of other conditions. The possibility that the amoebic infection may not be the primary cause of any or all of a patient's complaints should be borne in mind. This is particularly true when intestinal bleeding or other complaints or findings continue after a reasonable amount of antiamoebic therapy has been employed.

If a patient has been treated two times for amebiasis and the laboratory reports still indicate that *E. histolytica* is present, the validity of the laboratory findings should be questioned. Similarly, if clinical findings or complaints remain or recur after two courses of treatment with amebicides, the diagnosis should be reconsidered and another etiology sought. Serological procedures for amebiasis, such as those available in the United States through the services of the Center for Disease Control, Atlanta, Ga., can be very helpful in arriving at a correct diagnosis when diagnostic problems involving amebiasis and infections by other tissue-inhabiting parasites arise.

LOCATION OF PARASITES IN MAN

A listing of some of the parasites of man and their location in the body is given in Table 1.

LITERATURE CITED

1. Hunter, G. W., W. W. Frye, and J. C. Swartzwelder. 1966. A manual of tropical medicine. W. B. Saunders Co., Philadelphia.
2. Spencer, F. M., and L. S. Monroe. 1961. A color atlas of intestinal parasites. Charles C Thomas, Publisher, Springfield, Ill.

Chapter 65

Intestinal and Urogenital Protozoa

MARION M. BROOKE

INTRODUCTION

In the clinical laboratory, over a dozen species of intestinal and urogenital protozoa representing four groups of organisms (amoebas, flagellates, ciliates, and coccidia) must be considered (Table 1). Some are rarely encountered in the United States: *Entamoeba polecki*, *Balantidium coli*, *Enteromonas hominis*, and *Retortamonas intestinalis*. Six species, *Entamoeba histolytica*, *Balantidium coli*, *Giardia lamblia*, *Trichomonas vaginalis*, *Isospora belli*, and *Isospora hominis*, are capable of producing gastrointestinal or urogenital symptomatology, and one, *E. histolytica*, can produce extraintestinal complications. The pathogenicity of *Dientamoeba fragilis* is in question, but evidence is accumulating that it can be associated with clinical illness (24). Although the clinical laboratory in the United States should be competent to identify all of the species with the possible exception of *E. polecki*, *E. hominis*, and R. *intestinalis*, it should concentrate its attention on *E. histolytica*, *G. lamblia*, *T. vaginalis*, and *D. fragilis*.

The identification of the intestinal protozoa is based upon detailed morphology, as observed in several types of preparations with the use of various magnifications of the microscopy. Table 2 summarizes the morphological characteristics of the organisms, and Fig. 1 illustrates their classical features in permanently stained preparations. Figure 2 presents photomicrographs of representative organisms in wet mounts and stained smears of fecal specimens. For more complete descriptions and additional illustrations, the reader is referred to the excellent books by Burrows (12) and Spencer and Monroe (39).

The prevalence of the intestinal protozoa varies considerably in different population groups and is generally correlated with socioeconomic conditions. Higher rates are found in areas of poor sanitation, those without sewage systems and potable water, and in groups with poor personal hygiene, for example, patients in institutions for the mentally retarded. Today the prevalence rate of *E. histolytica* (etiological agent of amebiasis) in the general population of the United States is considered to be around 3 to 5% (11).

Since increased prevalence is correlated with poor sanitation and poor personal hygiene, the physician, while taking the case history, should ask questions concerning the home environment. Although person-to-person transmission of intestinal protozoa may not occur in a good home environment (10), several members of a family may be infected if the home environment is poor. The clinician must remember that most individuals infected with even the potentially pathogenic organism may not be experiencing any pathology or symptomatology.

As with most parasitic diseases, the symptomatology produced by pathogenic intestinal protozoa is too nonspecific to enable the physician to make an accurate clinical diagnosis (27). As a consequence, a clinical diagnosis without laboratory confirmation is rarely justified. The most reliable method of establishing a diagnosis is by direct examination of specimens to determine the presence of the parasite. Indirect (serological) methods are available for amebiasis, but at present their practical diagnostic value is primarily limited to extraintestinal complications (see Chapter 70).

The intestinal protozoa present special problems to the clinical laboratory because of their fragile nature and the necessity of identifying them on the basis of morphological details. Particular attention must be given to the handling of specimens during collection and examination to make certain that the diagnostic characteristics are maintained. Also, the laboratory director must be sure that the microscopists examining the materials are competent to identify the intestinal protozoa. Training in this area of microbiology is frequently neglected. A recently developed training aid in the laboratory diagnosis of amebiasis is programmed instruction (44). These self-instructional materials can teach basic fundamentals, but they must be supplemented with hours of practice at the microscope.

The urogenital protozoan *Trichomonas vaginalis* is identified by its characteristic morphology which is similar to that of the closely related intestinal flagellate *T. hominis*. The most distinctive features of *T. vaginalis* are its larger size (range, 8 to 30 μm; usual range, 12 to 18 μm), a shorter undulating membrane extending less than half the length of the body, and no free trailing posterior flagellum (Fig. 3). Differentiation of the two species by morphology is, however, unnecessary, since the flagellates can be identified by the source of the specimens (intestinal versus urogenital origins).

T. vaginalis may be found in the urogenital tracts of *both* women and men (42). It has been found in all races and climates, but the prevalence varies greatly with differences in socioeconomic conditions. There is no cyst, and transmission occurs in the trophozoite stage. Sexual intercourse is the method of transmission, although other means are implicated by findings of infections in infants and virgins. In women, *T. vaginalis* is frequently associated with vaginitis of various intensities. In men, infection of the urethra, prostate, and seminal vesicles is usually asymptomatic but may be responsible for irritating urethritis (14).

Most of the comments above concerning the intestinal protozoa—relationship with poor sanitation and personal hygiene, importance of laboratory confirmation of clinical diagnosis, care and collection of specimens, and the need for competent microscopists—apply equally well to the flagellate from the urogenital tract. Antibodies to the infection have been demonstrated, but serological tests are not used as a diagnostic procedure.

TABLE 1. *Intestinal and urogenital protozoa that may be found in specimens from patients in the United States*

Species of protozoa	Relative prevalence[a]	Pathogenicity
Amoebas		
Entamoeba histolytica	++	+
Entamoeba hartmanni	+	−
Entamoeba coli	++++	−
Entamoeba polecki	R	−
Endolimax nana	+++	−
Iodamoeba bütschlii	±	−
Dientamoeba fragilis	++	?
Ciliate		
Balantidium coli	R	+
Flagellates		
Giardia lamblia	++	+
Trichomonas vaginalis	+++	+
Trichomonas hominis	++	−
Chilomastix mesnili	±	−
Enteromonas hominis	R	−
Retortamonas intestinalis	R	−
Coccidia		
Isospora belli	R	+
Isospora hominis	R	+

[a] R = rare.

COLLECTION OF SPECIMENS

The clinical laboratory can expect to receive five types of specimens for examination for intestinal and urogenital protozoa: (i) feces, (ii) sigmoidoscopic materials, (iii) abscess aspirates, (iv) duodenal contents, and (v) urogenital materials. In each instance, it is important for the specimen to be ample and fresh when examined. In this regard, the clinical laboratory has a potential advantage over public health laboratories, since it can insist that collection procedures which meet laboratory requirements are followed. Preservatives may be used in the clinic and hospital, but their use is limited if the laboratory can be certain of having specimens brought to the laboratory immediately after collection.

The specimens should not be kept artificially warm under any circumstance. Many clinics attempt to maintain specimens at 37 C, but this practice only accelerates death and disintegration of the diagnostic stages, particularly in the case of the fragile trophozoites (23, 43). If a stool specimen cannot be examined immediately, it should be placed in a refrigerator, kept at room temperature, or preserved, rather than maintained at an elevated temperature. Specimens should not, however, be frozen (22).

In view of the importance of freshness, the specimen label, or diagnostic request slip, should indicate the date *and* time the specimen was collected from the patient so that the laboratory can determine the age of the specimen at the time of examination.

Collection of fecal specimens

In hospitals, or clinics, specimens may be collected in clean, dry bedpans, if care is taken not to contaminate the feces with urine, which might destroy any protozoan trophozoites present. The bedpan may be covered and used to transport the specimen, or the specimen can be transferred to a container. In either case, it is desirable to submit the whole fecal specimen so that satisfactory gross and microscopic examinations can be made. A half-pint waterproof, paper carton with an overlapping lid is recommended for the routine collection of specimens. The patient may defecate directly into this type of carton, and the label indicating identifying information, date, and hour of passage may be placed on the carton itself. Collecting feces from toilet bowls is unsatisfactory because the feces

TABLE 2. *Differential morphology of protozoa found in stool specimens of humans*[a]

A. Amoebas—trophozoites

Species	Size (diameter or length)	Motility	Nucleus			Cytoplasm	
			No.	Peripheral chromatin	Karyosomal chromatin	Appearance	Inclusions
Entamoeba histolytica	10–60 μm Usual range: 15–20 μm, commensal form[b]; over 20 μm, invasive form[c]	Progressive with hyaline, fingerlike pseudopods.	1 Not visible in unstained preparations.	Fine granules. Usually evenly distributed and uniform in size.	Small, discrete. Usually centrally located, but occasionally is eccentric.	Finely granular.	Red blood cells occasionally. Noninvasive organisms may contain bacteria.
Entamoeba hartmanni	5–12 μm Usual range: 8–10 μm	Usually nonprogressive, but may be progressive occasionally.	1 Not visible in unstained preparations.	Similar to *E. histolytica*.	Small, discrete, often eccentric.	Finely granular.	Bacteria.
Entamoeba coli	15–50 μm Usual range: 20–25 μm	Sluggish, nonprogressive, with blunt pseudopods.	1 Often visible in unstained preparations.	Coarse granules, irregular in size and distribution.	Large, discrete, usually eccentric.	Coarse, often vacuolated.	Bacteria, yeasts, other materials.
Endolimax nana	6–12 μm Usual range: 8–10 μm	Sluggish, usually nonprogressive with blunt pseudopods.	1 Visible occasionally in unstained preparations.	None	Large, irregularly shaped. (Blotlike.)	Granular, vacuolated.	Bacteria.
Iodamoeba bütschlii	8–20 μm Usual range: 12–15 μm	Sluggish, usually nonprogressive.	1 Not usually visible in unstained preparations.	None	Large, usually central. Surrounded by refractile, achromatic granules. These granules are often not distinct even in stained slides.	Coarsely granular, vacuolated.	Bacteria, yeasts, or other material.
Dientamoeba fragilis	5–15 μm Usual range: 9–12 μm	Usually nonprogressive. Pseudopodia are angular, serrated, or broad lobed and hyaline, almost transparent.	2 (In approximately 20% of organisms only 1 nucleus is present.) Nuclei invisible in unstained preparations.	None	Large cluster of 4–8 granules.	Finely granular, vacuolated.	Bacteria.

TABLE 2—*Continued*
B. Amoebas—cysts

Species	Size	Shape	Nucleus			Cytoplasm	
			No.	Peripheral chromatin	Karyosomal chromatin	Chromatoid bodies	Glycogen
Entamoeba histolytica	10–20 μm Usual range: 12–15 μm	Usually spherical.	4 in mature cyst. Immature cysts with 1 or 2 occasionally seen.	Peripheral chromatin present. Fine, uniform granules, evenly distributed.	Small, discrete, usually centrally located.	Present. Elongate bars with bluntly rounded ends.	Usually diffuse. Concentrated mass often present in young cysts. Stains reddish-brown with iodine.
Entamoeba hartmanni	5–10 μm Usual range: 6–8 μm	Usually spherical.	4 in mature cyst. Immature cysts with 1 or 2 nuclei often seen.	Similar to *E. histolytica*	Similar to *E. histolytica*	Present. Elongate bars with bluntly rounded ends.	Similar to *E. histolytica*.
Entamoeba coli	10–35 μm Usual range: 15–25 μm	Usually spherical. Occasionally oval, triangular, or other shapes.	8 in mature cyst. Occasionally, supernucleated cysts with 16 or more are seen. Immature cysts with 2 or more occasionally seen.	Peripheral chromatin present. Coarse granules irregular in size and distribution, but often appear more uniform than in trophs.	Large, discrete usually eccentric but occasionally centrally located.	Present, but less frequently seen than in *E. histolytica*. Usually splinterlike with pointed ends.	Usually diffuse, but occasionally well defined mass in immature cysts. Stains reddish-brown with iodine.
Endolimax nana	5–10 μm Usual range: 6–8 μm	Spherical, ovoidal or ellipsoidal.	4 in mature cysts. Immature cysts with less than 4 rarely seen.	None	Large (blotlike), usually central.	Occasionally granules or small oval masses seen, but bodies as seen in *Entamoeba* spp. are not present.	Usually diffuse. Concentrated mass seen occasionally in young cysts. Stains reddish brown with iodine.
Iodamoeba bütschlii	5–20 μm Usual range: 10–12 μm	Ovoidal, ellipsoidal, triangular or other shapes.	1 in mature cyst.	None	Large, usually eccentric. Refractile, achromatic granules on one side of karyosome. Indistinct in iodine preparations.	Occasionally granules present, but chromatoid bodies as seen in *Entamoeba* spp. are not present.	Compact, well-defined mass. Stains dark brown with iodine.

[a] From Brooke and Melvin (9).
[b] Commensal form—usually asymptomatic or chronic cases; may contain bacteria.
[c] Invasive form—usually in acute cases; often contain red blood cells.

TABLE 2—*Continued*

C. Flagellates—trophozoites

Species	Size and shape (*length*)	Motility	No. of nuclei	No. of flagella	Other features
Trichromonas hominis	Pear-shaped, 8–20 μm Usual range: 11–12 μm	Nervous, jerky.	1 Not visible in unstained mounts.	3-5 anterior 1 posterior	Undulating membrane extending length of body.
Chilomastix mesnili	Pear-shaped, 6–24 μm Usual range: 10–15 μm	Stiff, rotary.	1 Not visible in unstained mounts.	3 anterior 1 in cystostome	Prominent cytostome extending ⅓–½ length of body. Spiral groove across ventral surface.
Giardia lamblia	Pear-shaped, 10–20 μm Usual range: 12–15 μm	"Falling-leaf."	2 Not visible in unstained mounts.	4 lateral 2 ventral 2 caudal	Sucking disk occupying ½–¾ of ventral surface.
Enteromonas hominis	Oval, 4–10 μm Usual range: 8–9 μm	Jerky.	1 Not visible in unstained mounts.	3 anterior 1 posterior	One side of body flattened. Posterior flagellum extends free posteriorly or laterally.
Retortamonas intestinalis	Pear-shaped or oval, 4–9 μm Usual range: 6–7 μm	Jerky.	1 Not visible in unstained mounts.	1 anterior 1 posterior	Prominent cytostome extending approximately ½ length of body.

D. Flagellates—cysts

Species	Size	Shape	No. of nuclei	Other features
Trichomonas hominis	No cyst			
Chilomastix mesnili	6–10 μm Usual range: 8–9 μm	Lemon-shaped with anterior hyaline knob or "nipple."	1 Not visible in unstained preparations.	Cytostome with supporting fibrils. Usually visible in stained preparation.
Giardia lamblia	8–19 μm Usual range: 11–12 μm	Oval or ellipsoidal.	Usually 4 Not distinct in unstained preparations. Usually located at one end.	Fibrils or flagella longitudinally in cyst. Occasionally may be slightly visible in unstained cysts. Deep staining fibers or fibrils may be seen lying laterally or obliquely across longitudinal fibrils in lower part of cyst. Cytoplasm often retracts from a portion of cell wall.
Enteromonas hominis	6–8 μm Usual range: 4–10 μm	Elongate or oval.	1–4 Usually 2 lying at opposite ends of cyst. Not visible in unstained mounts.	Resembles *E. nana* cyst. Fibrils or flagella are usually not seen.
Retortamonas intestinalis	4–7 μm Usual range: 4–9 μm	Pear-shaped or slightly lemon-shaped.	1 Not visible in unstained mounts.	Resembles *Chilomastix* cyst. Shadow outline of cytostome with supporting fibrils extends above nucleus.

may be contaminated with coprozoic organisms, and the water may obscure the consistency of the specimen and destroy trophozoites of intestinal protozoa if they are present.

Collection of fecal specimens by catharsis

Specimens collected by catharsis are more likely to contain parasites than those passed normally (2). This difference is probably due to the evacuation of the cecal area where infections tend to flourish. Purged specimens have a disadvantage, however; they may contain only trophozoites of the amoebas, and these forms are notoriously difficult to identify. Furthermore, the cathartic may affect the appearance and activity of the organisms and thus interfere with identification. Before relying on this method of collection, the laboratory must be certain that the microscopists are thoroughly competent in this area.

If catharsis is employed, a saline cathartic such as sodium sulfate or buffered phosphosoda is recommended. Mineral oil is unsatisfactory, since the oil globules interfere with microscopic examination. Bismuth and magnesia compounds provide a crystalline debris that obscures the organisms and alters the appearance of trophozoites. In such instances, cultivation may help, since the unidentifiable organisms may produce progeny with more normal characteristics.

Upon catharsis, the patient should collect all passages in separate containers for immediate delivery to the laboratory. Since one cannot predict which of a series of specimens is most likely to contain organisms, each passage should be examined.

Collection of material by sigmoidoscopy

In suspected cases of amebiasis where stool specimens are negative, material for microscopy may be obtained by sigmoidoscopy. Furthermore, in the hospital and clinic, sigmoidoscopy is usually a regular part of the diagnostic regimen for patients with lower gastrointestinal complaints. In looking for intestinal amoebas, it is preferable not to use catharsis or a cleansing enema before sigmoidoscopy. The patient should not have received barium, as it may obscure evidence of amebiasis for several days.

If the patient has had a recent bowel movement when he reports to the clinic, sigmoidoscopy may be performed immediately. If a spontaneous bowel movement does not occur and catharsis is necessary, it is important to delay sigmoidoscopy for 2 to 3 h after purgation to permit the intestinal mucosa to recover from

TABLE 2—*Continued*

E. Ciliate and coccidia

Species	Shape and size	Motility	No. of nuclei	Other features
Balantidium coli Trophozoite	Ovoid with tapering anterior end; 50–70 µm or more. Usual range: 40–50 µm.	Rotary, boring.	1 large, kidney-shaped macronucleus. 1 small subspherical micronucleus immediately adjacent to macronucleus. Macronucleus occasionally visible in unstained preparation as hyaline mass.	Body surface covered by spiral longitudinal rows of cilia. Contractile vacuoles are present.
Cyst	Spherical or oval; 45–65 µm. Usual range: 50–55 µm.	—	1 large macronucleus visible in unstained preparations as hyaline mass.	Macronucleus and contractile vacuole are visible in young cysts. In older cysts, internal structure appears granular.
Isospora species (*I. belli* and *I. hominis*)	Ellipsoidal oöcyst; 25–30 µm long. Usual range: 28–30 µm. Immature oöcyst not usually seen in *I. hominis*. Sporocyst round or oval. *I. belli*, 12–14 µm. *I. hominis*, 14–16 µm.	Nonmotile	—	Mature oöcyst contains 2 sporocysts with 4 sporozoites each. *I. belli:* usual diagnostic stage is immature oöcyst with single granular mass (zygote) within. *I. hominis:* mature sporocysts, singly or in pairs, are usually passed in feces. Oöcyst wall not apparent.

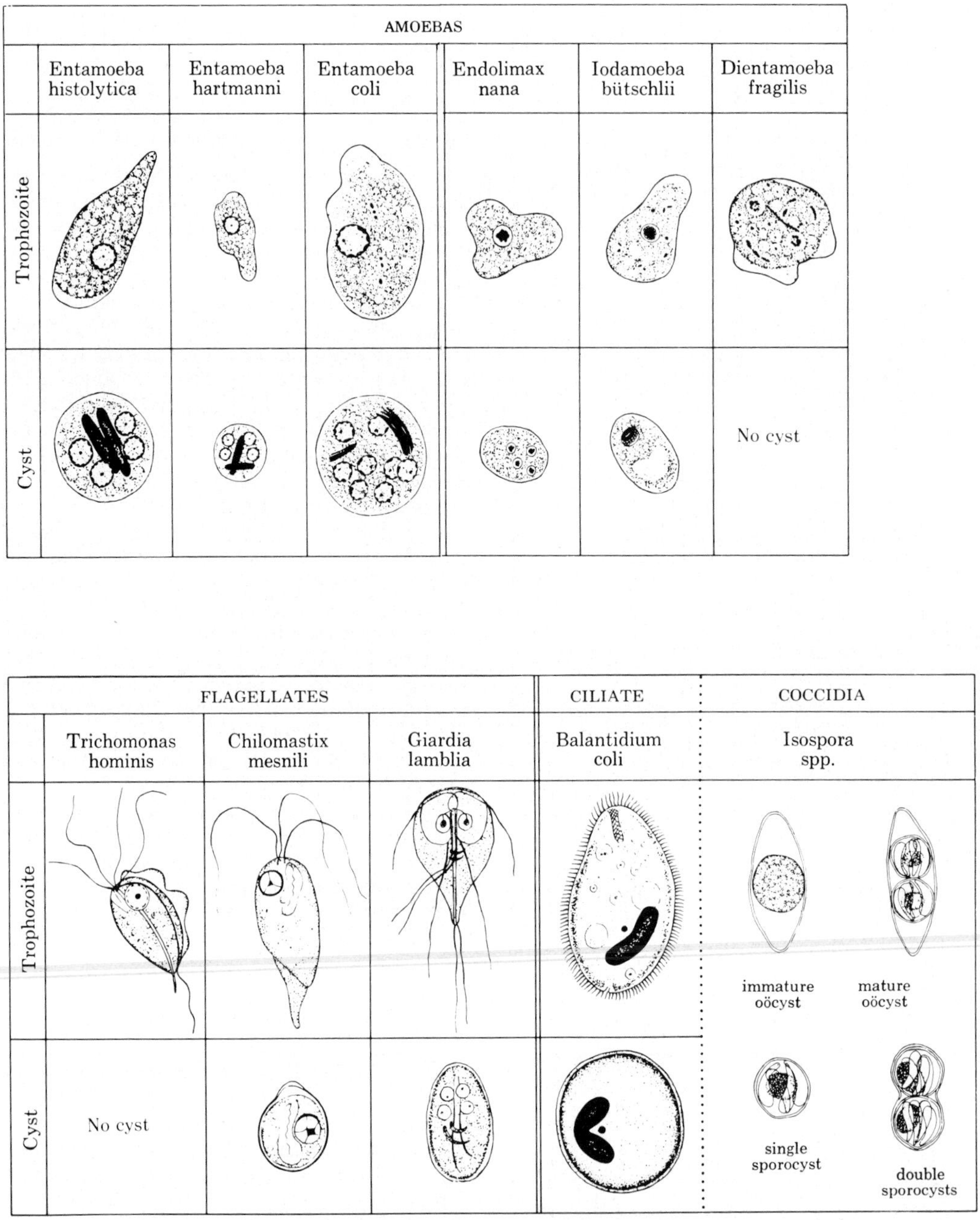

AMOEBAS						
	Entamoeba histolytica	Entamoeba hartmanni	Entamoeba coli	Endolimax nana	Iodamoeba bütschlii	Dientamoeba fragilis
Trophozoite						
Cyst						No cyst

FLAGELLATES				CILIATE	COCCIDIA	
	Trichomonas hominis	Chilomastix mesnili	Giardia lamblia	Balantidium coli	Isospora spp.	
Trophozoite					immature oöcyst	mature oöcyst
Cyst	No cyst				single sporocyst	double sporocysts

FIG. 1. *Protozoa found in stool specimens of humans (adapted from Brooke and Melvin, 1964).*

the trauma and to allow organisms to reappear. A cleansing enema is not advisable because it may remove organisms from the area which can be viewed through the sigmoidoscopy. A serological pipette (1 ml) with a small rubber bulb can be used to aspirate material from visible lesions and the mucosa. A curette or Volkman spoon may be used gently to scrape pathological areas of the mucosal wall, or a surgical instrument can be used to snip a biopsy of the mucosa. Generally, a long applicator stick with a cotton swab is not too satisfactory because it is difficult to obtain an adequate sample with it, and organisms may be trapped in the meshes of

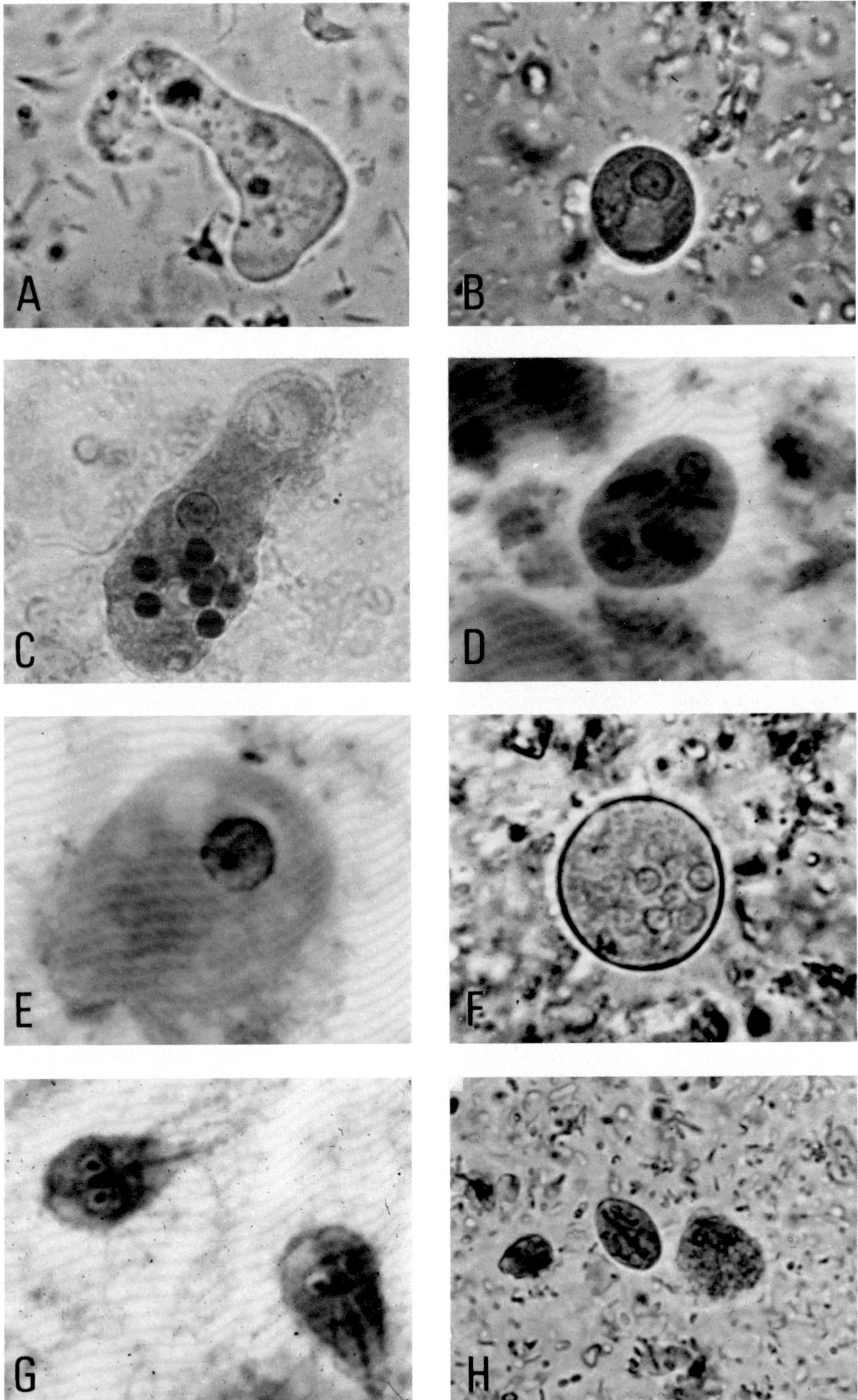

FIG. 2. *Photomicrographs of intestinal protozoa in fecal preparations. Oil immersion ×1,000. (A) Entamoeba histolytica, trophozoite showing directional locomotion. Saline mount. (Photograph courtesy of K. Juniper.) (B) E. histolytica, uninucleated cyst showing empty glycogen vacuole. Glycogen had leached out during preservation in Formalin solution. Iodine mount. (C) E. histolytica, trophozoite containing red blood cells. Trichrome stain. (D) E. histolytica, mature cyst showing two of four nuclei and chromatoid bodies. Trichrome stain. (E) Entamoeba coli, trophozoite containing a yeast cell. Trichrome stain. (F) E. coli, mature cyst showing six of eight nuclei. Iodine mount. (G) Giardia lamblia, trophozoites. Chlorazol black E stain. (H) G. lamblia, cyst. Iodine mount.*

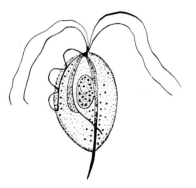

FIG. 3. *Trichomonas vaginalis.* (*Adapted from Brooke and Melvin, 1964.*)

the cotton. If an applicator stick is used, it should be dampened with saline.

Materials (except biopsied tissue) obtained by sigmoidoscopy should be placed on a slide and examined immediately. Preferably, this should be done at the bedside or in a room adjacent to the sigmoidoscopy room.

Collection of materials from abscesses and other lesions

Materials may be aspirated from a suspected extraintestinal lesion of amebiasis, particularly a liver abscess, to help promote healing and to assist in diagnosis. Clinical judgment must be exercised in deciding to aspirate (46), but any material obtained from such a procedure (or from open drainage or spontaneous rupture) should be carefully examined for trophozoites of *E. histolytica*. Cysts will not be present in such material.

Amoebae are difficult to find in abscess contents because they may not be present in all portions of the aspirate and, even when they are present, they are frequently partially immobilized or trapped in the thick coagulum. For these reasons, aspirated materials must be divided into several portions and treated in a special manner with proteolytic enzymes to help free the organisms (18). The details of this treatment are given below. Most of the amoebas in a liver abscess are in the peripheral areas of the lesion; therefore, the fluid withdrawn first from the more central region frequently will contain no organisms. The first material withdrawn is usually yellowish-white. The later portions, coming from the walls of the lesion, are brownish-red and are more likely to contain amoebas. Usually, the first time an abscess is aspirated, the "pus" is bacteriologically sterile. If more than 200 ml of exudate is aspirated, repeated drainage may be advisable (46). The later aspirates are more likely to contain demonstrable amoebae unless specific therapy has been instituted.

Materials from extraintestinal lesions should be placed in sterile tubes and taken to the laboratory immediately. If delay is unavoidable, or if the material must be shipped, some of the aspirated material should be preserved. Smears of the thick material can be made by pressing it between two microscope slides. The slides are separated by sliding them apart, and the resulting smears are fixed in Schaudinn's solution. The smears have to be transported to the laboratory in Schaudinn's fixative for staining. Aspirated materials can also be preserved in polyvinyl alcohol (PVA)-fixative (8).

In general, materials "coughed up" from lung lesions, or obtained from open abscesses and skin lesions, are handled in a similar manner. They are more likely, however, to contain bacteria.

Collection of duodenal contents

Usually, stool specimens from patients with giardiasis will reveal *Giardia lamblia*, but at times it may be neccessary to obtain materials from the duodenum in order to find the organism. The procedure is the same as for strongyloidiasis (*see* chapter 69). Again, the drainage material must be delivered to the laboratory immediately and examined while it is fresh.

Collection of urogenital materials for Trichomonas vaginalis

Usually, sterile cotton-tipped applicators are used to obtain specimens from the vagina suspected of *T. vaginalis* infection. Preferably, an unlubricated speculum should be used in obtaining the specimen, since the lubricant may present confusing artifacts to the microscopist. Vaginal discharge collected on the spoon-shaped depression of the speculum may be examined for the organism. Urethral discharge and urine specimens may also be collected from women.

In examining males for *T. vaginalis* infection, urethral discharge, urine, and prostatic secretions after prostatic massage should be collected. The first portion of a voided urine has the greatest likelihood of revealing the organisms.

After the specimens are collected, it is essential that they be examined immediately, before the organisms lose their motility. There should be *no delay* in getting the specimens to the laboratory or, preferably, the microscopy should be performed in the same area where the specimens are collected. The smears for permanently stained preparations may be made and culture tubes may be inoculated at the time of collection for later examination. However, they should be looked upon as secondary methods to the direct examination of wet mounts of clinical materials.

Collection of multiple specimens

Even in individuals known to be infected, a single specimen, regardless of its method of collection, cannot be relied upon to reveal the presence of parasites. Owing to the intermittent passage of the diagnostic stages and the fluctuation in numbers of organisms, multiple specimens from a clinically suspicious case may need to be examined to find intestinal and urogenital protozoa.

That a single normally passed fecal specimen (as opposed to a cathartic specimen) will contain only one-third to one-half of the species present is generally accepted. No agreement on the number of specimens that must be examined to rule out infections has been reached, but, from the practical standpoint, three specimens, collected over a period of several days, is a workable compromise. In the case of hospitalized patients, however, all fecal passages for a designated period of time should be submitted to the laboratory for examination in order not to prolong the hospital stay unnecessarily.

The series of normally passed fecal specimens should be collected before the patient is given a cathartic for two reasons: (i) cysts may predominate in the normal passage and can be identified with greater reliability than trophozoites, and (ii) for a week or more following purgation (or acute diarrhea), organisms in the passages may be extremely rare.

Preservation of fecal specimens for delivery to laboratory

Ideally, specimens collected in a hospital or clinic are immediately delivered to the laboratory. If an efficient delivery system is not available, however, or cannot be established, the specimens should be preserved so as to enable the laboratory to examine them for the various stages of parasites that may be present. Unless a specimen must be shipped or its examination otherwise delayed, the untreated fecal material is generally satisfactory for identifying protozoan cysts and for helminth eggs and larvae. Since trophozoites of intestinal amoebae disintegrate rapidly and laboratory confirmation of amoebic dysentery or amebiasis often is difficult, a portion of the specimen should be thoroughly fixed in PVA-fixative (8). This mixture of a water-soluble plastic and Schaudinn's fixative preserves and maintains the diagnostic characteristics of the fragile trophozoites and cysts, and is applicable particularly to central diagnostic and public health laboratories which receive specimens through the mails. Immediately, or weeks later, permanent stained films can be prepared from the preserved material. Trophozoites and cysts, if present, can be demonstrated by microscopic examination of the films with an oil immersion objective.

Preservation with PVA-fixative. The preparation of PVA-fixative is described in chapter 98. PVA powder is available commercially as Elvanol or Gelvatol Resin. When ordering the powder, specify the pretested powder for use in PVA-fixative. PVA-fixative solution also may be obtained commercially.

To obtain the full advantage of PVA-fixative as a preservative, specimens should be thoroughly mixed with the solution immediately after their passage from the patient and before the organisms lose their characteristic morphology.

On microscope slides. A drop of dysenteric stool or other material is placed on a microscope slide and mixed with three drops of PVA-fixative. With an applicator stock, the mixture is then spread (*not* smeared like a blood film) over approximately one-third of the glass surface, with care being taken to extend the smear to the sides of the slides to reduce later peeling, and allowed to dry *thoroughly* (preferably overnight at 37 C). Dried films remain satisfactory for staining for several weeks.

In vials. A quantity of specimen is thoroughly mixed in a vial containing three or more parts of PVA-fixative. Films for staining can be prepared immediately or weeks later by spreading two or three drops of the mixture over the surface of a microscope slide. Prepare the smear as described above. It is important not to make the films too thick and to allow them to dry thoroughly. If the specimen in the vial jells, it can be liquefied by heating in a water bath before the film is made.

PVA films are permeable to all commonly employed staining reagents. Therefore, they are handled in the same way as smears fixed in the conventional manner with Schaudinn's fixative, and may be stained by a variety of staining methods. Regardless of the staining procedure used, dried films are first placed in 70% alcohol containing iodine for approximately 20 min to remove mercuric chloride crystals. A distinct advantage of PVA-fixative is that it makes possible the successful staining of organisms occurring in fluid specimens such as diarrheic stools and the sediment of cultures (31). The solution serves as an adhesive as well as a preservative and prevents loss of organisms during the staining procedure.

Other preservatives such as MIF (38) and PAF-fixative (13) will preserve the trophozoites and cysts for wet mount examination, but these preservatives will not permit the preparation of permanently stained smears.

When collecting specimens for post-treatment examinations, the clinic or hospital may elect to have the patient mail his specimens to the laboratory rather than return in person. In this case, a *two-vial method* of preservation and of shipping, using (i) 5% Formalin and (ii) PVA-fixative, is recommended (8). This makes possible the recovery of all stages and types of organisms occurring in stools, since PVA-fixative serves primarily to preserve trophozoites of intestinal amoebae but is not entirely applicable to the diagnosis of protozoan cysts and helminth eggs.

If the laboratory is interested in attempting to culture amoebas, an egg-extract culture medium for transporting or shipping *E. histolytica* trophozoites in fecal specimens or sigmoidoscopic material has been developed (19). In this medium, trophozoites of *E. histolytica* and other amoebas may remain viable at room temperature for up to 4 days, thus permitting the laboratory to obtain cultures of the organisms for identification.

Although sputum, abscess aspirates, sigmoidoscopic materials, and urogenital materials can be preserved in PVA-fixative for subsequent processing, it is better to prepare smears from such materials and to place them in Schaudinn's or some other fixative for transporting to the laboratory.

METHODS OF EXAMINATION

Examination of fecal specimens

Macroscopic examination. Unfortunately, fecal specimens are frequently neglected in clinical laboratories until there is a "slack period" in the day. By that time, it may be too late to find identifiable intestinal protozoa. At the very least, each unpreserved specimen should undergo gross examination immediately upon its arrival in the clinical laboratory to determine the priority of its examination.

During the gross examination, the specimen should be inspected for (i) evidence of intestinal pathology (for example, blood and mucus), (ii) substances that interfere with examination (for example, barium or oil), and (iii) the consistency of the specimen. The consistency (or relative firmness) of the specimen can be designated as watery, loose, soft, or formed. The abnormalities and consistency observed should be recorded in the laboratory record. The initials W, L, S, and F can be used to indicate consistency. The age of the specimen in minutes and hours (from time of passage) should also be recorded. The consistency and age of the specimen determine the urgency of the examination and, in addition, this information will assist the laboratory director and practicing physician in better evaluating the results of the examination.

Since the more fluid specimens and those with blood and mucus are more likely to contain the fragile trophozoites, they should be examined first. Those containing barium, oil, and other interfering substances should be rejected as unsatisfactory for examination.

If the specimen cannot be examined immediately because of the pressure of other work, smears of the specimens should be made and placed in Schaudinn's fixative for staining at a later time, if indicated. Upon completing the gross examinations, those specimens that cannot be examined right away should be left at room temperature (preferably air-conditioned) or placed in a refrigerator. As previously stated, they should not be kept artificially warm (for example, in an incubator).

Microscopic examinations. Since identifying intestinal protozoa is dependent upon recognizing detailed morphological characteristics, the clinical laboratory must be equipped with a good binocular microscope and lamp. The microscope should have 5 and 10× oculars and three objectives: low power, 16 mm (10×); high-dry, 4 mm (44×); and oil immersion, 1.8 mm (98×). All lenses should be kept meticulously clean. A calibrated ocular micrometer is needed for accurate measurement of the organisms (*see* chapter 3). The microscope lamp, either the built-in or separate illuminator, should provide bluish-white light of variable intensity. Although a bright light is needed, its intensity should be adjustable because too much light obliterates organisms or obscures structural details.

Wet mount examinations

Generally, four types of techniques can be used to recover and identify intestinal protozoa: wet mount examinations, concentration procedures, permanently stained preparations, and cultivation procedures. Three general types of solutions are used in preparing wet mounts for the identification of intestinal protozoa: *physiological saline* for trophozoites and cysts, *iodine solution* for cysts, and a *temporary stain* for trophozoites. In physiological saline, the trophozoites and cysts will appear to be refractile and the trophozoites may exhibit characteristic movement. Because of these properties, organisms may be more easily spotted in saline than in any other type of preparation, even with a low-power objective. Even though no stain is present, some structures, such as the chromatoid bodies of the amoebic cysts, are more easily seen in saline than in other temporary mounts. Other structures such as nuclei may be invisible.

Iodine solutions are used primarily to stain the cysts in order to determine the number and structure of the nuclei. A weak rather than a strong iodine solution is best, for strong iodine tends to coagulate the fecal particles and to destroy the refractile nature of the organism. Several iodine solutions can be used satisfactorily. Two that have been widely used and are simply prepared are Dobell and O'Connor's (15) and Lugol's. The one recommended by Dobell and O'Connor is a weak iodine which should be prepared fresh about every 10 days for best results. Lugol's iodine *must be diluted* about five times with distilled water, as the full-strength solution is too strong. Lugol's iodine should be prepared fresh about every 3 weeks. The preparation of the iodine solutions is described in chapter 96. Gram's iodine, used in bacteriological work, is not satisfactory for staining protozoan cysts.

In a cyst correctly stained with iodine solution, the glycogen appears reddish brown, the cytoplasm is yellow, and the nuclei stand out as lighter refractile bodies. The location of the karyosomes may be more easily determined, but the chromatoid bodies are less visible than in saline solution. Since glycogen is a reserve food, it will not usually appear in older cysts.

Various staining solutions are available to help in the identification of amoebic trophozoites. Quensel's solution (41) perhaps has had the widest acceptance. Unfortunately, it is somewhat difficult to prepare and is not generally available commercially. Biological dyes like methylene blue and pyronine may be used for staining intestinal protozoa in wet mount preparations. The pH of the staining solution is a deciding factor in bringing out the morphological details of the nucleus (30), the optimal pH with an acetate buffer being 4.0 to 4.8. A good staining solution for amoebic trophozoites can be simply prepared by dissolving methylene blue in an appropriately buffered solution or by adding a buffer tablet to a solution of the dye. For staining trophozoites of *E. histolytica*, the exact pH is not critical, and the optimal range may vary with the buffer system employed. Directions for preparing acetate buffer with the pH range of 3.6 to 4.8 and for preparing a buffered methylene blue solution are given in chapter 96. Buffer tablets giving a range of 3.8 to 6.0 are available commercially.

In a preparation correctly stained with methylene blue, after about 5 to 10 min the trophozoite nuclei are stained blue with a lighter blue cytoplasm. The appearance is similar to that described for Quensel's stain and resembles a permanent hematoxylin-stained preparation. Inclusions in the cytoplasm are also stained. After a time, the organisms will become overstained and no longer identifiable. The preparation should be examined within approximately 30 min. *D. fragilis* does not stain well, nor do flagellate trophozoites or living cysts stain.

In preparing wet mounts for examination, a small portion of the specimen (feces, culture sediment, sigmoidoscopic material) is comminuted in a drop of solution on the surface of a microscope slide. The preferred slide size is 5 by 7.6 cm (2 by 3 inches), because these slides have adequate space for three mounts (saline, iodine, and stain) of the specimens. The wet mounts should be covered with glass of no. 1 thickness or plastic cover slips. To prevent evaporation and facilitate the use of the oil immersion objective, the cover slip should be sealed to the slide with equal parts of heated paraffin and petroleum jelly. A cotton swab can be used to apply the heated mixture to the edges of the cover slip.

The wet mounts are searched systematically with a 16-mm objective with reduced light to locate trophozoites and cysts. When organisms are found, the 4-mm and oil immersion objectives can be used to observe detailed morphology. In certain instances, by carefully studying a number of organisms in wet mount, final species identifications can be made. In other instances, however, only presumptive identifications will be possible. If no organisms are found, at least one complete mount should be searched thoroughly for 10 to 15 min.

Concentration procedures

Numerous studies have demonstrated the usefulness of concentration procedures in recovering cysts and eggs of intestinal parasites (16, 21). In the diagnosis of intestinal protozoan infections, concentration techniques are useful in revealing light infections in which cysts are present, but as yet no satisfactory method for concentrating trophozoites exists.

The zinc sulfate flotation technique (16) is an effective concentration procedure for the recovery of both protozoan cysts and helminth eggs and larvae from unpreserved specimens; however, operculated eggs and those of the schistosomes are not recovered by this method. Numerous laboratories have obtained good results with slight modifications of the original technique.

The Formalin-ether (FE) sedimentation technique (35) is likewise effective in concentrating both protozoan cysts and helminth eggs from unpreserved specimens. In addition, the technique can be performed satisfactorily on Formalin-preserved or MIF-preserved specimens. In comparative studies with the zinc sulfate flotation procedure, the FE sedimentation technique was considered better (36, 37). Generally, in comparison with the zinc sulfate method, in the FE concentration procedure the cysts appear more normal, particularly small cysts such as *E. nana* and *E. hartmanni*, and are, therefore, more easily identified. In addition, the FE sedimentation recovers a wider range of diagnostic stages (helminth eggs, including the schistosome and operculated eggs, as well as cysts) and the concentrations can be kept for a longer period without affecting the results of the examination. Since the sediments are preserved, most of the supernatant fluid can be poured off; the tubes are then stoppered to prevent drying and left for later examination. However, the FE technique is not as efficient as the zinc sulfate method for detecting *G. lamblia* and *I. bütschlii cysts* (or *H. nana* eggs).

The concentrates should be examined carefully in unstained wet mount preparations. Iodine mounts can be prepared to stain the contents of cysts.

Procedures for the concentration of fecal specimens are as follows.

Modified zinc sulfate concentration. (The preparation of zinc sulfate solution is described in chapter 96.)

1. Using two applicators, comminute a fecal sample about the size of a small pea in a Wassermann tube (100 by 13 mm) half filled with tap water. Make certain that all obvious particles are broken up and that an even suspension is formed.
2. Add additional tap water until the tube is two-thirds full.
3. Centrifuge for 1 min at approximately 2,500 rpm.
4. Pour off the supernatant fluid into a container holding a disinfectant, for example, cresol.
5. Repeat this washing only if the stool is extremely oily.
6. Add enough zinc sulfate solution to fill the tube half full.
7. Using an applicator, break up the packed sediment very thoroughly.
8. Add additional zinc sulfate solution to fill the tube within 1.3 cm of the top.
9. Centrifuge this suspension for 1 min at 2,500 rpm.
10. Without shaking or spilling the solution, carefully place the tube in a rack.
11. Slowly fill the tube brimful with zinc sulfate *without allowing any runover.*
12. Place a clean, grease-free no. 1 cover slip (22 by 22 mm) on top of the tube so that the under surface touches the meniscus. Leave undisturbed for about 10 min.
13. Deftly remove the cover slip with a straight, upward motion. A drop containing egg and cysts will adhere to the underside of the cover slip.
14. Lower this onto a drop of iodine stain placed on a clean 5 by 7.6 cm (2 by 3 inch) slide. Seal the preparation.
15. Examine under a microscope for eggs and cysts.

Formalin-ether concentration of fresh specimens. (Note: If permanently stained slides are to be made, the smears should be prepared before the specimen is used for concentration. If a portion of the specimen is to be preserved in PVA-fixative, this should be done before proceeding with the concentration procedure.)

1. Comminute a portion of the stool specimen in sufficient saline so that upon centrifugation 10 ml of emulsion will yield about 2 ml of sediment. A portion about the size of a walnut is usually enough. The suspension can be prepared in the carton in which it is submitted or in a beaker or flat-bottom paper cup.
2. Using a small glass funnel, strain about 10 ml of the emulsion through one or two layers of wet gauze into a 15-ml pointed centrifuge tube. With wide-mesh gauze, use two layers; with narrow-mesh material, use one layer. To conserve glassware, a cone-shaped paper cup with the point cut off can be substituted for the funnel.
3. Centrifuge at 2,000 to 2,500 rpm for 1 min. Decant the supernatant fluid.
4. Resuspend the sediment in fresh saline, centrifuge, and decant as before. This step may be repeated if a cleaner sediment is desired.
5. Add about 10 ml of 10% Formalin to the

sediment, mix thoroughly, and allow to stand for 5 min.

6. Add 3 ml of ether, stopper the tube, and shake vigorously in an inverted position for a full 30 s. Remove the stopper with care.

7. Centrifuge at 1,500 rpm for about 1 min. Four layers should result as follows: (i) ether at top, (ii) plug of debris, (iii) Formalin solution, and (iv) sediment.

8. Free the plug of debris from the sides of the tube by ringing with an applicator stick, and carefully decant the top three layers. Use a cotton swab to remove any debris adhering to the sides of the tube.

9. Mix the remaining sediment with the small amount of fluid that drains back from the sides of the tube (or, if necessary, add a small amount of Formalin or saline), and prepare iodine and unstained mounts in the usual manner for microscopic examination.

Formalin-ether concentration of Formalin-preserved specimens.

1. Stir the formalinized specimen thoroughly and, depending on the size and density of the specimen, strain a sufficient quantity through gauze into a 15-ml pointed centrifuge tube to give the desired amount of sediment indicated below.

2. Add tap water, mix thoroughly, and centrifuge at 2,000 to 2,500 rpm for 1 min. The resulting sediment should be about 1 ml.

3. Decant the supernatant fluid and, if desired, wash again with tap water.

4. Proceed with the addition of Formalin and ether as described above for the concentration of fresh specimens, steps 5 through 9.

Permanently stained preparations

Various workers (1, 7, 21, 29) have emphasized the importance of using permanently stained fecal smears for demonstrating and accurately identifying intestinal protozoa. During the examination of wet mounts, an experienced microscopist can on occasion make positive identification of certain species of intestinal protozoa, for example, *G. lamblia* and *E. coli* cysts. In many instances, however, and particularly in regard to *E. histolytica*, unless indisputably typical characteristics are observed, the identification should be considered only tentative. Confirmation in permanently stained smears in such cases is essential for the accurate diagnosis of infection with intestinal protozoa. Since the procedure need not be time-consuming, staining all specimens found to contain amoebae or questionable organisms is strongly recommended. In addition to aiding in the identification of organisms, the examination of permanently stained fecal smears, with an oil immersion objective, may reveal small organisms not found by other techniques. Experienced microscopists will find a 50× oil immersion objective useful for scanning and the 95×, for careful study. In most instances, a stained fecal smear should be examined for a minimum of 15 min.

Although many persons still prefer Heidenhain's iron hematoxylin procedure for critical work, a number of simpler staining techniques have been developed that can be completed in less than 1 h and are satisfactory for diagnostic work. The Wheatley trichrome method (26, 45) is very satisfactory and can be used for both fresh fecal specimens and those preserved in PVA-fixative. The chlorazol black E procedure (20, 24, 25), which combines both fixation and staining in a single step and does not require destaining, is a simplified procedure for clinical laboratories receiving fresh fecal material. However, PVA-fixed specimens do not stain well by this technique and are better stained by iron-hematoxylin or trichrome stains. The chlorazol black E stain could be of particular value in hospital and clinic laboratories where fresh specimens are usually obtained, since fewer steps are involved than in other procedures and since the steps require less attention. Specimens fixed in Formalin, MIF, and PAF-fixative cannot be used for satisfactory, permanently stained preparations. Two problems are involved: the fixation of such solutions is not satisfactory, and getting the liquid suspension to adhere to the slide during staining is difficult. In this case, PVA-fixative cannot be used as an adhesive, since it is not compatible with Formalin and a cloudy precipitate results. Arensburger and Markell (3) described a procedure for concentrating cysts, mixing the concentrate with a portion of the fresh fecal specimen, and staining smears made in the usual way for permanent preparations. If trophozoites are present in the fresh specimen, this procedure affords an opportunity to find them in the same smear. To date, no satisfactory procedure is available for concentrating trophozoites in fecal material for subsequent staining.

Permanently stained fecal smears afford the most satisfactory method of keeping positive evidence of intestinal protozoa identified in the laboratory. They also make it possible for the microscopist to consult with others on objects or organisms that are difficult to identify. In view of the infinite biological variations that the intestinal protozoa can exhibit and the many confusing artifacts encountered in fecal specimens, the microscopist should never hesitate to seek assistance from qualified specialists.

Stained slides also afford the best opportunity to observe carefully the cellular exudate in stool specimens, thus obtaining indirect evidence for the differentiation of amoebic and bacillary dysentery. For example, the presence of a large quantity of mucus, many pus cells (polymorphonuclear leukocytes, macrophages, lymphocytes, etc.), and degenerative inflammatory cells ("ring nuclei," "ghost cells") suggests bacillary dysentery, whereas the scarcity of these elements and the presence of the fragmented nuclear material (pyknotic bodies), cells with scarce cytoplasm ("mouse eaten" cells), and Charcot-Leyden crystals suggests amoebic dysentery. These and other aspects of the cellular exudate may be observed in saline wet mounts and temporary stained preparations (4).

Preparation of fecal smears

From fresh specimens. Using an applicator stick, make a thin smear of the fecal sample on a clean 2.5 by 7.6 cm (1 by 3 inch) slide. *If necessary*, dilute feces with physiological saline. Immerse slide immediately into Schaudinn's fixative. The smear must not be permitted to dry from the time it is made until it is mounted. *This is very important*. If the staining schedule must be interrupted, slides may be stored for long periods in the last 70% alcohol (step before staining).

From specimens preserved in PVA-fixative. With an applicator stick, 2 or 3 drops of the preserved specimen are spread (*not smeared*) over approximately one-third of the surface of a microscope slide. The films are allowed to dry thoroughly, either overnight in a 37 C incubator or at room temperature. It is important that the films dry thoroughly to prevent the material from washing off the slide during staining.

Trichrome stain for intestinal protozoa

The preparation of the reagents needed for the trichrome technique (Schaudinn's fixative solution, iodine alcohol, trichrome stain, destaining solution, and carbol-xylene) is described in chapter 96. The stain solution is stable and may be used repeatedly, the lost volume being replaced by adding stock solution. Staining over 15 smears daily (in 50 ml of stain) tends to weaken the stain. If the stain is allowed to stand and evaporate in open air for 3 to 8 h, its strength will return.

The staining of fresh and PVA-fixed material differs chiefly in that the latter requires increased time, and, since the material in the PVA solution is already fixed, the fixative step is omitted.

Staining procedure with fresh specimens.

1. Schaudinn's fixative, 5 min at 50 C, 1 h at room temperature.
2. Alcohol, 70%, plus iodine, 1 min.
3. Alcohol, 70%, 1 min.
4. Alcohol, 70%, 1 min.
5. Trichrome stain, 2 to 8 min.
6. Alcohol, 90% acidified (1 drop of glacial acetic acid in 10 ml of alcohol), 10 to 20 s or until stain barely runs from smear. Prolonged destaining in 90% alcohol (over 20 s) may differentiate organisms poorly, although larger trophozoites, particularly those of *E. coli*, may require slightly longer periods of decolorization.
7. Alcohol, 95 or 100%; rinse twice.
8. Alcohol, 100%, or carbol-xylene, 1 min.
9. Xylene, 1 min or until refraction at smear-xylene interface ends.
10. Mount with cover slip, using Permount, Balsam, or other mounting media.

Staining procedure with PVA films.

1. Alcohol, 70%, plus iodine, 10 to 20 min.
2. Alcohol, 70%, 3 to 5 min.
3. Alcohol, 70%, 3 to 5 min.
4. Trichrome stain, 6 to 8 min.
5. Alcohol, 90% acidified (1 drop of glacial acetic acid in 10 ml of alcohol), 10 to 20 s or until stain barely runs from smear.
6. Alcohol, 95%; rinse.
7. Alcohol, 95%, 5 min.
8. Carbol-xylene, 5 to 10 min.
9. Xylene, 10 min.
10. Mount with cover slip, using Permount, Balsam, or other mounting media.

Stain reactions (trichrome). The cytoplasm of thoroughly fixed and well-stained cysts and trophozoites is blue-green tinged with purple. Occasionally, *E. coli* cysts may stain slightly more purplish than cysts of other species. The nuclear chromatin, chromatoid bodies, and ingested red cells and bacteria stain red or purplish red. Other ingested particles, such as yeasts or molds, usually stain green, but variations frequently occur in the color reaction of ingested particles. Background material usually stains green, and a color contrast with the protozoa results. In contrast to preparations stained with hematoxylin, trichrome smears have a transparency which makes it possible to identify imbedded protozoa even in thicker smears. Protozoa and eggs are less subject to distortion, however, in thinner smears. Eggs and larvae usually stain red and contrast strongly with green background. Thin-shelled eggs often collapse when placed in mounting medium, although if the smear is examined immediately they may retain some diagnostic features.

Nonstaining cysts and those staining predominantly red are most frequently associated with incomplete fixation. Obtaining unsatisfactorily stained organisms from specimens submitted in PVA-fixative usually indicates incomplete fixation associated with poor emulsification. Thorough emulsification of preferably *soft* stools will yield critically stained cysts and trophozoites. Degenerate forms stain pale green. Organisms may also appear green if understained or overdestained.

Mononuclear and polymorphonuclear leukocytes, as well as *Blastocytis*, present the same diagnostic problems with this technique as with the technique using hematoxylin. The cytoplasm of pus and tissue cells, however, does stain more greenish than that of the protozoa.

Smears should be examined with an oil immersion lens. Occasionally, large protozoa may be detected with the lower power (10×) objective, and smaller forms, with high dry lenses. Details are more distinct, however, with oil immersion.

Chlorazol black E stain for intestinal protozoa in feces and in tissue

The preparation of the reagents needed for the chlorazol black E staining procedure (basic solution, stock chlorazol black E solution, and carbol-xylene) is described in chapter 96. The stock stain may be kept indefinitely, and stain dilutions may be used repeatedly. However, repeated use "wears out" the stain dilution, and when slides appear visibly red rather than greenish-black at the end of the staining period, the dilution should be discarded. Approximately 20 slides can be stained satisfactorily in a 50-ml coplin jar of diluted stain before deterioration makes change necessary. Deterioration of the stain is dependent on use (slides stained) and not on time, since satisfactory staining may be obtained with stain dilutions up to 30 days old if the number of slides stained has not been excessive. Slides that appear red can be restained in fresh stain.

Optimal dilution and staining time. The optimal dilution and staining time must be determined for each liter of fixative-stain. For this purpose, the series of dilutions and staining periods are suggested in Tables 3 and 4 for intestinal protozoa in feces and tissue, respectively. A solution producing good overnight staining does not appear to overstain when left for periods of several days.

TABLE 3. *Optimal dilution and staining times for chlorazol black E staining of intestinal protozoa in feces*

Dilution		Time (h)
Fixative-stain	Basic solution	
Undiluted	—	2–3
1	1	2–4 or overnight
2	1	2–4
1	2	2 or overnight
1	3	4 or overnight

TABLE 4. *Optimal dilution and staining times for chlorazol black E staining of intestinal protozoa in tissue*

Dilution		Time (h)
Fixative-stain	Distilled water	
Undiluted	—	4–6
1	1	4–8 or overnight
2	1	4–8
1	2	4 or overnight
1	3	8 or overnight

Trial smears and tissue sections should be stained with each dilution according to the techniques given below, and the optimal dilution and time should be selected for routine staining with the "batch" of stain concerned. More than one dilution-time combination may be satisfactory, and the choice of which to use will depend on the laboratory schedule and urgency of diagnosis. The range most commonly found satisfactory is a 1:2 dilution for 2 h or a 1:3 dilution for 4 h or overnight. However, for best results, the exact combination should be determined.

Staining procedure with fecal specimens. Smears from fecal specimens should be prepared in the usual fashion and placed *immediately* in the fixative-stain solution. Organisms preserved in PVA-fixative do not stain well with this procedure.

1. Fixative-stain dilution, 2 h or overnight (for routine use, use dilution and time predetermined from Table 3).
2. Ethyl alcohol, 95%, 10 to 15 s.
3. Carbol-xylene or 100% ethyl alcohol, 5 min.
4. Xylene, 5 min.
5. Mount in Permount or other suitable media.

Staining procedure for protozoa in tissue. Tissue slides are prepared following the usual histological procedures for fixing, embedding, sectioning, and preparing slides. The sections are treated in xylene and alcohol as usual to remove the paraffin and to prepare them for staining. Good stains have been obtained on sections of 5 to 7 μm thickness.

For staining protozoa in tissue with chlorazol black E, the fixative-stain is diluted with the distilled water (Table 4), rather than with the basic solution, and the staining time is twice as long as for fecal smears. The most commonly satisfactory time is about 6 to 7 h with the optimal dilution.

1. Fixative-stain 4 h or overnight (as determined from Table 4).
2. Alcohol, 95%, 10 to 15 s.
3. Carbol-xylene, 5 to 10 min.
4. Xylene, 5 to 10 min.
5. Mount in Permount or other suitable media.

Stain reactions (chlorazol black E). Protozoa in fresh fecal specimens stain green to gray-green; in older stools, organisms are gray to black. Nuclei, chromatoid bodies, karyosomes, and cell membranes stain dark green to black. Ingested red cells may vary from pink to black. *Entamoeba coli* cysts may stain pink or green, and, rarely, *E. histolytica* cysts stain faintly pink. Trophozoites in tissue have the same appearance as those in feces.

Cultivation procedures

Cultivation is time-consuming and requires special materials and equipment; therefore, it is not generally used routinely for the diagnosis of intestinal protozoa. However, it will give a greater number of positive results, provided the laboratory receives fresh specimens (32). It increases the number of organisms available for observation and can revive trophozoites that may have lost their diagnostic morphology. All intestinal protozoa can be cultured in a routine manner with the exception of *Giardia* and *Isospora*. These organisms require specialized techniques, but they will not be presented in this discussion. Although several satisfactory culture media for intestinal protozoa are available, modified Boeck and Drbohlav's medium, to which small quantities of penicillin and streptomycin have been added, has perhaps been most used (6, 32, 34, 40). Balamuth's egg infusion medium (5) is also satisfactory for diagnostic work. The preparation of these culture media is described in chapter 95. Additional details on procedure can be obtained from the references cited and from the manual of Melvin and Brooke (28).

Although *E. histolytica* tends to culture more easily than other species, no differential medium that will isolate this pathogen alone is available. Therefore, after amoebae have been successfully established in a culture, the necessity of differentiating the species by morphological characteristics still exists. Stained wet mounts will help, but permanently stained preparations should be made from the sediments for positive identification and realization of the full effectiveness of cultivation as a diagnostic procedure. The sediments of cultures revealing organisms or questionable objects are mixed in vials with PVA-fixative, and permanently stained films of the fixed sediments are prepared and examined carefully under an oil immersion objective (31). In a group of 878 fecal cultures, Norman and Brooke (31) increased the number of positive identifications by 85% through the examination of permanently stained sediments preserved in PVA-fixative.

Examination of other materials for intestinal protozoa

No delay in the examination of sigmoidoscopic material, abscess aspirates, sputum, and duodenal drainages should occur. Since these specimens can be expected to contain only trophozoites, wet mounts, permanently stained preparations, and cultivation can be used.

Wet mounts prepared from lesions should be sealed with heated paraffin-Vaseline (petroleum jelly) and carefully examined for a considerable period. *E. histolytica* trophozoites frequently take time to become acclimated to the preparation and become free from the coagulum. Care must be taken not to confuse the trophozoites with tissue elements and inflammatory cells. Definite, progressive locomotion should be observed for the microscopist to suspect *E. histolytica*, and final identification should be made from a permanently stained smear. The microscopist must be cautious in identifying amoebas in sputum, since the nonpathogenic *Entamoeba gingivalis* residing in the mouth may be present. *Giardia* in duodenal contents can generally be identified in wet mounts with ease, but permanently stained preparations should be made to record positive findings.

In the examination of aspirates of liver abscesses suspected of being caused by *E. histolytica*, the demonstration of amoebas in the thick pus removed from the abscesses frequently is difficult. Several factors contribute to this difficulty: (i) most of the organisms are in the peripheral area of the abscess and, often, relatively few are free in the abscess contents;

(ii) the organisms may be partially immobilized by coagulum; and (iii) since the fluid is sterile, amoebae will not grow in culture when the material is inoculated in the manner routinely used for stool cultures.

The Amoebiasis Research Unit, Durban, South Africa, has reported great success in using proteolytic enzymes in freeing the amoebas from the aspirates of liver abscesses. The following procedure incorporates recommendations from a unit publication (18) and from Elsdon-Dew (personal communication, 1960).

1. During aspiration, a minimum of two portions of exudate are removed. These are kept separate. The first portion withdrawn, usually yellowish-white, seldom contains amoebae and is not examined routinely. Later portions, which are reddish, are likely to include organisms. The final portion containing most of the material from near the wall is most likely to be positive. (Collapse of the abscess and inflowing blood is believed to release amoebas from the tissue.) Portions obtained on later aspirations, performed after appropriate rest periods, have a greater chance of revealing organisms.

2. Ten units of the enzyme Streptodornase are added to each 1 ml of thick pus, and the mixture is incubated for 30 min at 37 C with repeated shaking. This process frees the amoebae from the coagulum.

3. Centrifuge the mixture at 1,000 rpm for 5 min. The sediments may be microscopically examined in wet mounts or used to inoculate culture media.

4. In culturing the material, the egg slant medium overlaid with Locke's solution is conditioned by inoculation with *Clostridium perfringens*, since the aspirated material may be free from bacteria. This can be done at the time of inoculation with the amoebic pus, although it is preferable, if possible, to precondition the medium for 24 h at 37 C. Sterile rice powder is added when the medium is inoculated. Overlay with a mixture of equal parts of paraffin and petrolatum. Incubate the culture at 37 C, and examine for amoebae after 24 and 48 h.

Examination of urogenital materials for Trichomonas vaginalis

Microscopic examination of wet mounts of urogenital materials is the usual method employed for diagnosing infections of *T. vaginalis*, and cultivation is an effective supplemental procedure. Permanently stained preparations may reveal the presence of the organisms but are not satisfactory for routine diagnosis.

Wet mount examinations. Most of the procedures and precautions discussed above for intestinal protozoa apply to *T. vaginalis* except that there is no need to use temporary stains. Vaginal and urethral discharges and prostatic secretions are usually diluted with a drop of physiological saline solution in preparing wet mounts. Urine specimens and cultures are centrifuged at low speed for 1 min, and a drop of the sediments is removed for preparation of the mounts.

Wet mounts are examined with low power of the compound microscope and reduced illumination. The organisms appear as clear, actively motile structures about the size of pus cells. Presently, the organisms will begin to lose their jerky movement and their undulating membranes may become visible, particularly with higher magnification. Before and during the examination, specimens should not be chilled, since the lowered temperature may stop the organism's movement, which is so important in spotting and identifying the flagellate. Nevertheless, there is no need to bother with warm-stage equipment, since a reasonably warm room and heat from the microscope lamp will usually suffice.

Cultivation procedures. Although the culture media suggested for the intestinal protozoa may be used for *T. vaginalis*, Feinberg's medium is recommended, since it produces good growth, is easier to prepare, and keeps well (17). Preparation and use of this proteolyzed liver medium are described in chapter 95.

Because of the effectiveness of the cultivation for revealing infections due to *T. vaginalis*, it is advisable to use it routinely to supplement the examination of direct wet mounts of urogenital materials. This combination of techniques may almost double the number of positive results found on permanently stained smears (33).

Culture medium may be inoculated with vaginal and urethral discharges and prostatic secretions at the time of clinical examination and taken to the laboratory for incubation. Urine specimens should be centrifuged and the sediments used as the inocula. Cultures are generally examined after 24 and 48 h of incubation, and centrifugation of the cultures may be used to assist in detecting light infections.

Permanently stained preparations. Permanently stained smears of urogenital materials may reveal *T. vaginalis* infections although they are not recommended for routine diagnostic use. Stain preparations are usually unnecessary for confirmation of diagnosis but may be made for a permanent record. The trichrome stain described above or stains used primarily for other purposes may be satisfactory for the experienced microscopist to determine the presence of *T. vaginalis*. Some of the other stains are Gram's, Sellers', and Papanicolaou's. Permanently stained preparations alone should not be considered satisfactory for the diagnosis of *T. vaginalis*. For example, with Papanicolaou smears, false-positive and false-negative findings for *T. vaginalis* may approach 50% and should not be relied upon for the diagnosis of this parasite (33). The reduced proficiency of stained preparations results from the presence of confusing artifacts and distortion of the organism and its loss of motion. Furthermore, in reference to the Papanicolaou smears, great care should be exercised in the diagnosis of cancer in the presence of *T. vaginalis* infection, since the degenerative cellular changes produced by the flagellates may mimic carcinogenic change (14). This emphasizes the importance of confirming the diagnosis of *T. vaginalis* in wet mounts of clinical materials and culture sediments.

LITERATURE CITED

1. Anderson, H. H., W. L. Bostick, and H. G. Johnstone. 1953. Amebiasis—pathology, diagnosis, and chemotherapy. Charles C Thomas, Publisher, Springfield, Ill.
2. Andrews, J. 1934. The diagnosis of intestinal protozoa from purges and normally-passed stools. J. Parasitol. **20**:253–254.
3. Arensburger, K. E., and E. K. Markell. 1960. A simple combination direct smear and fecal concentrate for permanent stained preparations. Amer. J. Clin. Pathol. **44**:50–51.
4. Ash, J. E., and S. Spitz. 1945. Pathology of tropical diseases. W. B. Saunders Co., Philadelphia.
5. Balamuth, W. 1946. Improved egg yolk infusion for cultivation of *Entamoeba histolytica* and other intestinal protozoa. Amer. J. Clin. Pathol. **16**:380.
6. Boeck, W. C., and J. Drbohlav. 1925. The cultivation of *Endamoeba histolytica*. Amer. J. Hyg. **5**:371–407.
7. Brooke, M. M., A. W. Donaldson, and E. Brown. 1954. An amebiasis survey in a Veterans Administration Hospital, Chamblee, Georgia with comparison of technics. Amer. J. Trop. Med. Hyg. **3**:615–620.
8. Brooke, M. M., and M. Goldman. 1949. Polyvinyl alcohol-fixative as a preservative and adhesive for protozoa in dysenteric stools and other liquid materials. J. Lab. Clin. Med. **34**:1554–1560.
9. Brooke, M. M., and D. M. Melvin. 1969. Morphology of diagnostic stages of intestinal parasites of man. Pub. Health Serv. Publ. No. 1966, Center for Disease Control, Atlanta, Ga.
10. Brooke, M. M., D. M. Melvin, R. Sappenfield, F. Payne, F. R. N. Carter, A. C. Offutt, and W. W. Fraye. 1955. Studies of a waterborne outbreak of amebiasis. South Bend, Indiana. III. Investigation of family contacts. Amer. J. Hyg. **62**:214–226.
11. Burrows, R. B. 1961. Prevalence of amebiasis in the United States and Canada. Amer. J. Trop. Med. Hyg. **10**:172–184.
12. Burrows, R. B. 1965. Microscopic diagnosis of the parasites of man. Yale Univ. Press, New Haven.
13. Burrows, R. B. 1967. A new fixative and technic for the diagnosis of intestinal parasites. Amer. J. Clin. Pathol. **48**:342–346.
14. De León, E. 1971. Trichomoniasis, p. 124–138. *In* Raúl A. Marcial-Rojas (ed.), Pathology of protozoal and helminthic diseases. The Williams & Wilkins Co., Baltimore.
15. Dobell, C., and F. W. O'Connor. 1921. Intestinal protozoa of man. William Wood, Publisher, New York.
16. Faust, E. C., J. S. D'Antoni, V. Odum, M. J. Miller, C. Peres, W. Sawitz, L. F. Thomen, J. E. Tobie, and J. H. Walker. 1938. A critical study of clinical laboratory technics for the diagnosis of protozoan cysts and helminth eggs in feces. Amer. J. Trop. Med. **18**:169–183.
17. Feinberg, J. G., and M. J. Whittington. 1957. A culture for *Trichomonas vaginalis* Donne and species of *Candida*. J. Clin. Pathol. **10**:327–329.
18. Freedman, L., S. E. Maddison, and R. Elsdon-Dew. 1958. Moxenic cultures of *Entamoeba histolytica* derived from human liver abscesses. S. Afr. J. Med. Sci. **23**:9–12.
19. Gleason, N., M. Goldman, and R. K. Carver. 1960. An enriched egg extract medium for recovering viable *Entamoeba histolytica* trophozoites from fecal suspensions kept at room temperature for four days. Amer. J. Trop. Med. Hyg. **9**:46–49.
20. Gleason, N. N., and G. R. Healy. 1965. Modification and evaluation of Kohn's one-step staining technique for intestinal protozoa in feces or tissue. Amer. J. Clin. Pathol. **43**:494–496.
21. Goldman, M., and M. M. Brooke. 1953. Protozoans in stools unpreserved and preserved in PVA-fixative. Pub. Health Rep. **68**:703–706.
22. Goldman, M., and S. A. Johnson. 1950. Deep-freeze preservation of stool specimens containing intestinal parasites. J. Parasitol. **36**:88.
23. Gurevitch, J., and J. Delightish. 1947. Survival time of *Endamoeba histolytica* in feces. Harefuah **32**:60.
24. Hunter, G. W., W. W. Frye, and J. C. Swartzwelder. 1966. Manual of tropical medicine. W. B. Saunders Co., Philadelphia.
25. Kohn, J. 1960. A one stage permanent staining method for fecal protozoa. Dapim Refuiim Med. Quart. Israel **19**:160–161.
26. Markell, E. K. 1956. A comparison of three staining techniques for protozoan parasites as applied to PVA-preserved fecal specimens. J. Parasitol. **42**:478.
27. Markell, E. K., and M. Voge. 1971. Medical parasitology. W. B. Saunders Co., Philadelphia.
28. Melvin, D. M., and M. M. Brooke. 1969. Laboratory procedures for the diagnosis of intestinal parasites. Pub. Health Serv. Publ. No. 1969, Government Printing Office, Washington, D.C.
29. Meyer, K. F., and H. G. Johnstone. 1935. Laboratory diagnosis of amebiasis. Amer. J. Pub. Health **25**:405–414.
30. Nair, C. P. 1953. Rapid staining of intestinal amoebae on wet mounts. Nature (London) **172**:1051.
31. Norman, L., and M. M. Brooke. 1955. The effectiveness of the PVA-fixative technique in revealing intestinal amebae in diagnostic cultures. Amer. J. Trop. Med. Hyg. **4**:479–482.
32. Norman, L., and M. M. Brooke. 1955. The use of penicillin and streptomycin in the routine cultivation of amebae from fecal specimens. Amer. J. Trop. Med. Hyg. **4**:472–478.
33. Perl, G. 1972. Errors in the diagnosis of *Trichomonas vaginalis* infection. Obstet. Gynecol. **39**:7–9.
34. Reardon, L. V., and C. W. Rees. 1939. The cultivation of *Endamoeba histolytica* without serum. J. Parasitol. **25**(Suppl.):13–14.
35. Ritchie, L. S. 1948. An ether sedimentation technique for routine stool examinations. Bull. U.S. Army Med. Dep. **8**:326.
36. Ritchie, L. S., C. Pan, and G. W. Hunter III. 1952. A

Chapter 67

Blood and Hematopoietic Parasites

JOSEPH H. MILLER, LIONEL G. WARREN, STANLEY H. ABADIE, AND J. CLYDE SWARTZWELDER

MALARIA

The disease entity malaria is caused by protozoa of the genus *Plasmodium*. The four species concerned are *P. vivax*, *P. falciparum*, *P. malariae*, and *P. ovale*. The last species is relatively uncommon and will not be discussed. After the inoculation of humans with sporozoites by an infected mosquito, the parasite undergoes schizogony in the liver cells. This cycle continues for various periods of time, depending on the species and strain, but periodically parasites are released into the blood stream. These invade erythrocytes, and another schizogonic cycle ensues within the cell (Fig. 1). The *definitive diagnosis* is based on finding and identifying these erythrocytic stages. The parasites are easily found and identified in thick blood films. Thin blood films are useful for the detailed study of malaria parasites when they are known to be present but they are less efficient and impractical in the routine search for these organisms.

Methods of preparation of thick blood films

The practice of preparing thick and thin films on the same slide is not a satisfactory procedure because preparation techniques for staining differ.

Peripheral blood from a finger or ear lobe, or freshly drawn venous blood without an anticoagulant, must be used for the preparation of consistently good films. Once a puncture of the skin has been made, the area is wiped vigorously with dry cotton to remove disinfectants and other contaminants.

Method of staining (Wilcox [7]). A spherical drop is permitted to well up, and the surface of a chemically clean slide is touched to the top of this drop. The slide is inverted and the drop is "puddled" (stirred rapidly with the edge of a clean slide or applicator stick) to the size of a dime. A number of thick films may be placed on the same slide. The thickness of the film is optimal when the film "crawls" but does not form an immediate drop when the slide is held vertically.

The thick films are allowed to dry without heat until they no longer shine. Optimal staining results are to be expected only when thick films are processed within a short period after drying. A delay of 8 h or more may result in unsatisfactory films.

Thick films are immersed in distilled water until all hemoglobin is removed. Upon removal from the distilled water, films are immediately flooded with Giemsa stain (1 drop to 1 ml of phosphate buffer, pH 7) for 30 to 60 min. The films are washed briefly in buffered water to remove excess stain and allowed to dry without heat. For additional methods, see Walker (5).

Methods of preparation of thin blood films

The thin film is prepared in exactly the same way as for a routine differential blood count.

Method of staining. Thin films are fixed in absolute methanol for 1 min and allowed to dry. They are then flooded with Giemsa stain (1 part stain to 50 parts phosphate buffer at pH 6.4) and allowed to react for 30 to 60 min. The stain is flooded off with copious amounts of phosphate buffer, drained, and allowed to dry. For additional methods, see Walker (5).

Laboratory diagnosis of malaria

In patients suspected of having malaria, two or three thick smears should be taken at intervals of 6 to 18 h for 3 successive days. One hundred microscopic fields should be examined before a film is declared negative for parasites (5).

It is important to understand certain aspects of the erythrocytic shizogony of the three common species of malaria in order to diagnose blood films.

1. Merozopes of *P. falciparum* enter erythrocytes of any age and cause a physiological change in the plasma membrane of the erythrocyte which results in its becoming sticky. Therefore, intermediate stages of schizogony (late trophozoites and schizonts) are not ordinarily seen in the peripheral blood. These stages are in the erythrocytes adherent to the endothelial

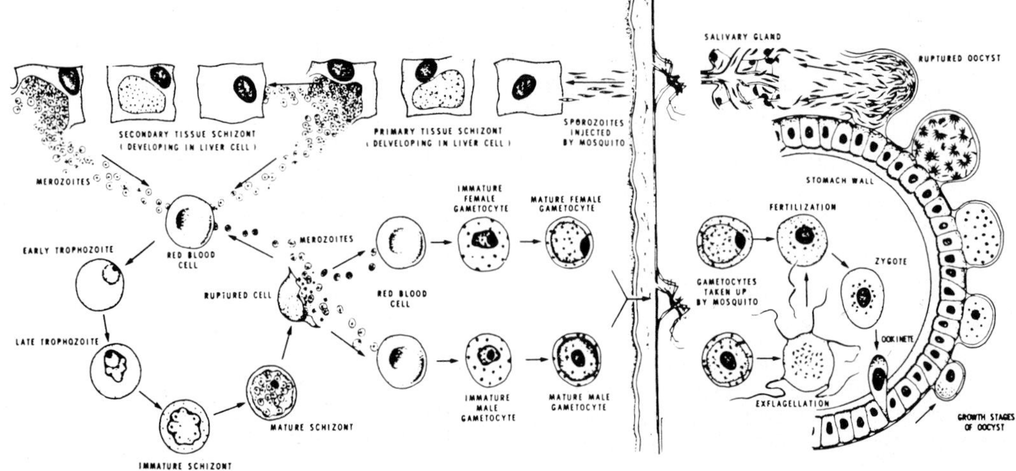

CYCLE IN MAN

CYCLE IN MOSQUITO

FIG. 1. *Schematic representation of typical malaria life cycle modified from Hunter, Frye, Swartzwelder* (2).

lining of blood vessels. In peripheral blood, usually only early trophozoites (ring stages) or characteristic crescent-shaped gametocytes, or both, are present.

2. Merozoites of *P. vivax* enter only young erythrocytes, whereas merozoites of *P. malariae* invade only mature erythrocytes. There is no physiological change in the plasma membrane of the erythrocytes parasitized by these species, and all infected cells circulate freely and continuously. All stages of the erythrocytic schizogonic cycle are present at all times, although the proportion of one stage to another (i.e., trophozoites to schizonts) varies with the period of time from the last paroxysm; i.e., immediately after a paroxysm young trophozoites will predominate, whereas just before a paroxysm schizonts will be most numerous.

The following keys and the description of morphological characteristics given in Table 1, to be used in conjunction with Fig. 2–7, will serve to differentiate and identify the several species of malarial parasites in thick and thin films.

Key to the Differential Diagnosis of Malaria in Thick Blood Films (*Fig.* 2–4)

1. *No intermediate stages present.* Usually only characteristic rings (rings, exclamation marks, swallows, comets, etc.) or crescent-shaped gametocytes, or both, present.—*P. falciparum.* (Gametocytes may be distorted or "round-up"; see Fig. 4.)
2. *Intermediate stages present.—P. vivax or P. malariae.*
   - A. *Cytoplasm of trophozoites is often irregular, with streamers; spidery appearance.* Fine golden pigment. Stippling occasionally seen around parasite.—*P. vivax.*
   - B. *Trophozoites are small, rounded, and compact.* Pigment dark and heavy.—*P. malariae.*

Key to the Differentiation of the Three Common Malaria Species in Thin Blood Films (*Fig.* 5–7)

1. *No intermediate stages present* (no late trophozoites or schizonts). Usually only characteristic rings (rodlike nucleus; rings located at periphery of red cell; binucleate rings; small rings; frequently multiple rings in a red cell) or crescent-shaped gametocytes, or both.—*P. falciparum.*
2. *Intermediate stages present* (late trophozoites and schizonts).—*P. vivax* or *P. malariae.*
   - A. *Parasitized red cells enlarged and pale;* trophozoites with irregular outlines; pigment fine; Schüffner's dots may be present.—*P. vivax.*
   - B. *Parasitized red cells normal in size and color;* growing forms compact; pigment coarse; no stippling of the red cells.—*P. malariae.*

Note: Schüffner's dots are *not* always present in *P. vivax* infection. Crescents are *not* always present in *P. falciparum* infection. Band forms are *not* always present in *P. malariae* infection.

HEMOFLAGELLATES

Trypanosomatidae

Leishmaniases and trypanosomiases. The hemoflagellates are members of the class Mastigophora of the phylum Protozoa. Some species may circulate in the blood stream. At times they may be present in muscle and lymph nodes. Other species primarily parasitize mononuclear cells of the hemopoietic organs, particularly the reticuloendothelial cells. Typically, hemoflagellates possess a flagellum during one or more of their stages and also an alternating phase in the intestine of some insects. The species of importance to man include: *Leishmania donovani*, *Leishmania tropica*, *Leishmania braziliensis*, *Trypanosoma gambiense*, *Trypanosoma rhodesiense*, and *Trypanosoma cruzi*. *L. donovani*, *L. braziliensis*, and *T. cruzi* are endemic in some area of the Americas. Additional species and subspecies names for the genus *Leishmania* may be found in the literature (1).

Hemoflagellates are characterized by (i) a single cell body, (ii) a nucleus, (iii) a kinetoplast consisting of a rodlike parabasal body and a blepharoplast, and (iv) an axoneme originating in the blepharoplast which in some forms extends beyond the anterior (i.e., flagellar) end of the body as a free flagellum. The hemoflagellates of man have four morphological types: trypaniform, crithidiform, leptomonad, and leishmaniform (Table 2). However, the various species of hemoflagellates may not show all of these morphological types during their life history. Species of *Leishmania* usually exist in the leishmaniform stage in humans and in the leptomonad stage in their insect host, and have neither crithidiform nor trypaniform stages. Species of *Trypanosoma* usually are found in the trypaniform stage in man and in the crithidiform stage in the insect host, and, with the notable exception of *T. cruzi*, which manifests all four morphological types, have no leptomonad or leishmaniform stage (Table 3.)

Collection and examination of tissues for hemoflagellates

Blood, marrow, and spleen pulp examination. Thick and thin blood films can be prepared as described for malaria diagnosis. Similarly, scrapings from cutaneous lesions and tissue aspirates obtained by puncture methods can be prepared as thin smears.

Culture methods. Diphasic blood-agar cultures (see chapter 95) can be useful in the diagnosis of all hemoflagellate infections. Diphasic blood-agar cultures should be inoculated with 2 ml of sterile heparinized venous blood. At least three cultures should be inoculated. Flagellates, if present, will usually appear within 3 to 7 days, but occasionally 1 month may be

TABLE 1. *Comparison of the morphological characteristics of malarial organisms in Wright-stained thin films (see Fig. 5–7)*

Characteristic	*P. falciparum*	*P. vivax*	*P. malariae*
Trophozoites	Signet rings, typically very small and delicate with vacuole; chromatin rod-shaped or as two-nuclear granules near each other or at opposite poles of the cytoplasm; sometimes at edge of corpuscle (applied forms); filamentous "tenue" forms seen	Signet rings of various sizes with vacuole and single chromatin dot	Rings of various sizes with vacuole and single chromatin dot; slow growth
Trophozoites	*Later stages usually not seen in peripheral blood* except in moribund cases; small, round or oval, with early clumping of pigment in a single black mass	Growing forms irregular in outline, amoeboid, delicate structure; vacuole retained during early stages	Vacuole soon disappears; *compact* forms; difficult to differentiate from gametocytes; occasionally band forms
Mature schizont ("rosette")	Distinctly smaller than a red blood cell; *usually not found in peripheral blood*	Larger than a normal red blood cell; may fill the enlarged blood cell	Slightly smaller than a normal red blood cell
Number of merozoites in mature schizont	Eight to 24 arranged about a central pigment mass; *usually not seen in peripheral blood*	Twelve to 24 irregularly arranged about a central pigment mass	Six to 12 regularly arranged around a central mass
Gametocytes	Crescentic or sausage-shaped; often apparently free in the blood; no vacuole; called "crescents"	Ovoid or round, larger than a normal red cell; no vacuole; compact	Round or slightly ovoid; size of a normal red blood cell; no vacuole; compact
Infected red blood corpuscles	Not enlarged, sometimes smaller than normal; in later stages paler, purple, or at times brassy	Enlarged and pale; occasionally slate-gray in color	Not enlarged; may be slightly contracted
Stippling	Maurer's dots or clefts (rare): at times coarse, irregular, basophilic mottling of red blood cells; not commonly seen	Schüffner's dots (eosinophilic) occasionally present	No stippling
Multiple infection of red blood cells	Common	Occasional	Rare
Pigment (hemozoin) in parasite	Blacker than others, as coarse granules or small clumps; tends to clump early	Yellowish-brown, small, fine granules or rodlets	Coarse, dark-brown granules, rods, or clumps

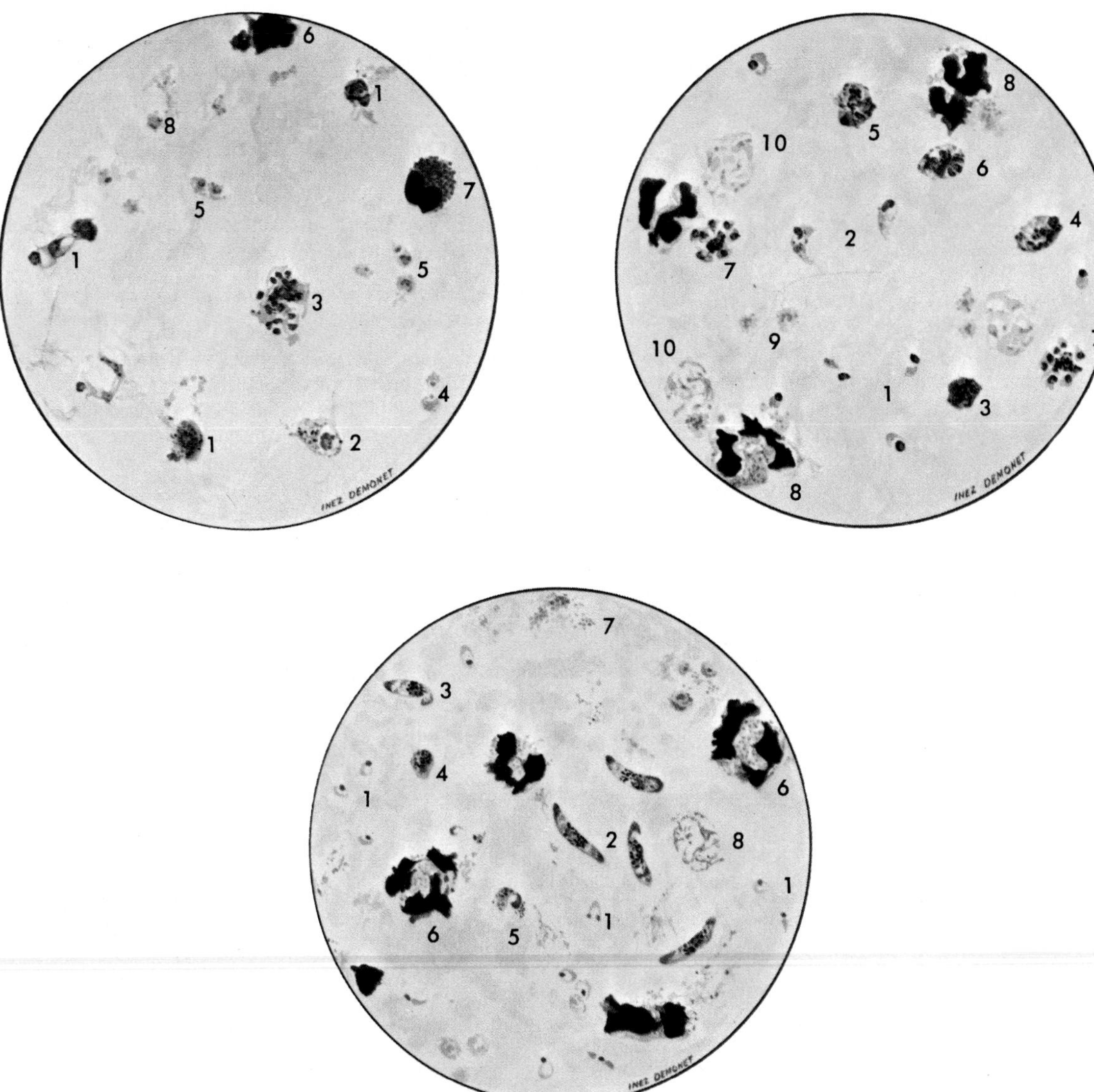

FIG. 2. (*top left*). *P. vivax—thick film.* (*1*) *Amoeboid trophozoites.* (2) *Schizont, two divisions of chromatin.* (3) *Mature schizont.* (4) *Microgametocyte.* (5) *Blood platelets.* (6) *Nucleus of neutrophil.* (7) *Eosinophil.* (8) *Blood platelet associated with cellular remains of young erythrocytes.*

FIG. 3. (*top right*). *P. malariae—thick film.* (*1*) *Small trophozoites.* (2) *Growing trophozoites.* (3) *Mature trophozoites.* (4, 5, 6) *Schizonts (presegmenting) with varying numbers of divisions of the chromatin.* (7) *Mature shizonts.* (8) *Nucleus of leukocyte.* (9) *Blood platelets.* (*10*) *Cellular remains of young erythrocytes.*

FIG. 4. (*bottom*). *P. falciparum—thick film.* (*1*) *Small trophozoites.* (2) *Gametocytes—normal.* (3) *Slightly distorted gametocyte.* (4) *"Rounded-up" gametocyte.* (5) *Disintegrated gametocyte.* (6) *Nucleus of leukocyte.* (7) *Blood platelets.* (8) *Cellular remains of young erythrocyte.*

FIG. 5. *Plasmodium vivax. Giemsa stain. ×2,000. (upper left) Young trophozoites. A, B, young ring forms; C, D, half-grown trophozoites. (upper right) E, F, G, trophozoites with nuclear chromatin ready to subdivide. (middle left) H, I, young schizonts showing first division of nuclear chromatin; J, K, older schizonts showing four or more subdivisions of nuclear chromatin. (middle right) Half-grown schizonts; L, M, N, schizonts showing 7, 8, and 10 nuclear subdivisions. (lower left) Mature schizonts; O, P, Q, mature schizonts showing complete subdivision of nuclear chromatin and clumping of malarial pigment. (lower right) Gametocytes or sexual forms; R, male gametocyte or microgametocyte, with diffuse nuclear chromatin; S, T, female gametocyte or macrogametocyte with compact chromatin.*

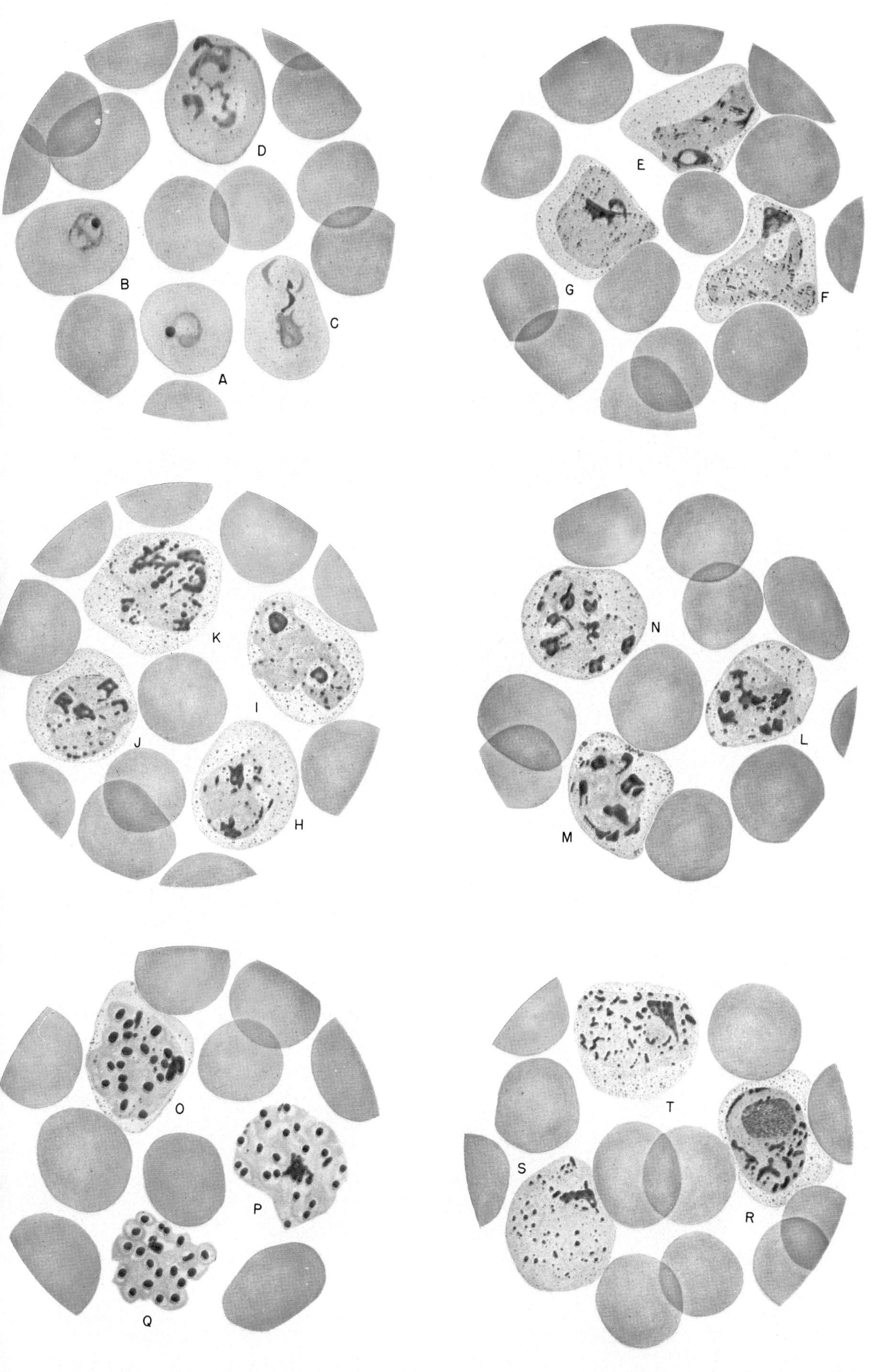
D
B
C
A
E
G
F
K
I
J
H
N
L
M
O
P
Q
T
S
R

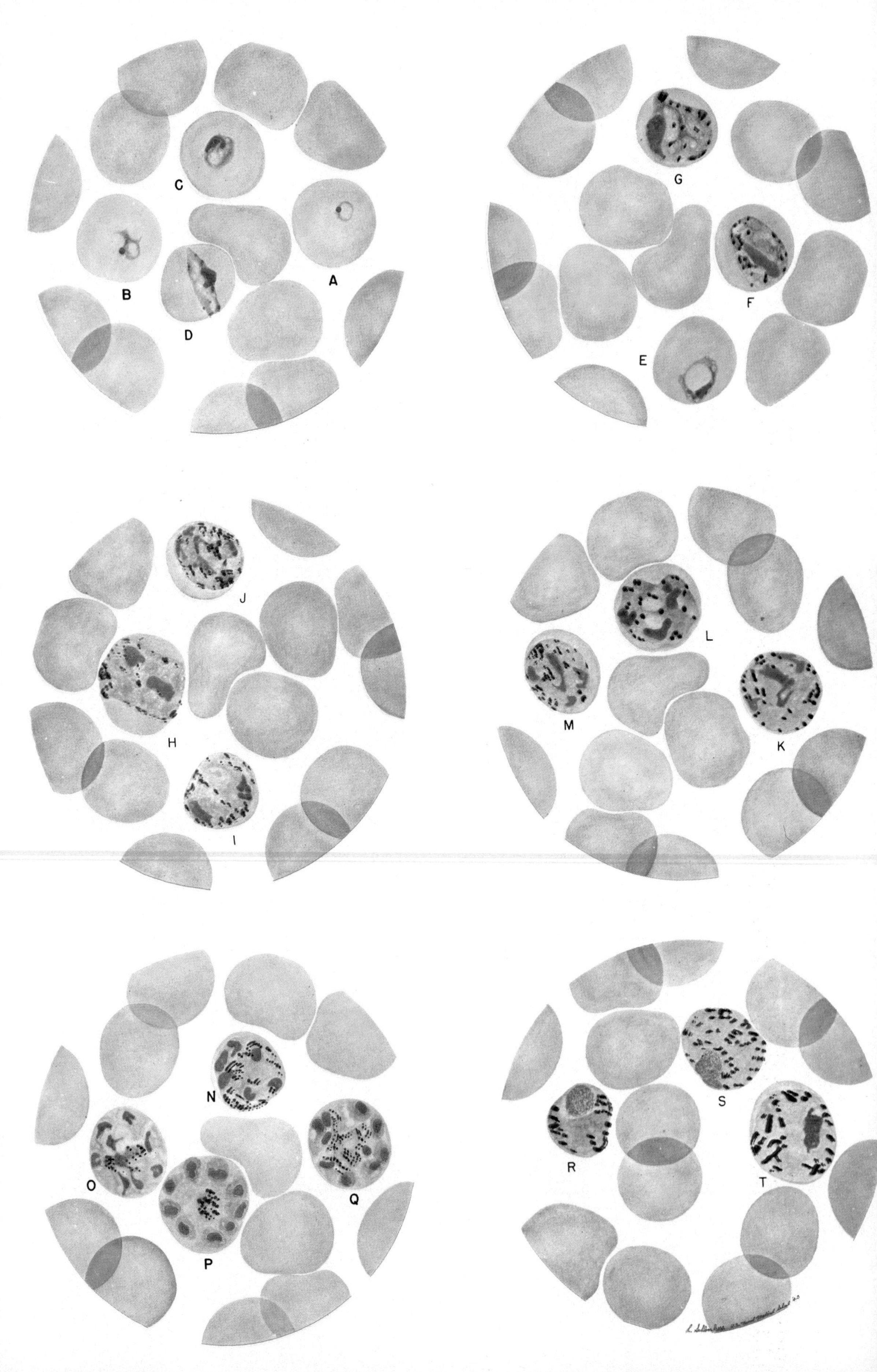
C
B
A
D
G
F
E
J
H
I
L
M
K
N
O
Q
P
S
R
T

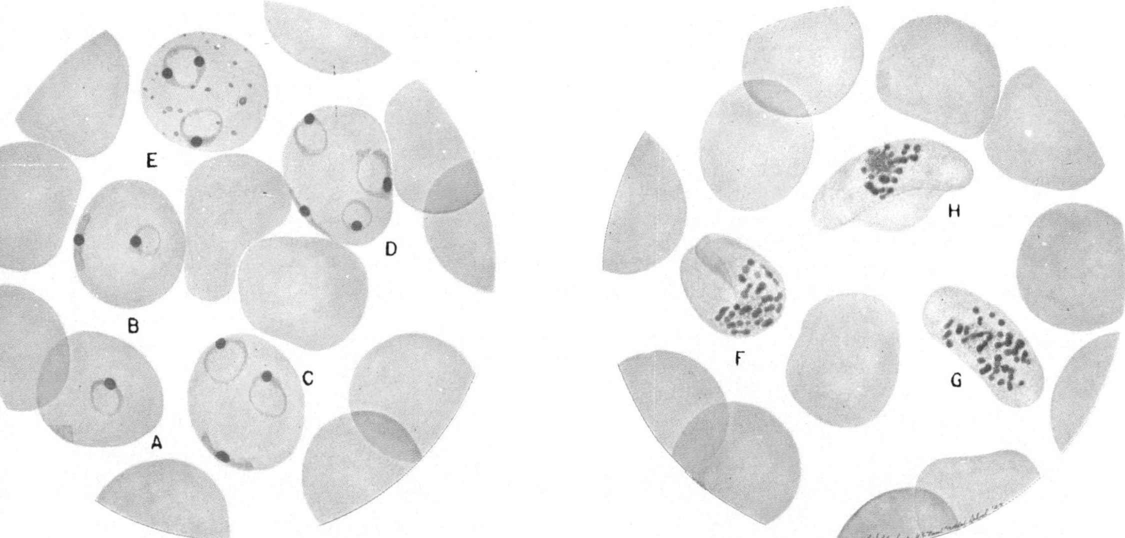

FIG. 7. *Plasmodium falciparum. Giemsa stain. ×2,000. (left) Trophozoites in peripheral blood. A, young ring forms; B, C, D, young trophozoites (note multiple infections of cells and appliqué forms); E, examples of oldest forms normally found in peripheral blood. (right) Gametocytes or sexual forms in peripheral blood. F, gametocyte folded over; G, microgametocyte or male gametocyte; H, female or microgametocyte. (Note diffuse chromatin in G and compact chromatin in H.)*

TABLE 2. *Morphological types of hemoflagellates*

Type	Appearance
Trypaniform (trypanosome)	Spindle-shaped (8 to 30 × 1 to 3 nm). Undulating membrane present. Free flagellum present. *Kinetoplast is posterior to the nucleus.*
Crithidiform	Spindle-shaped (10 to 20 × 3 nm). Undulating membrane present. Free flagellum present. *Kinetoplast immediately anterior to the nucleus.*
Leptomonad	Spindle-shaped (14 to 20 × 1.5 to 3.5 nm). *No* undulating membrane. Free flagellum. *Kinetoplast at extreme anterior (flagellar) end of body.*
Leishmaniform (Leishman-Donovan or L-D body)[a]	Ovoid or round (2 to 4 nm in breadth). *No* undulating membrane. *No* free flagellum. *Kinetoplast with short axoneme.*

[a] Leishmaniform bodies (Leishman-Donovan or L-D bodies) should not be confused with the Donovan bodies of *Granuloma inguinale* in tissue. *Histoplasma capsulatum*, a yeastlike organism producing histoplasmosis in humans resembles closely the leishmaniform bodies found in *Leishmania* and *T. cruzi* infections, but lacks a rodlike kinetoplast.

required. The culture can be examined by making a wet mount of a drop of the fluid overlay. Motile organisms can readily be seen in wet-mount preparations. For a permanent record, stained smears can be made from the fluid overlay. *Cultivation of hemoflagellates should always be done at room temperature (22 to 25 C), never at 37 C.*

Genus Leishmania

There are three major diseases of humans caused by species of the genus *Leishmania*: visceral leishmaniasis caused by *L. donovani*, cutaneous leishmaniasis caused by *L. tropica* and *L. braziliensis*, and mucocutaneous leishmaniasis caused by *L. braziliensis*. Although all

FIG. 6. *Plasmodium malariae. Giemsa stain. ×2,000. (upper left) Young trophozoite. A, B, C, progressively older ring forms; D, band trophozoite. (upper right) Half-grown trophozoite. E, ring form; F, G, mature trophozoites, (Note amount of pigment and compactness of cytoplasm.) (middle left) Young schizonts. H, band schizont; I, J, three- and five-nucleated schizonts. (Note large amount of pigment.) (middle right) Half-grown schizonts, K, L, M, four- to six-nucleated schizonts. (Note amount of pigment.) (lower left) Mature shizonts. N, O, P, Q, eight- to ten-nucleated schizonts ready to segment and release merozoites. (Note "daisy" forms.) (lower right) Gametocytes or sexual forms. R, S, male gametocytes or microgametocytes; T, female gametocyte or macrogametocyte.*

TABLE 3. *Leishmaniases and trypanosomiases*

Organism	Stages of parasites found in human infections			
	Leishmaniform	Leptomonad	Crithidiform	Trypaniform
Leishmania donovani	In man: parasites are intracellular in reticuloendothelial cells of visceral organs; occasionally seen in blood smears in mononuclear cells	In culture and insect host (sandfly)		
Leishmania tropica	In man: parasites located in reticuloendothelial cells of the skin	In culture and sandfly		
Leishmania braziliensis	In man: parasites located in reticuloendothelial cells of the skin and mucous membranes	In culture and sandfly		
Trypanosoma gambiense			In insect host (tsetse fly)	In man: blood stream, lymph nodes, spinal fluid, and brain; also in tsetse fly
Trypanosoma rhodesiense			In insect host and in culture	In man and in tsetse fly
Trypanosoma cruzi.	In man: heart muscle, lymph nodes, and other organs	In insect	In insect, tissue, and in culture	In man: blood stream, and other tissues; also in insect
Trypanosoma rangeli	In insect	In insect	In insect	In man: blood; also in insect

of these species, and perhaps certain others, present distinct clinical characteristics, the laboratory diagnosis depends upon the demonstration of the leishmaniform stage in human tissue. The various species are not distinguishable morphologically one from another. Ramanowski dyes (e.g., Giemsa stain) should be employed to stain material collected for the detection of *Leishmania*. Characteristically, these dyes stain chromatin of the nucleus and other nucleic acid-containing structures a brilliant red or violet, whereas the cytoplasm is stained a pale blue.

Leishmania donovani. *L. donovani* is the etiological agent of kala-azar, and occurs in the reticuloendothelial cells of the viscera, particularly the spleen, bone marrow, and liver. The diagnostic stages are as follows.

1. *L. donovani* has an aflagellar stage in man and a flagellate stage which can be detected in cultures. The aflagellar, or leishmanial, stage occurs and multiplies in the cytoplasm of reticuloendothelial cells. The leishmanial forms are seen in groups. Individually they appear as round or oval bodies ranging from 2 to 3 nm in major diameter (Fig. 8). Within these leishmanial bodies, two distinct chromatin-containing structures can be seen: the nucleus and the kinetoplast. The cytoplasm of the parasite often stains the same as the host cell cytoplasm, and only the nucleus and kinetoplast can be seen against a background of parasite-host cell cytoplasm.

2. The flagellar culture forms, or leptomonad stage, of *L. donovani* are spindle-shaped organisms measuring 10 to 20 nm in length, not including the length of the flagellum, which may equal the body length. The pale blue-staining cytoplasm contains a centrally placed nucleus and a kinetoplast located at one end of the spindle. The free trailing flagellum arises from the kinetoplast. Dividing forms, possessing two flagella, nuclei, and kinetoplasts, are frequently seen.

Diagnosis is made by the following procedures.

1. *Examination of thin blood smears.* Although leishmanial forms may be detected in monocytes circulating in the peripheral blood, the percentage of positives reported by this method is highly variable in different areas, and usually many films must be examined. Blood smears prepared for differential blood counts are suitable and may be stained with any Romanowski-type dye. Leishmaniform bodies may also be detected in thick blood films and should not be confused with malaria parasites.

2. *Cultivation of tissue or blood.* The culture of material obtained by puncture of bone mar-

row, liver, spleen, or glands may yield leishmanial bodies when other methods have failed. However, when the tissues are negative upon examination under a microscope, the cultures derived from these materials usually are negative. In contrast, the cultivation of peripheral blood may increase the probability of positive findings when direct examination of a blood smear proves negative. *Leishmania* spp. can be cultured on diphasic blood-agar medium (see Chapter 95).

3. *Examination of bone marrow smears*. This is one of the best methods of diagnosis of kala-azar. Bone marrow material obtained by gentle aspiration from a sternal puncture is placed upon a glass slide, and this material is used to prepare slides which are stained with Giemsa or some other Ramonowski dye. Bone marrow smears will detect about 80% of the positive cases.

4. *Examination of splenic pulp smears and other tissues*. Puncture of the spleen is ordinarily not employed as a diagnostic procedure in the United States as it is attended with danger. This danger is considered slight in kala-azar patients in the hands of an experienced operator (1). Splenic puncture should be done only when the organ is enlarged and projects some distance below the ribs. The procedure of splenic puncture should be preceded by careful blood examination for dyscrasias which might complicate or contraindicate the procedure; if leishmanial forms were detected, there would be no need for splenic puncture. The spleen pulp is smeared upon a glass slide and stained with a Romanowski dye by the usual procedures. The parasites will be found in the reticuloendothelial elements of the spleen pulp, and rarely in the blood from the spleen. Spleen puncture will detect 85 to 90% of positive cases. Diagnostic material may be obtained by aspirating pulp from an enlarged liver or juices from an enlarged lymphatic gland. However, these materials are not as effective diagnostically as bone marrow and spleen aspirates.

Leishmania tropica and Leishmania braziliensis. *L. tropica* and *L. braziliensis* are etiological agents of cutaneous leishmaniasis. *L. braziliensis* also may be associated with oronasal leishmaniasis (espundia).

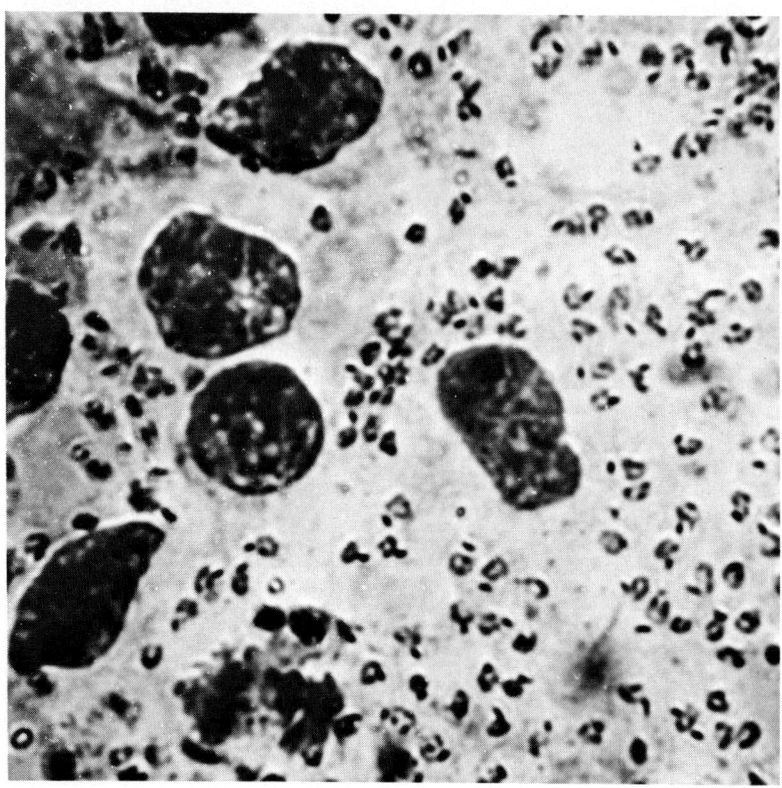

FIG. 8. *Leishmania donovani in stained smear from spleen puncture.*

The diagnostic stages of *L. tropica* and *L. braziliensis* are indistinguishable from *L. donovani* or from each other.

Examination of smears of tissue or aspirate obtained from lesion. The best procedure is to insert a fine hypodermic needle into the raised margin of the lesion and aspirate the interior of the lesion beneath the exudate layer. The aspirate is then fixed and stained for leishmanial bodies. Smears prepared directly from the surface of the lesions are seldom positive. Material obtained from biopsy at the base or side of the lesion should be spread upon a glass microscope slide by compressing the tissue with another glass slide and sliding the two halves of the sandwich in opposite directions. Both slides may then be fixed and stained for leishmanial bodies as described for *L. donovani*.

Cultivation of tissue or exudate. Material is obtained from the lesion as for the preparation of smears, but is inoculated into diphasic blood-agar cultures. The flagellar stages observed in cultures are identical to those seen in cultures of *L. donovani*.

Genus Trypanosoma

Three types of trypanosomiasis occur in humans: (i) African trypanosomiasis caused by *T. gambiense* and *T. rhodesiense*, (ii) Chagas' disease (pathogenic American trypanosomiasis) caused by *T. cruzi*, and (iii) benign American trypanosomiasis caused by *T. rangeli*. In all three types of trypanosomiasis, the flagellar trypanosome stage can be observed in the peripheral blood. The morphology of the bloodstream stage is diagnostic for each of the three types. In the case of *T. cruzi*, an aflagellar intracellular tissue stage also occurs. As in the case of the *Leishmania* species, trypanosomes are best stained with Romanowski dyes.

Trypanosoma gambiense and Trypanosoma rhodesiense. *T. gambiense* and *T. rhodesiense* are the etiological agents of West and East African sleeping sickness, respectively. In the diagnostic stage, they appear as polymorphic spindle-shaped flagellates which vary in length from 15 to 30 nm. Each possesses a more or less centrally located nucleus, and at one end is a kinetoplast from which the flagellum arises. All three structures stain deep red or violet with Ramanowski dyes. The flagellum runs from the kinetoplast at one end of the organism within an undulating membrane to the opposite end, and may terminate there or may continue as a free trailing flagellum. The kinetoplast in African trypanosomes appears as a small dot from which the flagellum arises. Dividing forms may be seen in smears (see Fig. 9).

Diagnostic procedures are as follows.

1. *Thick or thin blood films.* Typical trypanosome forms may be seen. Fresh unstained cover-slip preparations of blood may reveal sparse trypanosomes by their motility. However, the trypanosomes are frequently rare or impossible to find in the peripheral blood.

2. *Examination of fluid aspirated from an enlarged lymph gland.* A stained smear of fluid from an enlarged lymph node is the most reliable procedure for diagnosis in the early stages of the disease. Thick and thin films should be prepared from the lymph aspirate.

3. *Examination of cerebrospinal fluid.* The cerebrospinal fluid should be centrifuged (ca. $600 \times g$), and stained smears should be prepared from the sediment. Trypanosomes will be found even in early light infections by this technique.

4. *Cultivation on diphasic blood-agar medium.* Samples of blood or gland juices can be cultured in diphasic blood-agar medium. Usually, the African trypanosomes are difficult to isolate in culture. The forms seen in cultures are trypaniform stages and crithidial stages. The latter possess a kinetoplast situated close to the nucleus, but towards the free trailing flagellum end of the organism. A small undulating membrane will be present.

Trypanosoma cruzi. *T. cruzi* is the etiological agents of Chagas' disease. Its diagnostic stages are as follows.

1. *Trypaniform stage in blood.* The trypaniform stage of *T. cruzi* is about 20 nm long and usually has a free trailing flagellum. The kinetoplast is very large, ca. 2 nm in diameter, and in stained preparations appears to extend beyond the body of the parasite. The organism will assume characteristic U-, C-, or S-shaped configurations in fixed preparations. The latter features are diagnostic for this species. Dividing trypanosomes are *never seen* in *T. cruzi* infections (see Fig. 10).

2. *Leishmania stage in tissue cells.* The morphology of these stages is basically similar to those described for *Leishmania* spp. However, the organisms are somewhat larger, ranging from 3 to 4 nm in major diameter.

3. *Crithidial stages in cultures.* These are similar to those described above for *T. gambiense* and *T. rhodesiense*.

Diagnosis is made by the following procedures:

1. *Demonstration of trypanosomes in thick and thin blood films prepared during the febrile*

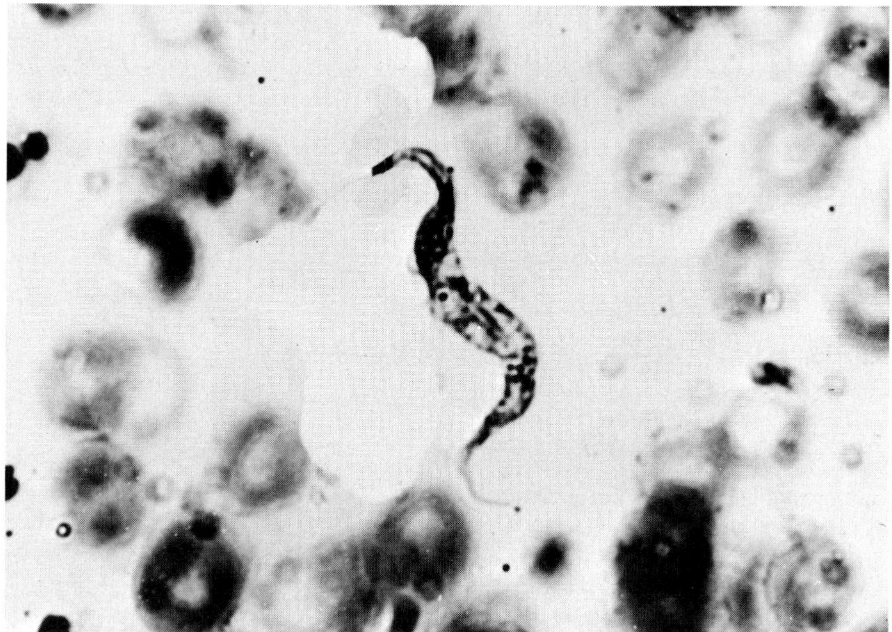

FIG. 9. *Dividing Trypanosoma gambiense in stained blood film.*

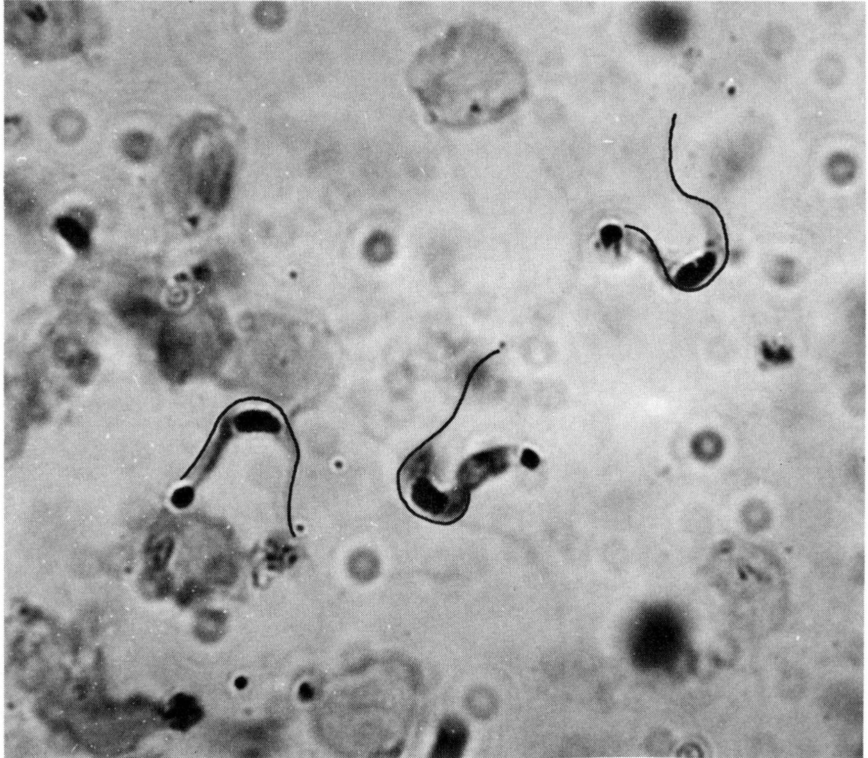

FIG. 10. *Trypanosoma cruzi in stained blood film exhibiting C, S, and U configurations.*

stage. Trypanosomes of *T. cruzi* are usually rare in blood films because they do not multiply in the peripheral blood. Examine wet blood films for motile forms; also examine Giemsa-stained films.

2. *Culture of blood and bone marrow aspirates on diphasic blood-agar medium*. This method yields about 30% of positives.

3. *Stained smears of bone marrow aspirates*. Smears will contain intracellular leishmaniform stages.

4. *Serology*. Complement fixation tests and indirect hemagglutination tests are available for presumptive diagnosis (see chapter 70).

5. *Xenodiagnosis*. Laboratory-bred triatomids, the insect transmitters, are fed on suspected cases, and the intestinal contents are examined 2 weeks later. This procedure is usually not available outside of Latin America. For details, consult Maekelt (4).

Trypanosoma rangeli. *T. rangeli* is the etiological agent of benign American trypanosomiasis. The trypaniform stage in peripheral blood measures about 30 nm in length; the nucleus is situated toward the free flagellum rather than in the center of the cell as in other trypanosomes. This species may occur in patients who also have *T. cruzi* infection; however, it can be differentiated from the latter by its small kinetoplast, and, when present, by dividing forms.

Forms obtained in diphasic culture of blood may be differentiated from *T. cruzi* by subculturing in brain heart infusion-sheep's blood medium (6; see chapter 95). *T. rangeli* will not subculture in the latter medium, but *T. cruzi* will (8). Therefore, a positive subculture in brain heart infusion-sheep's blood medium can be interpreted as positive for *T. cruzi*. Negative cultures are not significant, as some strains of *T. cruzi* culture with difficulty on brain heart infusion medium.

LITERATURE CITED

1. Craig, C. F. 1942. Laboratory diagnosis of protozoan disease. Lea & Febiger, Philadelphia.
2. Hunter, G. W., III, W. W. Frye, and J. C. Swartzwelder. 1966. A manual of tropical medicine, 4th ed. W. B. Saunders Co., Philadephia.
3. Lainson, R., and J. J. Shaw. 1972. Leishmaniasis in the New World: taxonomic problems. Brit. Med. Bull. **28:**44.
4. Maekelt, G. A. 1964. A modified procedure of xenodiagnosis for Chagas' disease. Amer. J. Trop. Med. Hyg. **13:**11–15.
5. Walker, A. J. 1963. Manual for the microscopical diagnosis of malaria. Pan American Health Organization. World Health Organization Scientific Publication No. 87.
6. Warren, L. G. 1960. Metabolism of *Schizotrypanum cruzi* Chagas. I. Effect of culture age and substrate concentration on respiratory rate. J. Parasitol. **46:**529–540.
7. Wilcox, G. 1960. Manual for the microscopical diagnosis of malaria in man. Public Health Serv. Publ. No. 796.
8. Zeledón, R. 1959. Differentiation of *Trypanosoma rangeli* and Schizotrypanum cruzi in a liquid medium, with notes on the nutrition of hemoflagellates. J. Parasitol. **45:**652.

Chapter 68
Helminths

STANLEY H. ABADIE, JOSEPH H. MILLER, LIONEL G. WARREN, J. CLYDE SWARTZWELDER, AND MARK R. FELDMAN

COLLECTION AND EXAMINATION OF STOOLS AND OTHER MATERIALS

General instructions

For accurate diagnosis, fecal specimens must be free from oil, barium, and bismuth, and should be examined shortly after evacuation. No preservative is necessary.

The patient should pass the stool into a bed pan if hospitalized. If the patient is not hospitalized, he should pass the stool directly into a wide-mouthed container, if possible. The patient may place a sheet of newspaper over the toilet seat and pass the stool onto the paper. With a tongue blade or suitable implement, place the stool in a container which is clean and dry. If mucus or blood is present, place this material in the container also. The container should be capped tightly to prevent leakage or drying.

Liquid and mucosanguineous stools should be examined as soon as possible after evacuation. Formed stools may be examined more leisurely or preserved for slightly longer periods by refrigeration.

Routine stool examination

Examination of a stool for parasites should not be considered complete unless gross examination, direct fecal smear, and Formalin-ether centrifugal concentration have been performed.

Gross examination. Gross examination should include a careful search for blood, mucus, and adult worms, e.g., pinworms or tapeworm proglottids, which might otherwise be overlooked.

Direct fecal smear. The following procedure provides a satisfactory smear. A glass slide (1.5 by 3 inches; 3.8 by 7.6 cm) should be used. A drop of physiological saline is placed on one half of the glass slide. A drop of iodine stain (see chapter 96) is placed on the other half of the slide. By means of a wooden applicator, a carefully selected quantity of the fecal material is transferred to the slide and spread *evenly* throughout the saline over an area the width of one cover slip (22 by 22 mm) on the slide. In selecting the material for the smear, one should look especially for blood and mucus. Also, it is desirable to select material from several portions of the stool specimen. Next, additional fecal material is smeared evenly in the drop of iodine stain. A cover slip is then applied to each side of the smear. When stools are examined microscopically, the two-cover slip preparation should *always* be employed.

Care should be taken to avoid certain errors which are frequently made in the preparation of direct fecal smears and which may invalidate the observed microscopic findings.

1. Smearing feces onto a dry slide instead of into the drops of saline and iodine stain, making the preparation useless for examination for helminths and intestinal protozoa.

2. Making preparations too thick, with the result that parasites are obscured in dense fecal masses; there should be no clumps of fecal material under the cover slips.

3. Making preparations too thin, with the result that parasites are not detected unless extremely numerous; the desired density of the fecal emulsion on the slide is often described as one which is uniform throughout and through which the print of a newspaper can easily be discerned after the cover slips are applied.

4. Failure to use cover slips, with the resultant drying of the smear, fogging and contamination of the lens, and rapid loss of the stain.

5. Employing tap water instead of physiological saline; tap water destroys or alters trophozoites.

6. Failure to employ both saline and iodine-stained preparations; both sides of the double fecal smear serve distinct purposes and complement each other.

7. Employing iodine stain which is too concentrated; the supernatant fluid of a 1% solution of potassium iodide, supersaturated with iodine crystals, provides a satisfactory stain which affords uniform results.

8. Employing iodine stain of too low concentration to provide a satisfactory stain; if the stain is too old, the iodine may have become

sublimated; if a drop of satisfactory iodine is left on the slide too long before the feces are smeared into it, or if there is delay in applying the cover slip, the material will not be stained satisfactorily.

9. Allowing slides to stand indefinitely before examination; the smears should be examined promptly after preparation and should not be allowed to dry on standing.

10. Use of a narrow slide (1 by 3 inches) such as is employed in work in hematology; the narrow slide does not provide adequate space for preparation; the smear may overrun the slide and interfere with the examination, as well as contaminate the microscope and the microscopist.

11. Employing oil immersion on direct fecal smears; low power (10×) and high dry (43×) objectives are preferable to oil immersion for wet smears.

Formalin-ether centrifugal sedimentation. The Formalin-ether sedimentation technique is an excellent concentration procedure for the detection and identification of protozoan cysts and helminth eggs and larvae of most intestinal parasites. The technique also is very useful for the examination of stools containing fatty substances which interfere with the performance of the zinc sulfate centrifugal flotation method. It is *not* satisfactory for trophozoites. The procedure for Formalin-ether centrifugal sedimentation is described in chapters 65 and 96, to which the reader is referred.

Other techniques

Scotch tape swab for the diagnosis of Enterobius vermicularis infection. The most satisfactory means of diagnosing pinworm infection is by the recovery of eggs or female worms from the perianal region, as only 5 to 10% of infected persons pass demonstrable eggs in their stools (Fig. 1).

1. Prepare a swab with a 9-cm strip of Scotch tape, 1.9 to 2.5 cm in width, and a standard 1 by 3 inch (2.5 by 7.6 cm) microscope slide. At one end of the tape, 0.5 cm is folded upon itself to provide a nonadhesive area for handling. The remainder is applied to the slide with the gummed side down, extending over the end and for about 1 cm on the undersurface of the slide.

2. Employ the swab in the morning before bathing or bowel movement.

3. Hold the slide against a tongue depressor 2.5 cm below the end, and lift the long portion of tape from the upper surface of the slide.

4. Loop the tape over the extended end of the depressor to expose the gummed surface. Hold the tape and slide against the depressor to provide tension and a firm support for the loop of Scotch tape.

5. Separate the buttocks and press the gummed surfaces against several areas of the perianal region.

6. Replace the tape on the side (to which it has remained attached on the undersurface), and smooth the tape with cotton or gauze.

7. Examine the swab microscopically for eggs (not adults) of *E. vermicularis*.

8. A drop of toluene or xylene may be added to the slide before replacing tape for clearing, if desired; however, the cells and detritus in uncleared preparations serve as a guide for focusing on the correct optical plane.

Stoll egg-counting technique. The Stoll-counting technique is employed primarily in hookworm infections but may be used in other

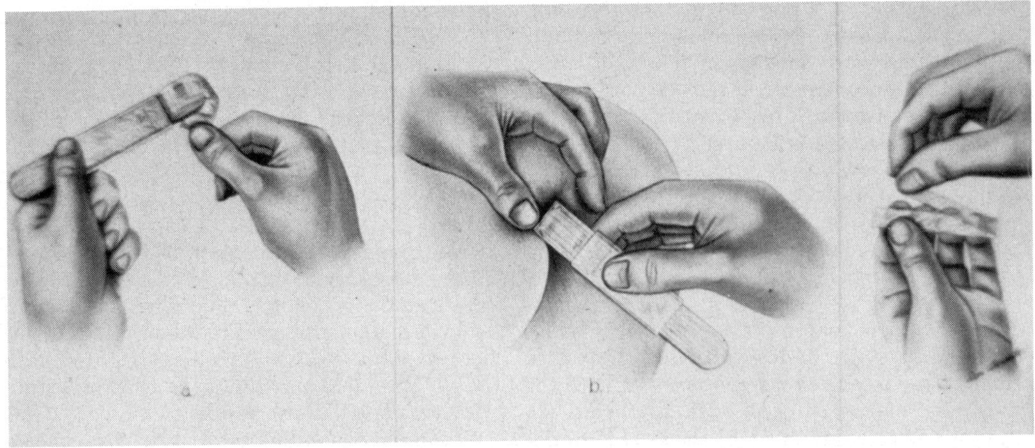

FIG. 1. *Scotch tape swab. Courtesy of A Manual of Tropical Medicine (1).*

helminthic infections. It is used to obtain a quantitative estimation of the number of worm eggs in a measured sample of feces (chapter 96).

Methods employed in the diagnosis of Strongyloides stercoralis infection. In addition to routine procedures, special methods are described for use when the routine examinations are negative. The routine procedures include examination of several stool specimens by direct smear and Formalin-ether concentration. The special methods are as follows.

Duodenal aspiration of rhabditiform larvae and embryonated eggs in suspended mucus fragments in sediment of deeply bile-stained aspirate is employed only if stool examinations are negative for *S. stercoralis* larvae and a diagnosis of strongyloidiasis is still considered (see procedure described below).

The Harada and Mori test tube cultivation method for nematode larvae is useful for demonstrations of larvae of *Ancylostoma duodenale*, *Necator americanus*, *Trichostrongylus orientalis*, and *Stronglyoides stercoralis*. Approximately 0.5 g of feces is smeared on a narrow sheet of filter paper (3 by 16 cm). About 5 cm of space on one end and 1 cm (for handling) on the other end are left unsmeared. The filter paper is placed in a test tube 18 cm in height and 2 cm in diameter, with the unsmeared end (5 cm) toward the bottom. A 2- to 3-ml amount of water is introduced into the tube; then the opening is covered with a piece of polyethylene sheet which is held in place by a rubber band. The tube is kept in an incubator at 24 to 28 C for about 10 days. Eggs of hookworm and certain other nematodes hatch on the filter paper, develop into infective larvae, crawl out of the feces, and migrate to the water. The tubes are examined under low-power magnification for presence of larvae. If larvae are present, fluid is removed with a pipette and the larvae are identified under higher magnification. Incubation for 8 days at 30 C provides the optimal condition for detection of *Strongyloides* larvae. Larvae usually are found much earlier than 8 days.

A third method is to place a layer of filter paper (cut circular to fit flat) in a petri dish. Moisten the paper with tap water. Mix stool with animal charcoal and water (*not saline*) to a consistency of paste and spread out on the filter paper in a petri dish. A portion of the mixture should be touching the petri dish cover when in place. Allow to stand at room temperature for about 48 h. Add a few drops of distilled water to the inside of the cover of the petri dish and to the surface of the fecal mixture. Then remove the fluid with a pipette. Examine the washings of the culture and of the inside of the cover for filariform larvae with notched tails.

Procedure for duodenal drainage

A standard Rehfuss tube with olive tip is used. The tube is passed (*through the mouth*), with the patient in a sitting position, until it reaches the stomach. The above location is indicated when the mark of *one ring* on the tube is at the level of the patient's lips. The stomach contents are then aspirated (with a 30-ml syringe). The patient is then placed in position on his right side. It is important that the patient lies on his side and not on his back or stomach. The patient is instructed to swallow the tube farther at a slow pace of approximately 2.5 to 5 cm every 5 to 10 min, until the mark showing *three rings* on the tube is at the patient's lips. Usually during this period, clear or cloudy gastric juice will flow; this may be discarded. After a period of time (which varies with each patient), a clear light-yellow material will be seen. The patient is then ready to be stimulated. Magnesium sulfate (33.3%) or olive oil may be used. Approximately 30 ml of 33.3% magnesium sulfate is introduced into the duodenum through the tube and allowed to flow back into a test tube immediately. If the entire procedure has been properly carried out, dark bile will follow the returning magnesium sulfate. The latter step may be repeated as often as is necessary to stimulate the bile flow.

If difficulty is encountered in introducing the tube into the duodenum, a few simple aids may be tried: (i) place a pillow under the patient to elevate the hips, or (ii) turn the patient on his left side for 5 to 10 min and then return the patient to the original position.

Two simple ways of determining the position of the tube are as follows. (i) The patient is given a small amount of water by mouth, and a syringe is attached to the free end of the tube. If water can be aspirated, the tube is in the stomach and must be returned to stomach depth (that is, withdrawn until the mark of *one ring* is at the level of the patient's lips). The progressive swallowing process outlined above should then be repeated. (ii) Attach a syringe to the free end of the tube and attempt to aspirate. If a vacuum is formed and you are unable to aspirate the fluid, it is safe to assume that the tube is in the duodenum or in the pylorus approaching the duodenum.

Examination of duodenal drainage fluid

Intestinal parasites may be found in A, B, or C bile, but are detected most frequently in C bile (darkest bile). In most instances, the parasites are located in the mucoid content of the bile. They should be sought in the *mucus suspended in the bile* and in the sedimented mucus. Some of the mucus usually settles to the bottom of the container upon standing for a few minutes. Because of the viscosity of bile, centrifugation is of no significant aid in this procedure. The dark bile-stained drainage fluid may be placed in a conical sedimentation jar or in a pilsener glass. Transillumination of the fluid, by placing a microscope lamp behind it, aids in making visible the suspended mucus fragments which should be examined microscopically. The floating and sedimented mucus may be removed for examination by use of a large-caliber pipette with a rubber bulb attached. The material is placed on a glass fecal slide and examined unstained under low power of the microscope. Several slides should be examined before the drainage fluid is considered negative.

The three parasites most frequently found are *Stongyloides stercoralis*, *Giardia lamblia*, and hookworm. If the material has just been obtained, the most frequent finding in cases of strongyloidiasis will be the active rhabditiform larva still encapsulated in the egg. These are usually found in the mucus. For a positive identification, the slide may be set aside at room temperature for 10 to 15 min, during which time the larvae will hatch. A drop of iodine may be added before examination so that the buccal cavity may be more readily visible. If the material to be examined has been standing for 15 to 30 min, the larvae will have already hatched, but will still be found in the mucoid fragments of the bile. In the case of *G. lamblia*, the trophozoites will be present. In hookworm infection, eggs in various stages of cleavage may be seen.

Examination of sputum for parasite eggs and larvae

Mix sputum and 3% sodium hydroxide solution in equal amounts. Centrifuge at high speed, and decant the supernatant fluid. Examine the sediment for eggs and/or larvae. Instead of sodium hydroxide, Clorox (full strength) may be added in quantity sufficient to liquefy sputum.

IDENTIFICATION OF THE HELMINTHS

Following are the distinguishing characteristics of the helminths, by means of which the several organisms may be identified.

Nematodes

Intestinal roundworms

Five important members of the class Nematoda which inhabit the intestinal tract of humans will be discussed.

Ascaris lumbricoides. *A. lumbricoides* is the largest of the intestinal nematodes of humans. The adult is white or pink in color and 20 to 30 cm or more in length. It has three anterior lips. The posterior extremity of the male is recurved. The mature female is larger than the male and has a pointed tail. The adults live in the lumen of the small intestine. Female worms may lay 200,000 or more eggs per day.

The eggs of *A. lumbricoides* are of two principal types, fertilized and unfertilized. The fertilized egg is round, oval, or elliptical. It measures 45 by 60 μm and is brown in color. The egg stains intensely with iodine. The outer mammillated membrane stains deeply; the inner translucent shell appears yellow. The fertilized egg contains a large, round, unsegmented embryo, with clear spaces at either pole (Fig. 2). The egg is immature when passed and becomes infective for humans only after maturing in soil. When the outer membrane is lacking, the egg is called decorticated.

The unfertilized egg is more elongate. It is often misshapen or distorted and contains yellow, globular material with no clear spaces at the poles. This egg is often mistaken for a plant cell (Fig. 2). Diagnosis is made by finding eggs in the stool or occasionally by finding adult worms passed spontaneously.

Trichuris trichiura. The adult worm is white and is 30 to 50 mm in length, with a long threadlike anterior portion. The posterior portion is bulbous, giving it a whiplike appearance. The posterior portion of the male is coiled like a watchspring. The adults live partially embedded in the wall of the large intestine. Adult females are capable of laying several thousand eggs per day.

Eggs of *T. trichiura* are brown (bile-stained), barrel-shaped, 22 by 50 μm, with a transparent, mucoid, polar plug at either end. The eggs have a double wall; the inner one is light and the outer one is dark. An embryo fills the egg. The eggs are immature when passed and become infective after maturing in the soil. Diagnosis is made by finding the characteristic eggs in the stool (Fig. 3).

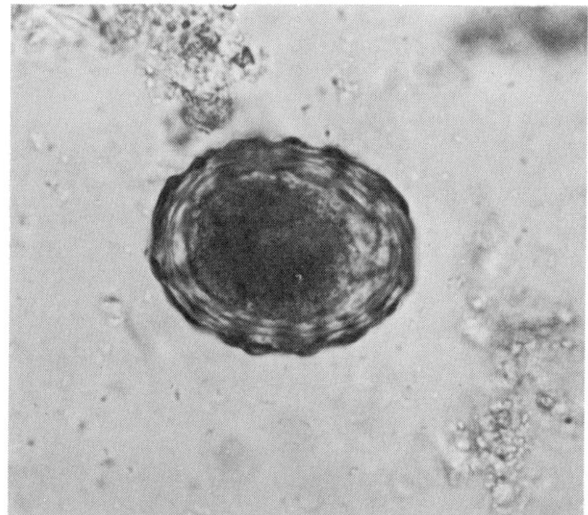

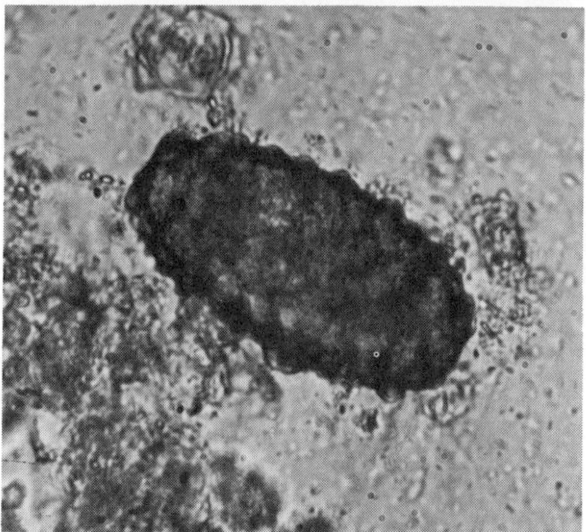

FIG. 2. *Fertilized (top) and unfertilized (bottom) eggs of Ascaris lumbricoides.* ×450.

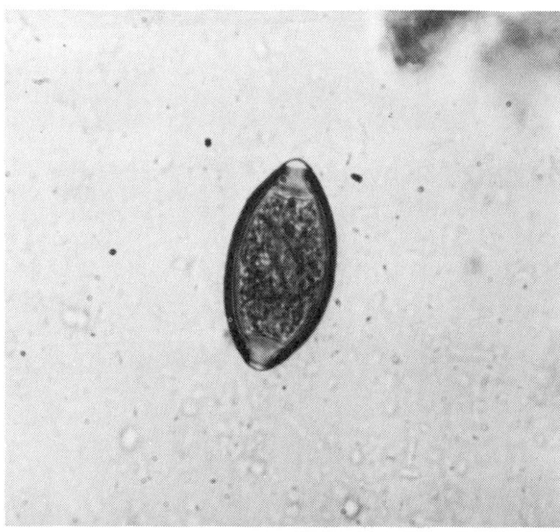

FIG. 3. *Trichuris trichiura egg.* ×450.

Necator americanus. The adult worm is creamy or grayish-white. It measures 9 to 12 mm in length. The mouth capsule has two pairs of semilunar cutting plates (no hooks or teeth). The posterior end of the female is bluntly pointed, and the male has a fan-shaped or bursate posterior end with barbed spicules. Adult hookworms are firmly attached to the mucosa of the small intestine.

Hookworm eggs are elliptical or oval, colorless or hyaline, and measure 40 by 60 μm with a single, thin transparent shell containing an immature segmented embryo (two- to eight-cell stage). The egg has a clear outer zone between the embryo and the egg shell. The egg is immature when passed in the stool, is not infective for man, and is the diagnostic stage.

The rhabditiform larva may be found in old stools. It is wormlike and about one high-power field long (20 by 400 μm), and is motile when living. The larva is colorless and has a granular appearance due to its internal structure. It has a *comparatively* long preesophageal groove with a muscular esophagus. The midgut, anus, and other structures may be visible. This stage is not infective for humans (Fig. 4).

Diagnosis is made by finding the characteristic eggs (and, rarely, larvae) in the stool (Fig. 5).

Ancylostoma duodenale. The adult has essentially the same appearance as *Necator* except that the mouth has two pairs of hooks or teeth and the spicules on the male lack barbs. The eggs and rhabditiform larvae are similar in appearance to those of *Necator*.

Strongyloides stercoralis. The parasitic female is filiform or threadlike and measures about 2 to 3 mm. It is usually embedded in the mucosa of the small intestine. The egg of *S. stercoralis* is rarely seen in the stool. It resembles an embryonated hookworm egg (containing an active larva). The rhabditiform larva is the diagnostic stage in the stool. It has a very short preesophageal groove. Otherwise, it resembles the rhabditiform larva of *Necator*. The rhabditiform larva is not infective for humans (Fig. 4).

Diagnosis ordinarily is made by finding the characteristic rhabditiform larvae in the stool or duodenal aspirate. If the stool has been allowed to stand for several hours, especially in warm water, filariform larvae of *S. stercoralis* may be present. They are longer and more slender than rhabditiform larvae and have a minutely notched tail, visible under high dry (43×)

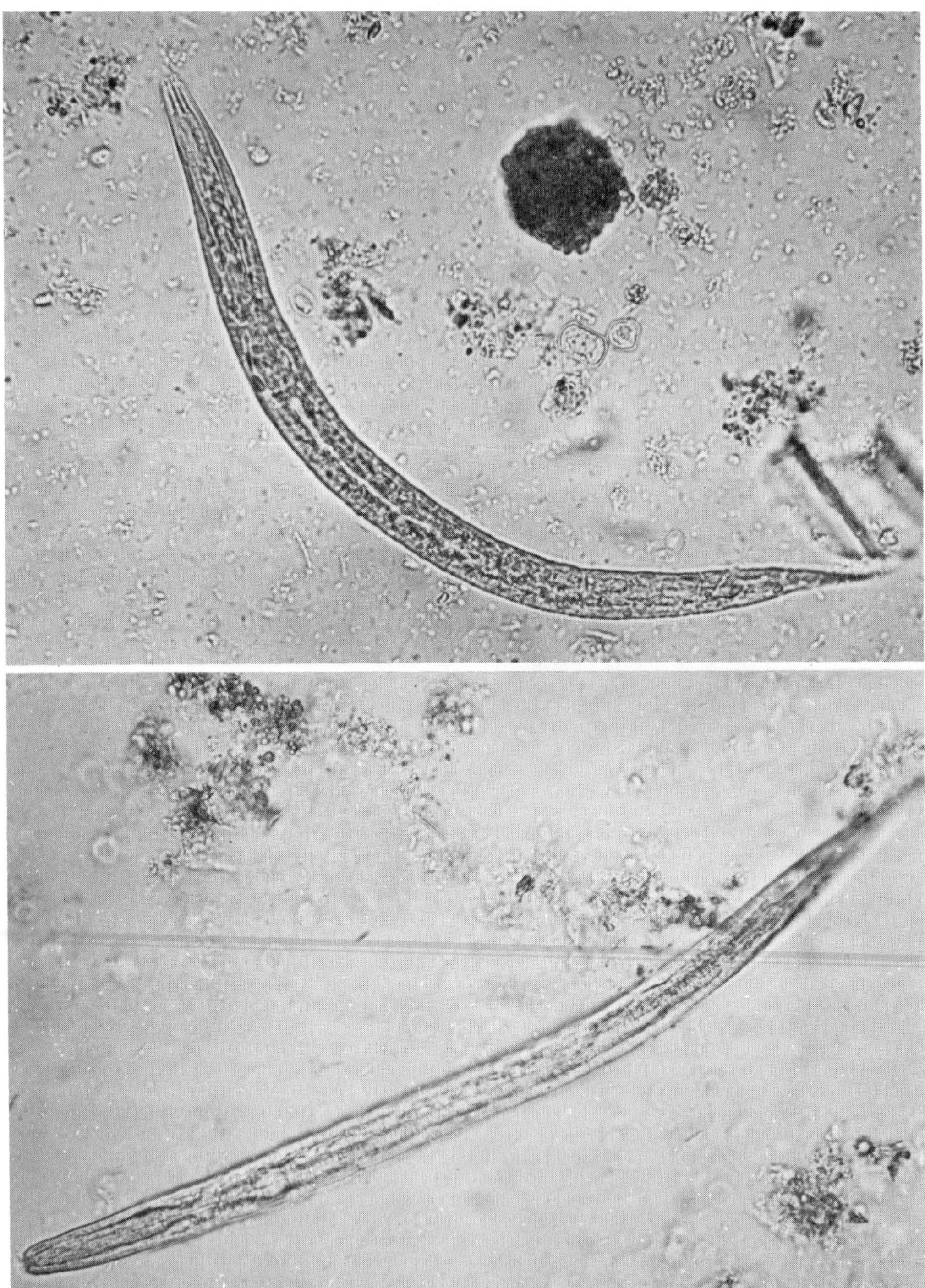

FIG. 4. *Rhabditiform larva of hookworm (top) and of Strongyloides stercoralis (bottom).* ×450.

magnification. Such stools should be handled with care because the filariform larvae are directly infective.

Enterobius vermicularis. The adult female is about 1.3 cm long, is white, and has the diameter of a common pin. It has lateral cuticular expansions on the anterior end called cephalic alae. The posterior end is long, clear, and pointed. The adult female contains thousands of eggs. The adult male is practically microscopic and plays no role either in the disease process or in diagnosis. Diagnosis is made by finding the characteristic egg (Fig. 5), or occasionally the adult female worm, on Scotch tape swabs.

Tissue roundworms

A number of species of nematodes principally inhabit the extraintestinal tissues of man.

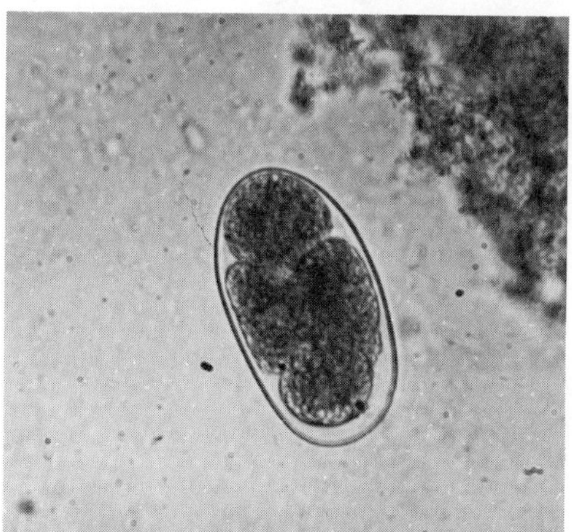

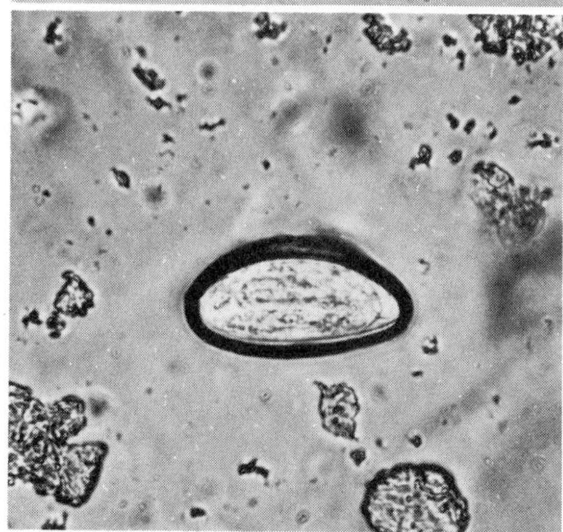

FIG. 5. *Hookworm egg (top) and Enterobius vermicularis egg (bottom).* ×450.

These include the filarial worms, *Wuchereria bancrofti*, *Brugia malayi*, *Loa loa*, *Dipetalonema perstans*, *Dipetalonema streptocerca*, *Mansonella ozzardi*, and *Onchocerca volvulus*, and also the guinea worm, *Dracunculus medinensis*, and the trichina worm, *Trichinella spiralis*. Several other species are normally parasitic in animals, but their larval stages may parasitize humans. These include: the dog and cat hookworm, *Ancylostoma braziliense;* the dog and cat ascarids, *Toxocara canis* and *Toxocara cati;* and the gnathostome, *Gnathostoma spinigerum*. These species belong to the following superfamilies: Filarioidea, Dracunculoidea, Trichuroidea, Strongyloidea, Ascaridoidea, and Spiruroidea.

Filarioidea. There are seven species belonging to the superfamily Filarioidea whose adults are parasitic in the lymphoid, connective, or subcutaneous tissues of humans. Adults produce larvae (microfilariae) that are found in the blood, subcutaneous tissue, or cutaneous tissue, depending upon the species.

Wuchereria bancrofti (Bancroft's filaria) and Brugia malayi (Brug's filaria). Diagnostic stage: typical sheathed microfilariae with nocturnal periodicity in peripheral blood, except for some areas of the South Central Pacific where the microfilariae of *W. bancrofti* are essentially nonperiodic or partially diurnal (Fig. 6).

Diagnostic procedures are as follows.

1. Demonstration of microfilariae (often microfilariae may not be demonstrable in the blood of cases of filarial disease with elephantiasis, or in early phases of the disease) in:
   a. Unstained thick wet blood films prepared at night and during the day. Examine for motile microfilariae.
   b. Thick blood films dehemoglobinized and stained with Giemsa or Wright stain.
   c. Knott's concentration technique: to 1 ml of venous blood, add 9 ml of 2% Formalin. Centrifuge at 1,500 rpm for 5 min. Pour off the supernatant fluid and examine the sediment.
   d. Chylous exudates.
2. Differential leukocyte count. Eosinophilia may be present during the early stage of infection. Later, the eosinophil percentage may be normal.
3. X-ray examination. In old infections some adult worms become calcified; the minute sites of calcification may be detected.
4. Serological tests; see chapter 70.

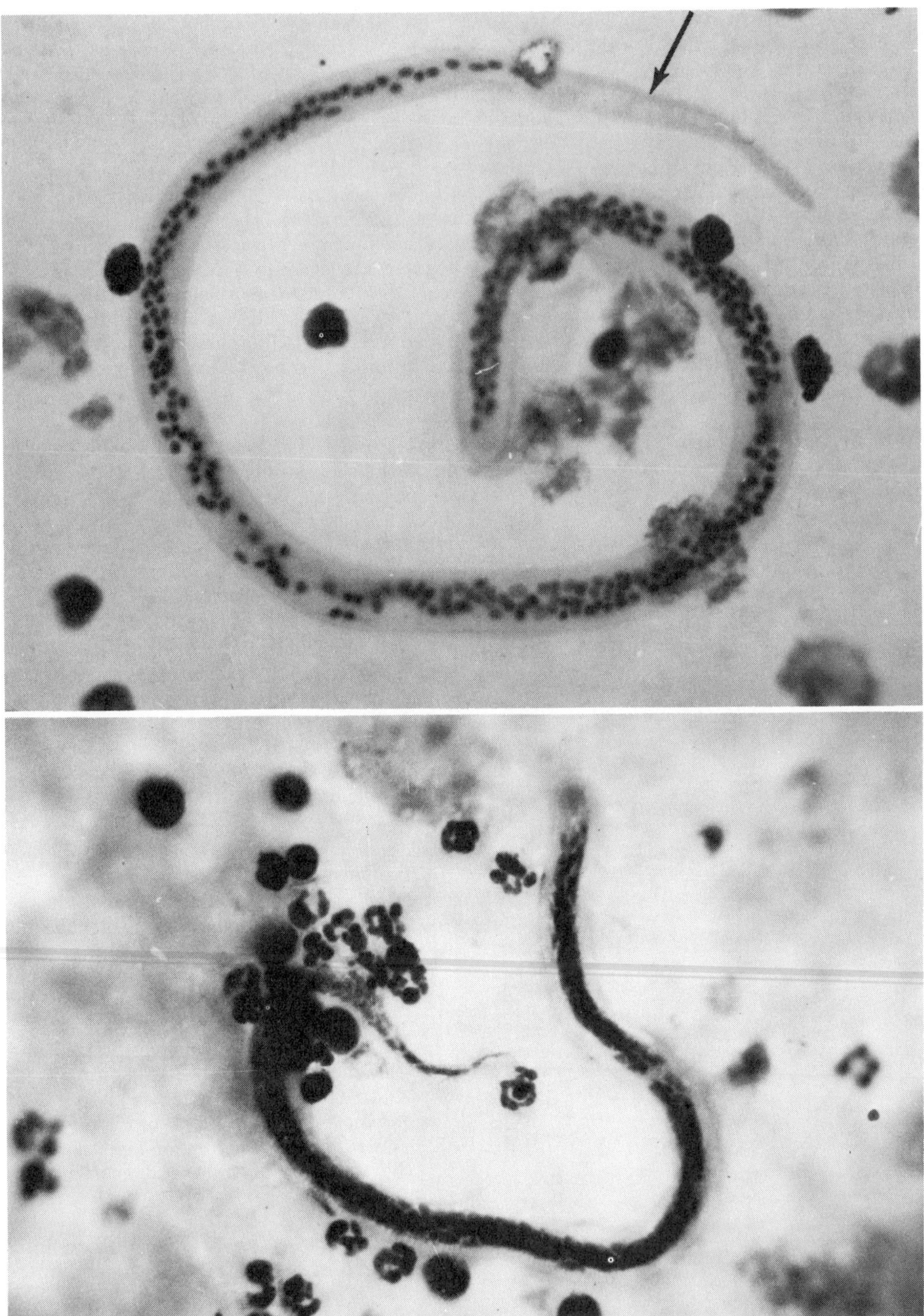

FIG. 6. *Sheathed (top) and unsheathed (bottom) microfilariae.* ×*1,000.*

Loa loa (eye worm). Diagnostic stages: microfilariae in peripheral blood; adult filariae visible or palpable in superficial sites.

Diagnostic procedures are as follows:

1. Demonstration of typical sheathed microfilariae with diurnal periodicity in unstained wet blood films, stained thick and thin blood films, and by concentration. Microfilariae may be demonstrated even though migrating adults have not been observed.

2. Demonstration of adult worms by surgical extraction when they are located in an operable site. The application of external heat attracts the worm to the surface of the body. The adult worm may be observed crossing the eye or its outline may be detected under the skin.

3. Differential leukocyte count to determine presence or absence of eosinophilia.

4. Demonstration of microfilariae in aspirate of the Calabar swellings.

5. Serological tests; see chapter 70.

Dipetalonema perstans (persistent filaria) and Mansonella ozzardi (Ozzard's filaria). Diagnostic stage: unsheathed microfilaria in peripheral blood.

Diagnosis is accomplished by demonstration of nonsheathed, nonperiodic microfilaria with typical morphology in peripheral blood. Motile microfilariae may be observed in wet blood films. Detail may be observed in Giemsa- or Wright-stained thick and thin dehemoglobinized blood films (Fig. 6).

Onchocerca volvulus (the blinding filaria). Diagnostic stages: unsheathed microfilariae in or from skin or onchocercomas; adult filaria coiled in subcutaneous onchocercomas.

Diagnostic procedures are as follows:

1. Demonstrate microfilaria in:
   a. Thin skin snips taken with a razor from area of nodules placed in warm saline under a cover slip. Snips may also be sectioned and stained.
   b. Expressed blood and lymph from scarification in area of nodule. Method employs several closely approximated superficial linear incisions into the skin to obtain blood and lymph. May be examined fresh or stained with Giemsa.
   c. Material aspirated from onchocercomas unstained or stained with Giemsa.

2. Excision of onchocercomas and demonstration of coiled adult worms either unstained or in stained tissue section.

3. Differential leukocyte count. Eosinophilia is frequently present.

Dipetalonema streptocerca. Diagnostic stage: unsheathed microfilariae in or from skin.

Diagnosis is made by demonstrating microfilariae in skin snips from upper torso, neck, and upper arms, or in expressed blood and lymph (refer to diagnostic procedures for *O. volvulus*).

The following key may be of assistance in the differentiation of the common microfilariae.

Key to the Common Microfilariae

In peripheral blood

Sheathed

a. Nuclei do not extend to tip of tail; usually nocturnal periodicity—*W. bancrofti.*

b. Nuclei extend to tip of tail in broken row with two terminal nuclei; nocturnal periodicity—*B. malayi.*

c. Nuclei extend to tip of tail in solid row; diurnal periodicity—*L. loa.*

Unsheathed

a. Nuclei extend to tip of tail, often in two rows—*D. perstans.*

b. Nuclei not extending to tip of tail—*M. ozzardi.*

In skin and subcutaneous tissues

Unsheathed

a. Tail slightly curved—*O. volvulus.*

b. Tail bent into shepherd's crook—*D. streptocerca.*

Dracunculoidea. The superfamily Dracunculoidea has a single representative, *Dracunculus medinensis* (Guinea worm), which infects humans. The adult is found in the deep connective and subcutaneous tissues. However, gravid females cause superficial lesions through which large numbers of larvae are discharged.

Diagnostic stage: larvae, 500 to 750 μm by 15 to 25 μm with a blunt anterior and a long attenuated posterior extremity.

Diagnostic procedures are as follows.

1. Fluid or washings from ulcerated areas are examined unstained for the presence of typical larvae.

2. A differential leukocyte count may demonstrate a moderate eosinophilia.

Trichuroidea. The superfamily Trichuroidea contains the family Trichinellidae with one species. *Trichinella spiralis* (trichina worm), parasitic in humans. Adult worms develop in the duodenal mucosa from larvae ingested in muscle tissue. Adult females discharge larvae which penetrate the intestinal lymphatics and enter the blood stream. Although many tissues are invaded, the larvae have a predilection for skeletal muscle for further development and encystment.

Diagnostic stage: coiled larvae in an ovoid capsule forming a cyst in skeletal muscle (Fig. 7).

Diagnostic procedures are as follows.

1. Serological techniques: see chapter 70. Excellent specific serological tests are available for the diagnosis of *T. spiralis* infection; therefore, biopsy (procedure 2) is not the method of choice.

2. Demonstration of encysted larvae in biopsy of deltoid, biceps, or gastrocnemius offers a specific although a delayed method of diagnosis since larvae may not be present in sufficient numbers before the second or even third week. Freshly excised muscle is compressed between glass slides and examined under a microscope. Pieces of muscle may also be placed in artificial peptic digest; the residue is then concentrated and examined for larvae. Pieces of muscle may also be processed with usual histological technique of sectioning and staining for demonstration of larvae.

3. Differential leukocyte count. A significant eosinophilia usually develops during the second week of the disease.

Strongyloidea. The infective larvae of the dog and cat hookworm, *Ancylostoma braziliense*, may penetrate the skin of humans and produce serpiginous tracts accompanied by intense pruritus. Other nematodes also have been incriminated in the production of this entity commonly called creeping eruption.

Diagnosis is limited almost entirely to clinical findings. However, in heavy infections where larvae may reach the lungs, they may be observed unstained in deep sputum samples. See previous section on Examination of sputum for parasite eggs and larvae.

Ascaridoidea. Two species from the superfamily Ascaridoidea have larval stages which migrate in human tissues other than the skin. The dog and probably less frequently the cat ascarid (*Toxocara canis* and *T. cati*) are the species involved. Some other animal nematodes also may produce this entity commonly known as visceral larva migrans.

Diagnosis is limited almost entirely to clinical findings. However, a high, sustained eosinophilia usually accompanies this infection. Serological techniques may be used; see chapter 70.

Spiruroidea. The larvae of one species from the superfamily Spiruroidea, namely, *Gnathostoma spinigerum*, are commonly associated

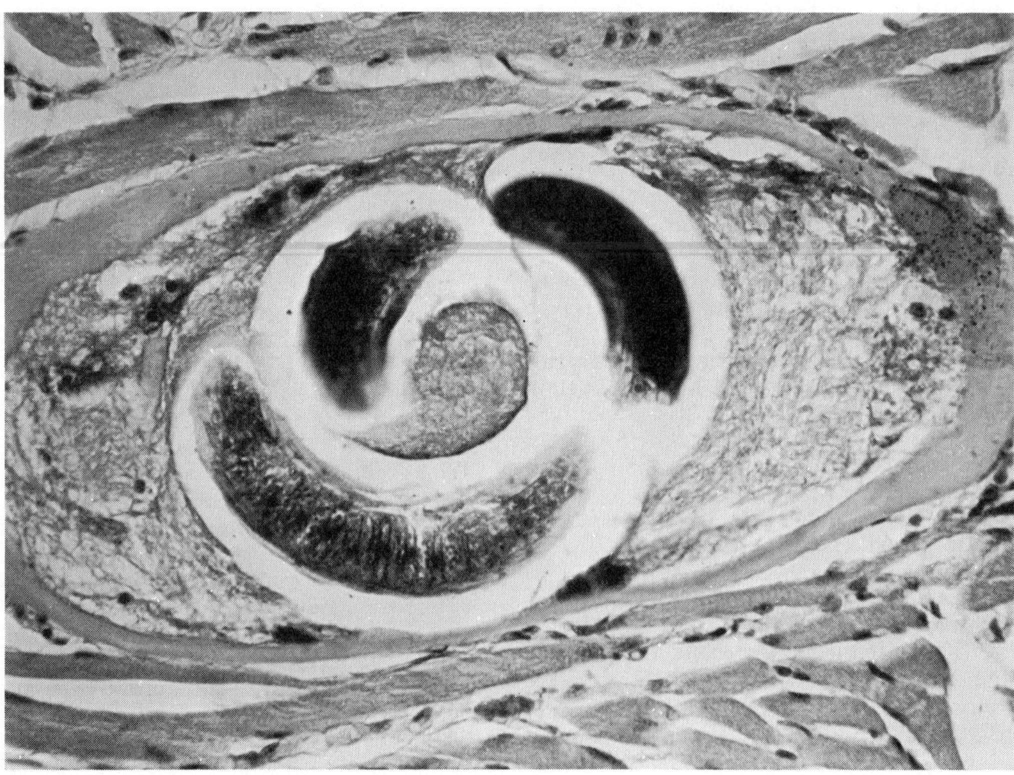

FIG. 7. *Trichinella spiralis in muscle.* ×450.

with a disease entity causing a cutaneous larva migrans in South East Asia. Other species have been incriminated in Japan.

Diagnosis is limited almost entirely to clinical findings of abscesses, cutaneous nodules, or subcutaneous tunnels of migrating larvae. Definitive diagnosis depends on recovery and identification of the parasite from the lesions.

Tapeworms

Common cestodes of the intestines

Four important members of the class Cestoda normally inhabit the intestinal tract of man: (i) *Taenia saginata*, (ii) *Taenia solium*, (iii) *Hymenolepis nana*, and (iv) *Diphyllobothrium latum*.

Taenia saginata (beef tapeworm). The adult worm averages from 2.75 to 4 meters in length (may reach up to 30 meters or more). It is flat, white or pink in color, and motile. The worm consists of the "head" or scolex, and immature, mature, and gravid proglottids. The scolex has four sucking cups and is unarmed (contains no hooks; Fig. 8). The gravid proglottids are longer than broad (2 by 1 cm or more). They contain 15 to 30 primary uterine branches on each side of the main uterine stem (Fig. 8). The proglottids must disintegrate to liberate eggs. The proglottids are more commonly seen in the stool than are the eggs. *Taenia* eggs are spherical, brown, and about 35 μm in diameter. They have a thick, dark-brown, radially striated wall, and contain a hexacanth embryo (contains six hooklets). The egg is not infective for humans. Diagnosis is made by finding either the characteristic egg (Fig. 9) or proglottid in the stool.

Taenia solium (pork tapeworm). The adult worm averages from 1.8 to 3 meters in length (may reach up to 7.6 meters). It is morphologically similar to *T. saginata* with two exceptions. The scolex is armed (contains hooks) and the gravid proglottids have 5 to 13 primary uterine branches on each side of the main uterine stem (Fig. 10). The egg is morphologically undistinguishable from that of *T. saginata*.

Hymenolepis nana (dwarf tapeworm). The adult worm measures from 2.5 to 3.8 cm in length. It has an armed scolex. The proglottids are very small, broader than long, and are very seldom observed in the stool. The egg is about 35 by 45 μm and colorless. It has both an inner and outer membrane and threadlike polar filaments. It contains a hexacanth embryo with prominent hooklets. This egg is infective for man. Diagnosis is made by finding the characteristic egg in the stool (Fig. 9).

Diphyllobothrium latum (fish tapeworm). The adult worm averages from 2.75 to 4.5 meters in length (may reach up to 18 meters) and is creamy white. The scolex (Fig. 11) is spatulate in shape, is unarmed, and has lateral suctorial grooves. The gravid proglottid is broader than long. The uterus is coiled in the center of the proglottid and is usually described as being rosette-shaped (Fig. 11). Unlike some other cestodes, this species lays eggs (does not rupture). The eggs are more frequently observed than the proglottids in the stool. The egg measures about 45 to 70 μm, is ovoid shaped, and has a "cap" or operculum. It is yellowish-brown in color and its contents are globular. The egg is immature when laid and is not infective for humans. Diagnosis is made by finding the characteristic eggs or proglottids in the stool (Fig. 12).

Tissue-inhabiting cestodes

Four members of the class Cestoda in which the larval stage infects humans are discussed: (i) *Echinococcus granulosus*, (ii) *Echinococcus multilocularis*, (iii) *Cysticercus cellulosae*, and (iv) *Sparganum* and *Spirometra* spp.

Echinococcus granulosus (hydatid worm, cause of unilocular hydatid disease). The adult worm is found in dogs. It is minute, usually consists of three proglottids, and has an armed scolex with sucking cups. The egg in the excreta of dogs is morphologically indistinguishable from those of *T. saginata* and *T. solium* and is infective for humans. Since the onchospheres are distributed through the body by the blood, hydatid cysts may develop in any organ. They are most commonly found, however, in the liver and lungs. Although puncture is *not* recommended as a diagnostic procedure, if it is done, diagnosis may be accomplished by identification of hooklets or scolices, or both, in the hydatid fluid recovered from the cyst (Fig. 12). Diagnosis is most often made by X-ray and serological tests (see chapter 70).

Echinococcus multilocularis (hydatid worm, cause of alveolar hydatid disease). The adult worm and egg are morphologically similar to those of *E. granulosus*. The adults are found normally in wild carnivores. Humans become infected with the larval stage. The liver is involved in over 90% of the human infections. Diagnosis may be accomplished by the use of serological tests and X-ray (see chapter 70).

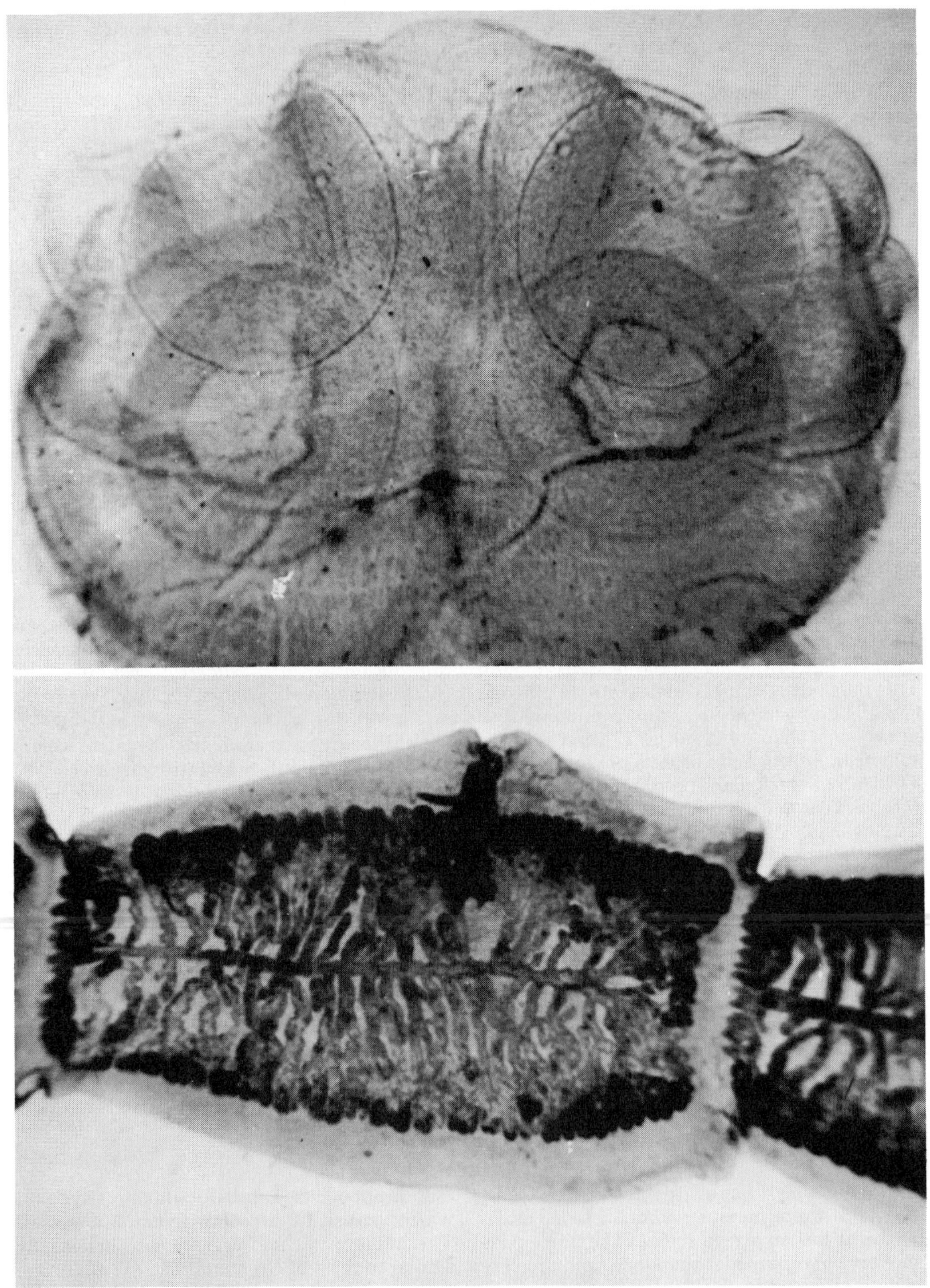

FIG. 8. *Scolex (top) and proglottid (bottom) of Taenia saginata.* ×450.

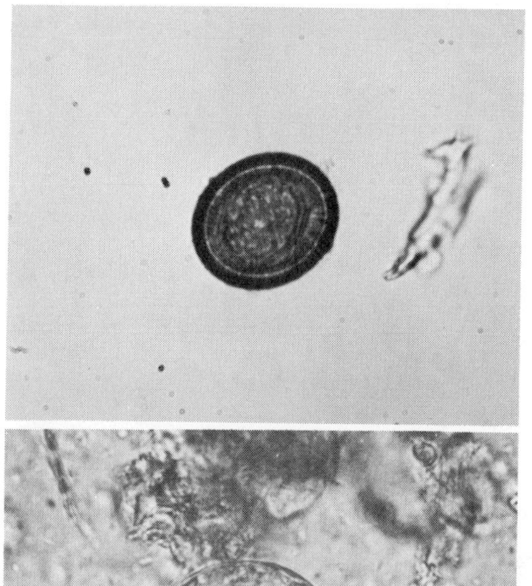

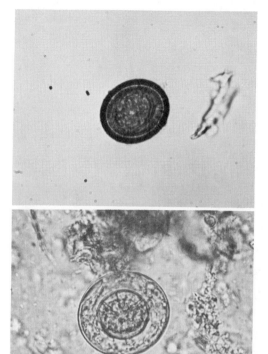

FIG. 9. *(top) Taenia egg. (bottom) Hymenolepis nana egg.* ×450.

Cysticercus cellulosae (larva of Taenia solium, the pork tapeworm. Cysticercosis is infection by the larval form of *T. solium*. Humans inadvertently serve as an intermediate host in this infection by ingesting the eggs of *T. solium*. The cysticerci may lodge in any tissue of the body. They are most frequently found in the skeletal musculature, brain, and eye. The heart, liver, lungs, and abdominal cavity may be involved. Diagnosis is made by X-ray of the soft tissues or by serological tests (see chapter 70).

Sparganum and Spirometra spp. (spargana, cause of sparganosis). Sparganosis is an infection caused by the presence of migrating larvae or spargana of several species of tapeworms related to *D. latum*, but requiring a final host other than humans. *Spirometra mansonoides* probably is the species involved in human infections in the United States. Localization occurs primarily in the subcutaneous tissue and muscle fascia. Diagnosis is usually accomplished by gross or histological examination of surgically removed specimens.

Less common cestodes of the intestine

Two additional cestodes which are found in man only infrequently are *Hymenolepis diminuta* and *Dipylidium caninum*.

Hymenolepis diminuta (rat tapeworm). The adult worm is 1.9 to 6.4 cm long and is normally found in rats. It has an unarmed scolex with sucking cups. The proglottid is small, broader than long, and is seldom seen in the stool. The egg is about 50 to 70 μm in diameter and has a yellowish outer shell and a thickened irregular inner border. It has a thick-walled hexacanth embryo with prominent hooklets but no polar filaments. The egg is not infective for humans. Diagnosis is made by finding the characteristic egg in the stool (Fig. 12).

Dipylidium caninum (dog tapeworm). The adult worm is about 10 to 40 cm long and is normally found in dogs. It has an armed scolex with sucking cups. The proglottids are elliptical or melon-shaped and are commonly passed in the stool. The egg is about 35 μm in diameter. It has a thin wall and contains a hexacanth embryo. Eggs are usually passed in packets cemented in a capsule in groups of 8 to 15. The egg is not infective for humans. Diagnosis is made by finding either the proglottid or typical egg packet in the stool (Fig. 13).

Trematodes

The adult trematodes infecting humans can be divided into two groups: (i) those living in the tissues (i.e., blood flukes, liver flukes, and lung flukes), and (ii) those residing in the intestine. All adult flukes oviposit a characteristic egg containing a ciliate larva (miracidium). The egg serves as the laboratory diagnostic stage. Some species produce operculate eggs, whereas others do not. The eggs are deposited in the tissue or lumen of the organ involved, and may reach the exterior in the urine, sputum, or feces.

Blood flukes

Schistosoma mansoni and Schistosoma japonicum. *S. mansoni*, and *S. japonicum* are the etiological agents of schistosomal dysentery, parasitic periportal cirrhosis, and secondary portal hypertension.

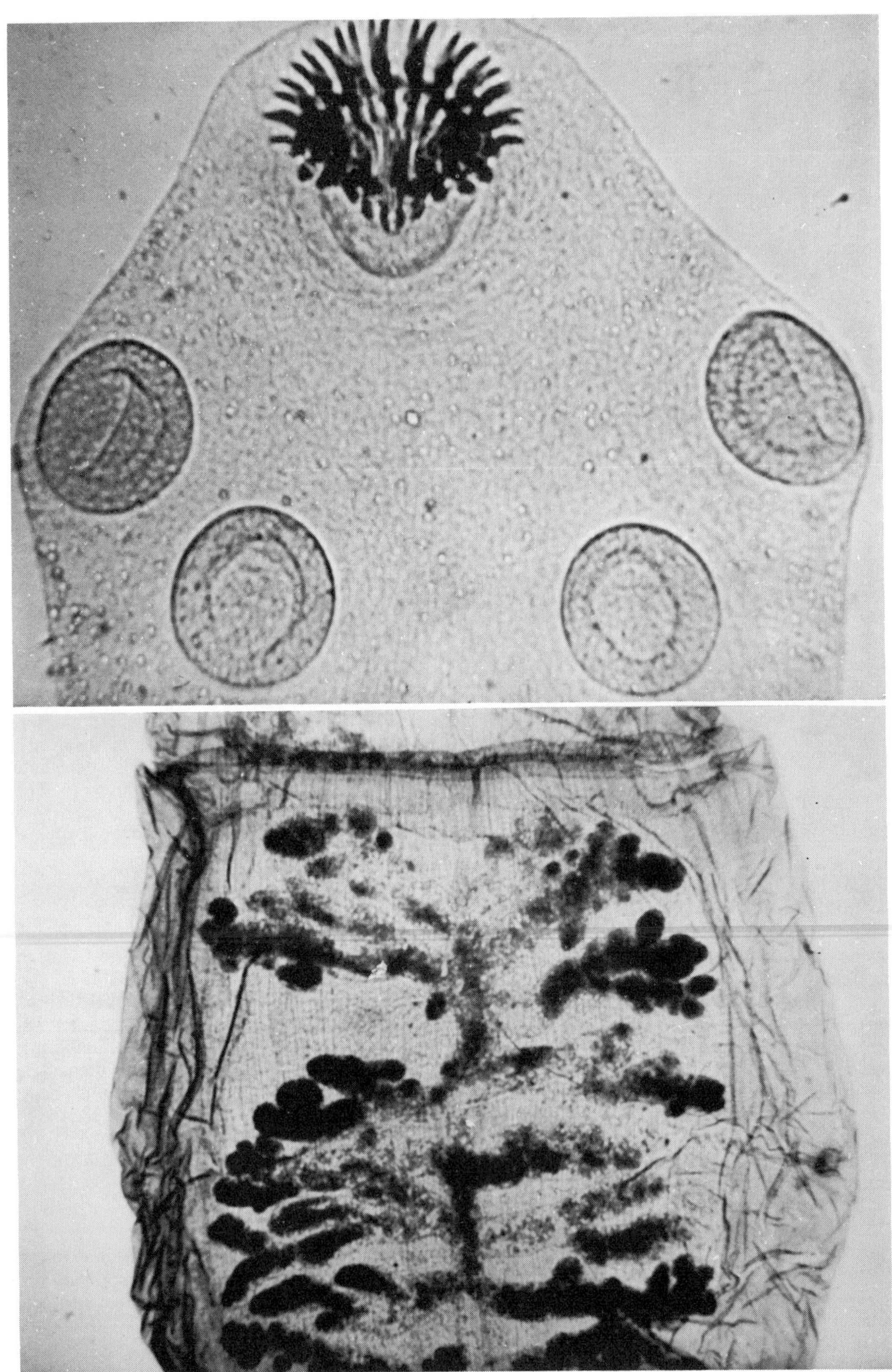

FIG. 10. *Scolex (top) and proglottid (bottom) of Taenia solium.* ×*450.*

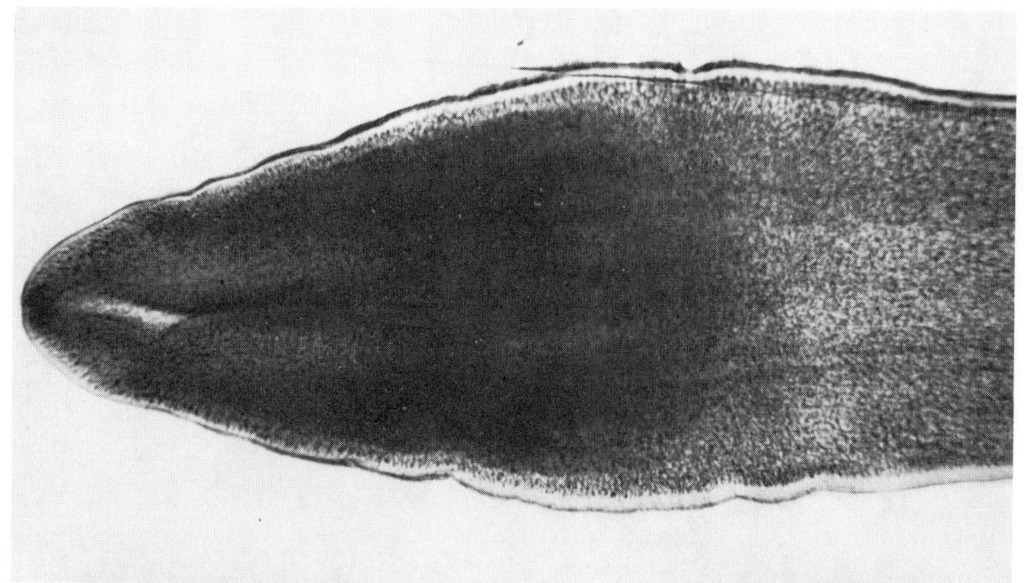

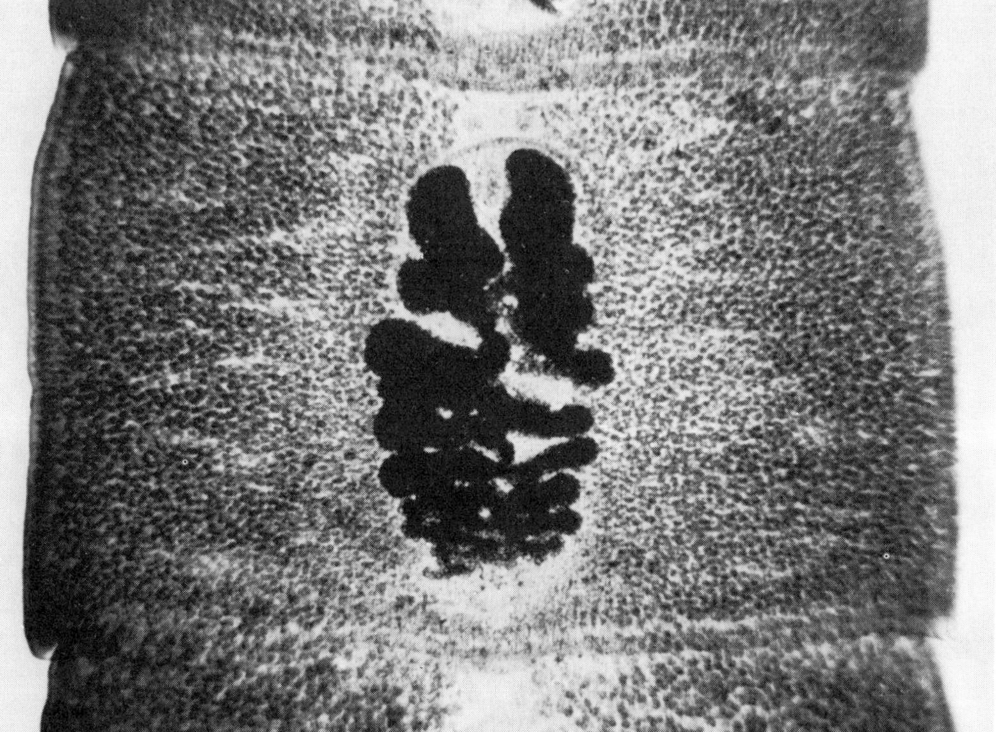

FIG. 11. *Scolex (top) and proglottid (bottom) of Diphyllobothrium latum.* ×*450.*

Diagnostic stage: nonoperculate egg possessing lateral spine or knob typical of respective species. *S. mansoni:* lateral spined egg; length, 114 to 175 μm; breadth, 45 to 70 μm (Fig. 14). *S. japonicum:* small lateral spine or knob which may not be seen; length, 70 to 100 μm; breadth, 50 to 70 μm (Fig. 14).

Diagnostic procedures are as follows.

1. Examination of stools by direct smear technique for typical eggs. It may be necessary to examine many stools in cases of early light infections, or in old chronic cases.

2. Examination of stools by Formalin-ether

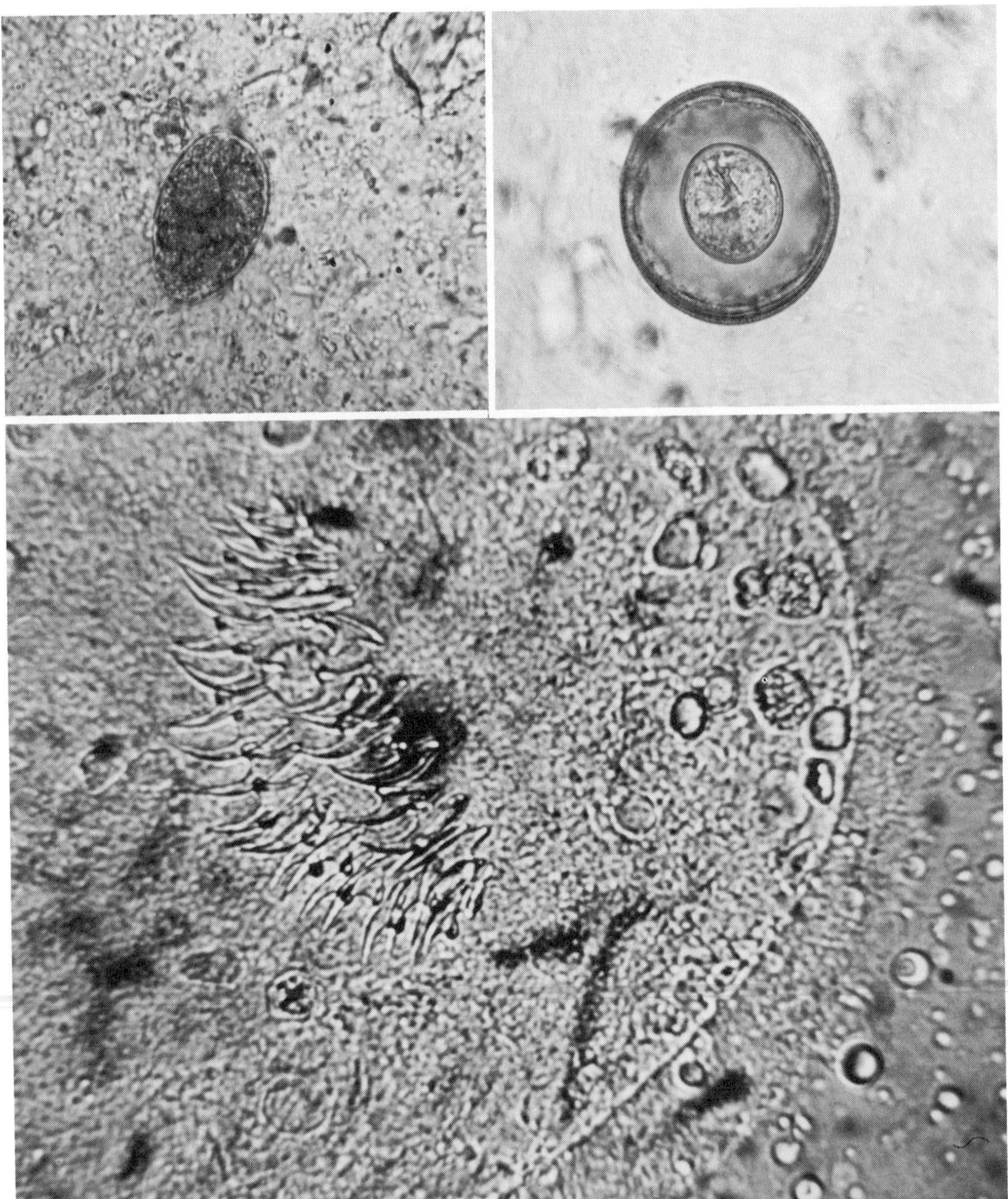

FIG. 12. (*top left*) *Diphyllobothrium latum egg.* (*top right*) *Hymenolepis diminuta egg.* (*bottom*) *Hydatid cyst with scolex and hooklets.* ×450.

technique. Although the Formalin-ether technique is generally satisfactory for the detection of trematode eggs, schistosome-infected patients often pass relatively few eggs in their stool. Therefore, a special modification of the Formalin-ether technique has been devised by Hunter et al. (2). The latter procedure is more complex but also more efficient than the routine Formalin-ether technique. The techniques recommended here are essential for concentrating trematode eggs, because these eggs will not float and cannot be detected by flotation techniques.

3. Sigmoidoscopic examination and biopsy. Erythematous nodular lesions and submucosal plaques may be observed in early cases of intestinal schistosomiasis. Later, papillomas

may develop. Aspiration, scraping, and biopsy of suspicious lesions in the large bowel may reveal eggs of the parasites. The rectal biopsy tissue fragments should be immediately immersed in water for 3 to 5 min. The hydrated tissue is then compressed between two slides; a drop of water is added to the tissue film, and another slide is used as a cover. The "sandwich" is pressed gently and examined under low power for eggs. Nonviable eggs will appear dark, whereas viable eggs will be translucent and contain motile larvae (miracidia). The tissue obtained may be sectioned and stained by the usual techniques. Sigmoidoscopic examination is inferior to stool sedimentation in early cases, but may be very helpful in late cases when few eggs are extruded into the lumen.

4. Serology. Presumptive diagnosis can be made with cholesterol lecithin slide flocculation test or fluorescent-antibody techniques. These procedures are described in chapter 70.

Schistosoma haematobium. *S. haematobium* is the etiological agent of schistosomal hematuria and schistosomal carcinoma of the bladder.

Diagnostic stage: nonoperculate egg possessing terminal spine (Fig. 14); length, 112 to 170 μm; breadth, 40 to 70 μm.

Diagnosis is accomplished by examination of urine for eggs. The typical terminal-spined eggs are most frequently found in the last few drops of urine at the end of micturition, particularly if there is blood present. The urine sample may be concentrated by centrifugation, or by allowing the particulate matter to settle. The sediment should be examined under low-power microscopy.

Liver flukes

Fasciola hepatica. *F. hepatica* is the etiological agent of parasitic biliary cirrhosis, and pharyngeal fascioliasis (halzoun).

Diagnostic stage: operculate egg, measuring 150 by 90 μm, which is found in stools, biliary drainage, or duodenal drainage (Fig. 14).

Diagnostic procedures are as follows:

1. Demonstration of typical operculate egg by direct fecal smear or concentration technique. Several examinations should be made following a positive finding to rule out spurious presence of eggs resulting from ingestion of infected cattle liver.

2. Examination of bile-drainage fluid. The

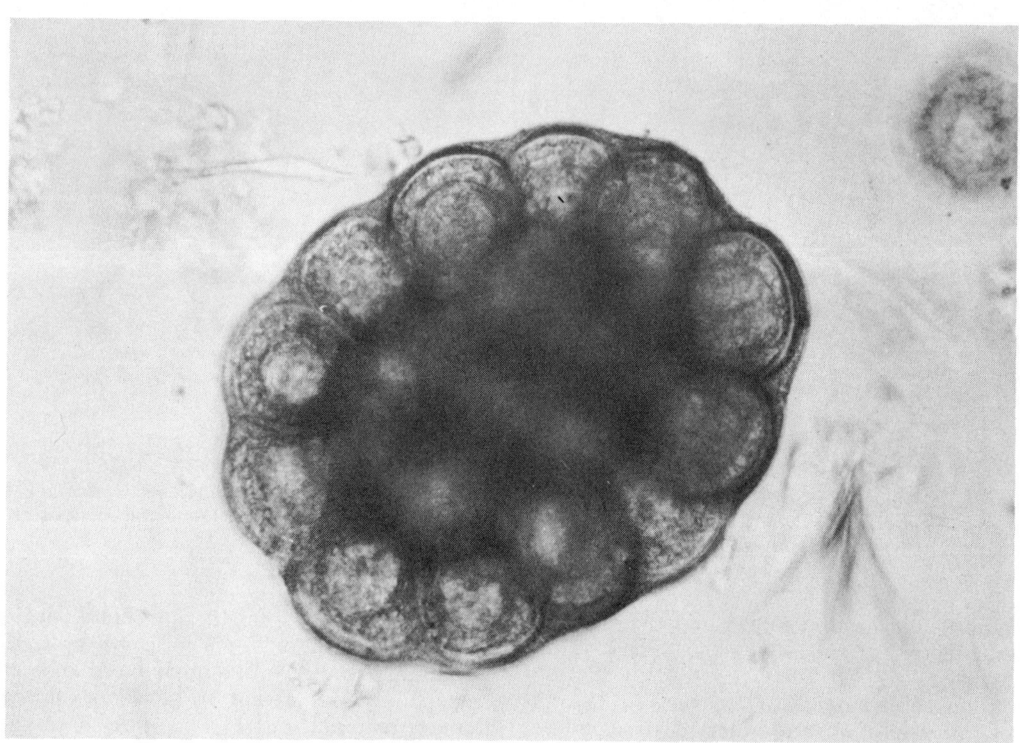

FIG. 13. *Dipylidium caninum egg packet.* ×450.

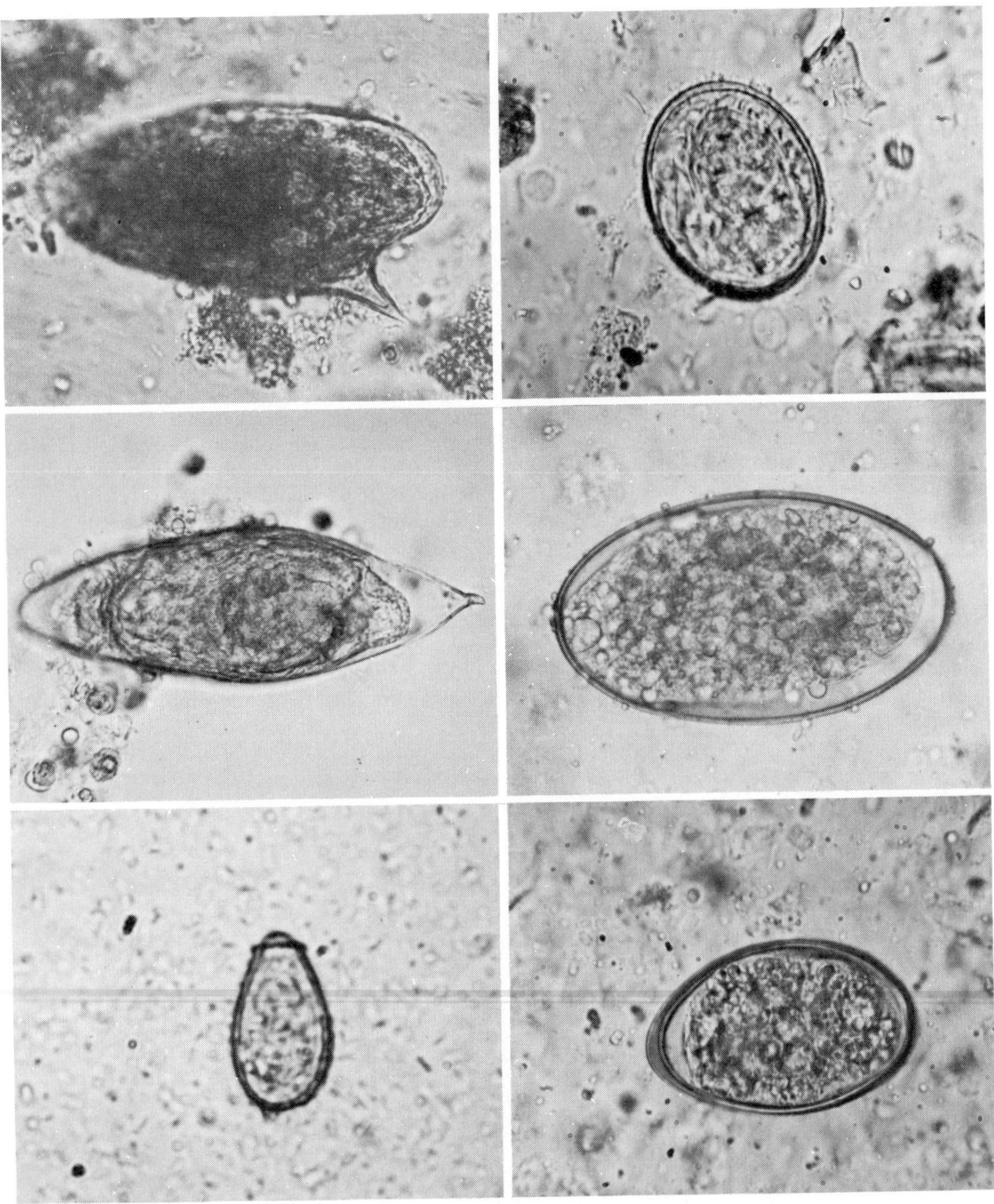

FIG. 14. (*top left*) *Schistosoma mansoni* egg. (*top right*) *Schistosoma japonicum* egg. (*middle left*) *Schistosoma haematobium* egg. (*middle right*) *Fasciola hepatica* egg. (*bottom left*) *Clonorchis sinensis* egg. (*bottom right*) *Paragonimus westermani* egg. ×450.

fluid should be centrifuged and the sediment examined.

Clonorchis sinensis. *C. sinensis* is the etiological agent of oriental biliary cirrhosis.

Diagnostic stage: small, operculate, ovoid egg, measuring 27 to 35 μm in length by 12 to 19.5 μm in breadth, with a pronounced knob at anopercular end. Found in stools or biliary drainage material (Fig. 14).

Diagnostic procedures are the same as those described for *F. hepatica.*

Lung fluke

Paragonimus westermani. *P. westermani* is the etiological agent of parasitic hemoptysis, oriental lung fluke infection.

Diagnostic stage: ovoid, operculate, golden-brown egg measuring 80 to 120 μm in length by 50 to 60 μm in breadth. The eggs do not contain a developed larva (Fig. 14).

Diagnosis is based on direct smear examination of sputum or feces. (Procedures employed in handling and concentrating sputum samples have been described. Procedures for concentrating stools are the same as previously described for schistosome eggs.) Occasionally, cutaneous abscesses containing adult flukes may be encountered. Eggs may be found in the exudates of such abscesses.

Intestinal fluke

Fasciolopsis buski. *F. buski* is the etiological agent of intestinal fluke infection.

Diagnostic stage: ovoid, operculate egg measuring 130 to 140 μm in length by 80 to 85 μm in breadth. The eggs are immature when laid.

Adult worms are large intestinal flukes, 50 to 75 mm long. The adults are fleshy, broadly ovate, and possess a spined integument. They can be readily differentiated from *F. hepatica* by the lack of branching of the intestinal caeca.

Diagnostic procedures include gross examination of stool for adult worms and direct smear examination of stools and Formalin-ether concentration technique for eggs. The eggs of *F. buski* may be confused with *F. hepatica.* The latter are smaller, but the operculum of *F. hepatica* is larger than that of *F. buski.*

LITERATURE CITED

1. Hunter, G. W., W. W. Frye, and J. C. Swartzwelder. 1966. A manual of tropical medicine. W. B. Saunders Co., Philadelphia.
2. Hunter, G. W., III, E. P. Hodges, W. G. Jahnes, L. S. Diamond, and J. W. Ingalls, Jr. 1948. Studies on schistosomiasis. II. Summary of further studies on methods of recovering eggs of *S. japanicum* from stools. Bull. U.S. Army Med. Dept. **8**:128–131.

Chapter 69

Arthropods Affecting Humans

JEROME P. VANDERBERG AND BERNARD V. TRAVIS

INTRODUCTION

The Arthropoda constitute the largest of the animal phyla. They are characterized by a segmented body with the segments generally grouped in two or three more or less distinct body regions, several pairs of jointed appendages (from which the phylum gets its name), a rigid chitinous exoskeleton which is periodically molted and renewed as the animal grows, and certain characteristic internal organs. Three classes among the arthropods may be of particular interest to the clinical microbiologist.

Class Arachnida

Representatives. Mites, ticks, spiders, scorpions.

Characterization. Lacking antennae and with four pairs of legs (three pairs in first-stage larvae).

Medical importance. May be venomous or, as in the case of mites and ticks, serve as vectors of disease.

Class Insecta

Representatives. Lice, bugs, fleas, flies, etc.

Characterization. As adults, a single pair of antennae and three pairs of legs; usually one or two pairs of wings.

Medical importance. May be venomous or parasitic, or act as vectors of disease.

Class Pentastomida (Linguatulida)

Representatives. Tongue worms.

Characterization. Adults are elongate, legless, wormlike parasites divided externally by prominent rings; mouth associated with two pairs of fanglike hooks. Larvae have two pairs of short segmented legs.

Medical importance. Strictly endoparasitic, encysted in tissues. Diagnosed either postmortem or from sections of biopsied tissue.

Other classes

In addition to the above, members of other classes may have medical importance. Thus, some species of the class Crustacea are intermediate hosts and vectors of the parasitic helminths *Dracunculus*, *Diphyllobothrium*, and *Paragonimus*. Also, centipedes (class Chilopoda) may produce a venomous bite, and millipedes (class Diplopoda) may secrete an irritating fluid from pores on their body surface.

The clinical microbiologist may be confronted with problems created by arthropods in any of several ways.

1. He may come in contact with a disease transmitted by arthropods, such as mosquito-borne encephalitis or tick-borne spotted fever.
2. He may see a patient showing the results of attack by arthropods, such as stings of wasps, bees, and hornets; dermatitis produced by urticating and vesicating insects; or sensitization caused by bites of lice, fleas, bugs, or biting flies.
3. He may come directly in contact with arthropods parasitizing a patient, such as ticks, lice, fleas, or tissue-invading fly larvae.
4. He may be confronted with nonparasitic arthropods that have accidentally become associated with people.
5. Finally, he may be asked to determine whether arthropods actually are present in submitted material in a suspected case of entomophobia, that is, when a psychologically disturbed patient has the illusion of being attacked by arthropods.

This chapter will be concerned with the third and fourth types of problems, i.e., cases when a person brings in for identification an arthropod that he has found, or when a parasitic arthropod is found during the examination of a patient.

It is not uncommon for arthropods to be brought into a clinical diagnostic laboratory for identification. Because of the great number and variety of arthropods, very often an accurate specific diagnosis can be made only by a specialist in the particular field. However, it is possible for anyone with a basic amount of biological training to identify the major groups of arthropods that are apt to be seen in the laboratory (Fig. 1), and in some arthropod groups to identify a specimen as to genus and species with reasonable confidence (5–7, 10, 14, 17, 18).

The laboratory should be in a position to

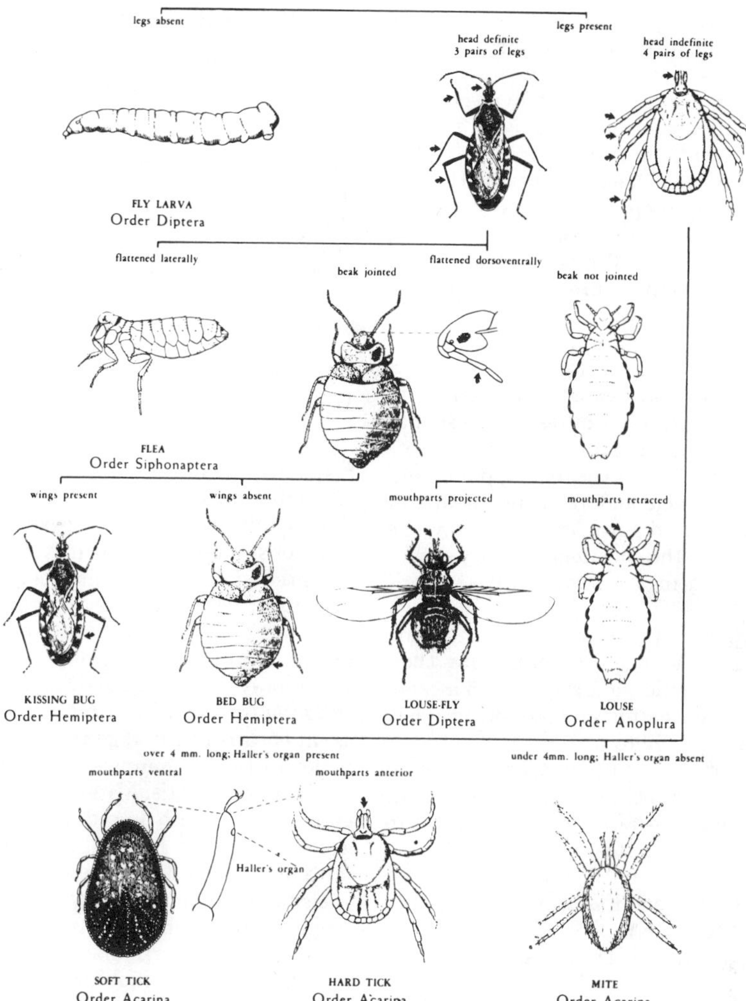

FIG. 1. *Pictorial key to groups of human ectoparasites (C. J. Stojanovich and H. G. Scott; U.S. Dept. of Health, Education, and Welfare, Center for Disease Control, Atlanta, Ga.).*

determine whether the arthropods submitted for identification are capable of parasitizing humans or are merely nuisance-type pests. If no one is available to make a proper identification, the laboratory personnel should at least be aware of how to pack the specimens properly and where to send them for identification.

HANDLING OF SPECIMENS

Most arthropods can be preserved and then shipped through the mail in 70% alcohol. Inasmuch as specimens may be damaged by being buffeted by air bubbles in transit, care should be taken to fill the container with as much fluid as possible. The vial should be carefully packed to prevent breakage.

Insects with many bristles or scales, such as adult flies, mosquitoes, or moths, are best sent dry. They may be packed between layers of cellucotton or soft tissue paper in a pill box which is then firmly packed in a mailing container. (Avoid absorbent cotton, since fibers may become entangled in the specimen.) A taxonomist receiving these dry specimens can later rehydrate them in a saturated atmosphere and properly mount them on insect pins. Specimens sent loosely in a container or envelope will generally break up and become worthless for identification.

Small ectoparasites such as mites, fleas, and lice can be carefully studied only after clearing and mounting on slides. They may be shipped in alcohol to an appropriate specialist for mounting and identification, or they may be mounted in the clinical laboratory.

Mites and lice can be mounted live (preferably) or directly from alcohol in any of several commercially available combination clearing and mounting agents. One of the best is Hoyer's mounting medium, prepared by mixing 50 g of distilled water, 30 g of gum arabic (flakes), 200 g of chloral hydrate, and 20 g of glycerol in this sequence at room temperature. The specimen is placed in a drop of medium on a slide, a cover slip is placed on top, and the side is heated gently until bubbles start to form. Mounted slides may also be heated in a warm oven (25 to 40 C) for 24 h. Blood-filled mites or lice should first be punctured, cleared for 5 to 10 min in 85% lactic acid, heated to near the boiling point, and washed free from acid before being mounted. Nonpermanent rapid preparations may be made by mounting the specimen directly in 85% lactic acid and heating the slide as with Hoyer's solution.

Fleas, because of their heavy sclerotization and because of the need to eliminate their internal organs, should be macerated in a caustic solution before clearing and mounting. They may be prepared as follows.

1. Place in 10% potassium hydroxide at room temperature for 12 to 14 h. (If time is important, puncture specimen with fine needle and heat to steaming for a few minutes.)
2. Place in water for 1 h.
3. Place in water acidified with a drop of 1 to 5% acetic acid for 30 min.
4. Dehydrate through graded series of alcohols to 95% alcohol (to 100% if xylol is to be used as clearing agent).
5. Clear in xylol, oil of wintergreen (methyl salicylate), oil of cloves, or beechwood creosote for 15 min.
6. Mount on a slide in permanent mounting medium.

A small curved forceps or a small wire loop may be placed under the specimen for moving it from one container to another. Liquids may be drawn off from a container by means of a medicine dropper, the tip of which has been screened with bolting cloth or a piece of old stocking.

When specimens are sent to a specialist for identification, as complete collection data as possible also should be submitted. Identification services usually are provided by departments of entomology in various natural history museums, colleges, or universities, or by medical entomologists associated with medical schools.

NONPARASITIC ARTHROPODS

Many nonparasitic arthropods may be closely associated with humans or human habitations (19). Some of the more common types which may be submitted to the diagnostic laboratory are (i) garden and greenhouse pests which may enter homes, hidden on fruit, vegetables, or flowers; (ii) insect pests of dried food products; (iii) insects attacking fibers, such as clothes moths and carpet beetles; and (iv) household pests such as cockroaches, ants, termites, and silverfish.

PARASITIC ARTHROPODS

Mites (1–3, 21)

A number of mites known to parasitize humans may be brought to the clinical microbiology laboratory for identification. Because of their small size, mites are generally difficult for the nonspecialist to identify. However, well-mounted specimens of the more common and important parasitic mites may be identified by reference to illustrations or to a picture key, as in Fig. 2. Some major groups of mite problems which may be encountered are as follows.

Sarcoptes scabiei (itch mite). Causative agent of sarcoptic mange or scabies. Adult mites make tortuous channels a few millimeters in length in epidermis. Mites may be picked out of end of burrow with a needle and mounted under a cover slip (see Fig. 2). Other species of itch mite may infest domestic animals.

Demodex folliculorum (follicle mite). Microscopic mites found in hair follicles and sebaceous glands, particularly around nose and eyelids. May be squeezed out of sebaceous glands, or more commonly are found in histological sections of skin. No well-established role in disease. Mites vermiform; annulate abdomen with no setae; eight stumplike legs.

Larvae of trombiculid mites (chiggers, red mites, harvest mites). Parasitic larval mites of family Trombiculidae (of the genera *Trombicula* and *Eutrombicula*). Mites often appear as tiny, almost microscopic reddish dots attached to skin. Three pairs of legs are present; adults have four pairs and are not parasitic. The characteristic bristles are branched and featherlike. Transmit scrub typhus.

Pyemotes (= Pediculoides) ventricosus (hay itch mite). Parasitize insect larvae which infest grains, straw hay, and other plant products. Mites may attack people who come in contact with these products. Resulting dermatitis may cover large portion of body. Abdomen of gravid female mite becomes enormously distended, resembling a small pearl.

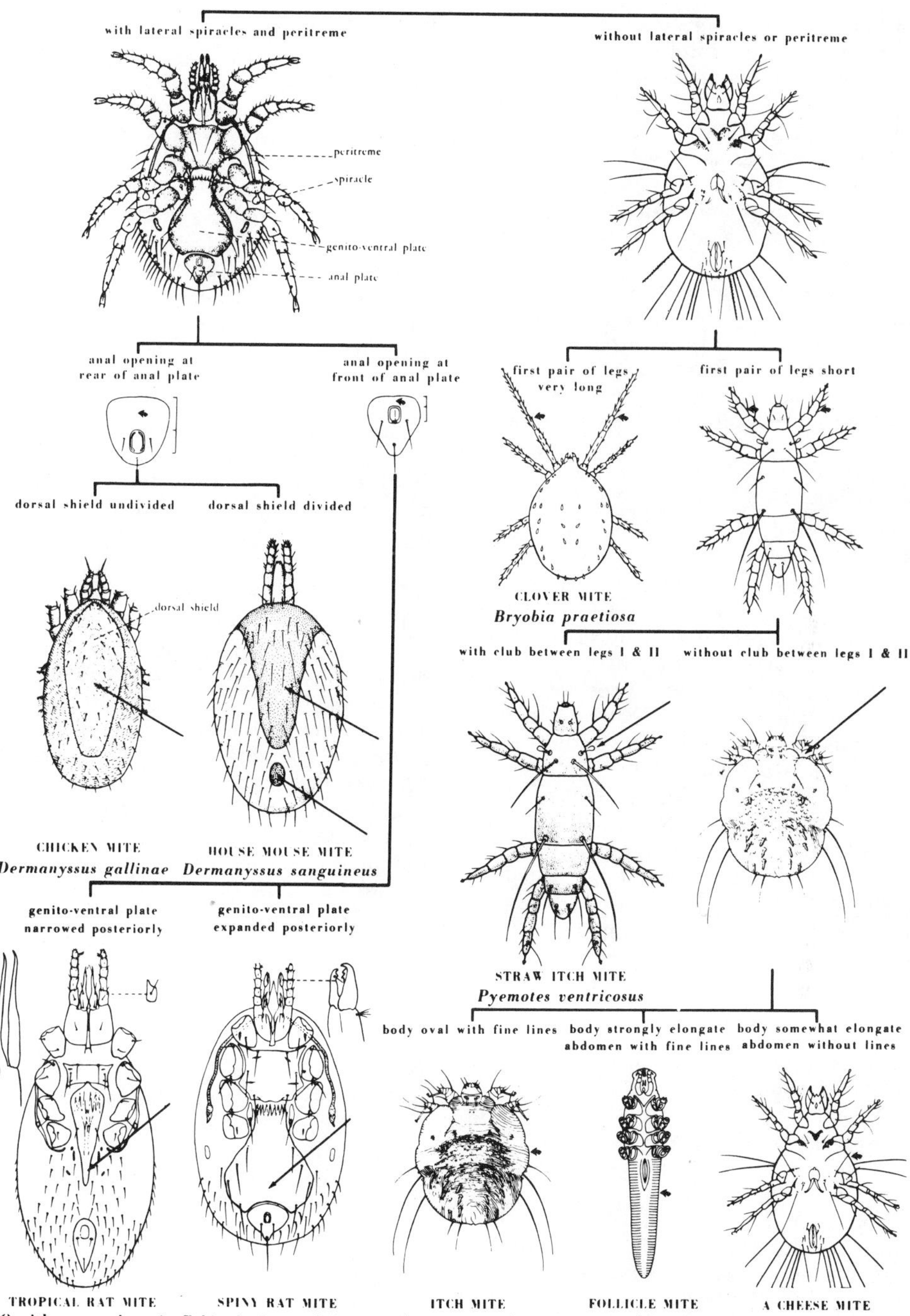

FIG. 2. *Pictorial key to some common species of mites of public health importance (H. G. Scott and C. J. Stojanovitch; U.S. Dept. of Health, Education, and Welfare, Center for Disease Control, Atlanta, Ga.).*

Mites of family Dermanyssidae. Mites of this family belong to a group characterized by lateral respiratory organs (peritremes) opening into spiracles at about the middle of the body (visible only in well-cleared specimens). Brown sclerotized plates are found on the body. Their shapes plus bristle characteristics are used in making identification. Generally parasites of rodents or birds, but may occasionally attack humans, causing a mild dermatitis.

Mites living in dry processed food (cheese mites, grain mites, dried food mites, grocer's itch mite). Mites belonging to several genera within families Acaridae (= Tyroglyphidae), Glycyphagidae, and Carpoglyphidae. Feed on stored products and may cause dermatitis in people coming in contact with infested products.

Bryobia praetiosa (clover mite). Pest of various agricultural crops. Nonparasitic, but often an annoying pest when large numbers of mites migrate into homes. Body with fanlike setae; four protuberances near head, each bearing a fanlike setae; newly hatched larvae are bright red.

Ticks (4, 11)

Ticks are closely related to mites, and indeed can be considered to be overgrown mites. They may be of medical importance by virtue of their transmission of diseases (spotted fever, relapsing, tularemia, and others) or by their production of a paralysis when they attach, particularly in the region of the head, back of the neck, or over the spinal column. Ticks are divided into two families: the hard ticks (Ixodidae), and the soft ticks (Argasidae). Hard ticks are characterized by a dorsal shield, the scutum, which covers almost the entire dorsal surface in the male, and only the anterior portion of the dorsal surface in the female. Some of the important ticks are shown in Fig. 3.

Argas persicus. An important pest of poultry. Will occasionally bite poultry workers.

Ornithodoros. Species of this genus are found in the southern United States, and in Pacific Coast and Rocky Mountain states. Primarily found in caves and in rugged mountain terrain. Vector of relapsing fever.

Amblyomma americanum. Infects deer, cattle, dogs, and birds in the southern United States, and will attack humans. Vector of spotted fever and tularemia.

Dermacentor. Members of this genus have prominent white markings on the scutum. *D. variabilis* is found east of the Rocky Mountains and along the Pacific Coast. It is a common pest of dogs, and freely attacks humans, particularly in rural and suburban areas. *D. andersoni* is found in the Rocky Moutain states in areas of low bushy vegetation. Both species are the chief vectors of spotted fever and the most important causes of tick paralysis in the United States.

Rhipicephalus sanguineus. An important house pest, attacking dogs but rarely humans. Identifiable by shape of the base of the head region (*basis capituli*) as shown in Fig. 3.

Fleas, order Siphonaptera (8, 9, 13, 15)

Fleas are small, wingless, highly sclerotized, laterally flattened ectoparasites (Fig. 1). Their long, well developed hind legs are an adaptation for jumping. Also characteristic of fleas are the backward-projecting spines and bristles, which enable the fleas to walk forward through hair or fur without becoming entangled. The presence or absence of various bristles or spines is important in identifying fleas as to species (Fig. 4).

Fleas, unlike lice, move more readily from host to host and generally have a wider range of hosts that they will attack. Those which bite humans usually come from infested pets or rodents.

Fleas have a complete metamorphosis consisting of egg, larval stages, pupa, and adult. Only the adults are parasites. They are vectors of bubonic plague and endemic (murine) typhus.

Lice, order Anoplura (20)

Lice (sucking lice) are small, wingless, dorsoventrally flattened ectoparasites. They can be distinguished from other ectoparasites by their specialized legs, each of which ends with a curved claw. This claw, together with a thumblike process, enables the lice to cling to hair and fibers of clothing.

Lice are very specific in the host species that they attack. The three kinds of lice found on humans are exclusively human parasites. These lice are as follows.

Body louse (Pediculus humanus humanus). Found primarily attached to fibers of clothing that come in close contact with skin. Eggs (nits) generally attached to clothing. Vector of epidemic typhus.

Head louse (Pediculus humanus capitus). Found primarily among hairs of head. Morphologically similar to body louse.

Crab or pubic louse (Phthirus pubis). Particularly found in pubic region, but may also attack other hairy parts of the body.

Because of the limited number of louse species which attack humans, identification is relatively easy and can be made by referring to Fig. 5.

Bugs, order Hemiptera

The most important of the bugs which attack humans are the bed bug, *Cimex lectularius*, and the assassin kissing bugs belonging to the family *Reduviidae* (Fig. 1). The adult bed bug is a flattened, reddish-brown insect, 4 to 5 mm long and 3 mm wide. The nymphal stages, which look like miniature adults, are yellowish-white. Bed bugs are nocturnal in their feeding habits,

PICTORIAL KEY TO SOME COMMON TICKS

capitulum visible from above, scutum present, family Ixodidae, HARD TICKS

capitulum
scutum
female
male

capitulum not visible from above, scutum absent, family Argasidae. SOFT TICKS

capitulum
ventral
dorsal

sutural line present

sutural line absent

Argas persicus FOWL TICK

Ornithodoros RELAPSING FEVER TICK

mouthparts short, about as long as basis capituli

mouthparts
basis capitulum

mouthparts much longer than basis capituli white spot on tip of scutum of female

mouthparts
basis capitulum

Amblyomma americanum LONE STAR TICK

scutum with white markings; basis capituli with parallel sides

scutum
male
female

Dermacentor variabilis and *D. andersoni* AMERICAN DOG TICK AND WOOD TICK

scutum without white markings; basis capituli produced laterally to form an angle

scutum
male
female

Rhipicephalus sanguineus BROWN DOG TICK

FIG. 3. *Pictorial key to some common ticks (H. D. Pratt; U.S. Dept. of Health, Education, and Welfare, Center for Disease Control, Atlanta, Ga.).*

hiding in cracks and crevices during the day. They are not known to be important in the transmission of disease. Occasionally, humans will be bitten by species of bed bugs that are normally parasites of birds or bats. Kissing bugs are of particular importance in the southwestern United States and in Central and South America, where they are vectors of Chagas' disease.

Myiasis (12, 16)

Invasion of the body by larval stages of flies is known as myiasis. Larvae of other insects, such as beetles and moths, may occasionally invade the intestinal or urogenital tracts, but such cases are rare compared to those in which fly larvae are involved. Eggs or larvae of myiasis-producing flies may be deposited on either broken or unbroken skin, or near body orifices. Infection of the gastrointestinal tract may occur by the ingestion of food contaminated with eggs or larvae.

Myiasis larvae should be killed by placing them in water near the boiling point for 3 to 5 min and then they should be preserved in 70%

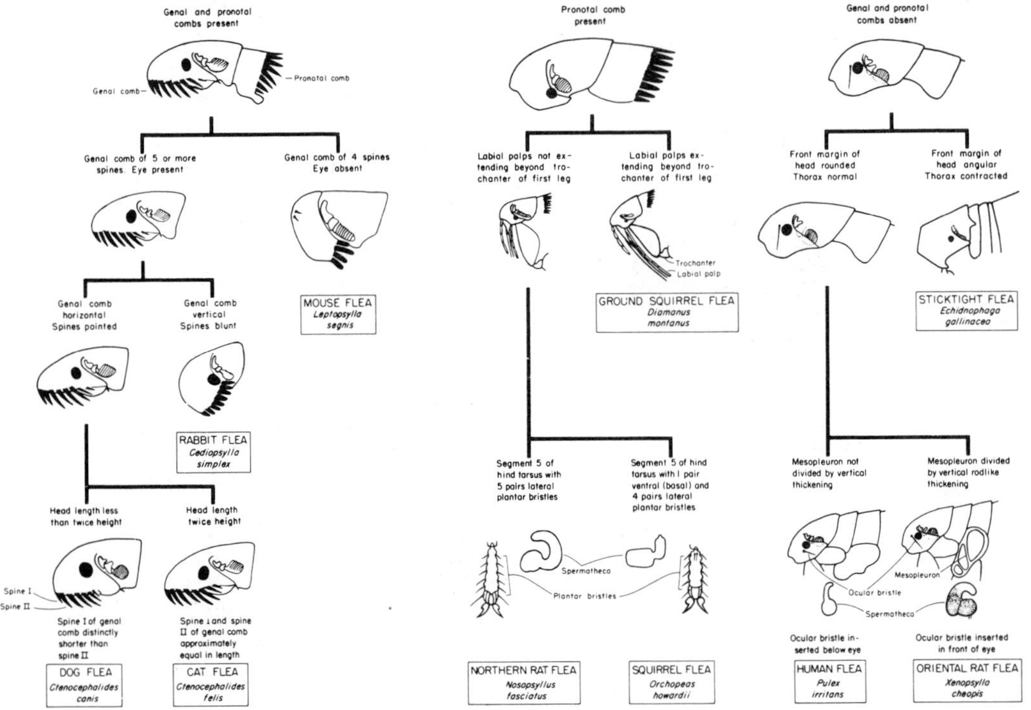

FIG. 4. *Pictorial key to some common fleas in the United States (H. D. Pratt; U.S. Dept. of Health, Education, and Welfare, Center for Disease Control, Atlanta, Ga.).*

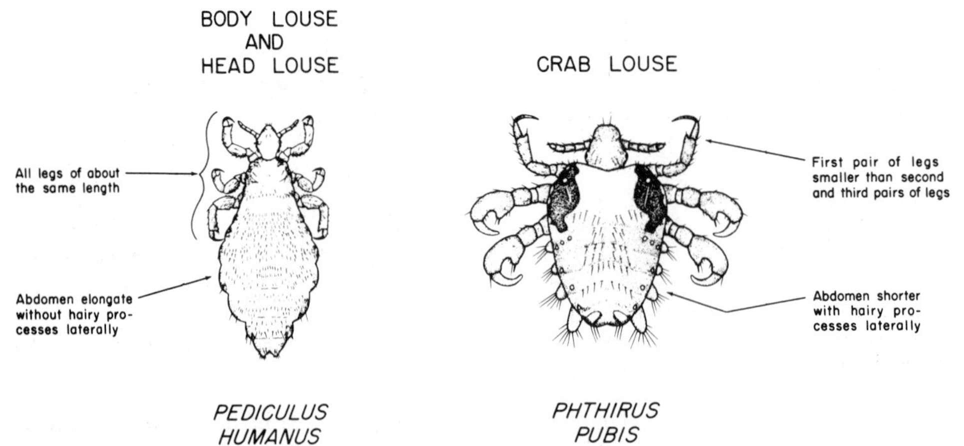

FIG. 5. *Lice commonly found on humans (U.S. Dept. of Health, Education, and Welfare, Center for Disease Control, Atlanta, Ga.).*

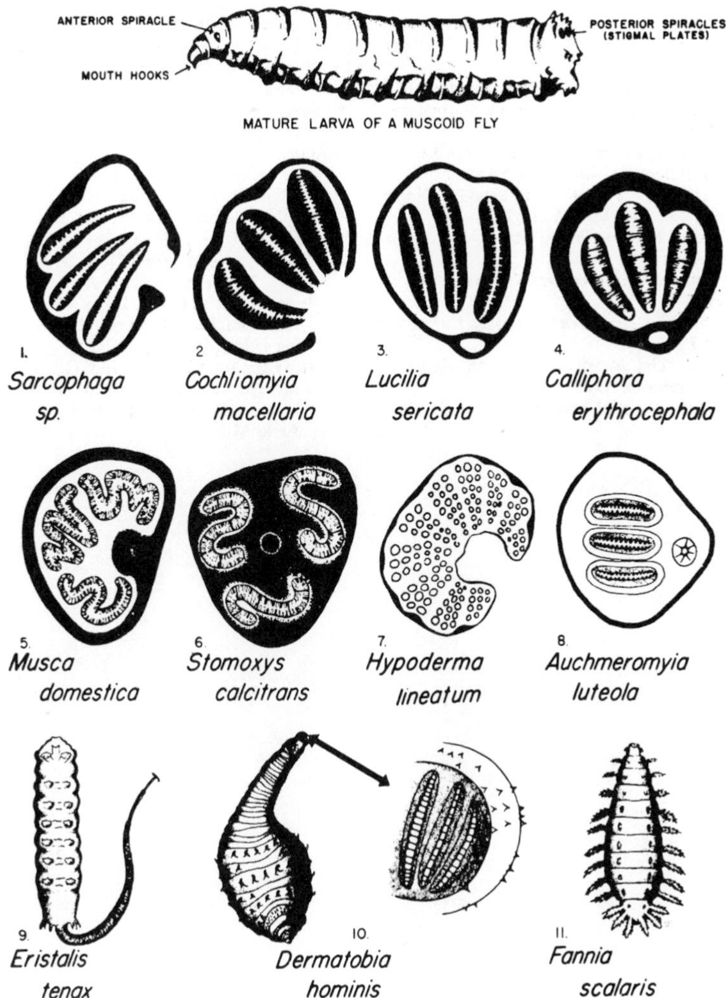

FIG. 6. *Key characters of myiasis-producing fly larvae (U.S. Dept. of Health, Education, and Welfare, Center for Disease Control, Atlanta, Ga.).*

alcohol. They may be examined in alcohol in a small glass container under the lower magnifications of a dissecting microscope.

A typical larva of a muscoid (house fly-like) fly is peg-shaped with one or two sclerotized mouth hooks at the anterior (narrow) end. One of the chief diagnostic characters used for identification is the structure of the paired plates surrounding the openings of the respiratory system at the posterior end of the larvae (Fig. 6).

If myiasis flies are still alive when received in the laboratory, it is often advisable to attempt to rear them to the adult stage so as to permit a more positive identification. Many of the tissue-invading larvae can be induced to complete their development in a vial containing ground beef. The vial should be tightly plugged to prevent other flies from depositing eggs or larvae in it. Adults which merge within the vial can be killed with chloroform or ether, and can be packed and shipped as discussed under Handling of specimens.

LITERATURE CITED

1. Baker, E. W., J. H. Camin, F. Cunliffe, T. A. Woolley, and C. E. Yunker. 1958. Guide to the families of mites. Contr No. 3, Institute of Acarology, College Park, Md.
2. Baker, E. W., T. M. Evans, D. J. Gould, W. B. Hull, and H. L. Kegan. 1956. A manual of parasitic mites of medical or economic importance. National Pest Control Association, Inc., New York.
3. Baker, E. W., and G. W. Wharton. 1952. An introduction to acarology. The Macmillan Co., New York.
4. Bequaert, J. C. 1946. The ticks, or Ixodoidea, of the northern United States and eastern Canada. Entomologia Amer. **25**:73–120.

5. Borror, D. J., and D. M DeLong. 1964. An introduction to the study of insects, 2nd ed. Reinhard and Co., New York.
6. Brues, C. T., A. L. Melander and F. M. Carpenter. 1954. Classification of insects, 2nd ed. Harvard Museum, Cambridge, Mass.
7. Emerton, J. H. 1961. The common spiders of the United States. Dover Publications, Inc., New York.
8. Ewing, H. E., and I. Fox. 1943. The fleas of North America. U S. Dept. Agr. Misc. Publ. 500.
9. Fox, I. 1940. Fleas of Eastern United States. Iowa State College Press, Ames.
10. Gertsch, W. J. 1949. American spiders. C. Van Nostrand Co., New York.
11. Gregson, J. D. 1956. The Ixodoidea of Canada. Can. Dep. Agr Sci. Serv. Publ. 930.
12. Hall, D. G. 1948. The blowflies of North America. Thomas Say Foundation, Baltimore.
13. Holland, G. P. 1949. The Siphonaptera of Canada. Can. Dep. Agr. Tech. Bull. 70
14. Horsfall, W. R. 1962. Medical entomology. The Ronald Press Co., New York.
15. Hubbard, C. A. 1947. Fleas of western Northern America. Iowa State College Press, Ames.
16. James, M. T. 1947. The flies that cause myiasis in man. U.S. Dep. Agr. Misc. Publ. 631.
17. James, M. T., and R F. Harwood. 1969. Herms' medical entomology. The Macmillan Co., New York.
18. Kaston, B. J., and E. Kaston. 1953. How to know the spiders. Wm. C. Brown Co., Dubuque.
19. Metcalf, C. L., W. Flint, and R. L. Metcalf. 1962. Destructive and useful insects. McGraw-Hill Book Co., Inc., New York.
20. Pratt, H. D., and K. S. Littig. 1961. Lice of public health importance and their control. U.S. Government Printing Office, Washington, D.C.
21. Strandtmann, R. W., and G. W. Wharton. 1958. A manual of mesostigmatid mites parasitic on vertebrates. Contr No. 4, Institute of Acarology, College Park, Md.

Chapter 70
Serodiagnosis of Parasitic Diseases

IRVING G. KAGAN AND LOIS NORMAN

INTRODUCTION

Serological tests for the diagnosis of parasitic diseases have been performed for over 60 years, and excellent summaries and bibliographies of parasitic antigen-antibody interactions have been published (29, 63, 88, 92, 93). Reviews of the serology of specific diseases, such as trichinosis (41, 49, 58), echinococcosis (43, 47), schistosomiasis (36, 46, 53, 77), ascariasis (81, 100), filariasis (42), cysticercosis (8, 80), Chagas' disease (15, 68), leishmaniasis (1), toxoplasmosis (30, 37), amebiasis (3, 21), and malaria (31), are available. Furthermore, interest in the field has been stimulated by the World Health Organization (109) and at several international congresses and seminars (35, 56).

In this chapter, we will not attempt to review the merits of all serological procedures for the diagnosis of each parasitic disease or to evaluate the general diagnostic serology of parasitic diseases. For some serological tests, there are almost as many variations as there are laboratories using the techniques. Kwapinski (61) should be consulted for a detailed discussion of serological methods.

Immunodiagnostic tests for 18 parasitic infections are shown in Table 1. Included are the particle agglutination tests (bentonite flocculation [BF], indirect hemagglutination [IHA], latex agglutination, and cholesterol-lecithin flocculation [CL] tests), the complement fixation (CF) test, precipitin tests, the indirect immunofluorescence (IF) test, and the diffusion tests (double diffusion in gels [DD] and immunoelectrophoresis [IE]). The methods described for performing the basic tests are those which have been found to yield fairly reproducible results at the Center for Disease Control (CDC). A list of antigens recommended for each test and a table of sources of commercially available antigens are given in the appendix.

TRICHINOSIS

Many tests are used for the diagnosis of trichinosis. A good test should be sufficiently sensitive and reproducible to measure increase or decrease in serum titer during the acute stage of infection, yet not so sensitive that it reveals residual circulating antibodies from past experience with the parasite. The BF test most nearly meets these prerequisities for a practical diagnostic procedure (44, 59, 75). The BF test, however, is not adequate for testing lightly infected pigs (89). The IF test is the only procedure that demonstrates antibodies in pigs infected with less than one larva per gram of diaphragm muscle tissue (54).

With the BF test, antibodies are detected after the third week of a clinical infection; with the CF test, also a good method, a little earlier. Titers obtained by BF rise rapidly for several weeks, until a peak is reached, and then drop slowly; specimens from almost all persons are negative 2 to 3 years after infection. The specificity of the BF test is very high (59, 75). The IF test is probably the most reactive diagnostic procedure (62, 95). The other tests available to the diagnostic laboratory, such as the latex agglutination (9. 74) and CL (6) tests, are good techniques that are particularly suitable for small laboratories because of their simplicity.

In the CDC laboratory, the BF test is the standard test performed for the diagnosis of trichinosis. Sera are titrated in twofold dilutions from 1:5, and a 1:5 titer is considered diagnostically significant. Rising titers in a series of serum samples from a patient are particularly important. Since no single test or single antigen will reveal all infections at all stages of the disease, a second test, preferably of a different type, is recommended for confirmation of low titers or to resolve questionable reactions. An evaluation of the BF test is given in Table 2.

ECHINOCOCCOSIS

The tests of choice in the diagnosis of hydatid disease are the IHA, IF, and IE tests. High titers in the IHA test are usually indicative of hydatid disease. Low titers are equivocal because they have been found in sera from patients with collagen diseases or liver cirrhosis (51). Hydatid cysts of the lung are detected less frequently with serological tests. Cross-reactions are ob-

TABLE 1. *Immunodiagnostic tests for parasitic diseases*[a]

Parasitic disease	Intradermal	Complement fixation	Bentonite flocculation	Indirect hemag-glutination	Latex	Indirect fluorescent antibody	Precipitin
Amebiasis	▲	●	▲	●	●	▲	○
Chagas'	○	●		●	○	●	○
African trypanosomiasis		▲		○		▲	●
Leishmaniasis	●	●		●	○	▲	●
Malaria		▲		▲	○	●	○
Pneumocystis		▲				▲	
Toxoplasmosis	●	●		●	○	●	
Ancylostomiasis	▲	○		▲	▲	○	
Ascariasis	▲	○	●	●		▲	▲
Filariasis	▲	●	●	●	○	▲	
Toxocariasis	▲	●	●	●		▲	○
Trichinellosis	●	●	●	●	●	●	●
Clonorchiasis	●	●		●			○
Fascioliasis	▲	●		●		▲	○
Paragonimiasis	●	●	○	○			
Schistosomiasis	●	●	▲	●	○	●	○
Cysticercosis	○	●		●	○	▲	○
Echinococcosis	●	●	●	●	●	●	▲

[a] Symbols: ●, evaluated; ▲, experimental test; ○, reported in the literature.

TABLE 2. *Sensitivity and specificity of the bentonite flocculation test for the diagnosis of trichinosis*

Human serum	No. positive/no. tested	Percent positive
Trichina	38/39	97
Echinococcus	0/28	0
Filaria	0/29	0
Ascaris-toxocara	0/21	0
Schistosoma	0/34	0
Protozoa	0/48	0
Bacteria-virus	0/46	0
Normal controls	0/30	0

served with cysticercosis antisera and echinococcus antigens (Table 3).

A combination of IHA and BF tests is routinely performed on all diagnostic sera in our laboratory. The IHA test is the more sensitive. The sensitivity of the serological tests has been found to vary from 82 to 88% for sera from individuals with liver cysts and from 33 to 50% for sera from patients with lung cysts (52). Specificity is high when only those sera with titers of 1:32 or higher by IHA and 1:5 or higher by BF are reported as positive. The BF test, introduced in 1959 (76), and the latex agglutination tests of Fischman (27, 28) are somewhat simpler to perform, and their specificity is about the same as that of the IHA test. Sensitivity is a little lower. Sera from healthy people are consistently negative with the echinococcus tests; however, the large number of reactive sera from people ill with other diseases makes the interpretation of low titers particularly difficult.

TABLE 3. *Sensitivity and specificity of indirect hemagglutination (IHA) and bentonite flocculation (BF) tests for the diagnosis of hydatid disease*

Human antiserum	Serological tests: IHA		Serological tests: BF	
	No. positive/no. tested	Percent positive	No. positive/no. tested	Percent positive
Hydatid disease				
Liver	52/59	88	50/58	86
Lung	6/18	33	9/18	50
Controls				
Cysticercus cellulosae	9/9	100	4/8	50
Taenia saginata	0/16	0	2/16	12
Cancer	0/16	0	2/15	13
Other parasitic diseases	5/126	4	8/113	7
Miscellaneous diseases	0/62	0	0/52	0
Normal	0/47	0	0/52	0

The immunofluorescence test can best be performed with scolices from viable cysts of human or animal origin (4). In the IE test, the identification of "Band #5" of Capron (14) is diagnostic for hydatid infection and may be useful in increasing the specificity of the serological test. Both the IF and IE tests are being evaluated as routine methods of diagnosis in many parts of the world.

SCHISTOSOMIASIS

The tests used in our laboratory for routine diagnosis are the CL, the BF, the CF, and the IF tests. The antigens include a delipidized cercarial antigen for the first two tests, delipidized adult antigen for the CF test, and cryostat sections of adult worms for the IF test. The CL test was adapted for the diagnosis of schistosomiasis by Anderson (5), and the sensitivity and specificity of this procedure were evaluated by Jachowski and Anderson (36) and Buck and Anderson (13). In our laboratory, the test showed a sensitivity of 77% for sera from patients with confirmed infections (55). The CL test cannot be performed with chylous or contaminated sera and has been found to be too nonspecific in seroepidemiological studies (13). To overcome this problem, a BF test was developed which showed a sensitivity of approximately 70% with sera from patients with proven cases of schistosomiasis (2). The BF test is positive with approximately 15% of nonschistosomiasis sera (46). Positive trichina antisera are positive in most schistosome tests. Results of the CF test correlate closely with active clinical infection, although Buck and Anderson (13) reported that it lacks sensitivity in children and in persons with chronic infections. The IF test is the most sensitive technique, and with sections of adult worms used as the antigen cross-reactions with trichina sera are decreased. Routine use of the IF test is increasing.

ASCARIASIS AND TOXOCARIASIS

Serological tests for the diagnosis of visceral larva migrans (VLM) have been less than satisfactory. Two antigens, a fraction from a Sephadex column of *Ascaris lumbricoides* perientic fluid (78) and an extract of *Toxocara canis* adults, are employed in the tests under evaluation. In spite of considerable cross-reactivity, a specific diagnosis may occasionally be reported on the basis of the difference in titers produced by the two antigens. In addition, *Ascaris* antibody can be absorbed with *Ascaris* antigen to reveal specific *Toxocara* antibody. A combination of two tests, IHA and BF, is used in routine diagnosis. Sera reacting in one test are usually reactive in both, but titer differences may contribute some information.

Serological results are often difficult to interpret and evaluate. False-negative reactions are a diagnostic problem, since sera from cases of ascariasis as well as from VLM may be negative serologically. Very few specimens are received from patients with proven VLM. Diagnosis is usually established on the basis of the clinical history. In many strongly presumptive cases of VLM, the serum is negative. A high titer is indicative of present infection or previous experience with the parasite. Serological diagnosis has been discussed by Kagan et al. (45, 48) and Jung and Pacheco (40).

Serological tests for the diagnosis of VLM require much more research and evaluation. Until more specific and sensitive antigens or tests have been prepared and evaluated, the diagnosis of VLM must be based on an interpretation of the combined laboratory and clinical findings in each case.

In our laboratory, the IHA and BF tests are performed. A titer of 1:32 or greater in the IHA or of 1:5 or greater in the BF test reaction is considered of diagnostic significance. Sensitivity with these techniques is not over 66%, and specificity is poor (Table 4). Tests with greater sensitivity are required for these infections.

FILARIASIS

IHA and BF tests, with antigen prepared from *Dirofilaria immitis* adults, are used routinely in our laboratory. The sensitivity of the tests varies with the clinical history of the patient, and the specificity may not be satisfactory (50, 64). In *Loa loa* and *Onchocerca volvulus* infections, titers can be very high. On the other hand, very low titers are the rule with *Acanthocheilonema perstans* infections. Sera from patients with eosinophilic lung may be positive. Because of the many reactions with low titers in sera from "sick" people, interpretation is difficult.

In our evaluation, 27 of 37 filariasis sera (73%) were positive by the IHA test (Table 4). Of 152 sera from missionaries with microfilaria in the blood, 64% were positive. In addition, 14% of the approximately 2,877 sera from individuals without microfilaria in the blood were positive. Obviously, the serology of filariasis requires further study and evaluation.

CYSTICERCOSIS

The serology of cysticercosis is of interest from both the medical and veterinary points of view. The paucity of sera from proven cases of human cysticercosis in the United States has made diagnostic tests difficult to evaluate. CF, IHA, and DD reactions have been used. Results obtained with the CF test have been inconsistent. Although comparisons are difficult because of the variations in methods and reagents used, some evidence indicates that the test lacks both sensitivity and specificity. In South Africa, workers (79, 80) have evaluated an IHA test and a DD test with sera from both human and pig cysticercosis. The IHA test yielded 85% positive results with sera from proven cases of cysticercosis in humans, 5% positive results with sera from African hospital patients, and 2% with blood donor sera. The test was more sensitive with serum than with spinal fluid. Of sera from patients with intestinal tapeworm (*Taenia saginata*), 17% were serologically reactive. The IHA test on hog serum was 100% positive with sera from animals condemned because of heavy infection with cysticercosis; only 26% of the sera from animals showing light infection were positive. Biagi et al. (8) in Mexico reported the best results with the IHA test. Cross-reactions with sera from patients with hydatid disease, *T. saginata*, and *Coenurus* infections have been found. In our laboratory, we have been able to test a small number of sera from patients with proven cases of cysticercosis. Using IHA tests with extracts of whole worms of *T. saginata* and cysticerci of *Taenia solium*, we observed good sensitivity in most instances. In one case, 3 months after a solitary cyst was removed from a 16-year-old girl, her serum became negative. In three other cases, serology following surgery was positive several months later but, in each instance, the surgeon was not able to remove all of the cyst. An evaluation of the IHA test with cysticercal antigen is shown in Table 4. Although an IHA titer of 1:4 may be considered positive with animal infections, higher dilutions may have to be used as a standard with human sera to eliminate false-positive reactions. We have found DD insensitive with both human and animal sera.

CHAGAS' DISEASE

The CF test is the most sensitive method for the diagnosis of Chagas' disease. In addition, an IHA test has been used (Table 4). This technique is not as specific as the CF test, but it can be readily adapted to epidemiological studies (15, 20, 32, 68).

A direct agglutination test, introduced recently by Vattuone and Yanovsky (103), is very sensitive with sera from patients with acute infections. This method employs trypsinized, Formalin-fixed epimastigotes. Evaluations indicate high reactivity with sera from patients with acute Chagas' disease and relatively good specificity with regard to cross-reactions with leishmaniasis.

LEISHMANIASIS

Visceral leishmaniasis can be serologically diagnosed quite adequately by IHA, IF, and CF tests. The diagnosis of cutaneous leishmaniasis, especially in the Americas, is more difficult. For diagnosis, the IHA test was employed with antigens of *Leishmania donovani*, *L. tropica*, and *L. brasiliensis*. Since the sensitivity of the IHA test was low, the IF test is being used routinely. Walton et al. (107) reported excellent results from an IF test with an amastigote antigen in cutaneous leishmaniasis. Preparing the amastigote antigen for the IF test from tissue cultures is, however, somewhat complicated. Using promastigote antigen in the IF test yields tests of poor sensitivity and specificity. Cross-reactions are obtained with sera from patients with Chagas' disease.

The direct agglutination test with trypsinized, Formalin-fixed promastigotes of the three *Leishmania* species, according to the method of Vattuone and Yanovsky (103), has proven to be slightly more sensitive than the IF test with sera from American leishmaniasis. This test shows promise.

TOXOPLASMOSIS

The extensive use of the methylene blue dye (MBD) test established a firm basis for the serological diagnosis of toxoplasmosis (83). For technical reasons, the trend is toward the use of other tests, especially the IHA and IF tests. Both utilize a killed antigen, are technically simple, pose no threat of infection to the laboratory worker, and are more economical to perform than the MBD test.

The IHA test for toxoplasmosis was introduced by Jacobs and Lunde (38) and is being used in our laboratory for routine diagnosis. Recently, we have also used this test in epidemiological studies (106).

The IF test is as sensitive and specific as the IHA and MBD tests, and in a "blind" evaluation its reproducibility was greater than 98% (96). The IF test can also be done with class-specific conjugates of the immunoglobulin M (IgM) type. Newborn babies whose sera are positive with an IgM conjugate are believed to have congenital infections.

In our laboratory, IHA titers of 1:64, 1:128, and 1:256 are considered to be of questionable clinical importance. These titers probably represent the low persistent antibody levels which are detectable in a large percentage of a "normal" population. Titers higher than 1:256 reflect recent experience with the parasite and may be of clinical significance. Titers obtained with the IF test are slightly lower than those obtained with the IHA test, and an IF titer above 1:64 may be clinically significant. A combination of two tests facilitates interpretation of the reactions. IHA and IF tests are a practical pair which utilize two kinds of antigen.

MALARIA

With the introduction of IF methods, interest in the serological diagnosis of malaria (24, 60, 105) has been renewed. Intensive work by Tobie et al. (102) and Collins et al. (18) has contributed much to the evaluation of this procedure. We have adapted for use in the IF test (98) a thick smear antigen prepared from washed, parasitized blood cells. Evaluation of this antigen indicates a false-positive rate of 1% at a titer of 1:16. Sensitivity of the test is 95% (99).

The IHA test has also been extensively used (22). Stein and Desowitz (94) described an IHA test in which they used Formalin and tannic acid-treated sheep red cells sensitized with antigen from *Plasmodium cynomolgi* and *P. coatneyi*. Mahoney et al. (69) prepared their antigen by disrupting the parasites in a French press and reported good results with the test. Rogers et al. (82), who used *P. knowlesi* antigen prepared by the method of Mahoney et al. (69), reported that the test is both sensitive and relatively specific for malaria. The IHA procedure revealed antibody titers of 1:16 or greater in 98% of sera from slide-proven cases of malaria and in less than 1% of sera from individuals without a history of malaria. Pyruvic aldehyde-sensitized cells (25), which enhance the usefulness and stability of the IHA test for malaria, have been evaluated by Meuwissen and Leeuwenberg (72).

AMEBIASIS

The CF test for amebiasis, although the oldest serological test, has generally been superseded by other techniques, particularly the IHA (57), DD (7, 65, 66), and IF methods (10, 39). With the advent of axenic cultivation of *Entamoeba histolytica* (23), improved soluble antigens have been made, and more reproducible and standardized tests have resulted. The sensitivity of all the tests varies with the type of infection (Table 5). For extraintestinal amebiasis, the sensitivity of the serological tests is very high. With sera from patients with acute amoebic dysentery, sensitivity is lower, and with

TABLE 4. *Sensitivity and specificity of the indirect hemagglutination test with six parasitic antigens*[a]

Human antiserum	Antigens					
	Ascaris	Toxocara	Echinococcus	Filaria	*T. cruzi*[b]	Cysticercus[c]
Ascaris-toxocara	14/21	8/21	1/20	6/22	0/21	4/23
Bacteria-virus	3/39	2/39	0/49	7/84	1/24	0/33
Echinococcus	3/19	0/19	20/20	3/35	0/25	15/21
Filaria	2/23	14/23	2/32	27/37	0/22	4/23
Protozoa	3/18	1/8	1/21	3/28	3/14	1/18
Schistosoma	2/28	1/28	0/24	9/41	1/24	8/29
Trichina	4/33	7/33	1/29	15/43	2/30	1/31
Normal controls	1/24	1/24	0/25	4/84	0/23	1/24

[a] Results show number positive/number tested.
[b] Sera from Chagas' disease, 11/11.
[c] Sera from cysticercus infections, 10/14.

TABLE 5. *Sensitivity and specificity of three serological tests in amebiasis as compiled from reports*

Human serum	Serological tests					
	Indirect hemagglutination		Double diffusion		Indirect immunofluorescence	
	No. tested	Percent positive	No. tested	Percent positive	No. tested	Percent positive
Amoebic abscesses	314	91	622	92	484	98
Amoebic dysentery	514	84	595	72	257	58
Asymptomatic cyst carriers	191	9	19	55	74	23
Patients with other diseases[a] and healthy people	658	2	198	10	1,667	1

[a] Including inflammatory bowel disease.

sera from asymptomatic carriers, still lower. Investigators using the IHA test have reported from 87 to 100% (33, 34, 73) positive in cases of liver abscess, and from 85 to 98% positive in acute amoebic dysentery. The diagnosis of asymptomatic carriers of *E. histolytica* cysts is very variable and appears to be dependent on the population from which the sample is drawn. The test was positive for 2 to 6% of the sera from noninfected controls and hospitalized patients sick with bacillary dysentery and other diseases. The percentage of serological reactors was as high as 44% in some endemic areas. The IF test appears to be almost as sensitive as the IHA test, but reports vary on its specificity (3). Agreement between the results of the DD and IHA tests is fairly good. IHA titers of 1:128 and above are reported as positive in our diagnostic laboratory.

SEROLOGICAL TESTS

Precipitin Tests

Diagnostic precipitin tests for parasitic diseases include the old "ring" test, microprecipitin reactions in which clumps of precipitate form about living larval or other life-cycle stages of parasites when they are incubated in serum containing antibodies, double diffusion in gels, and the newer immunoelectrophoresis and counterelectrophoreses methods.

Microprecipitin tests (70, 104)

A. Special equipment and reagents

Hanging-drop or "well" slides and cover slips

Sterile physiological saline and solutions of penicillin and streptomycin

Antisera—not chylous or cloudy; positive and negative control sera

Living *Trichinella spiralis* larvae, schistosome cercariae or eggs

B. Preparation of parasite antigens for microprecipitin reactions

Trichina larvae. Digest muscle of rats or mice infected for 1 to 2 months with *T. spiralis*. Wash in 1:10,000 merthiolated saline for not more than 5 min, then several times with sterile saline to remove the Merthiolate. Larvae can be used as long as they remain viable. Suspend clean, sterile larvae in sufficient sterile saline that a measured number (10 to 100) can be transferred in 1 drop.

Schistosome cercariae. Transfer several infected snails to a beaker of warm water (37 C) and incubate for 1 h to induce shedding of cercariae. Decant the fluid and concentrate cercariae by centrifugation if yield is low. Wash in fresh water and resuspend cercariae so that a drop contains from 30 to 50 organisms. Cercariae can be used after storage at 4 C for as long as 12 h.

Schistosome eggs. Collect eggs from infected hamster or mouse livers in 1.75% saline. Separate the eggs and debris by screening through fine mesh screens. The eggs are isolated by sedimentation. Wash eggs in 1.75% saline and suspend so that 1 drop contains approximately 100 eggs. The egg suspension can be stored in the cold for 12 to 24 h, if necessary.

C. Performance of microprecipitin tests (do not use merthiolated serum in these tests)

Circumlarval: trichina (70)

1. Transfer a drop of the antigen suspension containing not more than 100 washed, viable larvae (preferably 10 to 50) to the well of a hanging-drop slide.
2. Cover with about 0.5 ml of inactivated antiserum and mix gently with an applicator stick.
3. Place a cover slip over the well, seal with paraffin, and incubate in a moist chamber at 37 C.
4. Examine the slides with low magnification at 2-h intervals for 6 h for the appearance of a granular precipitate attached to the anterior end of the larvae.
5. Return to the incubator overnight. The next day the precipitates may have loosened and may be floating in the serum.

The percentage of larvae with precipitate and the size of the aggregates of precipitate should be noted and compared with the reactions of positive and negative control sera.

Cercarienhüllenreaktion (CHR): schistosomiasis (104)

This test is performed in the same way as the circumlarval test. Use 1 drop of cercariae containing 30 to 50 organisms and 1 drop of antiserum that has not been inactivated. To prevent bacterial contamination and to permit longer periods of observation, a small drop of penicillin G (4,000 units/ml) and streptomycin (0.5 mg/ml) can be added to the chamber. Incubate from 4 to 24 h at 22 C. Within this time, the cercariae will be immobilized and surrounded by a "membrane" of precipitate, if antibodies are present in the serum.

Results are read as follows: negative reaction, no envelope in 4 to 24 h; doubtful reaction, appearance of a fine envelope on the tails of a few cercariae; positive reaction, formation of a clearly defined envelope. A thin smooth membrane is a ± reaction. A thin, wrinkled membrane is a + reaction. A discrete, thick membrane is a 2+ to 3+ reaction. A heavy loose membrane is a 4+ reaction.

Circumoval precipitin test: schistosomiasis

This test is performed in the same manner as the circumlarval test. Use 1 drop of a suspension of eggs (about 100) in 1.75% saline and 1 drop or 0.05 ml of serum which has been inactivated at 56 C for 30 min. Incubate at 37 C for 24 h. Examine after 2 and 24 h, recording percentage of eggs showing precipitates, measuring length, and noting fingerlike shapes of the precipitate. Compare with negative and positive controls.

Weak reaction: precipitates 12.5 μm or less in

length. Moderate reaction: precipitates 25 μm in length. Strong reaction: precipitates 37.5 μm and over in length.

The circumoval precipitin reaction is considered more specific for the species of schistosomes than the CHR.

Gel diffusion tests (7, 14, 19, 65, 91)

Diagnostic precipitin tests in gels include the Ouchterlony type of double diffusion (DD), immunoelectrophoresis (IE), and countercurrent electrophoresis (CEP). They have been evaluated for amebiasis, echinococcosis, trichinosis, and Chagas' disease, Although their usefulness is somewhat limited by the larger quantities of concentrated antigen and the potent or concentrated antisera required, they permit identification of specific and nonspecific components, thus increasing accuracy of the tests. Techniques vary greatly. Described here are basic general methods which should be standardized in each laboratory for each disease.

A. Special equipment and reagents

Agar gels.

Glass slides (5 by 7.5 cm and 2.5 by 7.5 cm) coated with a thin film of dried agar of agarose.

Patterns and cutters. Slides can be cut with small "cork-borer" cutters. Mechanical IE cutters are recommended for IE slides.

Moist chambers and incubators 37 and 25 C.

Power supply and IE apparatus.

Staining solutions.

Veronal buffer solution.

Antigens. Saline or Veronal buffer extracts of parasites; concentrated hydatid fluid. Soluble antigens prepared for other serological tests can often be used after concentration 3- to 10-fold. Crude antigens must produce multiple bands with diagnostic sera and, in the case of hydatid antigen, include the diagnostic #5 band (14). Can be stored frozen or lyophilized and are usually very stable.

Antisera. Lyophilized or frozen positive and negative control sera of known reactivity which must also show any specific diagnostic bands. Diagnostic sera can be inactivated at 56 C for 30 min.

B. Preparation of media

For DD test:

Purified agar (Difco)	10.0 g
NaCl	5.0 g
Glycine	7.5 g
Merthiolate	0.1 g
Distilled water	1,000 ml

1. Dissolve all reagents except the agar in half the water.
2. Adjust the pH to 7.2 to 7.4 with small amounts of 0.1 M NaOH.
3. Dissolve the agar in the remaining water by carefully boiling over direct heat or in a boiling-water bath. (Freely flowing steam in an autoclave can be used to dissolve the agar, but do not use steam under pressure.)
4. Mix the two solutions, making sure the agar is completely dissolved; if necessary, use heat to make a uniform solution.
5. Dispense in 50- to 100-ml capped containers. Can be stored in the cold for several weeks without deterioration.
6. For use, melt containers of agar in a boiling-water bath and use the whole amount. Repeated heating can alter gel formation.

For IE and CEP tests:

Agarose	9 g
or Special agar-Noble	20 g
Distilled water	500 ml
Veronal buffer, ionic strength 0.075, pH 8.5	500 ml

1. Dissolve agarose or agar in the water heat.
2. Add Veronal buffer and heat to boiling to insure complete solution.
3. Prepare plates immediately or store as directed for purified agar medium.

Stock Veronal buffer, pH 8.5, ionic strength 0.075

Dissolve 5.53 g of barbital in approximately 500 ml of distilled water and 30.90 g of sodium barbital in a second 500 ml of distilled water. Mix and bring up to 2 liters in a volumetric flask. Add 0.4 g of Merthiolate crystals. Dilute with equal parts distilled water for use in the IE bath.

C. Preparation of other reagents

Buffered saline (PBS, pH 7.5) for dissolving the nonprecipitated proteins from the agar slides:

Mix 200 ml of Sorensen's 0.067 M phosphate buffer, pH 7.5, with 3,800 ml of 0.89% NaCl solution.

Staining solutions:

- 0.3% thiazine red R in 1% acetic acid or 0.1% amido black in 1% acetic acid
- 1% acetic acid
- 1% acetic acid and 1% glycerol
- 0.4% aqueous solution of bromophenol blue indicator; dilute to light purple with Veronal buffer for use

D. Preparation of slides

1. Clean 5 by 7.5 cm or 2.5 by 7.5 cm glass slides and coat with a thin layer of agar or agarose by swabbing the entire area with hot, melted 0.1% agar which has been prepared by diluting small amounts of the agar medium with distilled water.
2. Dry in the air or with low heat. Store in dust-free boxes for not less than 16 h before use. Can be stored indefinitely.
3. Place slides, coated side up, on a level surface and, with a pipette, transfer to each measured amounts of the desired hot, melted agar or agarose: 3 ml for 2.5 by 7.5 cm slides and 8 ml for 5 by 7.5 cm slides. Cover the whole area of the slide.
4. Allow to solidify at room temperature and store in moist chambers in a refrigerator. Slides should "set" overnight before use to insure maximal gelling. The thickness of the agar can be varied by using

different amounts of medium. Slides prepared carefully will be very smooth, uniform, and level.

Cutting slides

1. For DD, cut wells in a hexagon about a central well (Fig. 1A). Diameters of the wells and distances between wells must be uniform so that tests can be replicated. Recommended proportions: diameter of well, 8 mm, and space, 10 mm; diameter, 5 mm, and space, 6 mm; diameter, 3 mm, and space, 4 mm.

2. For IE, cut the antigen well near the center of the Noble agar slide (Fig. 1B-1) and nearer the cathode with agarose (Fig. 1B-2). Cut a small well for the indicator (bromophenol blue solution).

3. For CEP, cut parallel rows of wells as shown in Fig. 1C. Diameters of wells are 5 mm and the wells are 3 mm apart.

Aspirate the plugs of gel from the wells, but leave the gel in the antiserum slot cut in the IE slide until after electrophoresis. Seal the bottom edge of the wells with a minute drop of hot agar or agarose. Store in moist containers at 4 C or use immediately.

E. Performance of the double diffusion test

1. Fill the central well to the top with appropriate dilution of antigen.

2. Fill the six outside wells with unknown sera. Whenever possible, one well should contain a known positive serum. If the supply of reagents permits, run all unknown sera twice. When the sequence of the sera is changed, some weak reactions may be enhanced by being next to a strongly reacting antiserum.

3. Incubate in a moist chamber at 25 C for 3 days or at 37 C for 24 h.

4. Record lines as they appear.

5. Gently flush out remaining reactants from wells with distilled water. Cover slide with wet filter paper, making certain the wells are filled with fluid. Air-dry overnight.

6. Remove filter paper and soak out excess reactants from the gel in PBS, pH 7.5, for at least 4 h or overnight.

7. To stain: 10 min, distilled water; 10 min, distilled water; 15 min, thiazine red R stain; 10 min, 1% acetic acid; 10 min, 1% acetic acid; 10 min, 1% acetic acid plus 1% glycerol.

8. Air-dry slides and store for reference.

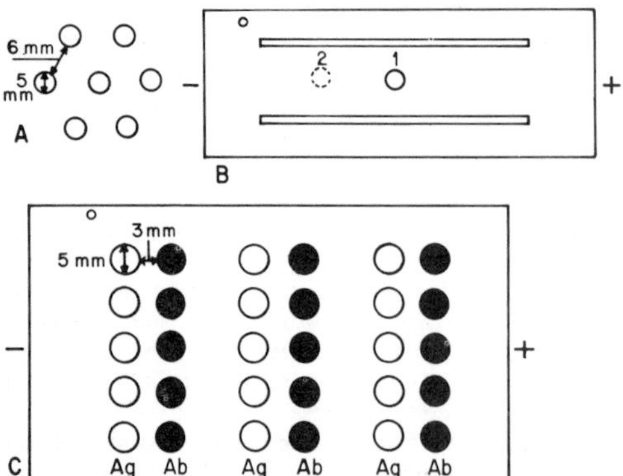

FIG. 1. *Patterns for cutting double-diffusion slides.*

F. Performance of immunoelectrophoresis test

1. Fill the IE bath with Veronal buffer, ionic strength 0.0375, pH 8.5, to the level recommended by the manufacturer.

2. Load the tray with cut agarose or Noble agar slides, and place filter-paper wicks in position.

3. Carefully fill antigen well. Place a drop of bromophenol blue solution in the indicator well.

4. Turn on power supply and adjust the current passing through the length of the slide to give a potential difference of 3 to 5 V per cm of agar.

5. When the indicator has reached the previously determined distance necessary for good separation—usually after 1.5 h—shut off machine and remove slides.

6. Remove agar from the trough and seal bottom edges with a small amount of hot agar or agarose.

7. Fill trough with antiserum. Incubate at room temperature in a moist chamber for 3 days and proceed as in steps 4 through 8 of the DD test description.

G. Performance of countercurrent electrophoresis test

Prepare IE bath and load slides as in steps 1 and 2 for the IE test. Fill wells on the cathodic side (labeled Ag in Fig. 1C) with antigen. Fill anodic wells (Ab, Fig. 1C) with the serum samples previously concentrated threefold by lyophilization. Turn on the power supply and allow current to pass through the slide until the bromophenol blue indicator has moved the desired distance. The optimal separation of reactants depends on the type of matrix, concentration of buffers in the matrix and bath, and the size of wells, as well as the type of IE apparatus employed. The machines should be initially standardized with some known antigen/antibody system, and the voltage necessary to produce good bands in 30 to 90 min without overheating the agar should be determined. Most of the parasitic CEP tests are run for 45 min. Remove the slides and examine for bands immediately. Wash out excess reactants and incubate slides for 1 to 3 h at room temperature. Reexamine for bands. Dry and stain slides as in steps 5 through 8 for the DD test.

Inert Particle Aggregation Tests

Tanned red blood cells, bentonite particles, polyvinyl latex particles, and cholesterol crystals have been employed as carriers of antigens in diagnostic tests for parasitic infections. Both test-tube and slide tests have been designed by which antibodies are measured qualitatively or quantitatively. Basic methods for indirect hemagglutination (IHA), bentonite flocculation (BF), and cholesterol-lecithin (CL) tests are fairly well standardized and can be used with several antigens. Latex tests are patterned after the rheumatoid arthritis test of Singer and Plotz (90). Since there is no single method for coating latex particles with parasitic antigens, methods for trichina and echinococcus antigens are described. CL tests require precise proportions of antigens and reagents. Although the CL tests for schistosomiasis and trichinosis are valuable tests, they should be performed with strict adherence to the methods described by their authors (5, 6) and are not included here.

Indirect hemagglutination test (13, 17, 25, 33, 38, 40, 57, 82, 94)

IHA tests in which tanned sheep or human red blood cells are used as the inert carrier of several parasitic antigens have been designed from the technique of Boyden (11). Tests for toxoplasmosis, amebiasis, malaria, hydatid disease, cysticercosis, and VLM are recommended. The technique is relatively simple to perform, and the test is very sensitive. The procedure can be varied and still demonstrate an antigen-antibody reaction. Cells treated with Formalin or glutaraldehyde have been used with slight adjustments in the IHA test.

A. Equipment and reagents

Equipment

Centrifuge, capable of 800 × *g*
Water baths, 56 C and 37 C
Graduated conical centrifuge tubes, 12 ml
Glassware: serological pipettes, flasks, graduates, 10 by 75 mm test tubes, dropping pipettes
Additional equipment for microtitration test: dropping pipettes of 0.05 and 0.025 ml; loops, 0.05 ml; U plates, vibrator

Reagents

Alsever's solution or 3.8% sodium citrate
Buffered saline
Normal rabbit serum
Tannic acid
Antigen
Positive serum of known titer and negative control serum
Erythrocytes—sheep or human "O"; allow cells to age at 4 C for at least 3 days before use

B. Preparation of reagents

Anticoagulating solutions

3.8% sodium citrate:

Sodium citrate	3.8 g
Distilled water	100.0 ml

(Sterilize at 15 psi pressure for 15 min and store at 4 C.)

Alsever's solution:

Dextrose	2.05 g
Sodium citrate	0.8 g
Sodium chloride	0.42 g
Citric acid	0.055 g
Distilled water	100.0 ml

(Sterilize by filtration and store at 4 C.)

Phosphate-buffered saline (PBS)

Stock solutions:	
0.15 M Na_2HPO_4	21.3 g/liter
0.15 M KH_2PO_4	20.4 g/liter
0.15 M NaCl	8.8 g/liter
PBS, pH 6.4:	
0.15 M Na_2HPO_4	32.3 ml
0.15 M KH_2PO_4	67.7 ml
0.15 M NaCl	100.0 ml
PBS, pH 7.2:	
0.15 M Na_2HPO_4	76.0 ml
0.15 M KH_2PO_4	24.0 ml
0.15 M NaCl	100.0 ml

Diluent: 1% normal rabbit serum (NRS)

Inactivate rabbit serum from healthy rabbits at 56 C for 30 min. Inactivated serum can be stored frozen and reinactivated for 10 min immediately before use.

Mix 1 ml of serum with 99 ml of PBS, pH 7.2.

If the diluent reacts with tanned sheep cells or sensitized sheep cells, discard it and replace with serum from nonreactive rabbit.

Preparation of tannic acid dilutions, 1:1,000 and 1:20,000

Immediately before use, prepare a fresh solution of 1:1,000 dilution of tannic acid by dissolving 10 mg of reagent-grade tannic acid in 10 ml of PBS, pH 7.2.

Dilute the 1:1,000 stock solution 1:20 for the 1:20,000 dilution used in the test (2.0 ml of 1:1,000 plus 38.0 ml of PBS, pH 7.2). If the cells show no tanning effect or if spontaneous agglutination occurs, several different concentrations of tannic acid must be tested to determine the optimal dilution for tanning a particular lot of cells.

C. Performance of indirect hemagglutination microtiter test

Preparation of tanned sensitized red cells

1. Wash sheep red cells suspended in Alsever's solution or 3.8% sterile sodium citrate three times with PBS, pH 7.2. Centrifuge at 800 × *g* for 5 min twice and for 10 min after the third wash. Adjust to a 2.5% suspension by adding 39 ml of buffered saline to each milliliter of packed cells.
2. Add an equal volume of 1:20,000 tannic acid solution; mix well. Incubate the mixture in a water bath at 37 C for 10 min.
3. Remove the tannic acid-treated cells from the water bath and centrifuge for 5 min at 800 × *g*. Decant the supernatant fluid. Wash once with PBS, pH 7.2, and resuspend the cells to a 2.5% suspension with PBS, pH 6.4.
4. Sensitize the tanned cells by adding an equal volume of the optimal dilution of antigen in PBS, pH 6.4, to the cell suspension. (Example: add 10 ml of antigen dilution to 10 ml of 2.5% cell suspension.) Incubate the mixture in a water bath at 37 C for 15 min. The optimal dilution must be predetermined for each lot of antigen by box titration of dilutions of positive sera of known titer, as shown below.
5. Remove the antigen-treated cells from the water bath and centrifuge for 5 min at 800 × *g*. Decant the

supernatant fluid and wash the cells twice with 1% NRS.

6. Adjust the cells to a 1.5% suspension in 1% NRS after a final pack by centrifugation at 800 × *g* for 10 min.

Determination of optimal concentration of antigen

1. Prepare four dilutions of antigen in PBS, pH 6.4 (example: 1:25, 1:50, 1:100, 1:150).

2. Sensitize cells with each dilution of antigen as described above in Preparation of tanned sensitized red cells, steps 4, 5, and 6.

3. Check one negative and one positive serum with each dilution by the test procedure given below. The lowest concentration of antigen giving the highest titer with the immune serum and no reaction with the negative serum is considered optimal.

Test procedure

Inactivate the serum specimens for 30 min at 56 C. Serial dilutions of the serum are made in 1% NRS.

1. Into microtitration U plates, transfer 0.05 ml of 1% NRS with a pipette dropper to all wells in which serum dilutions will be made.

2. With a microtitration loop, transfer 0.05 ml of the test serum to the first well containing 0.05 ml of 1% NRS.

3. Mix thoroughly and prepare 12 twofold serum dilutions by transferring 0.05 ml to each successive well, discarding the final 0.05 ml from the 12th well.

4. Place the plate on a vibrator. With pipette dropper, add 0.025 ml of 1.5% sensitized cell suspension to each serum dilution.

5. Allow the cells to settle for 2 or 3 h at room temperature.

6. Read the patterns of the cells on the bottom of the wells. A positive reaction (4+) is indicated by a mat or carpet of cells covering the bottom of the well. (In strong reactions, the edges can be folded.) A negative test is one in which the cells have settled to form a compact button or ring at the center of the well. Titer is the greatest dilution showing a 3+ or 4+ reaction depending on the test.

Controls

Diluent control. Transfer 0.05 ml of 1% NRS to several wells in a U plate and add 0.025 ml of the 1.5% suspension of sensitized cells. These reactions should be negative.

Serum control. Prepare a 1.5% suspension of unsensitized tanned cells in 1% NRS. Prepare a duplicate plate of serial dilutions of the sera to be tested, 6 wells for each serum instead of 12. To each well add 0.025 ml of unsensitized tanned cells. A negative reaction should be obtained with each serum. If the serum is reactive, it must be absorbed with sheep cells and retested.

D. Performance of indirect hemagglutination tube test

Preparation of tanned sensitized red cells

Washing and tanning. Wash sheep red cells in 3.8% sterile sodium citrate three times with PBS, pH 7.2 (centrifuge at 800 × *g* for 5 min each time). Adjust to a 2.5% suspension by adding 39 ml of PBS, pH 7.2, to each 1 ml of packed cells. Add an equal volume of 1:20,000 tannic acid (prepared from the stock 1:1,000 solution) in PBS, pH 7.2. Mix thoroughly. Incubate the mixture in a water bath at 37 C for 15 min. Remove tannic acid-treated cells from the water bath and centrifuge for 5 min at 800 × *g*. Decant supernatant fluid and wash once with PBS, pH 7.2.

Sensitizing. Decant the supernatant fluid. To a portion of packed tanned cells, add 5 volumes of the optimal dilution of antigen diluted in PBS, pH 6.4. (Example: to 0.2 ml of packed cells, add 1 ml of antigen dilution.) To a second portion to be used as cell controls, add 5 volumes of PBS, pH 6.4. Mix thoroughly and incubate the antigen-cell mixtures in a water bath at 37 C for 15 min. Add 1 volume of 0.4% normal rabbit serum diluted with PBS, pH 7.2, and centrifuge for 5 min at 800 × *g*. Wash one or two times with 0.4% NRS. Resuspend cells to a 2% suspension in 0.4% NRS.

Determination of optimal concentration of antigen

1. Prepare four dilutions of antigen in PBS, pH 6.4 (example: 1:10, 1:20, 1:40, 1:80).

2. Sensitize cells with each dilution of antigen.

3. Titrate one negative and one positive serum with each antigen-cell suspension. The highest concentration of antigen yielding the highest specific immune serum titer is considered optimal.

Test procedure

1. Make serial dilutions of the serum to be tested, using 1% NRS in PBS, pH 7.2, as follows: Prepare a rack with 10 by 75 mm test tubes (10 tubes for each serum). Add 0.5 ml of 1% NRS to all tubes except the first. To the first tube, add 0.98 ml of 1% NRS and 0.02 ml of the serum. For routine tests, this is the lowest dilution (1:50) tested. Mix well and prepare doubling dilutions by transferring 0.5 ml to each successive tube, discarding 0.5 ml from the last tube.

2. To each tube (0.5 ml of serum dilution), add 0.05 ml of sensitized cells.

3. Shake the rack to mix the cells thoroughly.

4. Allow the cells to settle for 2 to 3 h at room temperature; then read and record the patterns on the bottom of the tubes. (The patterns may be read after overnight settling at 4 C). The end point of a positive test is indicated by a mat or carpet of cells covering the bottom of the tube, equivalent to the 4+ reaction. In a negative test the cells have settled to form a compact button or ring. Diluent and serum controls and sera with known titers are included with each day's test.

Bentonite flocculation test

The BF test, initially developed with trichina antigen (12), has been adapted for the diagnosis of echinococcosis (27, 76), schistosomiasis (2), VLM (86), and filariasis (50). It is a slide flocculation test in which a small drop of antigen-coated bentonite particles is added to 0.1-ml samples of diluted serum. After 15 min of rotation, the degree of aggregation of the particles is estimated under low-power magnification. In a positive reaction, over 50% of the particles are in small-to-large floccules; less than 50% flocculation is a negative reaction.

A. Special equipment and reagents

Antigen solution in 0.85% saline

Suspension of standard-sized bentonite particles

Normal serum for negative control and positive serum of known titer (one serum of low and another of high titer are most satisfactory as positive control sera)

0.85% saline

0.1% thionin solution in distilled water

Tween 80 (Hilltop Laboratories, Inc., Cincinnati, Ohio; keep in refrigerator and do not use after expiration date on bottle)

Wax ring slides, as for Kline tests

Glass capillary pipettes calibrated to deliver 60 to 80 drops per ml (prepare very fine glass Pasteur pipettes from 3-mm glass tubing and calibrate; syringes with needles are not satisfactory)

Boerner-type rotating machine for slide flocculation tests

Dissecting microscope with 1× objective and 12× oculars

Water bath, 56 C

B. Preparation of reagents

Suspension of standard-sized bentonite particles

All glassware must be scrupulously clean and free from detergents.

1. Suspend 0.5 g of bentonite in 100 ml of glass-distilled water.
2. Homogenize in a Waring Blendor, or equivalent, for 1 min.
3. Transfer suspension to a 500-ml glass-stoppered graduate and add glass-distilled water to make 500 ml. Shake thoroughly.
4. Centrifuge in 50-ml centrifuge tubes for 15 min at 500 × *g*. (When an International centrifuge, size 1, type SB, with a head radius of 18 cm is used, 500 × *g* = 1,550 rpm.)
5. Pour off and save supernatant fluid; discard sediment.
6. Centrifuge supernatant fluid at 750 × *g* for 15 min (750 × *g* = 1,990 rpm).
7. Pour off and discard supernatant fluid.
8. Resuspend sediment in 100 ml of distilled water and homogenize in blendor for 1 min. This is the "stock" bentonite, which usually remains stable for at least 4 months without losing its adsorptive properties if stored at 4 C.

Suspensions of antigen-coated particles

Although an excess of antigen is needed to prepare stable stock antigen, some antigens can be too strong to coat the particles properly. Therefore, each fresh lot of antigen is titrated to determine the optimal dilution for the lot. Titration is carried out as described below, except that a series of dilutions of antigen is prepared instead of the "optimal dilution" mentioned.

Stock antigen. Mix 1 volume (10 ml) of optimal dilution of antigen with 2 volumes (20 ml) of bentonite suspension. Incubate at 4 C overnight (or several hours). Add 0.5 volume (5 ml) of a 0.1% thionin blue solution. Let the mixture stand for 1 h to stain the coated particles. This "stock antigen" can be used at least 3 months after preparation, if kept at 4 C.

Test antigen. Shake stock antigen suspension well and transfer 8 ml to a 15-ml conical centrifuge tube. Wash twice with 0.85% saline by centrifugation at 800 × *g* for 5 min (this step removes the nonadsorbed antigen).

Resuspend the sedimented particles in 4 ml of saline. At this stage, they will form into loosely aggregated clumps which must be dispersed by carefully adding an anionic detergent.

Prepare a fresh solution of Tween 80 by dissolving 0.5 ml in 99.5 ml of distilled water. Add 0.1 ml or less of the Tween 80 solution to the antigen. Shake well. Test with saline and normal serum (1:100), as described below under Performance of the bentonite flocculation test, steps 3-5. If the particles are still agglutinated, add additional small amounts of Tween 80 and retest until flocculation has entirely disappeared in the negative serum and less than 50% of the particles in saline are flocculated.

Test two positive control sera, one of high titer and one of low titer. If the titers of the positive control sera are more than one dilution lower than the expected titers, too much Tween 80 has been added. Although the excess can be washed away, it is better to discard the antigen and start with a new 8-ml portion of stock suspension.

The properly adjusted suspension of washed coated particles (test antigen) can be used for from 4 to 6 weeks when stored in the cold. *DO NOT FREEZE.*

Smaller or larger amounts of test antigen can be prepared by washing smaller or larger volumes of stock antigen. The final volume must be half of the original for optimal concentration of particles in each test.

C. Performance of the bentonite flocculation test

1. Sera to be tested should be inactivated for 30 min at 56 C.
2. Dilute serially each serum with 0.85% saline 1:5, 1:10, and 1:20. Positive sera are further diluted until flocculation is read as negative.
3. Pipette 0.1 ml of serum dilution into a well of a wax-ringed slide and add 1 drop of standardized test antigen (use a pipette that delivers 60 to 80 drops per ml).
4. Rotate the slide in a horizontal plane on a rotating apparatus for 15 min at 120 rotations per min.
5. Examine with dissecting microscope for presence of agglutination or flocculation.

D. Reading the test

Results are read as follows: 4+ reaction, all particles are agglutinated; 3+ reaction, 75% of the particles are agglutinated; 2+ reaction, 50% of the particles are agglutinated; 1+ reaction, 25% of the particles are agglutinated.

A 3+ or 4+ agglutination is considered positive. A 2+ or 1+ reaction is negative.

In each series of tests, saline control and negative and positive serum controls should be included.

Latex agglutination tests (9, 27, 28, 74)

Latex particles are coated with soluble parasitic antigens, and then are usually used in rapid slide diagnostic tests which are particularly useful in screen or field testing. They are only moderately sensitive tests. The size and concentration of the latex particles, the suspending buffers, and the concentration of antigens used to coat the particles all influence the preparation of satisfactory antigens. Only the trichina and echinococcus tests are described here.

A. Special equipment and reagents

Glycine-buffered saline
Suspensions of uniform-sized latex particles
Soluble antigens
Positive and negative control sera, inactivated at 56 C for 30 min; known titers
Spectrophotometer: Spectronic-20 or Coleman Junior type
Glass plates ruled into 2.5-cm squares
Dropping pipettes delivering 20 to 30 drops per cc
Wooden applicator sticks or toothpicks
Lighted viewing box

Preparation of glycine-buffered saline (GBS), pH 8.3

NaCl	9 g
$CaCl_2$	1 g
Glycine	7.51 g
Water	1,000 ml

Adjust to a pH of 8.2 to 8.4 with 1 N NaOH.

Preparation of standard latex suspension

Since suspensions of the 0.81-size latex particle are commercially available, it is used for preparing trichina and echinococcus reagents.

1. Prepare an estimated 1% (total solids) latex from the stock latex suspension in GBS, pH 8.3.
2. Measure the optical density of a 1:200 dilution of this 1% suspension (0.1 ml + 19.9 ml of GBS) in a Spectronic-20 colorimeter at a wavelength of 650 μm, or measure a 1:100 dilution in a Coleman Junior spectrophotometer at the same wavelength. An optical density of 0.28 ± 0.02 is optimal when 13 by 100 mm cuvettes are used in a Spectronic-20 colorimeter.
3. Adjust the stock latex suspension with sufficient GBS so that the optical density of a 1:200 dilution is optimal (0.28 ± 0.02). (The standard stock suspension is *not* the 1:200 dilution.)

The latex suspension can be stored at 4 C as long as it remains uncontaminated. It should not be frozen.

Preparation of sensitized particles

Trichina latex antigens:

1. Dilute 1 ml of Melcher's acid-soluble fraction (MASF) of trichina larvae (71) with 4 ml of GBS, pH 8.3. Add 5 ml of standard latex suspension. Incubate in a water bath at 37 C for 30 min and overnight at 4 C.
2. To 3 ml of Witebsky's boiled crude trichina antigen (108), add 2 ml of standard latex suspension. Incubate at 37 C in a water bath for 30 min and overnight at 4 C. Dilute by adding 1 ml of GBS, pH 8.3.

Echinococcus latex antigens:

Dialyze hydatid fluid against running water overnight, then concentrate by preevaporation to one-tenth or one-twelfth of the original volume.

Add 1 ml of concentrated hydatid fluid to 1.5 ml of standard latex suspension. Incubate at 37 C in a water bath for 30 min. Add 2.5 ml of GBS. Refrigerate overnight before use.

Since lots of antigens vary, titrate each new lot. They will be very near the proportions given above, but slightly different amounts or dilutions should be tested. The amounts of latex can also be varied slightly to prepare a suspension of coated particles that will be negative with normal serum, yet give the proper titers with known positive sera. Too little antigen permits flocculation of latex in negative sera. Excess antigen usually is indicated by negative or reduced reactivity with positive sera.

The coated particles will retain their reactivity for several weeks to several months if stored at 4 C (never frozen). Control sera must be tested with each day's run.

Performance of the slide test

1. Inactive sera at 56 C for 30 min.
2. Prepare serial dilutions of serum in GBS, 1:5, 1:10, 1:20, etc., for a quantitative test.
3. Place 1 drop of undiluted serum (or 1 drop of each dilution) in separate squares on a marked glass plate.
4. Add 1 drop of sensitized latex particles to each square and mix with a stick. Spread over an area about the size of a quarter.
5. Rotate the plate for 2 or 3 min by hand or on a mechanical rotator. Rotation by hand for 2 min is adequate for trichina tests; 3 min for echinococcus. Machine rotation at 180 rpm requires 5 min.
6. Read macroscopically for agglutination of particles. Use reflected light or a viewing box.

A negative test shows uniform turbidity and no flocculation, or slight granulation up to 1+ flocculation. A weakly positive reaction shows 2+ (usually fine) aggregation. A positive reaction shows 3+ or 4+ (complete) aggregation.

Complement Fixation Test

CF tests for parasitic diseases are the oldest, most widely employed, and most varied of all serological methods. Usually the CF technique used for syphilis serology is followed, but, without some modifications, it has not been entirely satisfactory with parasitic antigens. Both the quantitative-type test (67) and modified Kolmer tests have been successfully standardized; the results from different laboratories, however, are often not comparable. All tests employ the 50% hemolysis end point and require precise standardization of reagents and techniques. Since divergent results are caused as much by variation in techniques as by differences in antigens, a single standardized CF test is highly desirable. Such a test, the Laboratory Branch Complement Fixation (LBCF), has been devised by the CDC laboratories for viral, bacterial, and parasitic serological diagnosis. It has been used successfully for the diagnosis of Chagas' disease, malaria, pneumocystosis, toxoplasmosis, paragonomiasis, schistosomiasis, cysticercosis, and echinococcosis.

The LBCF test can be performed as a microtitration or a test-tube procedure. A 0.28% sheep cell suspension is prepared in Veronal-buffer-gelatin diluent and standardized (preferably) with a spectrophotometer. Five 50% units of complement are used in each test with optimal concentrations of antigen and sheep cell hemolysin. The first incubation period is 15 to 18 h at 4 to 6 C; the second incubation (after sensitized cells are added) is 30 min at 37 C. The percentages of hemolysis in the controls and in the tests are read. When controls are satisfactory, reactions showing 0 to 30% hemolysis are recorded as positive, and the remainder, negative. Anticomplementary sera are those reading less than 75% hemolysis in the serum control well without antigen.

Directions for the LBCF test are given in detail in *Public Health Monograph No. 74: Standardized Diagnostic Complement Fixation Method and Adaptation to Micro Test*. Single copies are available on request from the Public Inquiries Branch, U.S. Public Health Service, Washington, D.C. 20201.

Indirect Immunofluorescence Test (10, 26, 39, 60, 84, 85, 87, 96–98, 102, 105, 107)

The IF test has been investigated as a diagnostic technique for several parasitic diseases. including toxoplasmosis, malaria, trichinosis, schistosomiasis, and hydatid diseases. The detailed description of the IF test for toxoplasmosis serves as a general model for other antigen-antibody systems.

A. Special equipment and reagents

IF binocular microscope equipped with BG-12 exciter and OG-1 ocular filters or the equivalent; for malaria IF, a UG-1 or UG-2 exciter filter and a GG-9 ocular filter or the equivalent are essential

PBS, pH 7.6

Buffered glycerol, pH 9.0

Evans blue dye, 1% in PBS, pH 7.6

Antigen on slides

Fluorescein-conjugated antihuman globulins (must be free from specific toxoplasma antibody)

Antisera

B. Preparation of reagents

Stock buffer solution

Na_2HPO_4, anhydrous .... 12.36 g
NaH_2PO_4, H_2O .... 1.80 g
NaCl .... 85.00 g
Distilled water to a final volume of 1,000 ml

0.01 M PBS, pH 7.6

100 ml of stock buffer solution, 900 ml of distilled water. Check pH and adjust, if necessary.

Buffered glycerol

Prepare a 0.2 M Na_2HPO_4 solution by dissolving 28.4 g of anhydrous Na_2HPO_4 in 1,000 ml of distilled water; pH will be 9.0. Mix 1 volume with 9 volumes of glycerol.

C. Performance of the indirect immunofluorescence test (slide test)

The fluorescein-conjugated antihuman globulin should first be assayed with a positive control serum of known titer to determine the best dilution for use. The conjugate is diluted with PBS, pH 7.6, and Evans blue. (For example, for a 1:10 conjugate and 1:500 counterstain dilution, add to 0.1 ml of conjugate 0.2 ml of 1% Evans blue and 0.7 ml of PBS.)

1. Prepare serial fourfold dilutions of the serum to be tested in PBS, pH 7.6. Dilutions can be started at 1:16, because this is the lowest dilution that is considered significant. Fourfold dilutions of sera are preferred when making comparisons on a test-to-test basis, but twofold dilutions will give more information when comparisons of sera are to be made in the same test.
2. Remove antigen slides from freezer and wash in a gentle stream of distilled water.
3. Blot dry (facial tissue is satisfactory).
4. Place the slide on wet paper in a shallow pan with the smears up.
5. Cover each smear with a successive dilution of serum.
6. Cover the pan with a lid or aluminum foil and place in an incubator at 37 C for 30 min.
7. Rinse off serum dilutions with a gentle stream of distilled water, then dip several times in PBS bath.
8. Blot the smears dry and replace the slides in a pan on wet paper.
9. Cover the smears with the optimal dilution of antihuman conjugate diluted in Evans blue in PBS, pH 7.6.
10. Cover the pan and place in the 37 C incubator for 30 min.

11. Repeat washings as in step 7 with a final rinse in water.

12. Blot dry.

13. Place a small drop of buffered glycerol, pH 9, on the smear and cover with a cover slip.

14. Examine with the high-dry objective on a fluorescence microscope equipped with a BG-12 exciter and OG-1 ocular filter or the equivalent.

15. Prepare the following controls each time the test is performed: (i) saline, (ii) negative serum, and (iii) positive human serum of known titer. The positive serum is tested at four dilutions: one below, two above, and one at the known titer of the serum. For example, if the control serum has a titer of 1:1,024, using a fourfold dilution scheme, it should be tested at 1:256, 1:1,024, 1:4,096, and 1:16,384. The negative control serum can be tested only at 1:16.

When a large number of diagnostic sera are to be tested, they should be screened at 1:16 and 1:64 dilutions. If a serum is positive at 1:64, it should be retested at higher dilutions to determine its titer.

Frozen-sectioned antigens

Tests for schistosomiasis, echinococcosis, and filariasis generally employ cryostat sections of the adult or larval stages as antigen. The test procedure is the same as for toxoplasma except that the slides are not washed with water after being removed from the freezer. Instead they are allowed to dry and then immersed in acetone for 10 min.

D. Reading the toxoplasma immunofluorescence test

In the toxoplasmosis test, the reaction is negative when the organisms fluoresce reddish-purple (due to the Evans blue) with no yellow-green fluorescence around the periphery; the reaction is also considered negative when only the anterior ends of organisms fluoresce bright yellow-green with no extension of yellow-green around the posterior end. This "polar staining" will occur only with some sera and at lower dilutions, usually disappearing at a serum dilution between 1:16 and 1:64.

The reaction in toxoplasma serology is positive when yellow-green fluorescence extends around the entire periphery of the organism. This reaction can be intense enough (in lower dilutions of strong positive sera) to mask all internal red counterstain. In higher dilutions, the peripheral staining will become a thin, peripheral halo around an internal, red fluorescence.

The titer is the highest dilution at which more than half of the organisms exhibit the yellow-green fluorescence around their entire periphery. When fourfold dilutions are tested, the end point is usually sharply defined.

When reading the malaria IF test, both BG-12 and UG-1 or -2 exciter filters are used with the GG-9 ocular filter. Plasmodia are first located, with the BG-12 exciter filter, by refraction of blue light from the pigment; specific fluorescence is then evaluated by using the UG-1 or -2 exciter filter. Presence of at least 10% schizonts in the malaria antigen is recommended for greatest sensitivity.

In the malaria IF test, the reaction is positive when plasmodia can be distinguished against the background by their specific green fluorescence. Titers of reactions with schizonts always equal and often exceed titers observed with other life cycle forms. The reactions with schizonts therefore are used in determining titers of diagnostic sera.

E. Interpretation—toxoplasma immunofluorescence test

Serology serves only as an aid to diagnosis and can rarely be considered diagnostic in itself. The following observations should help the clinician interpret laboratory findings:

A titer of 1:16 to 1:64 usually reflects only some past exposure; however, it can signify early stages of disease when rising titers appear in later specimens of serum from the same patient.

A titer of 1:1,024 is very significant. The clinician should be advised to consider toxoplasmosis and should attempt to identify the disease by additional tests or isolation of the parasite from biopsied lymph nodes.

APPENDIX

A. Types of antigens recommended for parasitic serology

Test[a]	Disease	Extracts of parasites	Partially purified	Special
CF	Trichinosis	Saline-larvae	MASF[b]-larvae	
	Echinococcosis			Hydatid cyst fluid
	Schistosomiasis	Saline-adult and saline-cercariae	MASF-adults and delipidized adults (C)[b]	
	Cysticercosis		Delipidized adults and cysticerci	
	Chagas' disease	Maekelt extract-epimastigotes (67)		Exo-antigen (T)[b]
	Toxoplasmosis	Water-*T. gondii*		
	Amebiasis	Saline-axenic culture trophozoites (23)		
BF	Trichinosis	Saline-larvae	MASF-larvae	Metabolic products of larvae
	Echinococcosis			Hydatid cyst fluid
	Schistosomiasis		Delipidized cercariae (A)[b]	
	Ascariasis/ toxocariasis		Adults	
	Filariasis	Saline-adults *D. immitis*		
	Amebiasis	Saline-axenic culture trophozoites		
Latex	Trichinosis	Saline-larvae; saline-boiled larvae	MASF-larvae	
	Echinococcosis			Concentrated hydatid cyst fluid
CL	Schistosomiasis		Delipidized cercariae (A)	
IHA	Trichinosis		MASF-larvae	
	Echinococcosis			Hydatid cyst fluid
	Ascariasis/ toxocariasis		MASF-adults	Fraction of perientric fluid (78)
	Filariasis	Saline-adults *D. immitis*		
	Toxoplasmosis	*T. gondii* from peritoneal exudates		
	Amebiasis	Saline-axenic culture trophozoites		
	Malaria	Saline-*P. knowlesi* in monkey blood sediment		
	Cysticercosis		Delipidized adults and cysticerci	
IF	Trichinosis			Cuticles of larvae
	Schistosomiasis			Whole cercariae
	Toxoplasmosis			Whole organisms
	Malaria			Thick blood smears containing schizonts
	Pneumocystoses			*Pneumocystis carinii* cysts
Precipitin: DD, IE, CEP	Trichinosis	Saline-larval concentrate, 3 to 10×	MASF larvae concentrate, 5 to 10×	Metabolic concentrate, 3 to 10×
	Echinococcosis			Concentrated hydatid fluid (14, 91)
	Amebiasis	Saline-axenic culture trophozoites concentrate, 3×		

[a] CF, Complement fixation; BF, bentonite flocculation; CL, cholesterol-lecithin; IHA, indirect hemagglutination; IF, indirect immunofluorescence; DD, double diffusion; IE, immunoelectrophoresis; CEP, countercurrent electrophoresis.

[b] MASF, Melcher's acid-soluble fraction (71); A, Anderson type antigen (5); C, Chaffee type antigen (16); T, Tarrant et al. type antigen (101).

B. Partial listing of commercial parasitic antigens by manufacturer

Company	Disease	Type of reagent
Italdiagnostic, Rome, Italy	Echinococcosis	Latex test kit
	Toxoplasmosis	Latex test kit
	Toxoplasmosis	CF test antigen
ICN Chemical & Radioisotope Division, Irvine, Calif.	Toxoplasmosis	IF test kit
	Amebiasis	Agar gel test
Hyland Laboratories, Los Angeles, Calif.	Amebiasis	Countercurrent electrophoresis kit
	Chagas' disease	Countercurrent electrophoresis kit
	Trichinosis	Latex test kit
Behringwerke, Marburg, Germany	Chagas' disease	Latex test kit, CF test kit, IHA test kit
	Schistosomiasis	Skin test antigen
	Echinococcosis	Skin test antigen
	Toxoplasmosis	CF and latex test antigen and sera
Wellcome Reagents Ltd., Beckenham, Kent, England	Amebiasis	IF antigen
	Chagas' disease	IF antigen
	Echinococcosis	IF antigen
	Leishmaniasis	IF antigen
	Schistosomiasis	IF antigen
	Toxoplasmosis	IF antigen
	Trichinosis	IF antigen
	African trypanosomiasis (3 antigens)	IF antigen
Cooke Laboratory Products, Alexandria, Va.	Toxoplasmosis	IF test kit
Ames Co., Elkhart, Ind.	Amebiasis	Latex test kit
Electro-Nucleonics Laboratory, Inc., Bethesda, Md.	Toxoplasmosis	IF test kit
Canalco, Inc., Rockville, Md.	Toxoplasmosis	IHA, microhemagglutination test kit
Difco Laboratories, Detroit, Mich.	Trichinosis	Bentonite flocculation test reagents
ICL Scientific, Fountain Valley, Calif.	Trichinosis	Slide agglutination test
Cordis Laboratories, Miami, Fla.	Amebiasis	Countercurrent electrophoresis kit
Natural Veterinary Assay Laboratory, Tokyo, Japan	Toxoplasmosis	IHA sensitized cells

LITERATURE CITED

1. Adler, S. 1963. Immune phenomena in leishmaniasis, p. 235–245. *In* P. C. C. Garnham, A. E. Pierce, and I. Roitt (ed.), Immunity to protozoa. F. A. Davis Co., Philadelphia.
2. Allain, D. S., E. S. Chisholm, and I. G. Kagan. 1972. Use of the bentonite flocculation test for the diagnosis of schistosomiasis. Pub. Health Rep. **87**:550–559.
3. Ambroise-Thomas, P., and T. K. Truong. 1972. Fluorescent antibody test in amebiasis. Amer. J. Trop. Med. Hyg. **21**:907–912.
4. Ambroise-Thomas, P., and T. K. Truong. 1970. L'immuno-fluorescence dans le diagnostic serologique et le contrôle post-operataive de l'hydatidose humaine. I. Matériel et méthods. Cahiers Medicux Lyonnaise **46**:2955–2962.
5. Anderson, R. I. 1960. Serologic diagnosis of *Schistosoma mansoni* infections. I. Development of a cercarial antigen slide flocculation test. Amer. J. Trop. Med. Hyg. **9**:299–303.
6. Anderson, R. I., E. H. Sadun, and M. J. Schoenbechler. 1963. Cholesterol-lecithin slide (TsSF) and charcoal card (TsCC) flocculation tests using an acid soluble fraction of *Trichinella spiralis* larvae. J. Parasitol. **49**:642–647.
7. Atchley, F. O., A. H. Auernheimer, and M. A. Wasley. 1963. Precipitate patterns in agar gel with sera from

human amebiasis and *Entamoeba histolytica* antigen. J. Parasitol. **49**:313–315.

8. Biagi, F., F. Navarrete, A. Piña, A. M. Santiago, and L. Tapia. 1961. Estudio de tres reacciones serologicas en el diagnostico de la cisticercosis. Rev. Med. Hosp. Gen. Mexico City **24**:501–508.
9. Bloomfield, N., and G. W. Snook. 1962. Use of slide latex test for detecting trichinosis in hogs. Cornell Vet. **52**:569–581.
10. Boonpucknavig, S., and R. C. Nairn. 1967. Serological diagnosis of amoebiasis by immunofluorescence. J. Clin. Pathol. **20**:875–878.
11. Boyden, S. V. 1951. The adsorption of proteins on erythrocytes treated with tannic acid and subsequent hemagglutination by anti-protein sera. J. Exp. Med. **93**:107–120.
12. Bozicevich, J., J. E. Tobie, E. H. Thomas, M. H. Hoyem, and S. B. Ward. 1951. A rapid flocculation test for the diagnosis of trichinosis. Pub. Health Rep. **66**:806–814.
13. Buck, A. A., and R. I. Anderson. 1972. Validation of the complement fixation and slide flocculation tests for schistosomiasis. Amer. J. Epidemiol. **96**:205–214.
14. Capron, A., L. A. Yarzabal, A. Vernes, and J. Fruit. 1970. Le diagnostic immunologique de l'echinococcose humaine. Pathol. Biol. **18**:357–365.
15. Cerisola, J. A., M. Alvarez, H. Lugones, and J. B. Rebosolán. 1969. Sensibilidad de las reacciones serologicas para el diagnostico de la enfermedad de Chagas. Bol. Chil. Parasitol. **24**:2–8.
16. Chaffee, E. F., P. M. Bauman, and J. J. Shapilo. 1954. Diagnosis of schistosomiasis by complement fixation. Amer. J. Trop. Med. Hyg. **3**:905–913.
17. Chordi, A., K. W. Walls, and I. G. Kagan. 1964. Studies on the specificity of the indirect hemagglutination test for toxoplasmosis. J. Immunol. **93**:1024–1033.
18. Collins, W. E., G. M. Jeffery, E. Guinn, and J. C. Skinner. 1966. Fluorescent antibody studies in human malaria. IV. Cross reactions between human and simian malaria. Amer. J. Trop. Med. Hyg. **15**:11–15.
19. Crowle, A. J. 1961. Immunodiffusion. Academic Press Inc., New York.
20. Cuadrado, R. R., and I. G. Kagan. 1967. The prevalence of antibodies to parasitic diseases with sera of young army recruits from the United States and Brazil. Amer. J. Epidemiol. **86**:330–340.
21. de Blasi, R., and L. Magaudda-Borzi. 1958. Rivista sintetiche ecritiche la sierologia dell' amebiasi. Riv. Parassitol. **19**:267–296.
22. Desowitz, R. G., J. J. Saave, and B. Stein. 1966. Application of the indirect hemagglutination test in recent studies on the immunoepidemiology of human malaria and the immune response in experimental malaria. Mil. Med. (Suppl.) **131**:1157–1166.
23. Diamond, L. S. 1968. Techniques of axenic cultivation of *Entamoeba histolytica* Schaudinn, 1903 and *E. histolytica*-like amebae. J. Parasitol. **54**:1047–1056.
24. El-Nahal, H. M. S. 1967. Fluorescent antibody studies in the pre-erythrocytic schizonts of *Plasmodium berghei yoelli* and *Plasmodium cynomolgi* (larger strain). Trans. Roy. Soc. Trop. Med. Hyg. **61**:8–9.
25. Farshy, D. C., and I. G. Kagan. 1973. Use of stable sensitized cells in an improved indirect microhemagglutination test for malaria. Infect. Immunity **7**:680–682.
26. Fife, E. H., Jr., and L. H. Muschel. 1959. Fluorescent antibody technic for serodiagnosis of *Trypanosoma cruzi* infection. Proc. Soc. Exp. Biol. Med. **101**:540–543.
27. Fischman, A. 1960. Flocculation tests in hydatid disease. J. Clin. Pathol. **13**:72–75.
28. Fischman, A. 1960. A rapid latex test for hydatid disease. N.Z. Med. J. **59**:485–487.
29. Fulton, J. D. 1962. Diagnosis of protozoal diseases, p. 86–114. *In* P. P. H. Gell and R. P. A. Coombs (ed.), Clinical aspects of immunology. F. A. Davis Co., Philadelphia.
30. Fulton, J. D. 1963. Serological tests in toxoplasmosis, p. 259–272. *In* P. C. C. Garnham, A. E. Pierce, and I. Roitt (ed.), Immunity to protozoa. F. A. Davis Co., Philadelphia.
31. Garnham, P. C. C. 1967. Malaria in mammals excluding man, p. 139–204. *In* B. Dawes (ed.), Advances in parasitology, vol. 5. Academic Press Inc., London.
32. Goldsmith, R. S., I. G. Kagan, M. A. Reyes-Gonzáles, and J-Cedeño Ferreira. 1972. Seroepidemiologic studies in Oaxaca, Mexico. Search for parasitic antibody using the indirect hemagglutination test. Bol. Of. Sanit. Panamer. **6**:39–52 (English Ed.).
33. Healy, G. R. 1968. The use of and limitations to the indirect hemagglutination test in the diagnosis of intestinal amebiasis. Health Lab. Sci. **5**:174–179.
34. Healy, G. R. 1971. Laboratory diagnosis of amebiasis. Bull. N.Y. Acad. Med. **47**:478–493.
35. Jachowski, L. A. 1963. Immunodiagnosis of helminth infections. Amer. J. Hyg. Monograph Series No. 22, p. 112.
36. Jachowski, L. A., and R. I. Anderson. 1961. Evaluation of some laboratory procedures in diagnosing infections with *Schistosoma mansoni*. Bull. World Health Organ. **25**:675–693.
37. Jacobs, L. 1967. Toxoplasma and toxoplasmosis. p. 1–45. *In* B. Dawes (ed.), Advances in parasitology. vol. 5. Academic Press Inc., London.
38. Jacobs, L., and M. N. Lunde. 1957. A hemagglutination test for toxoplasmosis. J. Parasitol. **43**:308–314.
39. Jeanes, A. L. 1966. Indirect fluorescent antibody test in diagnosis of hepatic amoebiasis. Brit. Med. J. **5501**:1464.
40. Jung, R. C., and G. Pacheco. 1960. Use of a hemagglutination test in visceral larva migrans. Amer. J. Trop. Med. Hyg. **9**:185–191.
41. Kagan, I. G. 1960. Trichinosis: a review of biologic, serologic, and immunologic aspects. J. Infec. Dis. **107**:65–93.
42. Kagan, I. G. 1963. A review of immunologic methods for the diagnosis of filariasis. J. Parasitol. **49**:773–798.
43. Kagan, I. G. 1963. Seminar on immunity to parasitic helminths. VI. Hydatid disease. Exp. Parasitol. **13**:57–71.
44. Kagan, I. G. 1965. Evaluation of routine serologic testing for parasitic diseases. Amer. J. Pub. Health **55**:1820–1829.
45. Kagan, I. G. 1968. Serologic diagnosis of visceral larva migrans. Clin. Pediat. **7**:508–509.
46. Kagan, I. G. 1968. Serologic diagnosis of schistosomiasis. Bull. N.Y. Acad. Med. **44**:262–277.
47. Kagan, I. G. 1968. A review of serologic tests for the diagnosis of hydatid disease. Bull. World Health Organ. **39**:25–37.
48. Kagan, I. G., H. A. Fox, K. W. Walls, and G. R. Healy. 1967. The parasitic diseases of childhood with emphasis on the newer diagnostic methods. Clin. Pediat. **6**:641–654.
49. Kagan, I. G., and L. Norman. 1969. The serology of trichinosis, p. 222–268. *In* S. E. Gould (ed.). Trichinosis in man and animals. Charles C Thomas, Publisher, Springfield, Ill.
50. Kagan, I. G., L. Norman, and D. S. Allain. 1963. An evaluation of the bentonite flocculation and indirect hemagglutination tests for the diagnosis of filariasis. Amer. J. Trop. Med. Hyg. **12**:548–555.
51. Kagan, I. G., L. Norman, D. S. Allain, and C. G. Goodchild. 1960. Studies on echinococcosis: nonspecific serologic reactions of hydatid-fluid antigen with serum of patients ill with diseases other than

echinococcosis. J. Immunol. **84:**635–640.

52. Kagan, I. G., J. J. Osimani, J. C. Varela, and D. S. Allain. 1966. Evaluation of intradermal and serologic tests for the diagnosis of hydatid disease. Amer. J. Trop. Med. Hyg. **15:**172–179.
53. Kagan, I. G., and J. Pellegrino. 1961. A critical review of immunological methods for the diagnosis of bilharziasis. Bull. World Health Organ. **25:**611–674.
54. Kagan, I. G., and K. D. Quist. 1970. An evaluation of five serologic tests for the diagnosis of trichinosis in lightly infected swine, p. 271–277. *In* K. S. Singh and B. K. Tandan (ed.), H. D. Srivastava Commemoration Volume. India Veterinary Research Institute, Iznatnagar, U.P. India.
55. Kagan, I. G., D. W. Rairigh, and R. L. Kaiser. 1962. A clinical, parasitologic, and immunologic study of schistosomiasis in 103 Puerto Rican males residing in the United States. Ann. Intern. Med. **56:**457–470.
56. Kent, N. H. 1963. Seminar on immunity to parasitic helminths. I. Introduction. Exp. Parasitol. **13:**1–83.
57. Kessel, J. F., W. P. Lewis, C. M. Pasquel, and J. A. Turner. 1965. Indirect hemagglutination and complement fixation tests in amebiasis. Amer. J. Trop. Med. Hyg. **14:**540–550.
58. Kozar, Z. 1967. Investigation on trichinellosis with special reference to epidemiology and epizoology, immunodiagnosis of host parasite relationships, clinical and therapeutic aspects. Monograph. Published in Wroclaw, Poland.
59. Kozar, M., Z. Kozar, and K. Karmanska. 1964. The comparative evaluation of some agglutination tests in the diagnosis of trichinellosis. Wiad. Parazytol. **10:**717–737.
60. Kuvin, S. F., J. E. Tobie, C. B. Evans, G. R. Coatney, and P. G. Contacos. 1962. Fluorescent antibody studies on the course of antibody production and serum gamma globulin levels in normal volunteers infected with human and simian malaria. Amer. J. Trop. Med. Hyg. **11:**429–436.
61. Kwapinski, J. B. 1965. Methods of serological research. John Wiley & Sons, Inc., New York
62. Labzoffsky, N. A., R. K. Baratawidjaja, E. Kuitunen, F. N. Lewis, D. A. Kavelman, and L. P. Morrissey. 1964. Immunofluorescence as an aid in the early diagnosis of trichinosis. Can. Med. Ass. J. **90:**920–921.
63. Lumsden, W. H. R. 1967. The demonstration of antibodies to protozoa, p. 877–937. *In* D. M. Weir (ed.), Handbook of experimental immunology, F. A. Davis Co., Philadelphia.
64. McQuay, R. M. 1967. Parasitologic studies in a group of furloughed missionaries. II. Helminth findings. Amer. J. Trop. Med. Hyg. **16:**161–166.
65. Maddison, S. E. 1965. Characterization of *Entamoeba histolytica* antigen-antibody reaction by gel diffusion. Exp. Parasitol. **16:**224–235.
66. Maddison, S. E., S. J. Powell, and R. Elsdon-Dew. 1965. Application of serology to the epidemiology of amebiasis. Amer. J. Trop. Med. Hyg. **14:**554–557.
67. Maekelt, G. A. 1960. Die komplementbindungsreaktion der Chagaskrankheit. Z. Tropenmed. Parasitol. **11:**152–186.
68. Maekelt, G. A. 1964. Diagnóstico de laboratorio de las tripanosomiasis Americanas. Rev. Venez. Sanid. Asistencia Soc. **29:**1–18.
69. Mahoney, D. F., B. C. Redington, and M. J. Schoenbechler. 1966. Preparation and serologic activity of plasmodial fractions. Mil. Med. **131**(Suppl.):1141–1151.
70. Mauss, E. A. 1940. The *in vitro* effect of immune serum upon *Trichinella spiralis* larvae. Amer. J. Hyg., Sect. D **32:**80–83.
71. Melcher, L. R. 1943. An antigenic analysis of *Trichinella spiralis*. J. Infec. Dis. **73:**31–39.
72. Meuwissen, J. H. E. T., and A. D. E. M. Leeuwenberg. 1972. Indirect haemagglutination test for malaria with lyophilized cells. Trans. Roy. Soc. Trop. Med. Hyg. **66:**666–667.
73. Milgram, E. A., G. R. Healy, and I. G. Kagan. 1966. Studies on the use of the indirect hemagglutination test in the diagnosis of amebiasis. Gastroenterology **50:**645–649.
74. Muraschi, T. F., N. Bloomfield, and R. B. Newman. 1962. A slide latex-particle agglutination test for trichinosis. Amer. J. Clin. Pathol. **37:**227–231.
75. Norman, L., and I. G. Kagan. 1963. Bentonite, latex, and cholesterol flocculation tests for the diagnosis of trichinosis. Pub. Health Rep. **78:**227–232.
76. Norman, L., E. H. Sadun, and D. S. Allain. 1959. A bentonite flocculation test for the diagnosis of hydatid disease in man and animals. Amer. J. Trop. Med. Hyg. **8:**46–50.
77. Oliver-González, J., P. M. Bauman, and A. S. Benenson. 1955. Immunological aspects of infections with *Schistosoma mansoni*. Amer. J. Trop. Med. Hyg. **4:**443–454.
78. Oliver-Gonzales, J. P. Hurlbrink, E. Conde, and I. G. Kagan. 1969. Serologic activity of antigen isolated from the body fluid of *Ascaris suum*. J. Immunol. **103:**15–19.
79. Proctor, E. M., and R. Elsdon-Dew. 1966. Serological tests in porcine cysticercosis. S. Afr. J. Sci. **62:**264–267.
80. Proctor, E. M., S. J. Powell, and R. Elsdon-Dew. 1966. The serological diagnosis of cysticercosis. Ann. Trop. Med. Parasitol. **60:**146–151.
81. Rodriguez Burgos, A. 1961. Estudio immunologico sobre la somatoascaridiosis. Aportacion de un nuevo metodo para el diagnostico especie-especifico. Rev. Iber. Parasitol. **21:**463–504.
82. Rogers, W. A., Jr., J. A. Fried, and I. G. Kagan. 1968. A modified indirect microhemagglutination test for malaria. Amer. J. Trop. Med. Hyg. **17:**804–809.
83. Sabin, A. B., and H. A. Feldman. 1948. Dyes as microchemical indicators of a new immunity phenomenon affecting a protozoon parasite (Toxoplasma). Science **108:**660–663.
84. Sadun, E. H. 1963. Seminar on immunity to parasitic helminths. VII. Fluorescent antibody technique for helminth infections. Exp. Parasitol. **13:**72–82.
85. Sadun, E. H., R. I. Anderson, and J. S. Williams. 1962. Fluorescent antibody test for the serological diagnosis of trichinosis. Exp. Parasitol. **12:**424–433.
86. Sadun, E. H., L. Norman, and D. S. Allain. 1957. The detection of antibodies to infections with the nematode *Toxocara canis*, a causative agent of visceral larva migrans. Amer. J. Trop. Med. Hyg. **6:**562–568.
87. Sadun, E. H., J. S. Williams, and R. I. Anderson. 1960. A fluorescent antibody technique for the serodiagnosis of schistosomiasis in humans. Proc. Soc. Exp. Biol. Med. **105:**289–291.
88. Schiller, E. L. 1967. Progress and problems in the immunodiagnosis of helminthic infections. Advan. Clin. Chem. **9:**43–68.
89. Scholtens, R. G., I. G. Kagan, K. D. Quist, and L. Norman. 1966. An evaluation of tests for the diagnosis of trichinosis in swine and associated quantitative epidemiologic observations. Amer. J. Epidemiol. **83:**489–500.
90. Singer, J. M., and C. M. Plotz. 1958. Slide latex fixation test. J. Amer. Med. Ass. **168:**180–181.
91. Sorice, F., and L. Castagnari. 1970. Impiego della immunoprecipitazione elettroforetica nella diagnosi immunologica dell'idatidosé. G. Mal. Infet. Parassit. **23:**1–8.
92. Soulsby, E. J. L. 1962. Antigen-antibody reactions in helminth infections. Advan. Immunol. **2:**265–308.

93. Soulsby, E. J. L. 1967. The demonstration of antibodies to helminths, p. 938-966, *In* D. M. Weir (ed.), Handbook of experimental immunology. F. A. Davis Co., Philadelphia.
94. Stein, B., and R. S. Desowitz. 1964. The measurement of antibody in human malaria by a formalized sheep cell hemagglutination test. Bull. World Health Organ. **30:**45–49.
95. Sulzer, A. J., and E. S. Chisholm. 1966. Comparison of the IFA and other tests for *Trichinella spiralis* antibodies. Pub. Health Rep. **81:**729–734.
96. Sulzer, A. J., and E. C. Hall. 1967. Indirect fluorescent antibody tests for parasitic diseases. IV. Statistical study of variation in the indirect fluorescent antibody (IFA) test for toxoplasmosis. Amer. J. Epidemiol. **86:**401–407.
97. Sulzer, A. J., and I. G. Kagan. 1967. Indirect fluorescent antibody tests for parasitic diseases. III. Conjugate-antigen relationships in the tests for trichinosis and schistosomiasis. Amer. J. Med. Technol. **33:**1–8.
98. Sulzer, A. J., and M. Wilson. 1967. The use of thick-smear antigen slides in the malaria indirect fluorescent antibody test. J. Parasitol. **53:**1110–1111.
99. Sulzer, A. J., M. Wilson, and E. C. Hall. 1969. Indirect fluorescent antibody tests for parasitic diseases. V. An evaluation of a thick-smear antigen in the IFA test for malaria antibodies. Amer. J. Trop. Med. Hyg. **18:**199–205.
100. Taffs, L. F. 1961. Immunological studies on experimental infection of pigs with *Ascaris suum* Goeze, 1782. I. An introduction with a review of the literature and the demonstration of complement-fixing antibodies in the serum. J. Helminthol. **35:**319–344.
101. Tarrant, C. J., E. H. Fife, Jr., and R. I. Anderson. 1965. Serological characteristics and general chemical nature of the *in vitro* exoantigens of *Trypanosoma cruzi*. J. Parasitol. **51:**277–285.
102. Tobie, J. E., D. C. Abele, G. J. Hill, P. G. Contacos, and C. B. Evans. 1966. Fluorescent antibody studies on the immune response in sporozoite-induced and blood induced vivax malaria and the relationship of antibody production to parasitemia. Amer. J. Trop. Med. Hyg. **15:**676–683.
103. Vattuone, N. H., and J. F. Yanovsky. 1971. *Trypanosoma cruzi:* agglutination activity of enzyme-treated epimastigotes. Exp. Parasitol. **30:**349–355.
104. Vogel, H., and W. Minning. 1949. Hüllenbildung bei Bilharziacercarien im Serum Bilharzia-infizierter Tiere und Menschen. Zentralbl. Bakteriol. Parasitenk. Infektionskr. Hyg. Abt. I Orig. **153:**91–105.
105. Voller, A. 1962. Fluorescent antibody studies on malaria parasites. Bull. World Health Organ. **27:**283–287.
106. Walls, K. W., I. G. Kagan, and A. Turner. 1967. Studies on the prevalence of antibodies to *Toxoplasma gondii*. I. U.S. military recruits. Amer. J. Epidemiol. **85:**87–92.
107. Walton, B. C., W. H. Brooks, and I. Arjona. 1972. Serodiagnosis of American leishmaniasis by indirect fluorescent antibody test. Amer. J. Trop. Med. Hyg. **21:**296–299.
108. Witebsky, F., P. Wels, and A. Heide. 1942. Serodiagnosis of trichinosis by means of complement fixation. N.Y. J. Med. **42:**431–435.
109. World Health Organization. 1965. Immunology and parasitic diseases. World Health Organ. Tech. Rep. Ser. No. 315, p. 64.

Section IX

VIRUSES AND RICKETTSIAE

Chapter 71
Clinical Virology: Introduction to Methods

EDWIN H. LENNETTE, JOSEPH L. MELNICK, AND ROBERT L. MAGOFFIN

COLLECTION AND STORAGE OF SPECIMENS FOR VIROLOGICAL EXAMINATION

The laboratory diagnosis of viral infections is based upon three general approaches: (i) microscopic examination of infected tissues for pathognomonic changes or for the presence of viral material; (ii) isolation and identification of the viral agent; and (iii) demonstration of a significant increase in antibody titer to a given virus during the course of the illness.

Acute-phase blood specimens and materials for virus isolation must be collected within the first few days of illness. A brief clinical resumé should accompany the initial specimen from each patient, specifying date of onset, type of disease suspected, and the major clinical findings. The optimal time for collection of specimens is shown in Fig. 1, and the type of specimen to be collected for virus isolation in various forms of viral infection is shown in Table 1.

A number of other books on viral and rickettsial diseases are recommended as sources of additional information (1-9).

Blood specimens for serological tests

Blood is used for serological tests, but seldom for virus isolation. Acute- and convalescent-phase blood specimens must be examined in parallel to determine whether antibodies have appeared or increased in titer during the course of the illness. Collect the acute-phase blood as soon as possible after onset of the illness, no later than 5 to 7 days. Collect the convalescent-phase specimen 14 to 21 days or longer after onset.

Blood specimens should be collected aseptically, and the whole specimen (10 ml) should be sent immediately to the laboratory. There the serum is separated aseptically from the clot and may be held at 4 C pending completion of tests (up to several weeks) or at −20 C for longer storage. No anticoagulants or preservatives should be used, as they may adversely affect the results of serological tests. *Do not freeze* whole blood; this causes severe hemolysis and renders the specimen unsatisfactory for most serological tests. Submit each blood specimen as collected.

Specimens for virus isolation attempts

Collect specimens aseptically, preferably within 3 days, and no longer than 7 days, after the onset of illness. Collect postmortem specimens aseptically as soon as possible after death. Refrigerate all specimens promptly after collection. Specimens to be tested within 2 to 3 h may be kept at 4 C or on wet ice; for longer intervals, freeze specimens at −70 C. Recommended diluents or holding media for use in obtaining swabs, exudates, and washings for virus isolation are shown in Table 2. Do not add preservatives or fixatives. Label each specimen, giving patient's name, type of specimen, and date obtained.

Nasal washings

Nasal washings can be obtained by instilling 4 or 5 ml of sterile saline into each nostril with the head tilted back slightly; the head is then brought forward and the saline is allowed to flow into a small container held beneath the nose. Bovine serum albumin or gelatin (1%) should be added to the washing to stabilize the virus.

Nasal and pharyngeal swabs

A dry cotton swab may be used to swab each nostril, and the swab should be left in the nose a few seconds so that it absorbs as much secretion as possible. Throat swabs are best collected by rubbing the tonsils and back of the pharynx with a cotton swab, either dry or moistened with bacteriological broth.

Both the nasal and pharyngeal swabs are broken off just above the cotton tip and put into well-stoppered or screw-cap vials containing approximately 5 ml of nutrient broth with 1% bovine serum albumin or gelatin added. Other diluents may be used, such as tissue culture medium containing 2% fetal bovine serum or 1% gelatin, or tryptose-phosphate broth.

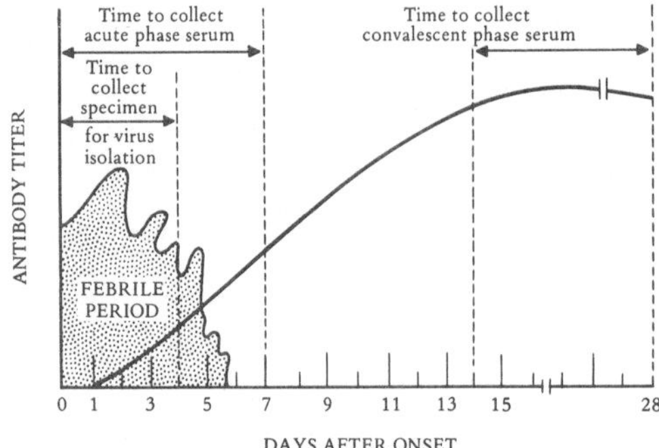

FIG. 1. *Optimal time for collecting specimen with regard to illness. Modified from Viral and Rickettsial Diseases, Physician's Handbook, 4th ed., Ontario Department of Health, Toronto, 1972.*

Throat washings or swab

For adults, have patient gargle with 10 ml of tryptose-phosphate broth (or other general purpose bacteriological broth) and spit into a clean paper cup. Then pour the fluid into a stoppered vial and seal with adhesive tape. For children, swab the throat thoroughly (using two swabs) as above under nasal swabs. Break off swab tips into 5 ml of bacteriological broth in a stoppered vial.

Mouth swabs

Mouth swabs are collected by rubbing a dry cotton swab over the inner side of both cheeks opposite the upper molars, and over the floor of the mouth anterior to the tongue. The swab is promptly rinsed in 2 ml of tissue culture medium for immediate assay, or in 2 ml of sorbitol diluent (50% sorbitol in distilled water) for specimens to be kept frozen at −70 C.

Eye exudates

For the collection of eye exudates, the palpebral conjunctiva is firmly rubbed with a sterile swab moistened with a suitable diluent. When possible, the exudate itself (pus) should be carried on the swab. The swab is then placed in a tube containing 2 to 3 ml of tissue culture medium or other diluent and is handled in the same manner as throat or rectal swabs. Scrapings from the conjunctivae or cornea should be collected only by an ophthalmologist or an adequately trained physician, and should be placed into a smaller volume of medium.

Vesicular fluids and skin scrapings

Vesicular fluids and cellular material from the base of lesions should be collected for viral isolation attempts during the first 3 days of the eruption; fluids collected later rarely yield virus. Vesicles are first washed gently with sterile saline and the fluids are aspirated with a 26- or 27-gauge needle attached to a tuberculin syringe, or with a capillary pipette. Fluids should be diluted immediately after collection in 1 or 2 ml of tissue culture medium or skim milk to prevent clotting. Alternatively, the cleansed vesicles may be opened and the fluids from several vesicles may be collected onto a swab which is then placed into 1 or 2 ml of nutrient broth, tissue culture medium, or skim milk. Cellular material from the base of the vesicles may be collected in addition to vesicular fluids for use in virus isolation attempts. The base of the opened vesicle is scraped with a scalpel blade, without producing bleeding, and the cellular material is placed in holding medium together with the vesicular fluid. Fluids or swabs in holding medium should be stored at −70 C until they can be examined in the laboratory.

Smears of vesicular lesions

For direct examination for pathognomonic changes or for fluorescent-antibody staining, it is of utmost importance to obtain a sufficient quantity of infected epithelial cells from the base of the lesion. Vesicular fluids generally are not suitable for direct examination. Material should be collected from fresh lesions containing no purulent material. In addition to material for smears, vesicular fluids and scrapings should always be taken for virus isolation attempts.

Smears prepared in the following manner may be used for Giemsa staining or for fluorescent-antibody staining. The vesicle is incised peripherally with a scalpel. The top of the lesion is lifted back and excess fluid is removed by gentle blotting. The base of the lesion is then scraped thoroughly with a scalpel blade; gross bleeding should be avoided. Cellular material collected on the edge of the blade is spread smoothly over two separate 5- to 10-mm areas on clean microscope slides, and the smears are air-dried. For examination by fluorescent-antibody staining, a minimum of three smears should be prepared so that suitable controls can be included in performing the test.

Stools and rectal swabs

In the case of stools, collect one or two specimens, 24 to 48 h apart. A 2- to 4-g specimen is adequate. Place in a 1-oz (28-ml) screw-capped glass jar; desiccation should be avoided, but no holding medium is used.

TABLE 1. *Specimens for virus isolation and types of serological tests employed for diagnosis*

Clinical manifestations and common etiological agents	Source of specimen for virus isolation		Serological tests[a]	
	Clinical	Postmortem	Usual	(Special)
Upper respiratory tract infections				
Rhinovirus Mycoplasma Parainfluenza	Throat swab or nasal secretions	—	NA CF CF, HI	(Nt)
Adenovirus Enterovirus Reovirus	Throat swab and feces	—	CF, HI, Nt NA HI, Nt	(Nt, HI)
Lower respiratory tract infections				
Influenza Adenovirus Parainfluenza Mycoplasma	Throat swab and sputum	Lung, bronchus, trachea	CF,HI CF, HI, Nt CF CF	
Pleurodynia				
Coxsackievirus	Feces and throat swab	—	NA	(Nt)
Cutaneous and mucous membrane diseases				
Vesicular				
Smallpox and vaccinia Herpes simplex Varicella-zoster	Vesicle fluid and scrapings	Lung, liver, spleen, brain	CF, HI CF, Nt CF	(FA) (FA) (FA)
Enterovirus	Vesicle fluid, feces, and throat swab	—	NA	(Nt, HI)
Exanthematous				
Measles Rubella	Throat swab	—	CF, HI HI, CF	(Nt, FA) (Nt)
Enterovirus	Feces and throat swab	—	NA	(Nt, HI)
Central nervous system infections				
Enterovirus	Feces and CSF[b]	Brain tissue, intestinal contents	NA	(Nt, HI)
Herpes simplex Mumps	Throat swab and CSF	Brain tissue	CF CF, HI	(Nt, FA) (Nt)
Lymphocytic choriomeningitis	Blood and CSF	Brain tissue	CF	(FA)
Arboviruses				
Western equine encephalitis Eastern equine encephalitis Venezuelan equine encaphalitis	Blood and CSF	Brain tissue	CF, HI CF CF	(Nt) (Nt) (Nt)
California encephalitis St. Louis encephalitis Japanese B encephalitis	Usually not possible to isolate virus from clinical specimens	Brain tissue	CF CF CF	(Nt) (Nt) (Nt)
Rabies	Saliva	Brain tissue	Nt, FA	
Parotitis				
Mumps	Throat swab	—	CF, HI	

TABLE 1—*Continued*

Clinical manifestations and common etiological agents	Source of specimen for virus isolation		Serological tests[a]	
	Clinical	Postmortem	Usual	(Special)
Severe undifferentiated febrile illnesses Colorado tick fever Yellow fever Dengue	Blood	Liver, spleen, lung, brain	CF CF CF	
Congenital anomalies Cytomegalovirus	Urine and throat swab	Kidney, lung, other tissues	CF	(FA)
Rubella	Throat swab and CSF	Lymph nodes, lung, spleen, other tissues	HI, CF	(Nt, FA)
Hepatitis Virus B (HB Ag)	Agent not recoverable	Agent not recoverable	CF, CIEP, RIA	

[a] Usual indicates types of serological tests commonly performed; (Special) indicates serological tests which may be used for special studies, not feasible for routine diagnosis. NA, Serological tests either not available or generally not feasible as routine diagnostic procedure; Nt, neutralization; CF, complement fixation; HI, hemagglutination inhibition; FA, fluorescent antibody; CIEP, counterimmunoelectrophoresis; RIA, radioimmunoassay.

[b] Cerebrospinal fluid.

TABLE 2. *Holding media for specimens for virus isolation*

Type of specimen[a]	Method of medium prepn
Swabs, exudates, cellular scrapings, or washings, e.g.: Nasal Nasopharyngeal Throat Mouth Skin or mucous membrane lesions Eye exudate Rectal	*Buffered tryptose phosphate broth with gelatin* Tryptose phosphate broth ... 2.95 g $Na_2HOP_4 \cdot 7H_2O$ ... 2.06 g $NaH_2PO_4 \cdot H_2O$ ... 0.08 g Gelatin ... 0.5 g Phenol red (optional) ... 0.002 g Distilled water ... 100.00 ml Dispense in 3.5-ml amounts in screw-cap vials. Autoclave at 15 psi for 15 min.
	Hanks balanced salt solution (BSS) with gelatin Hanks BSS ... 100.00 ml Gelatin ... 0.5 g Dispense in 3.5-ml amounts in screw-cap vials. Autoclave at 15 psi for 15 min; pH approximately 7.0.
For recovery of cytomegalovirus: Urine Throat washing	*70% sorbitol* Sorbitol ... 70.00 g Distilled water, to ... 100.00 ml Sterilize by membrane filtration. Store in 5- to 10-ml amounts at 4 C. For use, mix an equal amount of the sorbitol solution with an equal amount of specimen.

[a] Holding media are not used for feces (other than swab), spinal fluid, or organ samples such as brain, lung, kidney, etc. These should be refrigerated or frozen without preservative or holding media; see instructions for each specimen.

Rectal swab specimens are obtained by inserting a dry cotton-tipped applicator stick at least 5 cm into the anal orifice, rotating the stick, and then withdrawing it. If possible, some fecal material should be obtained on the cotton. Immediately after collection, the swab is swirled vigorously in 3 ml of tissue culture medium (containing 500 units of penicillin and 500 μg of streptomycin per ml) until a slightly turbid solution is obtained. Before the swab is discarded, as much fluid as possible is expressed from the cotton by pressing against the inside of the container above the fluid line.

Stool or rectal swab specimens are stored in the frozen state at as low a temperature as is available.

Urine

Urine samples are particularly important for the detection of cytomegalovirus. Clean-voided specimens collected in conventional containers yield satisfactory results provided that penicillin (500 units/ml), streptomycin (500 μg/ml), and nystatin (200 units/ml) are added as soon as possible after collection. Since the rate of virus isolation increases with frequency of sampling, two or three consecutive samples should be examined whenever possible.

Spinal fluid

Collect 3 to 5 ml in a sterile screw-capped vial or stoppered glass tube. (Seal stopper with adhesive tape.) It is imperative that spinal fluids be frozen immediately after collection and maintained at −70 C until tested, as many viruses are extremely labile in this medium.

Autopsy or biopsy specimen

Collect fresh, unfixed tissues from the probable sites involved using a separate sterile instrument to cut and remove each sample. Samples should be about 1.3 by 1.3 cm; place each specimen in a separate jar and label appropriately. In cases of central nervous system involvement, submit samples of medulla, midbrain, temporal lobe cortex, and cervical and lumbar spinal cord. A 5- to 7.5-cm segment of descending colon, with fecal contents retained by ligation, should be included for the recovery of enteroviruses. For influenza or other respiratory diseases, include specimens of trachea, carina, and lung. Heart muscle, liver, and kidney are less common sources of virus, but may be included if involvement is suspected. Both biopsy and autopsy specimens should be kept at 4 C and processed as soon as possible after collection. If delay is unavoidable, specimens can be kept frozen for a limited period at −70 C. Do not fix tissues in Formalin, embalming fluid, or other preservatives, as this renders them useless for purposes of virus isolation or fluorescent-antibody tests.

PROCESSING OF SPECIMENS FOR VIRUS ISOLATION ATTEMPTS

Throat, nasal, and mouth swabs

Frozen specimens are best thawed by placing them under cold, running tap water. When thawing is complete, fluid from the swabs should be expressed into the transport medium by firmly pressing the swabs along the side of the tube until no further liquid is seen running down the side of the tube. The swabs may then be discarded. The specimen is then thoroughly mixed prior to withdrawal of the sample for inoculation (the volume of sample is dependent upon the number of tissue culture tubes, animals, or embryonated eggs to be used). This sample *only* should be treated with antibiotics and antifungal agents prior to inoculation; the remaining, untreated portion of the specimen is dispensed in 1.0-ml amounts into flame-sealed glass ampoules or tightly sealed screw-capped vials for storage at −70 C. If gross particulate matter is visible, it should be removed by the method described below for rectal swabs.

Antimicrobial treatment of the sample to be used for virus isolation is as follows. To the swab material, an antibiotic and antifungal solution is added to give a final concentration of 200 to 500 units of penicillin per ml, 200 to 500 μg of streptomycin per ml, and 50 to 100 units of nystatin per ml. This mixture should be allowed to stand for 30 to 60 min at 4 C before being inoculated into the appropriate host system.

Throat and nasal washings

The technique described above for swabs is also employed for the antimicrobial treatment of throat and nasal washings (gargles). However, if gross particulate or mucoid material is visible, the specimen should be centrifuged with glass beads. This procedure is described below in the section on rectal swabs.

Rectal swabs

The processing of rectal swabs for virus isolation is essentially the same as that for throat swabs, with the following modifications. After the swabs have been expressed and discarded, the material is transferred to a centrifuge tube containing sterile glass beads. An appropriate-sized rubber stopper is put in place and taped securely. The centrifuge tube should be shaken briefly to break up large particles and then centrifuged for 30 min at 3,000 to 4,000 rpm in a refrigerated centrifuge. After centrifugation, as much supernatant fluid as possible is removed without disturbing the glass beads. This fluid is then dispensed as described above. Antimicrobial treatment varies from that employed for throat swab material only in that the final concentration of antimicrobial agents is higher. Add antimicrobial agents to give the following final concentrations: penicillin, 1,000 units/ml; streptomycin, 1,000 μg/ml; and nystatin, 100 units/ml.

Stool

Approximately 20 ml of an appropriate tissue culture diluent such as medium 199 or Hanks balanced salt solution (BSS) should be placed in a thick-walled screw-capped centrifuge tube containing 20 to 30 sterile glass beads. Approximately 2 g of stool is added to this tube by use of an ordinary tongue blade. An appropriate-sized rubber stopper is then inserted and taped in place. The mixture is vigorously shaken until all large particles of stool are broken up and then is centrifuged for 30 min at 4,000 rpm in a refrigerated centrifuge. The supernatant fluid is then removed and treated as described above for rectal swab extracts.

Body fluids

Most body fluids, such as cerebrospinal fluid and pleural fluid, need not be treated with antimicrobial agents prior to inoculation unless bacterial contamination is suspected or the patient's clinical course so indicates. If bacterial contamination is suspected, the method described for treatment of pharyngeal secretions should be employed.

As most specimens of urine *not* obtained by catheterization *contain* bacteria, it is recommended that prior to inoculation urine be treated with antimicrobial agents by the methods described above.

Autopsy and biopsy specimens

Ideally, 20% suspensions of tissues are desirable. However, biopsy specimens are sometimes quite small and tissue suspensions less concentrated than 20% must be used. The concentration chosen would depend on the volume of inoculum needed.

Tissue suspensions can be prepared with a sterile mortar and pestle or, when soft tissues such as liver or brain are being processed, with a glass tissue grinder. The tissue specimen is placed in a sterile petri dish and weighed on a beam balance. If the specimen weighed 2 g, one would prepare 10 ml of a diluent (Hanks BSS) containing 1,000 units of penicillin and 100 μg of streptomycin per ml. This is the *total* amount of diluent to be used throughout this procedure to prepare a 20% suspension.

After being weighed, the tissue is cut into small pieces (approximately 5 mm^3) by use of sterile forceps, scalpel, or scissors, and the minced tissue is placed into the mortar. A small quantity of sterile sand is added, followed by a small portion of the diluent, and grinding is initiated. Sufficient diluent is added to give a homogeneous paste. The remaining diluent is then added to the mortar and mixed with the tissue paste by use of a Propipette. The suspension is transferred to a 50-ml screw-capped centrifuge tube by use of a 10-ml wide-tipped pipette. After centrifugation at 4 C for 30 min at approximately 2,000 rpm, the supernatant fluid is removed and dispensed into appropriate-sized sterile vials for immediate use or for freezer storage.

SEROLOGICAL TESTS

The various serological tests employed in diagnostic virology (neutralization, hemagglutination-inhibition, fluorescent-antibody staining) are described in the several chapters dealing with specific viruses. Because of its length, and to save space and avoid repetition, a description of the complement fixation (CF) test is given in this introductory chapter.

COMPLEMENT-FIXATION TEST

The CF procedure described here is designed primarily for detection of antibodies and rises in antibody titer in paired sera. The techniques involved are simple, but they do require skill which can be gained only by practice. Rigorous attention to detail is necessary to obtain reliable and reproducible results.

The CF test comprises essentially two steps: (i) a primary reaction which involves antigen, antibody, and complement, and (ii) a secondary hemolytic reaction in which hemolysin-sensitized erythrocytes (RBC) act as an indicator of the amount of complement remaining after the primary reaction is complete.

The modified Kolmer CF test employing overnight (18 h) fixation at 4 C has been found to possess satisfactory sensitivity for the measurement of viral and rickettsial antigens and antibodies. The microtechnique described below is more widely applicable than macromethods. It is advantageous not only from the standpoint of conserving reagents, but also from the standpoint of space required for performing and incubating the tests and ease of performance.

The test is carried out in disposable molded plastic plates (available commercially), 12 by 83 by 130 mm, containing eight rows of 12 round-bottom cups. Each cup has a working capacity of 0.125 ml, which is the total volume employed in each test. Serum dilutions are carried out directly in the cups by use of stainless-steel diluters calibrated to transfer 0.025 ml. The other reagents are added with dropper pipettes calibrated to deliver 0.025 or 0.05 ml per drop. The plates may be sealed with 7.6-cm plastic tape.

Reagents

Diluents

Either Veronal-buffered saline or Kolmer saline may be employed as a diluent for the reagents. Mg^{2+} and Ca^{2+} are required for hemolysis, and these cations are supplied in the following formulas.

Veronal-buffered saline. For optimal results, recrystallize diethylbarbituric acid as follows. Add 1 lb (454 g) of commercial salt to 1 quart (0.95 liter) of hot absolute ethyl alcohol, filter while hot, cool in an ice bath, and recover crystals in a Büchner filter-funnel. Prepare sodium barbiturate from commercial barbitone by making a saturated solution of barbitone in absolute ethyl alcohol at 22 C and adding alcoholic sodium hydroxide (one part saturated aqueous NaOH and nine parts alcohol) with constant stirring until the mixture becomes slightly alkaline. Chill and recover precipitated sodium barbiturate.

To prepare Veronal-buffered saline, dissolve 85.0 g of NaCl and 3.75 g of Na-5,5-diethylbarbiturate in about 1,400 ml of distilled water. Dissolve 5.75 g of 5,5-diethylbarbituric acid in about 500 ml of hot distilled water. Mix the two solutions, cool to room temperature, and add 5.0 ml of a stock solution made of 10.0 g of $MgCl_2 \cdot 6H_2O$ and 4.0 g of $CaCl_2 \cdot 2H_2O$ in 100 ml of distilled water. Add distilled water to make 2,000 ml. (This stock solution will keep indefinitely at 4 C.)

For use, make a precise fivefold dilution, which results in an isotonic solution. This working solution should be at pH 7.3. It should be discarded at the end of each working day. Addition to the working solution of gelatin or bovine serum albumin to a final concentration of 0.1% helps to prevent spontaneous lysis of RBC.

Kolmer saline. Kolmer saline is 0.85% saline containing 1.0 ml of the following magnesium-calcium solution per liter: $MgCl_2 \cdot 6H_2O$, 10.0 g; $CaCl_2 \cdot 2H_2O$, 4.0 g; and distilled water to 100.0 ml (store at 4 C). This saline solution is used for the dilution of all reagents in the test.

Sensitized cell suspension

Sheep cells. Blood should be collected aseptically in Alsever's solution (24.6 g of glucose, 9.6 g of sodium citrate [dihydrate], and 5.04 g of NaCl dissolved in 1,200 ml of distilled water, adjusted to pH 6.1 with citric acid, and sterilized by filtration). Use one part blood to one part Alsever's solution, and age the RBC under sterile conditions at 4 C for 24 h. After this stabilization period, the RBC will remain constant in their susceptibility to lysis by complement and antibody for 10 weeks if stored at 4 C. Gentle treatment is essential to avoid hemolysis.

Wash sheep RBC by suspending them in saline and then centrifuging them for 8 min at 2,000 rpm three successive times. Pack the cells in a graduated centrifuge tube by centrifuging them for 10 min at 2,000 rpm. Prepare a 2% suspension of the cells in saline in a volume sufficient for the entire test. Lyse 0.8 ml of the cell suspension in 3.2 ml of distilled water for colorimetric standardization. Determine the optical density of the resulting hemoglobin solution at 550 nm in a Coleman Junior spectrophotometer using a 12 by 75 mm cuvette. Adjust the cell suspension to an optical density of 0.47.

Hemolysin. Anti-sheep cell hemolysin is available commercially. The use of sera from rabbits immunized with boiled sheep cell stromata (anti-Forssman) has been recommended. Such antisera have the advantage of providing a constant level of hemolytic activity even if used in large excess, while at the same time possessing a high ratio of hemolytic to agglutinating activity.

Prepare a 1:100 stock solution of hemolysin as follows: mix 94.0 ml of saline and 4.0 ml of 5.0% phenol in saline; add 2.0 ml of hemolysin, 50% in glycerol (stored at 4 C).

For titration (perform in 13 by 100 mm tubes), prepare dilutions of hemolysin as shown in Table 3. Titrate the hemolysin as follows. Mix 0.2 ml of hemolysin dilution (1:6,000 to 1:25,000), 0.1 ml of 1:30 complement (0.2 ml of complement + 5.8 ml of saline), 0.2 ml of 2.0% sheep cell suspension, and 0.5 ml of saline. As a cell control, use 0.2 ml of sheep cell suspension and 0.8 ml of saline. Shake and incubate the hemolysin titration in a water bath at 37 C for

TABLE 3. *Dilutions of hemolysin for use in titration*

Dilution	Saline diluent (ml)	Hemolysin to be added	
		Dilution	Volume (ml)
1:1,000	4.5	1:100	0.5
1:6,000	5.0	1:1,000	1.0
1:8,000	7.0	1:1,000	1.0
1:10,000	9.0	1:1,000	1.0
1:15,000	0.5	1:10,000	1.0
1:20,000	1.0	1:10,000	1.0
1:25,000	1.5	1:10,000	1.0

30 min and then read. The highest dilution of hemolysin which shows *complete* hemolysis represents 1 unit. Use 2 units in the test. (*Example:* If the 1:10,000 dilution shows complete hemolysis and the 1:15,000 dilution shows partial hemolysis, 1 unit would be represented by a 1:10,000 dilution. Therefore, 2 units would be contained in a 1:5,000 dilution of hemolysin.)

Prepare the proper dilution of hemolysin in a volume sufficient for the entire test. Sensitize cells in sufficient volume for the complement titration (see below) by pouring diluted hemolysin into an equal volume of the cell suspension and rapidly pouring the mixture back and forth several times. Allow the sensitized cells to remain at room temperature for at least 10 min before use.

Hold the remaining cell suspension and hemolysin at 4 C, and mix equal volumes together the following morning for completion of the test.

Complement

Lyophilized guinea pig serum for this purpose is available commercially. Fresh whole guinea pig serum may also be employed. The fresh material, if stored at −65 C in sealed glass containers, will keep its original complement titer for many weeks. Stored at 4 C, undiluted or as a 50% solution in glycerol, it will retain its titer for at least 1 month. It is important that the complement be free from the antibodies under study to avoid the apparent anticomplementary activity of the homologous antigen which will result if they are present. Antibodies to a variety of rickettsial and viral agents have been found in guinea pig complement, including Rocky Mountain spotted fever, rickettsial pox and psittacosis, myxoviruses, and reoviruses. It is therefore important to pretest lots of complement for such incidental antibodies prior to their use in the CF test.

Titrate guinea pig complement in the presence of each test antigen. (Restore lyophilized complement to the original volume in the diluent supplied by the producer.) Perform the titration in 13 by 75 mm tubes, using the volumes of reagents shown in Table 4. Shake the tubes, incubate them in a water bath at 37 C for 30 min, and then add 0.2 ml of sensitized cells to all tubes. Shake, incubate at 37 C for an additional 30 min, and read. The tube containing the least amount of complement showing complete hemolysis represents 1 unit. Use 2 *exact* units in the test. (*Example:* If 0.09 ml of a 1:60 dilution of complement equals 1 exact unit, then 0.18 ml of the 1:60 dilution of complement equals 2 exact units; $60/0.18 \times 0.1 = 1:33$ dilution of complement.)

Antigen

Standardize antigens by testing serial twofold dilutions of antigen against serial twofold dilutions of immune serum to determine the optimal dilution of antigen which gives fixation. This procedure, often referred to as a "box" titration, is illustrated in Table 5.

Some antigens are inherently anticomplementary; i.e., they bind or destroy complement by themselves. This anticomplementary activity may be reduced in some cases by treatment with fluorocarbons or by the addition of inactivated guinea pig serum to a final concentration of 5%.

Make serum dilutions by use of 0.025-ml diluters. Prepare dilutions of antigen in tubes and, starting with the highest dilution, add 0.025 ml of each dilution to the appropriate wells. Include complement controls for each antigen dilution (testing antigen dilutions against 2.0, 1.5, 1.0, and 0.5 units of complement). Add 0.025 ml of saline to the serum control wells and to the complement controls. To the test proper and the 2-unit complement control, add 0.025 ml of complement diluted to contain 2 units; add 0.025 ml of the appropriate complement dilutions to the complement controls containing 1.5, 1.0, and 0.5 units (see Table 7 for preparation of these complement dilutions).

Mix the contents of the wells by rubbing the

TABLE 4. *Titration of complement*

Reagent	Volume (ml) of reagent to be added to tube no.							
	1	2	3	4	5	6	7	8
Antigen (diluted to 2 units)	0.10	0.10	0.10	0.10	0.10	0.10	0.10	0.10
Complement (1:60)	0.12	0.11	0.10	0.09	0.08	0.07	0.06	0.05
Saline diluent ...	0.08	0.09	0.10	0.11	0.12	0.13	0.14	0.15

TABLE 5. *Titration of antigen*

Antigen dilution	Immune serum dilutions					Negative serum, 1:8	Complement control (units of complement)			
	1:8	1:16	1:32	1:64	1:128		2.0	1.5	1.0	0.5
1:2	4[a]	4	4	0	0	0	0	0	±	4
1:4	4	4	4	1	0	0	0	0	0	4
1:8	4	4	4	2	0	0	0	0	0	4
1:16	4	4	4	2	0	0	0	0	0	4
1:32	4	4	2	0	0	0	0	0	0	4
1:64	1	0	0	0	0	0	0	0	0	4
Serum control	0	0	0	0	0	0	—			
Control (uninfected) antigen	0	0	0	0	0	0	0	0	0	4
Previous lot of specific antigen	4	4	4	0	0	0	0	0	0	4

[a] Degree of fixation.

bottom of the plate gently. Incubate overnight at 4 ot 6 C. Warm the plates for 15 min at room temperature; add 0.05 ml of the sensitized cell suspension to each well. Mix on a vibrating shaker and then incubate at 37 C for 15 to 30 min, or until the complement controls show proper clearing.

The highest dilution of antigen showing 3+ or 4+ fixation with the highest dilution of immune serum is generally regarded as 1 unit (1:16 dilution in the above example). (For practical purposes, the unit is sometimes greater than this; for example, if a 1:32 dilution of antigen gives 3+ or 4+ fixation with a 1:256 dilution of immune serum, and a 1:64 antigen dilution gives 3+ fixation with a 1:128 serum dilution, the unit may be considered as 1:64.) Use 2 units of antigen in a volume of 0.025 ml.

Early detection of specific antibodies in cases of rickettsial disease may be facilitated by use of 8 instead of the customary 2 units of antigen.

Stocks of CF antigens for the diagnosis of spotted fever, Q fever, rickettsialpox, and murine typhus, as well as standard guinea pig reference sera, are maintained by the Center for Disease Control, Atlanta, Ga. Currently, these materials are made commercially by just one company in the U.S.

Specificity of CF antigens for detection and differentiation of *Rickettsia typhi* and *R. prowazeki* antibodies can usually be restored or improved by washing the antigen. Washing is accomplished by centrifugation at 20,000. × *g* for 20 min, discarding the supernatant fluid, and resuspending the pellet in 0.15 M NaCl containing 1:10,000 Merthiolate (final concentration).

Serum

Because a nonspecific reaction may be encountered with high concentrations of serum, use an initial serum dilution of 1:4 or 1:8 in the test. Inactivate the initial serum dilution for 30 min in a water bath at 60 C. In every run, include a serum with a known titer to each antigen as a positive control.

Sera may also exhibit anticomplementary activity. This is often caused by bacterial or chemical contamination, including anticoagulants and preservatives. Several methods have been described for the removal of anticomplementary activity from sera. Addition of a small piece of dry ice to an anticomplementary serum has been found useful in some cases. Serum from severely hemolyzed blood specimens may be made suitable for serological examination by passage through a small Sephadex G-75 or G-100 column. The antibody comes out ahead of the hemoglobin.

Test Proper

The scheme for the performance of the microtiter CF test is shown in Table 6.

Add 0.05 ml of the initial serum dilution to a well for each test antigen; add 0.025 ml to a well for each uninfected control antigen and to a well for the serum (anticomplementary) control. Prepare successive twofold serum dilutions for the test antigen sets using 0.025-ml diluters.

Dilute test antigens to contain 2 units and add 0.025 ml to appropriate wells. Add 0.025 ml of control antigen to the appropriate well and 0.025 ml of saline to the serum control wells.

Dilute complement as follows and add to the test. Dilute complement in cold saline to contain 2 exact units. Dilute further for the complement controls as shown in Table 7. Add 0.025 ml of the dilution of complement containing 0.5 unit to the appropriate wells; continue by adding 0.025 ml of the dilutions containing 1.0 and 1.5 units. Add 0.025 ml of the initial complement dilution (2 units) to the 2-unit

TABLE 6. *Scheme for performance of the microtiter complement-fixation test*

Wells	Serum (ml)	Saline diluent (ml)	Antigen (ml)	Nonspecific antigen[a] (ml)		Complement (ml)		Sensitized cells (ml)	
Serum under test	0.025[b]	—	0.025	—	Shake and add	0.025	Overnight incubation at 4 to 6 C followed by 15 min at room temp.	0.050	15 to 30 min at 37 C
Serum control (test for anticomplementary activity)	0.025[c]	0.025	—	—		0.025		0.050	
Serum nonspecific antigen control	0.025[c]	—	—	0.025		0.025		0.050	
Reagent controls									
Complement controls for specific (and nonspecific) antigens	Complement (units)								
	2.0	0.025	0.025	—[d]		0.025		0.050	
	1.5	0.025	0.025	—		0.025 (3:4)		0.050	
	1.0	0.025	0.025	—		0.025 (1:2)		0.050	
	0.5	0.025	0.025	—		0.025 (1:4)		0.050	
Hemolytic control	—	0.050	—	—		0.025		0.050	
Sheep cell control	—	0.075	—	—		—		0.050	

[a] Uninfected tissue prepared and diluted in the same manner as the specific antigen.
[b] Series of wells each containing 0.025 ml of a serial dilution of serum.
[c] Initial serum dilution of 1:4 or 1:8.
[d] Complement controls should also be run with nonspecific antigen.

TABLE 7. *Dilution of complement for the complement controls*

Complement, 2 units (ml)	Cold saline diluent	Final dilution of complement (units)
1.5	0.5	1.5
1.0	1.0	1.0
0.5	1.5	0.5

complement control wells. Add 0.025 ml of saline to all of the complement controls. Add 0.025 ml of the initial complement dilution (containing 2 units) to the remainder of the test.

Mix by rubbing the bottom of the plates gently. Cover plates and incubate overnight at 4 to 6 C. On the following day, warm the plates for 15 min at room temperature; add 0.05 ml of sensitized cells, mix, and incubate at 37 C for 15 to 30 min, or until the complement controls show proper clearing.

Explanation of complement controls

The wells containing 2.0 and 1.5 units of complement should show complete hemolysis. The wells containing 1.0 unit should show complete or nearly complete hemolysis, and the wells containing 0.5 unit of complement should show no hemolysis. If the wells containing 0.5 unit show hemolysis, an excess of complement was used in the test. If those containing 2.0 and 1.5 units do not show *complete* hemolysis, insufficient complement was used.

When the complement controls show the proper degree of hemolysis, remove the plates from the incubator. If the complement controls are insufficiently cleared after the initial incubation period, continue incubation, examining the controls at frequent intervals during the succeeding 15 min. After removing the plates from the incubator, hold them at 4 to 6 C until the unlysed cells have settled and the tests are ready to read. Settling of the cells may be facilitated by centrifugation of the plates in special carriers.

LITERATURE CITED

1. Behbehani, A. M. 1972. Human viral and rickettsial diseases. A handbook of laboratory diagnosis for practicing physicians. The Univ. of Kansas School of Medicine, Kansas City.
2. Busby, D. W. G., W. House, and J. R. MacDonald. 1964. Virological technique. Little, Brown & Co., London.

3. Grist, N. R., C. A. C. Ross, E. J. Bell, and E. J. Stott. 1966. Diagnostic methods in clinical virology. Blackwell Scientific Publications, Oxford, England.
4. Hoskins, J. 1967. Virological procedures. Appleton-Century-Crofts, New York.
5. Hsiung, G. D. 1973. Diagnostic virology, revised edition. Yale Univ. Press, New Haven.
6. Kalter, S. S. 1963. Procedures for routine laboratory diagnosis of virus and rickettsial diseases. Burgess Publishing Co., Minneapolis.
7. Lennette, E. H., and N. J. Schmidt (ed.) 1969. Diagnostic procedures for viral and rickettsial infections, 4th ed. American Public Health Association, Inc., New York.
8. Swain, R. H. A., and T. C. Dodds. 1967. Clinical virology. The Williams & Wilkins Co., Baltimore.
9. Virus Laboratory. 1972. Viral and rickettsial diseases. Physicians handbook, 4th ed. Virus Laboratory, Ontario Department of Health, Toronto.

Chapter 72

Influenza Virus

WALTER R. DOWDLE AND MARION T. COLEMAN

CLINICAL BACKGROUND

Influenza is an acute respiratory disease which characteristically occurs in epidemic form (5). It is transmitted through droplets and direct personal contacts. After an incubation period of 1 to 3 days, the disease usually begins abruptly with chilliness followed by fatigue, headache, and myalgia. Fever appears early and may persist for 2 to 4 days. Constitutional symptoms are more striking with influenza than with other respiratory diseases. A slight nonproductive cough may be present, but coryza and pharyngitis are rare. Physical findings are consistent with those of an acute febrile illness. Recovery from uncomplicated influenza begins 3 to 4 days after onset, although complaints of weakness and fatigue may persist for 1 week or longer. Pulmonary complications of viral or bacterial origin may occur. Fatal complications are most frequent in the aged or in patients of any age with chronic debilitating illnesses.

One of the major distinguishing characteristics of influenza is its epidemic nature. Epidemics of influenza type A may occur every 2 to 3 years, or at any time with the advent of a new subtype. Outbreaks of type B are less frequent and usually occur every 4 to 6 years. Epidemics in a particular geographic area appear abruptly and may run their course in 2 to 3 weeks. (Influenza type C is associated with subclinical or mild common coldlike illness and does not cause recognizable epidemics.)

Influenza may not always follow the classic clinical course or occur in epidemic patterns. Sporadic cases, particularly among children, may be difficult to recognize when viewed against a background of other febrile and respiratory diseases in the community, For this reason, laboratory diagnosis is essential.

DESCRIPTION OF AGENT

Influenza viruses are spherical with a diameter of 80 to 120 nm. Filamentous forms which may reach several nanometers in length are frequently seen. The surface of the virus is composed of repeating spikelike subunits consisting of hemagglutinin and a virus-coded enzyme, neuraminidase. These two morphologically distinct structures are 8 to 10 nm long and are spaced 7 to 8 nm apart. They extend from an external lipid bilayer membrane which, in turn, surrounds a protein matrix and a helical nucleocapsid containing ribonucleic acid. The hemagglutinin enables the virus to agglutinate red blood cells (RBC) from a variety of species and to adsorb RBC to infected cell cultures. The neuraminidase hydrolyzes neuraminic acid residues from mucoproteins and is responsible for elution of the virus from RBC. The essential function of the enzyme in virus infection or replication is not known.

The infectivity of influenza viruses is destroyed by heating at 56 C, exposure to lipid solvents, low pH (<3), ultraviolet irradiation, and formaldehyde. Infectivity may be preserved by lyophilization or by storage at −70 C.

Influenza viruses are classified as orthomyxoviruses and are divided into three types, A, B, and C. These types may be distinguished by their internal ribonucleoprotein and matrix proteins, which are antigenically identical for all strains of a given type. The external hemagglutinin and neuraminidase antigens are unstable and frequently undergo variation. Differences among these antigens constitute the basis for the influenza virus nomenclature system recommended by the World Health Organization (19). Each strain designation provides the following information: (i) a description of the antigenic type of ribonucleoprotein (A, B, or C); (ii) the host of origin (not specified for strains isolated from man); (iii) geographic origin; (iv) strain number; and (v) year of isolation. For influenza A viruses, an antigenic description follows the strain designation and includes, in parentheses, an index describing the antigenic character of the hemagglutinin (H) and neuraminidase (N) subtypes. For example, the major human subtypes are A/PR/8/34(H0N1), A/FM/1/47-(H1N1), A/Singapore/1/57(H2N2), and A/Hong Kong/1/68(H3N2).

A number of other H and N subtypes are also recognized among type A viruses isolated from horses, pigs, and birds. These are designated by host of origin, such as A/equine/Prague/

1/56(Heq1Neq1) and A/tern/S. Africa/61 (Hav5-Nav2). Certain N subtypes are shared among strains isolated from different species. For example, the neuraminidase of A/turkey/Canada/63(Hav2Neq2) is similar to that of A/equine/Miami/1/63(Heq2Neq2).

Because each H and N subtype may encompass strains possessing considerable degrees of antigenic heterogeneity, the geographic origin, number, and year of isolation of each strain provides important additional information. The full description permits the designation of selected strains as representative of antigenic groupings within a subtype. Also, the listing of the geographic origin and year of isolation provides some guide as to its probable antigenic relationships with other strains.

No formal divisions into subtypes have been made for types B and C, although antigenic variation has occurred extensively among B strains and, to a lesser extent, among C strains. The H and N antigens of the current type B strains are clearly different from their predecessors of the 1940s and 1950s, but there has been considerable antigenic overlap through the years and distinct lines of demarcation are difficult to define.

COLLECTION AND STORAGE OF SPECIMENS

Two types of specimens are collected for the diagnosis of influenza: throat and nasal specimens for virus isolation and paired blood specimens for serological examination. Specimens for virus isolation should be collected within the first 3 days after onset of disease. Although throat garglings and nasal washings may be used successfully, throat and nasal swabs are generally more convenient for the physician and less objectionable to the patient. Throat swabs are obtained by rubbing the posterior of the tonsils, the soft palate, and the back wall of the lower pharynx with two dry cotton applicators. Swabs may also be taken from the nasal mucosa. After the specimens are collected, the cotton tips of applicators are broken off into a single screw-cap vial containing 5 ml of tryptose phosphate broth with 0.5% gelatin. Specimens for virus isolation should be kept cold (4 C) at all times. If they are not to be inoculated within 48 h after collection, specimens should be sealed and stored in dry ice or under mechanical refrigeration (−70 C).

Blood specimens for serological diagnosis are drawn by venipuncture during the acute stage of the disease, usually at the time a throat swab is collected, and again 2 to 3 weeks later during the convalescent stage. Sera collected aseptically from the blood clots need not be refrigerated during transport to the laboratory, but should be stored at 4 or −20 C.

In fatal cases of suspected influenza pneumonia, virus isolation should be attempted from lung tissue, tracheal mucosa, and blood. Tissue specimens, about 1 to 2 cm^3, and heart blood, about 1 ml, should be collected as soon as possible on autopsy and frozen at −70 C in sterile screw-capped containers.

DIRECT EXAMINATION

As early as 1956, Liu (10) showed that 71% of influenza A and 38% of influenza B infections could be diagnosed by direct fluorescent-antibody staining of nasal epithelial cells. Workers in other countries have also reported successful use of the technique (16). Although it has not been used extensively, fluorescent-antibody staining may be useful for rapid diagnosis of influenza virus infections.

CULTIVATION (ISOLATION) OF INFLUENZA VIRUSES

Influenza virus types A and B may be grown in embryonated hen's eggs and in kidney cell cultures from embryonic chickens, human embryos, hamsters, calves, and rhesus and green monkeys. The embryonated egg and rhesus monkey kidney tissue cultures appear to be the most sensitive hosts for isolation. Influenza C has been isolated only in the embryonated egg.

Inoculation of primary rhesus monkey kidney as well as the amniotic and allantoic sac of the embryonated egg is recommended for isolation of the maximal number of type A and B strains. The ease with which viruses of both types can be isolated has varied through the years. In general, monkey kidney has been superior to eggs for isolating influenza B, but the degree of superiority has varied. Experience with influenza A suggests even wider variability, and for this type eggs usually are more sensitive.

Prior to inoculation, the throat and nasal specimens are treated with an equal volume of tryptose phosphate broth containing 0.5% gelatin, 1,600 units of penicillin, and 800 μg of streptomycin sulfate per ml. The mixture is clarified by centrifugation in the cold at approximately 1,500 × g for 15 min. Tissues collected on autopsy are ground in a sterile mortar with a small amount of alundum and prepared as a 10% suspension in the same treatment medium described above.

Embryonated eggs

Ten- to 11-day-old embryonated eggs are swabbed with 70% alcohol directly over the air sac, and a small hole is punched in the shell in the center of the area. The egg is placed on a candler, with the air sac up, and rotated to locate the embryo. A 23-gauge, 3.8-cm needle attached to a 1-ml syringe is inserted into the amniotic sac with a jabbing motion. The needle is in the correct position when the embryo can be moved with the needle. A 0.2-ml amount of inoculum is injected into the amniotic cavity. The needle is withdrawn slightly, and an additional 0.2 ml is injected into the allantoic cavity. The hole in the shell is sealed with "model airplane cement" or wax. Two or three eggs are inoculated per specimen. Eggs are incubated at 33 C for 3 to 4 days.

Seven-day-old embryonated eggs are inoculated intra-amniotically and incubated at 33 C for 5 days to isolate influenza C.

Eggs are chilled overnight at 4 C to minimize bleeding during harvesting. The area over the air sac is swabbed with 70% alcohol. The egg shell is broken away to the level of the allantoic membrane, and the membrane is pulled away with sterile forceps. The allantoic fluid is harvested with a pipette or syringe and the amniotic fluid, with a short 20- to 22-gauge needle attached to a 1-ml syringe.

Undiluted samples of both fluids are tested in 0.05-ml (microtiter) quantities for the presence of virus by adding equal volumes of 0.4% guinea pig RBC or 0.5% chicken RBC. (RBC should be collected at a ratio of 1 volume of whole blood to 4 volumes of Alsever's solution. RBC suspension in Alsever's solution may be held as long as 1 week under refrigeration. Just prior to use, the RBC are washed three times with phosphate-buffered saline, pH 7.2, centrifuged at 1,000 rpm [about 250 × *g*] for 10 min, and resuspended to a concentration of 0.4% for guinea pig cells and 0.5% for chicken cells [7].) The fluid-RBC mixtures are incubated at 4 C for several hours or until control cells have settled.

Chicken RBC are the cells of choice for hemagglutinin assays once the virus has been adapted to eggs. However, guinea pig or human type O RBC may be more sensitive for detecting virus in early egg or tissue culture passage.

Two or three blind amniotic passages may be necessary in some instances to increase the titer of the virus to the level at which hemagglutinin is detectable. Once the virus has adapted to growth in the allantoic cavity, amniotic inoculation is no longer necessary.

Rhesus monkey kidney cells

Inhibition of influenza viruses by nonspecific substances in cell culture media containing serum may be avoided by washing the monolayers twice with Hanks balanced salt solution (BSS) before replacing the growth medium with 1 ml of serum-free Eagle's minimal essential medium (MEM). Two or three tubes are inoculated with 0.3 ml of the antibiotic-treated specimen and incubated at 33 C. They are observed microscopically each day to detect viral cytopathic effect (CPE). The appearance of CPE and production of hemagglutinins can be hastened by placing the tubes on a roller drum. In the absence of serum, frequent adding or changing of medium is required to maintain the cell cultures.

Tubes should be harvested as soon as CPE is detected. In the absence of CPE, tubes are harvested between the 7th and 14th days. Medium from one tube is transferred to the remaining one or two tubes and replaced with 1 ml of Hanks BSS. A 0.2-ml amount of fresh 0.4% guinea pig RBC is added, and the tube is returned to a slanted position. The cell sheet is examined for hemadsorption after 10 min and again after 30 min of incubation at room temperature. Uninfected control tubes should be tested to rule out nonspecific adsorption (4).

If a culture is positive for hemadsorption, a hemagglutinin titration should be performed on the pooled medium with 0.4% guinea pig RBC at 4 C. If the specimen is negative for hemadsorption or if the hemagglutinin titer is less than 8, the harvested material should be repassaged.

Most influenza B isolates are detected during the 3rd to 7th day of the first passage by hemadsorption or hemagglutination. CPE may also be evident. Cells become progressively granular, swollen, and round; later they become pyknotic and fragmented, and the cell sheet is eventually destroyed. Influenza A virus grows less vigorously in cell culture. The CPE, consisting of slowly vacuolating or lacy cells which degenerate and detach from the glass, is difficult to detect and may not become apparent until late in the second passage. Hemadsorption of varying degree is generally detected on the first passage, well in advance of an obvious CPE.

IDENTIFICATION

Influenza viruses may be identified by hemagglutination-inhibition (HI) hemadsorption-inhibition (HAdI), neutralization, or complement fixation (CF) tests.

Hemagglutination-inhibition test

Fluids from eggs or monkey kidney cell cultures containing hemagglutinin are titrated with 0.4% guinea pig RBC or human "O" RBC and 0.5% chicken RBC. Select the RBC giving the highest hemagglutinin titers for use in the HI test.

Hemagglutinin titration. The following procedure is described for the use of microtiter equipment. Beginning with a 1:10 dilution of the virus in 0.01 M phosphate-buffered physiological saline (PBS), pH 7.2, prepare twofold serial dilutions, in duplicate, in 0.05-ml volumes. Add 0.05 ml of chicken or guinea pig RBC to each well in the series. Include one well for each RBC suspension as a cell control (diluent plus RBC). Mix and incubate at room temperature until the cells settle. Consider the highest dilution of virus causing agglutination as the titration end point; that dilution contains 1 hemagglutination unit (HA unit) per 0.05 ml.

Preparation of test antigen. The HI test is performed with the most sensitive RBC system (chicken or guinea pig) and a test antigen preparation containing 4 HA units in 0.025 ml. Since 0.025 ml of the HA end point dilution would contain only 0.5 HA unit, the proper dilution of virus to be used in the HI test is determined by dividing the HA titer by 8. For example, if the HA titer is 160 with titration volumes of 0.05 ml (by definition 0.05 of the end point dilution contains 1 unit), then a 1:20 dilution would contain 8 HA units in 0.05 ml or 4 HA units in 0.025 ml.

To control possible errors in dilution and to confirm the HA titer, retitrate the test or working virus dilution. Prepare a row of six wells, each containing 0.05 ml of diluent. Add 0.05 ml of the working dilution of virus (8 HA units) to the first well and make the twofold dilution series through five wells. To the sixth well add 0.05 ml of diluent in place of virus. This will serve as the cell control.

Add 0.05 ml of the appropriate RBC suspension to all wells and mix; allow the contents to settle. The cell control and the last two wells should show compact buttons of normal settling. Agglutination in the first three wells of the series indicates that the working dilution contains 8 HA units of virus per 0.05 ml or 4 HA units per 0.025-ml volume to be used in the HI test. Adjust the virus concentration of the working dilution, if necessary, by adding PBS (if more than three wells show agglutination) or by adding virus (if fewer than three wells show agglutination). If adjustment of working antigen dilution is required, confirm its HA titer by retitration as just described.

Serum treatment. Many influenza isolates are highly sensitive to serum factors which may nonspecifically inhibit agglutination. Such inhibitors in human, chicken, and most rabbit sera can be successfully removed by treatment with the receptor-destroying enzyme (RDE) of *Vibrio cholerae* (2). Successful destruction of inhibitors in other animal sera varies with the virus to be tested and may require treatment with potassium periodate (3) or kaolin (6). RDE treatment is performed as follows. Add 4 volumes of RDE (100 units per ml) to each volume of serum. Incubate the mixture overnight in a water bath at 37 C. Add 3 volumes of 2.5% sodium citrate and incubate the mixture at 56 C for 30 min. Add 2 volumes of PBS to yield a final 1:10 dilution of treated serum. To avoid nonspecific agglutination of RBC, adsorb the treated serum at a rate of 0.1 ml of 50% RBC to 1 ml of the 1:10 serum dilution. Allow adsorption to proceed for 1 h at 4 C, and remove RBC by centrifugation. If chicken cells are used, adsorption is usually unnecessary and should be undertaken only if serum control wells (PBS substituted for virus) indicate nonspecific agglutination.

HI tests. Prepare twofold dilutions of treated reference antiserum from 1:10 through 1:5,120 in 0.025-ml volumes. Add 0.025 ml of the test virus suspension containing 4 HA units to each well. To test for RBC agglutinins in the serum, add diluent instead of antigen to a well containing the lowest dilution of serum. Also prepare cell controls (PBS only) and antigen controls (PBS and antigen) for each test. Shake and incubate for 30 min at room temperature.

Add 0.05 ml of RBC to each well, shake, and incubate at room temperature until the cell control shows the button of normal settling. The HI titer is defined as the dilution factor of the highest dilution of serum which completely inhibits agglutination. Complete inhibition is determined by tilting the plates and observing the "tear-shaped" streaming of cells which flow at the same rate as cell controls.

Hemadsorption inhibition test

Since all human myxoviruses may be isolated in rhesus monkey kidney and all exhibit the property of hemadsorption, it is impractical to attempt to identify the virus by HAdI unless there is sufficient evidence to narrow the possibility to only one or two suspected types. Such evidence may consist of the type of CPE, its rate of appearance, hemadsorption patterns, or epidemiological information. In general, specific antisera are employed to best advantage in the HI test. HAdI is less sensitive than HI; a serum with an HI titer of less than 80 may fail to inhibit hemadsorption of recent isolates which show slight changes in antigenic composition. The HAdI test is useful, however, in some instances: during a known epidemic where the identification of type A or type B isolates simply needs to be confirmed, or in the event that the hemagglutinin titer is too low to perform the HI test. The HAdI test is performed as follows.

Treat antisera with RDE in the same manner as described for the HI test. Wash infected monkey kidney cell cultures twice with Hanks BSS. Add 0.2 ml of the RDE-treated serum diluted 1:10 and then add 0.6 ml of Hanks BSS. Incubate the cultures for 30 min at room temperature with the entire cell sheet covered; add 0.2 ml of 0.4% guinea pig RBC suspensions to each tube. Reincubate the cultures at room temperature for 30 min and examine microscopically for the presence of hemadsorption. The isolate is identified by the serum that prevents hemadsorption.

Neutralization test

Influenza viruses may be identified by neutralization tests performed in either eggs or primary rhesus monkey kidney cell cultures. Mix equal volumes of 100 to 300 infectious doses of virus and serial twofold dilutions of reference antisera, incubate for 1 h at room temperature, and inoculate into the appropriate test system. Test allantoic harvests from eggs for the presence of hemagglutinins and record inhibition. Examine cell cultures for inhibition of hemadsorption. Neutralization test results generally parallel those obtained by the HI test. Neutralization procedures are more complex and only rarely yield additional information over that obtained by the HI test.

Neuraminidase-inhibition test

A complete description of the influenza A viruses requires characterization of the neuraminidase as well as the hemagglutinin antigens. Although neuraminidase subtypes may be distinguished by double immunodiffusion tests (see below), more precise antigenic analysis requires examination by the neuraminidase-inhibition test.

The basis of the test is the ability of virus antineuraminidase antibody to inhibit enzymatic release of *N*-acetyl neuraminic acid (NANA) from fetuin substrate. Neuraminidase activity is assayed by incubating serial dilutions of virus overnight in the presence of fetuin. Free NANA released into the medium by the action of the enzyme is converted to a chromophore by the addition of periodate and thiobarbituric acid and its concentration is determined by spectrophotometric analysis.

Neuraminidase-inhibiting antibody is assayed by mixing virus suspensions of the required potency with serial dilutions of normal and test sera before incubation overnight with fetuin. Free NANA is determined and the inhibitory effect of the sera is calculated. The recommended procedures are described in detail in a publication of the World Health Organization (1).

Complement fixation test

Influenza viruses may be typed as A, B, or C through identification of their ribonucleoprotein (RNP) antigen by the CF test. This test is most useful in the event of a major change in the composition of the surface (hemagglutinin and neuraminidase) antigens of a new variant, or if strains are encountered which are poorly reactive in the HI test.

The strain-specific CF test may be used for studying the antigenic relationships of viral surface components. It is particularly useful for the study of viruses which, in the HI test, are either nonsensitive to antibody or highly sensitive to nonspecific serum inhibitors. Reference antisera must be free from antibody to the type-specific antigens. Methods for preparing antigens and antisera for use in the type-specific and strain-specific CF test have been described elsewhere (9).

Immuno-double-diffusion test

The potential of the immuno-double-diffusion (IDD) test for rapid identification of type and subtype of influenza virus isolates has recently been recognized. When virus concentrates are disrupted with detergents such as sodium dodecyl sulfate (SDS) or sodium *N*-lauroyl-sarcosinate and placed in wells adjacent to specific potent antisera, precipitin lines form which correspond to the RNP, the matrix protein (M), the hemagglutinin (HA), and the neuraminidase (NA; 12, 14). The detergent may have a deleterious effect on the formation of precipitin lines with the surface antigens (HA and NA) of some strains, but experience with the type-specific RNP and M antigen has been uniformly good.

The major obstacle to the general use of the test has been the unavailability of potent specific antisera.

RECOMMENDED PROCEDURES

Influenza viruses are usually the only human myxoviruses isolated in 10- to 11-day-old embryonated eggs. Although mumps virus will grow in eggs, it is rarely isolated under the above conditions. When hemagglutinins are detected in egg fluids, the virus may be identified directly by HI tests with antisera prepared against current influenza A and B (or C, if indicated) strains. Failure of the influenza virus antisera to inhibit hemagglutination suggests that the egg fluids may be contaminated with hemagglutinating bacteria, avian mycoplasma, Newcastle disease virus of chickens, or Sendai virus (parainfluenza type 1) of mice. Another possibility is that the hemagglutinating agent may be a new antigenic subtype of influenza virus. In this event, the virus is identified by the type-specific CF or IDD test.

Identification of influenza viruses in monkey kidney cell cultures is more complex. A presumptive identification of type B may be made from its characteristic CPE. Serological confirmation of its identity may be obtained quickly by the HI test. The CPE, if any, of type A isolates usually cannot be readily differentiated from that of parainfluenza viruses which may be isolated under the same conditions and may also cause hemagglutination.

Identification of the hemagglutinating agent is dependent upon serological tests, preferably the HI test. Commercial antisera or antisera produced against crude allantoic fluid harvests of current type A or B strains are adequate for identifying antigenically related isolates. Such antisera may be prepared in chickens by intravenous injection of 5 ml of infected allantoic fluid containing a minimum of 160 HA units/ml. Animals are exsanguinated 9 to 10 days later. Since chicken serum cannot be used satisfactorily in the CF test, some workers prefer ferret antiserum, which may be employed in CF as well as HI tests. Ferrets are infected by intranasal instillation of 1 ml of allantoic or amniotic fluid containing at least 10^4 infectious virus particles. Ferrets must be kept under strict isolation since they are highly susceptible to infection with influenza viruses. Preimmunization serum should be tested to rule out prior infection.

Such chicken and ferret antisera are suitable diagnostic reagents, but they contain antibodies to both the hemagglutinin and neuraminidase and therefore are not satisfactory for determining the precise antigenic composition of the isolate. Hemagglutination by certain viruses may be inhibited by neuraminidase antibody, presumably through steric hindrance of the hemagglutinin, and may therefore indicate false antigenic relationships. The HI titers of neuraminidase antibody are often low and unpredictable, but they may be exaggerated by inadequate destruction of nonspecific inhibitors in the reference sera. The possibility that inhibition may occur is sufficient reason to question the results of antigenic analyses performed by the HI test under conditions where antineuraminidase antibody is present. Hemagglutinin-specific and neuraminidase-specific antisera may be produced by using influenza recombinants possessing genetically segregated surface antigens (15) or by using isolated hemagglutinin subunits (18). The recommended procedure for performing the neuraminidase inhibition test is described elsewhere (1). Tests for antigenic characterization of influenza strains are not normally performed in the diagnostic laboratory. Strains requiring antigenic analysis may be forwarded to a designated reference center (World Health Organization International Influenza Center for the Americas, Center for Disease Control, Atlanta, Ga. 30333).

SEROLOGICAL DIAGNOSIS

The serological diagnosis of influenza is based upon demonstration of a fourfold or greater increase in antibody titer between acute and convalescent sera. This may be measured by the type-specific CF test with RNP antigens or by the HI test with antigens carefully selected as similar to currently prevalent strains. The CF test is often used because of its wide applicability in the virus laboratory. Unlike the HI test, the CF test is influenced neither by antigenic variability of prevalent strains nor by nonspecific inhibitors. However, of the two, the HI test is agreed to be the most sensitive test for serological diagnoses.

A quantitative, single-radial-diffusion test for hemagglutinin and neuraminidase antibodies has also been described (13). In some laboratories, this test may be the most convenient method for serological diagnosis.

The CF test may be performed as described for the LBCF test (17) or by various methods used in different laboratories; influenza antigens may be readily standardized in the procedure used for the diagnosis of other virus diseases. RNP antigens and control sera for type A and type B influenza viruses may be obtained from commercial sources or prepared in the laboratory. (Antigens are prepared by allantoic inoculation of 10- to 11-day-old eggs. After incubation at 33 C for 48 h, eggs are chilled overnight, and the chorioallantoic membranes are removed and washed in sterile PBS. Membranes are ground in a mortar with sterile alundum and suspended in 1.0 ml of PBS per membrane, or they are homogenized mechanically. The mixture is then centrifuged at 250 × *g* for 15 min, and the supernatant fluid is decanted. Hemagglutinin is adsorbed by mixing

1 volume of packed chicken RBC with 15 volumes of chilled supernatant fluid. RBC are removed by centrifugation. The RBC adsorption procedure is repeated until the supernatant fluid fails to agglutinate chicken RBC. The supernatant fluid contains the RNP antigen. Type A and B antigens, together with control antigens similarly prepared from uninoculated eggs, are used for the assay of antibody in acute and convalescent sera.) Sera for control of the CF test with RNP antigens are prepared by intranasal inoculation of guinea pigs or ferrets (8).

The HI test for serological diagnosis is performed in the same manner as described previously for virus identification, except that acute and convalescent sera are titrated simultaneously against known reference virus antigens.

EVALUATION, INTERPRETATION, AND REPORTING OF RESULTS

The laboratory diagnosis of influenza is based upon the isolation and identification of the virus and/or the demonstration of a fourfold or greater increase in antibody titer, usually by the CF or HI test (Fig. 1). The identity of the isolate should be reported only as to type, unless tests have been performed with hemagglutinin- or neuraminidase-specific antisera to characterize the antigens fully. If the virus was identified with influenza A hemagglutinin-specific antisera, then the H subtype of the virus may be included, for example A/Georgia/1/74(H3N-).

In the absence of virus isolation, caution should be exercised in the interpretation of serological results. A fourfold or greater increase in antibody titer measured in the CF test with RNP antigen is interpreted only to mean infection, or vaccination, with type A or type B influenza virus. Since the RNP antigen is identical for all viruses of a given type, this technique does not provide information identifying the subtype causing the disease.

Results of HI tests on patients' sera should be similarly interpreted. The specific antigen used for diagnostic serology does not necessarily identify the infecting virus. Anamnestic responses frequently occur, depending on the previous immunological experience of the patient. For example, an increase in antibody response to a current infection with a virus of subtype H3 might be measurable with subtype H2 antigens if the individual had been infected with these viruses earlier in life. For maximal diagnostic efficiency, antigens that closely resemble currently prevalent strains and antigens of recently prevalent strains may both be included in the HI test.

Two different subtypes of human influenza A viruses are not known to circulate within a population simultaneously. Once a virus has

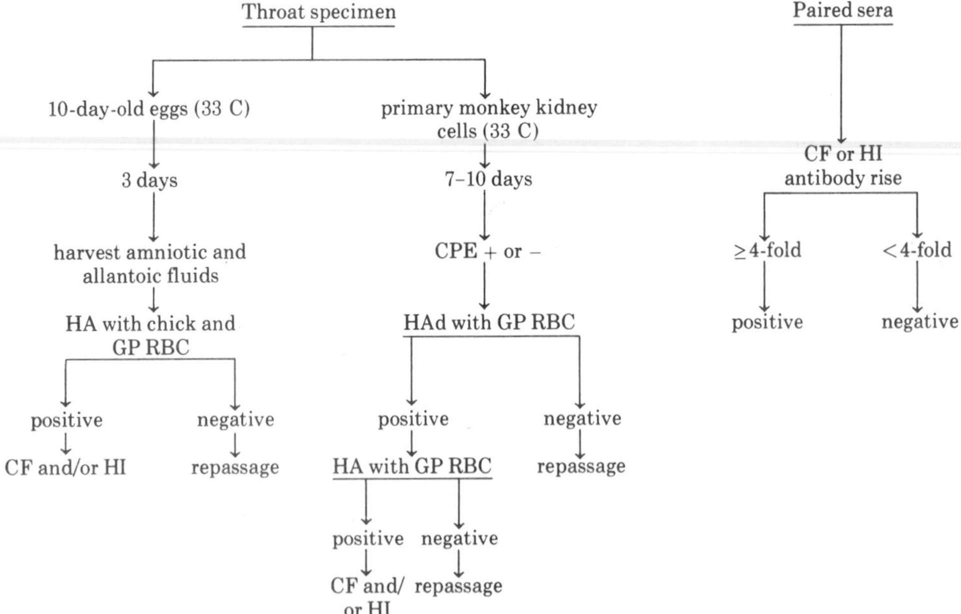

FIG. 1. *Flow chart for laboratory diagnosis of influenza. GP, guinea pig; HA, hemagglutination; HAd, hemadsorption.*

been isolated and identified during an epidemic, subsequent cases are presumed to be due to an antigenically similar virus and may be diagnosed by serological means.

In epidemic situations when influenza is suspected, a rapid presumptive diagnosis can often be made by examining single serum specimens from selected individuals. Sera are collected from 10 or more patients who are in the acute stage of the disease and from the same number of age-matched cohorts who experienced the same symptoms 10 or more days earlier. All sera are tested simultaneously for influenza A and B hemagglutinin or RNP antibody titers. If the epidemic was caused by influenza, the geometric mean antibody titer for type A or B should be significantly higher (by the *t* test) in the latter group than in the former (11). If the rise in antibody titer is fourfold or greater, the difference may be considered significant without resorting to statistical analysis. A diagnosis made on this basis should be confirmed subsequently by conventional methods of virus isolation and serological diagnosis with paired sera.

LITERATURE CITED

1. Aymard-Henry, M., M. T. Coleman, W. R. Dowdle, W. G. Laver, G. C. Schild, and R. G. Webster. 1973. Influenzavirus neuraminidase and neuraminidase-inhibition test procedures. Bull. W.H.O. **48:**199–202.
2. Burnet, F. M., and J. D. Stone. 1947. The receptor-destroying enzyme of *V(ibrio) cholerae*. Aust. J. Exp. Biol. Med. Sci. **25:**227–233.
3. Communicable Disease Center. 1958. Influenza surveillance report no. 38, March. Communicable Disease Center, Atlanta, Ga.
4. Dowdle, W. R., and R. Q. Robinson. 1966. Non-specific hemadsorption by rhesus monkey kidney cells. Proc. Soc. Exp. Biol. Med. **121:**193–198.
5. Dull, H. B., and W. R. Dowdle. 1973. Influenza. *In* P. E. Sartwell (ed.), Maxcy-Rosenau preventive medicine and public health, 10th ed. Appleton-Century-Crofts, New York.
6. Hammon, W. McD., and G. E. Sather. 1969. Arboviruses, p. 227–280. *In* E. H. Lennette and N. J. Schmidt (ed.), Diagnostic procedures for viral and rickettsial infections, 4th ed. American Public Health Association, Inc., New York.
7. Hierholzer, J. C., M. T. Suggs, and E. C. Hall. 1969. Standardized viral hemagglutination and hemagglutination-inhibition tests. II. Description and statistical evaluation. Appl. Microbiol. **18:**824–833.
8. Lief, F. S. 1963. Antigenic analysis of influenza viruses by complement fixation. VII. Further studies on production of pure anti-S serum and on specificity of type A S antigens. J. Immunol. **90:**172–177.
9. Lief, F. S., and W. Henle. 1959. Methods and procedures for use of complement-fixation technique in type- and strain-specific diagnosis of influenza. Bull. W.H.O. **20:**411–420.
10. Liu, C. 1956. Rapid diagnosis of human influenza infection from nasal smears by fluorescein-labeled antibody. Proc. Soc. Exp. Biol. Med. **92:**883–887.
11. National Communicable Disease Center. 1968. Rapid diagnosis of influenza epidemics, p. 23–25. *In* Influenza-respiratory disease surveillance report no. 84, September. National Communicable Disease Center, Atlanta, Ga.
12. Schild, G. C. 1972. Evidence for a new type-specific structural antigen of the influenzavirus particle. J. Gen. Virol. **15:**99–103.
13. Schild, G. C., M. Henry-Aymard, and H. G. Pereira. 1972. A quantitative single-radial-diffusion test for immunological studies with influenza virus. J. Gen. Virol. **16:**231–236.
14. Schild, G. C., and Pereira, H. G. 1969. Characterization of the ribonucleoprotein and neuraminidase of influenza A viruses by immunodiffusion. J. Gen. Virol. **4:**355–363.
15. Schulman, J. L., and E. D. Kilbourne. 1969. Independent variation in nature of influenza virus: distinctiveness of the hemagglutinin. Proc. Nat. Acad. Sci. U.S.A. **63:**326–333.
16. Tateno, I., O. Kitamoto, and A. Kawamura. 1966. Diverse immunocytologic findings of nasal smears in influenza. N. Engl. J. Med. **274:**237–242.
17. U.S. Public Health Service. 1965. Standardized diagnostic complement fixation method and adaptation to micro test. Pub. Health Monogr. No. 74, U.S. Pub. Health Serv. Publ. No. 1228.
18. Webster, R. G., and W. G. Laver. 1972. Studies on the origin of pandemic influenza. I. Antigenic analysis of A2 influenza virus isolated before and after the appearance of Hong Kong influenza using antisera to the isolated hemagglutinin subunits. Virology **48:**433–444.
19. World Health Organization Committee. 1971. A revised system of nomenclature for influenza viruses. Bull. W.H.O. **45:**119–124.

Chapter 73

Parainfluenza and Respiratory Syncytial Viruses

VINCENT A. FULGINITI AND MARLENE STAHL

CLINICAL BACKGROUND

The parainfluenza viruses (PIVs) and respiratory syncytial virus (RSV) constitute the most important viral pathogens for infants and children (4, 7, 8, 10). They are among the most common and the most virulent respiratory viruses that produce significant clinical disease in this age group.

The clinical syndromes produced by PIVs and RSV are similar, differing only in the relative etiological role played by the specific virus type. These viruses can affect the entire respiratory tract resulting in the following recognizable clinical syndromes: the common cold, pharyngitis, acute laryngotracheobronchitis (LBT or croup), bronchitis, pneumonia, broncho-pneumonia, and bronchiolitis (9, 10, 18, 19). Infections outside the respiratory tract are rare. A rash may be associated with RSV infection, and on occasion PIVs may be associated with infection or disease in other organs (liver, central nervous system, parotid glands; 9, 10, 22). For practical purposes, one need not consider diseases other than respiratory diseases when attempting to identify these agents.

The most susceptible individual is the very young infant. First-contact infection often results in severe disease, usually of the lower respiratory tract, which may be life-threatening (11). Transplacental antibody does not appear to afford protection against infection with RSV or PIV type 3. In fact, there is some suspicion that passive serum antibody in the absence of secretory antibody may predispose to severe lower tract disease (11). Exact mechanisms of immunity for both agents are not known with certainty. Secretory antibody (of the 11*S* immunoglobulin A [IgA] class) appears to be of major importance (29). Stimulated by natural infection or by live virus immunization by the respiratory route, the presence of this type of antibody is associated more closely with resistance to reexposure to the agent than is circulating 7*S* IgG antibody. Reinfection is common, but the disease produced is much milder than primary, first-contact infection, often amounting to little more than a common cold. The role of cell-mediated immunity (lymphocyte-associated) is largely unexplored and, therefore, unknown.

One aspect of the immune response is worthy of note here. Very young infants infected with RSV may produce no antibody detectable by the currently available complement-fixing (CF) or neutralizing antibody tests (18, 23). This leads to an underestimation of the contribution of RSV to clinical syndromes when serological techniques alone are employed.

RSV is the most frequent cause of bronchiolitis in young infants. It accounts for two-thirds to three-fourths of all such cases (18, 23). PIV type 3 can also produce this syndrome consisting of low-grade or no fever, marked respiratory distress associated with obstruction of the small airways manifested by wheezing, and variable upper respiratory tract symptoms (rhinorrhea, otitis media, etc.).

Both RSV and the PIVs can produce viral bronchopneumonia and together constitute the major cause of this syndrome in infants and young children (10, 18, 23).

The PIVs, particularly type 1, produce acute laryngotracheo-bronchitis (croup syndrome). Most all cases of croup, particularly in epidemics, are due to one of the PIVs (10, 19, 20).

RSV and the PIVs are seasonal in occurrence. The PIVs generally occur in fall and early winter and RSV occurs in late winter and early spring (10, 18, 23). Individual epidemics may show greater variability, and sporadic cases of infection can occur all year long.

DESCRIPTION OF THE AGENTS

Parainfluenza viruses

Discovered in 1953, the PIVs belong to the paramyxovirus group (7, 10). There are four known types, numbered 1 through 4. They are ribonucleic acid viruses with helical symmetry and are wrapped in a lipoprotein envelope through which project the hemagglutinin moieties. They are 150 to 250 nm in size. As paramyxoviruses, they are sensitive to ether and to temperatures greater than 37 C, resistant to freezing in the presence of protein, and acid-sensitive (pH 3.0).

The human PIVs are antigenically distinct from influenza but share common antigens among themselves and with other human myxoviruses (mumps, Newcastle disease virus). Antigenic relationships have also been observed with animal myxoviruses, principally with the simian group of agents (SV5, SV40), the murine agents (Sendai), and others like shipping fever virus (1, 6, 10).

Types 1, 2, and 3 are major pathogens for humans and are single serotypes (10). Clear distinction from one another is easily demonstrated despite shared antigens and cross-reactivity in serum containing antibody derived from a single type. Type 4 is a relatively minor human pathogen and consists of at least two subtypes, A and B (6).

All types contain a hemagglutinin for fowl and mammalian erythrocytes (10, 16). The hemagglutinin is a surface antigen composed of the hemagglutinating projection and fragments of lipoprotein membrane. Intimately bound is neuraminidase.

The PIVs are broadly infective for a variety of laboratory animals and tissue cultures (10, 12). Monkey kidney tissue culture and certain human diploid cell strains support the growth of PIVs as do some heteroploid human cell lines. Most investigators prefer primary monkey kidney tissue culture because of its greater sensitivity. The embryonated egg also supports PIV growth, usually in the amniotic cavity, although allantoic growth has been accomplished. However, embryonated eggs are not recommended for isolation from clinical materials.

Respiratory syncytial virus

RSV is most likely a paramyxovirus based upon its physical characteristics (13, 17). It is a ribonucleic acid virus and the ribonucleoprotein core has a helical configuration. The core is surrounded by an envelope with surface projections. However, particles observed by electron microscopy are pleomorphic, varying in both size and shape. Variations in size from 90 to 860 nm have been noted.

Either sensitivity is characteristic, implying lipid composition, at least in part; however, the exact chemical composition has not been determined. The virus is relatively stable at low temperatures (4 C), but infectivity is rapidly lost at both extremes (55 C and below freezing). Acid sensitivity, pH ≤ 3, is characteristic.

RSV appears to be an antigenically distinct group of agents, sharing antigens with no other known group (3, 7). Heterogeneity within RSV strains is evident by differential reactivity with animal sera prepared against specific strains, but human sera do not show these differences.

Despite its classification as a probable paramyxovirus, no hemagglutinating activity has been detected.

The animal host range is broad, with inapparent infection the rule except in the human. Virus growth in the embryonated egg has not been demonstrated. Continuous cell lines, such as HEp-2 and HeLa, human diploid cell strains, or rhesus monkey kidney cells, readily support RSV growth. The characteristic cytopathic effect (CPE), detailed below (3, 23), is best observed in continuous cell lines of human origin. Although the tissue culture systems indicated are generally sensitive to RSV, there is great variability and each system must be tested for its sensitivity.

COLLECTION AND STORAGE OF SPECIMENS

The most useful materials for isolation of PIVs and RSV are respiratory secretions (9, 10). These are best obtained by swabbing the mucosal surfaces available. In our experience, in young infants and children the yield in terms of isolation is improved by increasing the quantity of material collected and by utilizing both naspharyngeal and oropharyngeal swabbing. The most important steps in successful isolation of PIVs and RSV are the appropriate collection, transport, and handling of the specimens.

Swabs of the mucosa are obtained by adequate movement of a cotton or similar absorbent material over the affected area. Attempts should be made to include the watery or mucoid material in the respiratory tract. I prefer to twirl the swab in place in order to wrap such tenacious secretions around the swab. In older children and adults, throat washings or gargles with appropriate medium should be utilized whenever possible.

A balanced salt solution containing protein should always be used for optimal recovery rates. Such preparations as veal infusion broth or Hanks BSS with 0.5% gelatin or bovine serum albumin (BSA) added are preferred. Antibiotics are added to collection medium to achieve a final concentration of 250 units of penicillin, 250 mg of streptomycin, and 5 mg of amphotericin B per ml. We have chosen not to add antibiotics to medium used for gargling to minimize the risk of adverse reactions in sensitized persons. Swabs can be immersed in antibiotic-containing medium.

Transportation to the laboratory is a critical step. If possible, specimens should have brief transit time and immediate inoculation without intermediate freezing. In situations not permitting this optimal method, cool the specimens in ordinary ice chips *without* freezing the medium. RSV is very sensitive to freezing, and reduction in isolation rates is to be expected if the specimen is frozen (15). PIVs are less sensitive to freezing but, since both RSV and PIVs are usually sought from similar clinical syndromes, it is best not to freeze the specimens. If a long period of time is anticipated between collection and inoculation of the specimen, storage at 4 C for 4 to 5 h will best preserve the infectivity of both RSV and PIVs. If longer periods of storage are necessary, then rapid freezing and storage in sealed containers at −60 C is desirable. It should be recognized that freezing will reduce chances of recovery of RSV, and in some instances specimens initially containing RSV will be interpreted as negative.

DIRECT EXAMINATION

Two methods used for direct identification of PIVs and RSV in clinical specimens are electron microscopy and the fluorescent-antibody procedure. Both are of limited usefulness for the ordinary laboratory facility and therefore offer little of practical value (14, 21, 22).

Identification of PIV type 1 by electron microscopy has been described. In this technique, a small drop of suspect fluid is placed into a drop of water on a waxed surface. A copper grid coated with Formvarcarbon is touched to the drop and quickly removed, a drop of 2% potassium phosphatungstate at pH 7.0 is added, excess fluid is absorbed by a filter paper, and the drop-grid is air-dried. Direct examination will reveal characteristic myxovirus particles (14).

Fluorescent-antibody techniques have been employed for identification of both RSV and PIV in respiratory specimens (21, 22). High-titered specific antiserum is prepared in a suitable animal host, usually by repeated inoculation of large amounts of the inactivated virus. Neutralizing antibody activity of the sera approximates 1:640 or greater for the PIVs and 1:1,024 for RSV. The antisera are then conjugated with fluorescein isothiocyanate and purified by Sephadex and diethylaminoethyl cellulose column chromotography. Absorption by appropriate animal and human organ powders to remove nonspecific staining is carried out. The conjugate is best stored in small quantities at −70 C.

Nasopharyngeal secretions obtained early in the course of infection are smeared onto acetone-cleaned glass cover slips and are air-dried (21). The best fixation for RSV and PIV is at room temperature in acetone for 10 min. One drop of the appropriate conjugated-antibody is placed on the dried smear, incubated in a moist chamber at 37 C for 30 min, rinsed with phosphate-buffered saline, dried, mounted on a glass slide in 0.5 M carbonate-bicarbonate buffered glycerine (pH 9.0), and examined by fluorescence microscopy. A satisfactory optical system is a Zeiss microscope mounted with a HBO 200 W Osram mercury vapor lamp and a combination of UG5 (II) exciter filter and 65/47 barrier filter inserted into the optical path. An equally satisfactory filter system employs a BG-12 (III) exciter and a 50/44 barrier filter. Positive results consist of fluorescence observed in exfoliated cells from a patient suspected of having RSV or PIV infection. Control observations should always be performed on cells without the addition of fluorescent antibody and on cells from patients not infected with RSV or PIVs. Indirect fluorescent-antibody microscopy has also been described for PIVs (21). In both techniques, false-positive and false-negative results have been observed.

CULTIVATION OF AGENTS

Parainfluenzaviruses

Inoculation of specimens into rhesus monkey kidney (RMK) tissue culture monolayers, maintained with 1.5 to 2.0 ml of Eagle's minimal essential medium (MEM) and 2% fetal bovine serum (FBS) or a mixture of equal volumes of medium 199 and Eagle's MEM, with 2% FBS, is the best system for isolation of PIVs (8, 10). Contamination of RMK with simian parainfluenza virus (SV5) can be controlled by adding 0.2% hyperimmune rabbit serum. Others have used vervet monkey kidney or human embryonic kidney or lung cell cultures maintained with 1.5 to 2.0 ml of Eagle's MEM in Earle's salts and 1 to 2% FBS. Our practice is to employ two or three tubes containing cell monolayers and to inoculate 0.1 to 0.2 ml of the specimen per tube. The cell monolayers can be maintained at 33 to 36 C, preferably in a roller drum apparatus to increase the rate of PIV type 4 isolation. PIVs do not usually produce a CPE; however, type 2 or 3 will occasionally produce some degree of CPE on primary isolation. Detection of viral growth for each virus type is usually accomplished by hemadsorption with guinea pig red blood cells (RBC).

The cell cultures are examined for hemadsorption on approximately the 5th, 10th, and 14th days (8, 10) of incubation. If the cell cultures are in good condition, an additional examination can be made at 21 days. More frequently, a blind passage is performed in the second week and tests for hemadsorption are carried out again.

For use in the hemadsorption test, guinea pig RBC are prepared as a 10% suspension in Alsever's solution. These can be obtained commercially and can be stored in Alsever's solution for 7 to 10 days at 4 C. Just prior to testing, they are diluted in isotonic saline after three washing cycles and packing to a final concentration of 0.4%. To each culture tube containing 1.0 ml of medium is added 0.2 ml of the 0.4% suspension. The tubes are then held horizontally for 30 min at 4 C to permit RBC contact with the cells. (Type 4 virus requires 25 to 37 C for optimal hemadsorption.) The tubes are individually read at low magnification (10 × 6 or 10 × 10). Adsorption of the RBC to the cell monolayer is usually quite evident, but one can be certain by rotating the tube gently to dislodge RBC simply lying on the surface. Weak reactions may be difficult to interpret and may require subsequent tissue culture passage.

Some laboratories prefer to wash the monolayer *prior* to addition of the erythrocytes. After washing with Hanks BSS or maintenance medium, the RBC are added alone or into fresh medium. This step is preferred by some to prevent hemagglutination with free virus in the medium from interfering with detection of hemadsorption. An alert technician will examine the fluid for the presence of hemagglutination. If found, the cell monolayer must be washed and the hemadsorption test must be repeated. After each test for hemadsorption, the medium containing the RBC is removed and replaced with fresh maintenance medium to prevent nonspecific hemadsorption.

Respiratory syncytial virus

Isolation of RSV is fraught with difficulty. Attention must be paid to detail to insure that the system employed will isolate RSV if present in the specimen and to insure equal sensitivity of the system from time to time. Despite straightforward techniques and textbook assurances of the ease of growth of RSV, it is not unusual for a laboratory to encounter problems during its initial attempt to isolate RSV.

The best tissue culture systems for primary recovery are HEp-2 or WI-38 (human diploid) maintained with Eagle's MEM supplemented with 1 to 2% FBS. Cultures may be incubated at 33 to 35 C in a stationary rack (2, 3, 17). Various passages of the same cell strain may differ in sensitivity; therefore, it is good practice to inoculate known RSV into cell cultures along with the unknown specimens as a check on current sensitivity. Failure of the stock virus to produce CPE invalidates negative observations among the unknowns. With the HEp-2 system, it is best to inoculate the cell culture before a complete monolayer develops, so that overgrowth of cells which may interfere with RSV isolation is avoided. Monolayer cell cultures are prepared by seeding tubes with 50 to 60 thousand cells per ml and changing to maintenance medium after 2 days of incubation at 35 to 37 C.

Serum used in maintenance media may contain RSV neutralizing antibody (especially bovine and equine). Each batch should be tested for such activity before it is used in RSV isolation attempts.

Virus growth is detected by the characteristic syncytia formation in HEp-2 cells (3, 25). Adjacent cells become fused, forming an irregular large cell with multiple nuclei. These giant cells stand out from the surrounding cell sheet and are refractile. In the WI-38 cell system, one usually observes a destructive CPE rather than the syncytia formation which is characteristic in the HEp-2 cells.

IDENTIFICATION OF ISOLATES

Parainfluenzaviruses

Once hemadsorption is demonstrated in an infected cell monolayer, one can employ a variety of techniques for specific identification, ranging from fluorescent-antibody staining to hemagglutination-inhibition (9). The test most commonly employed in our laboratory is the hemadsorption-inhibition (HAdI) test (8).

Animal sera specific for PIV types 1 to 4 are used for typing by the HAdI technique. It is common to test simultaneously for other hemadsorbing agents such as mumps and influenza types A and B. Equal volumes of undiluted receptor-destroying enzyme (RDE) and undiluted type-specific sera are mixed and incubated overnight at 37 C. For satisfactory removal of inhibitors from serum, the RDE preparation should have a titer of 1:128 or greater when tested with parainfluenza type 3 (5). On the day of the test, the RDE-treated sera are inactivated for 30 min at 56 C in a water bath and further diluted 1:5 in isotonic saline or maintenance medium. The infected cell monolayers are washed three times with BSS and then 0.8 ml of the diluted RDE-treated serum is added. After 30 min of incubation at room temperature, 0.2 ml of 0.4% guinea pig RBC is added and the cultures are reincubated at 4 C for 30 min. Generally, an antiserum must have a hemagglutination-inhibition (HI) titer of 1:160 to 1:320 before it will effectively prevent hemadsorption when used at a dilution of 1:10. Positive identification consists of inhibition of hemadsorption by a specific antiserum when compared with controls.

One may also use an HI test in which type-specific sera and supernatant fluid from infected cultures are employed. Similarly, a CF test can be employed.

For those isolates exhibiting CPE, serum neutralization tests may be employed with the use of 100 $TCID_{50}$ of the virus (10).

Respiratory syncytial virus

The usual syncytial CPE in HEp-2 cells is sufficiently characteristic to permit presumptive identification of RSV (3, 17, 25). Many laboratories will end their identification attempts at this point. With the possible exception of PIV type 3, no other commonly encountered respiratory tract virus produces giant cell and syncytium formation in human heteroploid cells comparable to that produced by RSV. Specific identification is always advisable when possible.

Animal sera specific for RSV should be diluted in BSS so that, when mixed with an equal volume of supernatant fluid from infected HEp-2 cell cultures, the mixture contains between 10 and 20 antibody units (25). (One unit of antibody is usually considered to be equivalent to the highest dilution of serum which neutralizes 50% of the cell cultures infected with a standard dose of virus.) Some experience is necessary to determine the exact amount of virus-containing supernatant fluid to use; most laboratories use a 1:2 dilution if the cell sheet shows 3+ to 4+ CPE. The virus-serum mixture is incubated at room temperature for 1 h and then 0.1 to 0.2 ml is inoculated into each of three HEp-2 monolayer cell cultures. Examination of these cultures and simultaneous observation of infected control monolayers (equal volumes of virus and maintenance medium handled exactly as above) is continued for 1 week. Lack of CPE in cell cultures inoculated with the serum-virus mixture as opposed to those inoculated with the medium-virus mixtures indicates specific neutralization. With some isolates, one does not achieve complete neutralization with this technique. Some strains may be encountered which are not as readily neutralized by immune serum prepared to the prototype strain as they are by homotypic antiserum. In those cases, a significant delay in appearance of CPE can be cautiously interpreted as a positive result; alternatively one can titrate the virus and employ exactly 100 $TCID_{50}$ in an attempt to identify the isolate more definitively.

Alternative methods for identification include (i) utilizing infected cell culture fluids in the CF test against animal immune RSV serum or acute and convalescent human sera previously tested for RSV CF antibody content and (ii) the use of fluorescein-labeled animal antisera for identification of RSV antigens in infected cells (22, 26). Schieble and associates described a satisfactory technique for this purpose (26).

SEROLOGICAL METHODS

General

Both PIVs and RSV evoke serum antibody in infected individuals. Usually, a fourfold rise in antibody observed between sera taken early during clinical symptoms and in convalescence (2–3 weeks later) is diagnostic of specific infection. Several viral and epidemiological characteristics may influence interpretation of serological results.

As has been noted, PIVs share antigens among themselves and with certain other myxoviruses (8, 10). Thus, low levels of HI antibody to a given type may be present in acute sera and thus represent cross-reacting antibody. Since infection with PIV usually results in a $\geq 4\times$ rise in HI antibody to the infecting virus type, the low-level cross-reacting HI antibody does' not pose a serious problem. However, heterologous increases in titer are occasionally observed, and one must always perform simultaneous titrations against the four types of PIV, mumps, and influenza viruses to be reasonably certain of specificity. The virus to which the titer rise is greatest is assumed to be the primary infecting agent. This task is made simpler if a specific agent has been identified in the patient or if neutralization tests are employed.

Low levels of RSV antibody are frequently encountered and most often represent prior infection (4, 25). One must remember that reinfection is a common characteristic of RSV disease. Significant increase in antibody titer ($\geq$4 times rise) indicates current infection.

Frequently the timing of serum collection cannot be attuned to the clinical process. As a result, paired sera are collected late in the illness. One then may observe a *decline* in titer of 4 times. We have interpreted this to mean acute infection, but I am unaware of solid data to support this conclusion. Of course, if one identifies a virus from the patient and follows serum titers serially, one can observe a rise and decline of the proportions utilized diagnostically.

Single serum titers are almost impossible to interpret with certainty as to their significance in relation to specificity of infection. For the most part, we refuse to test single sera for this reason.

Once again, the reader is reminded that young infants may not demonstrate an increase in antibody titer despite recovery of the virus during an acute illness (18, 23). Thus, lack of serological evidence for infection in this age group does not rule out RSV as a cause for the illness.

Parainfluenza viruses

Three antibody tests are available: the HI antibody test, the neutralizing antibody test, and the CF antibody test. Our laboratory employs the HI antibody procedure for all sera and only occasionally will resort to neutralizing antibody for diagnostic purposes. We never use the CF test in routine diagnostic work.

Antigens for PIV types 1, 2, and 3 can be prepared by harvesting monkey kidney tissue culture at the point of near-maximal hemadsorption. Pools of supernatant fluids are treated in our laboratory by the Tween-80 and ether method of viral disruption to increase the hemagglutinin titer (16). The procedure is to dissolve 0.125 ml of Tween-80 in 2 ml of maintenance medium. Add the dissolved Tween-80 to the virus suspension in a volume of 0.1 ml for each 5 ml of virus. Mix by shaking at room temperature for 5 min. Ether is then added to a final concentration of 33.3%. Mix well by shaking at 4 C for 15 min. This mixture is centrifuged at 2,000 rpm for 30 min, and the aqueous phase is removed and placed into an open container to allow the ether to evaporate. Treated antigen can be stored at 4 C. Untreated antigens are stored in sealed ampoules in small quantities at −70 C.

Serum is treated prior to testing to remove nonspecific inhibitors. Equal volumes of undiluted RDE (0.1 ml) and serum are incubated at 37 C overnight. Eight volumes of 0.01 M PBS at pH 7.2 are added to give a 1:10 dilution. Inactivation of serum is done just prior to testing by incubation at 56 C for 30 min. Some sera contain agglutinins for guinea pig RBC; these agglutinins may be removed by prior absorption for 1 h at 4 C with such cells at a final concentration of 5%.

One can use a microtechnique in Microtiter plates or a macrotechnique in Kahn tubes (27, 28). The principles are identical; we will describe the microtechnique, which is most widely employed.

Serial twofold dilutions of the virus in 0.05-ml amounts are prepared in a Microtiter plate to which are added equal volumes of 0.4% guinea pig or human erythrocytes to determine the hemagglutinin titer. The end point is the highest dilution of antigen which produces partial agglutination of the erythrocytes. Partial agglutination is a small button of unagglutinated cells surrounded by agglutinated cells. The amount of virus needed to provide 4 units of hemagglutinin in 0.025 ml, for use in the HI test, is determined by dividing the titer obtained in this titration by 8.

The actual performance of the HI microtiter technique is as follows:

1. The antigen control is performed in triplicate by adding 0.05 ml of PBS to three rows of five wells and to three RBC control wells. The Microtiter "V" plates are used. Add 0.05 ml of the test antigen diluted to contain 8 hemagglutinating units per 0.05 ml to the first well in each row of five wells. Make serial dilutions using 0.05-ml microdiluters. The five wells then contain 4, 2, 1, 0.5, and 0.25 units of antigen. Add 0.05 ml of 0.4% erythrocyte suspension to the wells containing diluted antigen and the RBC control wells. The 4- and 2-unit wells should show complete agglutination; the 1-unit, partial agglutination; and the 0.5- and 0.25-unit, no agglutination.

2. A standard reference serum of known titer is incorporated into each test to verify specificity and sensitivity of the test.

3. An RBC control, consisting of 0.05 ml volumes of PBS and 0.4% erythrocytes, is included in each test.

4. A serum control is included for each serum tested; the 1:10 dilution of RDE-treated serum is added to an equal volume of PBS (0.025 ml of each).

5. Human sera may contain agglutinins for guinea pig erythrocytes. These agglutinins should be removed by prior adsorption for 1 h at 4 C with a 5% suspension of guinea pig erythrocytes. The dilutions of the absorbed and RDE-treated sera are made by adding 0.025 ml of PBS to all dilution wells except those for the initial (1:10) serum dilution. Add 0.05 ml of the 1:10 dilution of treated serum to the first well and then make serial twofold dilutions using 0.025-ml microdiluters. The antigen, diluted to contain 4 hemagglutinating units, is added to the serum dilutions in 0.025-ml amounts and mixed. The virus-serum mixtures are incubated at room temperature for 1 h. Guinea pig RBC (0.4%) are added to each well with an 0.05-ml

dropper or by pipette in 0.05-ml amounts. The resultant mixture is shaken and incubated at 37 C (some prefer room temperature; both should be tried initially and the temperature which gives the clearest end point should be selected). We use the serum controls and RBC control cups to determine the appropriate time to read the test—usually 60 min is required but occasionally a longer interval is necessary. Titers are read as the highest dilution of serum which completely inhibits hemagglutination (button of unagglutinated RBC in bottom of cup).

Respiratory syncytial virus

Many techniques for determination of RSV neutralizing antibody have been explored. It appears that the technique used is highly individualized to the particular laboratory and requires some experience to obtain consistent and reliable results. We currently employ a microtiter neutralizing antibody test as the procedure of choice (27, 28). In principle, the neutralizing antibody test is designed to determine the lowest concentration of serum (highest dilution) that is required to neutralize a standard dose of virus, usually 100 tissue culture infectious doses ($TCID_{50}$). One $TCID_{50}$ is defined as the lowest concentration of virus (highest dilution) that is required to infect 50% of the inoculated cell cultures. To estimate the dilution of virus equivalent to 100 $TCID_{50}$ for use in the neutralization test, a virus titration must be performed.

Virus titration

1. Make 10-fold dilutions of virus in 2-ml volumes using Eagle's MEM as diluent.
2. Add 0.025 ml of each virus dilution from the tubes to three or four wells in a flat-bottom Microtiter tissue culture plate.
3. Add 0.025 ml of HEp-2 cells at a concentration of 150,000 cells/ml to the wells containing diluted virus and also to three or four wells containing 0.025 ml of diluent. The latter wells are reserved as cell controls to establish the viability of the cells.
4. Add 0.05 ml of MEM containing 5% FBS to the virus titration wells and cell control wells.
5. Place loose lids over the plates and incubate in a 5% carbon dioxide atmosphere at 35 C.
6. After approximately 3 days, the Microtiter plates are examined with the aid of an inverted microscope for the characteristic CPE of RSV.
7. The virus titer is determined by the method of Reed and Muench (24). The virus titer is then used to estimate the virus dilution containing 100 $TCID_{50}$.

Neutralization test

1. Make a 1:10 dilution of each serum to be tested in Eagle's MEM and inactivate at 56 C for 30 min.
2. Make serial twofold dilutions in 0.025-ml amounts with microdiluters. Test each serum in triplicate. To determine the effect of the test sera on cell growth, serum controls are required and are prepared by adding 0.025 ml of the 1:10 dilution of each test serum to three wells containing 0.025 ml of diluent.
3. Add 0.025 ml of the virus dilution containing 100 $TCID_{50}$ to all serum dilution wells *except* the serum control wells.
4. Add 0.025 ml of Eagle's MEM containing 5% FBS to all wells.
5. Incubate at room temperature for 1 h.
6. Add 0.025 ml of the 150,000 HEp-2 cells/ml.
7. A virus control titration (as described above) must accompany the neutralization test and is used to determine the exact virus concentration ($TCID_{50}$) used in the neutralization test.
8. Cover each Microtiter plate and place in a CO_2 incubator at 35 C.
9. The accompanying virus titration is periodically examined with an inverted microscope for typical CPE of RSV. When the virus titration indicates that approximately 100 $TCID_{50}$ are present in the test virus dose (usually 3 days), the neutralization test is read. The serum titer may be expressed as the highest dilution of serum which completely inhibits the CPE of the test virus dose.

EVALUATION AND REPORTING

The objective of the virus laboratory is to assist the clinician in identifying the etiology of the patient's infection. Ideally, the report should include the results of attempts at isolation of the agent and serological testing. In addition, an interpretation of the results based upon the theoretical nature of the laboratory tests frequently proves most helpful. The goals are to indicate to the clinician (i) the results of the test and (ii) whether this means etiological identification is established, suspected, uncertain, or unknown.

Isolation of the specific agent is the best evidence of infection. Since PIVs or RSV are seldom, if ever, found in a healthy carrier, isolation is presumptive evidence of etiological association with disease. Additionally, these agents have a brief residence in the respiratory tract and one does not see a long "carrier state" after an acute illness. However, the difficulties in insuring adequate collection, transport, and storage of specimens frequently results in failure to isolate a virus. Often the laboratory has no way of knowing the reliability of collection, storage, and transport. Thus, the negative result of attempts at isolation is often mistakenly equated by the physician with absence of the agent. It is our practice to indicate that specimens for isolation should be supplemented by appropriate blood specimens to increase the possibility of specific etiological identification. We request an acute-ph•se (as early in the course of illness as possible) and a convalescent-phase blood specimen (at least 2 to 3 weeks after the first specimen).

Diagnosis of PIV infection is made more difficult by heterologous antibody increases, especially in HI antibody titers. The laboratory must perform the battery of HI antibody testing indicated in the text in order to differentiate homologous from heterologous antibody titer increases.

Most laboratories utilize the HI antibody test for serological diagnosis of PIV infection. If the laboratory is equipped for and experienced in neutralizing techniques (HAdI) and performs these in quantity and routinely, it may prefer to handle all serum specimens in this way. However, for most laboratories this undertaking is needlessly complex and expensive when contrasted to HIA testing. Since both HIA and neutralizing antibody develop in parallel during the acute illness, we prefer the simpler and less expensive HIA.

Isolation of RSV remains the best single test for identifying the etiology of such infections, especially in young infants.

Serological diagnosis of RSV infection presents several problems. First, young infants may appear to have no response regardless of the isolation of RSV during an infection (18, 23). The exact reason for this phenomenon is unknown, but it may be related to the relative insensitivity of our present serological techniques.

Another problem is the disparity between CF and neutralizing antibody titers. In our laboratory, we have noted that only 50% of sera in which CF antibody is detected contain neutralizing antibody. Kim and co-workers also observed this phenomenon (18). They reported that 91% of infants receiving RSV vaccine had $\geq 4\times$ rises in CF antibody but the same sera only demonstrated a 43% incidence of $\geq 4\times$ rises in neutralizing antibody. A similar but smaller disparity was noted for natural infection (94% CF to 75% neutralizing antibody). Thus, if one performed CF tests during an infection, a titer rise might be detected, whereas neutralizing antibody would not increase. At this point, it is unclear whether this is simply related to insensitivity of the neutralizing antibody technique or oversensitivity of the CF technique.

A final serological problem is related to reinfection in the presence of serum antibody. The laboratory will encounter individuals in whom the acute serum contains antibody and in whom a rise is detected. Thus, it is important to measure paired sera in evaluation of illness.

LITERATURE CITED

1. Abinati, F. R., R. M. Chanock, M. K. Cook, D. Wong, and M. Warfield. 1961. Relationship of human and bovine strains of myxovirus para-influenza 3. Proc. Soc. Exp. Biol. Med. **106**:466–469.
2. Anderson, J. M., and M. O. Beem. 1966. Use of human diploid cell cultures for primary isolation of respiratory syncytial virus. Proc. Soc. Exp. Biol. Med. **121**:205–209.
3. Armstrong, J. A., H. G. Pereira, and R. C. Valentine. 1962. Morphology and development of respiratory syncytial virus in cell cultures. Nature (London) **196**:1179–1181.
4. Beem, M. 1967. Repeated infections with respiratory syncytial virus. J. Immunol. **98**:1115–1122.
5. Burnet, F. M., and J. D. Stone. 1947. Receptor destroying enzyme of V. *cholera*. Aust. J. Exp. Biol. Med. Sci. **25**:227–233.
6. Canchola, J., A. J. Vargosko, H. W. Kim, R. H. Parrott, E. Christmas, B. Jeffries, and R. M. Chanock. 1964. Antigenic variation among newly isolated strains of parainfluenza type 4 virus. Amer. J. Hyg. **79**:357–364.
7. Chanock, R. M., and L. Finberg. 1957. Recovery from infants with respiratory illness of a virus related to chimpanzee coryza agent (CCA). II. Epidemiologic aspects of infection in infants and young children. Amer. J. Hyg. **66**:291–300.
8. Chanock, R. M., K. M. Johnson, M. Cook, D. C. Wong, and A. Vargosko. 1961. The hemadsorption technique, with special reference to the problem of naturally occurring simian parainfluenza virus. Amer. Rev. Resp. Dis. **83**:125–129.
9. Chanock, R. M., H. W. Kim, A. J. Vargosko, et al. 1961. Respiratory syncytial virus. I. Virus recovery and other observations during 1960 outbreak of bronchiolitis, pneumonia, and minor respiratory diseases in children. J. Amer. Med. Ass. **176**:647–653.
10. Chanock, R. M., R. H. Parrott, K. M. Johnson, A. Z. Kapikian, and J. A. Bell. 1963. Myxoviruses: parainfluenza. Amer. Rev. Resp. Dis. **88**:152–166.
11. Chanock, R. M., R. H. Parrott, A. Z. Kapikian, H. W. Kim, and C. D. Brandt. 1968. Possible role of immunologic factors in pathogenesis of RS virus lower respiratory tract disease. Perspect. Virol. **6**:125–139.
12. Chanock, R. M., D. Wong, R. J. Huebner, and J. A. Bell. 1960. Serologic response of individuals infected with parainfluenza viruses. Amer. J. Pub. Health Nat. Health **50**:1858–1865.
13. Coates, H. V., D. W. Ailling, and R. M. Chanock. 1966. An antigenic analysis of respiratory syncytial virus isolates by a plaque reduction neutralization test. Amer. J. Epidemiol. **83**:299–313.
14. Doane, F. W., N. Anderson, K. Chatiyanonda, R. M. Bannatyne, D. M. McLean, and A. J. Rhodes. 1967. Rapid laboratory diagnosis of paramyxovirus infections by electron microscopy. Lancet **2**:751–753.

15. Hambling, M. H. 1964. Survival of the respiratory syncytial virus during storage under various conditions. Brit. J. Exp. Pathol. **45:**647–655.
16. John, T. J., and V. A. Fulginiti. 1966. Parainfluenza 2 virus: increase in hemagglutinin titer on treatment with tween-70 and ether. Proc. Soc. Exp. Biol. Med. **121:** 109–111.
17. Jordan, W. S., Jr. 1962. Growth characteristics of respiratory syncytial virus. J. Immunol. **88:**581–590.
18. Kim, H. W., J. O. Arrobio, C. D. Brandt, B. C. Jeffries, G. Pyles, J. L. Reid, R. M. Chanock, and R. H. Parrott. 1973. Epidemiology of respiratory syncytial virus infection in Washington, D.C. Amer. J. Epidemiol. **98:** 216–225.
19. Lewis, F. A., N. I. Lehmann, and A. A. Ferris. 1961. The hemadsorption viruses in laryngo-tracheobronchitis. Med. J. Aust. **48:**929–932.
20. McLean, D. M., R. D. Bach, R. P. B. Larke, and G. A. McNaughton. 1963. Myxoviruses associated with acute laryngotracheobronchitis in Toronto 1962–63. Can. Med. Ass. J. **89:** 1257–1259.
21. Marks, M. I., H. Nagahama, and J. J. Eller. 1971. Parainfluenza virus immunofluorescence. Pediatrics **48:** 73–78.
22. Nagahama, H., J. J. Eller, V. A. Fulginiti, and M. Marks. 1970. Direct immunofluorescent studies of infection with respiratory syncytial virus. J. Infect. Dis. **122:**260–271.
23. Parrott, R. H., A. J. Vargosko, H. W. Kim, C. Cumming, H. Turner, R. J. Huebner, and R. M. Chanock. 1961. Respiratory syncytial virus. II. Serologic studies over a 34-month period of children with bronchiolitis, pneumonia, and minor respiratory diseases. J. Amer. Med. Ass. **176:**653–657.
24. Reed, L. J., and J. Muench. 1938. A simple method for estimating fifty percent end-points. Amer. J. Hyg. **27:**493–497.
25. Ross, C. A. C., E. J. Stott, S. McMichael, and I. A. Crowther. 1964. Problems of laboratory diagnosis of respiratory syncytial virus infection in childhood. Arch. Gesamte Virusforsch. **14:**553–562.
26. Schieble, J. H., E. H. Lennette, and A. Kase. 1965. An immunofluorescent staining method for rapid identification of respiratory syncytial virus. Proc. Soc. Exp. Biol. Med. **120:**203–208.
27. Schmidt, N. J., E. H. Lennette, and M. F. Hanahoe. 1966. A micro-method for performing parainfluenza virus neutralization tests. Proc. Soc. Exp. Biol. Med. **122:**1062–1067.
28. Sever, J. L. 1962. Application of a microtechnique to viral serological investigations. J. Immunol. **88:**320–329.
29. Smith, C. B., R. H. Purcell, J. A. Bellanti, and R. M. Chanock. 1966. Protective effect of antibody to parainfluenza type I virus. N. Engl. J. Med. **275:**1145–1152.

Chapter 74
Adenoviruses

BERNARD PORTNOY AND MARGARET A. SALVATORE

CLINICAL BACKGROUND

The clinical expressions of adenovirus infections vary from pharyngitis clinically indistinguishable from that caused by the group A, beta-hemolytic streptococci (7) to pneumonia (16), conjunctivitis, and keratoconjunctivitis (8). Additional clinical syndromes include undifferentiated upper respiratory infections (7), "influenza-like" illnesses, and, especially in infants and children, laryngotracheobronchitis (croup), bronchiolitis, and pneumonia (33). Adenovirus types 3, 4, and 7 are most frequently responsible for epidemics of acute respiratory disease in military recruits, and types 1, 2, 3, and 5 are most often encountered in pediatric patients (34). Acute follicular conjunctivitis, seen mainly in adults, is most commonly caused by type 3 or 7 (1, 3, 20, 21, 47). The major cause of epidemic keratoconjunctivitis in the United States is type 8 (23).

The adenoviruses represent the first group of agents of human origin which have been shown to be oncogenic (12). This property, however, has only been demonstrated in laboratory rodents. Although there has been a report of the isolation of the human adenovirus from a neoplasm in a child (28), there is no conclusive evidence that these viruses are oncogenic for man. Nevertheless, this oncogenic characteristic has led to a further grouping of these agents as highly oncogenic, moderately oncogenic, and non-oncogenic. The serotypes most commonly implicated in the causation of human disease (types 1, 2, 4, 5, and 6) fall into the non-oncogenic category.

DESCRIPTION OF AGENT

The first member of the adenovirus group was isolated (1953) from human adenoid tissue removed at adenoidectomy (41), and independently from the throat washing of an army recruit with primary atypical pneumonia (17). First designated APC (2, 22, 42), ARD (9, 13), or RI (17) viruses, the adenoviruses of human origin include 31 serotypes that are related by a major cross-reactive complement-fixing (CF) antigen (14). Although type-specific CF antigens can be demonstrated (14), serotyping is usually accomplished by neutralization and/or hemagglutination-inhibition (HI) tests (35, 44). Their major physiochemical properties include ether and chloroform resistance (42), relatively high pH stability (11, 42), a deoxyribonucleic acid core, icosahedral symmetry, and the ability to replicate in various tissue cultures of human and simian origin (42). They are approximately 65 to 80 nm in diameter.

COLLECTION AND STORAGE OF SPECIMENS

Adenoviruses can be isolated from pharyngeal secretions, eye exudates, stool, body fluids, including blood, and tissues obtained at biopsy or autopsy. The type of isolation specimen chosen would, in general, depend upon the clinical syndrome for which a viral etiology is being sought.

Types of isolation specimens and their collection

The techniques for the collection, shipment and storage of pharyngeal secretions, blood, body fluids, stool, and tissues described in Chapter 71 are generally applicable to the adenoviruses. However, several procedures and techniques are worthy of special note. Specifically, isolation rates of adenoviruses from throat washings or throat swabs have been shown to be comparable in adult patients (39).

Eye exudates can be obtained in the following manner. The palpebral conjunctiva is firmly rubbed with a sterile swab moistened with a suitable diluent. When possible, the exudate itself (pus) should be carried on the swab. The swab is rinsed and then is extracted in a tube containing 2 to 3 ml of medium and handled in the same manner as a throat or rectal swab. Scrapings obtained from the conjunctivae or cornea should be obtained only by an ophthalmologist or an adequately trained physician and should be placed into a smaller volume of medium.

DIRECT EXAMINATION

Although examination of adenovirus-infected tissues (e.g., lung or tissue cultures) is useful, one cannot make a definitive etiological diagnosis in this manner. The results obtained by light microscopy are usually used as confirmatory evidence of adenovirus infection after virus isolation and specific serotyping.

Light microscopy

The cytopathic effect (CPE) in tissue cultures characteristic of an adenovirus can be seen with a scanning lens (approximately 50× to 100×) and consists of marked rounding and the aggregation of affected cells into "grapelike clusters" (22). However, the clumping of affected cells is not a constant feature. Some cytoplasmic stranding or "bridging" may occur, giving a weblike appearance to the tissue culture monolayer. The characteristic cytopathology is most evident when the agents are propagated in continuous cell lines of human origin, e.g., HEp-2, HeLa, and KB. Primary tissue cultures such as monkey kidney and human amnion produce characteristic changes similar to the continuous lines but at a much slower rate. Highly concentrated adenovirus inocula may produce a gross CPE in a few hours. This change is not due to viral replication but to "the cell detaching" or penton antigen (29, 40).

Adenoviruses in continuous cell lines also initiate an unusual production of acid resulting from increased glycolysis and the accumulation of organic acids (10, 22). The change in color of the pH indicator (red-purple to yellow) *early* in tissue culture infection is characteristic of this group and may be helpful in differentiating it from other viruses. Ultimately, virus replication will destroy the cells and the pH will rise.

Fluorescent-antibody staining

The fluorescent-antibody technique is useful for the detection of adenoviral antigens in infected cells (32). Its primary purpose is to localize antigenic material at specific sites. Fluorescein-labeled antibody molecules are placed in contact with homologous antigens in tissue cells, depositing the labeled antibody onto antigenic sites. When these treated cells or smears are viewed under a fluorescence microscope, the labeled antibody appears yellow-green at locations where the antigen is present. This technique is successful only when high-titered antisera and active antigens are employed. The limited number of studies to date have not assessed its real value relative to the diagnosis of adenovirus infections.

Electron microscopy

The intranuclear inclusion bodies associated with adenovirus infection appear as symmetrical arrays of viral particles when observed by electron microscopy (46). Adenovirus particles measure approximately 65 to 80 nm in diameter. The outer coat has icosahedral symmetry (a surface formed by 20 equilateral triangles) with the outer capsid containing 252 capsomers, each with a diameter of 5 to 7 nm.

Certain antigenic properties of adenoviruses have been associated with their morphological subunits (31). The major subunits of the capsid, the 240 nonvertex capsomers, are identical with the cross-reactive CF antigen (also called the hexon antigen). The 12 vertex capsomers represent the "cell detaching" or penton antigen. The fibers emanating from the vertex capsomers represent the type-specific CF antigen. The hemagglutinin of the adenoviruses is also represented by the penton fiber complex.

Hemotoxylin and eosin stains

When infected cell cultures are stained with hemotoxylin and eosin, they reveal characteristic eosinophilic and basophilic intranuclear inclusions (5). The nuclei are typically enlarged, but the patterns of the inclusions may vary. For example, types 3, 4, and 7 produce sharp-edged crystal-like masses which are not associated with types 1, 2, 5, and 6 (4).

CULTIVATION (ISOLATION) OF AGENT

Host systems

Tissue cultures constitute the only practical system for the cultivation and/or isolation of adenoviruses. Indeed, the lack of pathogenicity for laboratory animals, with the exception of type 5 for baby hamsters (30), is generally accepted as an identifying criterion for this virus group. Although the adenoviruses can replicate in a wide variety of tissue cultures of simian and human origin, the most sensitive tissue cultures employed are those derived from primary or diploid cultures of human embryonic cells, e.g., human embryonic kidney (HEK) cells, or continuous cultures of human neoplastic tissues, such as HeLa, HEp-2, and KB. Different lots of these tissue cultures vary in their ability to support the replication of the adenoviruses, and the choice of any particular lot or type can only be determined by individual trial and error.

Cultures and media of choice

The tissue culture of choice for the isolation of adenovirus from clinical specimens is generally accepted to be primary or diploid cultures of HEK cells. The basis for this consensus lies in its relative ease of maintenance, its reduced variability in lot sensitivity, and its capability to allow replication of all antigenic types rapidly with the production of typical cytopathological changes.

For ease of maintenance and the reduction or elimination of refeeding cultures, Leibovitz Medium No. 15 is recommended. Eagle's minimal essential medium with 2% bovine serum can also be used, but maintenance of HEK on this medium requires refeeding every 4 to 5 days. Regardless of the choice, antibiotics must be added to preclude the growth of bacterial or fungal contaminants. The combination most commonly used is penicillin (250 units/ml), streptomycin (250 μg/ml), and amphotericin B (30 μg/ml).

If HeLa, KB, or HEp-2 is selected for use, it is important to pretest each lot for sensitivity to adenovirus isolation. The cultures should be maintained on medium 199 (in Earle's balanced salt solution) with 5% chicken or fetal bovine serum (inactivated at 56 C for 30 min). Leibovitz Medium No. 15 with 5% fetal bovine serum (inactivated at 56 C) can also be used.

These tissue culture lines and media are available, ready for use, from several commercial sources.

Procedure of choice

The inoculation of tissue culture with clinical specimens for adenovirus isolation does not differ from techniques used for other virus types. However, if HEK cells on Leibovitz medium are to be used, the cultures should be placed on maintenance medium 48 h prior to use. This procedure allows the cells to acclimate to the change in carbohydrate metabolism and precludes the use of those cultures which do not maintain a healthy appearance.

Clinical specimens can be inoculated directly into duplicate or triplicate tissue culture tubes in 0.2-ml portions. Uninoculated controls must always be available. Throat and rectal swabs can also be placed into 4 ml of maintenance medium, thoroughly washed, and pressed against the glass. The swab is then discarded and 1.0 ml of the inoculum is placed into each of duplicate tissue culture tubes previously drained of media. The excess inoculum can then be quick-frozen and stored.

After inoculation, the tissue culture tubes are incubated in stationary racks at 37 C and observed daily for development of CPE. If heteroploid continuous cell lines such as HeLa are used, pathological changes may not be observable for 96 h. HEK cells frequently demonstrate CPE within 48 h. As a rule of thumb, the lower numbered adenovirus serotypes (1 to 7), with the exception of type 4, replicate more quickly than the higher numbered counterparts. If spontaneous degeneration of monolayers occurs before the development of definitive CPE, a blind passage may be necessary. The inoculum for this second passage is prepared by freezing and thawing the tissue culture tubes to release the cells into the supernatant fluid or by scraping the walls to achieve the same result. If no CPE develops during this passage, the specimen should be considered negative.

IDENTIFICATION OF ADENOVIRUSES

The criteria necessary for an agent to be classified as an adenovirus are as follows: (i) group-specific antigenicity, (ii) production of characteristic CPE in tissue culture, (iii) exclusive development in the nucleus, and (iv) the retention of infectivity after exposure to ether or chloroform. In practice, all of these criteria need not be met. The common identification methods are described below.

Methods of choice

Type-specific identification may be accomplished by a number of methods. The first 28 numbered adenoviruses, with the possible exception of type 18, agglutinate the erythrocytes of certain mammalian species and can therefore not only be typed by the HI test but can also be grouped by their reactions to specific red cells (25, 35, 36). Adenovirus types 29, 30, and 31 have not as yet been classified in specific hemagglutination groups. The most commonly used technique remains the tissue culture neutralization test, which employs pools or specific types of adenovirus antisera (usually prepared in rabbits) to block completely or significantly diminish the cytopathogenic effect of 100 $TCID_{50}$ of virus. When multiple adenovirus serotypes are prevalent in a community, this is the test of choice because of its relative simplicity. The neutralization test may also be adapted to a colorimetric technique based upon the ability of the adenovirus to initiate increased glycolysis and the production of unusual amounts of acid (27). The incorporation of a pH indicator, phenol red, into the medium allows an indirect measurement of the degree of acid production by a simple color change from red-purple to yellow. This procedure is most useful when large numbers of isolates are to be typed, as it eliminates the more tedious microscopic examination for CPE.

If tissue culture tests are not feasible, the CF test with the use of group-specific antisera may be a useful tool to classify the isolate as belonging to the adenovirus group. Specific serotyping would require either the HI or neutralization test.

Hemagglutination-inhibition test

For typing purposes, adenoviruses can be divided into four groups on the basis of their reactions with two types of erythrocytes: those from rhesus monkeys and those from the laboratory rat, *Rattus norvegicus* (25, 35, 36). Viruses in group I include types 3, 7, 11, 14, 16, 20, 21, 25, and 28. These viruses agglutinate only rhesus or grivet monkey erythrocytes. Members of group II (types 8, 9, 10, 13, 15, 17, 19, 22, 23, 24, 26, and 27) agglutinate rat erythrocytes. Some of these types will also agglutinate monkey erythrocytes but at a lower titer. The adenoviruses classified in group III (types 1, 2, 4, 5, and 6) partially agglutinate rat cells, but in this case agglutination patterns are complete or almost complete in the presence of heterotypic immune serum. Adenovirus types 12 and 18 were originally classified in group IV on the basis of the fact that hemagglutinins had not been demonstrated for these two serotypes. Schmidt et al. (43) have observed that type 12 adenovirus may agglutinate rat erythrocytes. As noted earlier, adenovirus types 29, 30, and 31 have as yet not been classified, although type 31 will probably be grouped with types 12 and 18 based on its oncogenic potential (19).

Individual rhesus monkeys and rats vary in the ability of their erythrocytes to be agglutinated by certain adenovirus serotypes. Screening of erythrocytes from these animals is therefore necessary so that animals whose cells give satisfactory reactions will be selected. It may also be necessary to screen rats for the ability of their red cells to form suitable sedimentation patterns. Further, it should be emphasized that some rat erythrocytes tend to agglutinate spontaneously, and this should be noted prior to the choice of an animal donor.

Preparation of reagents. Antigens can either be prepared in the laboratory or obtained commercially. Antigens can be grown in KB, HEp-2, or HeLa cells. It has been recommended by Rosen (36) that cultures be inoculated with a dilution of seed virus that will not destroy the monolayer in less than 72 h of incubation. After this time, fluid from infected cultures can be used as the antigen either before or after freezing and without further treatment. Monkeys are bled from the femoral vein; anesthetized rats, from the heart. A syringe containing a small amount of Alsever's solution as an anticoagulant is suggested (36). The blood obtained in this manner is stored in Alsever's solution in a ratio of approximately 10 ml of blood to 50 ml of Alsever's solution. Before the red cells are used, they are washed three times in a dextrose-gelatin-Veronal (DGV) solution (36) and can be kept as a 10% suspension in DGV for at least 1 week. A 0.75% suspension is used in the test. If spontaneous agglutination occurs, the addition of normal rabbit serum to the cells should eliminate the problem. The dilution of rabbit serum required is determined by adding 0.2-ml quantities of red cells to 0.4 ml of serial twofold dilutions of normal rabbit serum and allowing the cells to settle at 37 C. The highest dilution of serum causing a compact button of sedimented cells is the dilution chosen. (Typing sera can be prepared in rabbits by the same procedure described in the section on Neutralization Tests.)

Treatment of sera. Nonspecific inhibitors should be removed from all sera (animal or human) to be used in any HI test. Absorption with kaolin is very satisfactory for this purpose (37). This procedure is described in Chapter 71.

Typing procedure. Each prototype antiserum should be titrated against the prototype antigens within its group to determine whether any cross-reactions are present. Major cross-reactions have been found between types 7, 11, and 14 in group I, and between types 8 and 9, 10 and 19, and 15 and 22 in group II (38). The virus serotypes can be distinguished, however, by testing against serial dilutions of sera. Suspected adenovirus isolates are tested at a 1:20 dilution against rhesus or rat blood cells. Since partially agglutinating types often have a prozone, five serial twofold dilutions starting at 1:20 are made against rat cells (with 1:100 type 6 serum [HI $\geq$320] as a diluent). Under the above conditions, 95% of the isolates should agglutinate. If no reaction occurs, the isolate may be a type 6 (inhibited by the type 6 antiserum used in the diluent) or a type 12 or 18, which would not agglutinate either species. After an isolate has been found to hemagglutinate, it is tested in an HI test against antisera in the appropriate group with the use of 4 hemagglutination (HA) units of the unknown virus against at least 4 units of typing antiserum. The antigen is titrated by making serial twofold dilutions in 0.5-ml amounts into 13 × 100 mm tubes. A 0.5-ml amount of a 0.75% erythrocyte suspension is added. The tubes are shaken and allowed to stand for 1 h at 37 C. The first tube showing 50% agglutination of cells is considered to contain 1 HA unit. The HI tests are performed by the macro- or micromethod.

When using the macromethod, one begins by adding 0.2 ml of antigen containing 4 HA units to 0.5-ml amounts of serial twofold dilutions of kaolin-treated serum. The mixtures are shaken and allowed to stand for 1 h at room temperature; then 0.5 ml of the red cell suspension is added. The initial dilution of each serum is tested for its ability to agglutinate the erythrocytes in the absence of antigen and serves as a serum control. After incubation at 37 C for 1 h, the last dilution which completely inhibits agglutination (a compact button of uniformly sedimented erythrocytes) is considered to be the HI inhibition titer and contains 1 unit of antibody.

Microtiter HI test. Serum dilutions are made with 0.025-ml loops in conical (V-shaped) cups.

Four units of antigen as determined by macrotitration are added in 0.025-ml volumes.

Appropriate red cells (0.5 or 0.75%) are added in 0.025-ml volumes.

Tests are incubated for 1 h at 37 C.

HI antibody titrations of human sera. The same procedure described above for adenovirus typing is used for titration of adenovirus HI antibody in human sera. In this case, the antigen is known but the type and titer of HI antibody are not.

As one check on the reliability of the test, every HI antibody titration should be accompanied by a repeat hemagglutinating antigen titration.

Complement fixation test

The possession of a major, cross-reactive antigen capable of fixing complement in the presence of antibody to all adenovirus types affords a simple procedure for the diagnosis of adenovirus infection—the CF antibody test. The demonstration of a fourfold or greater increase in CF antibody in paired acute and convalescent sera is evidence of recent infection with one of the adenoviruses. The specific adenovirus serotype responsible for infection cannot be determined by this test. HI and/or neutralization antibody titrations, preferably accompanied by virus isolation, are necessary for this information.

The CF test may be performed by either macrotiter (test tube) or microtiter (45) methods. The differences would be only in equipment and quantities of reagents used. The basic principles of the serological tests are unchanged. However, the microtiter method has the distinct advantage that quantities of required reagents and sera are reduced, resulting in a great savings of both time and money. The step-by-step procedures for this test are recorded elsewhere in this *Manual.*

Preparation of CF antigen. The group CF antigen can be prepared by the method of Hilleman and Werner (17) or obtained commercially.

Treatment of sera. All sera should be heat-inactivated at 56 C for 30 min. No further treatment is necessary. A starting dilution of 1:8 is recommended because of the frequency of nonspecific reactions at lower dilutions.

Neutralization tests

The neutralization test, based on the ability of the virus to produce CPE in tissue culture and the inhibition of cellular destruction by type-specific hyperimmune animal antisera or the patient's own serum antibody, is one of the simplest of routine laboratory procedures.

Preparation of typing antisera in rabbits. The supernatant fluid of tissue cultures showing 3+ to 4+ CPE is removed after two freeze-thaws and centrifugation at 2,000 rpm for 15 min. Each rabbit is immunized with 1.0 ml of the supernatant fluid administered intravenously on a weekly schedule for 3 or 4 weeks; the rabbits are bled 10 days after the final injection.

Incorporation of typing antisera into test. Pools containing two or more specific types of adenovirus antisera or a monotypic antiserum can be employed. However, initial typing procedures in which serum pools are used are most economical and functional. The selection of sera to be incorporated into the pools may be arbitrary. However, certain combinations may be necessary to rule out heterologous neutralization. High-titered type 2 antiserum, for example, may neutralize type 1 adenovirus to a certain degree. Therefore, by combining types 1 and 2 in one pool and type 1 in an additional pool, interpretations previously difficult can be made. Further, the types of antisera in a pool may be dictated by the serotypes most prevalent in the community. Typing pools are prepared by mixing appropriate amounts of each serum diluted with Hanks balanced salt solution (HBSS) to contain a minimum of 4 antibody units per 0.2 ml of the pool. Pools are heat-inactivated at 56 C for 30 min. An example of serum pools used to identify the more common adenoviruses which may be isolated from the respiratory tracts is noted below:

Pool	*Types included*
A	2, 1, 5, 7
B	3, 1, 6, 7
C	4, 5, 6, 7
D	normal rabbit serum

Interpretation:

Neutralization by pool A only	= type 2
by pools A + B but not pool C	= type 1
by pools A, B, + C	= type 7
by pools B + C but not pool A	= type 6
by pools A + C but not pool B	= type 5
by pool B only	= type 3
by pool C only	= type 4

A more complete set of pools could be designed to utilize the same "elimination" principle.

Patient's paired sera. If paired acute- and convalescent-phase patients' sera are to be tested for the presence of type-specific antibody, sera are heat-inactivated and dilutions ranging from 1:5 to 1:640 are made in HBSS. Equal volumes of each dilution are added to the virus dose and incubated for 1 h at room temperature prior to inoculation.

Neutralization test protocol. The neutralization test protocol in which tissue culture tubes are used is not specific for the adenoviruses and can be found in Chapter 71.

Colorimetric neutralization test (24, 27)

HeLa cell cultures grown in Eagle's basal medium supplemented with 10% inactivated horse or human sera are utilized. The S3 clone HeLa cell line developed by Puck and associates can also be employed. The cells selected should have a relatively slow rate of metabolism. For all components of the test and for all serum and virus dilutions, a special metabolic medium of the following composition is used:

Rabbit serum (inactivated at 56 C for 30 min)	5.0 ml
Glucose, 20% solution	1.5 ml
Medium 199 in Eagle's balanced salt solution 2.5 ml of 8.8% $NaHCO_3$/100 ml	100 ml
Penicillin	100 units/ml
Streptomycin	100 μg/ml
Nystatin	20 units/ml

Make up cell suspension to contain 160,000 to 180,000 cells/ml as determined by a hemocytometer count. Set up a flask on a magnetic stirrer with constant agitation by a "plastic-coated" bar.

Dilute the unknown virus to contain 100 $TCID_{50}$/0.25 ml. The infectivity titer of the virus to be used must exceed $10^{-2.5}$ if clear-cut metabolic inhibition is to be seen.

Make up typing serum dilutions to contain 20 antibody units/0.25 ml of the specific adenovirus typing serum desired. Serial twofold dilutions ranging from 1:10 to 1:640 of patient's paired sera are to be titrated. Test results on patient's sera should be interpreted with caution because of the large number of heterotypic responses found, especially in adults (6, 15).

Pipette 0.25 ml of each typing serum into three 13 × 100 mm tubes.

Add 0.25 ml of virus to two of the three serum tubes. (Third tube acts as a serum toxicity control; 0.25 ml of medium is added to this tube in place of the virus dilution.)

Shake the tubes and allow them to stand at 4 C for 2 h.

After 2 h, add 0.25 ml of the cell suspension dispensed with a Cornwall pipette.

Two sets of four tubes labeled "cells before" and "cells after" comprising cells dispensed first and last during the test serve as cell controls.

Add 0.5 ml of sterile mineral oil to seal tubes (viscosity, 350).

The tests are read when both sets of cell controls show a pH of 7.0 or less. This is determined by comparison with a set of blanks containing 1% phenol red in phosphate-buffered saline, pH 6.8 to 7.8, at pH intervals of 0.2.

Approximately 8 days of incubation are required. A pH of 7.3 or higher = virus activity and no antibody; pH 7.2 or less = neutralization of virus and antibody.

Other methods

Although in limited use, there are two other procedures for the identification of adenoviruses. The rapid slide agglutination test demonstrates specific antibody levels in human sera that can be correlated with neutralization titers. This procedure requires the special preparation of specific adenovirus antigens absorbed onto charcoal particles which can be agglutinated by type-specific adenovirus antiserum (26).

If only small amounts of material are available and group identification of adenoviruses is required, the gel-diffusion precipitation test can be used (48).

SEROLOGICAL DIAGNOSIS

The serological diagnosis of adenovirus infection can be accomplished by use of the same techniques noted for the identification of the specific agent. In this case, the antigen is known whereas the titers of antibody in the patient's sera are unknown. So that valid interpretations of results can be made, the acute serum should be collected early in disease (1 to 4 days after onset), and the convalescent serum should be separated from the acute by at least 2 weeks. Further, titrations for adenovirus antibodies should be performed simultaneously on both acute and convalescent sera. A minimum of a fourfold rise in antibody is indicative of recent infection.

The most accurate procedure is the neutralization test, although the HI test is practically as sensitive and is less expensive. Although not as specific as the neutralization or HI test, the CF test is the most convenient serological procedure for the detection of adenovirus infection. As all adenoviruses possess a common cross-reactive CF antigen, any type of adenovirus may be used as the antigen. The CF test has the disadvantage of underestimating the number of actual adenovirus infections, but the fact that its use can detect infections due to any of the adenoviruses makes it the most popular serological technique in use today.

SKIN TEST

There is no skin test material available for the identification of adenovirus infections.

EVALUATION, INTERPRETATION, AND REPORTING OF RESULTS

The isolation of an adenovirus from a patient's excreta or secreta in the absence of a significant increase in antibody is *insufficient* evidence that the patient was infected with the isolated adenovirus. This is especially true of the adenoviruses because they are agents which can remain in a "latent" stage in normal, healthy children and adults. Indeed, the first adenovirus was isolated from adenoid tissue (41) removed from a child without respiratory disease. Thus, before a disease can be associated with adenovirus infection, the following criteria must be met: (i) isolation of a virus with evidence of a significant increase (four-fold or greater) in CF, HI, or neutralizing antibody (prototype or homologous), or (ii) a significant increase in HI, CF, or prototype neutralizing antibody in the absence of an isolate.

If isolation specimens are not available or isolation attempts have been negative, the demonstration of a significant increase in antibody is sufficient to associate adenovirus infection with disease. The demonstration of a falling titer or the presence of any level of adenovirus antibody in a *single* serum is not sufficient evidence of infection for the disease in question. It is merely indicative of past infection and cannot be considered serological confirmation of adenovirus infection even if an adenovirus has been isolated.

As noted previously, the most commonly used serological procedure is the CF test. The human response to this antigen, especially in adults, is generally group-specific and has been the basis of many useful seroepidemiological studies (35). Early investigators of adenovirus infections in infants and young children (2) reported that the CF antibody response in them was not as sensitive an indicator of infection as it was in young adults (18). Although different serotypes are usually involved, this age-related difference in CF antibody response has been further documented by more recent studies (35, 44). In one study, only 60% of adenovirus infections among infants and children with lower respiratory disease were accompanied by a significant CF antibody response (34). Thus, it is recommended that the CF antibody test be complemented by isolation and neutralizing or HI antibody studies to avoid underestimating the frequency of adenovirus infections.

LITERATURE CITED

1. Beale, A. J., F. Doane, and H. L. Ormsby. 1957. Studies on adenovirus infections of the eye in Toronto. Amer. J. Ophthalmol. **43**:26–31.
2. Bell, J. A., W. P. Rowe, J. I. Engler, R. H. Parrott, and R. J. Huebner. 1955. Pharyngoconjunctival fever. Epidemiological studies of a recently recognized disease entity. J. Amer. Med. Ass. **157**:1083–1092.
3. Bennett, F. M., B. B. Law, W. Hamilton, and A. MacDonald. 1957. Adenovirus eye infections in Aberdeen. Lancet **2**:670–673.
4. Boyer, G. S., F. W. Kenny Jr., and H. S. Ginsberg. 1959. Sequential cellular changes produced by types 5 and 7 adenoviruses in HeLa cells and in human amniotic cells. J. Exp. Med. **110**:827–844.
5. Boyer, G. S., C. Leuchtenberger, and H. S. Ginsberg. 1957. Cytological and cytochemical studies of HeLA cells infected with adenoviruses. J. Exp. Med. **105**:195–216.
6. Culver, J. O., E. H. Lennette, and L. Green. 1959. Serologic reactions in adenovirus disease. I. Delayed complement-fixing antibody response. J. Lab. Clin. Med. **53**:241–246.
7. Dascomb, H. E., and M. R. Hilleman. 1956. Clinical and laboratory studies in patients with respiratory disease caused by adenoviruses (RI-APC-ARD agents). Amer. J. Med. **21**:161–174.
8. Dawson, C., and R. Darrell. 1963. Infections due to adenovirus type 8 in the United States. I. An outbreak

of epidemic keratoconjunctivitis originating in a physician's office. N. Engl. J. Med. **268:**1031–1034.

9. Dingle, J. H., H. S. Ginsberg, G. F. Badger, W. S. Jordan, Jr., and S. Katz. 1954. Evidence for the specific etiology of "acute respiratory disease (ARD)". Tran. Ass. Amer. Physicians **67:**149–155.
10. Fisher, T. N., and H. S. Ginsberg. 1957. Accumulation of organic acids by HeLa cells infected with type 4 adenovirus. Proc. Soc. Exp. Biol. Med. **95:**47–51.
11. Ginsberg, H. S. 1956. Characteristics of the new respiratory viruses (adenoviruses). II. Stability to temperature and pH alterations. Proc. Soc. Exp. Biol. Med. **93:**48–52.
12. Ginsberg, H. S. 1972. Adenoviruses. Amer. J. Clin. Pathol. **57:**771–776.
13. Ginsberg, H. S., G. F. Badger, J. H. Dingle, W. S. Jordan, Jr., and S. Katz. 1955. Etiologic relationship of the RI-67 agent to "acute respiratory disease (ARD)". J. Clin. Invest. **34:**820–831.
14. Ginsberg, H. S., H. G. Pereira, R. C. Valentine, and W. C. Wilcox. 1966. A proposed terminology for the adenovirus antigens and virion morphological subunits. Virology **28:**782–783.
15. Grayston, J. T., C. G. Loosli, P. B. Johnston, M. E. Smith, and R. L. Woolridge. 1956. Neutralizing and complement fixing antibody response to adenovirus infection. J. Infect. Dis. **99:**199–206.
16. Hilleman, M. R. 1956. Acute respiratory illness caused by adenoviruses, a military problem. U.S. Armed Forces Med. J. **7:**1717–1725.
17. Hilleman, M. R., and J. H. Werner. 1954. Recovery of new agent from patients with acute respiratory illness. Proc. Soc. Exp. Biol. Med. **85:**183–199.
18. Hilleman, M. R., J. H. Werner, H. E. Dascomb, and R. L. Butler. 1955. Epidemiologic investigations with respiratory disease virus RI-67. Amer. J. Pub. Health **45:**203–210.
19. Huebner, J. J. 1967. The problem of oncogenicity of adenoviruses. First International Conference on Vaccine Against Viral and Rickettsial Diseases of Man. Sci. Publ. No. 147, Pan Amer. Health Organ., p. 73–80.
20. Huebner, R. J., and W. P. Rowe. 1957. Adenoviruses as etiologic agents in conjunctivitis and keratoconjunctivitis. Amer. J. Ophthalmol. **43:**20–25.
21. Huebner, R. J., W. P. Rowe, and R. M. Chanock. 1958. Newly recognized respiratory tract viruses. Annu. Rev. Microbiol. **12:**49–76.
22. Huebner, R. J., W. P. Rowe, T. G. Ward, R. H. Parrott, and J. A. Bell. 1954. Adenoidal-pharyngeal-conjunctival agents. A newly recognized group of common viruses of the respiratory system. N. Engl. J. Med. **251:**1077–1086.
23. Jawetz, E., P. Thygeson, L. Hanna, A. Nicholas, and S. J. Kimura. 1957. The etiology of epidemic keratoconjunctivitis. Amer. J. Ophthalmol. **43:**79–83.
24. Johnston, P. B., J. T. Grayston, and C. G. Loosli. 1957. Adenovirus neutralizing antibody determination by colorimetric assay. Proc. Soc. Exp. Biol. Med. **94:**338–343.
25. Kasel, J. A., P. A. Banks, R. Wingand, V. Knight, and D. W. Alling. 1965. An immunologic classification of heterotypic antibody responses to adenoviruses in man. Proc. Soc. Exp. Biol. Med. **119:**1162–1165.
26. Klein, M., A. Deforest, and J. Satz. 1967. Charcoal as a carrier in a rapid slide agglutination test for the detection of antibodies to adenoviruses. J. Immunol. **98:**707–709.
27. Lennette, E. H., B. J. Neff, and V. L. Fox. 1957. A colorimetric method for the typing of adenoviruses. Amer. J. Hyg. **65:**94–109.
28. McAllister, R. M., B. H. Landing, and C. R. Goodheart. 1964. Isolation of adenoviruses from neoplastic and non-neoplastic tissues of children. Lab. Invest. **13:**894–901.
29. Pereira, H. G. 1958. A protein factor responsible for the early cytopathic effect of adenoviruses. Virology **6:**601–611.
30. Pereira, H. G., A. C. Allison, J. S. F. Niven. 1962. Fatal infection of newborn hamsters by an adenovirus of human origin. Nature (London) **196:**244–245.
31. Pereira, H. G., and R. C. Valentine. 1967. Morphological and antigenic sub-units of viruses. Brit. Med. Bull. **23:**129–132.
32. Philipson, L. 1961. Adenovirus assay by the fluorescent cell-counting procedure. Virology **15:**263–268.
33. Portnoy, B. 1965. Pediatric virology—a review. Calif. Med. **102:**431–445.
34. Portnoy, B., M. A. Salvatore, B. Hanes, D. I. Hammer, J. M. Leedom, A. Jambazian, and H. L. Eckert. 1967. The sensitivity of the complement fixation test for the detection of adenovirus infections in infants and children with lower respiratory disease. Amer. J. Epidemiol. **86:**362–371.
35. Rosen, L. 1961. Hemagglutination-inhibition antibody responses in human adenovirus infections. Proc. Soc. Exp. Biol. Med. **108:**474–479.
36. Rosen, L. 1960. A hemagglutination-inhibition technique for typing adenoviruses. Amer. J. Hyg. **71:**120–128.
37. Rosen, L. 1960. Serologic grouping of reoviruses by hemagglutination-inhibition. Amer. J. Hyg. **71:**242–249.
38. Rosen, L., J. F. Hovis, and J. A. Bell. 1962. Further observation on typing adenoviruses and a description of two possible additional serotypes. Proc. Soc. Exp. Biol. Med. **110:**710–713.
39. Rosenbaum, M. J., M. Friedman, and M. Lieberman. 1959. A comparison of two sampling methods for the isolation of adenovirus. J. Lab. Clin. Med. **54:**966–969.
40. Rowe, W. P., J. W. Hartley, B. Roizman, and H. B. Levy. 1958. Characterization of a factor formed in the course of adenovirus infection of tissue cultures causing detachment of cells from glass. J. Exp. Med. **108:**713–729.
41. Rowe, W. P., R. J. Huebner, L. K. Gilmore, R. H. Parrott, and T. G. Ward. 1953. Isolation of a cytopathogenic agent from human adenoids undergoing spontaneous degeneration in tissue culture. Proc. Soc. Exp. Biol. Med. **84:**570–573.
42. Rowe, W. P., R. J. Huebner, J. W. Hartley, T. G. Ward, and R. H. Parrott. 1955. Studies of the adenoidal-pharyngealconjunctival (APC) group of viruses. Amer. J. Hyg. **61:**197–218.
43. Schmidt, N. J., C. J. King, and E. H. Lennette. 1965. Hemagglutination and hemagglutination-inhibition with adenovirus type 12. Proc. Soc. Exp. Biol. Med. **118:**208–211.
44. Schmidt, N. J., E. H. Lennette, and C. J. King. 1966. Neutralizing, hemagglutination-inhibiting and group complement-fixing antibody responses in human adenovirus infections. J. Immunol. **97:**64–74.
45. Sever, J. L. 1962. Application of a microtechnique to viral serological investigations. J. Immunol. **88:**320–329.
46. Trentin, J. J., Y. Yabe, and G. Taylor. 1962. The quest for human cancer viruses, a new approach to an old problem reveals cancer induction in hamsters by human adenovirus. Science **137:**835–841.
47. Tyrrell, D. A. J., D. Balducci, and T. E. Zaiman. 1956. Acute infections of the respiratory tract and the adenoviruses. Lancet **2:**1326–1330.
48. Yin-Coggrave, M. 1962. Identification of adenoviruses by microprecipitin agar-gel diffusion. Lancet **1:**1273–1275.

Chapter 75
Mumps Virus

FRIEDRICH W. DEINHARDT AND GRACE J. SHRAMEK

CLINICAL BACKGROUND

Mumps virus is responsible for parotitis epidemica (mumps) with secondary involvement of testes (11), the central nervous system, and, more rarely, the pancreas, ovaries, myocardium, and other organs (4). The incubation period ranges from 16 to 21 days. Infections occur generally by droplets via the upper respiratory route. Virus is excreted in saliva and urine from several days before onset of symptoms until 2 to 5 days after the beginning of the disease. Between 40 and 50% of all infections are silent. Immunity following overt or inapparent infection appears to be lifelong. Attenuated live and inactivated virus vaccines are available, but the latter should be used only in cases where the administration of a live vaccine is contraindicated.

DESCRIPTION OF AGENT

Mumps virus is a member of the myxovirus group, subgroup paramyxovirus (18). It is a ribonucleic acid virus with helical symmetry; particle size varies considerably, the average diameter being approximately 150 to 200 nm. Infectivity is destroyed by ether, heating at 56 C for 20 min, ultraviolet irradiation, and treatment with 0.1% Formalin (9).

Virus preparations agglutinate red blood cells (RBC) of fowls, humans, and other species (1). They contain a hemolysin (14), viral (V) and soluble (S) complement-fixing (CF) antigens (8, 10), and skin test antigens (5). Only one distinct antigenic type is known, but some antigenic cross-reactivity exists with other paramyxoviruses, particularly parainfluenza type I (Sendai) and Newcastle disease viruses. Mumps virus can be isolated and grown in various cell cultures and in embryonated hens' eggs (9). (Amniotic inoculation is used for primary isolation, and the virus can generally be adapted to the allantoic cavity after 5 to 10 amniotic passages.) Hemagglutinins and CF antigens are, however, best produced in embryonated hens' eggs. Mumps virus rapidly loses its pathogenicity for man during adaptation to growth in avian tissues and is generally nonpathogenic for man after 15 to 20 passages in avian host cells.

COLLECTION AND STORAGE OF SPECIMENS

The specimens to be examined include swabs obtained from the area around Stensen's duct, saliva, and urine. Spinal fluid should be examined if central nervous system disease is present. Specimens should be collected at the onset of disease or within 5 days of illness.

Swabs

Place swabs in 2 ml of a buffered salt solution, i.e., Hanks balanced salt solution (BSS), pH 7.0 to 7.2, containing 2% horse serum, chicken serum, fetal calf serum, or human serum albumin (*caution:* bovine serum may contain inhibitors) or, if serum or albumin is unavailable, 0.5% gelatin. Centrifuge the specimen at $1{,}000 \times g$ for 10 min, and treat the supernatant fluid with antibiotics (1,000 units of penicillin, 1,000 μg of streptomycin, 50 μg of amphotericin B per ml) for 60 min at room temperature. Store the specimen at 4 C if it is to be used within 24 h; if it cannot be inoculated within that period of time, store it at −65 C. Inoculate a suitable host system as soon as possible.

Saliva

Collect saliva into buffered salt solution and treat as above.

Urine

Collect first-voided morning urine. Clarify by centrifuging 15 to 25 ml of the sample at $1{,}000 \times g$ for 10 min at 4 C, and concentrate the supernatant fluid by centrifuging at 30,000 rpm for 60 min. Resuspend the pellet in one-tenth the original volume of Hanks BSS containing 2% serum, as described for swabs. Treat with antibiotics as described above and inoculate.

Spinal fluid

Collect spinal fluid aseptically and inoculate directly (add 2% serum if specimen is stored before inoculation).

Transport media

See description above (Swabs).

Temperature

Add 2% serum (see above, Swabs) or 0.5% gelatin to virus preparations. Mumps virus is stable at −65 C for months or years, at −20 C for a few weeks, and at 4 C for several days. Freeze preparations rapidly in dry ice-alcohol. Repeated freezing and thawing should be avoided. Specimens should be refrigerated at 4 C until they are delivered to the laboratory. If they are not inoculated within 24 h, they must be frozen. Specimens mailed to another laboratory must be sent in dry ice.

CULTIVATION

Cell cultures of primate origin, chick embryo fibroblast cell cultures, and embryonated hens' eggs (6) can be used for isolation of virus. Best results are obtained with primary monkey kidney (7, 15) or human embryonic kidney cell cultures grown in Eagle's basal medium (BME) in Hanks BSS supplemented with 10% fetal calf serum (see below).

Procedure of choice

Seed primary monkey or human kidney cells (150,000 to 200,000 cells/ml) or cells of tissue culture cell lines (40,000 to 80,000 cells/ml) in standard culture tubes in 1-ml amounts of growth medium FC_{10}, BMEI-H (inactivated fetal calf serum, 10 parts; BME improved [contains nonessential amino acids and pyruvate] in Hanks BSS, 90 parts; with a final addition of 2 ml of 7.5% $NaHCO_3$ per 100 ml, 100 units of penicillin per ml, 50 μg of streptomycin per ml, and 5 μg of amphotericin B per ml). Remove medium when islands of actively growing cells have formed, inoculate with 0.2 to 0.4 ml of specimen, and incubate for 30 to 60 min at 36 C. Add 1 ml of maintenance medium FC_{10}, BME-E (inactivated fetal calf serum, 10 parts; BME in Earle's BSS, 90 parts; with a final addition of 3.0 ml of 7.5% $NaHCO_3$ per 100 ml, 100 units of penicillin per ml, 50 μg of streptomycin per ml, and 5 μg of amphotericin B per ml) and incubate in a stationary position at 36 C for 6 to 7 days. The addition of 0.2 to 1% simian virus antiserum to media used for monkey cell cultures is recommended to prevent the growth of latent hemadsorbing simian viruses. Ingredients for these media or media ready for use are available commercially. Other tissue culture media in common use may be substituted; however, do not use calf serum.

Cytopathic effects (CPE) such as giant cell formation and rounding of cells (7) do not occur regularly enough to be of diagnostic value. A hemadsorption test is the simplest and most reliable assay for the presence of mumps virus in cell cultures (17). (*Caution:* As cells, particularly those of monkey kidney, may contain other latent hemadsorbing viruses, always test several uninoculated control cultures for hemadsorption.)

The hemadsorption test is performed as follows. Remove cell culture media. Add 0.2 ml of a precooled 1% chick RBC, guinea pig RBC, or human O RBC suspension in Veronal-buffered saline (VBS). Incubate at 4 C for 45 min in a slanted position so the RBC are in contact with the cell monolayer. Wash two or three times with 1- to 2-ml volumes of cold buffered saline or Hanks BSS. Examine the cultures microscopically for hemadsorption of RBC to the infected cells. Adherence of RBC to the inoculated cells indicates presence of virus.

If, however, more rapid detection of virus is desired, the indirect fluorescent antibody (FA) technique can be used about 3 days postinfection. The details of this procedure are given below (Identification of Agent).

Alternate procedure

Inoculate the amniotic cavity of three or four 8-day-old embryonated hens' eggs with 0.2 ml of specimen. Incubate inoculated eggs for 6 days at 36 C; then harvest and test individually the amniotic fluids from each of the eggs.

To determine the presence of virus in the amniotic fluids, set up a hemagglutination test as follows (12). Place 0.2-ml amounts of egg fluids in small round-bottomed test tubes or plastic hemagglutination plates. Add 0.2 ml of a 1% suspension of chick, guinea pig, or human O RBC in VBS, and shake the tubes or plates well. Include an RBC control (RBC and VBS only). Refrigerate the tubes or plates at 4 C for 45 min, and then read for hemagglutination of red cells (agglutinated RBC form a lattice covering the entire bottom of the tubes; nonagglutinated cells settle in a small button at the deepest point of the tube).

IDENTIFICATION OF AGENT

Methods of choice

Virus isolated in cell cultures is best identified by a hemadsorption-inhibition (HAdI) test, by a neutralization test (3), or by FA techniques. Virus isolated in embryonated hens' eggs is most rapidly identified by a hemagglutination-inhibition (HI) test or by demonstrating mumps CF antigens in the infected egg fluids. A neutralization test in eggs has been described in the literature but is cumbersome and can give irregular results. Infected egg materials may also be used for a neutralization test in cell cultures.

Hemadsorption-inhibition test

Remove media from inoculated cell cultures, and add 1.5 to 2 ml of appropriate dilutions of specific and negative control sera in Hanks BSS (the dilution of the specific serum should contain at least 4 to 8 hemadsorption-inhibiting units per ml, and this serum dilution should not cross-react with other paramyxoviruses). The highest dilution of serum showing inhibition of hemagglutination contains 1 unit of antibody. Incubate for 1 h at 36 C; then remove the serum dilution, add 0.2 ml of 1% RBC suspension, and continue as described above for the hemadsorption test.

Inhibition of hemadsorption in the cell cultures pretreated with specific antiserum but not with the control serum identifies the agent as mumps virus.

Hemagglutination-inhibition test

Determination of hemagglutination unit. Prepare twofold serial dilutions of the infected amniotic or allantoic fluid in 0.4-ml volumes of VBS, pH 7.2. Add 0.2 ml of a 1% chick, guinea pig, or human O RBC suspension in VBS, shake well, and refrigerate at 4 C for 45 min. The highest dilution showing hemagglutination contains 1 hemagglutination unit/0.4 ml. The dilution of virus containing 4 units in 0.2 ml is used for the HI test.

Procedure for HI test. Prepare twofold serial dilutions of mumps antiserum ranging from two dilutions before to two dilutions after the known end point. Transfer 0.2-ml portions of these dilutions to tubes, and add to each 0.2 ml of virus containing 4 hemagglutination units. Include virus, RBC, and serum controls. The virus dilution calculated to contain 4 hemagglutinating units should be further diluted through four twofold steps and tested for hemagglutination. Complete agglutination in the first three tubes in this series confirms that 4 hemagglutinating units were used in the HI test. Shake the tubes well and incubate them for 1 h at 37 C or overnight at 4 C. Add 0.2 ml of a 1% suspension of the same RBC used before, shake the tubes well, and refrigerate them at 4 C for 45 min.

Inhibition of hemagglutination by the mumps antiserum to approximately the same titer previously established with a mumps reference strain and absence of hemagglutination in the RBC and serum controls identify the agent as mumps virus.

Neutralization test

Freeze-thaw infected tissue cultures two or three times (freeze rapidly in dry ice-alcohol; thaw in a water bath). Centrifuge the cultures at 1,000 × *g* for 10 min to remove cell debris. Use egg fluids without treatment or dialyze them against phosphate-buffered saline (PBS). Add 2% serum (see above, section on Swabs, under Collection and Storage of Specimens) after dialysis. Freeze in 1- to 2-ml portions at −20 C or, if possible, at −65 C.

Use one portion for determination of virus titer. Inoculate 10-fold dilutions into the same susceptible host system which will be used for final identification, and evaluate the presence or absence of virus in the cell cultures or embryonated eggs inoculated with the various virus dilutions after 5 to 7 days of incubation at 36 C. The highest dilution which still infects 50% of the inoculated hosts is considered to contain one 50% infecting dose (ID_{50}).

Mix equal volumes of virus from a second portion (stored frozen during the virus titration) diluted to contain approximately 10^2 ID_{50}/ml with a dilution of a specific mumps antiserum containing at least 4 to 8 neutralizing antibody units and shake well. The highest dilution of serum showing neutralization of virus contains 1 unit of antibody. Incubate the mixture overnight at 4 C, or for 60 min at 37 C. Inoculate cell cultures or the amniotic cavity of embryonated hens' eggs with 0.2 ml of the serum-virus mixture. Include as a control the appropriate host system inoculated with dilutions of 10^{-1}, 10^{-2}, and 10^{-3} of the non-neutralized portion of the virus dilution used in the test. Also include four to six uninoculated controls. Incubate for 6 to 7 days at 36 C. Determine presence of virus by hemadsorption of test and control cell cultures or hemagglutination of harvested fluids of test and control embryonated hens' eggs.

Presence of virus in the infected controls and absence of hemadsorption or hemagglutination in the hosts inoculated with the virus-antiserum mixture and uninoculated controls identify the agent as mumps virus.

Fluorescent-antibody test

Cell cultures inoculated with clinical specimens can be examined for virus 3 to 5 days postinfection by the indirect FA technique.

The medium from control and infected cell monolayers is decanted and washed one or two times with PBS, pH 7.2. The cells are then trypsinized off the wall of the culture vessel, centrifuged, and washed once with PBS. Resuspend the cell pellet in a small amount of PBS

(0.5 ml) and prepare several smears on microscope slides (Corning, 0.97 to 1.06 mm thick) with a Pasteur pipette. Air-dry and fix in cold acetone for 10 min. The indirect FA staining procedure as described in Chapter 71 is carried out with the use of specific mumps antisera at a predetermined dilution and fluorescein-conjugated antiserum prepared against the animal species of the specific serum, also at a predetermined dilution. The test is positive for mumps virus if fluorescence is observed in cells stained with specific mumps antisera but not in the cells stained with control sera or with the conjugate only.

SEROLOGICAL DIAGNOSIS

Determination of complement-fixing serum antibodies

Mumps viral (V) and soluble (S) antigens for serum antibody determination are commercially available or can be prepared and titrated by the following procedure.

Preparation of antigens. Inoculate 8-day-old embryonated hens' eggs with mumps virus adapted to grow in the allantoic cavity. Harvest the allantoic fluids and chorioallantoic membranes 5 to 6 days after inoculation. Test for the presence of virus by performing a hemagglutination test on the individual allantoic fluids.

To prepare V antigen, pool hemagglutination-positive allantoic fluids, centrifuge them at 1,000 × *g* for 10 min to clarify, and dialyze them overnight against PBS, pH 7.2.

To prepare S antigen, wash the chorioallantoic membranes thoroughly two or three times in PBS, pH 7.2, and homogenize the membranes in a Waring blender for 3 to 5 min. Clarify the suspension by centrifugation at 1,000 × *g* for 10 min. Centrifuge the suspension at 35,000 × *g* for 30 min to sediment viral particles containing V antigen. Check the supernatant fluid (S antigen) for hemagglutinating activity. One 30-min centrifugation at 35,000 × *g* should remove all hemagglutinating activity from the supernatant fluid, but this step should be repeated if the control test indicates any residual hemagglutinating activity. (If a high-speed centrifuge is not available, the hemagglutinins may be removed from the S antigen by adsorption with chick RBC as follows. Add an approximately equal volume of loosely packed chick RBC to S antigen preparation. Shake the mixture and let it stand for 45 min at 4 C. Centrifuge at 1,000 × *g* for 10 min at 4 C; harvest the supernatant fluid and check for hemagglutinating activity. Repeat adsorption if residual hemagglutination is present.)

Control antigens are prepared in a similar manner from the allantoic fluid and chorioallantoic membranes of uninfected eggs. Merthiolate at a final concentration of 1:10,000 can be added to all antigens as a preservative. Stock antigens should be kept frozen at −20 C in small portions.

Titration of antigens. Block titrations of V and S antigens against known mumps antisera are performed with each new batch of antigens. Increasing twofold dilutions of antigen (1:2 to 1:512) are reacted against dilutions of antisera with known S and V titers. The highest dilution of antigen which gives 3+ or 4+ fixation (i.e., little or no hemolysis by remaining free complement) with the highest dilution of antiserum is considered 1 unit of antigen. Two units are used in the CF test. V and S antigens will show a certain degree of cross-reactivity, but the optimal dilution used in the final CF test should be free from reactivity with the heterologous antibody.

Determination of CF serum antibodies. Perform the actual diagnostic CF test as described in Chapter 71.

Determination of neutralizing serum antibodies by hemadsorption

Prepare twofold serial dilutions of inactivated sera (56 C, 30 min) in Hanks BSS, and add equal volumes of mumps virus containing 5 × 10^2 to 1 × 10^3 ID_{50}/ml. Shake the mixtures well, and incubate them overnight at 4 C. Inoculate 0.2 ml into cell cultures on maintenance medium and incubate the cultures for 6 to 7 days at 36 C. Primary monkey or human kidney cells, chick embryo fibroblasts, and HEp-2, HeLa, or other diploid or heteroploid cell cultures give equally good results, but diploid or heteroploid cell cultures should be pretested by a standard virus titration for susceptibility to mumps virus (3, 7, 13). Set up a hemadsorption test as described above.

The highest dilution of serum preventing the multiplication of mumps virus (i.e., cultures show no hemadsorption) is considered the end point.

Determination of serum antibodies by hemagglutination-inhibition

Prepare twofold serial dilutions of inactivated serum in VBS, pH 7.2. Sera often contain nonspecific inhibitors which should be removed by treatment with $NaIO_4$. (Add 0.15 ml of freshly prepared 0.1 M $NaIO_4$ to 0.5 ml of the serum, allow the mixture to stand for 30 min at 37 C, and then add 0.15 ml of 40% glucose solution. The volume of the serum is then brought to 1 ml by the addition of a buffered salt solution.) Add equal volumes of mumps virus containing 4 hemagglutination units and shake well. Incubate the virus-serum mixtures for 1 h at 37 C or overnight at 4 C. Include serum, virus, and RBC controls. Add 0.2 ml of 1% chick, guinea pig, or human O RBC suspension in VBS and shake well. Refrigerate at 4 C for 45 min.

No hemagglutination indicates the presence of antibody; hemagglutination indicates no antibody. The highest dilution of serum inhibiting hemagglutination is considered the end point.

Determination of neutralizing serum antibodies by interference

This test method is useful only for large scale epidemiological studies. The hemadsorption method is preferable for routine diagnostic laboratories evaluating small numbers of sera in any given test.

Prepare tube cultures by seeding 100,000 Earle's L (MCN) cells (3) per tube in 1 ml of growth medium ES_{10} MS_{60} 199_{30} (inactivated horse serum, 10 parts; Scherer's maintenance solution, 60 parts; medium 199, 30 parts; with a final addition of 0.5 ml of 7.5% $NaHCO_3$ per 100 ml, 100 units of penicillin per ml, 50 μg of streptomycin per ml, and 5 μg of amphotericin B per ml). Inoculate cultures 1 to 2 days after seeding of cells. Prepare twofold serial dilutions of inactivated sera (56 C, 30 min) in Hanks BSS, and add equal volumes of mumps virus containing 5×10^2 to 1×10^3 ID_{50}/ml. Shake the mixtures well, and incubate them overnight at 4 C. Inoculate 0.2 ml of the virus-serum mixtures into MCN cells (use two cultures per serum dilution), and incubate the inoculated cultures for 7 days at 36 C. Include serum, virus, and cell controls. Refeed cultures with medium ES_{10} MS_{60} 199_{30} containing 5×10^2 to 1×10^3 ID_{50} of vesicular stomatitis virus (VSV)/ml (use the same formula as above, but increase the amount of 7.5% $NaHCO_3$ to 3 ml/100 ml; the medium must have a pH of 7.4 as VSV does not grow at an acid pH.) Incubate the cultures for 48 h at 36 C.

Complete destruction of MCN cells by VSV indicates no interference due to the inhibition of the outgrowth of mumps virus by the presence of antibody. No CPE indicates the presence of interfering mumps virus and, hence, the absence of antibody. The highest serum dilution inoculated into cultures still showing a 2+ to 4+ CPE by VSV (i.e., lack of mumps virus multiplication and, therefore, no interference with VSV) is taken as the end point.

Determination of serum antibodies by radioimmunoassay

Radioimmunoassay (RIA) techniques which have recently been developed for the differentiation of early 19*S* and late 7*S* antibodies (2) can also be used for differentiation among a current infection, infection in the past, vaccination, or an anamnestic response. Although currently only a research tool, RIA techniques will probably be used more generally in the future.

Preparation of specific mumps antisera

Human sera with known titers of neutralizing HI, HAdI, and V or S CF antibodies may be used for titration of CF antigens or as controls in other serological procedures. It is, however, generally advisable to prepare specific antisera in guinea pigs.

Inoculate live mumps virus into guinea pigs by either the intranasal route (0.2 ml) or the subcutaneous route (0.5 to 1.0 ml). Inoculate a second dose 3 to 4 weeks later to obtain maximal neutralizing HI, HAdI, and V and S CF antibodies 14 days after the second inoculation.

To prepare antisera with anti-S antibody with no or very low anti-V antibody, inoculate guinea pigs intranasally and bleed them 7 to 10 days later. A low anti-V titer can be eliminated by dilution.

To prepare antisera containing only anti-V antibody, inoculate guinea pigs subcutaneously with ultraviolet- or Formalin-inactivated virus, or pool human convalencent sera from which the anti-S titer has disappeared. (As guinea pig sera may contain antibodies against other paramyxoviruses, such sera must be checked for specificity if they are to be used for virus identification.)

Hemagglutination, hemadsorption, neutralization, HI, HAdI, and CF tests can all be adapted to micromethods with the use of plastic plates (16), but micromethods are suggested only for large-scale work in laboratories in which micromethods are used as standard established procedures.

Skin test

Skin test antigen is commercially available; control material is not. Control antigen can be prepared as follows. Remove allantoic fluid from leukosis-free uninoculated 14-day-old embryonated hens' eggs. Centrifuge the allantoic fluid at 2,000 rpm for 10 min to clarify, dialyze overnight against PBS (pH 7.2), and heat-inactivate at 60 C for 1 h. Test the antigen for sterility before use. Add Merthiolate (1:10,000 concentration) as a preservative.

The test and control antigens are injected intradermally in 0.1-ml amounts in opposite forearms. Read the tests after 24 to 48 h for areas of erythema or induration, or both.

INTERPRETATION OF LABORATORY RESULTS

Isolation of mumps virus is diagnostic for a current infection because a carrier state with prolonged excretion of the agent is unknown.

A serological diagnosis can be made by showing a fourfold or greater antibody rise by any of the described methods (HI, CF, or neutralization).

Although HI is the simplest method, it is unfortunately the least reliable. Cross-reactions with other paramyxoviruses are most pronounced in this test system, and low titers may be due to nonspecific inhibitors (even after adsorption or $NaIO_4$ treatment).

CF tests give specific and reliable results and may provide a tentative diagnosis from examination of the first serum sample since S antibodies often develop early in the disease and rise faster than V antibodies. V antibodies, on the other hand, persist for years after the infection, whereas S antibodies decline rapidly a few months after the infection. An acute serum having a high S and low V or high S and high V titer therefore indicates current or very recent infection, whereas a serum with only a V titer indicates an infection in the past.

Neutralizing antibodies are generally not measured for the diagnosis of disease but give the best serological evidence of past infection. They remain elevated for many years after the infection, and even a titer as low as 1:2 in the absence of measurable CF antibodies almost certainly indicates past infection. RIA techniques may in the future become the method of choice, replacing the CF, HI, and neutralization procedures.

The skin test should always be used in conjunction with a control antigen and never in persons with a known allergy to egg protein. Erythema or induration of an area with a diameter of 1.0 to 1.5 cm or larger in the absence of reaction with the control antigen indicates a past infection with mumps, even though neutralizing antibodies may no longer be demonstrable. However, the inaccuracies inherent in any skin test also apply to the mumps skin test and must be considered in the interpretation of the results. Because of these inaccuracies, the skin test is not widely used as a diagnostic test.

LITERATURE CITED

1. Cabasso, V. J., and H. R. Cox. 1955. Hemagglutination behavior of mumps virus strains of different origin. Proc. Soc. Exp. Biol. Med. **88:**370–372.
2. Daugharty, H., D. T. Warfield, W. D. Hemingway, and H. L. Casey. 1973. Mumps class-specific immunoglobulins in radioimmunoassay and conventional serology. Infect. Immunity **7:**380–385.
3. Deinhardt, F., and G. Shramek. 1964. Development of an attenuated mumps virus vaccine. I. Determination of neutralizing serum antibodies against mumps virus. J. Immunol. **93:**462–465.
4. Deinhardt, F., and G. Shramek. 1969. Immunization against mumps. Progr. Med. Virol. **11:**126–153.
5. Enders, J. F., S. Cohen, and L. W. Kane. 1945. Immunity in mumps. II. The development of complement-fixing antibody and dermal hypersensitivity in human beings following mumps. J. Exp. Med. **81:**119–135.
6. Habel, K. 1945. Cultivation of mumps virus in the developing chick embryo and its application to studies of immunity to mumps in man. Pub. Health Rep. **60:**201–212.
7. Henle, G., and F. Deinhardt. 1955. Propagation and primary isolation of mumps virus in tissue culture. Proc. Soc. Exp. Biol. Med. **89:**556–560.
8. Henle, G., S. Harris, and W. Henle. 1948. The reactivity of various human sera with mumps complement-fixation antigens. J. Exp. Med. **88:**133–147.
9. Horsfall, F. L., Jr., and I. Tamm. 1965. Viral and rickettsial infections of man, 4th ed. J. B. Lippincott Co., Philadelphia.
10. Hummeler, K. 1957. Mumps complement fixing antibodies in guinea pigs. J. Immunol. **79:**337–341.
11. Krugman, S., and R. Ward. 1960. Infectious diseases of children, 2nd ed. The C. V. Mosby Co., St. Louis, Mo.
12. Levens, J., and J. Enders. 1945. The hemagglutinative properties of amniotic fluid embryonated eggs infected with mumps virus. Science **102:**117–120.
13. Moore, E. A., L. Sabachewski, and H. W. Toolan. 1955. Culture characteristics of four permanent lines of human cancer cells. Cancer Res. **15:**598–602.
14. Morgan, H. R., J. F. Enders, and P. F. Wagley. 1948. A hemolysin associated with the mumps virus. J. Exp. Med. **88:**503–514.
15. Schur, V. V., and A. W. Holmes. 1965. Virus susceptibility of marmoset kidney cell cultures. Proc. Soc. Exp. Biol. Med. **119:**950–952.
16. Sever, J. L. 1962. Applications of a microtechnique to viral serological investigations. J. Immunol. **88:**320–329.
17. Vogel, J., and A. Shelokov. 1957. Adsorption-hemagglutination test for influenza virus in monkey kidney tissue cultures. Science **126:**358–359.
18. Wilner, B. I. 1965. A classification of the major groups of human and other animals viruses, 3rd ed. Burgess Publishing Co., Minneapolis, Minn.

Chapter 76
Measles Virus

FRANCIS L. BLACK

CLINICAL BACKGROUND

The laboratory is rarely needed to diagnose typical measles. Clinical criteria are usually enough. The total number of measles cases in this country has been considerably reduced by the availability of a highly effective vaccine, but the fact of fewer cases sometimes makes individual cases of greater epidemiological interest. The vaccine virus has also introduced new diagnostic questions regarding its own role in specific cases. Other questions concern the role of measles virus in cases of encephalitis.

A rare but serious form of measles virus infection is subacute sclerosing panencephalitis (SSPE). Disseminated sclerotic areas occur in the brain, especially in the white areas. These may contain measles viral antigen and virus substructures but no complete infectious virus. The disease seems to be a late sequel of measles resulting from persistent virus some years after initial infection.

There has long been association between elevated measles antibody titers and multiple sclerosis. Etiological relationships are not clear, but specific tests for measles antibody may be helpful in characterizing this disease.

DESCRIPTION OF AGENT

The etiological agent of measles is an enveloped ribonucleic acid-containing virus 120 to 160 nm in diameter. It is morphologically indistinguishable from the paramyxoviruses and may be considered a member of this group. Its nucleocapsid ribonucleic acid is predominantly comprised of a single 6.4×10^6 molecular weight species, although variable amounts of smaller species may be associated with the virion (4). There is a single 6×10^4 molecular weight nucleocapsid protein in the 18-nm (diameter) helical structure. Five other polypeptides, two of them glycosylated, are found in the virion.

Unlike the parainfluenza viruses, measles virus has a long, 12-h, eclipse period and causes extensive pathological changes in the nucleus. Of practical significance in diagnostic tests is its hemagglutinin, which reacts only with erythrocytes from old-world monkeys, and does not elute at 37 C.

Antigenic differences between measles virus strains have not been reported, nor have cross-reactions between measles and any other human virus been detected. Serological cross-reactions between measles virus and related animal viruses (canine distemper and rinderpest viruses) are not troublesome because of virus host specificity. The virus is labile (half-life of 2 h at 37 C in tissue culture media) but withstands freeze-thawing well in protein-containing media and is stable on storage at −60 C or lower.

COLLECTION AND STORAGE OF SPECIMENS

Choice of specimens

For virus isolation, serum or plasma should be collected on or before the first day of rash. Whole blood or buffy coat is generally preferable to serum and may be useful if collected early in the course of infection. Urine may be infectious up to 7 days after onset of rash. Urinary sediment is usually a better source of virus than the supernatant fluid.

For serological diagnosis, an initial specimen of serum or plasma should be obtained as early as possible. Two specimens taken as little as 2 days apart during the first week after rash will usually show a titer change, and even a single specimen taken during the first month may yield relevant results. Cerebrospinal fluid (CSF) is also useful in certain diagnoses.

Smears from nasal swabs may be useful in identifying sluffed infected cells by the fluorescent-antibody (FA) technique if they are collected within 1 or 2 days of onset of rash.

Brain tissue obtained by biopsy or promptly postmortem is required for diagnosis of SSPE.

Transport and storage

Materials to be used for isolation should not be frozen but held at 4 C. Except for blood and blood fractions, they should be covered or mixed with a buffered balanced salt solution with 2 to 10% calf serum. Brain specimens for isolation from suspected SSPE patients should not be stored but cultured immediately. Serological specimens may be held frozen at −20 C but are also stable for extended periods at 4 C. Nasal smears should be fixed by dipping in acetone and held at −20 C. For microscopy of brain specimens, separate tissue slices should be fixed (i) by freezing, (ii) in 1% buffered glutaraldehyde or 2% osmium tetroxide, and (iii) in Formalin.

DIRECT EXAMINATION

Examination of nasal smears by standard histological methods may show giant cells of distinctive pathology, but a high proportion of negative results limits the value of this technique. Indirect FA staining of these smears greatly increases both specificity and sensitivity (10). Appropriate measles antisera prepared in rabbits are commercially available, and are preferable to paired human pre- and post-measles vaccine specimens, which may be used for this test.

Histological examination and electron microscopy of brain specimens for SSPE are research procedures, and the reader is referred to the original references (5, 7, 8, 11). Intranuclear Cowdry A-type inclusions in various cells, but especially the oligodendroglial, are characteristic of the disease but not always demonstrable. The FA technique is probably the single most useful method for diagnosing SSPE (6). Measles antibody in the patients' serum has usually combined with antigen in the SSPE lesion in situ. Therefore, misleading results may be obtained if virus identification is attempted with the use of human antimeasles serum as an intermediate serum in the indirect FA test; the fluorescein-labeled anti-human globulin may combine with the antigen-γ G complexes in the tissue even if the intermediate, specific antimeasles serum is omitted. To circumvent this problem, an animal-derived antimeasles serum and appropriately tagged antibody must be used, or the bound antibody must be extracted with 3 M NaSCN (7). A direct test with tagged antimeasles globulins produced in animals may also be used, but this may be less sensitive.

CULTIVATION OF AGENT

Isolation of measles virus from natural cases is a slow and demanding procedure, and it is normally reserved for research situations. Primary human kidney cell cultures are the only fully tested and entirely satisfactory system for isolation of virus from patients with measles. *Cercopithecus* or Macaque monkey kidney cells are probably equally sensitive, but monkey-derived measles virus may occur as a contaminant of primary cultures and cause confusion. Other primary human cultures such as amnion cells may be useful but are slightly less sensitive. Human diploid cell strains and monkey cell lines such as Vero or BS-C-1 probably offer the most satisfactory alternative to primary human kidney, but little work has been done on comparative susceptibility.

For isolation of virus from SSPE, brain tissue must be cocultivated with a susceptible indicator culture. HeLa cells have been used successfully, but Vero or BS-C-1 may be preferred (5, 8). Cell fusion with inactivated Sendai virus has been used, but is not always necessary.

Vaccine virus and at least some SSPE strains have wider host ranges than the common wild strains, growing readily in HeLa and other cell strains. Vaccine strains also grow in chick embryo fibroblasts. The titer of virus in blood and in throat swabs during the normal vaccine virus reaction is low, and negative results may not indicate absence of infection.

IDENTIFICATION

Syncytial lesions are the most common manifestation of measles virus during primary isolation (Fig. 1). Nuclei may form a ring around a granular mass of cell organelles in the center of the giant cell or may be distributed throughout the fused cytoplasm. A negative hemadsorption test with red blood cells of nonsimian origin may be useful in distinguishing measles virus from other paramyxoviruses. Type A Cowdry intranuclear inclusions and polygonal eosinophilic cytoplasmic inclusions are common but not invariable evidence of measles in primary cell cultures.

Some virus strains cause cells to contract into long, narrow, and often branched forms. Epithelial cell cultures may then take on the appearance of disorganized fibroblastic cultures (Fig. 2).

Measles virus strains may be identified by FA staining or by neutralization (see below). Low-passage virus rarely produces sufficient hemagglutinin or complement-fixing antigen to permit the use of these procedures for identification.

Vaccine strains can usually be distinguished from wild virus by their ability to grow and produce cytopathic effects in chick embryo fibroblast cultures. SSPE isolates have been reported to kill mice and newborn hamsters when injected intracerebrally (11) and not to infect simian virus 40-transformed cells (8) in contrast to wild strains, but too few isolates have been tested to know how general these characteristics may be.

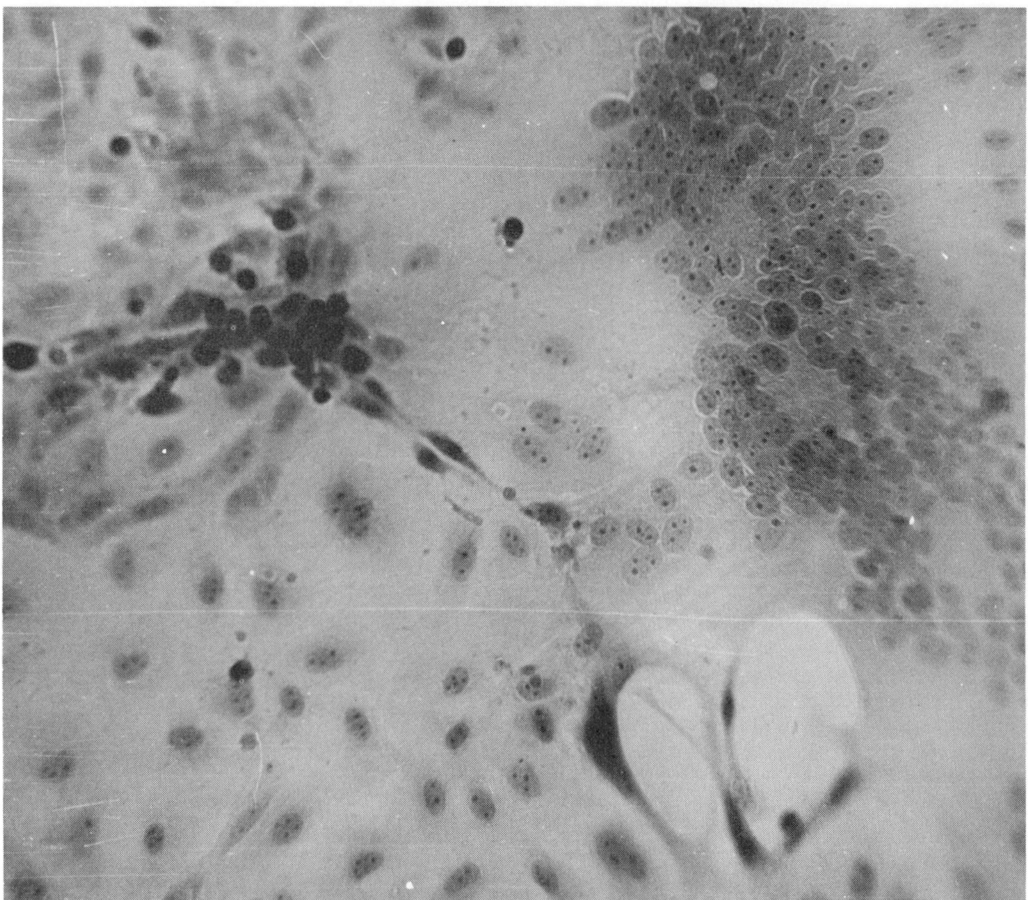

FIG. 1. *Measles cytopathology. Vero stable green monkey kidney cell line showing syncytial lesion caused by measles virus.*

SEROLOGICAL DIAGNOSIS

Hemagglutination-inhibition test

The hemagglutination-inhibition (HI) test is generally the most useful and rapid, giving specificity and sensitivity comparable to the neutralization test and somewhat greater than the complement-fixation (CF) test.

Treatment of sera. Mix 1 volume of serum with 9 volumes of 14% (wt/vol) kaolin in phosphate-buffered (pH 7.4) isotonic saline (PBS) and let stand for 20 min at room temperature. Sediment kaolin at 2,000 rpm and discard. Add washed, packed monkey red blood cells in a volume corresponding to one-fourth that of the serum and let stand for 1 h at 4 C. After removal of cells by centrifugation (2,000 rpm) in the cold, the serum is ready for testing. If it is desired to test undiluted serum or to retain the γ-M antibodies, other methods of separating nonspecific inhibitors of hemagglutination may be used. The immunoglobulins may be precipitated by mixing the serum with one-half volume of saturated $(NH_4)_2SO_4$, letting the mixture stand at 4 C for 1 h, centrifuging at 2,000 rpm for 20 min, and resuspending the pellet in PBS.

Antigens. Virus strains vary in initial titer and vary in the increase in titer that can be obtained by treatment. A suitable strain should be selected and retained. Various primate cell culture lines and strains such as Vero or HEp-2 provide suitable systems for propagating the virus. Harvest may be made by one to three freeze-thaw cycles at a time when viral cytopathology involves a majority of the cells. The best of such preparations may contain 64 hemagglutinating units per 0.1 ml, but many virus pools with lower potency are usable.

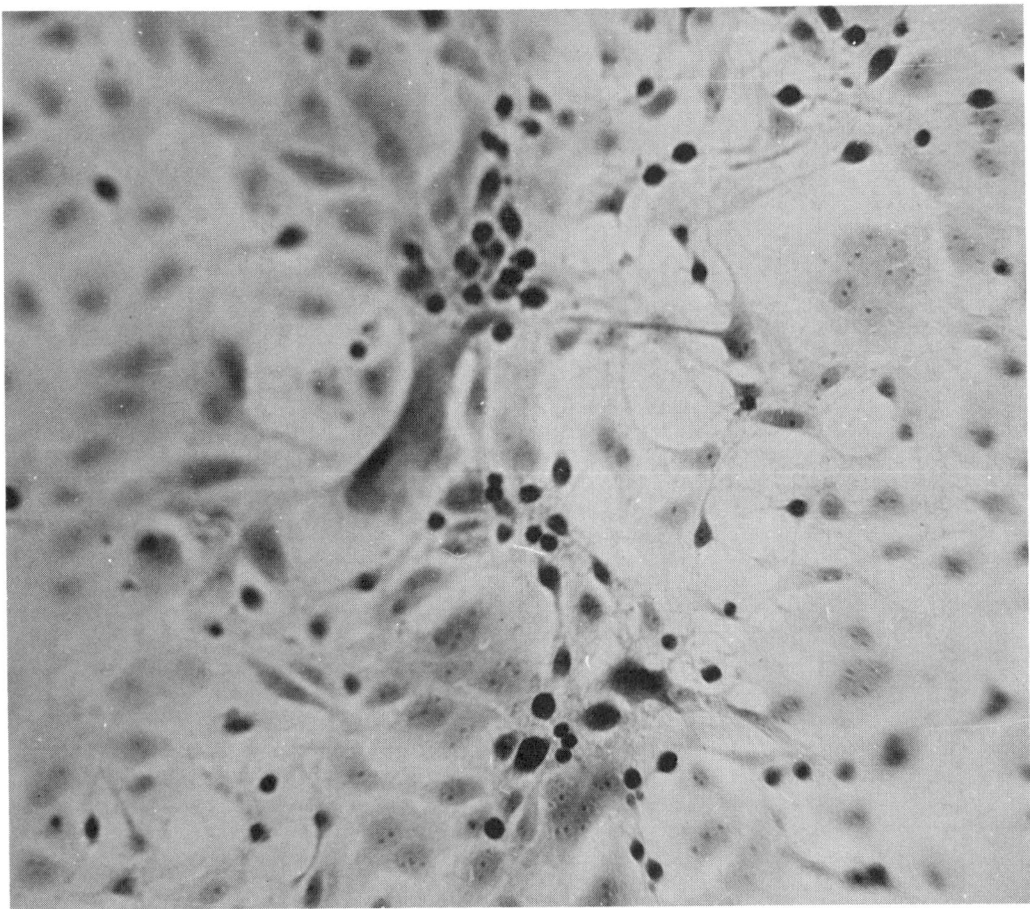

FIG. 2. *Measles cytopathology. Vero cells showing spindle shapes caused by measles virus.*

Antigen titers may be increased up to fourfold by treating antigen with Tween 80 and ether or by ultrasonic vibration. For the former treatment, add to the antigen Tween 80 (Atlas Chemical Industries, Wilmington, Del.) to a final concentration of 0.13% and stir for 15 min. Add one-half volume of anesthetic-grade ether; stir for 15 min in an ice bath. Remove the ether phase by centrifugation; ether dissolved in the aqueous phase is removed by bubbling nitrogen gas through the preparation. Alternatively, expose antigen to 10 min of sonic vibration with the 4-mm probe of a Biosonik instrument (Bronwill Scientific, Rochester, N.Y.) at 25% power, or to comparable treatment with another instrument. These treated antigen preparations exhibit increased sensitivity to inhibition and give higher serum HI values.

Cells. Red blood cells from old-world monkeys must be used. Variation in sensitivity within the *Cercopithecoidea* (catarrhines) are small, but genus *Cercopithecus* is preferred. Collect red cells in Alsever's solution or 0.1% heparin and wash several times by centrifugation in PBS. Use as a 1% suspension in PBS.

Test procedure. Prepare serial twofold dilutions of extracted sera in PBS, placing 0.1-ml portions in test tubes (10 by 75 mm), or prepare dilutions in 0.05-ml volumes in U-shaped microtiter cups. Add an equal volume of antigen diluted in PBS to contain three hemagglutinating units and incubate for 1 h at 37 C. Then add one volume of 1% red blood cells, shake, and allow to settle at 37 C. Read the pattern of cells on first settling or after reshaking and resettling. The results obtained on first settling generally give a slightly higher serum titer, but after reshaking the pattern may be clearer.

If microtiter plates are used, any static charge should be removed by a preliminary alcohol rinse or should be neutralized by incorporating 1% bovine serum into the diluent.

The test may be carried out at room temperature rather than 37 C with a small loss in sensitivity. Overnight incubation of serum and antigen at 4 C gives little increase in sensitivity.

Test for γ-M antibody

γ-M antibody (19*S*) is present for about 30 days after infection with wild or vaccine strains of measles virus. Its presence is therefore indicative of recent infection.

Centrifugation. Place a continuous or five-step 6 to 18% sucrose gradient in nitrocellulose horizontal-centrifuge tubes (e.g., Spinco SW50L). Layer 0.3 ml of a 1:2 dilution of serum in PBS (previously absorbed with monkey red cells) on top of the gradient and centrifuge for 4 h at 190,000 × *g* or for 8 h at 95,000 × *g*. Collect fractions dropwise through a needle hole placed in the bottom or by use of a commercial fractionator. γ-G antibody will peak in the upper half of the tube and γ-M, if present, will peak in the lower half, with a broad saddle of intermediate sizes between. The identity of each fraction may be confirmed by determining its sensitivity to 2-mercaptoethanol (2-ME) as described below.

Sensitivity to reduction. Add 0.1 volume of 1 M 2-ME to serum absorbed with red blood cells or fractionated by centrifugation as described above. Let the mixture stand for 30 min at 37 C.

Titrate treated and untreated serum in parallel by HI. γ-M antibody is inactivated by 2-ME, whereas γ-G antibody is not.

Complement-fixation test

The CF test is slightly less sensitive than HI or neutralization, but few immune persons have titers less than four, and this test may be more convenient than the others in laboratories where the technique is routine. The standard procedure described in chapter 71 may be used on either a conventional or a microtiter scale. Antigen is commercially available or may consist of selected, untreated or heat-inactivated, measles-infected tissue culture (HEp-2, Vero, etc.) fluids.

Hemolysis-inhibition test

Various measles strains carry variable amounts of hemolytic activity which seems to be related to a distinct antigenic site on the virus. This activity is blocked, probably sterically, by HI antibody, and hemolysin-inhibition (HLI) titers usually parallel HI titers. However, occasional specimens showed relatively high serum HLI titers (9), and high CSF titers by the HLI test have been found in specimens from multiple sclerosis patients (13). For the HLI test, virus released from cells without freeze-thawing and without Tween-ether or sonic treatment is concentrated by dialysis against polyethylene glycol (Carbowax 6000, Union Carbide). This is titrated by incubating with one-fourth volume of 10% *Cercopithecus* red blood cells for 3 h at 37 C. Lysis is measured in the supernatant fluid by optical density at 540 nm. A standard amount of measles hemolysin is then incubated with serial serum or CSF dilutions for 1 h at 22 C and lysis is measured as before.

Other tests

Various other serological tests may be used. None of these offer special advantage except to the laboratory that uses the method routinely for other purposes and wishes to integrate measles tests into a standard procedure.

Neutralization tests may be carried out with any tissue culture-adapted strain either by looking for cytopathology (CPE) in cultures of primate cells or by plaque reduction on primary or serial diploid *Cercopithecus*-derived cultures (2). If the CPE method is used, a challenge of more than 100 TCD_{50} may be used, and observations are terminated when a control titration shows pathology at a 10^{-2} dilution of the test dose. This shortens the process considerably over waiting for a true end point. Plaque reduction is considerably more sensitive than the CPE method. A satisfactory overlay may be prepared by use of the high magnesium modified Earle's solution of Georgiades et al. (3).

The indirect FA technique may be used with slides carrying measles-infected cells to provide a sensitive test for measles antibodies, and gel immunodiffusion methods may be used for the same purpose. Both of these methods offer research opportunities for resolution of specific components of the reaction.

SKIN TESTS

Positive skin reactions are demonstrable with concentrated measles antigen, but these have never been developed for diagnostic purposes, nor is any licensed antigen preparation available.

EVALUATION

The pattern of antibody development in measles is highly characteristic (2; Fig. 3). Neutralizing, HI, and complement-fixing antibodies appear very soon after appearance of the rash or about 10 days after vaccination. Normal individual variation in this timing is not more than 1 to 2 days in children. Adults may exhibit longer incubation periods, but antibody develops as consistently when the rash appears. All titers reach peak values in about 10 days after rash (or 20 days after infection), decline slightly over 6 months, and remain nearly stable thereafter. This pattern means that, to show an increase in titer, the first specimen must be collected within a few days of onset of rash; a second specimen may then show a significant change even if collected soon thereafter. The later decline is too small and too protracted to offer a satisfactory alternative sequence for serodiagnosis.

The difficulty in obtaining appropriately spaced specimens increases the need for reliable conclusions based on single specimens. The tests for γ-M and reduction-sensitive antibody (which includes γ-M and some smaller species) have helped fill this need. In a primary infection with wild or attenuated virus, these antibodies appear at about the same time (Fig. 4) as the γ-G. Reduction-sensitive antibodies never greatly exceed the γ-G concentration, so titer reduction may be no more than twofold; nevertheless, by careful control with untreated sera and by the use of sucrose gradient separations, reliable data can be obtained. It is not unusual for late-phase sera to show a small increase in titer after treatment with 2-ME.

Occasionally, a sharply rising γ-G titer is encountered without reduction-sensitive antibody. This happens on reinfection of persons whose initial encounter with the virus was aborted by maternal or artificially administered antibody and sometimes on re-exposure of vaccinated individuals. It may be unaccompanied by the usual measles virus-related symptoms (13). Atypical measles in persons infected after previous immunization with killed vaccine has posed a diagnostic problem, but removal of the killed product from the market and passage of time seem to have eliminated this form of disease. Persons with a history of immunization with killed vaccine may demonstrate a secondary-type antibody response.

Serum titers against measles are characteristically higher in SSPE patients than in persons recently convalescent from measles and average 10 times higher than in specimens from persons more than 1 year after measles. This is true whether the HI, CF, FA, or neutralization test is used (1). All tests exhibit considerable variation around their mean, and a higher titer is not

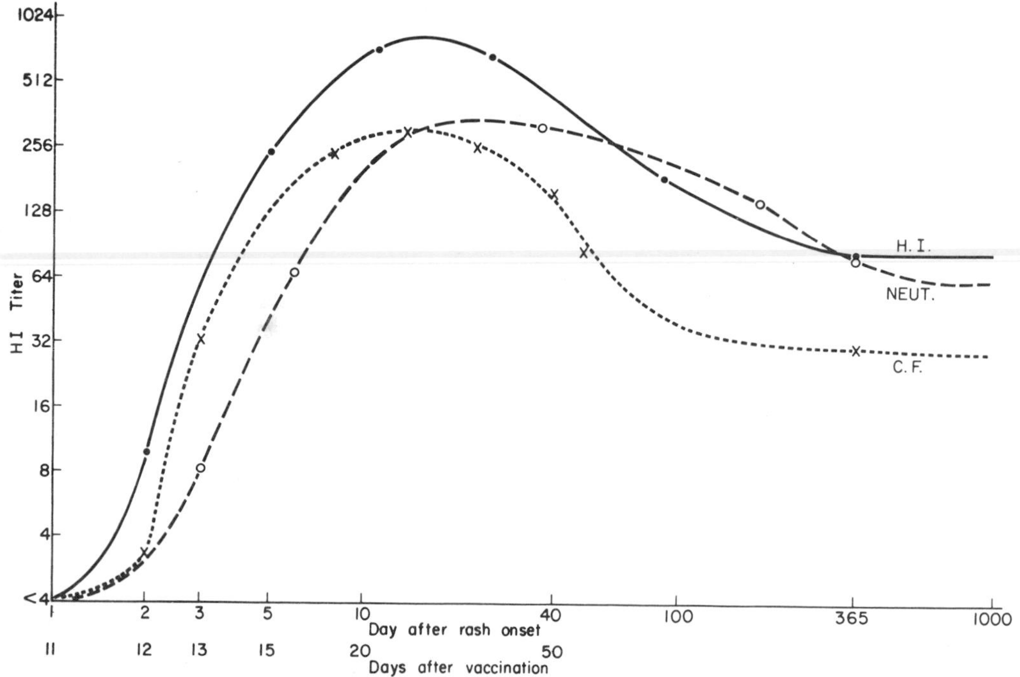

FIG. 3. *Time relationships of measles antibody titer changes. CF titers are based on data obtained after natural infection and other titers on postvaccination studies, but the results would be similar regardless of the mechanism of infection. Note logarithmic time scale.*

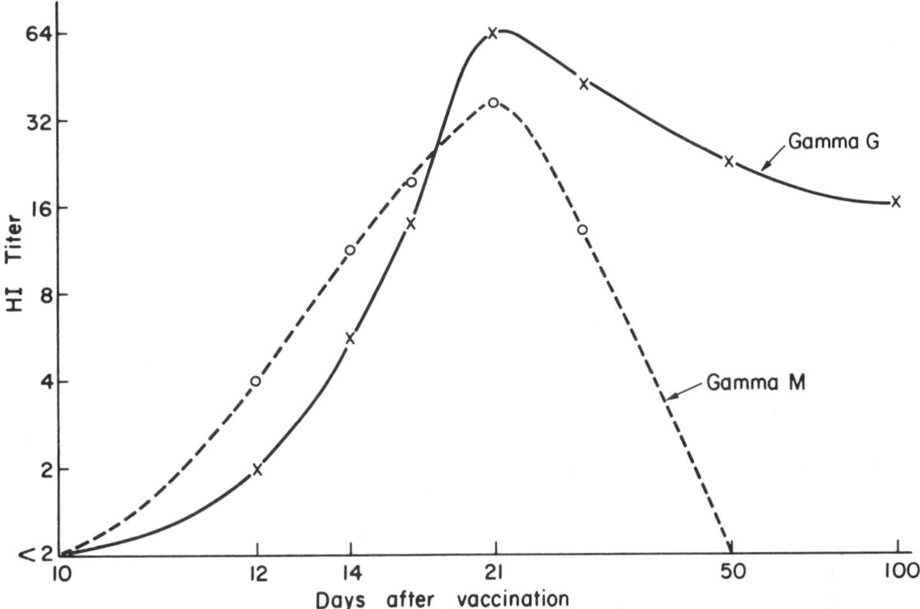

FIG. 4. *Time relationships of the appearance and decline of measles HI. γ-G and γ-M antibodies after infection with attenuated virus.*

diagnostic by itself. Coupled with other symptoms, though, an HI titer over 1,000 without a recent history of measles can be a helpful indication of SSPE.

Measles antibody in the CSF is suggestive of severe neurological disturbance. This is especially true if it can be shown that the measles CSF titer is specifically elevated relative to the serum titer by comparison with CSF and serum titers to some other common antigen (12). Elevated CSF titers are regularly found in SSPE and commonly in multiple sclerosis.

LITERATURE CITED

1. Adels, B. R., C. Gajdusek, C. J. Gibbs, Jr., P. A. Albrecht, and N. G. Rogers. 1968. Attempt to transmit subacute sclerosing panencephalitis and isolate a measles related agent, with a study of the immune response in patients and experimental animals. Neurology **18**(Pt. 2):30–50.
2. Black, F. L., and L. Rosen. 1962. Patterns of measles antibodies in residents of Tahiti and their stability in the absence of re-exposure. J. Immunol. **88**:725–731.
3. Georgiades, J., T. B. Stim, R. W. McCollum, and J. R. Henderson. 1965. Dengue virus plaque formation in rhesus monkey kidney cultures. Proc. Soc. Exp. Biol. Med. **118**:385–388.
4. Hall, W. W., and S. J. Martin. 1973. Purification and characterization of measles virus. J. Gen. Virol. **19**:175–188.
5. Horta-Barbosa, L., D. A. Fuccillo, J. L. Sever, and W. Zeman. 1969. Subacute sclerosing panencephalitis: isolation of measles virus from a brain biopsy. Nature (London) **221**:974.
6. Lennette, E. H., R. L. Magoffin, and J. M. Freeman. 1968. Immunologic evidence of measles virus as an etiologic agent in subacute sclerosing panencephalitis. Neurology **18**(Pt. 2):21–27.
7. Meulen, V. ter, G. Enders-Ruckle, D. Müller, and G. Joppich. 1969. Immunohistological, microscopical and neurochemical studies on encephalitis. III. Subacute progressive panencephalitis. Virological and immunological studies. Acta Neuropathol. **12**:244–259.
8. Meulen, V. ter, M. Katz, and D. Müller. 1972. Subacute sclerosing panencephalitis: a review. Curr. Top. Microbiol. Immunol. **57**:1–38.
9. Norrby, E., and Y. Gollmar. 1972. Appearance and persistence of antibodies against different virus components after regular measles infection. Infect. Immunity **6**:240–247.
10. Noskova, J., and A. Novak. 1971. Fluorezenz- und zytologische Diagnostik der Masern. Zentralbl. Bakteriol. Parasitenk. Infektionskr. Hyg. Abt. I. Orig. **216**:158–162.
11. Oyanagi, S., L. B. Rorke, M. Katz, and H. Koprowski. 1971. Histopathology and electron microscopy of three cases of subacute sclerosing panencephalitis (SSPE). Acta Neuropathol. **18**:58–73.
12. Payne, F. E., and J. V. Baublis. 1971. Measles virus and subacute sclerosing panencephalitis. Perspect. Virol. **7**:179–192.
13. Salmi, A. A., E. Norrby, and M. Panelius. 1972. Identification of different measles virus-specific antibodies in the serum and cerebrospinal fluid from patients with subacute sclerosing panencephalitis and multiple sclerosis. Infect. Immunity **6**:248–254.
14. Schluederberg, A. 1965. Modification of immune response by previous experience with measles. Arch. Gesamte Virusforsch. **16**:347–350.

Chapter 77

Rubella Virus

WILLIAM E. RAWLS AND DONALD A. PERSON

CLINICAL BACKGROUND

The clinical entity recognized today as rubella was first described in the German literature over 200 years ago and was termed *roetheln*. Following the rubella epidemic of 1940 in Australia, Gregg established the relationship between congenital anomalies of infancy and maternal rubella (5). Infection with rubella virus in childhood or adulthood results in a self-limited, benign disease characterized by mild upper respiratory symptoms, an erythematous rash, and suboccipital lymphadenopathy (see Fig. 1). Complications of arthralgias and arthritis which may follow disappearance of the rash are most commonly found in young women. Severe complications such as encephalitis and thrombocytopenic purpura occur rarely. Infection of the fetus during the first trimester of pregnancy, and to a much lesser degree the second or third trimesters, may result in congenital rubella. Congenital rubella is characterized by neurosensory deafness, heart anomalies, cataracts, growth retardation, and encephalitic symptoms, occurring alone or in various combinations. In neonates so affected, the virus frequently can persist for 6 to 9 months after birth. Excretion of the virus beyond the first year of life is uncommon (17).

The incubation period of rubella is 14 to 21 days. Antibodies to the virus appear as the rash fades and initially both immunoglobulin G (IgG) and IgM antibodies can be detected. Antibodies of the IgM class do not persist beyond 4 to 6 weeks, whereas IgG antibodies usually persist for the lifetime of the patient. Reinfection with the virus can occur but is almost always asymptomatic and can be detected by a rise in antibodies which are of the IgG type. The attenuated virus vaccines induce the production of IgM and IgG antibodies similar to that observed with natural infections except that the titers are not as high, especially the complement-fixing (CF) antibody. Reinfection rates with wild virus are greater among vaccinees than among persons previously infected under natural conditions.

DESCRIPTION OF AGENT

Rubella virus has been classified as a togavirus, although it is not antigenically related to other viruses. The genetic information is contained in a single strand of ribonucleic acid with a molecular weight of about 3×10^6. The virion is surrounded by a lipid envelope and is comprised of three polypeptides which have been identified by polyacrylamide-gel electrophoresis. Two virus-associated antigens can be detected by immunoprecipitation. In addition to infectivity and immunoprecipitating antigens, a hemagglutinating antigen and a soluble and a sedimentable CF antigen are associated with the virus.

Morphologically, rubella virus is a spherical particle with a diameter of about 60 nm. The virus contains a dense core surrounded by a lipid bilayer. Replication occurs in the cytoplasm of the cell, and the virus matures by budding into cytoplasmic vesicles or from the marginal plasma membrane. The virus is destroyed by trypsin and lipid solvents but not by repeated freezing and thawing or by ultrasonic treatments.

COLLECTION AND STORAGE OF SPECIMENS

In patients with acquired rubella, the virus is most readily isolated from throat and nasal secretions (see Fig. 1). Isolation rates are highest during the exanthum. Although the virus has been isolated from serum, circulating lymphocytes, and areas of involved skin, specimens from these sources are usually not needed for diagnostic purposes. Amniotic fluid, however, may be used to diagnose intrauterine infection. (Some pregnant women who are suspected of having experienced rubella in the first trimester report to their physicians later than 4 to 6 weeks after the illness. Amniotic fluid for virus isolation can be safely obtained at 16 or more weeks of gestation.) Rubella virus is readily isolated from most fetal and neonatal tissues obtained at autopsy. The virus can be isolated from urine, feces, and throat swabs during the neonatal period in congenitally infected infants. As the infant grows older, the specimens of choice are throat swabs and cerebrospinal fluid (14). Isolation rates are highest at birth and decline with increasing age of the patient.

Samples are collected and suspended in 2 ml of a balanced salt solution containing 1% bovine albumin, 200 units of penicillin/ml, and 200 μg of streptomycin/ml. The virus is quite stable in this medium and can be stored at -20 C for up to 2 months or at -70 C for longer periods. No appreciable loss of infectivity occurs at the latter temperature over a period of 1 year. If the specimen is to be sent to a distant laboratory, it should be shipped frozen on dry ice.

ISOLATION AND IDENTIFICATION OF THE VIRUS

African green monkey kidney (GMK) cells used for virus isolation and assay are prepared as detailed elsewhere (10). For virus isolation, four tubes containing GMK cell monolayers are drained of medium; 0.2 ml of the specimen is inoculated into each tube and allowed to adsorb for 1 h at 36 C. A 1-ml amount of maintenance medium is then added to each tube, and the tubes are incubated in stationary racks at 36 C for 1 week. Uninoculated GMK cells serve as controls. At the end of the incubation period, two inoculated and two control tubes are challenged with echovirus 11 by adding 10^2 to 10^3 50% tissue culture infectious doses ($TCID_{50}$) to the culture medium of the tubes. The proper concentration of echovirus 11 is determined by prior titration. Challenged tubes are observed daily for typical enterovirus cytopathic effects (CPE). The presence of rubella virus is indicated by complete destruction of the control cells with little or no CPE in the inoculated tubes. Absolute identification of the isolate requires specific neutralization of the interference with rubella antibody.

Specific neutralization of the rubella virus can be accomplished with rubella antiserum raised in rabbits (12, 21). The medium from the inoculated cultures which were not challenged with echovirus 11 is pooled, and serial 10-fold dilutions are made in maintenance medium (undiluted to 10^{-5}). Drained GMK tubes (three per dilution) are inoculated with 0.1 ml of each dilution. After a 1-h adsorption, 1 ml of maintenance medium is added to each tube and the cultures are incubated for 7 days at 36 C. All cultures are then challenged with echovirus 11 and observed for CPE. The dilution of virus containing one 50% inhibitory dose (ID_{50}) is calculated. Preimmune and immune rabbit sera are diluted 1:4 in maintenance medium, and the virus stock is diluted in the same medium to contain 50 ID_{50}/0.1 ml. Then 0.5 ml of the diluted virus is added to 0.5 ml of the diluted preimmune serum and, likewise, 0.5 ml of the diluted virus is added to 0.5 ml of the diluted immune serum. After 1 h of incubation at room temperature, 0.2 ml of each of the mixtures is inoculated into three GMK tubes. The tubes are incubated at 36 C for 7 days, challenged with echovirus 11, and observed for the development of enterovirus CPE. Destruction of the GMK monolayers inoculated with the isolate and immune serum, and protection of the monolayers inoculated with the isolate and preimmune serum, positively identifies the isolate as rubella virus.

Specimens with low concentrations of rubella virus may produce little or partial interference in the culture tubes initially inoculated. Passage of the culture fluid from these cultures may be necessary to demonstrate the virus. Fluid from the cultures which were not challenged with echovirus 11 should be inoculated into an additional four tubes of GMK cells. Additional control tubes are also included. These tubes should be incubated for an additional 7 days. Two inoculated tubes and two control tubes are then challenged with echovirus 11 and observed for CPE. The absence of interference with the echovirus CPE on passage of fluid from tubes which did not demonstrate interference initially confirms the absence of an interfering agent; if virus is not revealed after such a passage, its presence is rarely revealed by further passages.

Rubella virus produces CPE in a limited number of established cell lines. A number of laboratories now use RK13 cells for isolation of the virus, which induces CPE in these cells. The RK13 cells are apparently as sensitive as GMK cells for rubella isolation and provide the advantage of direct neutralization for identification of an isolate. Furthermore, an indirect immunofluorescence staining method has been shown to be specific and sensitive for the identification of rubella virus isolates in these cells (21).

A convenient method for isolating rubella virus from fetal or maternal tissues is to explant minced tissue specimens and allow sufficient time for the outgrowth of cells. When the cells have formed monolayers, the extracellular fluids can be harvested and tested for the presence of an interfering agent as described above. This method is more sensitive for viral isolation than is the use of tissue suspensions or homogenates.

With the recent introduction of rubella virus vaccine strains, the differentiation of wild virus from vaccine rubella virus acquires significance. At present, no convenient laboratory procedure is readily available to distinguish the viruses.

SEROLOGICAL DIAGNOSIS

Serological techniques for detection of antibodies to rubella virus provide the method of choice for laboratory diagnosis. A serum obtained when the patient has the rash and a convalescent serum obtained 7 to 10 days later can be used to demonstrate a rise in antibody titer; this can be accomplished quicker and with less expense than isolation of the virus. Antibodies can be assayed by several techniques including hemagglutination-inhibition (HI), neutralization, complement fixation, fluorescent-antibody staining, and precipitation in agar gel.

Hemagglutination-inhibition

Of the various serological methods, the HI test is the most useful. It is sensitive, reliable, and readily adapted for routine use. The test requires careful attention to details and monitoring of reagents for good reproducibility. When the test is properly performed, the presence of antibodies correlates well with resistance to developing rubella. The test can thus be used to evaluate the need for vaccination in individuals and in determining which pregnant women are at risk of giving birth to an infant with congenital rubella.

Although the basic principles of the HI test are as originally described (22), a number of modifications have been introduced; however, none of these modified techniques has gained universal acceptance. The source of the antigen, choice of indicator erythrocytes, pH of reagents, and methods for removal of the β-lipoprotein inhibitor, which is present in most human sera, are among the variables. The interested reader may wish to examine published reports of these modifications (3, 9, 11, 13, 19). The following is a description of the method which has been used routinely in our laboratory during the past several years.

The hemagglutinating antigen is prepared in cultures of BHK21 cells. Monolayers of cells are grown in 16- or 32-oz (ca. 450- or 900-ml) prescription bottles. The medium is drained from the cells, and 5 to 10 ml of rubella virus stock which contains 10^5 or more ID_{50} per ml is added. The virus is allowed to adsorb for 3 h at 36 C, and then the monolayers are covered with Eagle's medium containing 2% fetal bovine serum that has been adsorbed with kaolin. The medium is changed after 24 h of incubation at 36 C. After 3 to 7 days of incubation, the medium is harvested and tested for hemagglutinating activity. Fresh medium can be added to the cultures, and additional harvests can be made at 48-h intervals after hemagglutinating activity appears.

An alternate method of preparing hemagglutinating antigen which avoids the necessity of using kaolin-adsorbed fetal bovine serum entails alkaline extraction of infected BHK21 cells. This technique is the same as that described below for preparation of CF antigen.

Erythrocytes to be used in the hemagglutination and HI tests are obtained from 1-day-old chicks, adult pigeons, or geese. The erythrocytes are collected in Alsever's solution and can be stored at 4 C for 1 week without loss of sensitivity. On the day the erythrocytes are to be used for tests, they are washed three times in dextrose-gelatin-Veronal (DGV) buffer (2). After the final wash, the packed erythrocytes are resuspended in an equal volume of DGV buffer, making a 50% suspension. A portion of this suspension is further diluted in a solution of 0.4% bovine albumin in phosphate-buffered saline, pH 6.4 (PBS-BA; 2), to yield a 0.25% suspension of cells.

The hemagglutination and HI tests can be conveniently performed in Microtiter disposable plates. The rubella hemagglutinating antigen is titered by making serial twofold dilutions of the antigen in 0.025 ml of PBS-BA to which 0.025 ml of the same diluent is subsequently added. To each well of the plate is then added 0.05 ml of a 0.25% suspension of erythrocytes. Higher titers of hemagglutinating activity are obtained if the test is performed at 4 C on an ice slurry. The plates are kept at 4 C for 1 to 1.5 h and then are read for hemagglutination. The highest dilution that produces a pattern of complete hemagglutination is considered 1 hemagglutinating unit.

To perform the HI test, the serum must first be adsorbed with kaolin and erythrocytes. To 0.2 ml of the test serum is added 0.8 ml of PBS-BA and 1 ml of a 25% suspension of kaolin; the mixture is allowed to stand at room temperature for 20 min with frequent agitation. The kaolin is then sedimented by centrifugation in a clinical centrifuge, and 0.1 ml of a 50% suspension of erythrocytes is added to the supernatant fluid. After 30 min of incubation at 4 C, the erythrocytes are sedimented by centrifugation, and the supernatant fluid, which represents a

1:10 dilution, is removed. Further serial twofold dilutions of the serum are made in 0.025-ml amounts of PBS-BA. To these dilutions are added 4 hemagglutinating units in a volume of 0.025 ml. The serum-antigen mixtures are incubated for 2 h at 4 C, after which 0.05 ml of a 0.25% suspension of erythrocytes is added to each well. The hemagglutination pattern is read after 1 h at 4 C, and that dilution of serum which completely inhibits hemagglutination is taken as the end point. Each test should be controlled by the inclusion of a hemagglutinating antigen titration, serum at the lowest dilution tested with erythrocytes and 0.025 ml of PBS-BA instead of antigen, and known positive and negative sera.

Neutralization test

The immune status of an individual can also be assessed by utilizing a neutralization test similar to that described above for the identification of rubella virus isolates. It is carried out in GMK cells and is based on the ability of rubella antibody to neutralize the interference of echovirus 11 CPE. Virus stocks are prepared in BHK21 or GMK cells and titrated to determine infectivity. Stock virus is diluted in maintenance medium containing 10% normal rabbit serum to contain 30 to 50 ID_{50}/0.1 ml. The test sera are diluted in the same medium in twofold steps from 1:8 to 1:128. Equal volumes of virus and the serum dilutions are mixed and incubated for 1 h at room temperature. After incubation, 0.2 ml of each of the virus-serum mixtures is inoculated into each of three tubes containing monolayers of GMK cells and allowed to adsorb for 1 h at room temperature; then 1 ml of maintenance medium is added. After 7 days of incubation at 36 C, the cell cultures are challenged with 10^2 to 10^3 $TCID_{50}$ of echovirus 11. The tubes are reincubated at 36 C and observed daily for CPE. A rubella virus titration is included as a control to assure that the quantity of virus used in the test proper was optimal. The end point is that dilution of serum which allows the appearance of enterovirus CPE in two or more tubes.

Several other neutralization tests have been used in various laboratories. The modified hemadsorbtion-negative (HAd^-) plaque reduction test has simplified the precise quantitation of rubella antibody. The test methods have been described in detail (16). Briefly, BSC1 cells are grown to confluence in plastic petri plates, and stock rubella virus is titrated, inoculated, and allowed to adsorb to the monolayers. After incubation in a 5% CO_2 atmosphere at 36 C for 72 h, each plate is superinfected with approximately 10^7 to 10^8 plaque-forming units (PFU) of Newcastle disease virus (NDV; as assayed in chick embryo fibroblast cells) and then reincubated for 18 h. The extracellular fluids are drained, and a 0.5% suspension of sheep red blood cells (SRBC) in saline is added. After 10 to 20 min, the monolayers are again drained, and the clear plaques (HAd^- PFU) are counted with the use of an indirect light source. The SRBC adsorb to the NDV-infected cells, and clear areas represent rubella virus-infected cells which interfere with the replication of NDV. In the HAd^- plaque reduction test, test sera are serially diluted in twofold steps and mixed with equal volumes of stock rubella virus which is diluted to contain approximately 200 HAd^- PFU/0.2 ml. The mixture is held for 1 h at room temperature, and then 0.2 ml of each of the serum-virus mixtures is inoculated onto at least two BSC1 cell culture plates. The virus is allowed to adsorb for 1 h at 36 C and maintenance medium is added to the plates. The cultures are then handled as described above for the virus titration. A rubella virus titration, NDV-infected cells for hemadsorption, and uninfected cells should be included for control purposes. Similar plaque reduction techniques have been described in which other plaquing methods, such as the positive hemadsorbing plaques with pigeon RBC (20) or direct plaque formation in RK13 or SIRC cells (15), are used.

Complement fixation test

Rubella-infected BHK21 cells serve as a source of CF antigen. Monolayers of BHK21 cells are grown in 16- or 32-oz prescription bottles and infected with 5 to 10 ml of rubella virus stock containing 10^5 ID_{50}/ml. After a 1-h adsorption period, maintenance medium (Eagle's minimal essential medium containing 2% fetal bovine serum, 1.5 g of sodium bicarbonate/liter, and antibiotics) is added, and the infected cultures are incubated for 4 to 6 days at 36 C. The cultures are drained of medium and the cells are scraped from the glass. The cells are then pelleted by centrifugation at 1,500 rpm for 15 min and suspended in 0.1 M glycine buffer, pH 9.5, to give a 15% suspension. The suspension is then incubated for 6 to 8 h at 36 C, sonically treated for 5 min, and clarified by low-speed centrifugation. The supernatant fluid contains the CF antigen, which usually titers 1:16 to 1:64 (18). The antigen is stable for long periods at −70 C. The standard CF test described elsewhere (chapter 71) is used for the detection of antibodies to rubella virus.

Immunofluorescence test

Cells infected with rubella virus produce antigens in their cytoplasm. These antigens are specific for the virus and can be used to identify an isolate or to quantitate antiviral antibodies. Antibodies to rubella virus are quantitated by infecting cells with rubella virus and by the indirect method of staining for antibodies to the antigens. The technique is rapid and inexpensive and allows quantitation of IgG and IgM antibodies; however, its use is limited to those laboratories proficient in the immunofluorescence techniques.

The present method of choice employs smears of acutely infected BHK21 cells. BHK21 cells contained in 8-oz prescription bottles are infected with rubella virus, incubated at 36 C for 3 to 5 days, and trypsinized. The infected cells are washed and resuspended to a concentration of about 2×10^7 cells/ml. Uninfected BHK21 cells handled in the same way serve as controls. Drops of the cell suspensions are placed on standard microscope slides and air-dried. The cells are then fixed with acetone for 10 min at room temperature and dried. Such cell preparations can be stored frozen (−60 C) for as long as 3 weeks (8). One drop of each serial twofold dilution of the test serum is added to separate smears of infected and uninfected cells. After incubation for 1 h at 37 C, the smears are washed three time with PBS. The smears are then covered with one drop of fluorescein-labeled antihuman globulin (details of preparation and labeling are outlined in chapter 71). To detect IgM antibody, specific anti-IgM antibody is used. The labeled antibody is allowed to react for 1 h and the smears are then washed three times with PBS. The smears are dried, cover slips are applied, and they are then examined with a fluorescence microscope. Antibody containing sera results in a specific fluorescence in the cytoplasm of the infected cells; the highest serum dilution which produces specific fluorescence is taken as the antibody end point. Some authors have found that dilutions of the test sera and fluorescein-labeled antihuman globulin in a 20% suspension of normal beef brain or mouse brain will reduce overstaining (8). Alternative sources of antigen for immunofluorescence are chronically or acutely infected cells which are grown on cover slips (1).

Special methods

The presence of IgM antibodies to rubella virus has diagnostic significance. Antirubella virus antibodies of the IgM class can be detected by immunofluorescence as described above, by degradation with 2-mercaptoethanol (3), or by physical separation of IgM from IgG by density gradient centrifugation (23). The last technique has been found to be the most satisfactory in our laboratory (4).

A density gradient is prepared by layering 1.5-ml amounts of 40, 25, and 10% (wt/vol) solutions of sucrose in PBS in a 5-ml Lusteroid tube. The gradient is equilibrated by overnight diffusion in a refrigerator. The test serum is diluted 1:4 in PBS and adsorbed with pigeon RBC (0.2 ml of serum is mixed with 0.6 ml of PBS and 0.1 ml of a 50% suspension of RBC). A 0.5-ml volume of the diluted serum is placed on top of the gradient. The gradient is then centrifuged at $157{,}000 \times g$ for 18 h. Six fractions of 0.8 ml each are collected by puncturing the bottom of the tube. The fractions are then tested for HI activity without further treatment or after dialysis against PBS to remove excess sucrose. IgM antibodies are present in the bottom two fractions, IgG antibodies separate primarily in the third and fourth fractions, and the nonspecific inhibitor is located at the top of the gradient.

Rubella precipitating antigens have been prepared, partially charactérized, and designated theta and iota. Both appear to be structural virion proteins, and theta antigen is apparently related to the rubella hemagglutinin. These antigens are not available for routine diagnosis; however, in specialized laboratories these precipitinogens have been used to measure precipitating antibody in patients with acquired infection and more recently in vaccinees. Certain vaccine strains induce almost no anti-iota precipitating antibody in the vaccinees, whereas natural infection and infection with other vaccine strains induce considerable anti-theta and anti-iota precipitins (7).

EVALUATION, INTERPRETATION, AND REPORTING OF RESULTS

Rubella virus produces essentially two clinical entities, congenital rubella and rubella acquired after birth. Establishing the diagnosis of rubella in the first trimester of pregnancy is of importance and may influence the decision to terminate the pregnancy. Because of the time required for isolation and identification of rubella virus, serological methods are preferred, especially the HI test. As shown in Fig. 1, antibodies to the virus appear promptly as the rash fades and reach peak titers in 10 to 20 days. When feasible, the acute serum should be obtained as early as possible in the disease, and

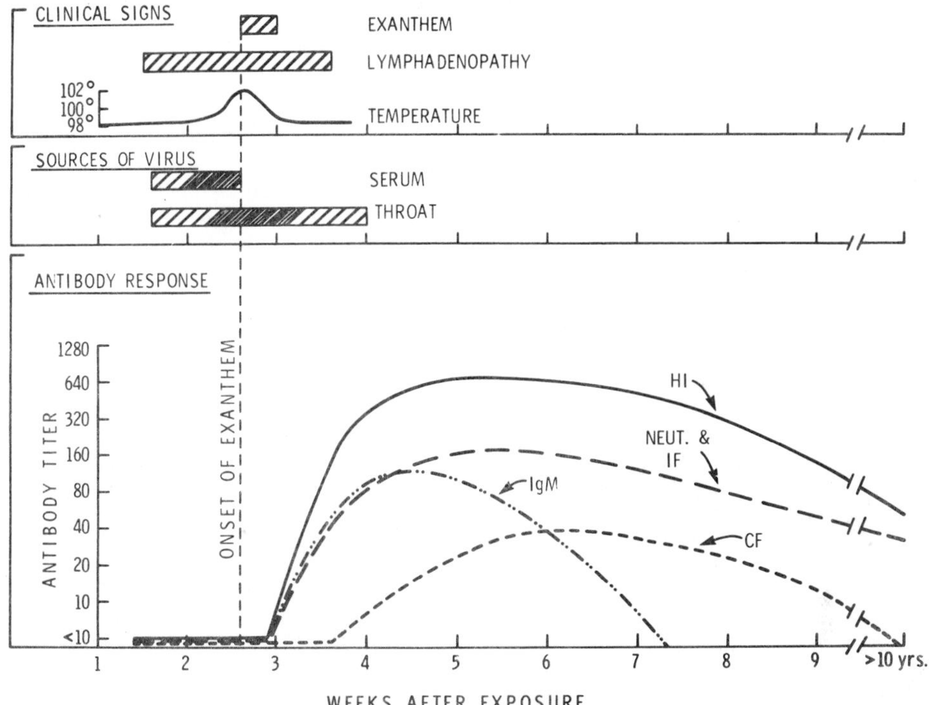

FIG. 1. *Features of a typical illness of postnatally acquired rubella. The incubation period is 14 to 21 days. Virus can be isolated from the serum prior to the onset of rash and from the throat for 1 week before to 1 week after the onset of the exanthem. Antibodies to the virus appear as the rash fades and reach maximal titers in 7 to 10 days (HI, hemagglutination-inhibition; Neut., neutralizing; IF, immunofluoresence; CF, complement fixation). Antibodies persist for life except those measured by CF. Antibodies of the IgM class are detectable for about 1 month after the rash fades.*

the convalescent specimen should be obtained as early as 5 to 7 days later. Acute and convalescent sera together with appropriate negative and positive controls must be run in the same test. A fourfold or greater rise in titer between acute and convalescent serum specimens is considered diagnostic of acquired rubella. Rubella antibodies measured by CF appear somewhat later, rise more slowly, attain a relatively lower maximal titer, and decline more rapidly than antibody measured by the other methods. Thus, the CF test may occasionally be useful for diagnosis because of the slower development of CF antibody. It should be recognized, however, that in practice very often, even with a relatively high HI titer in the acute serum, a substantially higher titer (fourfold or greater) can easily be demonstrated in the convalescent sample obtained from a patient with rubella virus infection (13).

In patients with a history compatible with rubella who are not seen until 2 or more weeks after the illness, it may be possible to establish the diagnosis by demonstrating IgM antibodies. This is rarely possible when more than 1 month has lapsed between the illness and the time of bleeding. In our laboratory, amniotic fluid is examined for rubella virus in women suspected of having had first trimester rubella more than 1 month prior to consulting a physician. Experience with this method of diagnosis has been limited, but in the case studied it has been found to be reliable.

Some persons exposed to rubella are found to have a rise in antibody titers, and this is thought to represent reinfection. Such persons rarely develop symptoms, and the risk of congenital malformations associated with reinfection appears to be minimal. The rise in antibody titers is due to an increase in IgG molecules, and a primary infection can be distinguished from a reinfection by evaluating the serum for the presence of IgM antibodies to rubella; these are absent in reinfection.

With the classical clinical manifestations of congenital rubella, isolation of the virus may be diagnostic. Congenitally infected infants may excrete the virus for many months, and repeated isolation attempts may be necessary to confirm the diagnosis. Serum specimens obtained shortly after birth may contain HI antibody quantitatively equal to or greater than maternal antibody. Maternal IgG antibodies are acquired transplacentally whereas IgM antibodies are not. It may be useful to attempt to demonstrate the immunoglobulin class of the infant's antiviral antibody. If it is primarily of the IgM class, active production of antibody by the infant is inferred and congenital infection is likely. Further, the persistence of HI antibody after 6 to 24 months of age, after the loss of passively acquired maternal antibody, is usually considered diagnostic for congenital rubella (6).

The HI test is the method of choice for determining an individual's immune status; the presence of antibody indicates past infection and immunity. Occasionally, individuals without HI antibodies at the lowest dilution tested will not respond to vaccination. Low levels of neutralizing antibodies can usually be demonstrated in the prevaccination serum, and repeated vaccinations to obtain a "take" are not indicated.

Results of routine serological procedures are reported as the titer of antibody with the method used. Special procedures in our laboratory are undertaken only after the requirements of the physician in the particular case and the limitations of the laboratory have been clearly communicated.

LITERATURE CITED

1. Brown, G. C., H. F. Maassab, J. A. Veronelli, and T. J. Francis, Jr. 1964. Rubella antibodies in human serum: detection by the indirect fluorescent antibody technique. Science **145**:943–945.
2. Clarke, D. H., and J. Casals. 1958. Techniques for hemagglutination and hemagglutination-inhibition with arthropod-borne viruses. Amer. J. Trop. Med. Hyg. **7**:561–573.
3. Cooper, L. Z., B. Matters, J. K. Rosenblum, and S. Krugman. 1969. Experience with a modified rubella hemagglutination inhibition antibody test. J. Amer. Med. Ass. **207**:89–93.
4. Desmyter, J., M. A. South, and W. E. Rawls. 1971. The IgM antibody response in rubella during pregnancy. J. Med. Microbiol. **4**:107–114.
5. Gregg, N. M. 1941. Congenital cataract following German measles in the mother. Trans. Ophthalmol. Soc. Aust. **3**:35–46.
6. Hayes, K., J. A. Dudgeon, and J. F. Soothill. 1967. Humoral immunity in congenital rubella. Clin. Exp. Immunol. **2**:653–657.
7. Le Bouvier. G. L., and S. A. Plotkin. 1971. Precipitin responses to rubella vaccine RA 27/3. J. Infect. Dis. **123**:220–223.
8. Lennette, E. H., J. D. Woodie, and N. J. Schmidt. 1967. A modified indirect immunofluorescent staining technique for demonstration of rubella antibodies in human sera. J. Lab. Clin. Med. **69**:689–695.
9. Liebhaber, H. 1970. Measurement of rubella antibody by hemagglutination inhibition. II. Characteristics of an improved HAI test employing a new method for removal of non-immunoglobulin HA inhibitors from serum. J. Immunol. **104**:826–834.
10. Melnick, J. L., and H. A. Wenner. 1969. Enteroviruses, p. 529–602. *In* E. H. Lennette and N. J. Schmidt (ed.), Diagnostic procedures for viral and rickettsial infections, 4th ed. American Public Health Association, Inc., New York.
11. Palmer, D. F., K. L. Herrmann, R. E. Lincoln, M. V. Hearn, and J. M. Fuller (ed.). 1970. A procedural guide to the performance of the standardized rubella hemagglutination-inhibition test. Center for Disease Control Immunology Series No. 2, Atlanta, Ga.
12. Parkman, P. D., F. K. Mundon, J. M. McCown, and E. L. Buescher. 1964. Studies of rubella. II. Neutralization of the virus. J. Immunol. **93**:608–617.
13. Person, D. A., and E. C. Herrmann, Jr. 1971. Laboratory diagnosis of rubella virus infections and antibody determinations in routine medical practice. Mayo Clin. Proc. **46**:477–483.
14. Phillips, C. A., W. E. Rawls, J. L. Melnick, and M. D. Yow. 1966. Viral studies of a congenital rubella epidemic. Health Lab. Sci. **3**:118–123.
15. Plotkin, S. A. 1969. Rubella virus, p. 364–413. *In* E. H. Lennette and N. J. Schmidt (ed.), Diagnostic procedures for viral and rickettsial infections, 4th ed. American Public Health Association, Inc., New York.
16. Rawls, W. E., J. Desmyter, and J. L. Melnick. 1967. Rubella virus neutralization by plaque reduction. Proc. Soc. Exp. Biol. Med. **124**:167–172.
17. Rudolph, A. J., and M. M. Desmond. 1972. Clinical manifestations of the congenital rubella syndrome. Int. Ophthalmol. Clin. **12**:3–19.
18. Schmidt, N. J., and E. H. Lennette. 1966. Rubella complement-fixing antigens derived from the fluid and cellular phases of infected BHK21 cells: extraction of cell-associated antigen with alkaline buffers. J. Immunol. **97**:815–821.
19. Schmidt, N. J., and E. H. Lennette. 1970. Variables of the rubella hemagglutination-inhibition test system and their effect on antigen and antibody titers. Appl. Microbiol. **19**:491–504.
20. Schmidt, N. J., E. H. Lennette, and J. Dennis. 1969. A plaque assay for rubella virus based upon hemadsorption. Proc. Soc. Exp. Biol. Med. **132**:128–133.
21. Schmidt, N. J., E. H. Lennette, J. D. Woodie, and H. H. Ho. 1966. Identification of rubella virus isolates by immunofluorescent staining, and a comparison of the sensitivity of three cell culture systems for recovery of virus. J. Lab. Clin. Med. **68**:502–509.
22. Stewart, G. L., P. D. Parkman, H. E. Hopps, R. D. Douglas, J. P. Hamilton, and H. M. Meyer, Jr. 1967. Rubella-virus hemagglutination-inhibition test. N. Engl. J. Med. **276**:554–557.
23. Vesikari, T., and A. Vaheri. 1968. Rubella: a method for rapid diagnosis of a recent infection by demonstration of the IgM antibodies. Brit. Med. J. **1**:221–223.

Chapter 78
Enteroviruses

C. A. PHILLIPS

CLINICAL BACKGROUND

In spite of the availability of effective vaccines, outbreaks of poliomyelitis still occur in unimmunized or poorly immunized populations. There are also a variety of other well-recognized clinical syndromes, such as paralysis, aseptic meningitis, encephalitis, myocarditis, pericarditis, pleurodynia, herpangina, acute respiratory tract infections, and hand-foot-and-mouth disease, caused by infection with other enteroviruses. In addition, enteroviruses may play a significant role in the etiology of such other entities as the newly described pandemic conjunctivitis (6), hemolytic uremic syndrome, pancreatitis, endocarditis, infantile diarrhea, and rapidly progressive glomerulonephritis. Although a viral infection may be strongly suggested by the results of some standard laboratory tests, such as a normal peripheral white blood count (usually less than 12,000), normal cell differential, and cerebral spinal fluid examination which shows no more than 500 white blood cells with a mild elevation in protein and a normal sugar, and by a clinical picture which includes fever, malaise, arthralgias and/or arthritis, photophobia with orbital pain, conjunctivitis, and rash, definitive diagnosis rests with the virology laboratory.

Recent reports have underlined the feasibility of providing enteroviral diagnostic services in large medical centers (3, 12). Rapid diagnosis can now be made, and cost estimates are reasonable. There is no question at all that the availability of these services improves patient care. By confirming viral diagnoses, particularly during epidemics, unnecessary antibiotic therapy is minimized and many unnecessary hospital admissions are avoided. The following section describes an approach to the diagnosis of enteroviral infections which can be implemented in most medical center laboratories.

DESCRIPTION OF AGENTS

The enteroviruses, which include the polioviruses, echoviruses, and coxsackieviruses (1), are members of the picornavirus group of viruses (5), which also includes the rhinoviruses. Many fine review articles are available in this area (9, 11). The enteroviruses are transient inhabitants of the human alimentary tract. They are small particles, 17 to 28 nm in diameter, which have a ribonucleic acid core, are ether- and acid-stable, and are stabilized to 1 h of heat at 50 C by molar $MgCl_2$ and other salts of divalent cations. There are presently 64 distinct serotypes: polioviruses 1–3, echoviruses 1–34 (echovirus 10 has been reclassified reovirus 1, echovirus 28 has been reclassified rhinovirus type 1A, and echovirus 34 is a prime strain of coxsackievirus A24), group A coxsackieviruses 1–24 (coxsackievirus A23 is identical to echovirus 9 and was never formally accepted as a new type), group B coxsackieviruses 1–6, and enterovirus 68 (13, 15). The agent associated with the newly described acute hemorrhagic conjunctivitis (6) and Toluca-1 virus (14) may further increase the number of enteroviruses. Enteroviruses differ from rhinoviruses in the following ways: (i) rhinoviruses are labile in acid solutions of pH 3.0 to 5.0; (ii) rhinoviruses are isolated more readily in cell cultures of human origin such as WI-38 (human embryonic lung), human embryonic kidney (HEK), and human aorta whereas most enteroviruses grow in primary monkey kidney tissue culture cells as well as in WI-38 and HEK, although it should be noted that many exceptions to this rule exist; (iii) rhinoviruses grow best when rolled at 33 C whereas enteroviruses grow best at 36 to 37 C; (iv) rhinoviruses are nonpathogenic for newborn mice whereas many enteroviruses are pathogenic for newborn mice and some of the group A coxsackieviruses grow best in newborn mice; (v) enteroviruses are stabilized to heat by the addition of molar $MgCl_2$ but this is not a consistent property of rhinoviruses; (vi) enteroviruses are shed most readily in feces and also in the throat whereas rhinoviruses are isolated almost entirely from nasal and pharyngeal swabs and washings. These properties of the viruses are obviously important in viral diagnosis.

COLLECTION AND STORAGE OF SPECIMENS

Specimens for enterovirus isolation should be collected as soon after the onset of clinical symptoms as possible. Being transitory inhabitants of the human alimentary tract, the viruses are most readily isolated from feces or rectal swabs and may be recovered from this source for up to 28 days after onset of clinical symptoms. They may also be isolated from throat swabs or washings for 7 to 10 days after the onset of clinical symptoms.

Fecal specimens are the most useful specimens for study and should be collected in 4- to 8-g amounts in leak-proof containers (ice cream cartons or screw-cap jars may be used). They can be held for several hours at 4 C; for longer periods before testing, they should be frozen (−20 C or colder). If stool is unavailable, rectal swabs should be obtained on moist, sterile cotton-tipped applicators. The swabs are placed in an appropriate carrier medium such as veal infusion broth with 0.5% crystallized bovine plasma albumin or 1% fetal calf serum and transported to the laboratory as soon as possible. Ideally, they should be kept at 4 C during transportation. If tissue culture or animal inoculation is to take place within 4 h of collection, swabs should be held at 4 C; if they are to be held longer, they should be frozen at −20 C or colder until inoculated. Any cell culture medium such as Melnick's medium A or B, or Hanks or Earle's balanced salt solution (BSS), may be used in place of veal infusion broth. Throat swabs are handled in a similar manner. It is worth noting that a charcoal medium has been developed for use in transporting specimens from the field to the laboratory (7). Swabs placed in this medium remain stable at ambient or refrigerator temperatures (4 C) for up to 72 h. I have found this medium to be very helpful and effective in field studies when specimens are inoculated within 72 h of collection. Recovery of virus after freezing is very poor.

If throat washings are to be tested, they should be collected by having the patient gargle with an isotonic solution such as phosphate-buffered saline. Patients should then expectorate this material into a sterile vessel for subsequent inoculation.

In cases of central nervous system disease, cerebrospinal fluid (CSF) specimens are most desirable and should be collected in a sterile tube within 5 days of the onset of clinical symptoms. They should be kept at 4 C if they are to be inoculated within 4 h or frozen at −20 C or colder if they are to be kept longer. Vesicular fluid, when available, can be collected in a sterile 1-ml syringe with a 26-gauge needle and eluted into 2 ml of BSS, or it can be obtained on a cotton-tipped applicator and handled as noted above for other swabs. Postmortem tissue specimens may occasionally be sent for examination; these should be placed in BSS and frozen until inoculated.

Serum specimens should be collected as early after onset of clinical symptoms as possible and again at approximately 14 to 28 days after onset of symptoms. Blood should be placed in sterile centrifuge tubes and stored at 4 C until clot retraction is adequate (2 to 24 h). After centrifugation, serum is used for antibody determinations. If virus isolation attempts are to be made from blood, heparinized blood should be used.

DIRECT EXAMINATION OF SPECIMENS

Although electron microscopy has a very real place in rapid viral diagnosis, particularly in differentiating herpes simplex and varicella-zoster from vaccinia, its role in enteroviral diagnosis is limited. A brighter hope for rapid diagnosis rests with immunofluorescence staining of viral antigens (18). A new technique which enables the rapid detection of viral antigens in CSF leukocytes is perhaps the most exciting recent development in this area (19).

CULTIVATION OF ENTEROVIRUSES

Isolation in tissue culture

Isolation of enteroviruses in tissue culture is the method of choice for making the diagnosis of infection. Most laboratories can isolate most of the common enteroviruses by using a combination of two tube culture systems including primary monkey kidney plus one human tissue culture system from among WI-38, HEK, HeLa, and human amnion cells. I prefer rhesus monkey kidney and WI-38 cells for routine enterovirus isolation studies. Tube cultures of monkey kidney, WI-38, HEK, and other cell lines are commercially available from several sources (Flow Laboratories, Rockville, Md.; Mogul Diagnostics, Grand Island, N.Y.; and Microbiological Associates, Bethesda, Md.). For most laboratories, it is probably most convenient to obtain cultures from one or more of these sources. For this reason, details of preparation of tissue cultures will not be described here. The reader is referred to other sources for these details (16).

Using at least two tissue culture systems as noted above, one should be able to isolate most of the enteroviruses. A few of the group A coxsackieviruses, however, require inoculation into newborn mice to be detected.

Since feces is the specimen most likely to yield enteroviruses, the following is offered as an example of how a specimen should be handled in the laboratory:

(1) A 4- to 8-g specimen is made into a 10% suspension in cold, sterile Hanks BSS. The suspension is agitated vigorously and allowed to settle at 4 C. The supernatant fluid is then clarified by centrifugation at 2,500 rpm for 10 min, separated, and treated with 1,000 units of potassium penicillin G and 1,000 μg of streptomycin sulfate per ml or with gentamicin in a final concentration of 200 μg per ml. After incubation at 25 C for 1 h the specimen is again clarified by centrifugation (2,500 rpm for 1 h at 4 C) and is now ready for inoculation.

(2) Tissue culture tubes of primary rhesus monkey kidney and WI-38 cells containing 0.9 ml of fresh maintenance medium are inoculated with 0.1 ml of the specimen. Maintenance medium consists of Melnick's medium B for monkey kidney and Eagle's medium for WI-38 with 2% fetal calf serum (inactivated at 56 C for 30 min), $NaHCO_3$, supplemental L-glutamine for WI-38 cells, and either 100 units of potassium penicillin G and 100 μg of streptomycin sulfate per ml or gentamicin in a final concentration of 200 μg per ml.

(3) Tubes are placed in an incubator and held stationary at 37 C.

(4) Tubes are observed on day 1 for evidence of early cytopathic effect (CPE) or toxicity and thereafter at least every other day for the appearance of typical CPE. This CPE is evidenced by rounding up and shrinking of cells and nuclear pyknosis. The cells may become refractile. This CPE usually begins at the periphery of the cell sheet and eventually involves the entire culture. *Note:* If toxicity of the inoculum is observed (usually evident within 24 h), a subpassage should be made as soon as possible.

(5) Cell cultures are observed for at least 14 days before being discarded. Cell sheets which remain in good condition may be kept for longer periods of observation or passed into new cultures for observation for an additional time period. If cultures are observed for any length of time, medium should be changed about every 4 days.

(6) Isolates may be passed to increase volume and infectivity titer before identification is attempted, or the original harvest may be of sufficient strength to type the isolate directly.

Since optimal management of patients is dependent upon early reporting of laboratory studies, a presumptive diagnosis is of great aid to the physician. This can be done in a surprisingly short period of time and is very accurate if there are experienced personnel in the laboratory. It is made on the basis of the typical picornavirus CPE.

Isolation in mice

In instances where a laboratory desires to attempt to isolate all possible enteroviruses, inoculation of newborn mice is indicated. This is particularly true of certain group A coxsackieviruses. It is best to use mice no more than 1 day of age. Fecal specimens, CSF, throat washings or 10% tissue suspensions should be inoculated by one of three routes: 0.02 ml intracerebrally, 0.05 ml intraperitoneally, or 0.03 ml subcutaneously. The mice should be observed for at least a 14-day period for the development of weakness, progressive flaccid paralysis, and death due to group A coxsackieviruses, or of weakness, tremors, and spastic paralysis due to group B coxsackieviruses.

Mice that develop signs of illness should be sacrificed. Using sterile techniques, remove brain and legs and make them into 20% suspensions. Skinned, eviscerated mouse torso may also be examined. These tissues are then used for further passage and identification procedures.

IDENTIFICATION OF ISOLATES

Usually it is possible to make a presumptive diagnosis of enteroviral disease based on the clinical history of the patient, the time of year when the specimen was obtained, the tissue culture system in which the isolate grew, and the characteristic CPE. Reporting a presumptive diagnosis of viral infection without waiting for the specific typing of the isolate is of real value in the clinical management of the patient.

Specific identification of the serotype rests with serum neutralization, and this is most readily accomplished by use of intersecting pools of hyperimmune sera (8, 17). These may be constructed in many ways, but the most economical one is the Lim-Benyesh-Melnick scheme. The Research Resources Branch (RRB) of the National Institute of Allergy and Infectious Diseases now has available, for all virus diagnostic laboratories, dried equine antisera pools consisting of 42 equine antisera combined into eight pools (10). Detailed directions for use of the pools are supplied by the RRB when pools are shipped. Combination pools are very convenient, but it is prudent to conserve these reagents. Therefore, if an epidemic due to a single serotype is in progress, use of the single hyperimmune serum to identify most isolates is clearly indicated. It should also be noted that it may not be in the best interest of the patient, the community, or the laboratory to attempt to type all isolates. At the present time, since no specific enterovirus therapy is available, it is probably sufficient in many instances for the physician to know simply that an enterovirus has been isolated.

It may be necessary to perform mouse neutralization tests to identify isolates which do not replicate in tissue culture systems. This may be done by titering a suspension of infected mouse torso or brain to determine its LD_{50} and mixing equal amounts of 100 LD_{50} of virus with 20 antibody units of either single or pooled sera. This mixture is incubated for 2 h at 37 C and then inoculated in 0.05-ml amounts intraperitoneally into newborn mice. Virus and serum controls should be included in each test. Mice should be observed for 1 to 14 days for the appearance of paralysis.

Hemagglutination-inhibition (HI) and complement fixation (CF) tests have also been used to identify enterovirus serotypes (11). Only about one-third of enteroviruses hemagglutinate red blood cells (RBC), and this limits the usefulness of this test for routine use. Likewise, not all enteroviruses can be identified by the CF test. For these reasons, these methods will not be described here in detail.

If a virus isolate cannot be identified, it may represent a new enterovirus, a mixture of viruses, or a virus other than an enterovirus. If there is uncertainty about the group to which an isolate belongs, determination of size, nucleic acid, ether stability, and acid lability should determine whether or not the isolate is an enterovirus (4).

SEROLOGICAL DIAGNOSIS OF INFECTION

Neutralization test

No rapid or inexpensive serological screening procedure is presently available to detect antibody titer rises to all 65 enteroviruses. The neutralization test is accurate and type-specific but requires the use of 65 antigens in tissue culture and mouse systems to screen completely for rises in antibody titer. It is really feasible for serological diagnosis only when a virus isolate from the patient is available, when an epidemic due to a single serotype is present, or when a clinical picture such as pleurodynia clearly implicates a small number of antigens such as the group B coxsackieviruses.

Paired sera collected from the patient as soon after the onset of symptoms as possible (acute serum) and 2 to 4 weeks later (convalescent serum) are diluted 1:2, 1:8, 1:32, 1:128, and 1:512 with BSS or maintenance medium. Twofold dilutions (1:2, 1:4, 1:8, etc.) may be preferred by some laboratories. A 0.5-ml sample of each serum dilution is then mixed with an equal amount of virus diluted to contain approximately 100 TCD_{50} per 0.1 ml, and the mixture is incubated for 2 h at 37 C. Virus-serum mixtures are then inoculated in 0.2-ml amounts into the appropriate tissue culture system, usually monkey kidney tube cultures containing 0.9 ml of Melnick's B medium containing $NaHCO_2$ and antibiotics as noted above. Two tissue culture tubes are usually used for each dilution. A control virus titration to determine TCD_{50} is always included. Virus is diluted in 10-fold steps, and 0.1 ml of each dilution is inoculated into monkey kidney tissue culture tubes containing 0.9 ml of Melnick's B medium. Tubes are incubated at 37 C and observed every 2 days for 7 to 10 days. Serum titers are calculated for the 50% end point per 0.1 ml of virus. A fourfold or greater rise in antibody titer is considered significant in making the diagnosis. It should be noted that neutralizing antibody may already be high at the time of onset of clinical symptoms, making interpretation of the test more difficult.

Other serological tests

Other serological tests which may be used include CF, HI, and passive hemmagglutination tests (2, 11). The CF test has limited value in diagnosing enteroviral disease because of major heterotypic cross-reactions among the antigens. Also, many individuals fail to develop homotypic CF antibody. The test has, however, been used successfully in the diagnosis of poliovirus infections. The HI test is relatively easy to perform, and patients who become infected with an enterovirus which hemagglutinates RBC do develop homotypic antibody. They also may develop heterotypic antibody, making the test somewhat nonspecific. The major drawback to the HI test, however, is that only about one-third of the known enteroviruses agglutinate RBC.

A new test, originally developed to screen for rises in antibody to rhinoviruses, has been found to be effective for detecting rises in antibody titer to the picornaviruses (2). This test, a passive hemagglutination test, relies on the use of a coupling reagent, chromic chloride, to attach proteins to indicator erythrocytes. This has made possible the hemagglutination of RBC by antigens which otherwise do not demonstrate this property. I have utilized this technique as a screening test using paired sera collected during an epidemic of coxsackievirus B5 and have found it to be very useful. More work on this test is needed before it can be recommended for diagnostic laboratories.

INTERPRETATION AND REPORTING OF LABORATORY RESULTS

Isolation of an enterovirus from feces or from throat swabs or washings does not necessarily indicate a causal relationship between the virus isolated and the clinical picture presented by the patient from whom the specimen was obtained. It may, in fact, be that the specimen was obtained from a clinically asymptomatic individual. Isolation of an enterovirus does indicate local infection in the sense that enteroviruses are not normal inhabitants of the gastrointestinal tract. Even the demonstration of a fourfold or greater rise in neutralizing antibody titer does not confirm a causal relationship between virus isolated and patient disease. When all factors are weighed, however, and bacterial or other microbial causes are eliminated, isolation of an enterovirus represents good presumptive evidence that the virus is, in fact, the causal agent. If virus is isolated from CSF in clinical aseptic meningitis or meningoencephalitis or from pericardial fluid in pericarditis, the diagnosis of enteroviral etiology is established. In interpreting laboratory results, it is probably best to consult with the physician caring for the patient and, with all of the data available, make a final judgment as to significance of results.

Reporting of results should be made as soon as possible and can be based on a presumptive diagnosis made by observing characteristic CPE in tissue culture. Typing of the agent should follow, but in most clinical situations the knowledge that a virus is associated with the clinical picture is the most useful information.

LITERATURE CITED

1. Committee on the Enteroviruses, N.F.I.P. 1957. The enteroviruses. Amer. J. Pub. Health Nat. Health **47**:1556–1566.
2. Faulk, W. P., G. N. Vyas, C. A. Phillips, H. H. Fudenberg, and K. Chism. 1971. Passive hemagglutination test for anti-rhinovirus antibodies. Nature N. Biol. **231**:101–104.
3. Herrmann, E. C. Jr., D. A. Person, and T. F. Smith. 1972. Experience in laboratory diagnosis of enterovirus infections in routine medical practice. Mayo Clin. Proc. **47**:577–586.
4. Hsiung, G. D. 1965. Use of ultrafiltration for animal virus grouping. Bacteriol Rev. **29**:477–486.
5. International Enterovirus Study Group. 1963. Picornavirus group. Virology **19**:114–116.
6. Kono, R., A. Sasagawa, K. Ishii, S. Sugiura, M. Ochi, H. Matsumiya, Y. Uchida, K. Kameyama, M. Kaneko, and N. Sakurai. 1972. Pandemic of new type of conjunctivitis. Lancet **2**:1191–1194.
7. Leibovitz, A. 1969. A transport medium for diagnostic virology. Proc. Soc. Exp. Biol. Med. **131**:127–130.
8. Lim, K. A., and M. Benyesh-Melnick. 1960. Typing of viruses by combinations of antiserum pools. Application of typing of enteroviruses (coxsackie and echo). J. Immunol. **84**:309–317.
9. Melnick, J. L. 1970. Enteroviruses: vaccines, epidemiology, diagnosis, classification, p. 87–118. *In* J. W. King and W. R. Faulkner (ed.), Critical reviews in clinical laboratory sciences, vol. 1. The Chemical Rubber Co., Cleveland.
10. Melnick, J. L., V. Rennick, B. Hampil, N. J. Schmidt, and H. H. Ho. 1973. Lyophilized combination pools of enterovirus equine antisera: preparation and test procedures for the identification of field strains of 42 enteroviruses. Bull. World Health Organ. **48**:263–268.
11. Melnick, J. L., and H. A. Wenner. 1969. Enteroviruses, p. 529–602. In E. H. Lennette and N. J. Schmidt (ed.), Diagnostic procedures for viral and rickettsial infections, 4th ed. American Public Health Association, Inc., New York.
12. Pearson, G., A. Valdmanis, J. D. Mann, M. E. Becker, and K. R. Wilcox Jr. 1972. The impact of viral diagnostic studies on medical practice: a report of the years' experience with enterovirus isolation in a hospital laboratory. Amer. J. Clin. Pathol. **58**:349–357.
13. Rosen, L., J. L. Melnick, N. J. Schmidt, and H. A. Wenner. 1970. Subclassification of enteroviruses and ECHO virus type 34. Arch. Gesamte Virusforsch. **30**:89–92.
14. Rosen, L., N. J. Schmidt, and J. Kern. 1973. Toluca-1, a newly recognized enterovirus. Arch. Gesamte Virusforsch. **40**:132–136.
15. Schieble, J. H., V. L. Fox, and E. H. Lennette. 1967. A probable new human picornavirus associated with respiratory disease. Amer. J. Epidemiol. **85**:297–310.
16. Schmidt, N. J. 1969. Tissue culture technics for diagnostic virology, p. 79–178. *In* E. H. Lennette and N. J. Schmidt (ed.), Diagnostic procedures for viral and rickettsial infections, 4th ed. American Public Health Association, Inc., New York.
17. Schmidt, N. J., R. W. Greenther, and E. H. Lennette. 1961. Typing of ECHO virus isolates by immune serum pools. The "intersecting serum scheme." J. Immunol. **87**:623–626.
18. Sommerville, R. G. 1968. Rapid diagnosis of viral infections by immunofluorescent staining of viral antigens in leukocytes and macrophages. Progr. Med. Virol. **10**:398–414.
19. Taber, L. H., R. R. Mirkovic, V. Adam, S. S. Ellis, M. D. Yow, and J. L. Melnick. 1973. Rapid diagnosis of enterovirus meningitis by immunofluroescent staining of CSF leukocytes. Intervirology **1**:128–135.

Chapter 79

Rhinoviruses

JACK H. SCHIEBLE

CLINICAL BACKGROUND

The etiological association of rhinoviruses with mild upper respiratory illness in man is well established. Several studies (8, 24, 27, 35) have shown that, in both experimental and naturally acquired infections, antibodies develop to the infecting virus strain and further that the presence of antibodies is generally protective. These and other similar studies have clearly demonstrated the causal relationship of rhinoviruses to the "common cold" syndrome. However, it is important to recognize that etiological distinctions between common cold illnesses cannot be made solely on clinical findings; many unrelated respiratory and nonrespiratory viruses have the potential of inducing clinically similar illnesses.

Characteristically in the common cold there is a prodomal irritation and stuffiness in the nose which is followed rapidly by a sometimes profuse watery discharge. There is frequently a sore throat with a dry cough and occasionally a slight febrile response may be noted. The duration of symptoms in naturally acquired infection ranges from 4 to 24 days, with the mean being 7 to 10 days (10). In one volunteer study the incubation period was found to be less than 24 h (15); however, in natural infections the incubation period varies between 1 and 5 days with a mean of 2 days. Virus shedding appears to begin with the onset of symptoms and may continue for as long as 1 week.

Rhinovirus infections are prevalent throughout the year and often peak during the fall. There are presently 90 different serological immunotypes, but no one type appears to be significantly more important than others in producing disease. For more detailed information on the clinical, pathological, and epidemiological aspect of rhinoviruses, the reader is referred to the excellent reviews of Hamre (9) and Tyrrell (33).

DESCRIPTION OF AGENT

Rhinoviruses are recognized as a separate virus group, and are classified as a subgroup of the human picornaviruses (14, 16, 34). In 1960, a systematic study (33) led to the development of cultural conditions which resulted in the isolation of rhinoviruses from a high proportion of patients with mild respiratory infections. Under these conditions, human embryo kidney cell cultures were maintained in medium of near neutral pH and incubated at 33 C in a roller apparatus. Use of these modified cultural conditions, in conjunction with methods used for the propagation of human fetal diploid cells (12), resulted in the isolation and characterization of numerous new rhinovirus immunotypes (8, 11, 22, 25, 26, 28, 35, 36).

The rhinovirus subgroup currently consists of 89 immunotypes and one subtype (17). Presently, there are additional candidate virus strains under study, and when these strains have been completely characterized the total number of rhinoviruses will probably be between 100 and 110 serological types (V. Hamparian, personal communication).

Rhinoviruses possess many of the biophysical and biochemical properties of enteroviruses and, since certain enteroviruses are frequently encountered in clinical specimens from respiratory disease, it is often necessary to distinguish between these two subgroups. The distinction is easily achieved by means of the acid stability test (5, 18). The infectivity of rhinoviruses is significantly reduced (95% or more) by exposure to pH 3.0 to 5.0 for 3 h at 25 C; such treatment has no effect on the infectivity of enteroviruses. The size of rhinoviruses has been estimated by Gradocol membrane filtration to range from 15 to 30 nm (5, 18); more precise measurements obtained by electron microscopy (1, 20) give diameters ranging from 20 to 25 nm. Rhinoviruses are resistant to 20% ether; hence, lipids are not an essential component of their structure (5, 10, 18). The infectious nucleic acid isolated from rhinoviruses is single-stranded ribonucleic acid (18, 23).

Classification within the rhinovirus group is based upon the serum neutralization reaction, and, although this has proved to be a satisfactory method for establishing a typing classification, some antigenic overlap has recently been observed between certain virus types. Within type 1 there are two subtypes, A and B, which give low-level reciprocal cross-reactions (16), and within type 22 a prime strain, which possesses broader antigenic reactivity than the prototype strain, has been described (29). In addition, low-level reciprocal cross-neutralization has been reported between types 9 and 32, 13 and 41, and 2 and 14 (3, 4). Recent studies in my laboratory have also shown a low reciprocal cross between types 29 and 44.

Complement fixation has been demonstrated with hyperimmune animal sera and human acute and convalescent sera; however, the reliability of the reaction with human sera is highly questionable because of the many heterotypic reactions which occur (2, 21). A direct hemagglutination test has recently been reported for 16 of 55 serotypes examined (32). Hemagglutination occurred preferentially with sheep erythrocytes at a pH of 8 to 9 and at either 4 C or room temperature.

COLLECTION AND STORAGE OF SPECIMENS

Specimens

The choice and method of specimen collection for rhinovirus isolation should be based upon those procedures which will give the highest yield of respiratory tract secretions. Rhinovirus isolations are usually made from nasal and pharyngeal swabs or from nasal washings. Although washings are reported to yield the greatest number of isolates, collection of such specimens is cumbersome, especially under field conditions. Generally, satisfactory rates of rhinovirus isolations are obtained by using a combination of nasal and pharyngeal swabs.

Collection and storage

Specimens should be collected within 3 days, and not later than 4 to 5 days, after the onset of symptoms. If possible, the specimen should be inoculated into cell cultures within 2 to 3 h of collection, and during the interval between collection and inoculation it is best to keep the specimen at approximately 4 C. If storage is necessary, the specimens can be frozen at −70 C in a mechanical freezer; if dry ice is used, the specimen must be stored in a flame-sealed glass ampoule, or other provisions must be made to prevent absorption of CO_2 by the specimen. This is especially important for storage of rhinoviruses which are inactivated at low pH.

The following procedures for specimen collection are recommended.

Nasal washings. Nasal washings can be obtained by instilling 4 or 5 ml of sterile saline into each nostril with the head tilted slightly back; the head is then brought forward and the saline is allowed to flow into a small container held beneath the nose. Bovine serum albumin or gelatin should be added at a final concentration of 0.5% to the washing to stabilize the virus.

Nasal and pharyngeal swabs. A dry cotton swab may be used to swab each nostril, and the swab should be left in the nose a few seconds to absorb as much secretion as possible. Throat swabs are best collected by rubbing the tonsils and back of the pharynx with a dry cotton swab. Both the nasal and pharyngeal swabs are placed in screw-cap vials containing approximately 3 to 5 ml of Tryptose phosphate broth with added bovine serum albumin or gelatin as described above.

DIRECT EXAMINATION

There are presently no procedures or tests for the direct examination of clinical specimens for the presence of rhinoviruses.

CULTIVATION (ISOLATION) OF AGENT

Host systems

Human diploid cell strains, WI-26 or WI-38, because of their sensitivity to rhinoviruses, availability, and ease of handling, are the cell system of choice and are widely used for the isolation of rhinoviruses (8, 22, 28). Cultures can also be readily prepared in the laboratory if human fetal tissue is available (30). Diploid cell strains are grown in Eagle's minimal essential medium (MEM) containing 10% fetal bovine serum. For maintenance, Leibovitz Medium No. 15 with 2% fetal bovine serum will maintain these cells for 2 to 3 weeks without a change of medium. Primary cultures of human embryonic kidney (10, 13) and a line of human aorta cells have also been used successfully (25). Many of these cell cultures can be obtained from commercial sources.

Inoculation of host cell system

For virus isolation attempts, respiratory tract specimens should be treated with antibiotics to suppress the growth of contaminating microorganisms. In this laboratory, a final concentration of 1,000 units of penicillin, 5,000 μg of streptomycin, and 10 μg of amphotericin B per ml has been found to be satisfactory for this purpose. The treated specimens are inoculated in a volume of 0.2 ml into two tube cultures of human fetal diploid cells. Inoculated cultures are incubated at 33 C in a roller apparatus revolving at approximately 12 revolutions per hour. The cultures are observed daily, or on alternate days, for cytopathic effect (CPE) for approximately 2 weeks. If no evidence of infection is observed, one blind passage may be carried out by inoculating 0.1 ml of the tissue culture fluids from the inoculated cultures into fresh cell cultures and observing the new cultures for about 7 days.

Evidence of infection

The growth of rhinoviruses in human fetal diploid cell cultures produces a CPE which can be easily seen under the low-power objective of a light microscope. Typical CPE induced by rhinoviruses is shown in Fig. 1. The first cellular changes are in the appearance of the fibroblast. The typically long slender cell becomes rounded or oval in appearance, and may swell in size, become refractile, and eventually lyse. These changes initially occur in discrete foci throughout the cell sheet but eventually involve all, or nearly all, of the cell sheet.

On occasion, adverse conditions in the cell culture may cause nonspecific changes in cellular morphology which may be confused with specific viral CPE. If this is suspected, a subculture should be carried out as described above. The additional passage not only serves as a check on the specificity of the viral CPE, but also serves to increase the virus titer. Some rhinoviruses require several passages before they become adapted to in vitro growth.

IDENTIFICATION OF AGENT

Neutralization test

A flow scheme for the identification of rhinoviruses is given in Fig. 2. Viruses causing a picornavirus-like CPE can be presumptively identified as either an enterovirus or a rhinovirus by determining their acid stability.

The acid stability test is performed by diluting the test virus 1:10 in Eagle's MEM prepared without sodium bicarbonate (pH 3.0) and also in the same medium buffered to pH 7.0 with tris(hydroxymethyl)aminomethane. Both mixtures are incubated at room temperature for 3 to 4 h. Infectivity titers of both the treated (pH 3.0) and control (pH 7.0) preparations are then determined by use of serial 10-fold dilutions prepared in Hanks balanced salt solution (BSS). Each virus dilution is inoculated in a volume of 0.1 ml into four human fetal diploid cell cultures and observed for 7 to 10 days for evidence of CPE. A virus is considered to be acid-labile if a 100-fold or greater reduction in infectivity titer occurs in the acid-treated preparation as compared to that of the virus control incubated at pH 7.0.

An alternate method is to mix equal volumes of virus-infected tissue culture fluids and 0.1 M sodium citrate-citric acid buffer, pH 4.0; for control purposes, equal volumes of virus suspension and 0.1 M sodium phosphate buffer, pH 7.0, are mixed. The conditions of incubation and assay are the same as those described above.

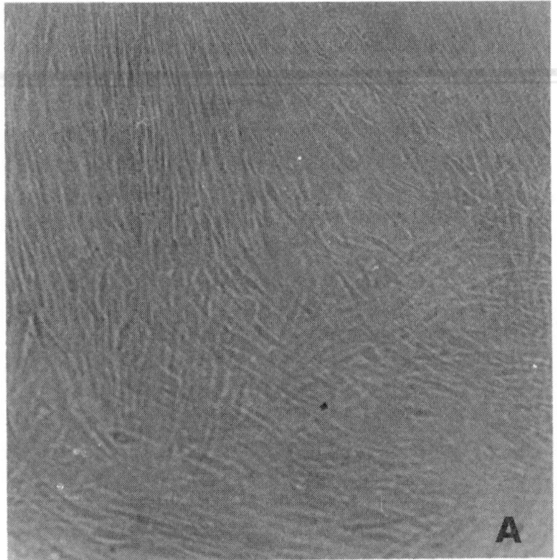

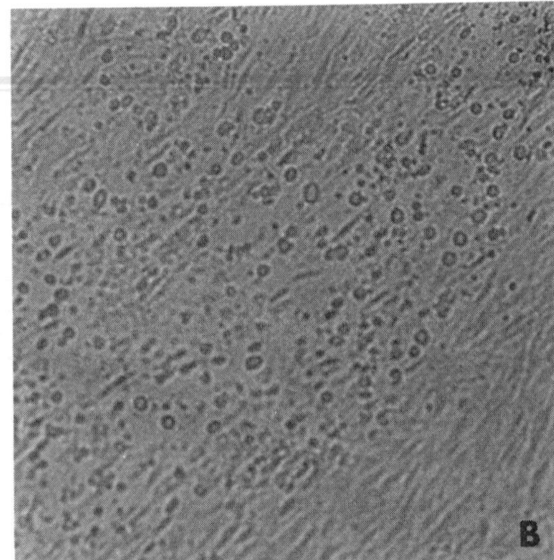

Fig. 1. *Human fetal diploid lung cells. (A) Uninfected. (B) Infected with rhinovirus type 2. ×160.*

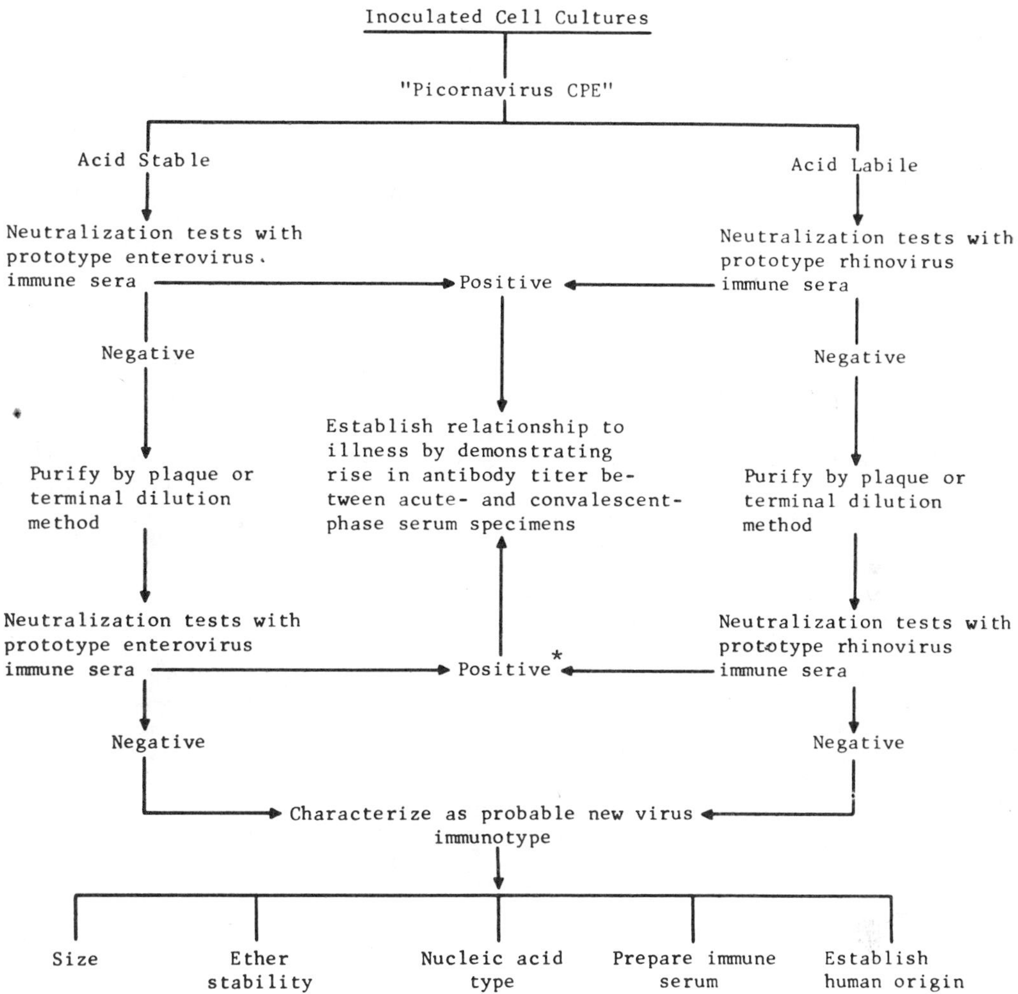

FIG. 2. *Identification of rhinoviruses.*

Acid-labile viruses which cause picornavirus-like CPE can be presumptively identified as rhinoviruses. Definitive identification, however, is based upon neutralization of the isolate by a type-specific rhinovirus immune serum. Identification of rhinoviruses is complicated by the existence of numerous serological types.

Specific identification by the serum neutralization test is greatly facilitated by use of combination or intersecting serum pools (19, 31). In the combination serum pools, a virus is identified by demonstrating neutralization in one, two, or three serum pools; in the intersecting serum scheme, identification is accomplished by demonstrating neutralization with two serum pools sharing a common virus type.

If the test virus is not neutralized by type-specific immune sera for the currently recognized rhinovirus serotypes, it is possible that the isolate may consist of two or more viruses, and therefore the isolate must be purified either by the plaque procedure (6) or by the terminal dilution procedure. For the latter procedure, half-log dilutions of the isolate are prepared in Hanks BSS, and each dilution is inoculated in a volume of 0.1 ml into 10 human fetal diploid cell cultures. The cultures are maintained for 14 to 18 days and observed for CPE. Three successive passages are made from the single positive culture at the limiting (highest) dilution or from the second of two cultures to exhibit CPE at the limiting dilution.

Viral aggregation may be an alternate reason for failure to neutralize a test virus, and although it is not a common problem with rhinoviruses it has been reported (7). Diluting one volume of the test virus with nine volumes of 1% deoxycholate is effective in disaggregating rhinoviruses.

The purified or disaggregated virus should be retested with immune serum for each of the prototype rhinoviruses as previously described. In the event that the test virus is not neutralized, the isolate may possibly represent a new immunological type. However, to establish the isolate as a candidate prototype virus, one must show it to be serologically distinct from the prototype rhinoviruses by reciprocal serum neutralization tests; i.e., in addition to showing that the purified virus isolated is not neutralized by immune sera to each of the prototype rhinoviruses, immune serum prepared with the new virus isolated must show no neutralizing activity for the known prototype viruses.

Viruses shown to be serologically distinct from prototype rhinoviruses should be characterized in terms of their biophysical and biochemical properties (see Fig. 2) prior to submission of the virus as a candidate virus. Details of the methods for these tests have been published (18, 25, 28, 34).

SEROLOGICAL DIAGNOSIS

Serological diagnosis of rhinovirus infection is at present impractical because of the large number of distinct virus types and the lack of a simple serological method for detecting rhinovirus antibody.

Hemagglutination and hemagglutination-inhibition have recently been reported for certain rhinovirus serotypes (32). However, hemagglutination was demonstrable for only 16 of 55 serotypes examined. Thus, until hemagglutination can be demonstrated for a significant number of additional serotypes, this test is presently not practical for the serological diagnosis of rhinovirus infection.

Complement-fixing antigens have been prepared by concentrating virus from infected tissue culture fluids. However, because of the numerous heterotypic reactions which occur with paired human sera, the complement fixation test is of little value in the serological diagnosis of natural rhinovirus infection.

The neutralization test is the only serological test available at this time which can be used for the measurement of rhinovirus antibody responses in man. Antibody responses to natural infection are frequently minimal, and the detection of small amounts of antibody requires that the neutralization test be carefully performed with a small test dose of virus (10 to 30 TCD_{50}). Acute-phase serum specimens should be collected as soon as possible after the onset of symptoms, and convalescent-phase specimens should be obtained approximately 3 weeks later. Sera are separated from the clot and stored at −20 C until needed for testing. The 50% end point neutralization test is performed as follows. All sera are inactivated at 56 C for 30 min. Equal volumes of the test virus dilution and twofold dilutions of serum in Hanks BSS are incubated at room temperature for 2 h, and 0.2-ml amounts of each serum-virus mixture are inoculated into two or four human fetal diploid cell cultures. These are examined for CPE after 2 or 3 days, when a simultaneous virus titration indicates that 10 to 30 TCD_{50} doses of virus are present in the test. Serum neutralization end points are calculated by the method of Reed and Muench and are expressed in terms of the initial serum dilutions. The test is considered positive or significant if there is a fourfold or greater rise in antibody titer to the homologous or infecting virus between the acute- and convalescent-phase serum specimens.

EVALUATION, INTERPRETATION, AND REPORTING OF RESULTS

The laboratory diagnosis of rhinovirus infection is dependent, in the absence of a simple serological method, upon the isolation of the virus. Rhinoviruses are recovered from respiratory tract specimens preferentially in human fetal diploid cells or primary culture of human embryonic kidney cell strains. Once isolated, the viruses can be adapted to heteroploid cells such as KB or HeLa. Adaptation to heteroploid cells usually results in higher virus titers, and infectious fluids from these cells yield potent antigens for use in immune serum production.

Of the many factors contributing to the successful isolation of rhinoviruses, the sensitivity or susceptibility of the host cells is of paramount importance. This may vary depending upon the particular embryo from which the cultures were derived or even with passage levels of the same cell strain.

The physiological condition of cells in culture can be influenced by the buffer capacity of the maintenance medium or the method of cultivation. Whole serum incorporated into the medium may contain nonspecific inhibitors or even specific antibodies to animal viruses which may share antigens with the viruses under study.

Isolates which produce a picornavirus CPE are readily identified as either enteroviruses or rhinoviruses depending on their acid stability. The test is reliable and simple to perform. It is important, however, that the isolate have an infectivity titer of at least $10^{-3.0}$ per ml before the acid stability test is attempted. This will not be a problem with most isolates, but in those few instances where virus titers are inadequate one or two rapid passages in cell cultures are usually sufficient to raise the titer to the minimal level.

In this laboratory, a preliminary report is made of an isolate as rhinovirus, type undetermined, for those isolates which induce picornavirus-like CPE and are acid-labile. A final report is filed when serotyping tests have been successfully completed.

Because of the numerous types of rhinoviruses, serotyping is not a simple procedure. The use of combination or intersecting serum pool schemes provides a relatively easy method for type-specific identification. However, since heterotypic neutralizing activity may be increased by pooling sera, it is advisable to verify the preliminary type identification by demonstrating neutralization of the isolate with approximately 20 antibody units of the individual immune serum.

LITERATURE CITED

1. Brown, E., J. F. E. Newman, and E. J. Stott. 1970. Molecular weight of rhinovirus ribonucleic acid. J. Gen. Virol. **8:**145–148.
2. Chapple, P. J., B. Head, and D. A. J. Tyrrell. 1967. A complement-fixing antigen from an M rhinovirus. Arch. Gesamte Virusforsch. **21:**123–126.
3. Cooney, M. K., and G. E. Kenny. 1970. Reciprocal neutralization cross-reaction between rhinovirus types 9 and 32. J. Immunol. **105:**531–533.
4. Cooney, M. K., G. E. Kenny, R. Tam, and J. P. Fox. 1972. Cross relationship among 37 rhinoviruses demonstrated by virus neutralization with potent monotypic rabbit anti-sera. Infect. Immunity **7:**335–340.
5. Dimmock, N. J., and D. A. J. Tyrrell. 1962. Physicochemical properties of some viruses isolated from common cold (rhinoviruses). Lancet **2:**536–537.
6. Fiala, M., and G. E. Kenny. 1966. Enhancement of rhinovirus plaque formation in human heteroploid cell cultures by magnesium and calcium. J. Bacteriol. **92:**1710–1715.
7. Gwaltney, J. M., Jr., and A. M. Calhoun. 1970. Viral aggregation resulting in the failure to correctly identify an unknown rhinovirus. Appl. Microbiol. **20:**390–392.
8. Hamparian, V. V., A. Ketler, and M. R. Hilleman. 1961. Recovery of new viruses (coryzaviruses) from cases of common cold in human adults. Proc. Soc. Exp. Biol. Med. **108:**444–453.
9. Hamre, D. 1968. Rhinoviruses, p. 1–76. *In* J. L. Melnick (ed.), Monographs in virology, vol. 1. Karger, Basel.
10. Hamre, D., and J. J. Procknow. 1961. Viruses isolated from common colds in the U.S.A. Brit. Med. J. **2:**1382–1385.
11. Hamre, D., and J. J. Procknow. 1963. Virologic studies on common colds among young adult medical students. Amer. Rev. Resp. Dis. **88:**277–281.
12. Hayflick, L., and P. S. Moorhead. 1961. Serial cultivation of human diploid cells strains. Exp. Cell Res. **25:**585–621.
13. Hobson, D., and G. C. Schild. 1960. Virological studies in natural common colds in Sheffield in 1960. Brit. Med. J. **2:**1414–1418.
14. International Subcommittee on Virus Nomenclature. 1963. Picornavirus Group. Virology **19:**114–116.
15. Jackson, G. G., H. F. Dowling, and W. J. Mogabgab. 1960. Infectivity and interrelationships of 2060 and JH viruses in volunteers. J. Lab. Clin. Med. **55:**331–341.
16. Kapikian, A. Z. (Chairman), et al. 1967. Rhinoviruses: a numbering system. Nature (London) **213:**761–762.
17. Kapikian, A. Z. (Chairman), et al. 1971. A collaborative report: rhinoviruses—extension of the numbering system. Virology **43:**524–526.
18. Ketler, A., V. V. Hamparian, and M. R. Hilleman. 1962. Characterization and classification of ECHO 28-rhinovirus-coryzavirus agents. Proc. Soc. Exp. Biol. Med. **110:**821–831.
19. Lim, K. A., and M. Benyesh-Melnick. 1960. Typing of viruses by combination of anti-serum pools. Application of typing of enteroviruses (coxsackie and echo). J. Immunol. **84:**309–317.
20. Mayor, H. D. 1964. Picornavirus symmetry. Virology **22:**156–160.
21. Mogabgab, W. J. 1962. 2060 virus (ECHO 28) in KB cell cultures. Characteristics, complement fixation and antigenic relationships to some other respiroviruses. Amer. J. Hyg. **76:**15–26.
22. Mufson, M. A., R. Kawana, H. D. James, Jr., L. W. Gauld, H. H. Bloom, and R. M. Chanock. 1965. A description of six new rhinoviruses of human origin. Amer. J. Epidemiol. **81:**32–43.
23. Nair, C. N., and K. Lonborg-Holm. 1971. Infectivity and sedimentation of rhinovirus ribonucleic acid. J. Virol. **7:**278–280.
24. Pelon, W., W. J. Mogabgab, I. A. Phillips, and W. E. Pierce. 1957. A cytopathogenic agent isolated from naval recruits with mild respiratory illness. Proc. Soc. Exp. Biol. Med. **94:**262–267.
25. Phillips, C. A., J. L. Melnick, and C. A. Grim. 1965. Characterization of three new rhinovirus serotypes. Proc. Soc. Exp. Biol. Med. **119:**798–801.
26. Phillips, C. A., J. L. Melnick, and C. A. Grim. 1968. Rhinovirus infections in a student population: isolation of five new serologic types. Amer. J. Epidemiol. **87:**447–456.
27. Price, W. H. 1956. The isolation of a new virus associated with respiratory clinical disease in humans. Proc. Nat. Acad. Sci. U.S.A. **42:**892–896.
28. Schieble, J. H., E. H. Lennette, and V. L. Fox. 1968. Rhinovirus: isolation and characterization of three new serologic types. Proc. Soc. Exp. Biol. Med. **127:**324–328.
29. Schieble, J. H., E. H. Lennette, and V. L. Fox. 1970. Antigenic variation of rhinovirus type 22. Proc. Soc. Exp. Biol. Med. **133:**329–333.

30. Schmidt, N. J. 1969. Tissue culture technics for diagnostic virology, p. 79–178. *In* E. H. Lennette and N. J. Schmidt (ed.), Diagnostic procedures for viral and rickettsial diseases, 4th ed. American Public Health Association, Inc., New York.
31. Schmidt, N. J., R. W. Guenther, and E. H. Lennette. 1961. Typing of ECHO virus isolates by immune serum pools. The "intersecting serum scheme." J. Immunol. **87**:623–626.
32. Stott, E. J., and R. A. Killington. 1972. Hemagglutination of rhinoviruses. Lancet **1**:1369–1370.
33. Tyrrell, D. A. J. 1968. Rhinoviruses, p. 68–124. *In* G. Gard, C. Hallauer, and K. F. Meyer (ed.), Virology monographs, vol. 2. Spring-Verlag Inc., New York.
34. Tyrrell, D. A. J., and R. M. Chanock. 1963. Rhinoviruses: a description. Science **141**:152–153.
35. Tyrrell, D. A. J., and R. Parsons. 1960. Some virus isolations from common colds. III. Cytopathic effects in tissue culture. Lancet **1**:239–242.
36. Webb, P. A., J. M. Johnson, and M. A. Mufson. 1964. A description of two newly recognized rhinoviruses of human origin. Proc. Soc. Exp. Biol. Med. **116**:845–852.

Chapter 80

Reoviruses

LEON ROSEN

CLINICAL BACKGROUND

As judged by serological surveys, reovirus infections of man are very common throughout the world, and apparently most are associated with either no, or only mild, clinical manifestations. Reoviruses have been isolated from patients with fever, exanthems, upper and lower tract respiratory disease, gastrointestinal disease (including steatorrhea), central nervous system disease, and hepatitis, but their importance as etiological agents of such illnesses is still unclear. Similarly, reoviruses (mainly type 3) have been isolated from tumor tissue of many patients with Burkitt's lymphoma, but as yet there is no convincing evidence that the association is of etiological significance (2).

DESCRIPTION OF AGENT

Reoviruses are approximately 70 nm in diameter and exhibit icosahedral symmetry. They have no envelope, are resistant to ether, contain a relatively large amount of double-stranded ribonucleic acid, and mature in the cytoplasm of cells. Recently it has been discovered that other viruses, many of which are biologically transmitted by arthropods, share these properties. However, the latter agents differ from the reoviruses in capsid architecture and acid lability, and it has been proposed (13) that they and the reoviruses be considered members of a group of viruses to be termed diplornaviruses. The reoviruses would be considered a subgroup within the diplornaviruses.

Mammalian reoviruses have an exceptionally wide host range and have been recovered from many different species. Isolates from both man and lower mammals can be classified into three serotypes which have been designated types 1, 2, and 3 (7). Strains of the same serotype from various mammals are indistinguishable from one another. Reoviruses which have been recovered from chickens are distinguishable from the three mammalian types. Because of their many unique properties, reoviruses have been studied extensively by molecular biologists and the literature on these agents is now voluminous. A comprehensive review is available of the data published on reoviruses prior to the end of 1966 (8).

COLLECTION AND STORAGE OF SPECIMENS

Most reoviruses recovered in both natural and experimental infections of man have been obtained from fecal specimens, either from stools or from rectal swabs. Isolates have also been reported from throat swabs, nasal secretions, urine, blood, cerebrospinal fluid, and various organs obtained at autopsy. Although virus excretion has been observed to continue for several weeks in some human infections, it is suggested that specimens be obtained as early as possible in the course of illness and, if possible, on several successive days.

The methods of collection and storage of specimens are described in chapter 71.

ISOLATION OF AGENT

Host systems

Mammalian reoviruses replicate and produce cytopathic effects (CPE) in a remarkably wide variety of cell cultures, including cultures derived from domestic animals as well as those of primate origin. The type of cell culture which has been the most widely used for recovery of reoviruses from clinical specimens is *Macaca* (rhesus) monkey kidney. In addition, KB cells, HeLa cells, human fibroblasts, stable human amnion lines, primary human kidney, primary *Cercopithecus* kidney, BSC-1 cells, and L cells, among others, have been used in experimental studies.

Primary *Macaca* kidney cell cultures are satisfactory for routine isolation, but primary human kidney should be used in very critical work when it is desired that the possibility of latent reovirus infection in the cells themselves be excluded. Reovirus type 1 has been recovered frequently from simian kidney cell cultures maintained for long periods of time, suggesting that the virus was present in a latent state in the cells. However, latent reovirus infection has not been encountered when *Macaca* kidney cells have been used as described below, nor has reovirus been recovered from uninoculated human kidney cell cultures, even when the latter have been maintained for long periods of time.

Reoviruses can sometimes be isolated directly in newborn mice, but few isolates have been obtained in this way and cell cultures are believed to be more sensitive. A possible source of error when mice are used is the presence of preexisting reovirus type 3 infection in most colonies of laboratory mice.

Conditions of incubation

Tube cultures of primary kidney cells are used when a confluent monolayer of cells has appeared. It is important that the cultures be washed free from serum before use, since it is likely that any mammalian serum present in the growth medium contains antibodies to one or more reovirus serotypes. Washing is accomplished by replacing the growth medium with three successive changes of 1 ml of Hanks balanced salt solution containing 100 units of penicillin and 100 μg of streptomycin per ml. After the last change, 1 ml of medium 199 or other suitable serum-free medium with the same concentration of antibiotics may be added as a maintenance medium.

The specimen is then inoculated into one or more culture tubes in 0.1-ml amounts. Tubes are incubated in a stationary state at 36 to 37 C and are observed microscopically every 2 or 3 days for 21 days. At the end of this time interval, 0.1 ml of the supernatant fluid of each tube is passed to a fresh culture tube which has been prepared in the same manner as the original tube. The passage tubes are incubated and observed for 7 days. Maintenance fluid is not changed on either the original or the passage tube, and the isolation tubes are ordinarily kept for 21 days, even though the cell sheet may have degenerated before then. However, if it appears from microscopic examination that cell degeneration is due to bacterial or fungal contamination, the isolation attempt is considered unsatisfactory.

The CPE typical of the reoviruses is often not seen in isolation tubes which are inoculated with relatively small amounts of virus. However, after 21 days, even a very small amount of virus usually will have increased to the extent that typical cytopathic change is seen in the passage tube. Even though the *Macaca* kidney cultures used in the isolation procedure could be maintained in better condition by periodic changing of the maintenance medium, such a procedure usually is not undertaken because of the increased risk of viral cross-contamination and because it is not necessary for the isolation of reoviruses.

Recognition of infection

Reoviruses usually can be distinguished from other viruses that are encountered in human fecal specimens by the nature of their CPE in unstained *Macaca* kidney cultures. The cells become granular and do not slough off the glass as readily as do cells affected by most enteroviruses. Often they remain fastened to the glass by a single process and flutter in the medium as the tube is agitated during microscopic examination. The typical effect is often confused by inexperienced personnel with nonspecific cellular degeneration. Doubtful cases can be resolved by additional cell culture passages. One way to gain experience is to observe the effect of various dilutions of a known reovirus in *Macaca* kidney cultures of good quality.

Reoviruses can also be recognized by the cytoplasmic inclusions visible by conventional microscopy in stained preparations of infected cell cultures and by their intra- or extracellular morphology when examined with an electron microscope.

IDENTIFICATION OF AGENT

Reoviruses are usually identified as to serotype by hemagglutination-inhibition (HI) techniques. All isolates so far described have the property of agglutinating human erythrocytes, although this phenomenon is sometimes difficult to demonstrate with strains of type 3. Isolates are tested for the presence and titer of hemagglutinin as follows.

Titration of hemagglutinins

Human type O erythrocytes are collected in Alsever's solution, by addition of 10 to 20 ml of blood to 50 ml of the solution. The cells are then washed three times in dextrose-gelatin-Veronal (DGV) solution and can be stored as a 10% suspension in this solution for at least 1 week. If the erythrocytes are to be used within 24 h after collection, they can be washed and stored temporarily in 0.85% NaCl.

Slightly higher titers have been reported when reoviruses are tested with human type A or AB erythrocytes rather than with type O erythrocytes (3), but the latter are more practical for use in HI tests with human sera.

To minimize variation in the number of erythrocytes employed in titrations of hemagglutinin and in HI tests, the concentration of cells is standardized by means of a spectrophotometer. The standard value is determined by allowing 0.2-ml amounts of various concentrations of human erythrocytes in 0.85% NaCl to settle at room temperature in test tubes (12 by 75 mm) with hemispherical bottoms. The lowest concentration of cells producing a solid button of cells after complete sedimentation is chosen as the standard. The optical density of this test preparation is determined at a wavelength of 490 nm on a spectrophotometer, and thereafter all erythrocyte suspensions are made up to this value. A simpler, but less satisfactory, technique is to prepare a 0.75% suspension of erythrocytes in 0.85% NaCl based on the packed-cell volume.

Supernatant fluid from infected tube cultures is tested for hemagglutination after the cell sheets have been completely destroyed by the virus and after the cultures have been frozen and thawed once. Fluid from two or more culture tubes is usually pooled (before testing) so that there is enough hemagglutinin to complete the identification procedure. Serial twofold dilutions of the fluid are prepared in 0.85% NaCl in 12 by 75 mm test tubes. Dilutions should range between 1:2 and 1:1,024, and each tube should contain 0.4 ml. The standard erythrocyte suspension is then added in 0.2-ml amounts. The tubes are shaken and the erythrocytes are allowed to settle at room temperature. The highest dilution of cell culture fluid which shows a 1+ pattern (4) of sedimentation is taken as the end point, and this tube is considered to contain 1 unit of hemagglutinin.

It is usually possible to demonstrate agglutination of human erythrocytes by strains of reovirus types 1 and 2 in any passage fluid from *Macaca* kidney cultures. Strains of type 3 sometimes have low titers or give negative results when first tested. Thus far, it has always been possible to obtain titers of hemagglutinin sufficiently high (20 units per ml) for purposes of identification for all strains of type 3 by testing additional passage levels. Hemagglutinin titers of type 3 strains are not necessarily increased with continued cell culture passage. Rather, it appears, for reasons unknown, that the multiplication of virus in one lot of cell cultures simply results in the production of a higher titer of hemagglutinin than does multiplication in another, grossly similar, lot of cultures.

Preparation of typing sera

Type-specific immune sera can be prepared in guinea pigs, chickens, and geese (1, 7). Since the sera of guinea pigs frequently contain HI antibodies against one or more reovirus serotypes, preimmunization sera should be tested against antigens of each of the three serotypes before animals of this species are employed for immune serum production.

Guinea pigs can be immunized by instilling 0.1 ml of undiluted cell culture fluid into each nostril of an anesthetized animal. The virus titer of the fluid is not critical, since reoviruses multiply in guinea pigs after intranasal inoculation. (It should be noted that the infected guinea pigs can transmit their infection to animals housed in the same cage.) Animals should be exsanguinated as soon as a trial bleeding indicates that a sufficiently high titer of homotypic HI antibody ($\geq$1:160) has appeared (usually 2 to 3 weeks after inoculation). The final serum also must be tested to determine whether the animal has responded with only a type-specific reaction. Some animals develop heterotypic antibodies. An immune serum is considered satisfactory if it has a homotypic HI titer of at least 1:160 and heterotypic titers of less than 1:10. The preimmunization serum of each animal yielding a satisfactory immune serum should be preserved for reference purposes, i.e., for use in the event that equivocal results are obtained in typing an isolate with the postimmunization serum. Considerable antigenic variation has been noted among strains of type 2, and it may be necessary to prepare several immune sera for this serotype with different strains used as antigens.

Preimmunization sera of chickens and geese which are to be used for immune serum production should also be tested for HI antibodies against mammalian reoviruses. Chickens can be immunized by a series of three intramuscular inoculations of 1 ml of undiluted cell culture fluid given 1 week apart, followed by exsanguination 1 week after the last inoculation. Geese can be immunized by an initial inoculation of 10 ml of cell culture fluid intraperitoneally and 5 ml intravenously, followed by 5 ml intraperitoneally on day 15, 5 ml intravenously on day 27, 2 ml intramuscularly on day 40, and exsanguination on day 50. Domestic fowl apparently do not transmit mammalian reoviruses to one another and can be housed in the same cage. However, as in guinea pigs, postimmunization sera should be tested for homotypic and heterotypic antibodies, and preimmunization sera should be preserved. Most mammalian species will respond with heterotypic antibodies when immunized with repeated parenteral inoculations of a single reovirus serotype.

Satisfactory immune sera can also be obtained by careful selection of sera from humans or cattle with naturally acquired antibodies (7). Individual sera are tested against antigens of each of the three serotypes until some are found which have the desired homotypic titers and do not have heterotypic titers.

Hemagglutination-inhibition test

The HI test for typing isolates is carried out as follows. The typing sera are adsorbed with kaolin by mixing a 1:5 dilution of serum in 0.85% NaCl with an equal volume of a 25% suspension of acid-washed kaolin in 0.85% NaCl (25 g of kaolin + 100 ml of saline solution) and allowing the mixture to stand for 20 min at room temperature. The mixture is then centrifuged briefly to sediment the kaolin, and the decanted supernatant fluid is considered a 1:10 dilution of serum. After this treatment, the sera are adsorbed with human type O erythrocytes to remove any agglutinins for this type of cell which might be present. This is done by adding 0.1 ml of a 50% suspension of erythrocytes to each 1.0 ml of the 1:10 dilution of serum and allowing the mixture to stand for 1 h at approximately 4 C. The supernatant fluid is then decanted and is ready for use. The sera are not inactivated.

It is known that kaolin removes some antibody from serum, and alternative methods of removing nonspecific serum inhibitors have been proposed (6, 11). However, the other methods are more complicated, and it has not been demonstrated that they offer any advantages from a practical point of view.

The HI test is set up by adding 0.2-ml amounts of hemagglutinin diluted in 0.85% NaCl to contain 20 units per ml (4 units per 0.2 ml) to 0.2-ml amounts of serial twofold dilutions of serum in 0.85% NaCl. Each serum is used from a dilution of 1:10 to, or beyond, its end point. The mixtures are shaken briefly and are then allowed to stand for 1 h at room temperature before the addition of 0.2-ml amounts of the standard erythrocyte suspension. The erythrocytes are allowed to settle at room temperature, and the titer of a serum is taken as that dilution which completely inhibits agglutination. The lowest dilution of each serum used is tested for the presence of erythrocyte agglutinins by substituting 0.2 ml of saline solution for the antigen. An antigen titration is also included in the test.

An isolate is considered typed if it is inhibited at a titer of at least 1:40 by one of the typing antisera, and not at a dilution of 1:10 by the others. Because of the antigenic heterogeneity of type 2 strains (5), it may sometimes be necessary to prepare an antiserum against the isolated strain to demonstrate a relationship to this serotype.

SEROLOGICAL DIAGNOSIS AND INTERPRETATION

Most diagnostic serology of reovirus infections has been done with the HI test. Not only is this procedure simpler in general than either the neutralization test or the complement fixation (CF) test, but the latter two procedures are also less satisfactory for diagnostic purposes in reovirus infections for the following reasons. In the neutralization tests, a relatively large amount of test virus is required to attain CPE before the tissue cultures degenerate spontaneously. Consequently, small amounts of antibody are difficult to detect. In the CF test, it is difficult or impossible to detect CF antibodies in the convalescent sera of many infected individuals. In other words, both tests are less sensitive than the HI test. When CF antibodies are present, they apparently are group-specific rather than type-specific.

A microneutralization test for reoviruses has been described as somewhat more sensitive than the conventional tube neutralization test (12) but does not appear to offer any particular advantage for the diagnosis of human infection. A method for preparing relatively potent reovirus CF antigens has also been described (10), but the use of such antigens in the diagnosis of human infection has not been reported.

It has been possible to demonstrate a fourfold or greater rise in homologous HI antibody in practically all natural or experimental reovirus infections which have been observed in man. Individuals infected with reovirus type 3 almost invariably show only a homotypic HI response, whereas those infected with types 1 or 2 often develop heterotypic antibody also (9). The heterotypic titers are usually, but not always, lower than the homotypic titers.

HI antibodies are present 21 days after the experimental infection of man, but may appear earlier. Ordinarily they can be detected for at least 1 year after natural infection, and they probably persist for much longer periods of time. Since reovirus antibodies are very common in human sera, it is essential that paired sera be employed for diagnostic purposes. A fourfold or greater rise in titer is considered a positive result.

HI tests are carried out by a technique similar to that already described for typing reovirus isolates. The test antigens are prepared with representative strains or with homotypic strains in the manner described previously. All sera are adsorbed with kaolin, but it is usually not necessary to adsorb human sera with erythrocytes.

Paired sera are always run in the same test and are usually titrated in twofold dilutions from 1:10 through 1:320 against 4 units of hemagglutinin of each of the three serotypes. Because of the antigenic heterogeneity of type 2 strains, it may be necessary to use more than one antigen of this type. If available, an antigen prepared from a strain isolated from the patient would be the most satisfactory in type 2 infections. This procedure has not been found necessary for types 1 and 3.

LITERATURE CITED

1. Behbehani, A. M., L. C. Foster, and H. A. Wenner, 1966. Preparation of type-specific antisera to reoviruses. Appl. Microbiol. **14**:1051–1053.
2. Bell, T. M. 1967. Viruses associated with Burkitt's tumor. Progr. Med. Virol. **9**:1–34.
3. Brubaker, M. M., B. West, and R. J. Ellis. 1964. Human blood group influence on reovirus hemagglutination titers. Proc. Soc. Exp. Biol. Med. **115**:1118–1120.
4. Chanock, R. M., and A. B. Sabin. 1953. The hemagglutinin of St. Louis encephalitis virus. I. Recovery of stable hemagglutinin from the brains of infected mice. J. Immunol. **70**:271–285.
5. Hartley, J. W., W. P. Rowe, and J. B. Austin. 1962. Subtype differentiation of reovirus type 2 strains by hemagglutination-inhibition with mouse antisera. Virology **16**:94–96.
6. Mann, J. J., R. D. Rossen, J. R. Lehrich, and J. A. Kasel. 1967. The effect of kaolin on immunoglobulins: an improved technique to remove the nonspecific serum inhibitor of reovirus hemagglutination. J. Immunol. **98**:1136–1142.
7. Rosen, L. 1960. Serologic grouping of reoviruses by hemagglutination-inhibition. Amer. J. Hyg. **71**:242–249.
8. Rosen, L. 1968. Reoviruses, p. 73–107. *In* Virology monographs, vol. 1. Springer-Verlag, New York.
9. Rosen, L., H. E. Evans, and A. Spickard. 1963. Reovirus infections in human volunteers. Amer. J. Hyg. **77**:29–37.
10. Schell, K., R. J. Huebner, and H. C. Turner. 1966. Concentration of complement fixing viral antigens. Proc. Soc. Exp. Biol. Med. **121**:41–46.
11. Schmidt, N. J., J. Dennis, and E. H. Lennette. 1964. Studies on filtrates from cultures of a psychrophylic *Pseudomonas sp.* which inactivate nonspecific serum inhibitors for certain hemagglutinating viruses. J. Immunol. **93**:140–147.
12. Schmidt, N. J., E. H. Lennette, and M. F. Hanahoe. 1966. Microneutralization test for the reoviruses. Application to detection and assay of antibodies in sera of laboratory animals. Proc. Soc. Exp. Biol. Med. **121**:1268–1275.
13. Verwoerd, D. W. 1970. Diplornaviruses: a newly recognized group of double-stranded RNA viruses. Progr. Med. Virol. **12**:192–210.

Chapter 81

Arboviruses

ROBERT E. SHOPE

CLINICAL BACKGROUND

The arboviruses are a heterogeneous group of animal viruses, usually biologically transmitted by hematophagous arthropods (mosquitoes, ticks, *Phlebotomus*, *Culicoides*). One or more of the following syndromes may be associated with human infection: fever, encephalitis, hemorrhagic fever, rash, acute arthritis, hepatitis, or hemolytic-uremic syndrome. Subclinical infection is common. The virus may be recovered from blood, and occasionally from cerebrospinal fluid or throat washings. At autopsy, it may be recovered from the central nervous system, liver, and spleen. However, isolation attempts are frequently unsuccessful, and diagnosis must depend on serological tests.

DESCRIPTION OF AGENTS

Important new world human pathogens include the viruses of eastern, western, Venezuelan, St. Louis, Powassan, and California encephalitis, yellow fever, dengue, Oropouche, Caraparu, Guaroa, Chagres, and Colorado tick fever. These viruses contain ribonucleic acid and are spherical or bullet-shaped; most have an essential lipid envelope.

The laboratory host of choice is the baby mouse. Other, less susceptible hosts are wet chicks, hamsters, primary tissue cultures (chick embryo, hamster kidney), and cell culture lines (Vero, BHK-21, HeLa).

Arboviruses pass 0.22-μm, and in many cases 0.1-μm, membrane filters or equivalent. They are readily heat-inactivated, and most of them agglutinate chick and goose red cells. Most are inactivated by sodium deoxycholate (SDC), di-ethyl ether, and chloroform.

Serological grouping is done by use of polyvalent sera in complement-fixation (CF), hemagglutination-inhibition (HI), and neutralization tests. Typing is done by use of type-specific sera in these same tests. Arboviruses embrace five taxonomic groups (Alphavirus, Flavivirus, Bunyavirus, Rhabdovirus, and Orbivirus) defined by physical characteristics including appearance by electron microscopy, but these groupings are not generally useful to the diagnostic laboratory.

COLLECTION AND STORAGE OF SPECIMENS

Virus isolation is usually successful only if specimens are obtained within the first few days of illness. For virus isolation, collect blood, cerebrospinal fluid, and brain or other organs aseptically; refrigerate specimens at 4 C. Separate serum from clot. Heparanized (0.16 mg/ml) whole blood or homogenized clots are satisfactory for virus isolation and are preferable to serum for some viruses (Colorado tick fever). If immediate inoculation of specimen is not possible, store material at −60 C or colder. Store in sealed ampoules if dry ice is used. Collect throat washings in 0.75% bovine albumin in phosphate buffer (BAP), prepared from 0.12 M NaCl, 0.02 M sodium phosphate buffer, and bovine albumin (fraction V) powder (final pH 7.2).

For antibody study, collect acute-phase and 3-week or later convalescent-phase sera, and store at 4 C or colder. Specimens may be shipped without refrigeration.

For long-term virus storage, add 50% normal serum or 7.5% BAP, and store at −60 C or colder. Freeze-drying is excellent for preservation of both virus and antibody.

ISOLATION OF VIRUS

Preparation of specimen

Mince the tissue with scissors and grind in a mortar or tissue grinder, or use a homogenizer. Make a 10% suspension in 0.75% BAP, and centrifuge it at 2,000 rpm for 10 min. If bacterial contamination is suspected, centrifuge the suspension for 1 h at 10,000 rpm in the cold (4 C) or add penicillin (1,200 units/ml) and streptomycin (10 mg/ml). Serum and cerebrospinal fluid are inoculated without preparation or dilution.

Mouse inoculation

The mouse is the animal of choice. Inoculate 0.015 ml intracerebrally into one or two litters of 1- to 4-day-old Swiss mice from a colony as free as possible of contaminating murine viruses. Observe the animals for 21 days for illness (lethargy, nonfeeding, tremor, loss of equilibrium, alopecia, paralysis, apnea, cyanosis, hyperexcitability, clonus, circling) or death. Kill such mice by exsanguination (ether and chloroform inactivate arboviruses) and passage a pool of liver and brain intracerebrally until mice uniformly sicken. Test harvested tissues from each passage for bacterial sterility.

Alternative laboratory hosts

If wet chicks are used, inoculate them subcutaneously; inoculate baby hamsters intracerebrally. Monolayer cell cultures in tubes, i.e., chick embryo, hamster kidney, Vero, BHK-21, HeLa, LLC-MK_2, and others, should be inoculated with 0.1 ml and observed for cytopathic effect (CPE); cell cultures under agar should also be inoculated with 0.1 ml and observed for plaques (3, 8, 9, 14).

If dengue virus is suspected and mice do not sicken, make a blind passage of brain tissue on the seventh to ninth day, and test survivors for humoral antibody or resistance to intracerebral challenge with mouse-adapted dengue virus. For detection of dengue virus in cell cultures, challenge with an enterovirus (6) if there is no CPE.

Reisolation of the virus is important to rule out laboratory contamination or a murine virus. Alternatively, it is necessary to show antibody rise in an infected natural host to prove the validity of the isolation.

IDENTIFICATION OF VIRUS

Characterization of isolate

Pathogenicity for laboratory hosts, incubation periods, infectivity titers by various routes of inoculation, filterability, and sensitivity to chemicals may aid in identification. A comprehensive listing of these properties for 257 arboviruses is available elsewhere (11–13).

The World Health Organization Regional Reference Centre for Arboviruses at the Vector-borne Diseases Branch of the Center for Disease Control (P.O. Box 2087, Fort Collins, Colo. 80521) and the International Centre at the Yale Arbovirus Research Unit (60 College St., New Haven, Conn. 06510) do special diagnostic tests, accept presumed arboviral isolates for identification, and offer consultation and technical training.

Sodium deoxycholate test

Inactivation by SDC is a reliable method of ruling out enteroviruses such as encephalomyocarditis virus, mouse encephalomyelitis virus, and coxsackievirus, but not myxoviruses, poxviruses, rabiesvirus, lymphocytic choriomeningitis virus, and herpes simplex virus. For the SDC test, prepare a 10% virus (usually brain) suspension in 0.75% BAP, and centrifuge at 10,000 rpm for 1 h at 4 C. Mix the supernatant fluid with an equal volume of 1:500 SDC in 0.75% BAP, and mix equal volumes of virus and BAP as a control. After incubating both mixtures for 1 h at 37 C, prepare 10-fold dilutions of SDC and control mixtures, and inoculate them intracerebrally into baby mice. A reduction of titer of 1 $\log_{10}$ or more is significant. Include an SDC test of a known arbovirus and an enterovirus as a control. Enteroviruses may give a higher titer in SDC than in the control. Arboviruses of the Orbivirus taxon (Colorado tick fever) are relatively insensitive to SDC.

Inactivation of arboviruses by ether or chloroform is equally satisfactory in distinguishing them from enteroviruses.

SEROLOGICAL IDENTIFICATION

Principle

Compare the new virus by the neutralization, CF, and HI tests with viruses known, or suspected to be, in the geographic region of isolation (2). Initially, test the new virus against polyvalent sera (prepared with agents known to exist in the geographic area). (Polyvalent sera are available from the Research Resources Branch, National Institute of Allergy and Infectious Diseases, Building 31, Room 7A-30, Bethesda, Md. 20014.) Once grouping is accomplished, test the virus with type-specific sera against viruses in the group. For definitive identification, the new virus and homologous immune serum must be compared in reciprocal cross tests with type strain reagents.

Mouse-pathogenic viruses which might be isolated in the United States and for which sera should be prepared are listed in Table 1.

Preparation of immune serum

The animal of choice is the mouse. Alternatively, guinea pigs, rabbits, monkeys, or horses are used. Mice are preferred because they are susceptible to most arboviruses, they do not usually produce mouse tissue antibody, and the serum is useful in CF, HI, and neutralization tests. Immunize mice with uncentrifuged, infected 10% mouse brain suspension in saline according to the following schedule: 0.2 ml intraperitoneally (ip) on days 1 and 30; bleed on day 37 (alternative schedule: 0.2 ml ip on days 1, 3, 10, 15 and 20; bleed on day 27). For polyvalent (grouping) sera, immunize with a mixture of viruses (polyvalent inoculum). For type-specific sera, use a single virus inoculum.

TABLE 1. *Mouse-pathogenic viruses occurring in the United States (including Puerto Rico and the Virgin Islands)*

Group	Virus
Group A	Venezuelan encephalitis Eastern encephalitis Western encephalitis
Group B	Cowbone Ridge Modoc St. Louis encephalitis Powassan Dengue-3 U.S. bat salivary gland Montana *Myotis* leukoencephalitis Yellow fever[a]
Supergroup Bunyamwera	Tensaw Cache Valley California (and several closely related viruses) Trivittatus Buttonwillow Mermet Patois Pahayokee Shark River Mahogany Hammock Gumbo Limbo Lokern Main Drain Bocas
Group vesicular stomatitis (VS)	VS-Indiana VS-New Jersey
Group Turlock	Turlock
Other groups and ungrouped	Hart Park Colorado tick fever Hughes Silverwater Bluetongue Epizootic hemorrhagic disease of deer Farallon Kern Canyon Lone Star Mono Lake Yaquina Head Sawgrass
Nonarbovirus, SDC-sensitive	Tamiami Lymphocytic choriomeningitis Herpes simplex Poxviruses Newcastle disease Rabies

[a] May be recovered from individuals inoculated with live, attenuated virus vaccine.

If the virus is lethal ip, inactivate a 10% brain suspension by incubation for 1 h at 37 C in 0.1% β-propiolactone in normal saline.

Neutralization test

The constant serum-virus dilution method, with inoculation of baby mice intracebrally, is uniformly applicable to all arboviruses. Other types of neutralization tests vary as to the age of the animal, route of inoculation, and temperature and time of incubation used (7, 10). (The constant virus-serum dilution test is commonly used in tissue culture studies.) Use 1- to 4-day-old Swiss mice and randomize the babies. Inoculate them intracerebrally with 0.015 ml/mouse. Use 0.75% BAP as diluent. Prepare virus stock as a 10 or 20% brain (liver and serum used in some cases) suspension from sick mice. Centrifuge the stock virus at 10,000 rpm for 1 h at 4 C.

Titrate part of the supernatant fluid under test conditions, and store the remainder at −60 C.

Make serial 10-fold virus dilutions, changing pipettes with each dilution. The number of dilutions to be used is determined from pretitration of the stock virus. In the run, include control negative and control positive sera with the test sera. Each serum is tested undiluted against several 10-fold dilutions of the virus. Shake the serum-virus mixtures and incubate them for 1 h at 37 C. Hold mixtures in an ice bath during inoculation, and inoculate at least six mice intracerebrally per dilution. Record deaths over a 2-week period, or at least until 3 days after the last death. Calculate the log LD_{50} for each test and control serum by the method of Reed and Muench. The log neutralization index (LNI) is the difference between the log LD_{50} of the control negative serum and the test serum.

Sera stored for long periods may lose neutralizing capacity. This is restored by performing the test ip or by inactivating the test serum and adding accessory factor (normal *rhesus* or human serum freshly collected) in a volume equal to that of the test serum.

Complement fixation test

See chapter 71 for details of the procedure.

Antigen preparation. Sucrose-acetone-extracted mouse brain (or liver) is the preferred antigen because it is useful in both CF and HI tests (4). Alternatively, 10% brain in Veronal buffer can be used as a CF antigen.

Use a hood for safety. Prepare brains (20%, wt/vol) in 8.5% sucrose by use of a blender, and express the mixture through an 18-gauge needle into 20 volumes (20 times the volume of the sucrose suspension) of chilled acetone. Shake thoroughly, and then decant the acetone. Immediately add 20 volumes of acetone and shake again; the sediment should appear as a finely dispersed particulate. Let stand for 1 h at 4 C without shaking. Carefully decant the acetone and dry the sediment (vacuum pump for 1 h).

Rehydrate the powder with normal saline in a volume twice the original brain weight, and centrifuge at 10,000 rpm for 30 min. The supernatant fluid is the antigen.

Each test should have the following controls: (i) for each serum dilution, 1 drop each of serum, dilute complement (2 units/0.025 ml), and Veronal buffer to detect anticomplementary activity in serum; (ii) for each serum dilution, 1 drop each of serum, complement, and normal antigen, 1:4 (or unrelated antigen), to detect mouse tissue reactivity of serum; (iii) for titration complement, eight wells containing 2 drops of complement from master tubes and 1 drop of 1:4 antigen to detect any anticomplementarity or procomplementarity of the antigen.

For identification of isolates, antigen made from the new isolate is used in two dilutions: the optimal dilution, as determined in grid titration with homologous serum (usually 1:32 to 1:64), and the lowest dilution (most concentrated antigen) which is not significantly anticomplementary (usually 1:4). The antigen is tested with polyvalent sera to determine the group, and then with type-specific sera to determine type. Definitive identification involves reciprocal cross CF tests, with the use of antigen and serum of the new isolate and antigen and serum of the type virus in a checkerboard scheme.

Fluorescent-antibody test

The indirect fluorescent-antibody (FA) test is used for Colorado tick fever (5) and may be adapted for other arboviruses. BHK-21 cell cultures are inoculated with virus; after 24 h, cells are removed from the culture vessel with 0.25% trypsin in phosphate-buffered saline (PBS), pH 7.5, and cells are concentrated to give 2.0×10^7 cells per ml. Smears of 0.05 ml of cells are placed on microscope slides, air-dried, fixed in acetone at room temperature, air-dried again, and stored at −65 C.

Test serum and known positive and negative control sera are inactivated at 56 C for 30 min, diluted serially in a 20% suspension of beef brain in PBS, pH 7.3, and then added to virus-infected cell smears. Test serum is added to uninfected cells as a control. Slides are incubated at 36 C for 20 min, rinsed briefly in PBS, washed twice for 10 min in PBS, pH 7.3, and rinsed in distilled water. Rabbit anti-species-specific serum conjugated to fluorescein isothiocyanate is added to the slide and incubated for 20 min at 36 C; the slide is washed in PBS and distilled water, and then is dried and examined for specific staining.

Hemagglutination and hemagglutination-inhibition

Antigen preparation. The sucrose-acetone antigen described in the section on CF is used. Alternatives are (i) acetone extraction of mouse or hamster serum (4); (ii) 10% brain in borate-saline buffer (BSB), pH 9.0; or (iii) sonic-treated sucrose-acetone antigens (1). Sonic treatment utilizes uncentrifuged sucrose-acetone antigen and a Sonifier with a probe microtip in a 16 by 160 mm glass tube immersed in an ice bath at −10 C (salt-water-ice mixture stirred magnetically). Sonic treatment is conducted at a 20-W output, with the use of four cycles of 2 min each and 2 min of rest between cycles. Avoid freezing the antigen during this procedure.

Chemical reagents. BSB, pH 9.0 (0.05 M borate-0.12 M NaCl), plus 0.4% bovine albumin (Armour fraction V) is used as diluent of antigens and sera; 0.15 M NaCl-0.2 M Na_2HPO_4 mixed with 0.15 M NaCl-0.2 M NaH_2PO_4 in the proportions shown in Table 2 is used as adjusting diluent for addition of cell suspensions.

Treatment of sera (4). Test sera are extracted with acetone for removal of nonspecific inhibitors of viral hemagglutinins. Dilute the serum 1:10 in 1% bovine albumin in demineralized water; then express the diluted serum through a 23-gauge needle into 12 volumes (referred to volume of diluted serum) of chilled acetone and shake. After 5 min, centrifuge *lightly* (bring to 1,200 rpm on an International PR-2 centrifuge or equivalent and turn off). Excessive centrifugation packs the sediment and hinders subsequent extraction. Decant the acetone, replace it immediately with 12 volumes of chilled acetone, and shake. Centrifuge for 5 min in the cold at 2,500 rpm. Decant the acetone. Spread the sediment over the surface of the tube and dry it for 1 h (vacuum pump).

TABLE 2. *Composition of adjusting diluents used for addition of cell suspensions*[a]

Final pH[b]	0.15 M NaCl-0.2 M Na_2HPO_4 (%)	0.15 M NaCl-0.2 M NaH_2PO_4 (%)
5.75	3.0	97.0
6.0	12.5	87.5
6.2	22.0	78.0
6.4	32.0	68.0
6.6	45.0	55.0
6.8	55.0	45.0
7.0	64.0	36.0

[a] Adapted from Clarke and Casals (4).

[b] Final pH is that pH realized by mixing equal volumes of adjusting diluent and BSB, pH 9.0.

Several sera may be dried simultaneously in a vacuum jar. Rehydrate to 1:10 original serum volume with BSB, pH 9.0, and let stand overnight at 4 C.

Red cell agglutinins (if present) are removed by mixing diluted serum 1:50 with packed cells (1 part cells, 49 parts 1:10 serum); keep at 4 C for 20 min with occasional shaking. Centrifuge at 1,800 rpm for 10 min at 4 C. The supernatant serum is used in testing.

Preparation of red cells (4). Goose or chick red blood cells are washed and stored not longer than 2 weeks in a solution of dextrose-gelatin-Veronal (recrystallized Veronal, 0.58 g; gelatin, 0.60 g; sodium Veronal, 0.38 g; $CaCl_2$, 0.02 g; $MgSO_4 \cdot 7H_2O$, 0.12 g; NaCl, 8.5 g; dextrose, 10.0 g; made up to 1 liter and autoclaved) as an 8% suspension and are diluted 1:24 in adjusting diluent (see above) just before use.

Hemagglutinin titrations. Plastic microplates (nondisposable or disposable) and dropping pipettes with 18-gauge needle (as described for CF tests in chapter 71) are used in hemagglutinin and HI tests. Serial twofold antigen dilutions made in tubes are transferred to plates, 1 drop per well. Rows of antigen dilutions are made to correspond to different pH values (for instance, pH 5.75, 6.0, 6.2, 6.4, etc.). For each pH used, 1 drop of diluent (BSB with 0.4% bovine albumin) is added to each well, and 2 drops are added to the control well. Cells are suspended in adjusting diluents corresponding to the desired final pH values, and 2 drops of cell suspension are added to each well. The plates are shaken by tapping their corners on a table top. Then the cells are allowed to settle (about 30 min) at room temperature or 37 C. Results are recorded in four grades: complete, nearly complete, partial, and no agglutination.

One unit is contained in the antigen dilution which gives complete or nearly complete agglutination; 4 to 8 units are used in the test. That pH which gives adequate titer and is on the alkaline side of optimal pH (to increase sensitivity of HI test) is chosen for the HI test.

HI test. Serial twofold dilutions of serum, 1 drop per well, are added to plates, followed by 1 drop of antigen per well. Serum controls (test serum plus diluent) and control positive serum are included in each test. The antigen titration is repeated with each test. The test is incubated overnight (16 h) at 24 C (the HI test is more sensitive with incubation at 24 C than at 2 C). Red cells in appropriate pH adjusting diluent are added, 2 drops per well, and the test is read as above. Complete inhibition is considered positive. Serum controls must show no agglutination. For identification of a new isolate, reciprocal cross HI testing is needed to establish identity with the type virus.

SEROLOGICAL DIAGNOSIS

Neutralization test

Test undiluted sera with 10-fold virus dilutions. A difference of 1.7 log LD_{50} between the acute- and convalescent-phase sera is of diagnostic significance.

Complement fixation test

Use antigen in two dilutions, namely, optimal, as determined in grid titration with homologous serum, and the most concentrated which at the same time is not significantly anticomplementary (for example, antigen dilutions 1:64 and 1:4). A fourfold rise in antibody titer between the acute- and convalescent-phase sera is of diagnostic significance.

Hemagglutination-inhibition test

Two to eight antigen units are used. Test the sera in twofold dilutions starting at 1:10. A fourfold rise in antibody titer between acute- and convalescent-phase sera is diagnostically significant.

Fluorescent-antibody test

For diagnosis of illness, rabbit anti-human globulin antiserum is used. A fourfold rise in antibody titer between the acute- and convalescent-phase sera is of diagnostic significance.

INTERPRETATION OF LABORATORY RESULTS

Definitive diagnosis can be made only with isolation and identification of virus. Presumptive diagnosis can be made on a diagnostically significant rise in antibody titer between acute and convalescent blood specimens; however, antibody may be heterologous (related to virus of same group). High titers of CF (≧1:32) or HI (≧1:320) antibody in a single convalescent specimen, or a fall in antibody titer during convalescence, is indicative of recent infection but must be interpreted cautiously. Isolation of virus and serological diagnosis may indicate association of the virus with clinical illness but are not proof of causation.

LITERATURE CITED

1. Ardoin, P., and D. H. Clarke. 1967. The use of sonication and of calcium-phosphate chromatography for preparation of group C arbovirus hemagglutinins. Amer. J. Trop. Med. Hyg. **16:**357–363.
2. Casals, J. 1961. Procedures for identification of arthropod-borne viruses. Bull. W.H.O. **24:**723–734.

3. Chamberlain, R. W., R. K. Sikes, and R. E. Kissling. 1954. Use of chicks in eastern and western equine encephalitis studies. J. Immunol. **73:**106–144.
4. Clarke, D. H., and J. Casals. 1958. Techniques for hemagglutination and hemagglutination-inhibition with arthropod-borne viruses. Amer. J. Trop. Med. Hyg. **7:**561–573.
5. Emmons, R. W., D. V. Dondero, V. Devlin, and E. H. Lennette. 1969. Serologic diagnosis of Colorado tick fever. A comparison of complement-fixation, immunofluorescence, and plaque-reduction methods. Amer. J. Trop. Med. Hyg. **18:**796–802.
6. Halstead, S. B., P. Sukhavachana, and A. Nisalak. 1964. Assay of mouse adapted dengue viruses in mammalian cell cultures by an interference method. Proc. Soc. Exp. Biol. Med. **115:**1062–1068.
7. Hammon, W. McD., and T. H. Work. 1964. Arbovirus infection in man, p. 268–311. *In* E. H. Lennette and N. J. Schmidt (ed.), Diagnostic procedures for viral and rickettsial diseases, 3rd ed. American Public Health Association, Inc., New York.
8. Karabatsos, N., and S. M. Buckley. 1967. Susceptibility of the baby hamster kidney-cell line (BHK-21) to infection with arboviruses. Amer. J. Trop. Med. Hyg. **16:**99–105.
9. Lennette, E. H., M. I. Ota, H. Ho, and N. J. Schmidt. 1961. Comparative sensitivity of four host systems for the isolation of certain arthropod-borne viruses from mosquitoes. Amer. J. Trop. Med. Hyg. **10:**897–904.
10. Schmidt, N. J., and E. H. Lennette. 1965. Appendix: Basic techniques for virology, p. 1189–1231. *In* F. L. Horsfall, Jr., and I. Tamm (ed.), Viral and rickettsial infections of man, 4th ed. J. B. Lippincott Co., Philadelphia.
11. Taylor, R. M. 1968. Catalogue of arthropod-borne viruses of the world. Government Printing Office, Washington, D. C.
12. The Subcommittee on Information Exchange of the American Committee on Arthropod-borne Viruses. 1970. Catalogue of arthropod-borne viruses of the world. Amer. J. Trop. Med. Hyg. **19:**1082–1160.
13. The Subcommittee on Information Exchange of the American Committee on Arthropod-borne Viruses. 1971. Catalogue of arthropod-borne and selected vertebrate viruses of the world. Amer. J. Trop. Med. Hyg. **20:**1018–1050.
14. Webb, P. A., K. M. Johnson, R. B. Mackenzie, and M. L. Kuns. 1967. Some characteristics of Machupo virus. causative agent of Bolivian hemorrhagic fever. Amer. J. Trop. Med. Hyg. **16:**531–538.

Chapter 82

Rabiesvirus

HARALD NORLIN JOHNSON

CLINICAL BACKGROUND

Rabies is an acute infectious disease of the central nervous system caused by a virus belonging to the rhabdovirus group. The virus is often present in the saliva of rabid animals and consequently is most commonly transmitted by bite. Infected dogs, cats, foxes, coyotes, skunks, and bats are the most common sources of human infection. The incubation period is usually from 1 to 3 months, but may vary from 10 days to at least 8 months.

The capacity of the virus to invade and multiply in the salivary glands, lungs, kidneys, pancreas, and mammary glands permits it to maintain a cycle of infection in wildlife not associated with encephalitis. The ecology of the virus indicates that it is normally a parasite of the respiratory tract. The permanent hosts of rabiesvirus in the United States appear to be limited to the family *Mustelidae*, particularly spotted skunks and weasels. In Puerto Rico the mongoose is the most common wildlife host of rabies. Canine rabies is an example of aberrant parasitism, wherein the natural capacity of the virus to produce encephalitis becomes the means by which it can adapt to the host, that is, by increasing the tendency of the host to bite.

The generally held idea that rabies in man is always fatal is related to the lack of facilities at hospitals for testing for the presence of the virus, resulting in the absence of positive identification of the virus in the oral secretions during the acute phase of the disease in those that recover. The only definitive diagnosis in the past has been the isolation of the virus from the brain after death. Laboratory confirmation of the diagnosis of rabies from clinical specimens prior to death has been demonstrated, prolonged survival has been reported (5), and recovery from rabies in man has been proved by serological tests (8).

DESCRIPTION OF AGENT

Rabiesvirus is a ribonucleic acid virus. It is inactivated by lipid solvents, produces cytoplasmic inclusion bodies, and has an affinity for mucus-secreting tissues, especially those associated with the respiratory system. It has a complement-fixing (CF) soluble (S) antigen which can be separated from an infectious virus (V) antigen by high-speed centrifugation (6, 16). Erythrocytes of geese, chickens, guinea pigs, rats, sheep, monkeys, and humans are agglutinated by rabiesvirus under certain conditions (7).

On the basis of recent electron microscopy studies, rabiesvirus has been classified as a rhabdovirus (3, 14). This group includes vesicular stomatitis, Kern Canyon, Cocal, and Hart Park viruses. The rabiesvirus virion is found in matrices replacing normal cytoplasmic structures, in cytoplasmic vacuoles, or budding from the cell surface. In cross section, the virion is cylindrical, with a diameter of about 80 nm. In longitudinal section, it is about 180 to 200 nm in length and has a bacillary form. The virions occur singly or are arranged in closely packed arrays which tend to a geometric pattern. There are filamentous forms to >1,000 nm which exhibit breaks at about 200 nm. The surface of the virion is studded with protrusions 6 to 7 nm long (1, 2, 4, 9, 12, 13, 15).

COLLECTION AND STORAGE OF SPECIMENS

Specimens

The laboratory diagnosis of rabies from clinical specimens depends on isolation of the virus from sputum, saliva, throat swab, nasal swab, urine, or spinal fluid. A negative saliva test does not rule out rabies infection because the virus may fail to establish itself in the salivary glands or in other secretory organs. The virus may be present in the oral secretions during the first few days of the infection and then disappear. The demonstration of a significant rise in the titer of antibodies to rabiesvirus in the blood during the course of the infection, in the absence of passive or active immunization, is also a satisfactory method of diagnosis. Acute and convalescent blood serum specimens should be taken in all cases of suspected human rabies. Urine specimens should be collected and centrifuged; the sediment is then saved for virus studies. Stool specimens should be collected for examination for other viruses which can produce encephalitis.

In cases of rabies exposure by animal bite, it is helpful to know whether the submaxillary salivary glands contained rabiesvirus. These can be examined for rabiesvirus antigen by the fluorescent rabies antibody (FRA) test and by animal inoculation. If the submaxillary salivary glands are to be taken, they should be removed before opening the calvarium to avoid contamination of the salivary glands with virus obtained from the brain. Animal heads submitted after decapitation will have superficial contamination with virus released by severing of the spinal cord if the animal has rabies. A negative test for virus in the salivary glands does not eliminate the need for anti-rabies treatment; if the animal brain is positive, treatment must be given.

The single most important factor about rabies specimens is that they be taken with sterile instruments. Instruments used for one animal head must be sterilized by boiling or autoclaving before they are used for removal of another specimen. Separate sets of instruments must be used for each organ to be tested. The work surface must be covered with a waterproof disposable paper, such as an absorbent paper with polyethlene backing, so that the table top or work tray will not be contaminated. The sheeting must be changed with each specimen and then decontaminated by burning or autoclaving. If rabiesvirus is carried over from one animal specimen to another, a wrong diagnosis may result, leading to unnecessary treatment of persons suspected of having been exposed to rabies and to erroneous conceptions about the source of rabies in nature.

Collection

It is important that clinical specimens be collected early in the course of the disease. This is true for most virus infections, and best results are obtained when specimens are available from the first day or two of the disease. When called to collect specimens, it is important to bring several 5-ml screw-cap serum vials, each containing about 2 ml of a buffered cell culture maintenance medium, such as Eagle's minimal essential medium (MEM), and some sterile cotton swabs. Sputum can be collected by using an eyedropper pipette and rinsing the pipette in the medium, or by use of a cotton swab, in which case the swab is rotated in the medium and the fluid is expressed from the swab by rolling it against the side of the tube. The cotton swab and pipette must be discarded in a metal pan for sterilization. Nasal swab specimens are treated similarly. Spinal fluid specimens and urine specimens must be centrifuged, and the cell sediment is taken up in the maintenance medium. Stool specimens should be collected as for enterovirus studies. The acute-phase blood serum specimen should be taken as soon as convenient after the patient is admitted. A second specimen should be taken 2 days later, and further specimens are taken at intervals of a few days for the first 2 weeks. Rabiesvirus antigen has been found in the corneal cells of rabid animals, and corneal impressions should be taken in cases of suspected rabies. This is done by touching several standard glass slides, such as those used for the FRA test, to the cornea of the eye, after use of surface anesthesia.

It is essential that labels be typed and attached to the specimen vials before they leave the laboratory, giving the name of the patient, the date, time of day, and source of specimen. Adhesive labels which do not come off must be used.

Storage

If the specimens are to be tested within 24 h, it is best to keep them at 4 C. Avoid exposure to light and heat at all stages of handling. If the specimens are to be shipped, they should be refrigerated with dry ice. For prolonged storage, the specimens should be stored in flame-sealed glass ampoules at −60 C or colder. Screw-cap serum vials should be sealed with tape.

Postmortem specimens should be put into sterile plastic petri dishes or wide-mouth screw-cap bottles. Typewritten labels such as the self-sticking vinyl-coated labels are necessary so that the information does not become illegible on handling.

Wild animal specimens submitted for rabies examination should be correctly identified. For example, it is very important to know whether an animal is a striped skunk or a spotted skunk. Small mammals such as rodents and bats should be saved until the diagnosis is completed so that positive specimens can be held for identification. All bat specimens should be kept until identified because it is important to know how many of each species have been examined.

DIRECT MICROSCOPIC OBSERVATION OF SPECIMENS

The direct microscopic examination of brain tissue for rabiesvirus is one of the common laboratory procedures in public health laboratories. Although the FRA test has largely supplanted other methods of diagnosis, the examination for Negri bodies is still a valuable method of diagnosis and characterization of rabiesvirus strains.

Examination for Negri bodies

The Ammon's horn of the hippocampus is the best material for use in examinations for Negri bodies and for rabiesvirus antigen by the FRA test. It is also advisable to examine the cerebral and cerebellar cortex for Negri bodies and rabiesvirus antigen. When examining large brain specimens, cut through the Ammon's horn transversely with a pair of straight scissors, removing a cross section about 2 mm thick. Use this for preparation of impressions. This can be done by placing the section on one end of a tongue depressor. Holding a clean glass slide between the thumb and forefinger, apply the slide gently against the cut surface of the tissue that is exposed and remove it quickly. This leaves a thin film of tissue on the slide—a mirror image of the cross section. This type of specimen is suitable for staining with Seller's stain for Negri bodies, for routine histological stains, for staining with Giemsa stain as for malaria parasites, and for the FRA test. For smear preparations, cut out a portion of tissue about 1 mm in diameter from the Ammon's horn or other tissue, and place this near one end of a glass slide. Superimpose a second slide on the first, flatten the tissue by gentle pressure, and then draw the top slide lengthwise over the bottom slide, leaving a thin elongated smear on both slides. The thicker smear should be stained immediately with Seller's stain; the other is saved for the FRA test. The paraffin section method is not recommended for routine diagnostic demonstration of Negri bodies in animal brains. Postmortem tissue material from human patients should be fixed in Zenker's fixative. Add glacial acetic acid to a concentration of 5% just before use. For demonstration of Negri bodies, stain with eosin and methylene blue or with Giemsa stain. Tissue fixed in Formalin and stained with hematoxylin and eosin may show some of the cytoplasmic inclusion bodies of rabies, but, as the inner structure is not stained, this method is not applicable to the diagnosis of rabies.

The wet impressions or smears of brain tissue are fixed and stained at the same time by covering the tissue material with Seller's stain. This stain is a mixture of basic fuchsin and methylene blue. Each stock stain is prepared as a 1% solution in absolute acetone-free methanol. The basic fuchsin should be color index no. 677, and the methylene blue, color index no. 922 or equivalent. Store the stock stains in brown bottles in a cabinet where they are protected from light. To prepare the working stain solution, mix one part of the basic fuchsin and two parts of the methylene blue stock stain solutions, but do not filter the mixture. The stain is kept in a dropper bottle, and the staining process is done over a metal container which can be sterilized by boiling. While the tissue on the glass slide is still moist, cover it with Seller's stain and leave this on for 10 to 30 s. Then rinse the stain from the slide with 0.0067 M phosphate buffer (pH 7). After being air-dried, the preparation is ready for examination. Handle the slide as contaminated material, because it is possible that there may be some active virus left in the tissue.

The properly stained tissue should appear reddish-violet or purplish-blue, depending on the density of the tissue. The cytoplasm of the neurons will be blue or purplish-blue; the nuclei and nucleoli, a deeper blue; the stroma, rose pink; and nerve fibers, a deeper pink. Bacteria, if present, stain an intense blue, and erythrocytes stain a copper color. Negri bodies, the specific cytoplasmic inclusion bodies of rabies, are found in the cytoplasm of large neurons. The Negri body is a sharply defined spherical, oval, or elongated body, ordinarily 2 to 10 μm in diameter. Several inclusion bodies, usually of variable size, may be present in one neuron. The larger Negri bodies contain blue-staining granules or inner bodies, often arranged in concentric layers; the ground substance of the inclusion body is finely granular, takes the fuchsin stain, and appears cherry-red. In smear preparations, the Negri bodies often appear to be outside the neurons because the cytoplasm of the neuron has been ruptured. The intracellular location of Negri bodies need not be demonstrated, because the staining reaction with Seller's stain is characteristic and they may be identified outside as well as inside the neurons.

Cytoplasmic inclusion bodies which are caused by viruses other than rabiesvirus and which stain red with Seller's stain may be found in dog, cat, skunk, and mouse brains. For example, distemper virus causes inclusion bodies in infected dogs, and many of the wildlife viruses produce cytoplasmic inclusion bodies in mouse brain.

Fluorescent rabies antibody test

The FRA test, when used with proper controls, makes possible a prompt diagnosis in cases of animal rabies, and the accuracy of the test is equal to that of isolation of the virus by animal inoculation. In certain instances, the mouse inoculation test will fail because there is little or no infectious virus in the brain tissue as a result of inactivation of the virus by antibodies or by exposure to heat. Furthermore, some strains of rabiesvirus are of low pathogenicity. The FRA test will demonstrate rabiesvirus antigen when the infectivity has been lost, and this test is of particular value in identifying natural strains of rabiesvirus of low pathogenicity. The mouse inoculation test should be used for confirmation of the FRA test when this test shows only a ± or 1+ result so that it cannot be reported definitely positive, or when other circumstances warrant confirmation of the FRA test.

Rabies immune serum conjugate. The best results are obtained with the use of rabies immune serum from hamsters hyperimmunized with the CVS strain of fixed rabiesvirus prepared as homologous-tissue antigen (11). Commercial preparations of tagged serum or that prepared in the laboratory must be titrated to obtain the correct working dilution of the conjugate. For this purpose, prepare a stock of 20% normal mouse brain suspension in 0.01 M phosphate-buffered saline (pH 7.2 to 7.4). Store this at −60 C. Prepare twofold dilutions of the globulin-dye conjugate in the 20% normal mouse brain suspension, beginning with 1:10; test each twofold dilution for its staining quality for a control positive smear. The highest twofold dilution of the globulin conjugate which gives 4+ staining is used for the FRA test. An average conjugate will stain satisfactorily at a dilution of 1:40. A glaring yellow-green fluorescence is a 4+ reaction, a bright yellow-green fluorescence without glare is noted as 3+, a dull yellow-green fluorescence is 2+, and a very dim but still noticeable yellow-green fluorescence is 1+.

Staining smears with fluorescent antibody. Regular glass slides (25 by 75 mm) 0.9 to 1.1 mm thick are used for the FRA test. The impression or smear preparations are usually fixed in acetone at 4 C for 4 h or at −20 C overnight. In emergency situations, fixation for 10 min at room temperature gives satisfactory results, but the overnight test should be done also. Prepare a stock of mouse brains infected with street rabiesvirus and hold these at −20 C in 5-ml screw-cap serum vials. Prepare a set of slides sufficient to last for 1 month, air-dry them, and store them at −20 C in acetone. Be sure to keep the acetone level over the tissue specimen. As needed, take one of these slides for use as a positive control. It is also necessary to have a negative control prepared the same day from normal mouse brain.

Allow the slides to dry for 10 to 15 min after taking them out of the acetone. Place the slides on a tray covered with a sheet of moistened absorbent paper with polyethylene backing. *Handle all slides as contaminated material* and decontaminate the paper by burning or autoclaving when finished. Use forceps for handling slides. With an indelible ink marking pen, make a circle about 12 to 15 mm in diameter in the mid-portion of the tissue smear or around the impression, and allow to dry. With a pipette, drop about 0.1 ml of the appropriate dilution of the tagged antibody onto the tissue preparation so as to cover the inside of the marked circles including the inner one-half of the marking-pen line. Cover each tray with another tray inverted, or other suitable cover to keep slides moist, and place in an incubator at 37 C for 20 min. Place slides in a carrier and rinse for 10 min in each of two changes of 0.01 M phosphate-buffered saline (pH 7.2 to 7.4). Rinse again with distilled water. Set the slides in the carrier on a tray covered with a sheet of polyethylene-backed absorbent paper and air-dry them. Mount a no. 1 cover slip (22 by 40 mm) on the tissue preparation, using 25% glycerol in buffered saline. Use a standard microscope equipped with a source of ultraviolet light, with a Zeiss UG-2 excitor filter giving a peak transmission of 360 nm and a W2A or comparable barrier filter in the eyepiece. The presence of fluorescent rabiesvirus antigen in the specimen is diagnostic for rabies. The fluorescent material may vary from small particles <1 μm to masses 2 to 10 μm in diameter. Nerve cells may be outlined by the fluorescent material in them. Appropriate positive and negative controls should be used each time the test is performed, and specificity tests are needed when the fluorescence is only 1+ or uncertain (10, 11). A portion of every specimen tested must be saved for repeat tests if needed, or for forwarding to a reference laboratory.

ISOLATION AND IDENTIFICATION OF VIRUS

Host systems

The white laboratory mouse is the best experimental host for the isolation and identification of rabiesvirus. There are a number of rabiesvirus strains, such as the HEP Flury vaccine virus, which are nonpathogenic for mature mice. Some strains of rabiesvirus found in nature are much more pathogenic for infant mice than for adult mice. Therefore, to be able to demonstrate minimal amounts of virus, it is preferable to use 1- to 2-day-old infant mice as test animals.

Preparation of specimens. Saliva, nose and throat swab, urine, and spinal fluid specimens should be made up to 2 ml with physiological phosphate-saline solution containing 0.75% bovine albumin fraction V or 2% heat-inactivated horse, guinea pig, or hamster serum. After centrifugation at 2,500 rpm for about 10 min, a portion of the supernatant fluid is taken for reference and placed in an ampoule which is sealed and stored at −60 C. Antibiotics are added to the material to be tested, usually 1 mg of streptomycin and 1,000 units of penicillin per ml.

Autopsy specimens are ground in a mortar by use of an abrasive such as sterile alundum and are diluted to a 20% suspension in phosphate-buffered saline containing a stabilizer as noted above. A portion of each specimen must be saved for reference. Neutraglas 2-ml ampoules are suitable for this purpose, with 0.5 to 1.0 ml of the specimen placed in each ampoule.

Mouse inoculation test. It is essential that the mice be inoculated on a sheet of absorbent paper with polyethylene backing or a sheet of aluminum foil so as to avoid contaminating the work surface. Any droplets of virus left on the paper can then be decontaminated by burning or autoclaving the paper. A clean work surface must be used for each specimen so that virus is not carried over from one specimen to another. It is advisable to work on metal trays and to sterilize these by autoclaving when finished. A 0.25-ml tuberculin syringe and a 0.25- to 0.5-inch (0.6- to 1.3-cm) 27-gauge needle are used for inoculating mice. Working over the tray, fill the syringe by placing the needle point just inside the lip of the tube, and tip the tube until the fluid can be drawn up without contaminating the barrel of the syringe. Use screw-cap tubes so as to avoid contamination of the hands. It is recommended to have available a jar of sterile dental rolls, cut in half, for use in clearing the bubble from the syringe barrel after taking up the fluid. Using sterile 4.5-inch (11.4-cm) grasping forceps, pick up the section of dental roll, put this on the needle of the syringe, and with gentle pressure express the bubble. Place the cotton roll on the paper work surface and use the forceps to hold the infant mice for inoculation. Hold the syringe with the index finger on the plunger, and support the barrel between the thumb and third and fourth fingers. The forearm should rest on the table to stabilize the arm. Introduce the needle to a depth of 1 to 2 mm into the central part of the upper parietal area of the calvarium. The dose is 0.015 ml. No antiseptic is necessary or desirable over the inoculation site. In suspected cases of rabies, stool and throat swab specimens should also be tested in cell culture systems to rule out other virus infections.

If a specimen contains rabiesvirus, some of the infant mice inoculated with it usually show tremulous muscular activity, incoordination, or paralysis between 5 and 12 days after inoculation. It is customary to observe the inoculated infant mice for 28 days. The microscopic examination of mouse brains for Negri bodies and preferably also for rabiesvirus antigen by the FRA test is necessary to establish a diagnosis of rabies.

Cross-protection test

The cross-protection test is the most certain method of determining the relationship of two viruses. If immunization with one virus produces resistance to infection with another virus, they are classified as the same organism. Further classification as to strain depends on serological tests and tests of pathogenicity for various experimental hosts. Mice inoculated intracerebrally at the age of 4 to 6 weeks with the HEP Flury rabiesvirus strain do not sicken or die, but are resistant to infection with the more pathogenic varieties of rabiesvirus, injected by the same route. Use about 10^3 LD_{50} determined by preliminary titration in infant mice, and vaccinate a group of six female mice; set aside a control group of the same age and sex. At 1 month after vaccination, challenge the vaccinated and control mice by giving them an intracerebral inoculation of 0.015 ml of the 10^{-2} dilution of the unknown virus prepared from infected mouse brain and having a titer of more than 10^{-5}. Inoculate the control mice last. If the vaccinated mice survive and the control mice die, one can be certain that the unknown virus is rabiesvirus.

SEROLOGICAL DIAGNOSIS

Virus neutralization test in mice

The virus neutralization test is used for titration of antibodies in rabies hyperimmune serum to be used for the FRA test and for testing human sera for antibodies to rabies. It is necessary to have a standard virus for the neutralization test. The CVS strain of rabiesvirus is the standard reference virus. Prepare a 20% suspension of mouse brain from infant mice infected with a moderate dosage of this virus, for example, 10^3 to 10^4 LD_{50} of the virus. Use a diluent of 0.01 M phosphate-saline solution containing 0.75% bovine fraction V or 2% heat-inactivated guinea pig, hamster, or horse serum. Dispense in ampoules in amounts of 1 ml, flame-seal, and store at −60 C as stock virus. The use of a 20% suspension of brain tissue virus simplifies titration of the virus in normal and rabies-immune serum; that is, when 0.3 ml of serum has been added to each tube of a titration series, the addition of 0.3 ml of the 10-fold virus dilutions will give a final tissue-virus dilution of 1:10, 1:100, etc. When high-titer virus prepared from infant mouse brain is used, the titration series should include 10-fold dilutions through $1:10^8$. When the virus dilutions have been added to the serum tubes, mix the tube contents by gently agitating the rack holding the test tubes, and place the rack in an incubator at 37 C for a period of 1 h. Subsequently, place the rack of tubes in a refrigerator at 4 C for 1 h. The mixtures are then ready for testing by intracerebral inoculation in young adult mice. Complete the inoculation of the immune serum series before testing the normal control serum series. The use of an inoculum of 0.015 ml for both infant and adult mice has the advantage of allowing direct comparison of the titrations in infant and adult mice; however, in some laboratories an inoculum of 0.03 ml is used for adult mice. The important thing is to keep the inoculum dose constant for all titrations in a given host.

Another method for serum-virus neutralization is to test various dilutions of serum against a constant amount of virus. This method is recommended for testing the potency of rabies-immune serum and for testing the serum of persons to determine the immunity obtained after vaccination. Knowing the titer of the stock rabiesvirus, dilute this so that 0.015 ml will contain about 2×10^2 LD_{50}. When this is mixed with an equal volume of serum or serum dilution, 0.015 ml will contain about 10^2 LD_{50} of virus. The serum is ordinarily tested in twofold or fivefold dilutions.

Maximal neutralization is obtained in tests of fresh serum specimens. In testing serum specimens which have been stored for some time, it is advisable to add the so-called "fresh serum factor." When testing undiluted serum against 10-fold dilutions of the virus, the serum to be tested may be mixed with an equal amount of fresh hamster or guinea pig serum. When testing dilutions against a standard virus suspension, the first dilution of the serum can be made in fresh normal serum, and subsequent dilutions are made in phosphate-saline solution.

Infant mice are susceptible to certain strains of rabiesvirus given by intraperitoneal inoculation. The virus titer by this route is about 2 $\log_{10}$ less than that attained by intracerebral inoculation. Non-neuroadapted strains of rabiesvirus are suitable for use in the intraperitoneal serum-virus neutralization test in infant mice. The use of this route of inoculation increases the effectiveness of the neutralization of viruses by immune serum, and may demonstrate minimal antibody titers not revealed by the intracerebral neutralization test.

Indirect fluorescent-antibody test

The indirect fluorescent-antibody (IFA) test has proved to be very useful in studies of human sera following treatment with hyperimmune rabies antiserum (equine) and rabies vaccine. The test reveals the individual's active antibody response to vaccination rather than passive immunity, since there is no cross-reaction between equine and human gamma globulin. The test was done originally with smears or impressions of mouse brain infected with the standard CVS strain of rabiesvirus. There was considerable variation in the amount of rabies antigen in such preparations, and more consistent results have been obtained by using cell cultures infected with rabiesvirus. The technique to be described is that used currently at the California State Health Department, Viral and Rickettsial Disease Laboratory (10). Cultures of baby hamster kidney cells (line 0853) derived at this laboratory are grown in 8-oz (240-ml) prescription bottles with Eagle's MEM containing 10% fetal bovine serum (FBS) as the outgrowth medium (OGM). When a complete sheet of cells is obtained, the cell sheet is infected with Flury strain LEP rabiesvirus, derived from the dog vaccine by a single passage in infant mice. Each bottle receives an inoculum of 0.1 ml containing about 10^6 LD_{50} of the virus. This virus suspension is added to the 10 ml of Eagle's MEM containing 2% FBS, which is the maintenance medium (MM). Additional uninoculated cell cultures are changed to the MM for use as normal cells. On the third day after inoculation, the infected cell cultures are trypsinized and, as the cell sheet begins to slip, the trypsin solution is removed. Normal cells are mixed with infected cells to adjust the proportion of antigen-containing cells. The cells from three bottles of uninfected cells are mixed with the cells from one bottle of infected cells. This is done by adding 10 ml of buffered saline containing 2% FBS to one bottle of uninfected cells. After mixing, this same medium is used to take up the cells from the other uninfected bottles and the infected bottle. The mixture of normal and infected cells is then centrifuged. The cell sediment is carefully mixed with buffered saline containing 2% FBS, using increments of 1 ml, until a uniform suspension is obtained, which takes about 0.5 ml per bottle.

The final suspension of 2 ml of infected and normal cells is used to make a series of slides with three 5-mm spots, marked as for routine FRA tests. The inoculum is about 0.005 ml per spot. Twelve to 14 slides can be made with 0.1 ml. A series of slides of normal cells are prepared with two spots of cells on each slide. The cell preparations are then air-dried and fixed with acetone. If kept below −20 C, they will be satisfactory for 1 year. One normal and two infected cell slides are used for each serum to be tested: twofold dilutions of 1:4 and 1:8 for the normal cells, and from 1:4 to 1:128 for the infected cells, and an inoculum of about 0.05 ml of the serum dilution per spot. The slides are incubated for 20 min, washed twice in buffer solution, rinsed with distilled water, and air-dried. Antihuman gamma globulin (IGG) conjugate is added to each spot in a volume of about 0.05 ml. The slides are incubated again for 20 min, washed for 5 min two times, rinsed with distilled water, and air-dried. After mounting with 25% glycerol, the slides are read in the same manner as for FRA tests. Each lot number of the IGG must be titrated on rabies-infected cells. Twofold dilutions from 1:4 to 1:64 of a human serum containing antibodies to rabiesvirus are tested against the antihuman IGG in twofold dilutions from 1:10 to 1:80, with the use of rabiesvirus-infected cells as in the IFA test. The lowest dilution of the IGG which gives the strongest reaction in the positive slides and elicits a minimal reaction in the normal cells is used in the test as the working dilution. This is apt to be the 1:40 dilution. This test is used routinely in testing sera from people who have received prophylactic immunization against rabies and also for testing for the level of immunity in persons treated because of exposure to rabies.

Fluorescent focus inhibition test

The fluorescent focus inhibition test (FFIT) is given as done at the California State Health Department, Viral and Rickettsial Disease Laboratory (10). Microcultures of baby hamster kidney cells (line 0853) are prepared on the standard glass glides used for routine FRA tests. About 100 slides are placed on a paper surface, with two culture sites on each marked by 15-mm cover slips. The slides are sprayed with Fluoroglide (Chemplast Inc. [made of Teflon], Wayne, N.J.), after which the cover slips are removed. Disks of filter paper are used to cover the bottom of 150-mm petri dishes, and five of the prepared slides are placed in each dish. The covers are replaced and the dishes are sterilized by autoclaving. In preparation for the addition of the cells, the filter paper in the petri dishes is wet with sterile distilled water. The baby hamster kidney cells are dispersed in Eagle's OGM, and 0.1 ml is pipetted onto each of the clear spots on the slides. The seeded microcultures are incubated in a CO_2 incubator at 35 C for 48 h. The sera to be tested are inactivated at 56 C for 30 min, and twofold dilutions, from 1:4 to 1:128, are prepared in Eagle's MM. On the basis of a preliminary titration, the Flury LEP strain of rabiesvirus, obtained from infected infant mouse brain, is diluted in the Eagle's MM to give 100 to 400 plaque-forming units (PFU) per 0.1 ml, when mixed with an equal amount of the serum dilution. A volume of 0.2 ml of the virus suspension is added to 0.2 ml of the serum dilution. After being mixed by shaking, the tubes are incubated at 37 C for 90 min. The OGM is then aspirated from the microcultures with a vacuum suction system. Each serum-virus mixture is inoculated, in a volume of 0.1 ml, onto two microcultures. The cultures are incubated for 4 days at 35 C in the CO_2 incubator. The medium is then aspirated, and the slides are fixed in acetone, air-dried, and stained with conjugated rabies immune serum according to the routine FRA system. The controls consist of normal human serum diluted 1:4 and 1:8, and the three highest of the twofold dilutions of the hamster antirabies serum which neutralize the inoculum of 100 to 400 PFU of the rabiesvirus. The antibody titer end point is given as the highest dilution of a serum which is able to inhibit the development of fluorescent foci to only one to two in 20 to 40 high-power fields. There will be a few single infected cells representing secondary seeding in dilutions of sera which contain very little neutralizing antibody. The FFIT has shown good agreement with the standard neutralization test in mice.

Plaque reduction test

Certain strains of rabiesvirus will produce plaques in a test system of BHK-21/13S cells suspended in agarose. Titrations of rabiesvirus in normal and test sera are done in the usual twofold dilutions and inoculated in 0.1-ml amounts onto the petri dish containing the BHK-21/13S cells suspended in agarose. A final overlay of agarose containing 1:10,000 neutral red is done on the sixth or seventh day, and the plaques are counted after 4 h (17).

Complement-fixation test

The CF test, in which infant mouse brain antigen or BHK cell culture antigen is used, is applicable to the study of rabiesvirus strains. When used to determine antigenic response to vaccination, uninfected antigen prepared from the same host tissue as the vaccine antigen must be tested against the sera to establish that any reactivity with the specific test antigen is not due to the presence of host material. It is preferable to use a test antigen that is derived from a host source different from the one employed for the immunizing antigen. The technique of the CF test for rabies is the same as that given for routine use with viral and rickettsial agents (see chapter 71). It is possible to use a crude antigen derived from infected infant mouse brain. The presence of other viruses associated with some strains of rabiesvirus can be a cause for confusion in CF studies.

Hemagglutination-inhibition test

The hemagglutination-inhibition test which has been described needs further study before it will be practicable for routine use (7). The problem remains as to how to remove the nonspecific inhibitors in serum specimens from man.

INTERPRETATION OF LABORATORY RESULTS

The examination of brain tissue for Negri bodies will identify about 90% of the cases of rabies in dogs. However, rabies in wildlife, especially in skunks and free-living bats, is apt to be caused by strains of rabiesvirus which do not produce Negri bodies. The combined results of FRA tests, examinations for Negri bodies, and the inoculation of mice on a series of 4,200 specimens examined at the California State Health Department showed that 363 of the specimens were positive for rabies. Of these, 361 (99.4%) were detected by the FRA test, 357 (98.3%) by inoculation of mice, and 239 (65.8%) by the presence of Negri bodies (11). The relatively low rate of detection of the virus by Negri body examination is due to the large number of cases of skunk rabies which were included in this series.

The major problem encountered with the FRA test is the possibility that the animals used for the preparation of rabiesvirus immune serum are naturally immune to agents other than rabiesvirus, which may be found in specimens submitted for rabies examination. This is a good reason for using hamsters for the preparation of rabiesvirus immune serum. Even this laboratory-reared animal can be infected with mouse pneumonitis virus, parainfluenza virus, lymphocytic choriomeningitis virus, and reovirus. The demonstration of rabiesvirus antigen in organs other than the brain is complicated by certain organ-specific factors; that is, the virus that is formed in the brain is to a certain extent recognized as brain virus by the FRA test. Of course, the animals used for the production of hyperimmune serum are immunized with brain virus.

The neutralization test depends on the use of known negative and positive control sera. If the titer of the unknown virus is reduced 100-fold or more by rabiesvirus-immune serum as compared with the control serum, this is good evidence that the unknown virus is rabiesvirus.

LITERATURE CITED

1. Almeida, J. D., A. F. Howatson, L. Pinteric, and P. Fenje. 1962. Electron microscope observations on rabiesvirus by negative staining. Virology **18:**147-151.
2. Atanasiu, P., and J. Sisman. 1967. Rage. L'aspect morphologique du virion rabique. Bull. Off. Int. Epizoot. **67:**521-533.
3. Bennett, J. A., E. R. Rabin, R. D. Wende, and J. L. Melnick. 1967. A comparative light and electron microscope study of rabies and Hart Park virus encephalitis. Exp. Mol. Pathol. **7:**1-10.
4. Davies, M. C., M. E. Englert, G. R. Sharpless, and V. J. Cabasso. 1963. The electron microscopy of rabiesvirus in cultures of chicken embryo tissues. Virology **21:**642-651.
5. Emmons, R. W., L. L. Leonard, F. DeGenaro, Jr., E. S. Protas, P. L. Bazeley, S. T. Giammona, and K. Sturckow. 1973. A case of human rabies with prolonged survival. Intervirology **1:**60-72.
6. Ende, M. van den, A. Polson, and G. S. Turner. 1957. Experiments with the soluble antigen of rabies in suckling mouse brains. J. Hyg. **55:**361-373.
7. Halonen, P. E., F. A. Murphy, B. N. Fields, and D. R. Reese. 1968. Hemagglutinin of rabies and some other bullet-shaped viruses. Proc. Soc. Exp. Biol. Med. **127:**1037-1042.
8. Hattwick, M. A., T. T. Weis, C. J. Stechschulte, G. M. Baer, and M. B. Gregg. 1972. Recovery from rabies. A case report. Ann. Intern. Med. **76:**931-942.
9. Hummeler, K., H. Koprowski, and T. J. Wiktor. 1967. Structure and development of rabies virus in tissue culture. J. Virol. **1:**152-170.
10. Lennette, E. H., and R. W. Emmons. 1971. The laboratory diagnosis of rabies: review and prospective, p. 77-90. *In* Y. Nagano and F. M. Davenport (ed.), Rabies. University Park Press, Baltimore.
11. Lennette, E. H., J. D. Woodie, K. Nakamura, and R. L. Magoffin. 1965. The diagnosis of rabies by fluorescent antibody method (FRA) employing immune hamster serum. Health Lab. Sci. **2:**24-34.
12. Matsumoto, S. 1962. Electron microscopy of nerve cells infected with street rabiesvirus. Virology **17:**198-202.
13. Matsumoto, S. 1963. Electron microscope studies of rabiesvirus in mouse brain. J. Cell Biol. **19:**565-591.
14. Murphy, F. A., and B. N. Fields. 1967. Kern Canyon virus: electron microscopic and immunological studies. Virology **33:**625-637.
15. Pinteric, L., P. Fenje, and J. D. Almeida. 1963. The visualization of rabiesvirus in mouse brain. Virology **20:**208-211.
16. Polson, A., and P. Wessels. 1953. Particle size of soluble antigen of rabiesvirus. Proc. Soc. Exp. Biol. Med. **84:**317-320.
17. Sedwick, W. D., and T. J. Wiktor. 1967. Reproducible plaquing system for rabies, lymphocytic choriomeningitis, and other ribonucleic acid viruses in BHK-21/13S agarose suspensions. J. Virol. **1:**1224-1226.

Chapter 83
Herpes Simplex Virus

ERNEST C. HERRMANN, JR., AND WILLIAM E. RAWLS

CLINICAL BACKGROUND

A report that 21% of almost 4,100 consecutive viral isolations were herpes simplex virus (*Herpesvirus hominis*, HSV) suggests that it may be the most ubiquitous human pathogenic virus (13). A primary infection occurs, in both adults and children having no HSV antibody, which is commonly mild and frequently results in lesions anywhere on the human integument, including the genitalia, around or in the oral cavity (gingivo-stomatitis), the eye (keratitis), and the fingers (whitlow). Primary infections can produce fever, adenopathy, and pharyngitis, sometimes followed by a stomatitis that may be associated with lip lesions. A generalized infection can occur in the newborn, seriously involving the eyes, the central nervous system, and the skin, as well as other organs. Abraded or traumatized skin is more susceptible to infection than intact skin, and persons with exzema may acquire a serious generalized infection (Kaposi's varicelliform eruption). Some believe that HSV is a primary cause of pharyngitis (10, 38). A portion of the population having HSV antibody can have recurrent lesions, most commonly around the mouth, but again these eruptions also occur on other areas of the body, including the eye and genitalia. Recurrent lesions of the eye can lead to blindness if untreated.

HSV occurs as types 1 and 2, strains which are closely related yet biologically and serologically distinguishable. Type 1 is associated with skin lesions above the waist, encephalitis, stomatitis, eye infections, and some cases of generalized herpes simplex. Type 2 is found primarily in and on the genitalia and surrounding areas, can be venereally transmitted, and usually is the cause of generalized infections of the newborn. The relationship between the locale of herpetic lesions and HSV types is not, however, absolute. The reported association of type 2 to cervical carcinoma (32) has encouraged substantial interest in HSV as a cause of human cancer (21).

HSV disease can be confused with herpangina (caused by type A coxsackieviruses), varicella, zoster, and other diseases involving skin eruptions. It is important that HSV eye infections be accurately diagnosed, for ill-advised therapy with anti-inflammatory steroids may make this infection worse (19). HSV-induced encephalitis, which some think may not always be serious, is now believed to be more common than had been thought, and it is likely many cases have not been properly diagnosed (17). There is also a growing awareness that aseptic meningitis may be rarely caused by HSV, but when it is it may involve type 2. For further details of the relationship of HSV to human disease, the recent monograph by Juel-Jensen and MacCallum should be consulted (18).

DESCRIPTION OF AGENT

HSV is the prototype of the herpesvirus group, which includes varicella-zoster (V-Z) virus (chapter 85), cytomegalovirus (chapter 84), Epstein-Barr virus (chapter 89), and a number of viruses of subhuman animals. The central core of HSV is symmetrical (icosahedron) with 162 capsomeres, has an overall size of 100 nm, and contains deoxyribonucleic acid (DNA). The core is surrounded by an envelope derived from the host cell nuclear membrane, producing an overall, average particle size of 150 nm (130 to 180 nm depending on the host cell). The DNA-containing core is produced in the cell nucleus and is associated with intranuclear inclusions (Cowdry or Lipschütz type A). The envelope contains essential phospholipid, and therefore the virus is inactivated by lipid solvents. As with other viruses sensitive to lipid solvents, HSV is also inactivated by a pH less than 4, as well as being inactivated by 0.5 h at 56 C. HSV synthesis can be inhibited by a variety of specific and nonspecific DNA inhibitors (35).

The two serotypes of HSV share common antigens, and both can be neutralized by antisera produced to either type. Types 1 and 2 also have specific antigens and differ from each other in many biological characteristics, mostly of a quantitative nature (27). Only those differences that seem pertinent to diagnostic procedures will be mentioned.

COLLECTION AND STORAGE OF SPECIMENS

HSV can be readily obtained by touching a cotton-tipped swab to open herpetic skin lesions, to oral lesions, and to ulcers and inflammation present in cases of pharyngitis. The fluid obtained from an aseptically opened fresh vesicle provides a rich source of virus. Vesicle fluid can also be aspirated with a tuberculin syringe equipped with a 0.25-inch (0.6-cm), 25-gauge needle. Swabs of pharyngeal secretions may yield virus in cases of herpetic lesions around the mouth and among some cases of pharyngitis in which no oral or skin lesions are observed.

It has been the practice to homogenize biopsy or necropsy brain tissue in suspected cases of HSV encephalitis, producing a 10% tissue suspension. Although many HSV isolations have resulted from this procedure, recent work suggests that HSV can be isolated more efficiently by trypsinizing the tissues prior to inoculation into cell cultures; this can be done with frozen specimens (39).

HSV-1 can rarely be isolated from spinal fluid, and HSV-2 can occasionally be isolated from spinal fluids of patients with meningitis. Prior reports of HSV isolations from rectal swabs or feces must now be doubted, for herpesviruses are inactivated by the acid of the human stomach as are rhinoviruses and myxoviruses, which are not found in feces. HSV isolations from feces may be due to the presence of anal herpetic lesions or a herpetic vulvovaginitis, usually involving type 2. HSV (type 2) can be isolated from the urine of patients with cystitis and primary genital infections. The culturing of blood for HSV is rarely performed even in cases of generalized infections or in encephalitis, despite the fact that it has been isolated from blood (2). It is difficult to say whether this has been primarily an unsuccessful approach or just a neglected one.

HSV is now known to be hardier than respiratory syncytial virus but certainly less hardy than the picornaviruses. Highest isolation rates are obtained if a swab extract is inoculated into cell cultures on the day the specimen is taken. Freezing of a specimen prior to inoculation into cell cultures should be discouraged. HSV will survive transportation over long distances if chilled, *not frozen*, in a suspending medium free from protein (29). Stuart's salt-glucose medium, devised for transportation of swabs containing beta-hemolytic streptococci, is useful for transporting HSV-containing swabs (Culturette, Scientific Products; 34). Dry swabs produce fewer viral isolations than those that are moist. No matter what the suspending medium or the temperature, however, there will be a continued loss of virus titer with time. Prolonged storage of HSV should be at low temperatures (−60 C) after addition of 20% heat-inactivated serum (56 C for 0.5 h).

DIRECT EXAMINATION

Cells scraped from the base of herpes-like lesions may show changes characteristic of herpesviruses. In the Tzanck test, the cells are smeared onto a slide, fixed, and stained with Wright's or Giemsa's preparations (1). Syncytial giant cells (polykaryocytes) and "ballooning" cytoplasm are observed in lesions produced by either HSV or V-Z virus; thus, the test is of limited value in distinguishing between lesions caused by one of the two viruses. Cowdry type A intranuclear inclusions may be found in infected cells which are stained with hematoxylin and eosin (36); however, these inclusions may also be produced by either HSV or V-Z virus. Intranuclear inclusions are not invariably detected in infected tissues, and the failure to detect inclusions in HSV-induced encephalitis may be one reason this disease has been thought to be rare (17).

Cells obtained from lesions may also be fixed with acetone and stained with fluorescence-labeled antibody to HSV (7). This procedure can produce rapid (1.5 to 2 h), definitive determination of the virus involved in a skin eruption. In addition, vesicle fluids usually contain sufficient particles to be detected with ease by electron microscopy. The electron microscopist is unable to distinguish HSV from V-Z virus but can readily distinguish herpesvirus from poxvirus (23, 41).

VIRUS ISOLATION

Human embryonic lung fibroblasts (WI-38 strain) are the most convenient cells in which to isolate HSV types 1 and 2 (13). These cells are available from many commercial firms and are sensitive to a wide range of other viruses of importance to a viral diagnostic laboratory. They multiply well in Eagle's basal medium containing 10% fetal bovine serum (8) and maintain their morphology for weeks in the same medium (with somewhat higher buffering capacity achieved best by addition of 20 mM HEPES [*N*-2-hydroxyethylpiperazine-*N*′-2′-ethanesulfonic acid] buffer per ml) with no need for refeeding the cultures. Fetal bovine serum, which can be reduced to 2 to 5% in the maintenance medium, has no suppressive effect on the isolation of HSV type 1 or 2. Both types of HSV rapidly produce cytopathic effects (CPE) in this cell system.

If WI-38 fibroblasts are not available, another strain of human diploid fibroblast can be chosen. It must be noted, however, that there is a report that a few strains of fibroblasts can be resistant to HSV infection (3). Human embryonic kidney cells, which are available commercially both as tube cultures and as a cell suspension, are useful in isolating HSV and a variety of viruses, but they may lack some sensitivity for HSV when compared with fibroblasts (14). Primary rabbit kidney cells are popular for research and are suggested by some as the most sensitive cell for the isolation of HSV (43). Unfortunately, this cell type has not been shown to be useful for detecting the many other human viruses that are routinely isolated in human fibroblasts in a comprehensive viral diagnostic program. Human amnion cells have also been recommended for HSV isolation (18), but, among their other disadvantages, they too do not seem to have the general viral sensitivity of human embryonic fibroblasts.

HSV will at times, usually after 1 week or more of incubation, produce CPE in heteroploid cells such as HeLa and HEp-2, but these cells are generally inferior to human fibroblasts, as are rhesus monkey kidney cells (10). CPE in WI-38 cells, however, can be observed early after inoculation, with 57% of HSV isolates detected by the 4th day of incubation and 92% by the 6th day (12).

Typical CPE produced by HSV in WI-38 cell cultures involves rounding of the cells with giant cell formation. This classical CPE can be observed by seeking out those with typical "cold sores," obtaining a little vesicle fluid on a swab, and infecting cell cultures. The various phases of HSV-induced CPE can be preserved by filling the culture tube with a balanced salt solution containing 10% formaldehyde. Very advanced CPE can be confusing, however, in that its distinctive nature may be lost. In rare cases, with a vesical fluid rich in V-Z virus, WI-38 cells may show a generalized and advanced CPE sometimes confused with that caused by HSV (10, 12). Such confusion is most readily resolved by the subpassage of cell-free culture medium to fresh WI-38 cultures. V-Z virus will not subpassage in cell-free medium.

Despite a long history of HSV isolation by use of the dropped chorioallantoic membrane of embryonated chicken eggs, this method should be discouraged since type 1, the most common type, produces very small lesions and in about 25% of the infections it produces none at all (28, 31). In the past, mice were used for the isolation of HSV by injecting specimens intracranially, but it is known that certain strains of HSV lack the neurotropic potential to produce overt disease in mice. Even less convenient are rabbits, which can, however, be infected by inoculation of the eye.

IDENTIFICATION OF HERPES SIMPLEX VIRUS

HSV isolates are best identified by reaction with specific antisera. Such antisera are sold by at least one firm (Microbiological Associates, Inc.) and are also distributed in limited quantities by the Research Resources Branch of the National Institutes of Health. Antisera can readily be prepared in laboratory animals such as mice or rabbits. Antigen for inoculation consists of crude tissue culture harvest or of disrupted 10% suspensions of infected cells. Documented strains of HSV (American Type Culture Collection) are inoculated onto monolayers of cells and, after an adsorption period of 1 h, medium is added. The cultures are incubated at 37 C until 4+ CPE has developed. The cells are scraped into the medium with a rubber policeman and then pelleted by low-speed centrifugation. A 10% cell suspension in the culture supernatant fluid is made and the cells are sonically disrupted. Since both HSV types 1 and 2 may cause lethal infections in the animals, an initial intraperitoneal injection of virus which has been inactivated by ultraviolet light (10 min at 15 cm from a standard ultraviolet lamp) or by heat (56 C for 30 min) will reduce the loss of animals. One to two weeks after the injection with inactivated virus, further injections containing live virus mixed with adjuvant are given. Adjuvant with or without antigen will in time induce considerable ascites formation. From each mouse it is possible to obtain 20 to 100 ml of antibody-rich ascitic fluid (4).

Antisera prepared against HSV type 1 or 2 will contain cross-reacting antibodies. Type specification can be obtained by adsorption of the sera with heterologous virus. For adsorption, infected cells are prepared in a manner similar to that described for antigen preparation. The infected cells pelleted by centrifugation are resuspended in a minimal volume of fluid and disrupted; approximately 10^8 to 10^9 cells usually provide sufficient material to adsorb 1 ml of serum with an initial neutralizing titer of 1:100 to 1:1,000. The adsorbing material is mixed with the antisera and incubated for 1 h at 37 C and overnight at 4 C. The serum sample is clarified by high-speed centrifugation and then heated at 56 C for 30 min to inactivate residual virus. The adequacy of adsorption should be evaluated by assessing the neutralizing capacity of the adsorbed sera against the heterologous virus.

Identification of the HSV isolate can be confirmed by neutralization tests or by immunofluorescence. A simplified neutralization test is usually sufficient to identify HSV. The antibody titer of the antisera should be predetermined by using documented strains of virus. The pools of unknown isolate should be titered, and that dilution which contains approximately 100 TCD_{50} (50% tissue culture doses) per 0.1 ml should be mixed with an equal volume of serum diluted to contain about 100 antibody units (1 unit neutralizes 100 TCD_{50}). The virus-serum mixture is incubated for about 2 h at room temperature and then inoculated into two WI-38 cell cultures. Two WI-38 cell cultures inoculated with virus plus diluent instead of antiserum serve as controls. The development of CPE in the tubes is assessed daily and judged for the protective effect of the antiserum.

The fluorescent-antibody (FA) technique can also be used for rapid identification of HSV (24). The globulin fraction of high-titered sera is prepared and conjugated with fluorescein isothiocyanate. The specificity and titer of the labeled antibody should be determined by using cells infected with documented strains of HSV and uninfected cells. Cells scraped directly from the base of herpetic lesions can be smeared onto slides, fixed in acetone for 15 min at −20 C, and stained with one drop of the conjugate. The excess conjugate is removed after incubation at 37 C for 45 min by three washes in buffered saline and one wash in distilled water. The air-dried slide is then mounted with a cover slip and examined with a fluorescence microscope. Cells from cultures which have been inoculated with a specimen and which develop herpes-like CPE can be removed from the culture tube, smeared onto a slide, fixed in acetone, and stained in the same manner.

When adsorbed sera are used, typing of the HSV isolates can be accomplished by neutralization or by the FA technique. Greatest success with the FA technique has been obtained by using viable cells and staining the cell surface antigens. The cells from the infected culture are dispersed with trypsin, washed in buffered saline containing 2% fetal bovine serum, and resuspended to about 5×10^5 cells in 0.1 ml of the same solution. Conjugated adsorbed serum, 0.1 ml, is added to the cells and incubated for 1 h at 37 C. Excess conjugate is removed by three washes in the same medium. After the final wash, the cells are placed on a slide with a Pasteur pipette. A cover slip is added and sealed to avoid drying. The presence of cells producing rings of fluorescence, for type 1, or beads of fluorescence, for type 2, provides positive identification. There are many other characteristics which can be utilized to distinguish HSV type 1 from type 2 (27). These include FA testing of fixed cells (26) and kinetic neutralization tests (31, 32, 45), as well as others. The interested reader should examine other methodologies.

Isolates can also be examined for pH (20) and chloroform (6) sensitivity. The myxoviruses and herpesviruses are inactivated by low pH and chloroform. Most myxoviruses produce CPE and hemadsorption, and they are rarely confused with HSV (10). In addition, the classic clinical manifestations of some of the lesions produced by HSV raise the question as to the necessity of serological identification or typing of all HSV isolates. In a comprehensive viral diagnostic program, isolations of HSV are made, and this can provide the necessary familiarity to permit tentative identification of the isolates without definitive serological testing. It has been shown that, at a minimum, 95.5% of HSV isolates can be so reported prior to serotyping (12). However, where indicated, the HSV isolates should be definitively identified with appropriate antisera and typed.

SEROLOGICAL PROCEDURES

There are times, especially in cases of suspected HSV-induced central nervous system (CNS) disease, when the laboratory receives only serum specimens. In such cases, the complement fixation (CF) test would be the first choice for serological diagnosis, and the use of a micromethod would be convenient and sparing of reagents (37). All CF reagents, including HSV antigen and positive control sera, are readily obtained from commercial sources (Flow Laboratories; Microbiological Associates, Inc.). Although CF antigen can be prepared in eggs (42), there is a high incidence of nonspecific reactions; thus, tissue culture methods are more desirable. A description of the production of CF antigen is presented elsewhere (43).

The procedure for the CF test is described in this manual (chapter 71) as well as elsewhere (22, 37, 42). The adequacy of the HSV antigen should first be determined in a titration using both known negative and positive sera. The test proper would, of course, require at least two sera, one taken as early as possible in the course of the disease and a second taken no less than 2 weeks later. Both sera must be heated at 56 C for 0.5 h to destroy any complement activity. It is generally accepted that the second serum should have at least a fourfold greater CF antibody titer than the first serum. This, along with a compatible clinical picture, would be suggestive of an HSV infection. The diagnosis is somewhat strengthened if the rise in antibody is greater than fourfold and the acute serum has a very low titer (1:16 or less).

The neutralization test is a second choice for serological diagnosis. Documented strains of HSV should be used. The measurement of HSV neutralizing antibody is a precise technique involving a viral suspension containing 100 TCD_{50} mixed in equal proportions with twofold dilutions (to 1:2,048) of the patient's sera in cell culture medium. These mixtures are kept at 20 to 25 C for 2 h, and then each mixture is inoculated into two or three cell cultures in a volume of 0.1 ml per culture. The cell cultures used, of course, must not only be quite sensitive to HSV but must be the same cell type that was used to determine the virus concentration. Adequate cell culture controls should be inoculated with 0.1 ml of a 1:2 dilution of the same virus suspension used in the test and produced either by further dilution with cell culture media or a known negative serum. Titers of neutralizing antibody are those serum dilutions that prevent HSV CPE for 4 or 5 days after such effects are produced by the same virus dose in cultures containing no specific antibody. All sera from the same patient must be tested at the same time. Again, the diagnosis is strengthened if the first serum has little or no antibody and the second has substantial levels.

Both CF and neutralizing antibody persist for long periods, even for life. Second infections with HSV, however, do not cause significant increases in either antibody type. Neither procedure, as described, will differentiate between type 1 and 2 HSV infections. In all cases, a serological diagnosis would represent a diagnosis in retrospect. It is suggested that while awaiting the second or convalescent serum specimen the physician be encouraged to submit specimens from which either HSV or other viruses might be isolated so the diagnosis could be more swiftly determined.

There are other serological procedures that have been used for diagnosis, such as the FA method, red cell aggregation, and antigen-antibody precipitating reactions. For routine diagnosis, these techniques are somewhat demanding and offer no clear advantages over the described procedures. It has also been recommended that even when HSV has been isolated the diagnosis should be further confirmed by serological procedures. In most HSV infections, this is unnecessary, but it could be considered when the disease seems atypical.

INTERPRETATION OF RESULTS

Virus isolation is the method of choice in confirming the diagnosis of herpetic lesions. It has been shown that HSV can be readily isolated and promptly reported to the physician (12). Because recurrent herpes may develop during febrile episodes, the pertinence of virus isolation with respect to disease rests primarily upon the clinical circumstances associated with the particular patient.

Serological diagnosis of HSV infections is more limited. Significant increases in antibody titers are normally found only with primary infections, and this method is of little value in diagnosing recurrent disease or reinfections. In addition, patients with V-Z infections may have a rise in titer to HSV antigens in the CF test. In cases of CNS disease, there has been criticism of the serological approach because the results are obtained too late to be of other than academic interest, or they are misleading since rises in HSV antibody can occur without HSV being the cause of disease (17). For example, serological data indicating that HSV-induced aseptic meningitis was common do not agree with the rare detection of this virus in spinal fluids (9, 10, 13, 30). It now appears that the very common type 1 produces an encephalitis and the rarer type 2 may be associated with meningitis (2). Whether certain diseases can incidentally induce activity of a latent HSV, resulting in misleading data, or for whatever reason, there is growing concern about the serological diagnosis of CNS disease. A rise in antibody titer does not "prove" the pertinence of even a related viral isolation, as discussed in more detail elsewhere (11), but in reality just provides another clue to what the infection may have been.

CHEMOTHERAPY

A recent review contains information about a number of antiviral compounds that influence HSV infections (35). One such compound has long been marketed (5-iodo-2′-deoxyuridine, IUdR) for treatment of HSV eye infections. Further, this and other DNA inhibitors have produced therapeutic effects in humans and animals having HSV-induced disease other than of the eye. More recently, there has been substantial interest in treating superficial herpetic lesions with neutral red, proflavine, or toluidine blue (5, 44). HSV is apparently inactivated by the dye's interaction with guanine on exposure to light. In addition, there are suggestions that dilute acetic acid, lipid solvents, and dimethylsulfoxide also may have a therapeutic effect on herpetic lesions.

It would appear that HSV-induced disease is amenable to the chemotherapeutic approach, and this should increase demands for a rapid, accurate laboratory diagnosis. Even with HSV-induced encephalitis, greater diagnostic effort is being suggested so that therapy might be applied to this often fatal disease (17). In addition, the laboratory must now be concerned about the drug susceptibility of HSV as well as the possible emergence of drug-resistant strains, for it is well known that this virus can become quite resistant to IUdR by laboratory manipulation and there are also data suggesting that the type 2 strain (in some cell cultures) is more resistant to DNA inhibitors than is type 1 (31). If this latter observation is found true of human infections, then subtyping of HSV strains would be necessary for proper therapy to be undertaken. At present, however, there is a suggestion that the drug susceptibility of HSV subtypes is not so obvious in animal infections (40), nor is it clear that drug-resistant mutants occur in clinical situations (16).

If the future of antiviral drugs follows the history of bacterial chemotherapy, some thought must now be given to susceptibility testing of viruses against antiviral drugs, perhaps using some modification of the disk plate-plaque inhibition test (31). It is even probable that viral inhibitors will find usefulness in identification of virus isolates. These possibilities are likely not only to increase demands for laboratory diagnosis but also to alter a belief that diagnosis of viral disease is an academic exercise.

B VIRUS

B virus (*Herpesvirus simiae*), which is indigenous to Asian monkeys (15), is important because it can cause a highly lethal CNS infection in humans, when transmitted by monkey bites, saliva, or even tissues and cells so widely used in virus laboratories. B virus is the counterpart of HSV in humans and causes subclinical infections, as well as dermal, oral, or eye lesions in monkeys. Once infected, a human may show localized redness and vesicles, and may have pain at the site of virus entrance. Vesicles on the mucous membranes, pneumonia, diarrhea, abdominal pain, and pharyngitis have been reported, but in all cases an encephalopathy occurs which is frequently fatal, and most who survive have serious brain damage.

B virus is similar to HSV in morphology and size (33) and is also inhbited by agents that suppress DNA synthesis (25). It is assumed this is a typical herpesvirus with an envelope and hence is sensitive to lipid solvents and an acid pH. There is an antigenic relationship between HSV (type 1?) and B virus in that antiserum specific for the latter will also neutralize HSV to almost the homologous titer. Complement seems required for readily demonstrating this relationship. Antisera to the herpesvirus simian agent 8 (SA8) will neutralize either HSV or B virus. High-titered serum specific for HSV, however, has no effect on B virus and almost none on SA8 (15). This "one-way cross" antigenic relationship unfortunately affords those persons immune to HSV no protection against simian herpesviruses.

B virus is reported to be somewhat hardier than HSV; it will survive for a few weeks at 4 C, loses little titer when stored at −70 C, and is inactivated at 37 C within 7 days. It has been reported that B virus can be isolated in a number of cell and animal systems (43), but it differs from human herpesviruses because of its rapid destruction of monkey kidney cells in culture. The CPE produced is much like that caused by HSV on those infrequent occasions when the latter virus produces any CPE at all, resulting in rounded and giant cell formation (15).

In B virus-induced disease, which in humans always involves the CNS, there can be problems in isolating this dangerous virus. Nevertheless, attempts must be made to obtain proper specimens for viral isolation as well as serum samples with a view to accurate diagnosis, since therapy with DNA inhibitors, at the earliest possible time, seems necessary. Once isolated, B virus can be identified by the simple neutralization test described for HSV. Specific antiserum is available from the Research Resources Branch of the National Institutes of Health. B virus disease, of course, is rare in humans but certainly common in Asian monkeys; hence, those dealing with such animals might well profit from studies to see whether B virus is or was prevalent. Such investigations, including not only serology but virus isolation, might best be referred to those expert in handling this virus. Inquiries can be directed to the Center for Disease Control or similar agencies. The Lilly Research Laboratories have had extensive experience in studies of B virus. Both specific sera and virus are obtainable from the Research Resources Branch of the National Institutes of Health, but use of this virus requires a Public Health Service permit. B virus infections in humans or monkeys are a serious problem, and positive serological procedures, done as with HSV, should be given considerable weight, especially in cases of human infection where viral isolation would be difficult.

LITERATURE CITED

1. Blank, H., C. F. Burgoon, G. D. Baldridge, P. L. McCarthy, and F. Urbach. 1951. Cytologic smears in diagnosis of herpes simplex, herpes zoster and varicella. J. Amer. Med. Ass. **146**:1410–1412.
2. Craig, C. P., and A. J. Nahmias. 1973. Different patterns of neurologic involvement with herpes simplex virus types 1 and 2: isolation of herpes simplex type 2 from the buffy coat of two adults with meningitis. J. Infect. Dis. **127**:365–372.
3. Dausset, J., A. L. Florman, R. Bachvaroff, G. Y. Kanra, M. Sasportes, and F. T. Rapaport. 1972. *In vitro* approach to correlation of cell susceptibility to viral infection with HL-A genotypes and other biological markers. Proc. Soc. Exp. Biol. Med. **140**:1344–1349.
4. Fabiyi, A., and H. A. Wenner. 1965. Enterovirus antibodies in mouse ascites fluids after immunization. J. Immunol. **94**:257–261.
5. Felber, T. D., E. B. Smith, J. M. Knox, C. Wallis, and J. L. Melnick. 1973. Photodynamic inactivation of herpes simplex: report of a clinical trial. J. Amer. Med. Ass. **223**:289–292.
6. Feldman, H. A., and S. S. Wang. 1961. Sensitivity of various viruses to chloroform. Proc. Soc. Exp. Biol. Med. **106**:736–738.
7. Gardner, P. S., J. McQuillin, M. M. Black, and J. Richardson. 1968. Rapid diagnosis of herpesvirus hominis infections in superficial lesions by immunofluorescent antibody techniques. Brit. Med. J. **4**:89–92.
8. Hayflick, L., and P. S. Moorhead. 1961. The serial cultivation of human diploid cell strains. Exp. Cell Res. **25**:585–621.
9. Haynes, R. E., P. H. Azimi, and H. G. Cramblett. 1968. Fatal Herpesvirus hominis (herpes simplex virus) infections in children. Clinical pathologic and virologic characteristics. J. Amer. Med. Ass. **206**:312–319.
10. Herrmann, E. C., Jr. 1967. Experiences in laboratory diagnosis of herpes simplex, varicella-zoster, and vaccinia virus infections in routine medical practice. Mayo Clin. Proc. **42**:744–753.
11. Herrmann, E. C., Jr. 1970. The tragedy of viral diagnosis. Postgrad. Med. J. **46**:545–550.
12. Herrmann, E. C., Jr. 1971. Efforts toward a more useful viral diagnostic laboratory. Amer. J. Clin. Pathol. **56**:681–686.
13. Herrmann, E. C., Jr. 1972. Rates of isolation of viruses from a wide spectrum of clinical specimens. Amer. J. Clin. Pathol. **57**:188–194.
14. Higgins, P. G. 1966. The isolation of viruses from acute respiratory infections. IV. A comparative study of the use of cultures of human embryo kidney and human embryo diploid fibroblasts (WI.38). Mon. Bull. Min. Health Publ. Health Lab. Serv. **25**:223–229.
15. Hull, R. N. 1968. The simian viruses. Virology monographs, vol. 2, p. 22–25. Springer-Verlag, Berlin.
16. Jawetz, E., V. R. Coleman, C. R. Dawson, and P. Thygeson. 1970. The dynamics of *IUDR* action in herpetic keratitis and the emergence of *IUDR* resistance *in vivo*. Ann. N.Y. Acad. Sci. **173**:282–291.
17. Johnson, R. T., L. C. Olson, and E. L. Buescher. 1968. Herpes simplex virus infections of the nervous system. Problems in laboratory diagnosis. Arch. Neurol. **18**:260–264.
18. Juel-Jensen, B. E., and F. O. MacCallum. 1972. Herpes simplex, varicella and zoster. Clinical manifestations and treatment. Heineman Medical Books, Ltd., London.
19. Kaufman, H. E., and E. D. Maloney. 1962. IDU and hydrocortisone in experimental herpes simplex keratitis. Arch. Opthalmol. **68**:396–398.
20. Ketler, A., V. V. Hamparian, and M. R. Hilleman. 1962. Characterization and classification of ECHO 28-rhinovirus-coryzavirus agents. Proc. Soc. Exp. Biol. Med. **110**:821–831.
21. Klein, G. 1972. Herpesviruses and oncogenesis. Proc. Nat. Acad. Sci. U.S.A. **69**:1056–1064.
22. Lennette, E. H. 1969. General principles underlying laboratory diagnosis of viral and rickettsial infections, p. 1–65. Diagnostic procedures for viral and rickettsial infections, 4th ed. E. H. Lennette and N. J. Schmidt (ed.), American Public Health Association, Inc., New York.
23. Long, G. W., J. Noble, Jr., F. A. Murphy, K. L. Herrmann, and B. Lourie. 1970. Experience with electron microscopy in the differential diagnosis of smallpox. Appl. Microbiol. **20**:497–504.
24. Marks, M. I. 1971. Rapid identification of *Herpes simplex* virus in tissue culture by direct immunofluorescence. J. Lab. Clin. Med. **78**:963–968.
25. Miller, F. A. 1967. Inhibition of B virus in cell culture by 5-iodo-2′-deoxyuridine. Appl. Microbiol. **15**:733–735.
26. Nahmias, A., I. delBuono, J. Pipkin, R. Hutton, and C. Wickliffe. 1971. Rapid identification and typing of herpes simplex virus types 1 and 2 by a direct immunofluorescence technique. Appl. Microbiol. **22**:455–458.
27. Nahmias, A. J., and W. R. Dowdle. 1968. Antigenic and biologic differences in herpesvirus hominis. Progr. Med. Virol. **10**:110–159.
28. Nahmias, A. J., W. R. Dowdle, Z. M. Naib, A. Highsmith, R. W. Harwell, and W. E. Josey. 1968. Relation of pock size on chorioallantoic membrane to antigenic type of herpesvirus hominis. Proc. Soc. Exp. Biol. Med. **127**:1022–1028.
29. Nahmias, A., C. Wickliffe, J. Pipkin, A. Leibovitz, and R. Hutton. 1971. Transport media for herpes simplex virus types 1 and 2. Appl. Microbiol. **22**:451–454.
30. Olson, L. C., E. L. Buescher, M. S. Artenstein, and P. D. Parkman. 1967. Herpesvirus infections of the human central nervous system. N. Engl. J. Med. **277**:1271–1277.
31. Person, D. A., P. J. Sheridan, and E. C. Herrmann, Jr. 1970. Sensitivity of types 1 and 2 herpes simplex virus to 5-iodo-2′-deoxyuridine and 9-β-D-arabinofuranosyladenine. Infect. Immunity **2**:815–820.
32. Rawls, W. E., W. A. F. Tompkins, M. E. Figueroa, and J. L. Melnick. 1968. Herpesvirus type 2: association with carcinoma of the cervix. Science **161**:1255–1256.
33. Reissig, M., and J. L. Melnick. 1955. The cellular changes produced in tissue cultures by herpes B virus correlated with the concurrent multiplication of the virus. J. Exp. Med. **101**:341–351.
34. Rodin, P., M. J. Hare, C. F. Barwell, and M. J. Withers. 1971. Transport of herpes simplex virus in Stuart's medium. Brit. J. Vener. Dis. **47**:198–199.
35. Schabel, F. M., Jr., and J. A. Montgomery. 1972. Purines and pyrimidines. Chapter 4 *in* Chemotherapy of virus diseases, vol. 1 (D. J. Bauer, sect. ed.). International Encyclopedia of Pharmacology and Therapeutics, Section 61, p. 231–363, Pergamon Press, Oxford.
36. Scott, T. F. McN., C. F. Burgoon, L. L. Coriell, and H. Blank. 1953. The growth curve of the virus of herpes simplex in rabbit corneal cells grown in tissue culture with parallel observations on the development of the intranuclear inclusion body. J. Immunol. **71**:385–396.
37. Sever, J. L. 1962. Application of microtechnique to viral serological investigations. J. Immunol. **88**:320–329.
38. Sheridan, P. J. and E. C. Herrmann, Jr. 1971. Intraoral lesions of adults associated with herpes simplex virus. Oral Surg. Oral Med. Oral Pathol. **32**:390–397.
39. Shope, T. C., J. Klein-Robbenhaar, and G. Miller. 1972. Fatal encephalitis due to *Herpesvirus hominis;* use of intact brain cells for isolation of virus. J. Infect. Dis. **125**:542–544.
40. Sloan, B. J., F. A. Miller, and I. W. McLean, Jr. 1972.

Treatment of herpes simplex virus types 1 and 2 encephalitis in mice with 9-β-D-arabinofuranosyladenine. Antimicrob. Ag. Chemother. **3:**74–80.

41. Smith, K. O., and J. L. Melnick. 1962. Recognition and quantitation of herpesvirus particles in human vesicular lesions. Science **137:**543–544.
42. Sosa-Martinez, J., and E. H. Lennette. 1955. Studies on a complement fixation test for herpes simplex. J. Bacteriol. **70:**205–215.
43. Tokumaru, T. 1969. Herpesviruses, *Herpesvirus hominis*, *Herpesvirus simiae*, *Herpesvirus suis*, p. 641–700 E. H. Lennette and N. J. Schmidt (ed.), Diagnostic procedures for viral and rickettsial infections, 4th ed. American Public Health Association, Inc., New York.
44. Wallis, C., and J. L. Melnick. 1965. Photodynamic inactivation of animal viruses: a review. Photochem. Photobiol. **4:**159–170.
45. Wheeler, C. E., Jr., R. A. Briggaman, and R. R. Henderson. 1969. Discrimination between two strains (types) of herpes simplex virus by various modifications of the neutralization test. J. Immunol. **102:**1179–1192.

Chapter 84
Human Cytomegalovirus

MATILDA BENYESH-MELNICK

CLINICAL BACKGROUND

Cytomegaloviruses (CMV), previously known as salivary gland viruses, comprise a group of related but highly species-specific agents indigenous for man and numerous other mammals. In vivo and in vitro infection with these agents results in a characteristic cytopathology of greatly enlarged (cytomegalic) cells containing intranuclear and cytoplasmic inclusions. In man, CMV infection in the newborn is usually congenital and results in generalized (often fatal) cytomegalic inclusion disease (CID) involving the liver, lungs, brain, and blood-forming organs. Microcephaly, motor disability, and mental retardation are common sequelae in surviving infants. Acquired infection with CMV is widespread and usually asymptomatic. In children, acquired infection may result in subacute or chronic hepatitis. CMV infection has been associated with acquired hemolytic anemia and an infectious mononucleosis-like syndrome (but without a heterophile antibody response), often occurring after transfusion of fresh blood.

Patients with malignancies or antibody deficiencies, or those undergoing immunosuppressive therapy for organ transplantation, may develop cytomegalovirus pneumonitis or hepatitis and occasionally generalized disease; the relative importance of primary infection versus reactivation of a latent infection in such cases remains to be clarified. Prolonged virus excretion in the urine and saliva in the presence of a significant level of antibody is characteristic for both congenital and acquired CMV infection.

Recent studies suggest the possibility of venereal acquisition and transmission of CMV infection; the virus has been isolated from semen, as well as from cervical secretions of women in the last trimester of pregnancy or of nonpregnant women suspected of venereal disease.

DESCRIPTION OF AGENT

Cytomegaloviruses are deoxyribonucleic acid-containing viruses classified as members of the herpesvirus group. The virion consists of a 110-nm capsid with 162 capsomeres, surrounded by a lipid-containing (single or double membrane) envelope; the enveloped particles range in size from 180 to 250 nm. The virus is heat-labile (56 C for 30 min), unstable at pH below 5, ether-sensitive, and unable to withstand freezing and thawing in the absence of stabilizers. Cell-free virus can be stored at −90 C in the presence of 35% sorbitol without appreciable loss of infectivity. Virus-infected cells, suspended in Eagle's medium with 10% serum and 10% dimethyl sulfoxide (DMSO) can be maintained in a viable state for indefinite periods of time in liquid nitrogen (−190 C). Antigenically, human CMV is distinct from other members of the herpesvirus group and from CMV of other species. Although there is some antigenic variation among strains of human CMV, there is no convincing evidence as yet that more than one distinct serotype exists.

COLLECTION AND STORAGE OF SPECIMENS

Pathognomonic cytomegalic cells can be found in stained sediments of urine, saliva, and gastric washings of infants with generalized CID. However, the method of choice for the diagnosis of congenital or acquired cytomegalovirus infection remains the direct isolation of virus from urine or saliva. Virus can be isolated also from various body fluids (including milk, cervical secretions, and semen), liver biopsies, adenoid tissues, lymph nodes, and peripheral blood leukocytes, as well as from various tissues taken at autopsy.

Urine for exfoliative cytology

Urine samples should be collected only when generalized CID is suspected. Since the specific cells deteriorate rapidly, only freshly collected urine samples should be tested. Addition of an equal volume of 70 or 95% alcohol immediately after collection enhances cell preservation (19). Excretion of cytomegalic cells is known to be intermittent; thus, two or three consecutive samples should be examined.

Specimens for virus isolation

In view of the relative instability of CMV upon freezing, it is desirable that body fluids or tissue suspensions be tested fresh, within 2 to 4 h after collection. Until processed, specimens should be kept at 4 C. When freezing of specimens is mandatory, a sorbitol-containing diluent (equal volumes of 50% sorbitol [in distilled water] and tissue culture medium) should be used as the medium for collection of mouth or cervical swabs, for preparation of suspensions, or for addition to an equal volume of fresh urine. See Chapter 71 for details on collection of urine, swabs, and tissue specimens.

Blood specimens for serological diagnosis

Serological procedures with a single sample of a patient's serum are of limited value in the diagnosis of CMV infection. Persistent or rising complement-fixing (CF) antibody titers in infants over 6 months of age may be helpful in confirming congenital CMV infection. Studies indicate the appearance of, or a significant rise in, CF antibodies (often with concomitant virus isolation) in patients receiving kidney transplants (7) and in an infectious mononucleosis-like syndrome, often occurring after transfusion of fresh blood (16). Thus, for individual patients, the collection of several serum samples is necessary for any meaningful testing.

A recently developed indirect fluorescent-antibody (FA) test for CMV-specific immunoglobulin M (IgM) antibody (15, 18, 26) is gaining diagnostic value in determining recent CMV infections through the use of a single serum sample.

DIRECT MICROSCOPIC EXAMINATION OF SPECIMENS

Histopathology

Routine histological techniques permit the detection of the characteristic cytomegalic cells in surgical biopsies or tissues taken at autopsy. The absence of cytomegalic cells does not preclude cytomegalovirus infection. Often, virus can be isolated from tissue without demonstrable pathognomonic cells.

Exfoliative cytology

Pathognomonic cytomegalic cells with prominent intranuclear inclusions may be detected in the urine sediment of about 50% of infants with CID (2, 13), but after early infancy this procedure is of little value when compared with virus isolation. The procedure of choice is that of filtering fresh urine samples through a membrane filter (2). Filters are fixed and stained with hematoxylin-eosin or Papanicolaou's stain. Under a microscope, the cytomegalic cell is easily distinguished from other cells that may be present by its large size (10 to 40 μm), scanty but well-delineated cytoplasm, and large nucleus containing a prominent central inclusion separated from the peripheral marginated chromatin by a distinct clear zone ("halo"). Similar cells may be demonstrated also in saliva, gastric washings, and other body fluids.

ISOLATION OF AGENT

Host system

Whereas in vivo cytomegalovirus infection involves exclusively epithelial cells, in vitro the virus can be isolated and propagated only in human fibroblastic cells derived from various tissues, such as embryonic skin-muscle or lung tissue, testis, foreskin, or myometrium. Serially propagated diploid strains of embryonic skin-muscle or lung fibroblasts (such as WI-38) are used. The procedures described for diploid cell strains, or for trypsinization of primary monkey kidney tissue, can be used to derive cell strains from a local supply of human embryonic tissues (25).

Cells are grown in Eagle's minimal essential medium (prepared in Earle's balanced salt solution) with 10% fetal bovine or hypogammaglobulinemic calf serum, $NaHCO_3$ (0.075% for cells grown in stoppered vessels and 0.225% for cells grown in petri dishes in a 5% CO_2 atmosphere), and antibiotics (penicillin, 100 units/ml; streptomycin, 100 μg/ml; and nystatin, 25 units/ml). Prior to inoculation of specimens, the same medium but with 2 to 5% serum and 0.225% $NaHCO_3$ is used for maintenance of monolayers in both stoppered vessels and petri dishes. For preparing stained preparations, cell cultures in Leighton tubes with 11 $\times$ 22 mm cover slips are recommended.

Inoculation and observation of cultures

For virus isolation, the urine can be inoculated directly, or it may be first clarified by centrifugation at 2,500 rpm for 20 min. The use of sediment-enriched urine (10 ml of urine centrifuged and the sediment resuspended in 2 ml of the supernatant urine) increases the chance for virus recovery without a significant increase in contaminants, provided the specimens are treated with a sufficient amount of antibiotics (penicillin, 500 units/ml; streptomycin, 500 μg/ml; and nystatin, 100 units/ml) and tested within 1 to 4 h after collection. The samples are inoculated in 0.2-ml amounts into each of four culture tubes containing 2 ml of maintenance medium. The cultures are incubated at 37 C in stationary racks or roller drums. Since occasional urine samples may be toxic to the fibroblast monolayers, the maintenance medium is replaced 24 h after inoculation. Thereafter, the medium is changed twice a week at the time of microscopic examination for viral cytopathic changes (CPE). The frequent medium change allows for preservation of clear confluent monolayers throughout the observation period. This should be at least 30 days and preferably longer to insure the detection of small quantities of virus present in the inoculum. Uninoculated cultures are handled in the same manner and serve as controls.

Other body fluids, mouth or cervical swabs, and 10 to 20% suspensions of biopsy or autopsy specimens are also inoculated into each of four replicate cultures.

For biopsy specimens or tissues obtained at autopsy, the in vitro cultivation of cells from the specimen offers an advantage over the procedures for virus isolation from tissue suspension, in that it allows for the detection of minute amounts of virus that may be present in the tissues (2). Tissue should be processed as soon as possible after collection and no later than 24 h. (Frozen tissues are not suitable for cell cultivation.) Tissues are minced and dispersed by trypsinization according to the procedures used for monkey kidneys (25). The resulting cell suspension containing 5×10^5 viable cells/ml is seeded into appropriate vessels.

Within 3 to 5 days of primary seeding, the growth medium is replaced, and this procedure is repeated twice a week until complete monolayers are formed. For initiation of autopsy kidney cell cultures, Melnick's medium A with 0.038% $NaHCO_3$ has been found to yield better results than Eagle's medium (2). After 3 to 5 days of primary growth, the medium may be replaced with Eagle's medium.

Secondary and tertiary cultures are prepared by subcultivation of trypsin-dispersed 2- to 3-week-old complete monolayers at a ratio of 1:2. When sufficient cells are not available, an equal amount of freshly trypsinized human embryo fibroblasts is added to each culture. Primary, secondary, and tertiary cultures are kept for a 60-day period of observation by feeding with Eagle's maintenance medium twice a week after microscopic examination for viral CPE. Periodically, cover-slip preparations are retrieved for histological examination.

Evidence of infection in cell cultures

Fibroblast monolayers inoculated with virus-containing specimens or cell cultures from virus-infected tissues reveal specific CPE within several days, several weeks, or even later, depending upon the amount of virus present. Often secondary cell cultures from biopsy or autopsy specimens reveal the CPE before the primary cultures, and occasionally the latter remain negative (2).

Initially, the CPE consists of small, round or elongated foci of enlarged, rounded, refractile cells, easily distinguishable from the normal cell monolayer (Fig. 1). Often the affected cells reveal brownish refractile cytoplasmic granules. In monolayers fixed in Bouin's or Zenker's solution and stained with hematoxylin-eosin, the affected cells reveal enlarged distorted nuclei containing one or more large eosinophilic (amphophilic or basophilic, depending upon the staining technique) inclusions. The inclusions are finely granular and separated by a clear zone (halo) from the marginated chromatin on the clearly delineated nuclear membrane. The nucleoli are more basophilic than the inclusion and are usually found within the halo. Often an eosinophilic or amphophilic cytoplasmic lesion is found adjacent to the nucleus (Fig. 2). Multinucleated cells with intranuclear inclusions and a prominent cytoplasmic lesion are often encountered.

The spread of CPE in infected cultures is usually very slow. Since infectious CMV is mainly cell-associated, infection first spreads to the cells adjacent to the initial foci, followed by central focal degeneration, appearance of new foci, and eventual involvement of the entire monolayer—a process which may take several weeks or longer.

This process is greatly accelerated by trypsin dispersion of the cells in infected cultures. The fluids of culture tubes exhibiting about 20 to 30% CPE and containing ample amounts of normal fibroblasts are decanted, and the monolayers are washed and flooded with 2 ml of 0.25% trypsin solution. The trypsin is removed and the tubes are incubated for 5 min at 37 C in the residual trypsin. Immediately thereafter, 2 ml of growth medium is added to each tube, and the tubes are reincubated at 37 C. This allows for a uniform dispersion of the infected cells among the normal fibroblasts in the newly formed monolayers and faster progression of the CPE.

Virus passage and storage

The conventional methods of subcultivation of supernatant fluids or frozen-and-thawed infected cell cultures are not applicable for CMV. The virus is mainly cell-associated (especially during the early stages after isolation) and may not withstand freezing and thawing. Furthermore, even though infectious titers of well-adapted strains can be obtained in the order of

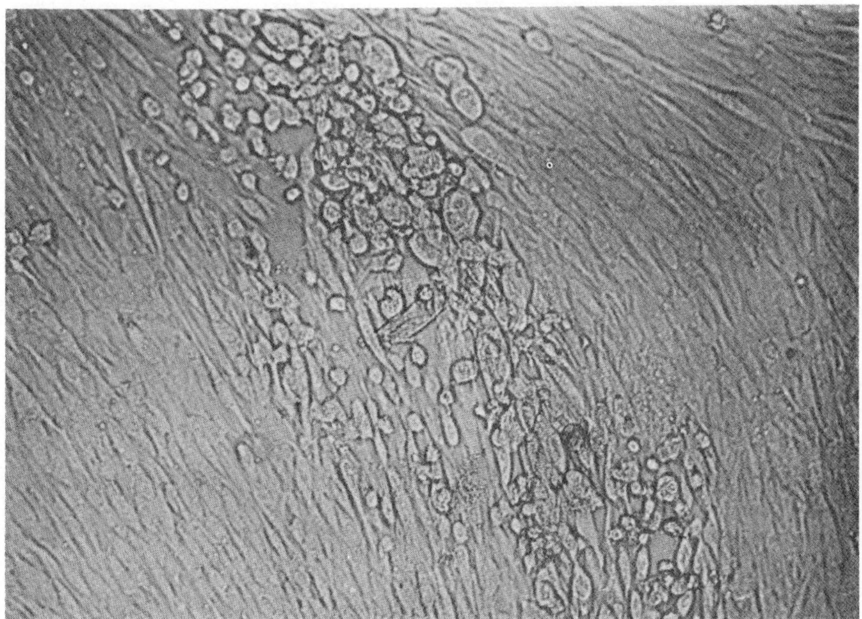

FIG. 1. *Cytopathic effect of cytomegalovirus in human embryonic fibroblasts. Unstained preparation; ×140.*

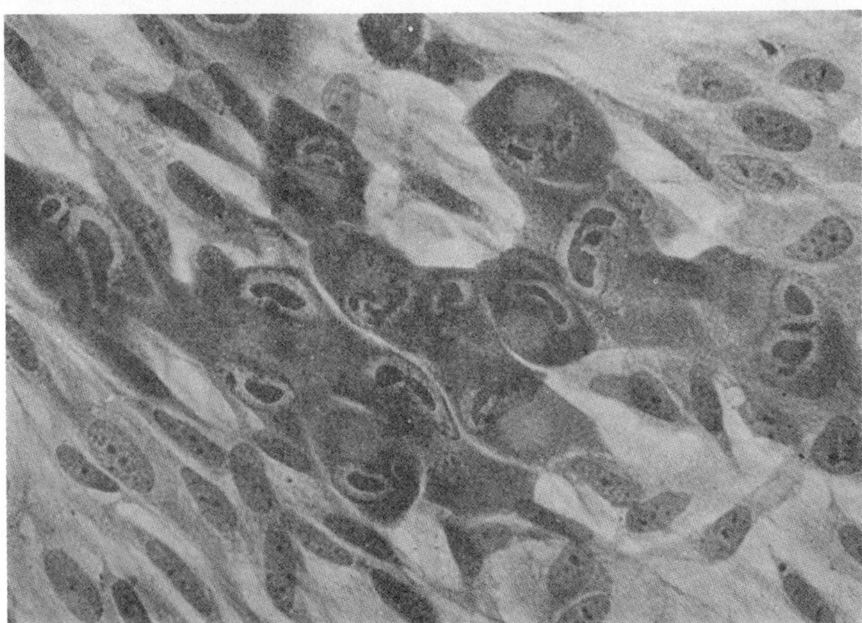

FIG. 2. *Cytopathic effect of cytomegalovirus in human embryonic fibroblasts. Hematoxylin and eosin; ×560.*

10^5 to 10^6 from homogenized infected cells, the initiation and progression of CPE with such virus is relatively slow; complete cell degeneration may not be achieved until the 10th day. Thus, passage inocula should contain intact infected cells. Infected cultures in which about 80% of the cells show CPE are trypsinized, and the resulting cell suspension is either adsorbed onto preformed normal monolayers or mixed with freshly trypsinized normal fibroblasts, the latter procedure yielding the best results (2, 28).

Infected cells can be stored in a viable state at

any time during subcultivation. Monolayers exhibiting about 80% CPE are trypsinized, and the cells are resuspended in Eagle's medium with 10% serum and 10% DMSO. The cell suspension can be stored at −90 C; however, infectivity is preserved more effectively upon storage in liquid nitrogen. Virus cultivation with stored infected cells is carried out by the procedures described above.

For quantitative laboratory work, cell-free virus stocks are prepared from disrupted infected cells and clarified by methods described (28). Unclarified virus preparations are unsuitable for quantitative virus assay. Samples of clarified virus suspension in equal volumes of 70% sorbitol (in water) can be stored at −90 C for long periods of time (over 12 months) without appreciable loss of infectivity. By use of this procedure, titers of 10^6 plaque-forming units (PFU)/ml of sorbitol-preserved virus stock can regularly be obtained.

Of the procedures available for titration of CMV, the most commonly used are the tube titration method, based on the cytopathic end point (32), and the plaque assay (22, 28, 33). The plaque assay, recently modified for use in disposable plastic trays (Linbro Disposotray model FB16-24TC) to employ lesser quantities of cells and other reagents (6), is recommended for laboratories in which CO_2 incubators are available; the test is more sensitive and is read at the end of 14 days as compared with 28 days required for the tube titration method. Other methods have been described: a 7-day immunofluorescence focus assay (23), a 3-day immunofluorescence single-cell assay (29), and a 2-day assay employing the enumeration of single cells with inclusion bodies in stained cover-slip preparations (10). Even though these methods are quantitative and require shorter periods of time, they offer little advantage over the plaque assay because they involve numerous cumbersome steps in inoculation and staining of cover-slip preparations, and high-power microscopy and sophistication are necessary for enumeration of infected cells.

IDENTIFICATION OF CYTOMEGALOVIRUS ISOLATES

Cytopathology and host range

The cytopathic changes induced by CMV and described above are considered pathognomonic for this agent and can be readily differentiated by the experienced worker from the changes induced by the other two members of the human herpesvirus group: varicella-zoster virus and herpes simplex virus. Furthermore, CMV can be propagated only in human fibroblasts, whereas varicella-zoster virus can also grow in epithelial cells and herpes simplex virus can be propagated in a wide variety of mammalian and avian cells as well as in embryonated eggs. Unlike CMV, varicella-zoster virus remains strictly cell-associated.

Serological identification

In many laboratories, the identification of suspected CMV isolates is based solely on the pathognomonic cytopathology and host range in tissue culture. However, it is desirable to confirm this with further serological identification. The most suitable and practical test for this purpose is the CF test. The test can be carried out by any of the standard procedures available (see Chapter 71). A microtechnique performed in plastic panels and utilizing 0.015 ml of the respective reagents is routinely used in this laboratory (20).

Standard animal antisera for typing of CMV by the CF test are not yet available; however, selected human sera are suitable. It is not clearly established whether more than one serotype of CMV exists, but it is generally found that the various strains of CMV share CF antigens (8, 19, 27). Sera of normal adults that react with the most widely used strain, AD169 (which appears to be more broadly reacting [8, 13]), also react with all other known CMV strains. For the test, a human serum is selected that is positive for a standard CMV antigen but free from CF antibody to herpes simplex and varicella-zoster viruses. Control sera include a human serum (or rabbit antiserum) positive for herpes simplex virus but negative for CMV, as well as a human serum positive for varicella-zoster virus but negative for CMV. All sera are inactivated at 56 C for 30 min, their titers are determined by a checkerboard titration with the respective standard antigen, and they are used at a dilution containing 4 units.

The antigen is prepared from the isolate to be tested by the procedures described below for preparation of CF antigen from standard CMV strains. Control antigen prepared from uninfected human embryonic lung cells (in which the isolate was grown) and a standard CMV antigen are included in the test. Veronal buffer-saline at pH 7.2 is used as diluent for all of the reagents, as well as to substitute for antigen or serum in controls for anticomplementarity of the reagents. The test employs 2 units of complement, 2 units of hemolysin, and a 2% suspension of sheep red blood cells (RBC).

Twofold dilutions of the antigen (usually starting with a dilution of 1:2) are mixed in

0.015-ml amounts with equal volumes of serum and of complement. After overnight incubation at 4 C, 0.015 ml of the sensitized sheep RBC is added, and incubation is continued for 1 h at 37 C. Antigen titer is expressed as the reciprocal of the highest dilution of antigen in which 75% or more of the sheep RBC are not hemolyzed (3+ to 4+). In the absence of anticomplementary activity, and the absence of reaction with the antigen from uninfected control cells, the unknown isolate can be identified as CMV if the antigen gives the reaction observed with the standard CMV antigen. There should be positive fixation with the CMV-positive serum and negative fixation with the sera containing antibody to the other two members of the herpesvirus group. Antigens prepared properly from the isolates usually yield titers of 1:16 to 1:64.

Animal antisera are now becoming available for identifying CMV isolates by neutralization tests. Human CMV-specific antisera have been prepared in guinea pigs (17), rabbits (1), primates bred in captivity and free from antibody to simian CMV (11), and in goats (12) after multiple inoculations with crude infectious virus. (Limited amounts of high-titered monkey and goat antisera to two strains of human CMV (AD169 and C87) are available as reference reagents through the Research Resources Branch of the National Institute of Allergy and Infectious Diseases.) Unlike with other herpesviruses or with simian CMV, the hyperimmunized animals produce mainly complement-requiring neutralizing (CRN) antibody, a fact to be contended with in neutralization tests with such antisera. So far, cross-neutralization tests with antisera to different strains of human CMV have not revealed wide antigenic differences; thus, the AD169 strain can be safely used to prepare antisera for identification of suspected CMV isolates.

In this laboratory's experience goats have proven to be the most suitable animals for immunization, as they are free of pre-existing cross-reacting antibody and yield large quantities of high-titer (1:1,000 to 1:3,000 in the presence of complement) antisera within a relatively short immunization period (12). The immunizing antigen consists of cell-free virus stocks prepared as described (2, 28); sorbitol-treated stocks (see above), kept frozen at −90 C, are suitable. Each inoculum should consist of approximately 10^6 PFU/ml in 5 ml given intraperitoneally (3 ml), intravenously (1 ml), and intramuscularly (1 ml of virus plus 1 ml of Freund's complete adjuvant). The animals are inoculated on days 0, 7, 14, 21, and 35, and are bled out 2 weeks after the last inoculation. All sera, including preinoculation samples, are kept at −20 C and heat-inactivated at 56 C for 30 min prior to testing.

For laboratories in which CO_2 incubators are available, the plaque reduction neutralization procedure (8, 22), modified to allow for the incorporation of complement (6, 11, 12) is recommended for determination of antibody titers in the hyperimmune sera. This method is less time-consuming and more precise than the tube neutralization test. Unheated guinea pig serum, free from nonspecific viral inhibitors, is employed as a source of complement and kept in small portions at −90 C. Eagle's medium free from $NaHCO_3$ [or tris(hydroxymethyl)aminomethane (Tris) buffer] with 5% heat-inactivated (56 C, 30 min) fetal bovine serum is used as diluent for all reagents. The test employs twofold dilutions of heat-inactivated (56 C, 30 min) test serum (first dilution, 1:8), unheated guinea pig serum, diluted to contain 5 full units of complement (usually a dilution of 1:8 or 1:16), and virus diluted to contain 600 PFU per 0.1 ml. Serum, complement, and virus (for tests in the presence of complement), or serum, diluent, and virus (for tests in the absence of complement) are mixed at a ratio of 2:1:1 (usually 0.4 ml + 0.2 ml + 0.2 ml, respectively). For virus controls, diluent is used to substitute for either serum or serum and complement. After 1 h of incubation at 37 C, 0.2 ml of each mixture is inoculated onto duplicate human embryo fibroblast monolayers in 60-mm plastic petri dishes, from which the medium has just been removed. The inoculum is allowed to adsorb for 1 h at 37 C, and 7 ml of Eagle's medium containing 2% methylcellulose, 5% fetal bovine serum, 0.15% $NaHCO_3$, and antibiotics is added. After 7 days of incubation at 37 C in a CO_2 incubator, 7 ml of the same medium but with 1.4% methylcellulose is added to each plate, and incubation is continued for an additional 7 days. (For tests in Disposotrays [6]), the volume of inoculum and overlay per well is reduced to 0.05 ml [one drop of a 1-ml pipette] and 1 ml, respectively.) Thereafter, the plates are transferred to 4 C for several hours, the overlay is sucked off, and the monolayers are stained with methylene blue (0.03% solution). Plaques are enumerated usually with a low-power dissecting microscope. Serum titers are expressed as the final serum dilution producing 60% plaque reduction, calculated on the basis of plaque counts in control cultures (300 PFU per plate; 75 PFU per well of dispostray) that have received the virus challenge dose alone. (An overlay medium consisting of Eagle's medium with 0.6% agarose [33] is being used in some laboratories instead of the methylcellulose overlay described here, with equivalent results.)

By the above-described test, properly prepared antisera yield, in the presence of complement, neutralization titers to the immunizing virus of 1:1,000 to 1:3,000 (in the absence of complement the antisera are either free from neutralizing activity or have maximal titers of 1:200); antisera prepared to strain AD169 neutralize equally well other strains of human CMV and are free from neutralizing antibody to herpes simplex virus (1, 6, 11, 12).

Thus, antisera to strain AD169 are suitable for identification of suspect CMV isolates. Antiserum to herpes simplex virus should be used as a control serum in the test. If the isolate is CMV, with the use of the above-described neutralization test in the presence of complement, a dilution of AD169 antiserum containing 10 antibody units (a 1:100 dilution of serum with a titer of 1:1,000) will neutralize the virus challenge dose (see above), whereas herpes simplex antiserum will not. If neutralization of CPE in tube cultures (5, 24, 32) is used as the assay method, 10^2 TCD_{50} of a suspect CMV isolate will be neutralized by the AD169 antiserum.

The indirect FA technique has been used for detection of CMV antigen (23). As with the CF test, identification of a suspected CMV isolate by this procedure requires the use of selected human sera that react with known CMV antigens but are free from antibody to herpes simplex virus or varicella-zoster virus.

SEROLOGICAL DIAGNOSIS

Several methods are available for quantitating CMV antibody: the most commonly used CF and neutralization tests and the more recently introduced FA test for the detection of IgG or IgM antibody. Two other indirect tests for measuring CMV antibody have been recently reported, an indirect hemagglutination-inhibition test (4, 9) and a platelet aggregation test (21); both tests are reported to be equal or surpass the CF test in sensitivity, but because of the more cumbersome methodology involved their use has been limited and can not be recommended for general use in a diagnostic laboratory.

Complement-fixation test

The CF test is the test of choice for routine diagnostic serology. Since the known CMV strains share CF antigens, the test can employ one standard antigen. The AD169 strain is recommended since it appears to have a broader reactivity than other strains (8, 13). More recent studies suggest that the use of additional strains, such as Davis and a local isolate, may be advisable for more precise serological surveys (30).

The methods used to obtain the CF antigen from disrupted infected cells vary slightly from laboratory to laboratory (3, 5, 17, 19, 27, 30, 31). To obtain potent antigen (titers of 1:16 to 1:64) free from anticomplementary activity, the following procedure is recommended. Since the supernatant fluids of infected cultures are usually free from CF activity (3), only the infected cells are used. Infected human embryo fibroblast monolayers in 16-oz (473-ml) bottles (about 5×10^6 cells) exhibiting about 80% CPE are used. The medium is decanted and the monolayers are washed twice with phosphate-buffered saline. The cells are dislodged from the glass either by incubating for 5 to 10 min with 10 ml of 0.2% trypsin or by scraping in 10 ml of Veronal-buffered saline at pH 7.2. The resulting cell suspension is centrifuged at 1,500 rpm for 15 min, the supernatant fluid is discarded, and the cell pack is resuspended in Veronal-buffered saline (1 to 2 ml per cell pack of one 16-oz bottle). The cells are disrupted by treatment for 2 min in a Raytheon ultrasonic oscillator at 10,000 kc/s (if such is not available, freeze and thaw the cell suspension three times), and the suspension is clarified at 800 rpm for 10 min; in some laboratories, prior to clarification, the suspensions are treated for 18 h at 37 C with isotonic glycine buffer at pH 10 (17). The resulting supernatant fluid containing the CF antigen is distributed in 0.5-ml amounts and kept frozen at −90 C. Control antigen from uninfected fibroblasts is prepared and stored in the same fashion. The antigen is used unheated. Anticomplementary activity which may be present in rare lots of antigen can be removed by treating at 56 C for 15 min without appreciable loss in viral antigen. The titer of the CF antigen is determined by checkerboard titration of the antigen against a known positive serum.

The CF test can be conveniently performed by the microtechnique in plastic panels (20). The test employs 2 units of complement, 2 units of hemolysin, and a 2% suspension of sheep RBC. Veronal-buffered saline at pH 7.2 is used as diluent for all of the reagents, as well as to substitute for antigen or serum in controls for anticomplementarity of the reagents. The antigen is used at a dilution containing 4 units. Test sera are inactivated at 56 C for 30 min, and serial twofold dilutions are mixed in 0.015-ml amounts with equal volumes of antigen and complement. After overnight incubation at 4 C, 0.015 ml of the sensitized sheep RBC is added, and incubation is continued for 1 h at 37 C. Serum titers are expressed as the reciprocal of the highest serum dilution in which 75% or more of the sheep RBC are not hemolyzed (3+ to 4+). A known positive serum and antigen prepared from uninfected cells are included as controls. In the absence of anticomplementary activity and the absence of reaction with the control antigen from uninfected cells, sera yielding titers of 1:8 or greater are considered positive for CMV antibody.

Neutralization tests

The several types of neutralization tests available for quantitating CMV neutralizing antibody are less likely to be used in routine diagnostic serology as compared with the CF test. It is not yet clearly established whether more than one serotype of CMV exists. A certain degree of heterogeneity has been suggested from neutralization tests with sera of infants with CID, in that sera of individual infants had higher antibody titers to the homologous virus they excreted than to heterologous strains (31). This is less apparent with sera of older children or adults. Until the question of strain differences is resolved, it is desirable that more than one of the known strains be used in the test; these should include the AD169 (24) and the Davis (32) strains, and preferably a local isolate.

For laboratories in which CO_2 incubators are available, the plaque reduction neutralization procedure (8, 22) is recommended. The test does not necessitate the incorporation of guinea pig serum since most human sera contain complement-independent antibody. Virus stocks are prepared in human embryonic fibroblasts and stored at −90 C. The titer of the stock is predetermined by the plaque assay (22, 28, 33). The test sera are inactivated at 56 C for 30 min prior to testing. A virus dilution containing 3×10^2 PFU/0.1 ml and fourfold dilutions of serum (starting at an initial dilution of 1:4 or 1:8) are each made in Eagle's medium free from $NaHCO_3$ (or Tris) containing 5% fetal bovine serum. A 0.4-ml amount of each serum dilution is mixed with 0.4 ml of virus. After 1 h of incubation at 37 C, residual infectivity is determined as described above for tests with animal antisera. Serum titers are expressed as the final serum dilution producing 60% plaque reduction, calculated on the basis of plaque counts in control plates that had received the virus challenge dose (0.2 ml of virus + diluent mixture) alone. Sera yielding titers equal to or greater than 1:8 are considered positive for antibody to CMV.

Neutralizing antibodies can also be measured by the inhibition of the CPE in tube cultures. The test most frequently used (32) employs the combination of about 10^2 TCD_{50} of virus and fourfold serum dilutions. Incubation of virus-serum mixtures for periods of 30 min to 1 h at room temperature or 4 C has been used by various investigators (5, 24, 32). The use of 1-h incubation at 37 C is recommended, provided the diluent in which the reagents are prepared contains 5% fetal bovine serum. Groups of three tube cultures are inoculated with 0.2 ml of the virus-serum mixtures. A parallel virus titration (0.1 ml of virus dilution per each of three tubes) is carried out to determine the exact dose of virus used in the test. Serum titers are expressed as the highest serum dilution inhibiting the CPE in all three cultures during an observation period of 28 days or longer (depending on the time necessary for the appearance of CPE in tubes receiving the virus challenge dose). Sera yielding titers equal to or greater than 1:8 are considered positive for antibody to CMV.

Other presently available methods for titration of CMV (10, 23, 29) have thus far had a more limited use in measuring neutralizing antibodies in human sera.

Indirect fluorescent-antibody test

CMV antigens are found in the nuclear and cytoplasmic inclusions of infected cells, and increasing numbers of laboratories are using the indirect FA test to quantitate antibodies in human sera specific for these antigens. Depending upon the reagents used, the test can preferentially detect IgG or IgM antibody, and in this respect it offers an advantage over the CF test, which measures only IgG antibody, and the neutralization test, which measures both types of antibody. However, successful interpretation of results hinges not only upon proficiency with immunofluorescence techniques but also upon careful discrimination of nonspecific reactions. Special attention should be paid to the localization of the FA staining—cytoplasmic staining in the absence of nuclear staining should be considered nonspecific.

Trypsinized suspensions of CMV-infected cells (15) or cover-slip preparations of CMV-infected monolayers (18, 26) have been used for the FA test; the latter procedure is recommended as it allows for better differentiation between nuclear and cytoplasmic staining. Human fibroblast cells are grown on cover slips and infected with CMV (stain AD169). When focal CPE is evident (monolayers with advanced CPE are harder to evaluate and their use should be avoided), the cover slips are removed, washed twice with phosphate-buffered saline (PBS), fixed in cold acetone for 10 min, and held at −20 C (or lower temperature) until used. Cover slips with noninfected cells are treated in the same way. Prior to staining, the cover slips are removed from the freezer, rinsed once with PBS, and air-dried at room temperature.

Human sera are tested in twofold dilutions, starting with a dilution of 1:8. Pretested FA-negative and FA-positive human sera are included as controls in each test. A drop of each serum dilution is applied to a cover slip of infected cells, and a drop of the first two dilutions is applied to cover slips of uninfected control cells. The cover slips are incubated in a humidified atmosphere at 37 C for 45 min (for test to detect IgG antibody) or for 90 min (for test to detect IgM antibody; this longer incubation compensates for the potential blocking effect of IgG antibody, when present). The cover slips are then rinsed three times (10 min each) with fresh PBS at pH 7.2 to 7.5 and allowed to react for 45 min at 37 C with a 1 drop of a working dilution (the highest dilution giving a 4+ specific staining, usually 1:10 or 1:20) of fluorescein isothiocyanate-conjugated goat or rabbit anti-human globulin; monospecific anti-IgG and anti-IgM globulins (obtained commercially or prepared as outlined in Chapter 76) are used for the test to detect IgG and IgM antibody, respectively. (In an alternate procedure, cover slips that had been exposed to the human test serum can be first allowed to react for 45 min at 37 C with a 1:30 dilution of unlabeled monospecific rabbit anti-human IgG or IgM globulin, followed by incubation for 45 min at 37 C with a 1:30 dilution of fluorescein-conjugated goat anti-rabbit globulin.) The cover slips are then rinsed three times with PBS, dried, mounted on slides in buffered glycerol solution (one part glycerol and four parts PBS, pH 7.2 to 7.5), and examined under a fluorescence microscope.

The degree of specific immunofluorescence is scored as 4+, 3+, 2+, and 1+, corresponding to strong yellow-green, bright-green, dull-green, and faint-green fluorescence, respectively. Cytoplasmic fluorescence in the absence of nuclear fluorescence should be considered nonspecific and excluded from consideration; the infected cells should not stain with the negative human control serum or with any of the antiglobulins used. The highest serum dilution showing 2+ or greater nuclear staining is considered as the indirect FA titer of the test human serum. In the absence of reactivity with uninfected control cells, test sera are considered positive for FA-IgG antibody when yielding a titer of 1:8 or greater. For FA-IgM antibody, a titer of 1:16 or greater is accepted as evidence of recent active infection; the alleged cross-reactivity that has been reported with EB virus and varicella-zoster virus (14, 31) does not occur at this dilution.

INTERPRETATION OF LABORATORY RESULTS

With the development of laboratory procedures for virus isolation, exfoliative cytology and histopathology of biopsy or autopsy material have become less useful in the diagnosis of CMV infection. The most reliable and sensitive method of establishing CMV infection is the direct isolation of the virus from the urine, throat, or other body fluids. However, with the exception of newborn infants with complete or partial manifestation of CID, virus recovery does not necessarily establish an etiological relationship to the existing disease. In older children, virus isolation in the presence of unexplained pneumonitis, acquired hemolytic anemia, and subacute or chronic hepatitis is suggestive of etiological relationship. The same is true for pneumonitis, hepatic involvement, or generalized CMV disease in patients with malignant disease or with immunological defects, or in patients undergoing immunosuppressive therapy for transplantations.

The recently described infectious mononucleosis-like syndrome occurring spontaneously or after transfusion of fresh blood has been accompanied by frequent CMV isolations from urine or leukocytes with concomitant appearance or increase in CF antibody to CMV. This suggests an etiological relationship between infection and disease. However, in both congenital and acquired infections, virus excretion may continue for prolonged periods of time, extending to many months. Furthermore, there is no information available as to whether different strains differ in pathogenic potential; thus, caution should be exercised in assessing the diagnostic significance of virus recovery from a single patient.

With the CF and neutralizing antibody tests, titers of 1:8 or greater in single serum samples tested are considered evidence of previous CMV infection. The CF test is recommended for seroepidemiological surveys because of the cross-reacting CF antigens of the different CMV strains. Until more knowledge is available on the possible heterogeneity of neutralizing antigens of different strains, the neutralization test must be considered of limited value. In population studies, there is usually a good correlation between the presence or absence of CF and neutralizing antibodies. However, the presence of neutralizing antibodies in the absence of CF antibodies has been observed.

A single CF test is of little diagnostic value in establishing CMV infection. It can be used as a screening test in infants suspected of CID. Less than 1% of normal infants from 6 months to 1 year of age have CF titers, in contrast to a nearly 100% incidence in infected infants. For the individual infant, persisting or rising antibody titers in tests with serial serum samples collected beyond the time of decline of maternal antibody are of diagnostic value. Since about 80% of adults over the age of 35 are seropositive, the interpretation of serial bleedings from individual patients may be difficult. However, the appearance of a fourfold or greater rise in CF antibody titers serves as serological evidence of CMV infection (7, 16).

The FA test for IgG antibody cannot be considered at present superior to the CF test as a diagnostic tool, as similar results are obtained by both tests. On the other hand, the FA test for IgM antibody is gaining value in the diagnosis of recent CMV infections through the use of a single serum sample. Since maternal IgM antibodies are not acquired transplacentally, finding of CMV-IgM antibody in infants with symptomatic CID is considered diagnostic for congenital CMV infection and correlates well with virus isolation; the test has been found less reliable in the diagnosis of asymptomatic infants (14, 15). Finding of IgM antibody in a single serum sample during postnatally acquired CMV infection is not considered at present indicative of primary infection since there is increasing evidence that CMV-IgM antibody tends to persist in slowly declining titers for periods of up to several months after acquisition (14, 18, 26). However, IgM titers of 1:16 or greater are indicative of recent infection (14, 18, 26, 31). When possible, the serological diagnosis of CMV infection should be confirmed by virus isolation.

LITERATURE CITED

1. Andersen, H. K. 1971. Serologic differentiation of human cytomegalovirus strains using rabbit hyperimmune sera. Arch. Gesamte Virusforsch. **33**:187–191.
2. Benyesh-Melnick, M. 1969. Cytomegaloviruses, p. 701–732. *In* E. H. Lennette and N. J. Schmidt (ed.), Diagnostic procedures for viral and rickettsial infections, 4th ed. American Public Health Association, Inc., New York.
3. Benyesh-Melnick, M., V. Vonka, F. Probstmeyer, and I. Wimberly. 1966. Human cytomegalovirus: properties of the complement-fixing antigen. J. Immunol. **96**:261–267.
4. Bernstein, M. T., and J. A. Stewart. 1971. Indirect hemagglutination test for detection of antibodies to cytomegalovirus. Appl. Microbiol. **21**:84–89.
5. Carlstrom, G. 1965. Virologic studies on cytomegalic inclusion disease. Acta Paediat. Scand. **54**:17–23.
6. Chiba, S., R. L. Striker, Jr., and M. Benyesh-Melnick. 1972. Microculture plaque assay for human and simian cytomegaloviruses. Appl. Microbiol. **23**:780–783.
7. Craighead, J. E., J. B. Hanshaw, and C. B. Carpenter. 1967. Cytomegalovirus infection after renal allotransplantation. J. Amer. Med. Ass. **201**:725–728.
8. Dreesman, G. R., and M. Benyesh-Melnick. 1967. Spectrum of human cytomegalovirus complement-fixing antigens. J. Immunol. **99**:1106–1114.
9. Fuccillo, D. A., F. L. Moder, R. G. Traub, S. Hensen, and J. L. Sever. 1971. Micro indirect hemagglutination test for cytomegalovirus. Appl. Microbiol. **21**:104–107.
10. Goodheart, C. R., and L. B. Jaross. 1963. Human cytomegalovirus. Assay by counting infected cells. Virology **19**:532–535.
11. Graham, B. J., Y. Minamishima, G. R. Dreesman, H. G. Haines, and M. Benyesh-Melnick. 1971. Complement-requiring neutralizing antibodies in hyperimmune sera to human cytomegaloviruses. J. Immunol. **107**:1618–1630.
12. Haines, H. G., R. Von Essen, and M. Benyesh-Melnick. 1971. Preparation of specific antisera to cytomegaloviruses in goats. Proc. Soc. Exp. Biol. Med. **138**:846–849.
13. Hanshaw, J. B. 1968. Cytomegaloviruses, p. 1–23. *In* S. Gard, C. Hallauer, and K. F. Meyer (ed.), Virology monographs no. 3. Springer-Verlag, New York.
14. Hanshaw, J. B. 1969. Congenital cytomegalovirus infection: laboratory methods of detection. J. Pediat. **75**:1179–1185.
15. Hanshaw, J. B., H. J. Steinfeld, and C. J. White. 1968. Fluorescent-antibody test for cytomegalovirus macroglobulin. N. Engl. J. Med. **279**:566–570.
16. Kääriäinen, L., E. Klemola, and J. Paloheimo. 1966. Rise of cytomegalovirus antibodies in an infectious-mononucleosis-like syndrome after transfusion. Brit. Med. J. **1**:1270–1272.
17. Krech, U., and M. Jung. 1969. The development of neutralizing antibodies in guinea pigs following immunization with human cytomegalovirus. Arch. Gesamte Virusforsch. **28**:248–250.
18. Langenhuysen, M. M. A. C., T. H. The, H. O. Nieweg, and J. G. Kapsenberg. 1970. Demonstration of IgM cytomegalovirus-antibodies as an aid to early diagnosis in adults. Clin. Exp. Immunol. **6**:387–393.
19. Medearis, D. N., Jr. 1964. Observations concerning human cytomegalovirus infection and disease. Bull. Johns Hopkins Hosp. **114**:181–211.
20. Melnick, J. L. 1969. Analytical serology of animal viruses, p. 411–514. *In* J. G. B. Kwapinski (ed.). Analytical serology of microorganisms. John Wiley & Sons, Inc., New York.
21. Penttinen, K., L. Kääriäinen, and G. Myllylä. 1970. Cytomegalovirus antibody assay by platelet aggregation. Arch. Gesamte Virusforsch. **29**:189–194.
22. Plummer, G., and M. Benyesh-Melnick. 1964. A plaque reduction neutralization test for human cytomegalovirus. Proc. Soc. Exp. Biol. Med. **117**:145–150.
23. Rapp, F., L. E. Rasmussen, and M. Benyesh-Melnick. 1963. The immunofluorescent focus technique in studying the replication of cytomegalovirus. J. Immunol. **91**:709–719.
24. Rowe, W. P., J. W. Hartley, S. Waterman, H. C. Turner, and R. J. Huebner. 1956. Cytopathic agent resembling human salivary gland virus recovered from tissue cultures of human adenoids. Proc. Soc. Exp. Biol. Med. **92**:418–424.
25. Schmidt, N. J. 1969. Tissue culture technics for diagnostic virology, p. 79–178. *In* E. H. Lennette and N. J. Schmidt (ed.), Diagnostic procedures for viral and rickettsial diseases, 4th ed. American Public Health Association, Inc., New York.

26. Schmitz, H., and R. Haas. 1972. Determination of different cytomegalovirus immunoglobulins (IgG, IgA, IgM) by immunofluorescence. Arch. Gesamte Virusforsch. **37**:131–140.
27. Stern, H., and S. D. Elek. 1965. The incidence of infection with cytomegalovirus in a normal population. A serologic study in Greater London. J. Hyg. **63**:79–87.
28. Vonka, V., and M. Benyesh-Melnick. 1966. Interactions of human cytomegalovirus with human fibroblasts. J. Bacteriol. **91**:213–220.
29. Waner, J. L., and J. E. Budnick. 1973. Three-day assay for human cytomegalovirus applicable to serum neutralization tests. Appl. Microbiol. **25**:37–39.
30. Waner, J. L., T. H. Weller, and S. V. Kevy. 1973. Patterns of cytomegaloviral complement-fixing antibody activity: a longitudinal study of blood donors. J. Infect. Dis. **127**:538–543.
31. Weller, T. H. 1971. The cytomegaloviruses: ubiquitous agents with protean clinical manifestations. N. Engl. J. Med. **285**:203–214, 267–274.
32. Weller, T. H., J. C. Macauley, J. M. Craig, and P. Wirth. 1957. Isolation of intranuclear inclusions producing agents from infants with illnesses resembling cytomegalic inclusion disease. Proc. Soc. Exp. Biol. Med. **94**:4–12.
33. Wentworth, B. B., and L. French. 1970. Plaque assay of cytomegalovirus strains of human origin. Proc. Soc. Exp. Biol. Med. **135**:253–258.

Chapter 85

Varicella-Zoster Virus

NATHALIE J. SCHMIDT

CLINICAL BACKGROUND

Varicella (chickenpox) and herpes zoster represent different clinical manifestations of infection with the same virus. Varicella occurs most frequently in children and is characterized by fever and a generalized vesicular exanthem. Herpes zoster generally occurs in adults and consists of a painful, circumscribed eruption of vesicular lesions with accompanying inflammation of associated dorsal root or cranial sensory nerve ganglia. It is generally considered that varicella constitutes the primary infection, whereas herpes zoster occurs in individuals with partial immunity resulting from a prior varicella infection. Whether herpes zoster infections result from reintroduction of the virus into the host or from reactivation of the latent virus has not been clearly established; however, the fact that herpes zoster does not exhibit the seasonal prevalence seen with varicella (late winter and spring) suggests that it is not caused by exogenous reinfection after exposure to varicella, but rather by activation of a latent virus.

There are several situations in which providing a specific laboratory diagnosis of varicella-zoster (V-Z) virus infection is crucial. These include (i) instances where there is a possibility of confusion with variola (smallpox); (ii) differentiating between generalized vesicular eruptions caused by V-Z, herpes simplex, or vaccinia viruses; (iii) differentiating between V-Z infection and vesicular eruptions caused by bacterial agents or hypersensitivity reactions; and (iv) furnishing a specific diagnosis of some of the less common manifestations of V-Z virus infections such as varicella pneumonia, encephalitic complications, and progressive varicella. The last is likely to occur in individuals who are on immunosuppressive therapy or have genetic defects in their immune response, and providing a specific diagnosis of V-Z infection in the patient or the patient's contacts may guide in the possible administration of zoster immune globulin (5, 6, 9).

DESCRIPTION OF AGENT

The V-Z virus has a morphology characteristic of members of the herpesvirus group. It has a diameter of 150 to 200 nm, and consists of an inner capsid, composed of 162 capsomeres, surrounded by an envelope composed of two or more membranes (1). The virus possesses an essential lipid, and thus is ether-sensitive. It is a deoxyribonucleic acid virus (12, 14, 15). To date, antigenic variation has not been noted between strains of V-Z virus. The virus appears to share minor antigens with herpes simplex virus (10, 17, 19, 23).

COLLECTION, SHIPMENT, AND STORAGE OF SPECIMENS

Specimens usually examined for V-Z virus or viral antigen are smears of vesicular lesions, vesicular fluids and scrapings, and tissues obtained at autopsy. Lung is the autopsy tissue from which V-Z virus is most frequently recovered. An acute-phase blood specimen should be taken as soon as possible after onset to be examined in parallel with a convalescent-phase specimen, collected at least 14 days later, in an effort to demonstrate a diagnostically significant increase in V-Z antibody titer.

Methods for collection of vesicular fluids and cellular material from the base of the lesions are described in Chapter 71.

Vesicular fluids

Vesicular fluids collected into capillary pipettes or syringes can be used for virus isolation attempts, electron microscopy, and gel diffusion tests, but fluids are unsatisfactory for immunofluorescent staining. Fluids collected onto swabs and placed in holding medium (see Chapter 71) may be used for virus isolation. Lesions more than 4 days old rarely yield infectious virus, but the fluids may give positive results by electron microscopy or immunodiffusion.

Smears of cellular material from the base of fresh lesions

Smears of cellular material from the base of fresh lesions are used for direct examination by fluorescent-antibody (FA) or histological staining. Since differentiation of V-Z, herpes simplex, and vaccinia by FA staining is accomplished by testing against FA conjugates to each of these viruses, and demonstrating staining with only a single conjugate, it is essential to prepare three smears of cellular material for FA examination. If insufficient material is available for this, what is available should be submitted for virus isolation or electron microscopy only. Cellular material should be placed in holding medium (see Chapter 71) for virus isolation attempts.

Crusts from lesions

Crusts from lesions do not yield infectious virus and are not suitable for FA staining, but if nothing else is available they may be used for examination by electron microscopy or gel diffusion.

Lung, liver, or skin tissue

Smears of autopsy tissue for immunofluorescent staining are prepared by excising three or four pieces of tissue about 10 to 15 mm in size, holding the tissue with forceps, and gently pressing the cut surface to the clean surface of a slide. A series of impressions is made over an area 30 to 40 mm in length. Three or four slides should be prepared from each specimen. The slides are allowed to dry at room temperature for 15 to 20 min and then are fixed in acetone for 10 min at room temperature. Suspensions of tissue are prepared for virus isolation attempts as described in Chapter 71.

Specimens for virus isolation attempts should be inoculated into suitable cell cultures as soon as possible after collection. If inoculation is to be delayed for no longer than 24 h, specimens may be transported, or held, in wet ice or a refrigerator. For longer periods of holding, dry ice temperatures are required. Refrigeration is not required for smears to be examined for viral antigen or intranuclear inclusions. It should be recognized that smears from vesicular lesions may be infectious, particularly in the case of vaccinia or smallpox materials, and suitable precautions should be taken in packing and storage to protect postal and laboratory personnel.

DIRECT EXAMINATION OF LESION MATERIAL

The examination of vesicular material for virus or viral antigen provides the most rapid diagnosis of V-Z virus infection, and it is particularly helpful in cases where smallpox is suspected. A differential diagnosis between herpesviruses and poxviruses may be made by cytological examination of smears from the base of vesicular lesions (2) or by electron microscopy of vesicular materials (13). These procedures do not, however, distinguish between V-Z virus and herpes simplex virus. Specific identification of V-Z virus or viral antigen in lesion materials can be accomplished by immunofluorescent staining (21) or gel diffusion tests (4, 13, 24).

Cytological examination of smears from the base of vesicular lesions

Smears of cellular material collected from the base of vesicular lesions are prepared as described in Chapter 71. They are fixed with methanol and stained with buffered Giemsa stain at pH 7.0 to 7.2 (2). Microscopy reveals the presence of multinucleated, giant epithelial cells with altered chromatin patterns (see Fig. 1); these are characteristic of infection with either V-Z virus or herpes simplex virus, and tend to rule out the possibility of infection with variola or vaccinia viruses.

Electron microscopy

Vesicular fluids are examined directly; crusts from lesions are ground in one or two drops of distilled water. When transportation of specimens to the laboratory presents a problem, heavy smears of fluids and crusts may be prepared on glass microscope slides and air-dried; material from the smears is reconstituted in a drop of water for examination by electron microscopy. A drop of the specimen is placed on a grid and blotted with filter paper. A drop of 3% phosphotungstic acid (prepared in distilled

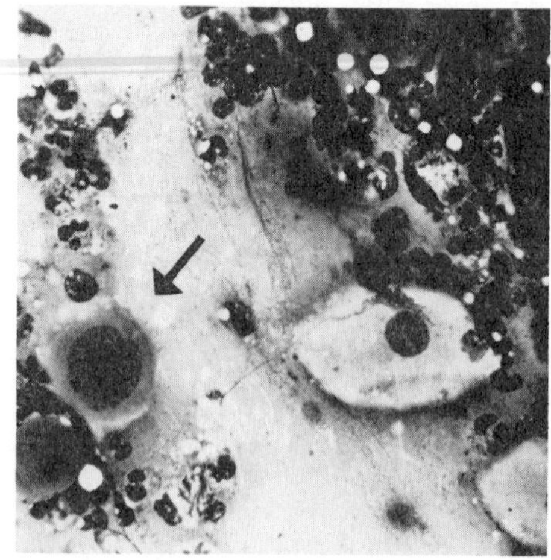

FIG. 1. *Giemsa-stained preparation of material from the base of a vesicular lesion. ×250. Arrow shows a giant cell with folded nucleus characteristic of varicella-zoster or herpes simplex infections.*

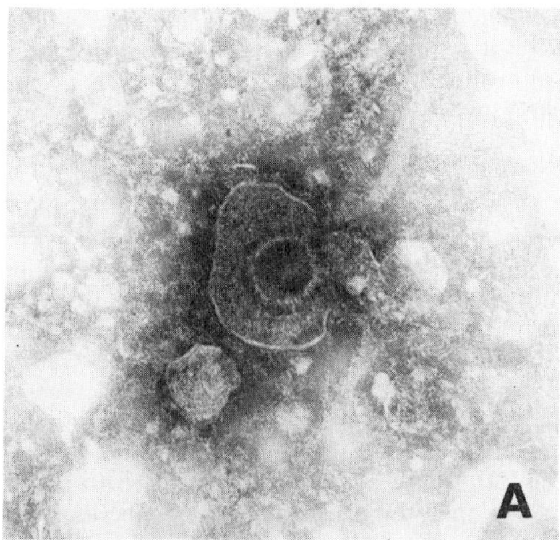

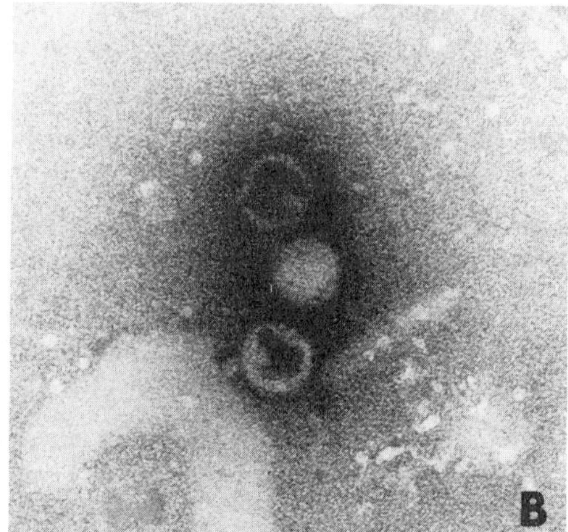

FIG. 2. *Electron micrograph of varicella-zoster virus in a preparation from a lesion scab. ×80,000. (A) Enveloped virus. (B) Naked nucleocapsids.*

water buffered to neutrality with 1 N KOH) is then added and blotted. The specimen should be examined in an electron microscope as soon as possible. The demonstration of virus particles with the typical morphology of herpesviruses (see Fig. 2) identifies the etiological agent as a member of this group and distinguishes it from viruses of the vaccinia-variola group, but it does not furnish a specific diagnosis of V-Z virus infection.

Immunofluorescent staining of smears from the base of vesicular lesions

Smears properly collected from the base of fresh vesicular lesions may be used for FA staining for the specific demonstration of V-Z antigen in the infected epithelial cells. It is essential that the smears contain a large number of infected cells, and three smears should be used to permit staining with conjugates to V-Z, herpes simplex, and vaccinia viruses. The direct method of staining, with the use of fluorescein-conjugated immune globulins from hyperimmune animal serum, is the most specific procedure. Direct FA staining is described below.

Immunodiffusion tests

Immunodiffusion tests have been used to a limited extent for specific demonstration of V-Z antigen in lesion materials (4, 13, 24). Either vesicular fluids or extracts of crusts (prepared in 0.25 to 0.50 ml Sorenson's phosphate buffer, pH 8.2) can be employed. The gel consists of 0.5% Ionagar No. 2 in Sorenson's phosphate buffer at pH 8.2 containing 0.1% free protamine; 2.5 ml of melted gel is spread onto a microscope slide and allowed to harden. Wells 2 mm in diameter are cut in the gel in a pattern of one central well surrounded by four peripheral wells. The center-to-center distance between the central and peripheral wells is 5 mm. Vesicular fluid or crust extracts are added to the center well. On one side of the center well, a positive vaccinia antigen is added to one well and vaccinia antiserum is added to the adjacent well. On the other side of the center well, a positive V-Z precipitating antigen is added to one well and a concentrated serum (reconstituted to one-tenth the original volume after lyophilization) from a patient with zoster is added to the adjacent well. The zoster serum should have no antibodies to herpes simplex virus. The slides are incubated in a humidified atmosphere at 25 C for 12 to 24 h.

A specimen containing V-Z antigen forms an immunoprecipitate only with the zoster serum, and the precipitate should show a reaction of identity with that formed by the zoster serum and the V-Z positive control antigen. A specimen containing vaccinia-variola antigen reacts only with the vaccinia antiserum and shows a reaction of identity with the vaccinia control antigen.

ISOLATION AND IDENTIFICATION OF VIRUS

Host systems

For isolation of V-Z virus from clinical materials, primary or diploid human cell cultures are the most sensitive host systems. In the event that smallpox is suspected, the material should also be inoculated onto the chorioallantoic membranes of 11- to 13-day-old embryonated hens' eggs.

In this laboratory, human fetal diploid kidney (HFDK) cells have been found to be highly sensitive for primary isolation of V-Z virus. Cell cultures are initiated with Eagle's minimal essential medium (MEM) containing 10% fetal bovine serum, and are maintained on 98% Leibovitz Medium No. 15 (or Eagle's MEM containing galactose rather than glucose) and 2% fetal bovine serum. Either of these media will maintain the cultures for 14 days without a fluid change, a period usually sufficient for the development of specific viral cytopathic effects (CPE). Rhesus monkey kidney (RhMK) cells are less sensitive than HFDK cells for isolation of V-Z virus (18). Primary human amnion (26) or primary human thyroid (7) cell cultures can be used for isolation of the virus, but the slower CPE produced in these cells may necessitate a fluid change during the incubation period.

V-Z virus has not been successfully propagated in small laboratory animals or in embryonated eggs.

Inoculation and incubation of cell cultures

Vesicular fluids and cell scrapings (collected in holding medium) or autopsy tissue suspensions are treated with an antibiotic solution to give a final concentration of 500 units of penicillin and 500 μg of streptomycin per ml or with gentamicin to give a final concentration of 100 μg per ml. Two cell culture tubes are inoculated with 0.25 ml of the specimen. A portion of the original specimen should be saved and stored at −70 C for retesting if necessary.

Inoculated cell cultures are incubated at 35 to 36 C in a roller drum and are examined microscopically for evidence of a viral CPE over a period of at least 14 days.

Evidence of infection in cell cultures

Figure 3 shows the characteristic CPE of V-Z virus in HFDK cells. Initially, the CPE consists of small, discrete foci of rounded and swollen refractile cells; these may appear from 3 to 14 days after inoculation of the cultures with clinical materials, but in most instances CPE is first apparent at 5 to 7 days. The foci of infected cells enlarge and may eventually involve most of the monolayer. In other cell culture systems the CPE may be somewhat slower to appear, and a medium change may be necessary to prevent nonspecific degeneration of the monolayer.

Subpassage and storage of virus

Infectious V-Z virus remains in close association with the host cell, and therefore it is necessary to use virus-infected cells, rather than culture fluids, as an inoculum for serial propagation of the virus. Trypsin-dispersed infected cells are most suitable for subpassage of V-Z virus (22). The medium is removed from cell cultures in which CPE involves 50 to 75% of the cell sheet, and 2 ml of 0.25% trypsin is added to each tube culture. The trypsin is flooded over the cell sheet and then removed. After incubation for 5 min at room temperature with the residual trypsin covering the cell sheet, the dispersed cells are suspended in the original volume of maintenance medium and inoculated into fresh cell cultures.

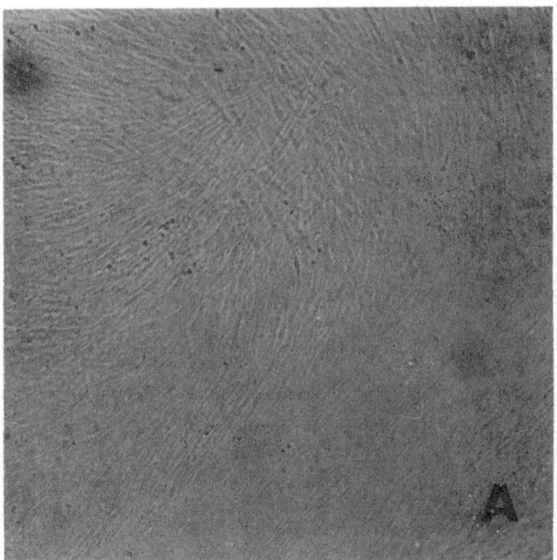

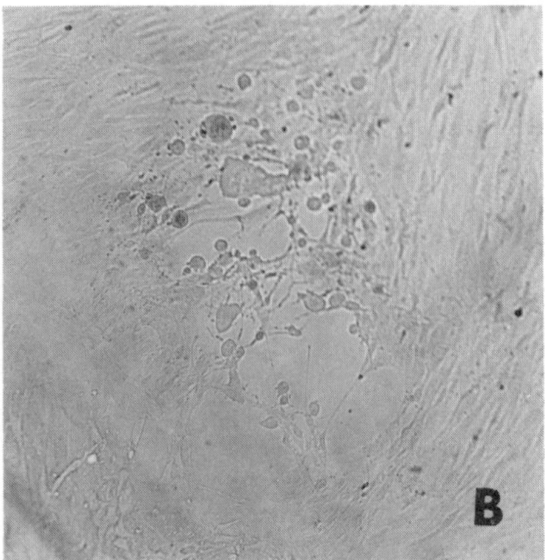

FIG. 3. *Cytopathic effect of varicella-zoster virus in human fetal diploid kidney cells.* ×*100. (A) Uninfected cells. (B) Virus-infected cells.*

Virus in infected cells can be stored in the frozen state if the viability of the cells is maintained through the use of dimethyl sulfoxide or glycerol in the medium (16). Infected cells are dispersed with trypsin as described above and then resuspended in Eagle's MEM containing 10 to 20% fetal bovine serum and either 10% dimethyl sulfoxide or 10% glycerol. Infectious virus can be recovered after 18 or more months of storage at −70 C, but infectivity is preserved more effectively by storage of the infected cells in liquid nitrogen.

IDENTIFICATION OF V-Z VIRUS ISOLATES

Presumptive Identification

Presumptive identification of V-Z virus may be made on the basis of a typical CPE, which progresses more slowly than that of herpes simplex virus. V-Z virus may also be differentiated from herpes simplex because it fails to produce a CPE in rabbit or hamster kidney cell cultures, whereas herpes simplex produces a rapid CPE. The source of the specimen and clinical manifestations of the illness should usually prevent confusion between V-Z and cytomegalovirus (CMV). However, if isolations are made from tissues, there might be a need to distinguish between these herpesviruses. V-Z virus grows well in epithelial cells, whereas CMV generally produces a cytopathic effect only in human fibroblast cells. The CPE produced by CMV is slower than that of V-Z virus. Further, human CMV strains fail to produce CPE in RhMK cells, but after initial isolation V-Z strains will generally do so.

Specific Identification

Specific identification of V-Z virus isolates is based upon demonstrating their reactivity with a known positive antiserum. Animal immune sera to V-Z virus are not generally available to most laboratories, and acute- and convalescent-phase sera from known cases of varicella are employed; identification is based upon the demonstration of a greater degree of reactivity (FA or complement fixation [CF]) of the isolate with the convalescent-phase serum than with the acute-phase serum. However, the use of human sera of uncertain antibody content for identification of viral isolates is not as reliable as is the use of specific animal immune serum. Human sera employed for identification of V-Z virus should be free from antibodies to the viruses from which it is important to distinguish V-Z, namely, herpes simplex, CMV, and vaccinia.

Specific identification of V-Z isolates is accomplished most readily by immunofluorescent staining with the use of the direct method. Alternative methods are indirect FA staining and the CF test.

Preparation of antisera to V-Z virus

(1) Rhesus monkeys can be immunized with V-Z virus propagated in RhMK cell cultures to produce an immune serum free from antibodies to foreign host proteins and suitable for use in immunofluorescent staining or CF tests (21). Monolayer cultures are prepared from freshly trypsinized RhMK cells in a growth medium consisting of 0.5% lactalbumin hydrolysate in Hanks' balanced salt solution (BSS) and 5% normal rhesus monkey serum. Serum-free Eagle's MEM is used as a maintenance medium for virus propagation.

The monkey kidney cell cultures can be infected with virus propagated in HFDK cells if the trypsin-dispersed, infected HFDK cells are washed at least five times in serum-free medium to remove traces of fetal bovine serum used for propagation and maintenance of the HFDK cells. The washed, infected HFDK cells are suspended in Hanks BSS in a volume of 2 ml for each tube culture trypsinized and are inoculated onto monkey kidney monolayers in a volume of 0.25 ml per tube culture. Cultures are incubated at 35 to 36 C and are harvested when they show 2+ to 3+ CPE. The culture material can be stored at −70 C until it is used for immunization.

Rhesus monkeys are inoculated intramuscularly with 4 ml of a mixture of equal parts of infected monkey kidney cell culture material and adjuvant (one part Arlacel A and nine parts Standard mineral oil, C.T. 70). A total of three injections are given at 2-week intervals, and the animals are bled 7 to 10 days after the last inoculation.

(2) Antisera to V-Z virus can also be produced in guinea pigs and rabbits by use of virus purified by density gradient centrifugation (11). Virus is propagated in human diploid fibroblast cells in 32-oz (ca. 900-ml) culture bottles. When the CPE involves 70 to 90% of the monolayer, the cells are scraped into 4 ml of phosphate-buffered saline (PBS), pH 7.4, and are disrupted by sonic oscillation. A sucrose gradient is prepared in a 34-ml tube by layering successively 80, 65, 50, 35, and 10% sucrose solutions; 5 ml of the virus preparation is put onto the gradient, and centrifugation is conducted in an SW-25 rotor at 20,000 rpm for 3.5 h. The band at the 50 to 35% sucrose interface contains the highest concentration of enveloped viral particles, and this

fraction is collected, dialyzed against PBS, and used as immunizing antigen.

Guinea pigs are inoculated by the intraperitoneal route with 0.2 ml of antigen on days 0, 2, 4, 7, 9, 11, and 18, and are bled 7 to 10 days after the last injection. Rabbits are inoculated by the intramuscular route, first with 2 ml of equal parts of antigen and Freund's adjuvant, and 27 days later with 1 ml of antigen without adjuvant. They are bled 50 days after the last inoculation.

Antisera produced in guinea pigs are suitable for use in CF tests. Immune globulins from rabbit sera can be separated by chromatography on diethylaminoethyl cellulose and conjugated with fluorescein isothiocyanate for use in direct immunofluorescent staining (11).

Preparation of fluorescein-conjugated immune globulins for use in direct immunofluorescent staining

The globulin fraction is separated from V-Z antiserum by precipitation with half-saturated ammonium sulfate at 4 C. The precipitate is dissolved in distilled water and reprecipitated until the supernatant fluid is clear. The final precipitate is dissolved in distilled water to 40% of the original serum volume and dialyzed against physiological saline. The protein concentration is determined by the biuret method, and the solution is diluted in physiological saline to a protein concentration of 2 to 3 g/100 ml. The pH of the globulin solution is adjusted to 8.7 to 8.8 by adding a volume of 0.5 M sodium carbonate-sodium bicarbonate buffer equivalent to 15% of the volume of globulin solution. (For preparation of the carbonate buffer, solution A contains 5.3 g of Na_2CO_3 in 100 ml of distilled water; solution B contains 4.2 g of $NaHCO_3$ in 100 ml of distilled water. To 100 ml of solution A, add 7 to 10 ml of solution B until the pH is 8.7 to 8.8, as indicated by a pH meter.) Fluorescein isothiocyanate powder is added in a ratio of 1.0 mg per 100 mg of protein, and the mixture is stirred gently overnight at 4 C. Uncoupled fluorescein is removed by passing the conjugate through a Sephadex G-50 column equilibrated with 0.01 M PBS, pH 7.2 to 7.5. The conjugate is stored at −20 C. As a control on the specificity of the immune conjugate, serum collected prior to immunization with V-Z virus is conjugated in the same manner.

The immune conjugate is titrated against smears of V-Z virus-infected cells to determine the appropriate "working dilution" for use in virus identification. The degree of specific immunofluorescence is graded as 1+, 2+, 3+, and 4+. A reading of 4+ indicates glaring yellow-green fluorescence; 3+ indicates bright green, but not glaring fluorescence; 2+ is dull green fluorescence; and 1+ and ± designate faint or questionable fluorescence, respectively. The "working dilution" of the conjugate is the highest dilution giving specific staining of 4+.

Direct immunofluorescent staining for identification of V-Z virus

Infected cell cultures are employed for FA staining when they show 2+ to 3+ degeneration. Cells from a set of three or four infected culture tubes are dispersed with trypsin and pooled. If only a single infected tube culture is available, the cells are mixed with those from two or three uninfected tubes to ensure an adequate volume of cells. Three or four uninfected tube cultures are trypsinized and pooled for control purposes. Cells from each set of cultures are suspended in 3 ml of PBS with 2% fetal bovine serum and then sedimented by light centrifugation. The supernatant fluids are removed, and the packed cells are thoroughly suspended in approximately 0.05 ml of PBS with 2% fetal bovine serum. Smears approximately 5 mm in diameter are made from the cell suspensions by placing small drops (approximately 0.005 ml) on microscope slides. Duplicate smears of each suspension are made on each of three slides to permit staining with three different conjugates. Three sets of smears of uninfected cells are prepared for controls. The smears are dried at room temperature, fixed with acetone at room temperature for 10 min, and then dried at room temperature.

A "working dilution" of V-Z immune conjugate, and also of herpes simplex and vaccinia conjugates for control purposes, is prepared in a 20% suspension of normal mouse or beef brain (prepared by blending brain tissue with PBS, pH 7.2, in a Waring Blendor for 5 to 10 min and storing the suspension at −20 C); this reduces overstaining and certain types of nonspecific staining. Each of the three conjugates is added to a smear of infected cells and a smear of uninfected cells, and the slides are incubated in a humidified atmosphere at 35 to 37 C for 20 min. Slides are rinsed twice in 0.01 M PBS, pH 7.2 to 7.5 (10 min each rinsing), and then in distilled water. They are allowed to dry and then mounted in buffered glycerol solution (one part glycerol and four parts PBS, pH 7.2 to 7.5).

Examination with a fluorescence microscope should reveal specific staining of 3+ to 4+ intensity in cells treated with the V-Z conjugate, but little or no staining in cells treated with the herpes simplex or vaccinia conjugates.

The uninfected cells should not stain with any of the conjugates. Cells from cultures showing advanced V-Z virus CPE contain stainable antigen in both the cytoplasm and nucleus.

Smears of epithelial cells from the base of vesicular lesions or smears of autopsy tissues are also examined for V-Z antigen by the above procedure, with the use of conjugates to V-Z, herpes simplex, and vaccinia viruses.

It should be recognized that immune conjugate prepared from monkeys are likely to contain antibodies to certain simian viruses, and, if the viral isolates are recovered in monkey kidney cells, the conjugates may give positive staining with cells containing the simian viruses as contaminants. This is indicated by the fact that uninfected monkey kidney cells from the same lot as the viral isolate show staining, and staining is also seen with the preimmunization conjugate. Since monkey kidney cells are not particularly sensitive for isolation of V-Z virus, this is not likely to present a serious problem. Antibodies to certain simian herpesviruses and poxviruses may show low levels of cross-reactivity with human viruses. These antibodies are generally not detected in monkey sera by the direct FA procedure, but they might be detectable by the more sensitive indirect staining procedure. The specificity of staining by monkey serum conjugates, or unconjugated sera used for the indirect procedure, should be demonstrated by failure of preimmunization serum to stain the V-Z virus.

Human convalescent-phase sera from herpes zoster infections have been conjugated for direct immunofluorescent staining of V-Z virus (8). However, for specific virus identification it is essential to use a human serum free from antibodies to herpes simplex, vaccinia, and CMV.

Indirect immunofluorescent staining for identification of V-Z virus

Indirect FA staining can be used for identification of V-Z virus isolates with the use of immune sera produced in animals together with serum obtained before immunization or, less desirably, acute- and convalescent-phase human sera from a known case of varicella (25). Human sera should be free from antibodies to herpes simplex and vaccinia. Identification is based upon the demonstration of a greater degree of staining of the virus-infected cells with the convalescent-phase serum than with the acute-phase serum. Ideally, the acute-phase serum should have an indirect FA titer of <1:10 against known V-Z virus-infected cells, and the convalescent serum should have a titer of at least 1:80.

A smear of infected cells is prepared as described above for each serum dilution to be tested, and smears of uninfected cells are prepared for the first two dilutions of each serum to serve as controls to detect possible nonspecific staining.

Preimmunization (or acute) and immune (or convalescent) sera are inactivated at 56 C for 30 min, and twofold dilutions (from 1:10 through 1:160) are prepared in a 20% suspension of normal mouse or beef brain. A drop of each serum dilution is applied to a smear of infected cells, and the first two serum dilutions are applied to uninfected cells for control purposes. The slides are incubated at 35 to 37 C in a humidified atmosphere for 20 min and then are washed twice in PBS, pH 7.2 to 7.5. A "working dilution" of fluorescein-conjugated anti-gamma globulin serum directed against the appropriate species is added to each smear. The conjugate is diluted in 20% normal mouse or beef brain suspension. After incubation at 35 to 37 C for 20 min, the slides are washed twice in PBS and mounted in buffered glycerol-saline solution. The highest dilution of serum showing staining of 2+ or greater is considered the indirect FA titer of the serum.

Identification of V-Z isolates by complement fixation

In laboratories lacking equipment for FA examinations, specific identification of V-Z virus isolates may be accomplished by preparing a complement-fixing antigen (20) from the isolate and testing it against known negative and positive V-Z sera, either pre- and postimmunization animal sera or acute- and convalescent-phase human sera. Again, the human sera must be free from antibodies to other human herpesviruses and vaccinia virus.

The isolate is propagated in bottle cultures of human fetal diploid cells (skin and muscle, lung or kidney). Eagle's MEM with 10% fetal bovine serum is used for growth medium, and Leibovitz Medium No. 15 with 2% fetal bovine serum is used for maintenance medium. Monolayer cultures are infected with trypsin-dispersed infected cells and incubated at 35 to 36 C. Viral CPE should involve the entire cell sheet by the 6th to the 8th day. At this time, the cultures are harvested, scraping adherent cells into the fluids.

The cells and fluids are separated by centrifugation at 2,000 rpm for 20 min, and the supernatant fluid is removed and discarded. The cells are resuspended in one-fiftieth of the original culture volume of Hanks BSS and sonically treated at 20 kc/s for 2 min; this material constitutes the antigen. Uninfected control antigen is prepared in the same manner from uninoculated cell cultures.

The antigen prepared from the isolate is run in a box titration (see CF procedure in Chapter 71) against known positive and negative V-Z serum, and identification is made on the basis of CF activity with the known positive serum and not the negative serum. The positive serum should not react with antigens for herpes simplex, CMV, or vaccinia.

SEROLOGICAL DIAGNOSIS

Complement fixation test

The CF test is the most widely applicable procedure for the serological diagnosis of V-Z virus infections. The value of the technique is limited to some extent by the fact that heterotypic CF antibody rises to V-Z antigen may occur in certain patients with herpes simplex infections who have experienced a prior infection with V-Z virus (10, 17, 19).

CF antigens for V-Z virus are prepared from infected human fetal diploid skin and muscle cell cultures by the procedure given above for preparation of CF antigen from isolates.

The technique for the CF test is described in Chapter 71.

For serodiagnosis of infection, acute- and convalescent-phase sera must be tested in parallel in the same run. Twofold dilutions of inactivated (56 C for 30 min) serum are tested against a dilution of V-Z antigen containing two antigenic units, and the lower serum dilutions are tested against a comparable dilution of uninfected control antigen and for possible anticomplementary activity. A fourfold or greater increase in CF antibody titer between the acute- and convalescent-phase serum specimen is considered diagnostically significant.

In chickenpox infections, CF antibodies for the V-Z virus are generally demonstrable by 7 to 10 days after appearance of the exanthem, and they reach peak titers at 2 to 3 weeks after onset of illness. The antibody response is generally more rapid in zoster infections, and CF antibodies may be present on the first or second day of the eruption.

Fluorescent-antibody staining

Serodiagnosis of V-Z virus infections may be accomplished by means of indirect FA staining. The patient's acute- and convalescent-phase serum specimens are tested against smears of V-Z virus-infected cells. The procedure is identical to that described above for identification of V-Z virus isolates. The test is more cumbersome and expensive to perform than the CF test, and it is no more specific than CF for distinguishing between V-Z and herpes simplex infections when titer rises are seen to both antigens (19).

Neutralization tests

Neutralizing antibody to V-Z virus can be assayed by use of a plaque reduction technique (19) with cell-free virus derived from infected human fetal diploid cells disrupted by sonic oscillation (3). However, this procedure is a research, rather than a diagnostic, tool.

EVALUATION AND INTERPRETATION OF RESULTS

Isolation of V-Z virus or demonstration of virus antigen in lesion material or autopsy tissues is diagnostic of a current infection.

The most rapid presumptive diagnosis of V-Z or herpes simplex infection can be made by electron microscopy of lesion materials or by Giemsa staining of cellular material from the lesions. This only identifies members of the herpesvirus group and does not distinguish between V-Z virus or herpes simplex virus. Specific identification of V-Z antigen can be made directly with lesion material by direct immunofluorescent staining or immunodiffusion tests.

Isolation of the virus is a relatively slow method, and is generally less sensitive than electron microscopy and the procedures used for identification of viral antigen; viable virus persists for a shorter length of time in vesicles and is more labile than the antigens which can be demonstrated by gel diffusion and FA staining. Specific identification of V-Z isolates is hampered by the lack of specific antisera in most laboratories. Pitfalls in the use of human sera for specific identification have been indicated. However, presumptive identification can be made on the basis of the typical V-Z CPE, failure of the virus to propagate in rabbit or hamster kidney cells, which distinguishes V-Z from herpes simplex, and ability of the virus to propagate in monkey kidney cells and human epithelial cells, which distinguishes it from CMV.

A fourfold or greater rise in CF antibody titer to V-Z antigen, in the absence of a fourfold rise to herpes simplex antigen, is diagnostic of a current V-Z virus infection. However, a high proportion (up to one-third) of individuals with current herpes simplex infections who have experienced a prior infection with V-Z virus show a heterotypic CF antibody response to the V-Z antigen, making a differential diagnosis between V-Z and herpes simplex difficult in the absence of clear-cut clinical findings. Individuals with herpes simplex infections who show heterotypic CF antibody titer rises to V-Z virus also show heterotypic rises by FA staining, and frequently in neutralization tests (19).

LITERATURE CITED

1. Almeida, J. D., A. F. Howatson, and M. G. Williams. 1962. Morphology of varicella (chicken pox) virus. Virology **16:**353–355.
2. Blank, H., C. F. Burgoon, G. D. Baldridge, P. L. McCarthy, and F. Urbach. 1951. Cytologic smears in diagnosis of herpes simplex, herpes zoster, and varicella. J. Amer. Med. Ass. **146:**1410–1412.
3. Brunell, P. A. 1967. Separation of infectious varicella-zoster virus from human embryonic lung fibroblasts. Virology **31:**732–734.
4. Brunell, P. A., B. H. Cohen, and M. Granat. 1971. A gel-precipitin test for the diagnosis of varicella. Bull. W. H. O. **44:**811–814.
5. Brunell, P. A., A. A. Gershon, W. T. Hughes, H. D. Riley, Jr., and J. Smith. 1972. Prevention of varicella in high risk children: a collaborative study. Pediatrics **50:**718–722.
6. Brunell, P. A., A. Ross, L. H. Miller, and B. Kuo. 1969. Prevention of varicella by zoster immune globulin. N. Engl. J. Med. **280:**1191–1194.
7. Caunt, A. E., and D. Taylor-Robinson. 1964. Cell-free varicella-zoster virus in tissue culture. J. Hyg. **62:**413–424.
8. Esiri, M. M., and A. H. Tomlinson. 1972. Herpes zoster. Demonstration of virus in trigeminal nerve and ganglion by immunofluorescence and electron microscopy. J. Neurol. Sci. **15:**35–48.
9. Judelsohn, R. G. 1972. Prevention and control of varicella-zoster infections. J. Infect. Dis. **125:**82–84.
10. Kapsenberg, J. G. 1964. Possible antigenic relationship between varicella/zoster virus and herpes simplex virus. Arch. Gesamte Virusforsch. **15:**67–73.
11. Kissling, R. E., H. L. Casey, and E. L. Palmer. 1968. Production of specific varicella antiserum. Appl. Microbiol. **16:**160–162.
12. Ludwig, H., H. G. Haines, N. Biswal, and M. Benyesh-Melnick. 1972. The characterization of varicella-zoster virus DNA. J. Gen. Virol. **14:**111–114.
13. Macrae, A. D., A. M. Field, J. R. McDonald, E. V. Meurisse, and A. A. Porter. 1969. Laboratory differential diagnosis of vesicular skin rashes. Lancet **2:**313–316.
14. Rapp, F., and D. Vanderslice. 1964. Spread of zoster virus in human embryonic lung cells and the inhibitory effect of iododeoxyuridine. Virology **22:**321–330.
15. Rawls, W. E., R. A. Cohen, and E. C. Hermann, Jr. 1964. Inhibition of varicella virus by 5-iodo-2′-deoxyuridine. Proc. Soc. Exp. Biol. Med. **115:**123–127.
16. Rosanoff, E. K., and C. P. Hegarty. 1964. Preservation of tissue cultured varicella virus in the frozen state. Virology **22:**284.
17. Ross, C. A. C., J. H. Subak-Sharpe, and P. Ferry. 1965. Antigenic relationship of varicella-zoster and herpes simplex. Lancet **2:**708–711.
18. Schmidt, N. J. 1972. Tissue culture in the laboratory diagnosis of viral infections. Amer. J. Clin. Pathol. **57:**820–828.
19. Schmidt, N. J., E. H. Lennette, and R. L. Magoffin. 1969. Immunological relationship between herpes simplex and varicella-zoster viruses demonstrated by complement fixation, neutralization and fluorescent antibody tests. J. Gen. Virol. **4:**321–328.
20. Schmidt, N. J., E. H. Lennette, C. W. Shon, and T. T. Shinomoto. 1964. A complement-fixing antigen for varicella-zoster derived from infected cultures of human fetal diploid cells. Proc. Soc. Exp. Biol. Med. **116:**144–149.
21. Schmidt, N. J., E. H. Lennette, J. D. Woodie, and H. H. Ho. 1965. Immunofluorescent staining in the laboratory diagnosis of varicella-zoster virus infections. J. Lab. Clin. Med. **66:**403–412.
22. Taylor-Robinson, D. 1959. Chickenpox and herpes zoster. III. Tissue culture studies. Brit. J. Exp. Pathol. **40:**521–532.
23. Trlifajová, J., J. Šourek, and M. Ryba. 1971. Antigenic relationship between varicella-herpes zoster and herpes simplex viruses studied by the gel precipitation reaction. Acta Virol. (Prague) **15:**293–300.
24. Uduman, S. A., A. A. Gershon, and P. A. Brunell. 1972. Rapid diagnosis of varicella-zoster infections by agar-gel diffusion. J. Infect. Dis. **126:**193–195.
25. Weller, T. H., and A. H. Coons. 1954. Fluorescent antibody studies with agents of varicella and herpes zoster propagated *in vitro*. Proc. Soc. Exp. Biol. Med. **86:**789–794.
26. Weller, T. H., H. M. Witton, and E. J. Bell. 1958. The etiologic agents of varicella and herpes zoster. Isolation, propagation and cultural characteristics *in vitro*. J. Exp. Med. **108:**843–868.

Chapter 86

Smallpox, Vaccinia, and Human Infections with Monkeypox Viruses

JAMES H. NAKANO AND PATRICIA G. BINGHAM

CLINICAL BACKGROUND

"'Could this be smallpox?' If this question occurs to the first physician seeing a case of severe prostration or acute skin eruption in a person who within two weeks has been exposed to travelers or to hospital personnel, half of the danger from smallpox could be averted." So wrote Louis Jacobs in the foreword to the 1966 reproduction of the book by Ricketts and Byles entitled *The Diagnosis of Smallpox*, originally published in 1908 (23). Jacobs' statement is even more important today. Physicians in the nonendemic areas, such as the United States, have less and less chance to see smallpox and develop clinical diagnostic acuity as the endemic areas for smallpox decrease. Furthermore, since compulsory smallpox vaccination has been abolished in many countries, it is more important than ever to prevent the spread of smallpox in an unvaccinated population. If the spread of smallpox is to be prevented and the disease is to be eradicated, rapid and accurate laboratory diagnosis is needed.

Variola, human monkeypox, and vaccinia are immunologically closely related but distinct poxviruses, each causing an exanthematous infection in humans. It is variola which causes smallpox, the most severe exanthematous communicable disease of humans. By 1971, smallpox was eradicated in South America, Indonesia, and all of the West African countries, but infections still occur in some parts of Africa and southeast Asia.

Smallpox is grouped into three types of illness based on differences in the degree of severity and the proportion of fatal cases occurring during an outbreak. Variola major, the severe type, with case fatality ratios of 15 to 40%, prevails in the Asiatic subcontinent; variola minor (alastrim, amass, Kaffir pox [17]), the mild form with fatalities of less than 1%, was most recently prevalent in South America and South Africa; variola intermediate, the intermediate type with case fatality ratios of 5 to 15%, reported by Bedson et al. (1), formerly prevailed in East Africa and Indonesia. The viruses causing these types of illnesses can be distinguished in the laboratory by their growth characteristics at certain supraoptimal temperatures.

According to Downie's 1951 description of the pathogenesis of smallpox (3), the virus enters through the mucosa of the upper respiratory tract, quickly passes to the lymphatic glands, and is carried by the bloodstream to the internal organs. During an incubation period of 7 to 17 days, the virus multiplies in the internal organs and overflows into the bloodstream, causing viremia. Widespread infection of the skin and mucous membranes follows, and skin lesions become apparent after an additional 2 to 3 days. As the lesions break down, virus is liberated, and the patient becomes highly infective. The immune response which follows determines to some extent the severity of the disease. The cause of death in persons in the late pustular stage, despite a high antibody titer, may be the late effects of earlier virus activity, some complicating disability, or a secondary infection.

The clinical picture of human disease caused by monkeypox, first recognized in Africa in 1970 (28), is similar to that of smallpox except that secondary infections in unimmunized household contacts are all but unknown to occur. The mode of transmission is not clearly understood, but intimate contact with monkeys has been apparent in some cases. Through 1973, only 17 cases had been identified, all in western and central Africa. Although outbreaks have occurred in monkeys and other mammals in captivity, the natural reservoir of the virus has not been elucidated.

Several different strains of vaccinia virus are used in vaccination. After vaccination, vaccinia infection may occur elsewhere on the skin and mucous membranes as a result of manual transfer of the virus from the vaccination site or following viremia. Rare but possible serious complications following vaccination include postvaccinal encephalitis, eczema vaccinatum, and progressive vaccinia (vaccinia gangrenosa).

DESCRIPTION OF AGENTS

The viruses of variola major, variola minor, variola intermediate, vaccinia, and human monkeypox, all of which are classified under the generic groups of poxvirus, also belong in the subgenus A, of which vaccinia is the representative type (26). They are double-stranded deoxyribonucleic acid viruses, are "brick-shaped" by electron microscopy, range in size from 250 to 300 mm long by 200 to 250 nm wide, and are morphologically indistinguishable from one another. They are stable in dried condition; variola viruses, especially in crusts, may survive at room temperature for many years. They are serologically closely related and can be identified as poxviruses belonging to one group by using the agar gel precipitation test with antivaccinia serum. The viruses produce soluble hemagglutinin. They grow on chick allantoic membrane and in tissue cultures.

COLLECTION AND STORAGE OF SPECIMENS

In the United States and its territories, all suspected cases of smallpox are, upon discovery, immediately reportable by telephone to the respective state or territorial health department.

All persons routinely handling specimens from patients with suspected smallpox must be vaccinated every 12 months. All laboratories located in geographic zones nonendemic for smallpox which handle specimens of suspected smallpox cases should be isolated from other work áreas, and all personnel in these laboratories must practice strict isolation techniques.

It is important to collect an amount of specimen sufficient to permit effective testing; use of too little specimen decreases the dependability of laboratory tests in the diagnosis of smallpox.

During the pre-eruptive phase of illness, blood collected with sterile anticoagulant can be used as a virus isolation source.

During the macular phase, at least four smears should be collected. These smears are made by lesion scrapings from the lower epithelial layers, with a no. 11 or 12 scalpel blade. Each smear made on a slide should be as small and as thick as possible. The slides should be shipped separately in a plastic slide holder with a tight-fitting cap, or several slides may be bundled together with a rubber band, with the individual slides separated by broken matches or tooth picks, and placed in a screw-capped metal container.

During the vesicular phase, a volume of vesicular fluid equivalent to at least two capillary tubes filled to a height of 10 mm should be collected. The tubes are sealed with clay or plastic cement. When the fluid is too viscous to permit collection in capillary tubes, as during the pustular phase, smears may be made on glass slides instead. Capillary tubes are placed in a tightly stoppered or screw-capped vial and then in a larger protective container, as described above.

During the crusting phase, no fewer than three crusts, each measuring about 5 mm in diameter, should be collected; for thorough testing, at least 12 crusts should be collected. All crusts should be shipped in a screw-capped vial. When smallpox is not definitely diagnosed in a patient suspected of having had fatal fulminating (hemorrhagic) smallpox because appropriate skin lesions could not be found, autopsy specimens, including clotted blood (cardiac) and sections from the lungs, liver, spleen, and kidneys, should be collected for virus isolation. The specimens should be shipped in separate screw-capped vials protected by larger containers. The sections of the organs should be shipped frozen, packed in dry ice, but the clotted blood should not be frozen.

The packaging and shipment of smallpox diagnostic specimens warrants special attention to avoid damage and leakage of the specimen in transit and possible accidental exposure of anyone enroute or at the destination. The *Interstate Quarantine Regulations* (42 CFR, Part 72.25, "Etiologic Agents," revised 30 July 1972) specify minimal packaging, labeling, and notification requirements to assure safe arrival and delivery.

Figure 1 illustrates proper packaging of a smallpox specimen. Clinical materials are placed in a primary container (test tube or screw-capped vial), which is securely closed and sealed with waterproof tape; this is then enclosed in a second durable, watertight container (secondary container). The space at the top, bottom, and sides between the primary and secondary containers should contain sufficient nonparticulate absorbent material (paper towel) to absorb the entire contents of the primary container if it breaks or leaks. Each set of primary and secondary containers is placed in an outer shipping container constructed of corrugated fiberboard, cardboard, or other material of equivalent strength. A copy of the laboratory record or other identifying information should be enclosed between the secondary con-

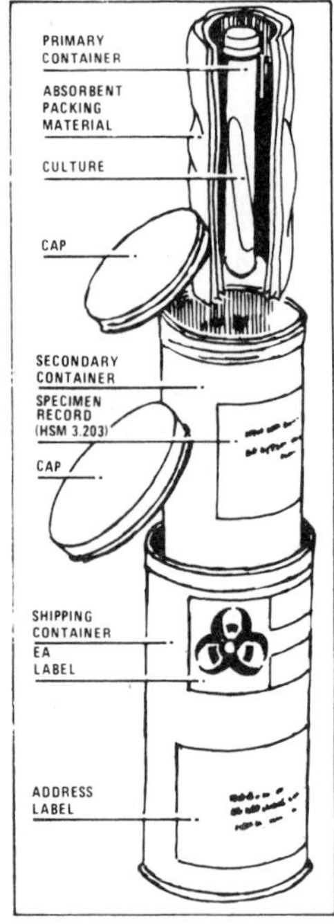

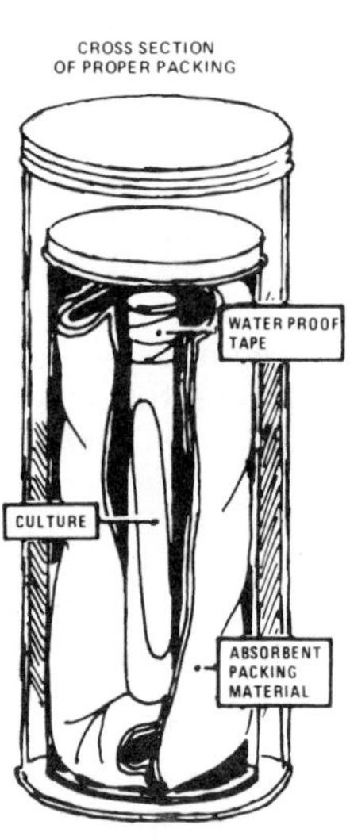

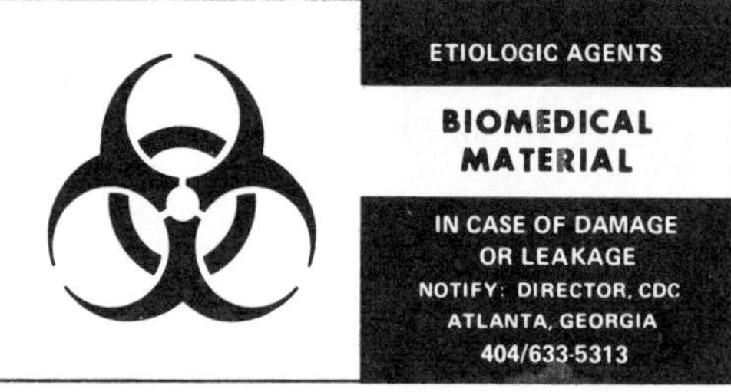

ETIOLOGIC AGENTS
BIOMEDICAL
MATERIAL
IN CASE OF DAMAGE
OR LEAKAGE
NOTIFY: DIRECTOR, CDC
ATLANTA, GEORGIA
404/633-5313

FIG. 1. *Illustration of proper packaging of etiological agents for shipment. The "Etiologic Agents" label shown at the bottom of the figure should be affixed to the outer shipping container.*

tainer and the outer shipping container. The "Etiologic Agents" label (Fig. 1) is affixed to the outer shipping container. Smallpox specimens should be transported by special air transportation system, registered mail, or an equivalent system which provides for the shipper to be notified immediately upon delivery.

In addition to the packaging, labeling, and transportation requirements of the *Interstate Quarantine Regulations*, the importation of smallpox specimens into the United States from abroad requires an authorizing permit issued by the Center for Disease Control (CDC). For more detailed information on importation permits and other requirements applicable to the shipment and receipt of smallpox specimens, write the CDC, Attention: Biohazards Control Officer, 1600 Clifton Road, Atlanta, Ga. 30333, or phone the CDC at 404-633-3311.

DIAGNOSTIC TESTS FOR SMALLPOX

Laboratory diagnostic tests for smallpox should produce accurate, easily interpreted results. They should be relatively quickly performed, simple, and direct. Seven methods that may be used for the laboratory diagnosis of smallpox are listed in Table 1. The first four methods, namely, electron microscopy, agar gel precipitation (AGP), chick chorioallantoic membrane (CAM) culture, and tissue cultures, have been shown over the past 7 years (1966–1973) at the CDC to be the combination of choice, giving the most dependable results with the least confusion. Each of these methods will be discussed in detail. The other three methods, stained smears, fluorescent-antibody (FA) tests, and complement fixation (CF), do not provide additional advantages to the laboratory diagnosis. They are not used routinely, but, for completeness, they will be referenced.

Serological tests are not generally employed in the definitive diagnosis of smallpox, but they may be useful when specimens for direct detection of viruses are not available.

TABLE 1. *Accepted methods for the laboratory diagnosis of smallpox, vaccinia infection, and human monkeypox*

Method	Accomplishment
Preferred methods	
Electron microscopy	Direct demonstration of virus
Agar gel precipitation	Antigenic identification
Chick chorioallantoic membrane culture	Growth of variola, vaccinia, human monkeypox, and herpes simplex viruses, with definitive pock characteristics
Tissue culture	Growth of variola, vaccinia, human monkeypox, and herpes simplex viruses, with definitive CPE characteristics
Other methods	
Stained smear	Demonstration of elementary bodies
Fluorescent antibody	Demonstration of virus-antibody complexes
Complement fixation	Demonstration of virus-antibody complexes; antigenic identification

Electron microscopy

The electron microscopy method described here is essentially that described by Long et al. (12) and requires the following equipment and reagents: 400-mesh grids coated with Formvar, platinum-tipped forceps, plastic petri dishes (60 mm in diameter) lined with filter paper, 2.0% sodium phosphotungstate (pH 7.0), wax-coated glass microscope slides prepared by dipping the slides into melted paraffin wax, and glass capillary tubes with individual rubber microbulbs.

Preparation of grids with specimens. Vesicular fluid collected in capillary tubes, lesion fluid collected as smears, and ground scab suspensions are all excellent sources of virus for examination by electron microscopy.

Capillary tubes containing vesicular fluid are nicked with a file, and the sealed ends are removed. A microbulb is attached to one end of the tubes, and two drops of the fluid are squeezed out to form a single larger drop on a wax-coated slide. If a fibrin plug is present in the fluid, it is included in the drop on the slide. An equal-size drop of phosphate buffer, pH 7.2, 0.01 M, is delivered in close proximity to the vesicular fluid, and the two drops are mixed with a clean capillary tube and microbulb to give an approximate 1:2 dilution. A drop of 2.0% sodium phosphotungstate is placed on another section of the same wax-coated slide. Two electron microscope grids coated with Formvar are placed first on the drop of the diluted vesicular fluid, coated side down, and allowed to float for about 30 s. The grids are then transferred to the drop of 2.0% sodium phosphotungstate and allowed to float there for 30 to 60 s. The grids are then placed, coated side up, on filter paper lining a small petri dish and labeled as the 1:2-diluted specimen. Subsequent dilutions of 1:4 and 1:8 are made in a similar manner, and two grids are prepared for each dilution. Undiluted vesicular fluid is not usually used because it would make the grids too dense for examination.

When lesion fluid collected as smears is used to prepare grids, the smears are softened with two drops of the buffer, and a suspension is made by the sucking-expelling action of a capillary tube equipped with a microbulb. Two or three smears are used to provide sufficient material. The suspension thus prepared is used, without further dilution, to prepare grids.

Scabs are ground with the buffer in a thick-walled glass tissue grinder. The volume of buffer added depends on the size and the number of scabs. About 0.3 to 0.5 ml of the buffer is used for each scab approximately 5 mm in diameter; smaller scabs are diluted with less volume and larger scabs with somewhat more. The suspension prepared in this manner is considered undiluted, and subsequent twofold dilutions are made from it on the wax-coated slide. Two grids are prepared for each dilution, as described for the vesicular fluid.

The grids and contaminated containers must be rendered noninfectious before they are taken out of the isolation laboratory for electron microscopy. To accomplish this, the small petri dish containing the prepared grids is placed open (base dish right side up, and the cover dish upside down) in a larger dish containing a shallow volume of 5% sodium hypochlorite and exposed for 30 min to ultraviolet light at a distance of 2.5 cm from the light source (General Electric Germicidal Lamp [G15T8], 15 W, with specification of 2.95 W/ft^2 at the exposure distance of 5 cm) in a pass-through box. The effectiveness of the ultraviolet light source must be checked at weekly intervals.

Examination. Initially, the grids are examined for density at a magnification of about 2,000 to 3,000 times. A grid too dense indicates that too much material has been put onto the grid, and a grid not dense enough indicates that too little material has been used. Either condition greatly diminishes the reliability of the test. Those grids which are found to have a satisfactory density are then scanned at a magnification of 10,000 to 20,000 times. Scanning at 10,000 rather than 20,000 times gives more thorough coverage, but requires that the operator be thoroughly experienced in detecting the virions of viruses of the pox and herpes groups. Once a virion is found, the detailed structure of the particle is examined at a higher magnification of 50,000 to 184,000 times.

Figure 2(*3*) illustrates the "C" form of poxvirus described by Harris and Westwood (9; the type 1b form of Nagington and Horne [18]) found in most scabs collected from patients with smallpox. Figure 2(*1*) illustrates the "M" form of Harris and Westwood (type 1a of Nagington and Horne) most prevalent in vesicular fluid from patients with smallpox. Figure 2(7) shows the naked capsids of herpes-type viruses, the most abundant form in scabs collected from patients with chickenpox. The typical enveloped virions of herpes-type viruses [Fig. 2(5)] also occur, but they are more abundant in vesicular fluid.

In examining grids, one must learn to differentiate nonviral particles that resemble poxvirus or herpesvirus from the real viral particles. Nonviral particles that resemble the "M" and

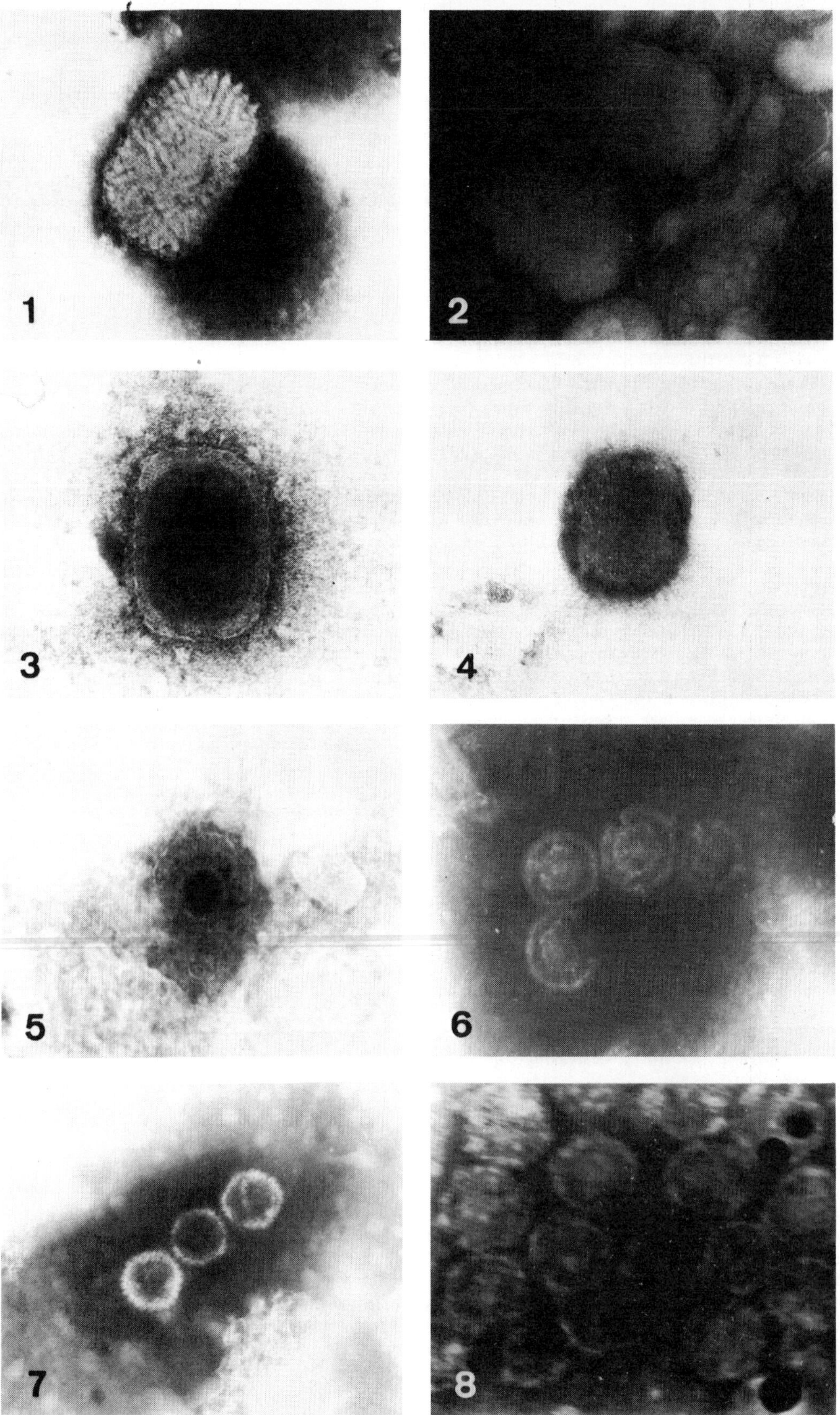
1
2
3
4
5
6
7
8

"C" forms of poxviruses are illustrated in Fig. 2(*2*) and 2(*4*).

What is the reliability of electron microscopy for the detection of viruses in specimens collected from patients with suspected smallpox? Of the specimens from 1,066 patients examined by our laboratory since 1966, a total of 367 were identified as variola or human monkeypox by the combination of electron microscopy, CAM, and AGP methods. Of the 367 positive specimens, 351, or 95.6%, were detected by electron microscopy alone. It was apparent that an even higher percentage of positive specimens could have been detected by electron microscopy alone if the quantity of vesicular, pustular, or crust material in all specimens had been adequate.

Of the specimens from the 1,066 patients with suspected smallpox, 282 were identified as varicella-herpes viruses by electron microscopy. This constituted the entire number identified as such. Varicella-herpes viruses are relatively labile as compared with poxviruses, and, since many specimens received were scabs or vesicular fluids which were not fresh, virus isolation was generally impossible. Electron microscopy remained the only dependable method for the detection of these viruses.

Stained smears

Stained smears can be examined by light microscope if no electron microscope is available, but this type of examination certainly does not equal electron microscopy in reliability. For details, consult Downie and Kempe (4), who describe and evaluate Gutstein's method (8) and Gispen's modification of Morosow's silver method (7).

Fluorescent-antibody test

Although several reports describe the use of FA tests for the diagnosis of smallpox, the technique is not considered reliable enough for routine diagnosis and is not recommended (21).

Chick embryo chorioallantoic membrane culture

Preparation of eggs. Fertile hen's eggs must be incubated at 38 to 39 C for 11 to 13 days to be useful for isolating and identifying the viruses of variola, vaccinia, and most known strains of human monkeypox. Lower incubation temperatures render the CAM less sensitive or totally insusceptible to poxviruses at the recommended time of 12 days.

Excellent photographic illustrations of methods for preparing an embryonated egg for inoculation may be found in the *WHO Guide to the Diagnosis of Smallpox* (27).

With the embryonated eggs in a rack, blunt ends up, a small hole is made in the shell and shell membrane of each egg over the air space by rotating the pointed end of a hand punch. (An electric-powered punching device has also been discussed [14].) Each egg is then candled to determine the embryo's viability; while the egg is being candled, a small hole is made with the hand punch (with rotary motion) through the shell at a spot over the CAM in an area without large blood vessels. Care is taken at this time *not* to puncture the shell membrane. All eggs are then placed with the CAM "hole" side up on a rack. The shell dust is blown away, and a drop of sterile phosphate-buffered saline (0.01 M PBS, pH 7.2: Na_2HPO_4 [anhydrous], 1.096 g; $NaH_2PO_4 \cdot H_2O$, 0.315 g; NaCl, 8.5 g; distilled water to 1,000 ml) is placed over the CAM hole. A sterile tip of a bent disposable blood lancet or a curved pen nib is inserted through the drop of PBS at an angle of about 20° to the horizontal and passed directly under the shell as far as it will go. The lancet handle is then raised towards the vertical; this motion tears the shell membrane, and the drop of PBS is drawn inside as the CAM falls. The eggs are candled to confirm the creation of a new air space above the dropped CAM. If the new air space is not found, slight suction is applied with a rubber bulb over the hole at the original air space on the blunt end of the egg. If the CAM still does not drop to create a new air space, the egg should be discarded. The eggs are returned to the incubator and inoculated within 2 h.

Preparation and inoculation of specimens. Blood which has been collected with sterile anticoagulant is centrifuged at 1,500 rpm. The plasma is drawn off by pipette and bulb first, and then the buffy coat (layer of white blood cells) is drawn off separately with the same pipette. Each is mixed 1:2 with McIlvaine's buffer, pH 7.8, 0.004 M (see appendix), contain-

FIG. 2. *Electron micrographs of particles at the original magnification of about 109,000 times. (1) "M" form of variola. (2) Nonviral particles resembling the "M" form of variola. (3) "C" form of variola. (4) Nonviral particles resembling the "C" forms of variola. (5) Typical varicella-herpes group virus with envelope, from vesicular fluid. (6) Particles found in a scab, may be varicella-herpes virus capsids, each surrounded by a degenerated contracted envelope; further search revealed typical enveloped virions on the same grid. (7) Varicella-herpes group virus capsids without the envelope. (8) Particles perhaps similar to those in Fig. 2(6).*

ing 500 units of penicillin, 500 μg of streptomycin, and 250 units of neomycin sulfate per ml. The plasma and the white cell suspension are inoculated separately, each into a set of four eggs. Each egg is inoculated with 0.1 ml directly onto the CAM by a disposable tuberculin syringe equipped with a 25-gauge 5/8-inch (1.6-cm) needle.

The scab suspension, vesicular fluid suspension, or smear suspension made for the preparation of electron microscope grids is also used to inoculate eggs. Each suspension is diluted 1:10, 1:1,000, and 1:10,000, with McIlvaine's buffer containing the antibiotics. Four eggs are inoculated with each dilution, as described above, and rocked back and forth for better distribution of the inoculum over the CAM. The holes in the shell are then sealed with a drop of plastic cement. The three dilutions of each specimen may be inoculated with one syringe, provided the highest dilution is inoculated first.

As a routine procedure, the inoculated eggs are incubated at 35 C instead of 36 to 37 C to avoid the complicating effects which result from supraoptimal temperatures. Some eggs are opened for examination at 48 h, if necessary (see Harvesting, below), and the remainder are incubated for 72 h. Negative CAMs are passed again in eggs (blind passage).

To monitor the susceptibility of CAMs to the poxviruses, some of each lot of embryonated eggs should be inoculated with variola and vaccinia virus as controls. (Controls should always be inoculated *after* test specimens are inoculated to avoid cross-contamination.) The controls are necessary because it has been observed since 1966 that at times CAMs do not support the growth of variola, vaccinia, human monkeypox, or herpes simplex. Possible reasons are (i) eggs from a physiologically different flock of hens, (ii) use of unusual antibiotics in the flock, (iii) viral infection in the flock, causing infection of the embryo and interference, (iv) incubation of the eggs at a temperature lower than 38 C, resulting in physiologically less developed embryos than the normal 12-day-old embryos, (v) insufficient humidity during incubation, (vi) use of a too concentrated buffer solution to dilute the test specimens, and (vii) incubation of inoculated eggs at a supraoptimal temperature.

Although the exact cause of the variable susceptibility is uncertain, the effects are real, and they are manifested in several ways: (i) CAMs support no growth of control strains of variola, vaccinia, human monkeypox, and herpes simplex; (ii) inoculation of a control strain of vaccinia virus promotes growth of atypically small pocks; or (iii) when a "house standard" vaccinia is inoculated, the pock titer may be 0.5 to 1.0 $\log_{10}$ lower than usual, although the pock morphology is characteristic of vaccinia.

Harvesting. Inoculated eggs should be harvested in an isolation cabinet, and the cabinet should be disinfected after harvesting each specimen lot. A separate set of sterile forceps and scissors is used for each specimen.

When an early result is required, some of the eggs are opened and the CAMs are examined at 48 h instead of 72 h. To harvest, hold the egg with the inoculated CAM uppermost, insert sharp-pointed scissors into the hole in the blunt end, and cut the shell along the horizontal axis. Thus, the egg is cut into half. The lower half, containing the yolk and embryo, is allowed to drop into a discard pan; only the inoculated CAM should adhere to the top half of the egg shell. The CAM is peeled from the shell with forceps and placed in a large petri dish containing sterile saline. All eggs are harvested in a similar manner, with the CAMs from each inoculum dilution deposited in separate petri dishes. The CAMs are examined for pocks by using a magnifying glass under a strong light. Since pocks stand out better against a black background, the petri dishes containing the CAMs are placed on a wet, black counter top for examination.

Differentiation of virus on the basis of pock morphology. The viruses of variola and vaccinia, most strains of human monkeypox, and types 1 and 2 herpes simplex are differentiated primarily by the morphology by the pocks they form on the CAM. Varicella-zoster virus does not grow on the chick CAM.

Variola pocks at 72 h of incubation are about 1 mm in diameter, grayish-white to white, opaque, convex or dome-shaped, raised above the CAM, round, regular, smooth on the surface, not hemorrhagic, and of about the same size.

Vaccinia pocks at 72 h are 3 to 4 mm in diameter, flattened with central necrosis and ulceration, and sometimes slightly hemorrhagic.

Human monkeypox pocks at 72 h are about the same size as those of variola, but they are not as raised; most of the pocks have a pinpoint hole in the center and are sometimes hemorrhagic. Marrenikova reported that hemorrhage appears when the inoculated eggs are incubated at 34 C (16).

Herpes simplex type 1 pocks at 72 h are

pinpoint size, not raised, not opaque, not regular shaped, and, when many are present, are in a lattice-work arrangement.

Herpes simplex type 2 pocks at 72 h are about 1 mm in diameter, white, flat, and irregular in shape and size.

If there is any doubt in the identification of pocks formed by herpes simplex, the virus can be directly identified by the electron microscopy, CF, or agar gel test.

Pocks of various poxviruses and herpes simplex have been clearly illustrated in excellent colored photographs by Dumbell (5).

The CAM culture method is highly effective for detecting variola and human monkeypox, as shown by the CDC comparative tests. Of 1,066 specimens from suspect cases of smallpox, 367 (34.4%) were found to be positive by electron microscopy, CAM, and AGP combined. Of these 367, 327 (89.1%) were positive on the CAM, despite the fact that many of the specimens had been in transit for up to 2 to 4 weeks at relatively high ambient temperatures before testing. Furthermore, the occasional unpredictable variation in CAM susceptibility already described may have allowed some positive specimens to go undetected. Special care to avoid these two problems will increase the efficiency of the CAM method.

A number of pitfalls can, with foresight, be avoided. For example, when the eggs are candled, examine the pointed end of the eggs to determine whether the CAM is adequately developed into that area; eggs with an underdeveloped CAM should not be used because they may be less sensitive to poxviruses. In this same vein, Westwood et al. (25) reported that eggs with albumin sac encroachment on the dropped area of the CAM gave only about one-tenth of the vaccinia pock count of the control.

In examining the pocks on the CAM, one must be careful not to mistake nonspecific lesions for true pocks. Among the several causes for the appearance of nonspecific lesions, the most common is mechanical trauma. In addition, Westwood et al. (25) reported that isotonic sodium phosphate buffer, 0.122 M, used for inoculation induced a high incidence of nonspecific lesions.

Dumbell (5) reported that large doses of variola virus inactivated by heat or ultraviolet irradiation can cause a general thickening of the CAM and obscure the effect of a small amount of viable virus which may be present. We have observed similar effects when the CAM is inoculated with diagnostic specimens containing a very high virus titer; they could be avoided by diluting the specimens 10^{-3} or 10^{-4} before inoculation. CAMs showing the thickening effect should always be put through a second passage at several 10-fold dilutions in attempts to obtain definitive evidence of pock growth.

Tissue cultures

The use of tissue cultures is a necessary alternate virus isolation method for the CAM, in view of the periodic, unpredictable insensitivity of the CAM. The tissue cultures used are primary rhesus monkey kidney (MK) cells, infant foreskin fibroblast (FS-32) cells, and Vero cells. These cells are grown in round screw-capped tissue culture tubes.

The MK cells are grown in lactalbumin hydrolysate with 5% fetal calf serum and are maintained in lactalbumin hydrolysate without calf serum. FS-32 cells are grown in Kissling's (11) modification of Eagle's minimal essential medium (MEM) with 10% fetal calf serum and are maintained in Eagle's MEM with 2% fetal calf serum. Vero cells are grown in Eagle's MEM with 10% fetal calf serum and are maintained in Eagle's MEM without calf serum. (See appendix for composition of media.)

The MK cells and the FS-32 cells are used routinely for isolation of variola, vaccinia, and monkeypox viruses, and the FS-32 cells are used for isolation of varicella and herpes simplex viruses. The Vero cells are used to differentiate variola and human monkeypox on the basis of plaque characteristics, since these two viruses are sometimes difficult to differentiate by pocks produced on CAMs. The plaques formed by variola and vaccinia in Vero cells also differ from each other, but those of human monkeypox and vaccinia are not clearly different.

Specimen suspensions previously made for electron microscopy are prepared for tissue culture inoculation by diluting 1:2 with McIlvaine's buffer containing 4,000 units of penicillin, 2,000 μg of streptomycin, and 2,500 units of neomycin sulfate. Usually, 0.1 ml of this dilution is inoculated into each of three tubes of the tissue culture and incubated at 35.5 C. The inoculated cultures are examined daily for signs of cytopathic effect (CPE). Those which fail to show CPE are observed for 10 to 12 days and then passaged in additional cultures. A test is not declared negative until the second passage cultures are also observed for 10 to 12 days without evidence of CPE.

Monkey kidney cells. Variola virus in clinical specimens may evoke signs of CPE within 1 day in MK cells, with a rounding-up of the cells and the presence of hyperplastic foci. The CPE spreads rapidly when high-titered inoculum is used, and the cells will eventually slough off. Vaccinia and human monkeypox virus may also cause CPE in 1 day, evidenced by the rounding up of cells and the formation of foci. However, they will also form plaques in 2 to 3 days which measure 2 to 3 mm in diameter and usually show cytoplasmic bridging. Again, when a high-titered inoculum is used, the entire cell sheet becomes involved, and the cells will eventually slough off.

FS-32 cells. When inoculated with variola, cells fuse and form multinucleated foci in 1 to 3 days, with little cytoplasmic bridging. With vaccinia and human monkeypox, cells fuse and fall apart, forming large plaques and a meshwork of cytoplasmic bridging in 1 to 3 days. After inoculation with varicella-zoster virus, foci of small groups of swollen, rounded, refractile cells appear in 4 to 5 days. With herpes simplex virus, on the other hand, some degenerating cells may be rounded and others are fattened while elongated. Some cells become fused in 24 h, and CPE spreads rapidly.

Vero cells. Variola causes hyperplastic clumping of cells within 48 h, followed by the formation of small plaques. These plaques are easily differentiated from those of vaccinia and human monkeypox. Vaccinia produces large plaques within 48 h, with a noticeable amount of cytoplasmic bridging. Human monkeypox produces large plaques within 48 h with relatively clear centers surrounded by cells piled up along the edges.

As a general rule, tissue cultures inoculated with high-titered viral materials show CPE on the entire cell sheets so that no individual plaques can be discerned. Therefore, when tissue cultures are used to produce viral plaques that can be characterized morphologically, one must inoculate several dilutions of the stock viruses (or specimens) so that the plaques formed are properly separated on the cell sheets.

Animals

Rabbits and suckling mice are not generally used for isolating the exanthematous viruses, but they are useful in differentiating variola and human monkeypox (13).

Dermal reaction in rabbits. A 0.1-ml volume of human monkeypox virus with a titer of $10^{2.5}$ pock-forming units (PoFU)/ml, when inoculated intradermally on the shaved skin of a rabbit, produces a local hemorrhagic lesion about 15 mm in diameter; a similar inoculum of variola with a titer of $10^{6.5}$ PoFU/ml produces only a slightly visible reaction. In contrast, a 0.1-ml inoculum of human monkeypox virus with a titer of $10^{6.0}$ PoFU/ml causes a generalized illness in the rabbit, with secondary "satellite" exanthems in about 3 to 4 days.

Suckling mouse virulence test by footpad inoculation. Inoculation of 0.02 ml of human monkeypox virus with a titer of $10^{3.0}$ PoFU/ml into a hind footpad of 1-day-old suckling mice produces a generalized infection and 100% mortality by day 7, but the same volume of variola virus inoculated at a titer of $10^{6.0}$ PoFU/ml produces only local infection of the limb and occasional runting.

Agar gel precipitation test

Methods for the preparation of vaccinia antigen in CAM and hyperimmune antivaccinia serum in rabbits are described in the appendix. An end-frosted glass slide (75 by 25 mm) precoated with 0.2% purified agar (Difco) in distilled water, is prepared in the following manner for use as an agar gel slide. A line is drawn between the frosted and the clear area with a marking pen containing a fast-drying oil-base paint. The slightly raised line produced prevents the melted agar from running into the frosted area. A 1.5-ml amount of melted 1.0% purified agar in distilled water containing a 1:10,000 dilution of thimerosal is carefully delivered and spread onto the entire clear area of the slide. This forms a layer of agar about 2 mm thick. After the agar hardens, a plastic template with a pattern, as shown in Fig. 3, is used to punch out wells in the agar. Agar cores are removed by suction produced with a Pasteur pipette attached to a vacuum line. (The dimension of the template is such that the wells arranged in the pattern shown in Fig. 3 are each 4 mm in diameter and are 1 mm apart from each other.)

The original suspensions of specimens prepared for the electron microscopy test are used for the AGP test without diluting. (According to Dumbell and Nizamuddin [6], the limit of dilution of crusts is about 1:60 [wt/vol].) The specimen suspension to be tested is placed in wells 1 and 4, as shown in Fig. 3. The positive control vaccinia antigen is placed in well 2, and the normal rabbit serum in well 3. The antivaccinia rabbit serum is placed in the central well, C. The slide is then placed in a humid chamber and incubated at 35 C. Lines of precipitation (positive reaction) will occur within 2 to 4 h between the wells containing the specimen and the antivaccinia serum, if the specimen is from lesions of smallpox, vaccinia, or human mon-

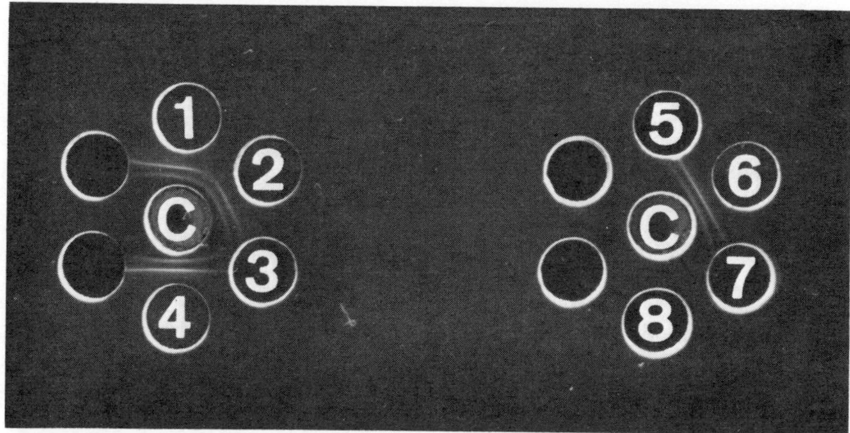

FIG. 3. *Agar gel precipitation tests. Left pattern represents positive results with an unknown specimen and right pattern represents negative results with an unknown specimen. (1 and 4) Positive unknown specimens; (5 and 8) negative unknown specimens; (2 and 6) positive control vaccinia antigen; (3 and 7) normal rabbit serum; (C) positive anti-vaccinia rabbit serum. Note the fusion of lines between wells 1 and C and wells 2 and C.*

keypox. The line(s) of precipitation formed between the wells containing the specimen and the antivaccinia serum must fuse or join (form a line of identity) with at least one of the lines between the wells of the positive control vaccinia antigen and the antivaccinia rabbit serum. Specimens are not considered negative unless diagnostic lines fail to appear by 24 h of incubation.

A specimen negative on first testing should be retested with antivaccinia rabbit serum diluted 1:2, 1:4, and 1:8, provided adequate specimen remains. The use of the diluted reagent antiserum in the test may result in an optimal antigen-antibody proportion and consequently give a positive result.

In evaluating the reliability of the AGP test for detecting pox-viruses, we found 288 (78.8%) of 1,066 specimens from patients with suspected smallpox positive by AGP versus 367 for electron microscopy, CAM, and AGP combined. The major reason that 21.2% were not detected was inadequate amount of specimen for testing. The next was probably degeneration of the soluble precipitating antigens brought about by the prolonged exposure of some of the specimens to high ambient temperatures during shipment. Dumbell and Nizamuddin (6) have shown that heating crust extracts at 60 C for 15 min greatly weakens AGP reactions.

Human convalescent smallpox serum should not be substituted for hyperimmune antivaccinia rabbit serum as a testing reagent. In human serum, antibodies other than those specific for vaccinia, variola, or human monkeypox may be present, in which case a precipitation line other than that against vaccinia may be observed and may confuse the diagnosis.

SEROLOGICAL DIAGNOSIS

Serological methods are almost useless for the diagnosis of smallpox because conditions under which the disease occurs demand more speed and accuracy than such procedures provide. The various serological procedures will not be described in detail, but the relative merits of each will be discussed briefly.

Four serological tests are applicable to the assay of antibodies evoked by smallpox, human monkeypox, and vaccinia infections: AGP (in which a patient's undiluted serum is tested instead of lesion material [Fig. 3]), CF, hemagglutination-inhibition (HI), and neutralization, with the use of tissue cultures such as LLC-MK_2 (10) or eggs. For the neutralization method with cell monolayers, the method described by Wulff et al. (29) is used; in this method, the cell monolayers are grown in tubes. The cells, however, are stained with a 1.3% solution of crystal violet in 10% Formalin instead of a 0.04% solution of neutral red in distilled water. Vaccinia virus is used as the test antigen in all four methods.

For the CF, HI, and neutralization tests, a fourfold rise in titer between acute and convalescent serum specimens is considered diagnostic. However, only a single serum specimen, taken late in the illness or during convalescence, may be all that is available. It is important to understand the limitations of the various tests when attempting to interpret the serological results obtained with such sera. For a single serum collected 8 or more days after the onset of symptoms of smallpox, the following range of results may be expected.

Agar gel precipitation test. After actual smallpox infection, the AGP test is generally clearly positive. On the other hand, sera from individuals recently vaccinated or revaccinated without a history of smallpox are rarely positive.

Complement fixation test. After smallpox infection, the CF antibody titer is usually greater than 1:20; the titer in specimens from individuals vaccinated or revaccinated without a history of smallpox is usually less than 1:20 or not detectable.

Hemagglutination-inhibition test. The HI titer is generally greater than 1:1,000. However, in some individuals without a history of smallpox, the titers resulting from vaccination or revaccination may be as high as 1:320, making diagnosis uncertain at best.

Neutralization test. The neutralization titers after smallpox infections are usually higher than in vaccinated individuals, but, since some vaccinated individuals do show high titers, results of tests of a single serum are not definitive and cannot be considered very helpful in diagnosis.

These shortcomings greatly limit the usefulness of serological tests in the diagnosis of the diseases except when a fourfold rise in titer is demonstrated. These tests are useful, however, for general serological surveys and special serological surveys to establish the fact of and date of past epidemic experience, in special studies of vaccination responses, and to establish the existence of subclinical infection in individuals.

EVALUATION OF SMALLPOX DIAGNOSTIC METHODS

Smallpox can be confidently diagnosed in the laboratory by the "four-test-combination" method, namely, the combined use of electron microscopy, AGP, CAM culture, and tissue culture methods for each specimen. The occasional shortcomings of one method are compensated for by the strong points of another. It must be emphasized, however, that an adequate amount of specimen is needed. Strongly positive specimens pose no problem; the problem is in making a negative diagnosis with confidence, and this cannot be done if the specimen received is inadequate.

In the past 2 years at the CDC, specimens from 345 patients with suspected smallpox from endemic and nonendemic areas were tested by the "four-test combination" method; 221 (64.1%) were found to be negative. All of these negative cases, under close surveillance, were confirmed beyond a reasonable doubt indeed to be negative for smallpox.

Traditionally, culturing on CAM has been thought to be the most sensitive and accurate single test for the laboratory confirmation of smallpox; however, the accumulated findings of many workers over the past 25 years have shown that electron microscopy methodology equals or surpasses the CAM method. The proficiency of electron microscopy for smallpox diagnosis was first demonstrated by Van Rooyen and Scott (24) and Nagler and Rake (20) in 1948; their findings were reinforced by more extensive investigations reported by Peters et al. in 1962 (22), Naginton and Macrae in 1965 (19), Cruickshank et al. in 1966 (2), Macrae et al. in 1969 (15), and, most recently, by the CDC.

On the other hand, electron microscopy has not been very reliable in detecting poxviruses in specimens from patients whose diseases were clinically diagnosed as vaccinia infection. In tests at the CDC, 30 of 77 specimens from patients with clinical vaccinia were found positive by combined CAM, tissue culture, and electron microscopy, and only 12 (40.0%) were found positive by electron microscopy alone, whereas 29 (96.7%) were found positive by culturing on CAM or in tissue culture. The AGP test was not used for these specimens, since the amount of specimen received was usually small.

Although the AGP test is not as sensitive as the electron microscopy, CAM, and tissue culture tests, the procedure is so simple and direct, and the results from positive specimens are obtained so rapidly, that it is a convenient companion for the electron microscopy test and a comfortable support for a positive electron microscopy result.

CAM culture is very sensitive, provided that the several pitfalls already discussed are avoided or dealt with appropriately. In addition to its sensitivity, the CAM culture method has a broad spectrum, permitting positive identification of variola, vaccinia, most known strains of monkeypox, and herpes simplex viruses. When test specimens are received in the laboratory in a fresh condition, viral inactivation should be minimal and the method should be highly reliable.

Tissue culture is an essential backup test for the CAM culture method. Its use in combination with the CAM culture method has amply confirmed its sensitivity.

APPENDIX

Growth medium for monkey kidney cells

10 × Hanks balanced salt solution	95 ml
Fetal bovine serum	50 ml
Glucose	1.0 g
Lactalbumin hydrolysate	5.0 g

Double distilled water added to 1,000 ml. Dissolve the lactalbumin hydrolysate in 800 ml of water with the aid of mild heat and stirring. Cool. Dissolve glucose in 100 ml of water and add to the lactalbumin hydrolysate solution while stirring. Add the serum and water to a volume of 1,000 ml. Sterilize by filtration. Before use, and sterile antibiotics and a sufficient volume of sterile 8.8% $NaHCO_3$ to give a pH of 7.2 to 7.4. Hanks balanced salt solution contains phenol red.

Maintenance medium for monkey kidney cells

50% Lactalbumin hydrolysate	100 ml
1 × Earle balanced salt solution	900 ml
22.6% Sodium acetate	5 ml
20% Glucose	5 ml
20% Yeastolate	5 ml

With necessary phenol red

Components sterilized by autoclaving before mixing. Add antibiotics and enough 8.8% sterile $NaHCO_3$ to give the desired pH.

Kissling's modification of Eagle's minimal essential medium (11)

For each liter of Eagle's MEM (see chapter 95), add 75 mg of glycine, 0.8 mg of thymidine, 6.8 mg of adenine, and 800 mg of galactose. The growth medium contains 10% fetal calf serum, and the maintenance medium contains 2% fetal calf serum.

McIlvaine's buffer 0.004 M, pH 7.8

Solution A = citric acid, 0.1 M ($H_3C_6O_7 \cdot H_2O$)

Solution B = Na_2HPO_4, 0.2 M (28.393 g/1,000 ml of water)

Combine 63.5 ml of solution A and 936.5 ml of solution B; this gives a solution of pH 7.6. Sterilize by membrane filtration.

To prepare 0.004 M buffer, pH 7.8, dilute 1.0 ml of the above pH 7.6 stock to 48.5 ml with sterile distilled water.

Vaccinia antigen produced on chorioallantoic membranes, positive control for agar gel precipitation

1. Obtain 20 CAMs, confluently infected with the Wyeth smallpox vaccine strain of vaccinia.
2. Place the 20 infected CAMs in a 250-ml Sorvall Omnimixer cup and homogenize for 3 min at full speed with the cup immersed in an ice-water bath.
3. Add 20 ml of sterile PBS and homogenize the mixture for 2 min with the cup immersed in an ice-water bath.
4. Add 1 part of Genetron 113 to 3 parts of the homogenate. Homogenize for 3 min with the cup immersed in an ice-water bath.
5. Centrifuge the mixture at 2,000 rpm for 10 minutes. Draw off and save the supernatant fluid. Add 1 part of 0.01% trypsin to 9 parts of the supernatant fluid, bringing the trypsin concentration to 0.001%. Mix and place in an incubator at 36 C for 1 h.
6. Dialyze the mixture against polyethylene glycol (20 M) to a final volume of 20 ml. Distribute in 1-ml portions and store at −20 C.

For normal CAM control, 20 uninfected CAMs are treated in the same manner.

Preparation of vaccinia antigen grown on rabbit skin (used to inject rabbit to produce antivaccinia rabbit serum)

1. Clip and shave the entire back of a 6-month-old or older New Zealand white rabbit.
2. Wash the shaved area, first with soap and water, then with 70% alcohol, to remove dirt and oil.
3. Scarify the animal's back with a 20-gauge needle with the point bent to form a burr. The scratchings should be about 5 mm apart, red but not bleeding.
4. With a gloved hand, rub the glycerinated vaccinia stock into the skin. (Vaccinia virus stock is the Lister strain which has been adapted to grow on rabbit skin.)
5. A confluent growth of the virus on the skin is obtained in about 3 to 5 days.
6. To harvest the growth: (i) anesthetize the rabbit with ether, (ii) exsanguinate by cardiac puncture, (iii) excise the portion of the skin with the confluent growth, and (iv) spread and tack down the hide on a wooden board.
7. Flood the hide with ether and allow to dry.
8. Scrape the crust and upper epithelial layers with a scalpel blade and save the "pulp." Keep the hide moist with McIlvaine's buffer 0.004 M, pH 7.8, while it is being scraped.
9. Homogenize the pulp with about 20 ml of McIlvaine's buffer in a 50-ml Sorvall Omni-mixer cup for 2 to 3 min. During this time, the cup should be immersed in the ice-water bath.
10. Centrifuge the mixture in a refrigerated centrifuge at 1,500 rpm for 10 min.
11. Discard hair and light debris and save the supernatant fluid.
12. Repeat steps 9–11 three more times, collecting the sediment at the end of each cycle.
13. Discard the sediment after the fourth extraction.
14. Pool the four samples of supernatant fluid and centrifuge at 2,000 rpm for 10 min; discard the sediment.
15. Centrifuge the supernatant fluid through a 40% (wt/wt) sucrose cushion.
16. Suspend the pellet of vaccinia virus in 10 ml of McIlvaine's buffer 0.004 M, pH 7.2, and add 10 ml of sterile glycerol (final glycerol concentrate of 50%). Store at −20 C.

Production of antivaccinia rabbit serum for agar gel precipitation

1. The antigen used is the Lister rabbit dermal vaccinia antigen with a titer of about 10^7 pock-forming units/ml.

2. First inoculation = 1.5 ml subcutaneously.

3. After 2 weeks, give second inoculation of 1.0 ml intravenously.

4. After 2 weeks, give third inoculation of 1.0 ml intravenously.

5. After 2 weeks, give fourth inoculation of 1.0 ml intravenously.

6. After 1 week, give fifth inoculation of 1.0 ml intravenously. Bleed out after 1 week.

A total of 8 weeks is required to prepare the serum.

LITERATURE CITED

1. Bedson, H. S., K. R. Dumbell, and W. R. G. Thomas. 1963. Variola in Tanganyika. Lancet **2**:1085–1088.
2. Cruickshank, J. G., H. S. Bedson, and D. H. Watson. 1966. Electron microscopy in the rapid diagnosis of smallpox. Lancet **2**:527–530.
3. Downie, A. W. 1951. Infection and immunity in smallpox. Lancet **1**:419–422.
4. Downie, A. W., and C. H. Kempe. 1969. Poxviruses, p. 281–320. *In* E. H. Lennette and N. J. Schmidt (ed.), Diagnostic procedures for viral and rickettsial diseases, 4th ed. American Public Health Association, Inc., New York.
5. Dumbell, K. R. 1968. Laboratory aids to the control of smallpox in countries where the disease is not endemic. Progr. Med. Virol. **10**:388–397.
6. Dumbell, K. R., and M. Nizamuddin. 1959. An agargel precipitation test for the laboratory diagnosis of smallpox. Lancet **1**:916–917.
7. Gispen, R. O. 1952. Silver impregnation of smallpox elementary bodies after treatment with xylol. Antonie van Leeuwenhoek J. Microbiol. Serol. **18**:107–108.
8. Gutstein, M. 1937. New direct staining methods for elementary bodies. J. Pathol. Bacteriol. **45**:313–314.
9. Harris, W. J., and J. C. N. Westwood. 1964. Phosphotungstate staining of vaccinia virus. J. Gen. Microbiol. **34**:491–495.
10. Hull, R. N., W. R. Cherry, and O. J. Tritch, 1962. Growth characteristics of monkey kidney cell strains LLC-MK_1, LLC-MK_2, and LLC-MK_2 (NCTC-3196) and their utility in virus research. J. Exp. Med. **115**:903–918.
11. Kissling, R. E., and D. R. Reese, 1963. Anti-rabies vaccine of tissue culture origin. J. Immunol. **91**:362–368.
12. Long, G. W., J. Noble, Jr., F. A. Murphy, K. L. Herrmann, and B. Lourie. 1970. Experience with electron microscopy in the differential diagnosis of smallpox. Appl. Microbiol. **20**:497–504.
13. Lourie, B., P. G. Bingham, H. H. Evans, S. O. Foster, J. H. Nakano, and K. L. Herrmann. 1972. Human infection with monkeypox virus: laboratory investigation of six cases in West Africa. Bull. W.H.O. **46**:633–639.
14. McCarthy, K., and K. R. Dumbell. 1961. Chorioallantoic inoculation of eggs: an improved method. Virology **14**:488–489.
15. Macrae, A. D., J. R. McDonald, A. M. Field, E. V. Meurisse, and A. A. Porter. 1969. Laboratory differential diagnosis of vesicular skin rashes. Lancet **2**:313–316.
16. Marennikova, S. S., E. M. Seluhina, N. N. Mal'Ceva, K. L. Cimiskjan, and G. Macevic. 1972. Isolation and properties of the causal agent of a new variola-like disease (monkeypox) in man. Bull. W.H.O. **46**:599–611.
17. Marsden, J. P. 1948. Variola minor, a personal analysis of 13,686 cases. Bull. Hyg. **30**:735–746.
18. Nagington, J., and R. W. Horne. 1962. Morphological studies of orf and vaccinia viruses. Virology **16**:248–260.
19. Nagington, J., and A. D. Macrae. 1965. Smallpox diagnosis and electron microscopy. Mon. Bull. Min. Health Pub. Health Lab. Serv. **24**:382–384.
20. Nagler, F. P. O., and G. Rake. 1948. The use of the electron microscope in diagnosis of variola, vaccinia, and varicella. J. Bacteriol. **55**:45–51.
21. Noble, J., Jr., and M. S. Loggins. 1970. Accuracy of smallpox diagnosis by immunofluorescence with a purified conjugate. Appl. Microbiol. **19**:855–861.
22. Peters, D., G. Nielsen, and M. E. Bayer. 1962. Variola. Die Zuverlassighest der elecktronen mikroskopischen Schnelldiagnostik. Deut. Med. Wochenschr. **87**:2240–2246.
23. Ricketts, T. F., and J. B. Byles. 1966. The diagnosis of smallpox. Baccliere, Tindall and Cassell Ltd. Reproduction for the U.S. Public Health Service.
24. Van Rooyen, C. E., and G. D. Scott. 1948. Smallpox diagnosis with special reference to electron microscopy. Can. J. Pub. Health **39**:467–477.
25. Westwood, J. C. N., P. H. Phipps, and E. A. Boulter. 1957. The titration of vaccinia virus on the chorioallantoic membrane of the developing chick embryo. J. Hyg. **52**:123–139.
26. Wildy, P. 1971. Classification and nomenclature of viruses. Monographs in virology, vol. 5. Karger, Basel.
27. World Health Organization. 1969. Guide to the laboratory diagnosis of smallpox for smallpox eradication programmes. World Health Organization, Geneva.
28. World Health Organization. 1972. Monkeypox (nine articles). Bull. W.H.O. **46**:567–639.
29. Wulff, H., T. D. Y. Chin, and H. A. Wenner. 1969. Serologic response of children after primary vaccination and revaccination against smallpox. Amer. J. Epidemiol. **99**:312–318.

Chapter 87

Chlamydiae (Psittacosis-Lymphogranuloma Venereum-Trachoma Group)

LAVELLE HANNA, JULIUS SCHACHTER, AND ERNEST JAWETZ

CLINICAL BACKGROUND

Chlamydiae infect many birds and mammals with well-defined disease patterns in each, including adenitis, enteritis, pneumonitis, keratoconjunctivitis, polyarthritis, urethritis, cervicitis, and abortion. Subclinical infection is the rule in the natural hosts. The principal diseases in humans include psittacosis, a respiratory infection usually transmitted to man from birds; lymphogranuloma venereum (LGV), a venereal disease occurring only in humans; and trachoma-inclusion conjunctivitis (TRIC), involving the eye and/or genital tract of humans.

DESCRIPTION OF AGENTS

Chlamydiae are nonmotile, gram-negative, obligate intracellular parasites, possessing a similar morphology and a common group antigen. They multiply in the cytoplasm of their host cells by a distinctive developmental cycle (13), forming characteristic intracellular microcolonies ("inclusions"). Because of their obligate intracellular parasitism, these organisms were once considered viruses. However, the chlamydiae differ from viruses in possessing *both* ribonucleic and deoxyribonucleic acids, in possessing bacterial type cell walls with mucopeptides containing muramic acid, in possessing ribosomes, in multiplying by binary fission, in possessing some metabolically active enzymes (e.g., carboxylases), and in being susceptible to many antimicrobial drugs. Chlamydiae can be regarded as gram-negative bacteria which lack some important mechanism for production of metabolic energy (13), and are therefore restricted to intracellular existence.

Developmental cycle

All chlamydiae share a general sequence of events in their reproduction. The infectious particle ("elementary body") is small, about 0.3 μm in diameter, with an electron-dense nucleoid. It is taken into the host cell by phagocytosis. A vacuole, derived from host cell surface membranes, forms around the small particle. This small particle is reorganized into a larger one ("initial body"), measuring about 0.5 to 1 μm and devoid of an electron-dense nucleoid. Within the membrane-bound vacuole, the large particle grows in size and divides repeatedly by binary fission. Eventually, the entire vacuole becomes filled with small particles derived by binary fission from large bodies to form an "inclusion" in the host cell cytoplasm. The newly formed small particles may be liberated from the host cell to infect new cells. The developmental cycles take 24 to 48 h.

Staining properties

Chlamydiae are large enough to be seen by light microscopy. They have distinctive staining properties (similar to those of rickettsiae) which differ somewhat at different stages of development. Single mature particles (elementary bodies) stain purple with Giemsa stain and red with Macchiavello or Giménez stain. The larger, noninfective bodies (initial bodies) stain blue or green. The Gram reaction of chlamydiae is negative or variable, and Gram stain is not useful in the identification of the agents.

Fully formed, mature intracellular inclusions are compact masses near the nucleus, stained dark purple with Giemsa stain because of the densely packed mature particles. If stained with diluted Lugol's iodine solution, the inclusions formed by some chlamydiae (mouse pneumonitis, LGV, trachoma, inclusion conjunctivitis, and others) appear brown because of the glycogen-like matrix which surrounds the particles.

Characteristics of host-parasite relationship

The outstanding biological feature of infection by chlamydiae is the balance that is often reached between host and parasite, resulting in prolonged, often lifetime, subclinical infection. Overt disease is the exception in the natural hosts of these agents, although epizootics occur. Spread from one host (e.g., avian) to another (e.g., human) more frequently leads to disease. Antibodies to several antigens of chlamydiae are regularly produced by the infected host. These antibodies appear to have little protective effect. Commonly, the infectious agent persists in the presence of high titers of antibodies. Treatment with effective antimicrobial drugs (e.g., tetracyclines) for prolonged periods may eliminate the chlamydiae from the infected host. Very early, intensive treatment may suppress antibody formation. Late or inadequate treatment with antimicrobial drugs may suppress disease but permit persistence of the infectious agent in tissues.

Immunization in animals or man fails to protect against infection. At best, immunization or prior infection induces some resistance which results in milder disease after challenge or reinfection (8).

Antigens

Chlamydiae possess two types of antigens (7), group antigens and specific antigens. Both are probably located in the cell wall. Group antigens are shared by all members of the group. They are probably lipopolysaccharides resembling those of gram-negative bacteria, and can be detected by complement fixation (CF; 3). Specific antigens remain attached to cell walls, after group antigens have been largely removed by treatment with fluorocarbon or deoxycholate. They are relatively labile, are alkali-soluble, and are shared by only a limited number of chlamydial types, but a given organism may contain several specific antigens. The specific antigens can be detected by immunofluorescence. A toxic factor exists in infectious chlamydiae in close association with antigens. This toxic factor can kill mice within 2 to 24 h after the intravenous injection of more than 10^8 infectious organisms. Specific neutralization of this lethal toxic factor permits limited antigenic typing of chlamydiae (1, 11), which apparently corresponds to the typing by immunofluorescence (20).

Classification

Chlamydiae are presently placed in the order *Chlamydiales*, family *Chlamydiaceae*, species *Chlamydia trachomatis* and *C. psittaci*. Historically, chlamydiae have been arranged according to their pathogenic potential and their host range. Chlamydiae can also be grouped according to the nature of the intracytoplasmic inclusion and according to their susceptibility to sulfonamides. *C. trachomatis* (trachoma-inclusion conjunctivitis, LGV, mouse pneumonitis, and others) produces a very compact inclusion which stains with iodine; it is inhibited by sulfonamides and cycloserine. *C. psittaci* (psittacosis-ornithosis, meningopneumonitis, feline pneumonitis, and others) produces diffuse inclusions which do not stain with iodine; it tends to be resistant to sulfonamides and cycloserine. Antigenic typing is possible by mouse toxicity protection tests (referred to above), by immunofluorescence, and for certain isolates by plaque reduction in cell culture, with the use of hyperimmune rooster sera (2).

Diagnosis of infection is supported by the laboratory examinations listed in Table 1.

PSITTACOSIS-ORNITHOSIS

The psittacosis-ornithosis group of infections includes chlamydial infections of psittacine birds and of man exposed to birds (psittacosis) as well as chlamydial infections of other avian species (ornithosis). Man is usually infected via the respiratory tract. Subclinical infection is common. If disease occurs, it may range from an atypical upper respiratory disease to a severe pneumonitis or sepsis (7).

The etiological agent *C. psittaci* typically is resistant to sulfonamides and cycloserine and does not produce an iodine-staining matrix in intracellular inclusions (4, 13). It shares group antigens with other chlamydiae, but perhaps can be separated from *C. trachomatis* (e.g., TRIC agents) by immunofluorescence (6, 21).

Collection and Storage of Specimens

Caution: The handling of infected specimens and the isolation of the infectious agents present a serious danger to laboratory workers. The agents may remain infectious in the dried state for years. Strict aseptic conditions must be

TABLE 1. *Laboratory methods of choice in etiological diagnosis of chlamydial infections*

Procedures	Psittacosis	LGV	TRIC
Direct microscopic examination (Giemsa, fluorescent antibody)	−	−	+
Isolation of agent			
Cell culture	+	±	−
Irradiated cell culture	+	+	+
Chick embryo yolk sac	+	+	+
Mice			
Intraperitoneal	+	−	−
Intracerebral	±	±	−
Serology (antibody titer rise)			
CF (group antigen)	+	+[a]	+
Fluorescent antibody	−	+	+
Skin test	−	±	−

[a] A single titer of 1:64 or higher supports the diagnosis of active LGV infection.

maintained, and inexperienced workers should not attempt these procedures.

Specimens to be examined include blood (heparinized or clotted), sputum, and tissues obtained at autopsy from bird or man, especially tissue from the spleen, liver, lung, and pericardial exudate. Serum is used for antibody determinations.

If bacterial contamination is suspected, the specimen may be treated with streptomycin (10 mg/ml) or other drugs (bacitracin, 1,000 units/ml; nystatin, 50 units/ml; neomycin, 0.5 mg/ml; or polymyxin, 0.1 mg/ml). These drug concentrations do not suppress chlamydial growth significantly.

Specimens for isolation may be kept at 4 C for several days; for longer periods, they are stored at −60 C or below. Serum for antibody determinations may be stored at 4 C or at −20 C.

Direct Examination

Fluorescence microscopy has not yet been applied to routine clinical diagnosis of human psittacosis infections. Chlamydiae are sufficiently large to be seen by light microscopy in smears from heavily infected bird tissues stained by the Giemsa or Macchiavello method. Stained smears from human sputum or tissues rarely reveal the infectious agent.

Isolation of Psittacosis-Ornithosis Agents

Ths host systems most commonly employed are yolk sacs of embryonated eggs, intraperitoneally inoculated mice, or cell cultures.

Embryonated eggs

Eggs must be from flocks receiving only antibiotic-free feed. Yolk sac inoculation, incubation, and harvest are performed as outlined at the end of this chapter. Up to three blind passages should be performed in the absence of egg deaths before isolation attempts are abandoned. Chlamydiae are sometimes seen microscopically in stained smears of yolk sacs harvested from live eggs, in the absence of deaths, but deaths usually occur in the next passage.

Mice

Mice to be used for the isolation of chlamydiae must be from a colony free from latent chlamydial infections, and they must be fed an antibiotic-free diet. The colony should be checked periodically for the presence of chlamydiae by three to five blind passages of spleen and lung suspensions. The susceptibility of mice to different strains of chlamydiae varies greatly.

The intraperitoneal route is employed most commonly. A suspension of the specimen (0.5 ml) is injected intraperitoneally into each of five mice. After 21 days, the mice are sacrificed, the spleens are harvested aseptically, and impression smears are made on sterile microscope slides. Smears are stained by the Giemsa or Macchiavello method. The spleens are pooled and ground to a paste with a mortar and pestle, with the use of an abrasive if necessary. A 20% suspension of tissue is made in sterile nutrient broth, and 0.5 ml is injected intraperitoneally into a second group of mice. Three blind passages should be performed before an isolation attempt is accepted as negative. If chlamydiae are present in dead or sacrificed mice, the spleen is large, with fibrin on the surface, and yields impression smears rich in elementary bodies. There may be ascitic fluid and foci of necrosis in the liver.

Subcutaneous injection is employed mainly when heavy bacterial contamination of the specimen is suspected. Bacteria may be localized at the site of subcutaneous injection, whereas psittacosis agent will reach the spleen and multiply there. Aseptic harvest of the spleen at 21 days then permits continued passage by the intraperitoneal route.

Intranasal instillation is employed mainly to detect subclinical chlamydial infection in a mouse colony by the blind passage of lung suspensions. After instillations of 0.03 ml into the nares of mice lightly anesthetized with ether, respiratory distress may develop within 3 to 10 days with consolidation of the lungs and death.

Intracerebral inoculation is a rapid and sensitive method for the detection of many psittacosis agents, but it is hampered by the frequent overgrowth of bacterial contaminants.

Cell culture

C. psittaci can be isolated by centrifugation onto irradiated cell monolayers (see below, Special Procedures). A series of dilutions must be inoculated, because high concentrations of chlamydiae may be rapidly toxic. Monolayers may be examined after 48 to 96 h for the presence of inclusions by immunofluorescence or Giemsa stains, but not by iodine stain.

Identification of Agent

The minimal criteria for proof of isolation of chlamydiae require serial transmission of the agent with microscopic evidence of the organisms in stained smears of yolk sac, or animal tissues or cells, and serological demonstration of the group antigen in passage material. A CF antigen can be prepared by boiling a 20 to 50% suspension in saline for 1 h. Further identification requires establishment of host range and immunological characterization (2, 16).

Serological Diagnosis

No reliable methods have been developed for the demonstration of neutralizing antibodies in human sera. A hemagglutination-inhibition test has been developed, with the use of certain chicken or mouse erythrocytes, but the test is subject to so many variations that it has not been employed in diagnosis.

Complement fixation

The CF test is the most widely employed serological test. It employs 4 units of an antigen such as that described in Special Procedures (see below). The antigen exhibits group reactivity and detects mainly group-reactive antibodies. The test may be performed by the CF technique described in Chapter 71 with mammalian sera, or by the method described by Meyer and Eddie (12) with many avian sera. Guinea pig complement is not bound by some avian sera, and therefore an indirect CF test may be necessary.

Serological diagnosis of psittacosis usually depends on a fourfold or greater rise in complement-fixing antibody titer during the period of illness, as evidenced by results obtained with paired sera. A single titer of 1:16 or higher is often considered significant, but there are marked variations in the titers encountered in different areas and in different population groups.

Treatment with antibiotics very early in the course of proven psittacosis-ornithosis infection may suppress the antibody response.

LYMPHOGRANULOMA VENEREUM

LGV is a venereal disease of man caused by chlamydiae closely related to TRIC agents. One to 3 weeks after sexual exposure, a small evanescent papule develops on genitalia or rectum. This heals but is followed by enlargement of inguinal (buboes) or perirectal lymph nodes which suppurate and may discharge pus through sinus tracts. Later, the chronic lymphadenitis leads to fibrosis, lymphatic obstruction, and rectal strictures. During the acute stage, there may be marked systemic involvement with fever, rashes, arthralgias, or, rarely, meningitis.

LGV chlamydiae are usually susceptible to inhibition by sulfonamides and cycloserine. The inclusions in infected cells stain with iodine. There are three or more immunological types.

Collection of Specimens

Specimens consist of pus aspirated aseptically from a fluctuant suppurative lymph node, biopsy tissue from an enlarged but not fluctuant lymph node, and cerebrospinal fluid. Serum is collected for antibody determinations. Streptomycin or neomycin may be added to the specimen to control the growth of bacterial contaminants. For other antimicrobial drugs and for storage conditions, see Psittacosis.

Direct Examination

Chlamydial particles are seen only with great difficulty in stained smears of pus. There is insufficient experience in their demonstration by immunofluorescence.

Isolation of LGV Chlamydiae

In the past, the most commonly employed host systems were the yolk sac of 7-day embryonated eggs or mice inoculated intracerebrally.

Cell culture

Irradiated cell cultures are now used more frequently and appear to provide a more sensitive method for isolation (14). For details of this procedure see Special Procedures. Serial dilutions of pus or of tissue homogenates should be inoculated, and one transfer should be made before the attempt is accepted as negative, because of toxicity for the cells.

Embryonated eggs

Eggs must be from flocks receiving only antibiotic-free feed. The method for yolk sac inoculation and harvest is outlined at the end of this chapter. Repeated blind passage of yolk sac material may be necessary to obtain an isolate manifest by stainable particles in yolk sac smears, by transmissible death of eggs, and by the presence of chlamydial group antigen in yolk sac suspensions (see section on Psittacosis).

Mice

Intracerebral injection was preferred in isolation attempts but does not appear to be as sensitive as cell culture or egg inoculation.

Intraperitoneal or subcutaneous inoculation of LGV into mice is not lethal and is not suitable for isolation attempts.

Serological Diagnosis

Neutralization tests

No reliable method has been developed.

Hemagglutination-inhibition tests

See the section on Psittacosis.

Complement fixation tests

The CF test is most widely used for the detection of group-reactive antibodies. The antigens are described under Special Procedures, and the technique of the test is described in Chapter 71. A fourfold rise in antibody titer during an illness compatible with LGV provides support for the diagnosis. Often, however, high titers of complement-fixing antibody are found early in the first serum specimen because active LGV infection has already been in progress for several weeks. A patient who received antimicrobial therapy soon after infection may not develop chlamydial antibodies.

Indirect immunofluorescence

Serum antibodies can be demonstrated, with the use of LGV-infected cell cultures as antigen. For more specific antibodies, the micro-immunofluorescence test developed by Wang (19) can be used.

Skin Test

The original Frei test consisted of the intradermal injection of heated pus aspirated from a human lymphogranuloma bubo. The antigen in use at the present time consists of lymphogranuloma chlamydiae, grown in yolk sac and partially purified. Uninfected yolk sac treated similarly serves as control. Amounts of 0.1 ml of these preparations are injected into the skin of the forearms. The test is read at 48 h. Edema and erythema are disregarded; only the size of the indurated papule is measured. A papule 6 mm larger than the control is considered to indicate a positive delayed sensitivity reaction to group antigen.

Some typical cases of lymphogranuloma venereum (proven by isolation) are serologically positive, yet skin test negative. It is believed that the skin reaction becomes positive within 2 to 3 weeks after infection and remains positive for many years. Early treatment may interfere with the development of a positive skin test. Since the skin test indicates only reactivity to the group antigen, infection with any chlamydiae (psittacosis, LGV, TRIC) may result in a positive reaction.

TRACHOMA-INCLUSION CONJUNCTIVITIS

TRIC chlamydial infections typically involve the eye, the urethra, and the cervix. Tissue reactions consist of hyperemia, exudate, follicular hypertrophy, and scarring. Neovascularization of the cornea may lead to pannus formation and opacity. Trachoma involves mainly the upper lid and is progressive, with gross lid deformity, whereas inclusion conjunctivitis involves particularly the lower lid and tends to regress spontaneously with little scarring. However, all types of eye lesions may follow venereal infection as well as endemic eye infection (9). One form of nongonococcal urethritis is caused by TRIC agents. Inclusion conjunctivitis of the newborn (inclusion blennorhea) results from venereally acquired cervical infection in the mother.

TRIC agents typically are susceptible to sulfonamides and cycloserine, form compact intracellular inclusions with an iodine-staining matrix, and infect mainly superficial epithelial cells. In cell culture, there is no spread to surrounding cells and no plaque formation. TRIC agents fall into nine or more immunological types.

Collection and Storage of Specimens

Scrapings of epithelial cells from conjunctiva, urethra, or cervix are obtained with a sterile platinum spatula or a swab, under local anesthesia.

For isolation in cell culture (5), the suspending medium consists of 0.2 M sucrose in 0.02 M phosphate buffer, pH 7.0 to 7.2, with antibiotics. For isolation in yolk sac, scrapings are suspended in 1 ml of buffered saline or broth with antibiotics as described in the section on Psittacosis. It is preferable to inoculate specimens onto susceptible host cells immediately. Storage at 0 to 4 C for up to 24 h reduces infectivity somewhat, but often still permits recovery of the chlamydiae. If more prolonged storage is required, scrapings may be kept at −60 C or below for weeks or months with some loss of infectivity.

Smears for microscopy must be prepared immediately and air-dired. Fixation and storage are discussed below.

Direct Examination

The typical TRIC intracytoplasmic inclusion is found in easily accessible epithelial cells of the conjunctiva or the genital tract. Therefore, direct microscopic examination of specimens is more contributory in TRIC infections than in psittacosis or LGV, but still may be tedious, difficult, and insensitive.

Immunofluorescence appears to be the most sensitive method available now for the demonstration of inclusions and is highly specific (18). However, the technique requires an experienced observer. Sera from rabbits hyperimmunized with yolk sac-grown TRIC agent or human convalescent serum with a high titer of group antibodies against chlamydia can be fluorescein-labeled (see Chapter 71) for use in a direct test, or can be used with the appropriate fluorescein-labeled anti-rabbit or anti-human gamma globulin.

The scraping is spread on a microscope slide, air-dried, fixed in cold acetone (4 C) for at least 10 min, rinsed in phosphate-buffered saline (PBS), pH 7.1, and can be stored at 4 C for 2 to 3 days or at −20 C for months or years. At the time of examination, the scraping is thawed and air-dried at room temperature. For the direct test, fluorescein-labeled serum diluted in PBS is added and the slide is incubated in a moist chamber at 37 C. Plastic or glass petri dishes 14 to 15 cm in diameter containing filter paper saturated with water provide convenient chambers. After 30 min, the labeled serum is decanted and the slide is rinsed with occasional shaking in PBS for 15 min at room temperature. The saline is then shaken off, 90% glycerine plus 10% saline is added to the smear, and a cover glass is added. The entire area of the scraping is examined under oil at a magnification of 480 times with an appropriate light source, e.g., ultraviolet light. (Slides with etched circles will limit the area to be examined.) The typical TRIC inclusion should be a sharply defined mass, fluorescing with a yellow-green light, clearly within the cytoplasm of an epithelial cell, and not attached to or a part of the nucleus (Fig. 1). Inclusions are frequent in very active or severe infections, but are rare in chronic ocular infections.

Giemsa stain

When air-dried, the smear is fixed for at least 5 min in absolute methanol at room temperature and again dried. At this stage, it can be stored at room temperature indefinitely. The procedure for the Giemsa stain is described below. Microscopic examination at a magnification of 200 times, with 900 to 1,000 times magnification of suspected inclusions, is usually satisfactory. The inclusion may be made up of initial bodies, elementary bodies, or both. The initial bodies are bluish, round or oval particles; the elementary bodies are smaller, more dense, round particles which stain purple with Giemsa stain (Fig. 2). The particles are imbedded in a matrix which does not stain with Giemsa stain.

Iodine

In scrapings which have been air-dried, fixed in absolute methanol, and stained with Lugol's iodine, or 5% iodine in 10% potassium iodide, for 3 to 5 min, the matrix of inclusions may appear as a reddish-brown mass recognizable under magnification of 200 times. However, iodine-staining is demonstrable only in a limited phase of the reproductive cycle, and failure to locate iodine-staining inclusions in scrapings does not exclude the demonstration of inclusions in the same preparation by Giemsa or other stain. Iodine staining is not applicable to cervical

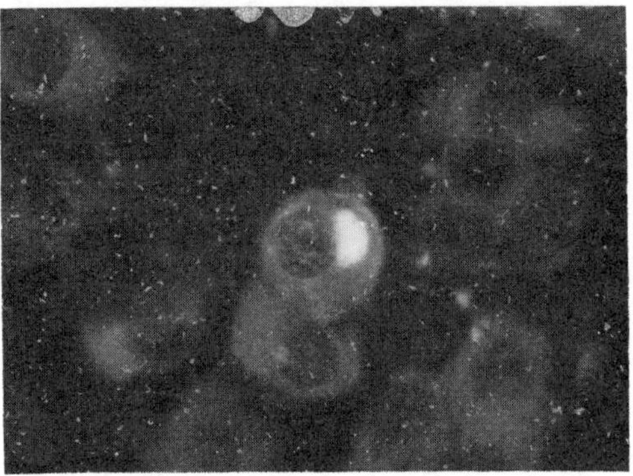

FIG. 1. *Typical intracytoplasmic TRIC inclusion in an epithelial cell from a conjunctival scraping. Immunofluorescent stain. The central epithelial cell contains a brilliantly fluorescing semilunar inclusion.*

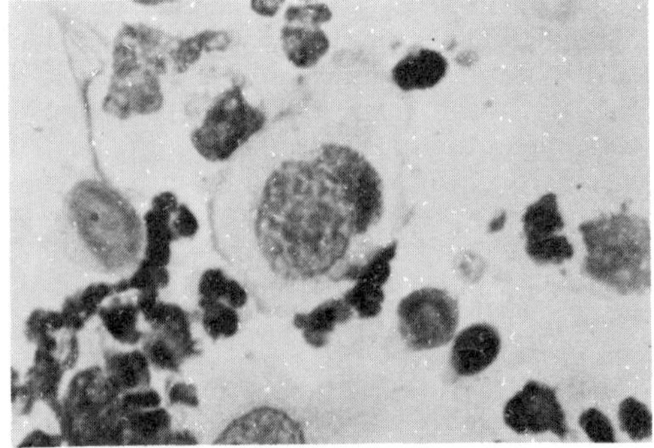

FIG. 2. *Typical intracytoplasmic TRIC inclusion in an epithelial cell from conjunctival scraping. Giemsa stain. A semilunar dense inclusion composed of many individual particles adjoins the nucleus of the epithelial cell. There are many polymorphonuclear cells in the field.*

specimens where there are normal glycogen-containing cells.

Isolation of TRIC Agents

The systems most commonly used for isolation of TRIC agents are cell cultures or yolk sacs of embryonated eggs. None of the common laboratory animals is susceptible.

Cell culture

TRIC agents do not readily infect cells in culture. Sensitivity is enhanced by (i) prior irradiation of the cells (5), (ii) prior treatment of the monolayer with diethylaminoethyl-dextran (10, 15), and (iii) centrifugation of the specimen onto the cell monolayer (5). The method is described in Special Procedures (see below).

Embryonated eggs

Yolk sac inoculation procedures are outlined at the end of this chapter. It is essential that inoculated eggs are incubated at temperatures not above 35 C. Repeated blind passages at 7 to 13 days are often required before chlamydiae are demonstrated.

An isolated chlamydial agent is identified as TRIC agent if (i) it produces typical compact iodine-staining inclusions in cell culture, or shows the characteristic appearance of elementary and initial bodies in yolk sacs; (ii) the agent is transmissible in susceptible cells or embryonated eggs but not in mice; and (iii) group and specific antigens are demonstrated by CF or micro-immunofluorescence, or it produces a follicular conjunctivitis in primates.

Serological Diagnosis

Complement-fixation test

TRIC agents share the heat-stable chlamydial group antigen, and group-reactive antibodies can be demonstrated by CF in many individuals after infection with TRIC agents. However, it has been shown (8, 17) that many individuals do not develop measurable levels of group antibody during acute infection, and that others who may possess antibodies against one of the chlamydiae at the time of infection do not show an increased titer during infection. There is no evidence that use of antibiotics during the course of the disease affects the level of antibody as has been reported in psittacosis and LGV.

Fluorescent antibody

A micro-immunofluorescence method offers a sensitive means of detecting TRIC antibodies with the added advantage that it may demonstrate some degree of antigenic type specificity. Wang and Grayston (21) have classified most isolates from classic trachoma infections as type A (limited to northern Africa and the eastern Mediterranean areas), B, or C; isolates from oculogenital infection are most commonly type D, E, or F. Other antigenic types (G, H, I) are recognized. At least three antigenic types of LGV exist. There appears to be little or no cross-reactivity between *C. trachomatis* and *C. psittaci*. (For the procedure, see Wang [19].)

In LGV and in oculogenital TRIC infections, 80 to 90% of serum specimens have antibody titers of more than 1:8, usually with considerable cross-reactivity. Sera from individuals with chronic trachoma are less likely to have demonstrable antibody. Prevalence of antibody ranges from 85% in endemic areas where disease is severe to less than 10% in Indian reservations of the American Southwest where disease is mild. Individuals infected with trachoma who have demonstrable levels of antibody are more likely to show monotypic responses, rather than broad cross-reactivity.

Skin Tests

Skin tests are not contributory in diagnosing TRIC infection.

SPECIAL PROCEDURES

Cell cultures

Stock cells. Confluent monolayers of cells (e.g., McCoy, Hela 229, or L 929) are subjected to 4,000 to 6,000 R (irradiation from any source). Five to 7 days later, 10^5 cells in 1 ml of growth medium (10% horse or fetal bovine serum in Eagle's minimal essential medium with glucose, 30 μmol/ml, and streptomycin, 50 μg/ml, vancomycin, 100 μg/ml, and nystatin, 25 μg/ml) are seeded onto cover slips. Round cover slips in 15-mm disposable plastic flat-bottom vials are satisfactory. After 1 to 2 days, when the monolayers are confluent, the tubes are ready for use.

Inoculation

Growth medium is replaced in two to four tubes with 0.1 to 1.0 ml of specimen. The tubes are centrifuged at 1,500 to 3,000 $\times$ g at 30 to 35 C for 1 h. The inoculum is replaced with fresh medium, and the tubes are incubated at 35 C for 2 to 3 days. One cover slip is then examined for presence of inclusions, with the use of Giemsa, iodine, or fluorescent-antibody stains (iodine will be positive only with *C.*

trachomatis). If the first cover slip shows inclusions, the cells in the second tube may be harvested for transfer.

As a substitute for irradiation, or to increase further the sensitivity of the technique, monolayers of cells may be washed twice with 1 ml of Hanks balanced salt solution containing 30 μg of diethylaminoethyl-dextran per ml (15). This treatment enhances infectivity by TRIC agents, but it does not appear to affect recovery of LGV agents (10).

The cell culture technique provides a relatively simple, fast method of demonstrating infectious chlamydiae. When large numbers of inclusions are apparent in the initial passage, the isolate can usually be established in cell culture (by use of the inoculation procedure described above) and at times becomes adapted to egg passage. However, when very few (less than 10) inclusions are seen on a cover slip, transfer is often unsuccessful. As a diagnostic procedure, it is very useful. Particularly when the iodine stain can be used (LGV and TRIC), inclusions can be recognized in the presence of heavy bacterial contamination.

Yolk Sac Inoculation of Embryonated Eggs

Eggs are preincubated at 38 to 39 C in saturated humidity for 7 days and then are candled. Viable embryonated eggs are inoculated with the specimen by injecting 0.2 to 1.0 ml into the yolk sac with a 22-gauge 1.5-inch (3.8-cm) needle. The hole in the shell is sealed, and incubation is continued at 35 C and saturated humidity. The eggs are candled daily. Deaths occurring during the first 2 to 4 days are considered nonspecific and the eggs are discarded. After the fourth day, the yolk sac may be harvested. The eggshell is disinfected with tincture of iodine and cracked with sterile forceps; the shell, shell membrane, and chorioallantoic membrane are removed in the area of the air sac. With a second pair of sterile forceps, the yolk is removed, excess yolk is stripped away, and impression smears are made on sterile slides. These smears are stained (Giemsa, Giménez, Macchiavello stains; see below) and are examined microscopically under oil immersion for the presence of chlamydiae.

Blind passage

Yolk sacs are harvested aseptically, weighed in a sterile dish, and are ground to a 50% suspension with mortar, pestle, and sand, or are shaken vigorously with sterile glass beads in a closed container to make a uniform suspension. This can be centrifuged for 30 to 60 min at 500 × *g* in a refrigerated centrifuge. The supernatant fluid is removed, tested for bacteriological sterility in thioglycolate broth, and injected into the yolk sacs of a second series of embryonated eggs. Three to six blind passages may be required before isolation of a chlamydial agent is established by egg death, microscopic findings, and presence of group antigen. Well-established psittacosis isolates kill eggs faster (4 to 5 days) than LGV or TRIC isolates (5 to 8 days).

Antigens for Complement Fixation Tests

Several antigens are available commercially, but higher titers can usually be obtained with antigens prepared from infected yolk sacs rich in infective particles as described below. Antigens have principally group-reactive properties. The preparation may involve the risk of airborne infection.

Antigen preparation

Although antigens extracted with ether or deoxycholate have been used, the following preparation is preferred. The starting material consists of pooled, infected yolk sacs containing large numbers of infective particles. The yolk sacs of 7-day embryonated eggs are inoculated with a chlamydial inoculum (e.g., psittacosis isolate 6BC), estimated to result in death of about 50% of inoculated eggs in 5 to 7 days. Eggs are candled daily and those dying early are discarded. When the 50% death end point is approached, the remaining eggs (recently dead or live) are refrigerated for 3 to 24 h. The yolk sacs are then harvested. If examination of random samples shows large numbers of particles, the yolk sacs are pooled. This preparation may be stored at −20 C until further processing.

The yolk sacs are ground in a mortar with sterile sand. Beef heart broth (pH 7.0) is added to make a 20% suspension, and the material is cultured for bacteriological sterility. The suspension is placed in a flask containing sterile glass beads and stored at 4 C for 3 to 6 weeks with daily shaking. It is then centrifuged at 2,000 rpm to remove coarse particles, transferred to a heavy sterile flask, and steamed at 100 C or immersed in boiling water for 30 min. After it has cooled, liquefied phenol is added to 0.5%. The antigen should then be refrigerated for at least 1 week before being used. It is stable for at least 1 year if not contaminated and should have an antigen titer of 1:256 or greater. A similar preparation from uninfected yolk sacs must be included as one of the controls.

Staining Reagents for Chlamydiae

Giemsa stain

Giemsa stain is prepared by dissolving 0.5 g of powder in 33 ml of glycerol at 55 to 60 C for 1.5 to 2 h. To this is added 33 ml of absolute methanol, acetone-free. The solution is mixed thoroughly and allowed to sediment, and then is stored at room temperature as stock. Dilutions of the stock stain are made with neutral distilled water or buffered water in a ratio of 1 part of stock Giemsa solution to 40 or 50 of diluent.

The smear is air-dried, fixed with absolute methanol for at least 5 min, and again dried. It is then covered with the diluted Giemsa stain, freshly prepared each day, for 1 h. The slide is then rinsed rapidly in 95% ethyl alcohol to remove excess dye, dried, and examined for the presence of the typical basophilic intracytoplasmic inclusion body.

Giménez stain

Stock carbol fuchsin contains 100 ml of 10% (wt/vol) fuchsin in 95% ethyl alcohol, 250 ml of 4% (vol/vol) aqueous phenol, and 650 ml of distilled water. This stock solution should be held at 37 C for 48 h before use; for the "working" solution, the stock is diluted 1:2.5 with phosphate buffer, pH 7.45 (3.5 ml of 0.2 M NaH_2PO_4, 15.5 ml of 0.2 M Na_2HPO_4, and 19 ml of distilled water). This working solution is immediately filtered and is filtered again before every stain. It is usable for 3 to 4 days.

Malachite green is used as 0.8% aqueous malachite green oxalate.

Procedure. The smear should be heat-fixed. The smear is stained as follows: stain with fuchsin for 1 to 2 min, wash with tap water; stain with malachite green for 6 to 9 s, wash with tap water; restain with malachite green for 6 to 9 s, wash thoroughly with tap water, and blot dry. In yolk sac smears, most elementary bodies will stain red against a greenish background.

Modified Macchiavello stain

The following solutions are used: basic fuchsin, 0.25 g in 100 ml of double-distilled water; citric acid, 0.5 g in 200 ml of double-distilled water; and methylene blue, 1.0 g in 100 ml of double-distilled water.

The smear is air-dried and fixed by heat. The basic fuchsin solution, freshly filtered, is dropped onto the film for 5 min and then drained. The slide is washed in tap water and rinsed briefly with the citric acid solution. The slide is then washed with tap water, stained with methylene blue for 20 to 30 s, again washed in tap water, and dried by blotting. Overexposure to citric acid will decolorize the elementary bodies and they will all stain blue. In a properly prepared slide, most of the elementary bodies will stain red. Initial bodies, if present, will appear blue. The background is pale blue.

LITERATURE CITED

1. Alexander, E. R., S. P. Wang, and J. T. Grayston. 1967. Further classification of TRIC agents from ocular trachoma and other sources by the mouse toxicity prevention test. Amer. J. Ophthalmol. (Ser. 3) **63:**1469–1478.
2. Banks, J., B. Eddie, M. Sung, N. Sugg, J. Schachter, and K. F. Meyer. 1970. Plaque reduction technique for demonstrating neutralizing antibodies for *Chlamydia*. Infect. Immunity **2:**443–447.
3. Dhir, S. P., S. Hakomori, G. E. Kenny, and J. T. Grayston. 1972. Immunochemical studies on chlamydial group antigens (presence of a 2-keto-3-deoxycarbohydrase as immunodominant group). J. Immunol. **109:**116–122.
4. Gordon, F. B., and A. L. Quan. 1965. Occurrence of glycogen in inclusions of the psittacosis-lymphogranuloma venereum-trachoma agents. J. Infect. Dis. **115:**186–196.
5. Gordon, F. B., and A. L. Quan. 1971. Isolation of chlamydia trachomatis from the human genital tract by cell culture: a summary, p. 476–484. *In* R. L. Nichols (ed), Trachoma and related disorders. Excerpta Medica, Amsterdam.
6. Hanna, L., and H. Bernkopf. 1964. Trachoma viruses isolated in the United States. VIII. Separation of TRIC viruses from related agents by immunofluorescence. Proc. Soc. Exp. Biol. Med. **116:**827–831.
7. Jawetz, E., J. L. Melnick, and E. A. Adelberg. 1972. Agents of the psittacosis-LGV-TRIC group (Bedsoniae, chlamydiae), p. 272. *In* Review of medical microbiology, 10th ed. Lange Medical Publications, Los Altos, Calif.
8. Jawetz, E., L. Rose, L. Hanna, and P. Thygeson. 1965. Experimental inclusion conjunctivitis in man. Measurements of infectivity and resistance. J. Amer. Med. Ass. **194:**620–632.
9. Jones, B. R. 1964. Ocular syndromes of TRIC virus infection and their possible genital significance. Brit. J. Vener. Dis. **40:**3–18.
10. Kuo, C., S. P. Wang, and J. T. Grayston. 1972. Differentiation of TRIC and LGV organisms based on enhancement of infectivity by DEAE-dextran in cell culture. J. Infect. Dis. **125:**313–317.
11. Manire, G. P., and K. F. Meyer. 1950. The toxins of the psittacosis-lymphogranuloma group of agents. III. Differentiation of strains by the toxin neutralization test. J. Infect. Dis. **86:**241–250.
12. Meyer, K. F., and B. Eddie. 1964. Psittacosis-lymphogranuloma venereum group (Bedsonia infections), p. 603–639. *In* E. H. Lennette and N. J. Schmidt (ed), Diagnostic procedures for viral and rickettsial diseases, 3rd ed. American Public Health Association, Inc., New York.
13. Moulder, J. W. 1966. The relation of the psittacosis group (Chlamydiae) to bacteria and viruses. Annu. Rev. Microbiol. **20:**107–130.
14. Philip, R. N., D. A. Hill, A. B. Greaves, F. B. Gordon, A. L. Quan, R. K. Gerloff, and L. A. Thomas. 1971. Study of chlamydiae in patients with lymphogranuloma venereum and urethritis attending a venereal diseases clinic. Brit. J. Vener. Dis. **47:**114–121.

15. Rota, T. R., and R. L. Nichols. 1971. Infection of cell cultures by trachoma agent: enhancement by DEAE-dextran. J. Infect. Dis. **124:**419–421.

16. Schachter, J. 1970. (Editorial) Recommended criteria for the identification of trachoma and inclusion conjunctivitis agents. J. Infect. Dis. **122:**105–107.

17. Schachter, J., C. R. Dawson, S. Balas, and P. Jones. 1970. Evaluation of laboratory methods for detecting acute TRIC agent infection. Amer. J. Ophthalmol. **70:**375–380.

18. Schachter, J., L. Hanna, M. L. Tarizzo, and C. R. Dawson. 1971. Relative efficacy of different methods for laboratory diagnosis in chronic trachoma in the United States, p. 273–288. *In* R. L. Nichols (ed), Trachoma and related disorders. Excerpta Medica, Amsterdam.

19. Wang, S. P. 1971. A micro immunofluorescence method. Study of antibody response to TRIC organisms in mice, p. 273–288. *In* R. L. Nichols (ed), Trachoma and related disorders. Excerpta Medica, Amsterdam.

20. Wang, S. P., and J. T. Grayston. 1970. Immunologic relationship between genital TRIC, lymphogranuloma venereum, and related organisms in a new microtiter indirect immunofluorescence test. Amer. J. Ophthalmol. **70:**367–374.

21. Wang, S. P., and J. T. Grayston. 1971. Classification of TRIC and related strains with micro immunofluorescence, p. 305–321. *In* R. L. Nichols (ed), Trachoma and related disorders. Excerpta Medica, Amsterdam.

Chapter 88

Rickettsiae

RICHARD A. ORMSBEE

INTRODUCTION

The important, naturally occurring rickettsial diseases in the United States are Rocky Mountain spotted fever, Q fever, and murine typhus. Consequently, the diagnosis of these diseases will be emphasized in this chapter.

Rickettsialpox occurs sporadically in cities but is considered to be a mild disease. The rapidity of international air travel and the lack of specific vaccines may permit the occasional, unwitting entry of individuals with scrub typhus, particularly from the Far East, or spotted fever group disease, particularly from the Indian subcontinent and some parts of Africa.

Rickettsial diseases of humans can be classified conveniently into four major groups, namely, typhus fevers, spotted fevers, Q fever, and trench fever. They are caused by various members of the family *Rickettsiaceae*. Rickettsiae are characterized by their ability to multiply in one or more arthropods and by their existence in natural reservoirs in one or several warm-blooded animal hosts (except for trench fever and epidemic typhus, for which the natural reservoir of infection is man). Effective therapy of human infections is usually provided by chloramphenicol and the tetracycline group of broad-spectrum antibiotics (questionably effective in Q fever).

The difficulties and dangers of working with live pathogenic rickettsiae are great enough to preclude such efforts in most clinical laboratories. Consequently, the reader is referred to the appropriate chapters in *Viral and Rickettsial Infections of Man* (16) and *Diagnostic Procedures for Viral and Rickettsial Diseases* (18) for the details of these procedures, and for clinical details also.

DESCRIPTION OF AGENTS

Rickettsiae essentially are highly fastidious bacteria. They are obligate intracellular parasites (except *Rickettsia quintana*), pleomorphic but typically rodlike in form, and often found in pairs in smears of infected cells. They possess double- or triple-layered limiting membranes which are susceptible to lysozyme digestion, but not to tryptic digestion, and they contain muramic acid and diaminopimelic acid in common with most bacteria, except the gram-positive cocci. They possess both synthetic and energy-yielding enzyme systems, contain ribonucleic and deoxyribonucleic acids, and multiply by binary fission. Characteristically, they vary in diameter; members of the spotted fever group are the largest, *Coxiella burneti* is the smallest, and members of the typhus group are intermediate. They also vary in their resistance to physical and chemical agents. *C. burneti* is more resistant than any other pathogenic rickettsia, indeed more resistant than most nonsporogenic microorganisms. Effective disinfection can be achieved with 2% formaldehyde, 1% lysol (a mixture of saponified aryl and alkyl derivatives of phenol), ethyl ether, and 5% H_2O_2. Other common antiseptics should not be relied upon.

A new agent, *R. canada*, has been isolated from the tick *Haemaphysalis leporispalustris* taken from a domestic rabbit in eastern Canada (20). This rickettsia is related antigenically to the typhus group. Koch's postulates, incriminating this organism unequivocally as a cause of human disease, have not yet been fulfilled. Serological data (4), however, strongly suggest that this rickettsia does cause human disease.

Table 1 lists the common rickettsial diseases of humans, their etiological agents, and other information descriptive of ecological characteristics of the rickettsiae and epidemiological features of rickettsial diseases.

COLLECTION, STORAGE, AND SHIPMENT OF SPECIMENS

For serological examination

In general, the only specimens pertinent to laboratory diagnosis are tissues obtained under aseptic conditions at autopsy, or blood samples. Laboratory diagnosis in most cases depends upon demonstration of specific antibodies in serum specimens and an increase in antibody titer as the disease progresses. Three samples of blood should be taken from the patient: one as

TABLE 1. *Rickettsial diseases of humans*

Disease	Etiological agent	Geographic distribution	Natural cycle		Mode of transmission to humans	Environmental associations
			Arthropod	Mammal		
Spotted fever group						
Rocky Mountain spotted fever	*Rickettsia rickettsi*	Western Hemisphere	Ixodid ticks	Rodents, dogs, foxes	Tick bite	Tick-infested terrain, houses, dogs
Boutonneuse fever	*R. conori*	Mediterranean, Black Sea, and Caspian Sea littorals, Middle East, India, Africa	Ixodid ticks	Dogs, rodents	Tick bite	Tick-infested terrain, houses, dogs
Rickettsialpox	*R. akari*	North America, USSR, Southern Africa, Korea	Mites	House mouse, other commensal rodents	Mite bite	Rodent- and mite-infested urban premises
Siberian tick typhus	*R. sibirica*	Armenia, Central Asia, Siberia, Mongolia	Ixodid ticks	Rodents	Tick bite	Tick-infested terrain, houses, dogs
Queensland tick typhus	*R. australis*	Australia	Ixodid ticks	Marsupials	Tick bite	Tick-infested terrain; rainy season
Typhus group						
Epidemic typhus	*R. prowazeki*	Worldwide	Human body louse	Humans	Infected louse feces into skin	Crowded filthy conditions, lousy population
Murine typhus	*R. typhi (mooseri)*	Worldwide	Flea	Rodents	Infected flea feces into skin	Rat- and flea-infested premises
Brill-Zinsser disease	*R. prowazeki*	North America, Europe	Recrudescences of latent epidemic typhus infection few to many years after primary attack. Stress may precipitate attack.			
Q fever	*Coxiella burneti*	Worldwide	Ixodid ticks	Rodents, cattle, sheep, goats	Inhalation of infectious aerosol, tick bite (?)	Animal husbandry, dairies, lambing pens, abattoirs
Trench fever	*R. quintana*	Europe, Africa, North America	Human body louse	Humans	Infected louse feces into skin	Crowded filthy conditions, lousy population
Scrub typhus	*R. tsutsugamushi*	Asia, Indian subcontinent, Australia, Pacific Islands	Trombiculid mites	Rodents	Mite bite	Chigger-infested terrain, secondary scrub, grass air fields, golf courses

soon as possible after onset of illness, one during the second week, and one during the fourth week after onset of illness.

For attempted isolation

If suspected material is to be injected into animals, the specimens should be injected within 30 min after making the suspensions, or else placed in a glass or plastic container, quickly frozen in an alcohol-dry ice bath, and stored at −70 C until used. Whole blood should be shell-frozen in an alcohol-dry ice bath. If possible, it is preferable to take a blood sample of 10 to 12 ml, allow it to clot, centrifuge it immediately, and freeze the clot and serum separately. The clot can then be injected as a 10% suspension in skim milk or brain-heart infusion (BHI) broth (100 g of Difco Skim Milk or 37 g of Difco Brain Heart Infusion dissolved in 1,000 ml of cold, distilled water, distributed in tubes or flasks, and sterilized in an autoclave for 15 min at 15 psi) (30). Use of other diluents may result in great loss of infectivity of rickettsiae present. The serum can be used for subsequent serological examination. Facilities permitting, a noncoagulated blood specimen may be taken with a syringe wet with USP heparin and injected immediately into susceptible animals. Blood specimens taken later than the first week of illness should routinely be separated into cells and serum (or plasma), which may by then contain antibodies. The cells should be resuspended in an equal volume of BHI or skim milk for injection into animals.

It is imperative that properly prepared frozen tissue and blood specimens be shipped to the reference laboratory by air in a properly insulated container with enough dry ice to maintain the inside temperature at −70 C for at least 24 h longer than the estimated length of time required for shipment. It is not sufficient that the sample merely be kept frozen. Once properly shell-frozen in an alcohol-dry ice bath, the specimen *must* be held at a constant −70 C until quickly thawed, by immersing the container in tepid water, immediately before injection into experimental animals. In addition, at the time of shipment the reference laboratory should be notified by telephone or telegram of time of departure of the shipment, airline and flight number, and adequate identification marks to enable the parcel to be individually spotted and retrieved at the receiving end. Neglect of any of these precautions may cause failure of the considerable efforts required to isolate and identify the rickettsiae.

If ticks, collected from the bodies or clothing of patients suspected of rickettsial disease, are to be examined directly for detection and identification of rickettsial infection (5), they should be shipped to the reference laboratory in a tightly stoppered receptacle which contains a pledget of moist cotton. Ticks are easily killed by desiccation.

DIRECT MICROSCOPIC OBSERVATION OF SPECIMENS

Smears of infected tissue may be made and examined directly for the presence of rickettsiae after appropriate staining. The stains commonly used are Giménez (13), Macchiavello (18), and Giemsa. Giménez stain is recommended. Rickettsiae (except for *R. tsutsugamushi*) stain brilliant red with Giménez stain, red with Macchiavello stain, purple with Giemsa stain, and gram-negative (but very poorly) with Gram stain. *R. tsutsugamushi* stains reddish-black with a modification of Giménez stain. None of these stains will reliably differentiate rickettsiae from bacteria.

Rickettsiae appear as pleomorphic coccobacillary forms and may vary in length from 0.25 to ≥2.0 μm within individual preparations. They are sometimes observed in chains or pairs. *C. burneti* is the smallest, with average dimensions of 0.25 by 1.0 μm. It is seen usually as a bipolar rod (as are the other rickettsiae) near cells or in the cytoplasm. Typhus group rickettsiae are a bit larger, averaging 0.3 by 1.2 μm, and also are typically found near cells or in the cytoplasm. The spotted fever rickettsiae are the largest and average 0.6 by 1.2 μm. They often may be found within the nuclei of infected cells, as well as in the ctyoplasm, and often are seen in pairs surrounded by a halo, as if encapsulated. Electron microscope studies of most of the pathogenic rickettsiae have been published (1).

The technique of the Giménez stain and preparation of the reagents are described in chapter 96.

Infected tissues or cells also may be directly examined by fluorescence microscopy. Specific antisera tagged with fluorescein isothiocyanate (FITC) have been successfully used to detect and identify pathogenic rickettsiae. (See below, section on Immunofluorescence tests.)

ISOLATION AND IDENTIFICATION OF RICKETTSIAE

As previously mentioned, the difficulties and dangers of working with most rickettsiae are such as to preclude attempts at isolation in animals or embryonated eggs by any except well-equipped research laboratories. If isolation and identification of a suspected rickettsial agent is deemed important, blood samples taken during the febrile period may be sent to a reference laboratory through the office of the local State Board of Health.

Tissue culture techniques have been successfully used for the primary isolation of spotted fever rickettsiae from infected ticks (29) and presumably could be used effectively in the primary isolation of rickettsiae from blood and other tissues. The appropriate use of FITC-tagged specific antiserum on infected monolayers of mouse L or primary chick embryo cells should provide direct identification of the agent, regardless of whether or not conditions were optimal for plaque formation. *R. rickettsi*, the agent of spotted fever, forms characteristic plaques in monolayers of primary chick embryo cells or Vero monkey cells within 7 to 8 days after inoculation.

SEROLOGICAL DIAGNOSIS

Rocky Mountain spotted fever and Q fever are the two rickettsial diseases most likely to be encountered in the continental United States. Others, however, do occur, either because of indigenous infections or, as a result of rapid air transport, because of infections acquired in other parts of the world. Thus, murine typhus, Brill-Zinsser disease, and rickettsialpox are endemic in the United States, and scrub typhus and boutonneuse fever are known to have occurred in the United States, although the infections were acquired in Asia and Africa, respectively. The clinical laboratory should be aware of these possibilities and should keep itself equipped to perform the initial serological tests which can classify the disease as belonging to the typhus fever, spotted fever, or Q fever groups. More definitive identification can then be secured by sending the appropriate serum samples to a reference laboratory.

Rickettsial diseases are acute illnesses of sudden onset. They are characterized by fever, severe headache, myalgia, chills, and pneumonitis. Except in Q fever, they are accompanied by a rash and disseminated focal peripheral vasculitis. Q fever may cause hepatitis, and chronic infection with *C. burneti* may result in fatal subacute endocarditis. Furthermore, *C. burneti* may heavily infect the placenta many months after recovery of the mother from Q fever. These aspects of rickettsial disease should be kept in mind by the laboratory diagnostician as well as by the clinician.

A complement fixation (CF) test for Q fever antibodies should be made routinely in cases of subacute endocarditis in which blood cultures from the patient are bacteriologically negative.

Complement fixation test

See chapter 71 for the CF test procedure.

Rickettsial agglutination test

A variety of rickettsial agglutination tests have been developed for diagnostic use in epidemic and murine typhus (18, 28) and in Q fever (11, 23). Agglutination tests with highly purified antigen are as sensitive as the CF test in detecting antibody and often are more specific. In addition, they have the virtue of being simple to perform. The major drawback at present is the lack of commercially available antigens suitable for agglutination tests. It is to be hoped that this notable lack will be remedied in the future.

Rickettsial agglutinating antigens are ordinarily prepared from infected chick yolk sac tissue, although satisfactory suspensions of *R. prowazeki* have been prepared from mouse lungs. Excellent antigen preparations of *C. burneti*, *R. rickettsi*, *R. prowazeki* and others have been made from tissue cultures of various cells.

Because agglutination techniques in general require more concentrated antigen suspensions, microtechniques have been developed which are less expensive of antigen. Babudieri's slide test (23) for Q fever antibodies employs 0.02-ml volumes of antigen and similar amounts of serum dilutions. These are mixed on microscope slides and incubated overnight at room temperature in a moist chamber. The slides are then dried, fixed in methanol, stained with Giemsa stain, and examined under a microscope. A similar technique has been used for titration of epidemic typhus, murine typhus, Q fever, and boutonneuse fever antisera. This technique has one major drawback in that agglutination artifacts often are produced by drying the slide, and considerable care needs to be taken to differentiate specific agglutination from nonspecific agglutination.

The capillary-agglutination test of Luoto (23) was developed for the detection of Q fever antibodies in milk and other opaque liquids. It is equally effective in detecting antibodies in sera of humans and animals. This test depends for its unique usefulness on purified suspensions of phase I *C. burneti* which have been stained with hematoxylin. I have used the technique extensively for detection of antibodies in animals' sera with unstained purified suspensions of *R. prowazeki*, *R. mooseri*, *R. conori*, and *C. burneti*. In this test, capillary tubes, 9 by 0.4

mm (inner diameter), are one-third filled with antigen by capillary attraction. Similar samples of test sera are next drawn in; the tubes are inverted and stuck into modeling clay in a vertical position with the antigen on the bottom. After incubation for 2 h at 37 C or 4 h at room temperature, clumping of the stained rickettsiae is visible macroscopically in tubes containing antibody. Results obtained are specific and reproducible. This is a particularly useful technique for field use. The antigen preparations are stable for long periods when stored at 4 C.

The agglutination-resuspension technique (23) for the detection of Q fever antibodies is even more rapid and more sensitive, and has produced reliable results with human and animal sera. In this test, the mixture of (phase I) antigen and antibody is incubated at 37 C for 30 min and then centrifuged briefly. Agglutination is demonstrated macroscopically by the formation of a sediment which does not readily resuspend in the supernatant fluid.

By far the most useful and practical agglutination test which has been developed is the microagglutination (MA) test (11) which employs the Microtiter equipment described in the section on the CF test in chapter 71. The MA test uses a 0.025-ml volume (containing 8 μg) of antigen and a similar volume of test serum. The plate is incubated overnight at room temperature, after which the agglutination pattern is read from the bottom like a hemagglutination test. Results indicate good reproducibility, titers as high as or higher than corresponding CF titers, and great economy of time and laboratory glassware. The purified antigens necessary for this test can be used interchangeably in the CF test. Differentiation of phase I and phase II antibodies against *C. burneti* is as sharp as in the CF test. The MA test also has been used successfully with antigens of *R. prowazeki*, *R. typhi*, *R. conori*, and *R. rickettsi*.

C. burneti in phase I is relatively easy to purify, and antigen preparations made from it are ordinarily stained with hematoxylin (Harris) to facilitate reading MA tests. Suspensions of *C. burneti* in phase II (egg-adapted) tend to agglutinate spontaneously, particularly if stained with hematoxylin (Harris). However, one can remove the phase I antigen from phase I rickettsiae by extraction with trichloroacetic acid (11) or by destruction with sodium periodate (26), thus converting the organisms to the phase II condition. Such "synthetic" phase II antigen does not spontaneously agglutinate even when stained with hematoxylin and constitutes a stable and sensitive antigen for the detection of phase II agglutinins. It is entirely comparable to the natural phase II antigen when used in the CF test.

Weil-Felix test

The Weil-Felix test (9) depends upon the agglutination of OX-19, OX-2, and OX-K strains of *Proteus vulgaris* by antibodies produced by typhus and spotted fever group rickettsiae. It is included here because the antigens and standard antisera are often more readily available than rickettsial antigens, notwithstanding the fact that its use has probably produced more erroneous and misleading results than any other serological test employed for the detection of rickettsial antibodies. Nevertheless, if the proper precautions are taken, the Weil-Felix test is capable of establishing useful presumptive diagnoses in diseases caused by the typhus and spotted fever groups of rickettsiae. Table 2 summarizes the usual reactions encountered in cases of rickettsial disease. Unfortunately, Weil-Felix reactions may vary widely from case to case of spotted fever, and therefore may be of little help either in detecting the disease or differentiating it from murine typhus.

Reagents. The procedures employed by Plotz (25) for the preparation of antigens and their use in tube agglutination tests will be given in outline. The slide test is not recommended for routine laboratory use.

Only the O or nonmotile variant is used. Purity of the strain should be checked frequently by streaking on a veal infusion-agar plate. After 24 h of incubation at 37 C, select smooth, nonspreading O-type colonies and transfer them to dry agar slants and broth. If the organisms then are found to be nonmotile, the culture may be used for antigen production. Maintain cultures on dry agar slants. Lyophilization helps to maintain a pure O variant.

Living or killed antigen may be used. The living antigen is prepared by suspending an 18- to 24-h agar culture in sufficient 0.85% NaCl to

TABLE 2. *Weil-Felix reactions in rickettsioses*

Disease	OX-19	OX-2	OX-K
Epidemic typhus	++++	+	0
Murine typhus	++++	+	0
Brill-Zinsser disease	Variable, often negative		0
Scrub typhus	0	0	+++
Spotted fever group	{ ++++	{ +	0
	+	+++	0
Q fever	0	0	0
Rickettsialpox	0	0	0

give a turbidity reading equal to tube 3 on the McFarland nephelometer scale or a reading of 179 with a no. 42 filter in a Klett-Summerson colorimeter. The killed antigen is prepared by growing an O strain on agar in Kolle flasks and harvesting the organisms at 18 to 24 h by washing off with 0.85% NaCl to form a heavy suspension to which 0.5% Formalin is added. This stock is then diluted to give the turbidity described above.

Commercial antigens and antisera are available, but certain precautions with their use must be observed. Sometimes commercial antigens are standardized against rabbit antisera from animals which have been immunized against the homologous strain of *Proteus*. Such rabbit sera will agglutinate *Proteus* regardless of whether or not the organisms comprising the antigen are sensitive to rickettsial antibodies. Such antigens have not been acceptably tested and should *not* be used in the Weil-Felix test. Such rabbit sera *cannot* be used as positive control sera in the Weil-Felix test. The only acceptable commercial antigens are those which have been standardized against the appropriate human convalescent serum. The only acceptable positive control sera are human convalescent sera. If these conditions cannot be met, do not use the Weil-Felix test. The results will mean nothing at best and cause confusion at the worst.

Test proper. The macroscopic agglutination test is performed by mixing 0.5-ml portions of antigen suspension and test serum. Serum dilutions of 1:10 to 1:640 (final dilutions, 1:20 to 1:1,280) should be tested. A control tube containing 0.5-ml portions of antigen in 0.85% NaCl and one containing positive serum should be included. The tubes are incubated in a water bath at 37 C for 2 h followed by incubation overnight at 4 C. Complete agglutination is shown by complete clearing of the supernatant fluid and the presence of large white masses in the bottom of the tube (4+). Partial agglutination is indicated by partial clearing of the supernatant fluid and the formation of smaller masses of agglutinated antigen in the bottom of the tube. Shaking the tubes does not resuspend the agglutinated antigen to give the even turbidity seen in the negative control. Reading the tubes can be facilitated by shielded illumination and viewing at a critical angle.

Immunofluorescence tests

Immunofluorescence (IF) tests have been developed for the direct identification of rickettsiae in infected tissues and fluids as well as for the detection and measurement of specific rickettsial antibodies.

The direct method is used for the identification of rickettsiae. In this method, specific antiserum is conjugated with FITC (24). This conjugate can then be used to stain the suspected organisms directly. This procedure has been used effectively for the identification of rickettsiae in hemolymph of ticks infected with *R. rickettsi* or other rickettsiae (5), the identification of *C. burneti* in infected cardiac tissue (21), and the enumeration of infected cells in tissue cultures (15).

In the indirect method, the specific antibody is allowed to fix to antigen. This complex in turn is allowed to react with FITC-conjugated antibody against the specific antiserum. This technique is most useful for the detection of rickettsial antibody but also can be employed for the detection and identification of antigen in infected tissues.

The indirect method of Weller and Coons as modified by Goldwasser and Shepard (14) has been used effectively by Elisberg and Bozeman for the diagnosis of scrub typhus and spotted fever (3, 8).

Essentially, the procedure is to allow the test serum to react with a suitable smear of yolk sac tissue heavily infected with the appropriate rickettsiae. After 30 min, excess serum is thoroughly rinsed away, and a drop of horse anti-human gamma globulin serum conjugated with FITC is applied to the slide. After 30 min, it is rinsed off and the slide is air-dried, mounted, and examined the same day under a microscope with ultraviolet (UV) light optics. A positive reaction results in the fluorescence of the rickettsiae in UV light. With this technique (as with the CF reaction), one can differentiate between sera from patients with murine and epidemic typhus fever.

The IF technique gives a broader (group) reaction with strains of *R. tsutsugamushi* than does the CF test, however. This is a definite advantage, because with CF antigens of *R. tsutsugamushi* the specificity is so marked that tests with antigens from several strains must be used to insure adequate testing of the suspect serum.

The direct IF technique is simple and relatively inexpensive. The main requirement is possession of high-titered specific antiserum. The indirect IF technique is neither simple nor inexpensive. Its use depends upon the availability of fresh, infected yolk sacs for making smears, and preservation of the smears at −70 C, because slide preparations of antigen are not yet available commercially. However, indirect immunofluorescence does possess attractive features, particularly in the diagnosis of scrub typhus. Refer to the review of Liu (19) and the manual of Cherry et al. (7) for further information.

Other tests

There are a number of other laboratory tests which are useful in research but which are of little practical use in the routine diagnosis of human disease. These tests include those for toxin neutralization, other neutralizations, antiglobulin sensitization, radioisotope precipitation (RIP), hemagglutination, and precipitins.

Toxin neutralization test. Injection into mice of suspensions of chick embryo yolk sac heavily infected with various members of the typhus and spotted fever groups of rickettsiae causes death within a few hours (28, 31). Death can be prevented by mixing the rickettsial suspension with antiserum prior to injection. This phenomenon has been employed to demonstrate antigenic relationships among members of the spotted fever group and to differentiate between the antibodies caused by murine and epidemic typhus rickettsiae; it is still used in the standard assay of epidemic typhus vaccine.

Other neutralization tests. Other neutralization tests have been used with many of the rickettsiae. Such tests are similar to the toxin neutralization test in principle and differ only in that the aim is to test the ability of a given serum to prevent typical rickettsial disease in laboratory animals rather than to prevent an acute toxic reaction. The techniques are costly in animals, laboratory space, and time, and therefore are employed only for special purposes.

Antiglobulin sensitization test. The antiglobulin sensitization test (18) essentially is a hyperagglutination test. It has been used for the detection and measurement of Q fever antibodies in human serum and for the detection of small amounts of antibody in bulk pools of cows' milk. Purified antigen is sensitized with the test serum and then treated with rabbit anti-human globulin to produce agglutination. The test is specific and results in much higher titers than those achieved by direct agglutination. It is of limited value as a diagnostic aid because of the relatively large amounts of purified antigen and time necessary to perform it.

Radioisotope precipitation test. The RIP test (12) is essentially a modification of the antiglobulin sensitization test, but differs in the method of detecting and measuring agglutination of the sensitized antigen. It has been used for the detection of Q fever antibodies (phase I) in human and animal sera (17).

The heart of the technique is the antigen tagged with a radioisotope. *C. burneti* may be tagged with ^{32}P while growing in chick embryo yolk sacs or with ^{131}I after being purified. In either case, a purified suspension of phase I *C. burneti* is sensitized with the suspect serum and then treated with the appropriate rabbit antiglobulin. The suspension is then centrifuged in a capillary tube lightly enough so that the antigen in negative control suspension is not sedimented. The upper and lower portions of the suspensions are then placed in planchets, and the radioactivity in both portions is measured in a Q-gas counter. A positive reaction is one in which most of the radioactivity is found in the lower portion of the capillary tube after centrifugation.

The RIP test gives specific results and is extremely sensitive. Titers against *C. burneti* as high as 1:32,000 have been recorded. Antibody levels which are not detectable by CF and direct agglutination techniques will give significant titers in the RIP test.

The RIP test is not easily adapted to the requirements of a routine diagnostic tool, and highly purified phase I antigen is required for its performance.

Hemagglutination test. Several attempts have been made to use erythrocytes coated with soluble rickettsial antigen as an indicator system for rickettsial antibodies. The most promising results have been those of Chang, Murray, and Snyder (6), who found that extracts of typhus and spotted fever group rickettsiae could be used to sensitize human O erythrocytes, which then could be agglutinated by convalescent human sera. These reactions were group-specific, like those with the soluble CF antigens produced from most rickettsiae. This system has been used to demonstrate hemagglutination-inhibition by antigens extracted from the tissues of mice infected with *R. mooseri*. None of the hemagglutination tests is of any practical value at present for the ordinary diagnostic laboratory, because of the requirements for purified antigen or suspensions of live rickettsiae or because of the time-consuming nature of the techniques.

Precipitin test. The precipitin reaction has been used in studies on soluble antigens of rickettsiae (16, 18). Again, there is the usual limitation in the requirement for large amounts of relatively pure antigen. Several workers have demonstrated the presence of specific, serologically active substances in the blood and urine of patients in acute stages of epidemic typhus, and this phenomenon was adapted to a slide test for early rapid diagnosis of the disease (27). The method has not been widely used and is not now routinely employed as a diagnostic test in the USSR where it was originally developed.

INTERPRETATION OF LABORATORY RESULTS

The single most important diagnostic aid in the identification of rickettsial disease is the demonstration of a rise in serum antibody titer when paired acute and convalescent sera are titrated simultaneously in the same test. Absolute antibody titers usually are of small diagnostic significance, whereas a rise in titer as the disease progresses is of the greatest importance in establishing a diagnosis. A significant rise in titer is defined as a fourfold increase. Sometimes only single serum specimens will be available for laboratory test. In such circumstances, although it is necessary to perform the appropriate tests for antibody, it is well to be conservative in assigning much significance to a positive finding. Certain rickettsial diseases, including Rocky Mountain spotted fever, Q fever, and murine typhus, are widespread in the United States and in certain areas there may be ecological "islands of infection" (2) in which a particular disease will have a much higher incidence than in the surrounding territory. The offending rickettsiae often produce inapparent infections or very mild disease from which the individual recovers without benefit of diagnosis or medical care. This is particularly, perhaps typically, true of *C. burneti* infections. To complicate the picture, vaccines against Rocky Mountain spotted fever have been used widely in the civilian population, and typhus vaccine has been employed routinely in the military population. Also, in the immigrant population, particularly in cities along the Atlantic seaboard, there are many individuals who have come from persisting endemic areas of typhus in Europe and Asia. Such individuals may still possess antibodies resulting from prior epidemic typhus disease, or they may become ill with Brill-Zinsser disease (recrudescent epidemic typhus) many years after recovery from the initial infection. These factors make it difficult to assess the significance of results from tests on a single serum specimen, particularly if the titer is low.

The time of appearance of serum antibodies produced in response to various rickettsiae is summarized in Table 3. Appearance of antibodies (particularly CF antibodies) may be delayed by broad-spectrum antibiotic therapy instituted early in the course of disease. Negative CF findings must therefore be interpreted cautiously if the patient has received such therapy.

TABLE 3. *Time of appearance of antibodies in serum from human patients*

Disease	Complement fixation	Weil-Felix	Agglutination
Spotted fever group[a]	8–10 days	5–12 days[a]	Unknown
Q fever	8–14 days	None	5–8 days
Epidemic and murine typhus	7–9 days	7–14 days	5–7 days
Scrub typhus	Unknown	10–14 days	Unknown

[a] Except for rickettsialpox in which Weil-Felix antibodies are not found.

Complement-fixation test

The lowest serum titer usually considered significant is 1:8 (original dilution), particularly if washed antigen is used. During convalescence from rickettsial disease, CF titers of 1:128 to 1:256 are often found. CF antibodies usually appear within 7 to 14 days after onset of disease. After convalescence, the titer slowly falls, but low levels may persist for several years.

The CF test is diagnostically useful in all rickettsioses, except scrub typhus in which the multiplicity of strains, which are mutually exclusive with respect to CF antigens, makes the test impractical except for a very few reference laboratories. Phase II Q fever antigen and group antigens for the typhus and spotted fever groups are commercially available. The available group antigens are actually partially group-specific and partially species-specific, and are composed of a mixture of soluble and particulate antigen. Caution must be used in interpreting results of tests with such antigens. Positive results are by themselves indicative only of infection with an anonymous member of the group, not with any specific member. Results should be so reported.

Commercial spotted fever group antigen is often made from *R. akari* rather than *R. rickettsi*. In most cases, but not invariably, the use of *R. akari* antigen will detect antibodies produced by *R. rickettsi*. At least two cases have been noted in which sera from patients with Rocky Mountain spotted fever gave good CF titers with *R. rickettsi* antigen but low or negative titers with *R. akari* antigen.

Q fever infections in humans produce two distinguishable CF antibodies (10). Phase II CF antibodies are produced initially; phase I CF antibodies (not phase I agglutinins) are produced irregularly several weeks or months later and remain at low levels, except in cases of subacute rickettsial endocarditis. In such cases, the invariable finding has been one of very high phase I CF antibody titers (1:256 to 1:2,048) and similarly high phase II CF titers (21). Patients with a diagnosis of subacute bacterial endocarditis with negative blood cultures should be examined routinely for Q fever antibodies. A similar stipulation applies to patients with hepatitis of unknown etiology.

Murine typhus in individuals previously given epidemic typhus vaccine may present an antibody pattern which is difficult or impossible to decipher by CF test, even by a reference laboratory with specific antigens available. Because of the presence of group antigens, the patient may give an anamnestic response to the group antigen and a primary response to the murine specific antigen. The result may be a higher CF titer with specific epidemic typhus antigen than with specific murine typhus antigen.

Brill-Zinsser disease, which results in the production primarily of immunoglobulin G (IgG; 7*S*) antibodies, can be distinguished from primary epidemic typhus, in which the major antibody present up to 21 days after onset is IgM (19*S*), by selective destruction of the 19*S* CF antibodies with the aid of heat and ethanethiol (22). This results in a drop in the CF titer of sera from patients with primary typhus but little change in the CF titer of sera from patients with Brill-Zinsser disease.

The CF test is the single most useful test now widely available for the detection and identification of rickettsial antibodies. It must be strongly emphasized, however, that the CF test can produce the most erroneous and misleading information of any laboratory test except the Weil-Felix. The details of the CF test must be rigorously and faithfully followed if reliable and reproducible results are to be forthcoming.

Agglutination test

Rickettsial agglutinin titers of 1:4 (phase I) and 1:8 (phase II) have been judged to be diagnostically significant in Q fever. Although phase II CF antibodies as well as phase I and II agglutinins appear early in the course of disease, phase I CF antibodies appear, if at all, only after several weeks, and never achieve high titers. (The known exception to this is in rickettsial endocarditis caused by *C. burneti*.) Diagnosis may be based, therefore, on a rise in phase I or phase II agglutinins or phase II CF antibodies. Agglutinins are demonstrable in 50% of patients in 5 to 7 days, in 92% within 14 days, and in 100% of patients within 30 days. In contrast, CF antibody is rarely detected within 7 days after onset, although 65% of patients have significant CF antibody levels by 14 days after onset, and 90% of patients are positive by 30 days. Both types of antibody may persist in high titer for many months after recovery from the acute disease. In general, agglutinin titers produced during the course of rickettsial disease appear earlier, rise earlier to higher titers, and decline on a time course comparable to that of CF antibodies. Thus, in patients with Q fever or in vaccinees, the agglutination test has been found to be more sensitive than the CF test in detecting early rises in specific antibody.

Antibodies to *C. burneti* do not cross-react with other pathogenic rickettsiae, and a rise in agglutinin titer is considered to be convincing evidence of Q fever infection (except in vaccinees).

Agglutinin titers of 1:32 have been considered to be diagnostically significant in persons ill with murine or epidemic typhus. Results in our laboratory with purified typhus antigens suggest that agglutinin titers $\geq$1:8 are significant, in that they have been confirmed by a rise in specific CF antibodies which appears, sometimes concurrently but usually in the following week, in clinically diagnosed cases of typhus fever. As in Q fever, agglutinins usually appear 5 to 8 days after onset of disease and reach titers comparable to or higher than CF antibody titers.

The rickettsial agglutination test appears to be consistently more species-specific than the CF test, even if the same antigen is used in both tests. Thus, it has been found possible to identify by agglutination test murine typhus infection in patients previously given epidemic typhus vaccine, although it was impossible to do this by CF test. Parallel tests by toxin neutralization and microagglutination of sera from individuals with laboratory-acquired infections of murine and epidemic typhus have been in close agreement. Both CF and agglutination tests can be used to distinguish Brill-Zinsser disease from primary epidemic typhus by the different susceptibilities of IgM and IgG antibodies to heat and ethanethiol (22) or 2-mercaptoethanol.

Agglutination tests for spotted fever antibodies have been little used, primarily because *R. rickettsi* and closely related species grow so poorly in embryonated eggs that the cost of producing diagnostic antigen from infected chick embryo yolk sacs for agglutinin measurements is prohibitive. The exploitation of modern tissue culture techniques may change this.

In any case, when agglutinating antigens made from *R. rickettsi* or other members of the spotted fever group have been used to measure agglutinins in sera from experimentally infected guinea pigs, the tests have been found to be quite species-specific and sensitive.

In addition to antigens or antigenic determinants unique to the typhus or spotted fever groups, there are other antigenic determinants which these two groups of rickettsiae share in common. This intergroup relationship has been revealed by simultaneous antibody rises to both *R. prowazeki* and *R. rickettsi* in the sera of persons who were convalescent from epidemic typhus fever. It is probable that the MA test is equally, if not more, effective than the CF test in detecting antibodies to common determinants. The possibility of concurrent rises in antibody titer to more than one species of rickettsiae, due to the existence of interspecific antigens, should be kept in mind when assessing the significance of serological findings.

The simplicity of the MA test (11) and the generally good reproducibility of results are strong recommendations for its general use when appropriate antigens become commercially available. Stocks of *C. burneti* antigen for the capillary agglutination test (23) are maintained by the Center for Disease Control (CDC), Atlanta, Ga. No antigens for the MA test are available from the CDC or any commercial source at this time.

Weil-Felix test

The Weil-Felix test is traditionally the convenient test which can be performed in any laboratory and often gives positive results which are later proven to be nonspecific. It is worth emphasizing again that reliable results depend upon the proper reagents and the proper controls, and that, even so, the test has limitations which must be kept in mind when the attempt is made to determine the significance of the results.

The lowest titer which may be considered significant is 1:160 (final dilution), and a rise in titer must be at least fourfold to be considered significant. Although Weil-Felix agglutinins never appear in the blood of many scrub typhus patients, they usually appear during the second week after onset of the disease. Weil-Felix agglutinins may appear somewhat earlier in spotted fever group disease, epidemic typhus, and murine typhus. Peak titers are usually found during the third week after onset.

Q fever and rickettsialpox do not give a positive Weil-Felix test. Brill-Zinsser disease gives variable and often negative results. In most cases, it is impossible to differentiate between typhus group and spotted fever group on the basis of the Weil-Felix reaction, and it is impossible to differentiate between murine and epidemic typhus with this test. Infections with *Proteus* and relapsing fever caused by spirochetes of the genus *Borrelia* also cause a rise in Weil-Felix agglutinins.

A fourfold rise in OX-2 and OX-19 agglutinins with a negative OX-K is presumptive evidence of typhus group or spotted fever group disease. Similarly, a rise in OX-K agglutinins only is presumptive evidence of scrub typhus infection.

Immunofluorescence test

The use of immunofluorescence as a means of identifying and measuring rickettsial antibody, as well as identifying rickettsiae in infected tissues, is a promising development in the diagnosis of rickettsial disease. Unfortunately, its use at present is restricted to reference and research laboratories which have facilities to prepare the necessary antigens and antisera, because these are not as yet commercially available.

The indirect IF test for antibody measurement in the diagnosis of Q fever, spotted fever, or murine typhus probably could not compete with either CF or MA test as a routine primary test. The technique does have the useful property of causing *R. tsutsugamushi* antigen of any strain to show its group-reactive quality. Thus, serum from a patient infected with a particular strain of *R. tsutsugamushi* will react in the indirect IF test with the group antigen of any other strain, in contrast to the CF test which is strain-specific. The IF test is thus the most reliable test available for the serological diagnosis of scrub typhus. Furthermore, the test can distinguish between sera from murine and epidemic typhus patients in most instances (3).

The direct IF test for specific identification of rickettsiae in ticks, other arthropod carriers, tissue cultures, or infected tissue has already shown its usefulness in assisting with presumptive clinical diagnosis in cases of spotted fever where a tick was found attached to the patient.

Although immunofluorescence techniques require a microscope with UV optics and the proper antigens or antisera are not available commercially, the technique is of real value in the serologists' armamentarium even though its use at present is confined to a few laboratories.

LITERATURE CITED

1. Anderson, D. R., H. E. Hopps, M. F. Barile, and B. C. Bernheim. 1965. Comparison of the ultrastructure of several rickettsiae, ornithosis virus, and *Mycoplasma* in tissue culture. J. Bacteriol. **90:**1387–1404.
2. Audy, J. R., and J. L. Harrison. 1951. A review of investigations on mite typhus in Burma and Malaya, 1945–1950. Trans. Roy Soc. Trop. Med. Hyg. **44:**371–395.
3. Bozeman, F. M., and B. L. Elisberg. 1963. Serological diagnosis of scrub typhus by indirect immunofluorescence. Proc. Soc. Exp. Biol. Med. **112:**568–573.
4. Bozeman, F. M., B. L. Elisberg, J. W. Humphries, K. Runcik, and D. B. Palmer, Jr. 1970. Serologic evidence of *Rickettsia canada* infection of man. J. Infect. Dis. **121:**367–371.
5. Burgdorfer, W. 1970. Hemolymph test. A technique for detection of rickettsiae in ticks. Amer. J. Trop. Med. Hyg. **19:**1010–1014.
6. Chang, R. S.-M., E. S. Murray, and J. C. Snyder. 1954. Erythrocyte-sensitizing substances from the rickettsiae of the Rocky Mountain spotted fever group. J. Immunol. **73:**8–15.
7. Cherry, W. B., M. Goldman, T. R. Corski, and M. D. Moody. 1960. Fluorescent antibody techniques in the diagnosis of communicable diseases. U.S. Pub. Health Serv. Publ. No. 729.
8. Elisberg, B. L., and F. L. Bozeman. 1966. Serological diagnosis of rickettsial diseases by indirect immunofluorescence. Arch. Inst. Pasteur Tunis **43:**193–204.
9. Felix, A. 1933. Serological types of typhus virus and corresponding types of Proteus. Trans. Roy. Soc. Trop. Med. Hyg. **27:**147–172.
10. Fiset, P. 1959. Serological diagnosis, strain variation and antigenic variation, p. 28–38. *In* Symposium on Q fever, Medical Science Publication No. 6, Walter Reed Army Institute of Research, Walter Reed Army Medical Center, Washington, D.C.
11. Fiset, P., R. A. Ormsbee, R. Silberman, M. Peacock, and S. H. Spielman. 1969. A microagglutination technique for the detection and measurement of rickettsial antibodies. Acta Virol. **13:**60–66.
12. Gerloff, R. K., B. H. Hoyer, and L. C. McLaren. 1962. Precipitation of radio-labeled poliovirus with specific antibody and antiglobulin. J. Immunol. **89:**559–570.
13. Giménez, D. F. 1964. Staining rickettsiae in yolk-sac cultures. Stain Technol. **39:**135–140.
14. Goldwasser, R. A., and C. C. Shepard. 1959. Fluorescent antibody methods in the differentiation of murine and epidemic typhus sera; specificity changes resulting from previous immunization. J. Immunol. **82:**373–380.
15. Hanon, N., and K. O. Cooke. 1966. Assay of *Coxiella burneti* by enumeration of immunofluorescent infected cells. J. Immunol. **97:**492–497.
16. Horsfall, F. L., Jr., and I. Tamm (ed.). 1965. Viral and rickettsial diseases of man, 4th ed. J. B. Lippincott Co., Philadelphia.
17. Lackman, D. B., G. Gilda, and R. N. Philip. 1964. Application of the radioisotope precipitation test to the study of Q fever in man. Health Lab. Sci. **1:**21–28.
18. Lennette, E. H., and N. J. Schmidt (ed.). 1969. Diagnostic procedures for viral and rickettsial diseases, 4th ed. American Public Health Association, Inc., New York.
19. Liu, C. 1969. Fluorescent antibody techniques, p. 179–204. *In* E. H. Lennette and N. J. Schmidt (ed.), Diagnostic procedures for viral and rickettsial diseases, 4th ed. American Public Health Association, Inc., New York.
20. McKiel, J. A., E. J. Bell, and D. B. Lackman. 1966. *Rickettsia canada*: a new member of the typhus group of Rickettsiae isolated from *Haemaphysalis leporispalustris* ticks in Canada. Can. J. Microbiol. **13:**503–510.
21. Mitchell, R., N. R. Grist, G. Bazaz, and A. C. F. Kenmuir. 1966. Pathological, rickettsiological and immuno-fluorescence studies of a case of Q fever endocarditis. J. Pathol. Bacteriol. **91:**317–323.
22. Murray, E. S., J. M. O'Connor, and J. A. Gaon. 1965. Differentiation of 19S and 7S complement fixing antibodies in primary versus recrudescent typhus by either ethanethiol or heat. Proc. Soc. Exp. Biol. Med. **119:**291–297.
23. Ormsbee, R. A. 1965. Q fever rickettsiae, p. 1144–1160. *In* F. L. Horsfall, Jr., and I. Tamm (ed.), Viral and rickettsial infections of man. J. B. Lippincott Co., Philadelphia.
24. Peacock, M., W. Burgdorfer, and R. A. Ormsbee. 1970. Rapid fluorescent-antibody conjugation procedure. Infect. Immunity **3:**355–357.
25. Plotz, H. 1944. The rickettsiae, p. 559–578. *In* J. S. Simmons and C. J. Gentzkow (ed.), Laboratory methods of the United States Army, 5th ed. Lea & Febiger, Philadelphia.
26. Schramek, S., R. Brezina, and J. Urvölgyi. 1972. A new method of preparing diagnostic Q fever antigen. Acta Virol. **16:**487–492.
27. Smorodintzeff, A. A., and R. V. Fradkina. 1944. Slide agglutination test for rapid diagnosis of pre-eruptive typhus fever. Proc. Soc. Exp. Biol. Med. **56:**93–94.
28. Snyder, J. C. 1965. Typhus fever rickettsiae, p. 1059–1094. *In* F. L. Horsfall, Jr., and I. Tamm (ed.), Viral and rickettsial infections of man. J. B. Lippincott Co., Philadelphia.
29. Wike, D. A., and W. Burgdorfer. 1972. Plaque formation in tissue cultures by *Rickettsia rickettsi* isolated directly from whole blood and tick hemolymph. Infect. Immunity **6:**736–738.
30. Wike, D. A., R. A. Ormsbee, G. Tallent, and M. G. Peacock. 1972. Effect of various suspending media on plaque formation by rickettsiae in tissue culture. Infect. Immunity **6:**550–556.
31. Woodward, T. E., and E. B. Jackson. 1965. Spotted fever rickettsiae, p. 1095–1129. *In* F. L. Horsfall, Jr., and I. Tamm (ed.), Viral and rickettsial infections of man, 4th ed. J. B. Lippincott Co., Philadelphia.

Chapter 89

EB Herpesvirus

PAUL GERBER

CLINICAL BACKGROUND

EB herpesvirus (Epstein-Barr virus, EBV) is one of the most ubiquitous viruses of man. Primary infection may occur in early childhood, and the incidence increases to 60 to 70% in young adults. Between 80 and 90% of adults possess antibodies to EBV.

Infections occurring in young children so far have not been associated with any recognizable illness. There is strong serological and clinical evidence that EBV infection of young adults may cause infectious mononucleosis (IM; 9). Recent findings indicate that EBV may be excreted orally by IM patients as well as occasionally by healthy, asymptomatic subjects (2, 7, 11).

Providing a laboratory diagnosis of recent EBV infection may be important in heterophile-antibody negative mononucleosis-like syndromes.

DESCRIPTION OF AGENT

EBV was discovered in 1964 by Epstein and Barr (4) in cultured lymphoblasts derived from Burkitt lymphomas. The agent is morphologically similar to herpesviruses. The viral capsid has an icosahedral structure composed of 162 capsomeres. Mature, enveloped particles measure 100 to 200 nm in diameter. This virus is ether-sensitive and heat-labile (56 C, 30 min) and contains deoxyribonucleic acid. Cell-free virus preparations in medium containing 5 to 10% fetal calf serum can be stored at −70 C for at least 1 year without appreciable loss of infectivity.

At present, only lymphoid cells of human or subhuman primates have been shown to be susceptible to EBV infection. Infection of peripheral lymphocytes results in morphological transformation of these cells into large immature blastoid cells, capable of rapid continuous growth in culture. Most of these cells are abortively infected and only a small fraction may contain infectious virus.

Infection of certain established human lymphoid cell lines (RAJI, NC_{37}) with EBV results in inhibition of the growth of these cells and the appearance of early EBV-determined antigens (EA) without productive virus synthesis (3, 10). EBV is antigenically distinct from other human or animal herpesviruses. Isolates derived from a variety of cells from malignant and normal patients appear to be antigenically indistinguishable.

COLLECTION AND STORAGE OF SPECIMENS

Pharyngeal swabs or throat washings are collected in medium 1640 (or any available tissue culture medium). Fetal calf serum in 2 to 5% concentration is added to the sample to enhance stability. Specimens should be placed on ice and frozen at −70 C as soon as possible. Oral excretion of EBV may be intermittent and it may be necessary to test consecutive samples. In my laboratory, urine samples obtained from IM patients contained no detectable EBV.

Blood samples for serological diagnosis

Acute and convalescent phase serum samples should be obtained and stored at −20 C.

DIRECT EXAMINATION

The amount of orally excreted EBV appears to be generally insufficient for detection by electron microscopy or by fluorescent-antibody (FA) techniques. Similarly, fresh leukocytes obtained from IM patients contain no detectable virus.

DETECTION OF AGENT

In the absence of a known permissive cell system for EBV, orally excreted EBV can be detected by the virus-induced morphological changes of cord blood lymphocytes (2, 7, 11). Human umbilical cord blood is aseptically collected with the use of 5 to 10 units of preservative-free heparin per ml. Leukocytes can be separated by spontaneous sedimentation of erythrocytes at 37 C. This process can be considerably enhanced by addition of two volumes of 3% dextran MW 228.000 or one-third volume of plasma gel (Roger Bellon Lab). The leukocyte-rich plasma is centrifuged at 250 × g for 10 min and resuspended in medium 1640 containing 20% fetal calf serum to a final concentration of 4 × 10^6 to 5 × 10^6 cells/ml. Samples of 1 ml are distributed to test tubes (15 by 100 mm) capped with Morton-type closures and are incubated in an upright position at 37 C in 5% CO_2 overnight. The throat washings or swab fluids are centrifuged at 4 C at 1,800 × g for 20 min to remove cellular debris. The supernatant fluids are passed through a 0.45-nm filter; if the volumes are too small for filtration, in most cases addition of an antibiotic mixture consisting of streptomycin (100 μg/ml), penicillin (100 μg/ml), tetracycline HCl (20 μg/ml), and mystatin (25 μg/ml) will effectively inhibit growth of microbial contaminants. After overnight incubation, the medium of the leukocyte cultures is removed carefully by aspiration and the cells are inoculated with 0.25- to 0.3-ml amounts of the samples, with the use of a minimum of four culture tubes per sample. In each isolation experiment, inoculated cell controls and a virus control group are included. The latter may consist of a known EBV-positive throat washing or an EBV preparation extracted from a virus-containing lymphoid cell line. After incubation for 1.5 h at 37 C to permit virus adsorption, 0.7 ml of growth medium is added to each tube and the cultures are maintained for 5 to 6 weeks with weekly refeeding. EBV-induced leukocyte transformation is signaled by a marked drop in pH of the medium and the appearance of cell aggregates consisting of large proliferating lymphoblastoid cells. These changes occur generally between 18 and 35 days. Uninoculated cells show a progressive decline in number and the absence of the morphological changes described above.

Cord blood leukocytes transformed by orally excreted EBV generally contain little or no detectable virus. However, the presence of the EB viral genome can be demonstrated by nucleic acid hybridization and complement fixation (CF) tests (7). Thus, this technique does not result in the isolation and propagation of the agent.

IDENTIFICATION OF AGENT

EBV-induced transformation of leukocytes can be specifically neutralized by sera of patients recovering from IM (8, 11). Equal volumes of throat washings and heat-inactivated sera diluted 1:2 to 1:8 are mixed and incubated for 1 h at 37 C. A control consisting of throat-washings plus a serum free from EBV antibodies is included in the test, as well as serum controls for observation of possible cytotoxic effects. The test is terminated when the cultures inoculated with the non-neutralized samples show leukocyte transformation.

SEROLOGICAL DIAGNOSIS

The FA and CF tests are the most practical procedures available at present. A neutralization test requiring about 1 week to complete has recently been described (13).

Fluorescent-antibody test

Two types of antibodies can be demonstrated by indirect immunofluorescence staining. For the detection of antibodies to the viral capsid antigens (VCA), acetone-fixed preparations of virus-positive lymphoid cells, e.g., HR_1K cells are used. Antibodies to the so-called early antigen (EA) of EBV (10) can be detected by immunofluorescence with cells containing EA. In my laboratory, EA-positive cells are prepared by treatment of a virus-free cell line, e.g., RAJI, with 10 μg of bromodeoxyuridine/ml for 7 days (6) or with 50 μg of iododeoxyuridine/ml for 3 days. Up to 10% of the treated cells contain EA-positive cells. Anti-VCA antibodies appear early in IM, do not show a significant increase, and may persist for years at slightly lower titers. By contrast, antibodies to EA generally appear during acute illness and decrease thereafter to low or nondetectable levels (10). Since there is no significant rise in antibodies following acute IM, these tests generally fail to distinguish past and recent EBV infections. Schmitz and Scherer (14) recently described an indirect FA test for the detection of immunoglobulin M (IgM) antibodies to EBV. The procedure consists of three steps: (i) acetone-fixed HR_1K cells containing about 20% EBV-positive cells are treated with various dilutions of the test serum for 3 h at 37 C; (ii) the cells are washed in phosphate-buffered saline (PBS) at 37 C for 60 min, and then rabbit anti-human IgM serum is added for 20 min at 37 C; (iii) after another washing in PBS (20 min at 37 C), fluorescein isothiocyanate-conjugated anti-rabbit globulin is applied for 15 min at 37 C, and the cells are washed and mounted for microscopy. According to these authors, EBV-IgM antibodies were found only during a period of 2 to 3 months after acute IM. Therefore, this test may be useful for diagnosis of recent EBV infection. Banatvala et al. (1) used the conventional indirect FA test to detect IgM antibodies to EBV in sera of IM patients. To increase the sensitivity of the test, they used the IgM fraction of sera obtained by sucrose gradient centrifugation.

Complement fixation test

Since CF antibody titers to EBV show no significant changes after onset of illness and tend to persist for years, the CF test has no diagnostic value and has been used mainly for sero-epidemiological studies (5). Crude EBV antigens can be obtained from sonically disrupted HR_1K cell suspensions. A negative control antigen can be prepared from a human lymphoid cell line "MOLT-4" (12) which appears to lack any detectable EBV genome.

Neutralization test

Recently, Rocchi et al. (13) described a neutralization test for EBV which is based on the observations that RAJI cells superinfected with EBV fail to form colonies. The procedure requires a supply of concentrated EBV and is therefore not suitable for use in routine diagnostic laboratories. Neutralizing antibodies appear later than FA (VCA) or CF antibodies during recovery from IM.

INTERPRETATION OF LABORATORY RESULTS

Detection of orally excreted EBV does not necessarily prove recent infection since some normal, asymptomatic carriers excrete this agent intermittently (7). At present, the most useful diagnostic test for recent EBV infection is the demonstration of IgM antibodies to the agent. The procedures described by Banatvala (1) or Schmitz (14) may be technically involved or tedious but are the only methods currently available.

LITERATURE CITED

1. Banatvala, J. E., J. M. Best, and D. K. Waller. 1972. Epstein-Barr virus-specific IgM in infectious mononucleosis, Burkitt lymphoma and nasopharyngeal carcinoma. Lancet **1**:1205–1208.
2. Chang, R. S., and H. D. Golden. 1971. Transformation of human leukocytes by throat washing from infectious mononucleosis patients. Nature (London) **234**:359–360.
3. Durr, F. E., J. H. Monroe, and R. Schmitter. 1970. Studies on the infectivity and cytopathology of Epstein-Barr virus in human lymphoblastoid cells. Int. J. Cancer **6**:436–449.
4. Epstein, M. A., B. G. Achong, and Y. M. Barr. 1964. Virus particles in cultured lymphoblasts from Burkitt's lymphoma. Lancet **1**:702–703.
5. Gerber, P., and S. M. Birch. 1967. Complement-fixing antibodies in sera of human and nonhuman primates to viral antigens derived from Burkitt's lymphoma cells. Proc. Nat. Acad. Sci. U.S.A. **58**:478–484.
6. Gerber, P., and S. Lucas. 1972. Epstein-Barr virus-associated antigens activated in human cells by 5-bromodeoxyuridine. Proc. Soc. Exp. Biol. Med. **141**:431–435.
7. Gerber, P., M. Nonoyama, S. Lucas, E. Perlin, and L. I. Goldstein. 1972. Oral excretion of Epstein-Barr virus by healthy subjects and patients with infectious mononucleosis. Lancet **1**:988–989.
8. Gerber, P., J. Whang-Peng, and J. H. Monroe. 1969. Transformation and chromosome changes induced by Epstein-Barr virus in normal human leukocyte cultures. Proc. Nat. Acad. Sci. U.S.A. **63**:740–747.
9. Henle, G., W. Henle, and V. Diehl. 1968. Relation of Burkitt's tumor-associated herpes-type virus to infectious mononucleosis. Proc. Nat. Acad. Sci. U.S.A. **59**:94–101.
10. Henle, W., G. Henle, and B. A. Zajac. 1970. Differential reactivity of human serums with early antigens induced by Epstein-Barr virus. Science **169**:188–190.
11. Miller, G., J. C. Niederman, and L. Andrews. 1973. Prolonged oropharyngeal excretion of Epstein-Barr virus after infectious mononucleosis. N. Engl. J. Med. **288**:229–232.
12. Minowada, J., T. Ohnuma, and G. E. Moore. 1972. Rosette-forming human lymphoid cell lines. Establishment and evidence for origin of thymus-derived lymphocytes. J. Nat. Cancer Inst. **49**:891–895.
13. Rocchi, G., and J. F. Hewetson. 1973. A practical and quantitative microtest for determination of neutralizing antibodies against Epstein-Barr virus. J. Gen. Virol. **18**:385–391.
14. Schmitz, H., and M. Scherer. 1972. IgM antibodies to Epstein-Barr virus in infectious mononucleosis. Arch. Gesamte Virusforsch. **37**:332–339.

Chapter 90

Hepatitis Viruses

F. BLAINE HOLLINGER

CLINICAL AND EPIDEMIOLOGICAL FEATURES

Viral hepatitis is a systemic disease primarily involving the liver. Most cases of acute viral hepatitis seen in children and adults are caused by one of two agents: hepatitis A virus (HAV), the etiological agent of hepatitis type A (infectious hepatitis or short-incubation hepatitis) and hepatitis B virus (HBV), which is associated with hepatitis type B (serum hepatitis or long-incubation hepatitis). Other well-characterized viruses which can cause hepatitis, such as yellow fever virus, cytomegalovirus, EB virus (infectious mononucleosis) and herpes simplex virus, are discussed in other chapters of this manual.

Table 1 presents the pertinent clinical and epidemiological features of viral hepatitis type A and type B. Both agents produce a characteristic, but indistinguishable, histopathological lesion in the liver. Clinical differentiation is rarely conclusive, and is extremely variable, ranging from asymptomatic (inapparent) infections through anicteric or icteric hepatitis to fulminant hepatitis and death. The prodromal or pre-icteric phase is frequently characterized by easy fatiguability, general malaise, myalgia, upper respiratory symptoms, an aversion to smoking, a maculopapular rash, arthralgia or polyarthritis, fever, and gastrointestinal complaints of anorexia, nausea, and vomiting. This is followed by right upper quadrant tenderness or pain associated with hepatomegaly and the onset of clinical jaundice. Patients with acute viral hepatitis usually recover completely. The frequency of fatal hepatitis is less than 1%.

Epidemiological and experimental observations indicate that hepatitis type A and type B are caused by two distinct etiological agents. The discovery of hepatitis B antigen (HB Ag or Australia antigen) by Blumberg and his associates and its specific relationship to HBV infections is now firmly established and serves to distinguish between the two types of infection (5). This has become increasingly important since it has been shown that viral hepatitis A, an enteric infection spread by close contact via the fecal-oral route, can also be transmitted parenterally (26), and viral hepatitis B, which occurs sporadically after parenteral inoculation of virus-infected blood or blood products, can also be spread by the oral route (13). Recognition of these lesser known transmission pathways has been beneficial in attempting to correlate a clinical classification of viral hepatitis with the presence or absence of HB Ag.

DESCRIPTION OF AGENTS (17)

The exact size of HAV is unknown, although it readily passes a 100-nm filter. It is remarkably resistant to heating (56 C for 30 min), acid, and disinfecting agents (chlorine, 1 ppm), and its infectivity can be preserved for years at −20 C. It does not appear to have essential lipids since infectivity remains after treatment with ether. The virus is destroyed by autoclaving (121 C for 20 min), by boiling in water for 1 min, or by dry heat (180 C for 1 h).

Three distinct morphological entities have been observed in sera from patients with hepatitis B infections (Fig. 1A). All share a common surface antigen (HB Ag) which appears to be a lipoprotein associated with some carbohydrate residues. These forms include small pleomorphic spherical particles measuring 20 nm in diameter, larger (42 nm), more complex double-shelled viruslike forms, and tubular or filamentous forms of varying length, but with a diameter similar to that of the smaller particles. The 27-nm rhinovirus-like inner core of the larger Dane particles appears to be devoid of HB Ag and may be the infectious virion (3). In contrast, the more numerous 20-nm particles probably represent excess virus coat protein. These particles have a buoyant density of 1.20 to 1.21 in CsCl and 1.16 to 1.18 in sucrose, a molecular weight of 3.5×10^6 to 6.0×10^6, and a sedimentation coefficient of approximately $40S_{20,w}$. Although the isolation of small amounts of nucleic acid has been reported, the results are conflicting and need to be confirmed.

HB Ag is resistant to ether, ordinary bacterial contamination, and heating at 60 C for 4 h. It is stable at pH 2.4 for at least 6 h at room

TABLE 1. *Epidemiological and clinical features of human hepatitis virus infections*[a]

Feature	Viral hepatitis type A	Viral hepatitis type B
Incubation period	15–50 days	43–180 days
Type of onset	Acute	Insidious
Principal age distribution	Children and young adults	All ages
Seasonal incidence	Autumn and winter	All year
Route of infection	Predominantly fecal-oral	Predominantly parenteral
Occurrence of virus/antigen		
Blood	Days	Months-years
Stool	Weeks-months	Present
Urine	?	Present
Clinical and laboratory features		
Fever > 38 C (100.4 F)	Common early	Less common
Duration of transaminase elevation	1–3 weeks	1–6 months or more
Immunoglobulins (IgM levels)	Significantly elevated	Normal to slightly elevated
Hepatitis B antigen (Au antigen)	Not present	Present
Immunity		
Homologous	Yes	Yes
Heterologous	No	No
Duration	Probably lifetime	Probably lifetime
Gamma globulin therapy	Regularly prevents or modifies hepatitis	Prevents or modifies hepatitis if specific HB immune serum globulin of sufficient potency is given

[a] From Melnick and Hollinger (17).

temperature and survives up to 40 freeze-thaw cycles. Antigenicity is also retained after storage at room temperature for 1 year or at −20 C for more than 15 years. Exposure of HB Ag for 3 min to equal volumes of sodium hypochlorite (0.5% for <1:10 dilutions of whole serum or 5% for whole serum) destroys antigenicity.

The infectious HBV readily passes a 50-nm filter and is stable at temperatures of −20 C or lower for over 20 years. Infectivity, but not antigenicity, is destroyed after heating at 60 C for 10 h. Both immunogenicity and infectivity are lost after direct boiling for 15 min or autoclaving for 1 min at 121 C.

HB Ag-containing particles are antigenically complex. Analysis has revealed that one specificity, *a*, is common to all HB Ag types. In almost all positive specimens, type specificity is conferred by finding one or the other of two mutually exclusive determinants, *d* or *y*, in association with the group *a* antigen. These virus-specific subtypes are useful as epidemiological markers. In the United States, the *ad* subtype is common in volunteer blood donors and in many cases of acute and chronic viral hepatitis except those associated with drug addicts, in which the *ay* subtype predominates. Two additional antigenic specificities, *w* and *r*, have been described in combination with the above subtypes. Most specimens collected in the United States contain the *w* subdeterminant.

COLLECTION AND STORAGE OF SPECIMENS FOR SEROLOGICAL TESTS

The stability of HB Ag obviates the need for extraordinary collection and storage procedures. Samples are frequently stored at 4 C until tested. If shipment over long distances is necessary, samples can be mailed at ambient temperatures. Antibody to HB Ag, designated HB Ab, is usually 7*S* immunoglobulin G (IgG) and is also quite stable. No loss of antibody titer has been observed in serum stored at 37, 4, or −20 C for 10 days. The use of anticoagulants or preservatives or the presence of hemolyzed blood will not adversely affect the radioimmunoassay, counterelectrophoresis, hemagglutination, or agar gel diffusion tests.

Low concentrations of HB Ag can occasionally be detected in saliva, pharyngeal washings, joint fluid, urine, and stool, and are usually associated with higher titers of HB Ag in the blood. It is probable that these sources are contaminated with small amounts of plasma.

Laboratory personnel should regard all specimens as potentially dangerous. Mouth pipetting, smoking, eating, or drinking in the laboratory should be strictly forbidden. In this laboratory, needles are placed in bottles and autoclaved before being discarded. All other materials are placed in discard pans and autoclaved at 121 C for 40 min. Work areas are decontaminated with 0.5% sodium hypochlorite

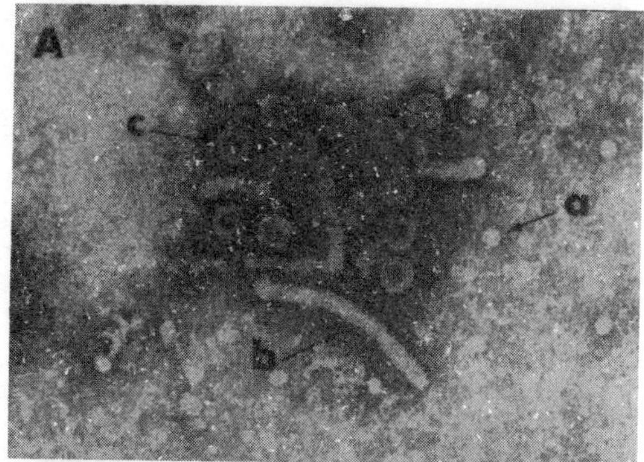

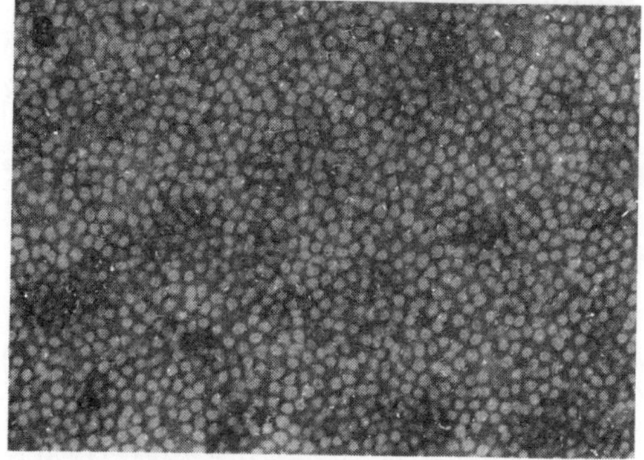

FIG. 1. *(A) Electron micrograph of serum showing the presence of three distinct morphological entities: (a) 20-nm pleomorphic spherical particles; (b) tubular or filamentous forms; and (c) large 42-nm double-shelled Dane particles. ×132,000. (B) Electron micrograph of a purified preparation of hepatitis B antigen showing the presence of 20- to 28-nm pleomorphic spherical particles. ×77,000. Electron microscopy by R. M. McCombs and J. P. Brunschwig.*

(1:10 Chlorox). Disposable gloves are worn when working with known infectious serum or plasma, and hand-washing procedures are strictly enforced. Additional safety recommendations are found in the WHO Technical Report (28).

DIRECT EXAMINATION

Fluorescent-antibody tests, electron microscopy, and immune electron microscopy have been used to examine liver biopsy material and serum specimens for the presence of HB Ag-containing particles (27). These tests are not applicable to rapid, large-scale screening of HBV infections by clinical laboratories. Electron microscopy of serum with the use of a negative staining technique is a valuable research technique for evaluating the relative proportions of the three morphological forms present. Its major disadvantage is that adequate demonstration requires a high concentration of particles, between 10^7 and 10^{10} per ml. By adding HB Ab to the sample (immune electron microscopy), the particles are caused to aggregate into an immune complex and can be concentrated by low-speed centrifugation, thereby enhancing the sensitivity of the procedure.

BIOLOGICAL INVESTIGATIONS

Lack of suitable tissue culture systems or animal models has hampered attempts to recover the etiological agents of hepatitis A and B from acute-phase serum. Chimpanzees may be naturally infected with HAV or HBV and can pass the disease to their handlers. Serial propagation of HBV has been reported in rhesus monkeys (16) and of HAV in certain species of marmosets (28). Attempts to isolate and propagate HBV or HAV in cell or organ cultures have been unsuccessful (28).

SEROLOGICAL IDENTIFICATION OF HEPATITIS B ANTIGEN AND ITS ANTIBODY

A number of serological techniques have been developed for the detection of HB Ag and its antibody, HB Ab. (Persons interested in obtaining information regarding commercially licensed test kits or reagents for detecting HB Ag or HB Ab may write to the Information Office, Bureau of Biologics, Food and Drug Administration, 5600 Fishers Lane, Bldg. 29, Rockville, Md. 20852, or call the Information Office at area 301 496-3343.) These methods include agarose gel diffusion (AGD), counter-electrophoresis (CEP), complement fixation (CF), passive hemagglutination (PHA) and inhibition, immune electron microscopy, red cell agglutination (RCA), platelet aggregation reaction, immune adherence, latex agglutination, and radioimmunoassay (RIA).

Each method offers certain advantages and disadvantages and differs markedly in sensitivity, specificity, simplicity, and expense. The more common procedures and their relative sensitivities are shown in Table 2. Five methods for detecting HB Ag or HB Ab which are used extensively in this laboratory as routine diagnostic procedures or for experimental research purposes are described in detail: AGD (subtyping), CEP (HB Ag and subtyping), RCA (HB Ag and subtyping), PHA (HB Ab), and RIA (HB Ag, HB Ab, and subtyping). The reader is referred to the Literature Cited for references to other techniques (17, 27–29).

TABLE 2. *Methods used to detect hepatitis B antigen and antibody (HB Ag and HB Ab), and their relative sensitivities as compared with agarose gel diffusion*

Assay method	HB Ag	HB Ab	Incubation time required for each test (h)
Agarose gel diffusion	1	1	24–72
Counterelectrophoresis	5	10	1
Complement fixation	10	1	18
Passive hemagglutination inhibition	10	—	3–6
Passive hemagglutination	—	4,000	3
Red cell agglutination	250	—	3
Radioimmunoassay	1,000	4,000	4–120

Preparation of reagents

The development of sensitive and specific detection systems for antigen or antibody requires the preparation of highly purified antigens and the production of antisera of high specificity, affinity, and avidity. In practice, it has been extremely difficult and perhaps impossible to prepare purified HB Ag which is totally devoid of contaminating normal human serum (NHS) proteins, especially albumin and gamma globulin. Whether this is because the proteins are simply contaminants of the purification procedure, are adsorbed to the particles, or are integral components of HB Ag is currently unknown. The purification method described below has resulted in some of the purest preparations encountered (Fig. 1B) and can be completed in 1 week. In this method (6), any existing antigen-antibody complexes are dissociated at pH 2.4 and then separated by high-speed centrifugation. Purification is enhanced because the low pH also denatures some of the human serum proteins. This step should be avoided if recovery of the large double-shelled Dane particles is desired, since these particles appear to be partially disrupted at low pH levels, apparently leaving the internal core intact. Tubular forms also disappear, but the 20-nm particles remain unchanged. This partial degradation of the Dane particles may actually be beneficial, since patients who are infected with hepatitis B apparently make antibodies to the 27-nm internal core which is antigenically distinct from HB Ag (3). If this observation is confirmed, preparations containing this antigen in addition to HB Ag may be more suitable as a reference reagent for testing or producing antibody (see heterogeneity of particles in Fig. 1B). Immunogenicity and radioisotopic labeling of these purified HB Ag preparations seems to be superior to that found with other methods of purification which lack a low pH step, suggesting that additional antigenic sites may be unmasked.

The production of potent HB Ab of high specificity and sensitivity is essential to the performance and reliability of any test procedure. As expected, low levels of anti-NHS are observed in almost all preparations of HB Ab when sensitive methods of detection are utilized (6). Criteria for assessing the purity of HB Ag should always be similar in sensitivity to the method being used; e.g., AGD should not be employed to determine whether anti-NHS contaminants exist if the antibody is to be used in an RIA test. Low levels of anti-NHS frequently remain unrecognized unless a two-dimensional titration is performed with NHS as the antigen. These contaminating antibodies to NHS components can be removed by adsorption to water-insoluble glutaraldehyde cross-linked preparations of NHS (4).

Hepatitis B antigen purification method (6)

Acid-citrate-dextrose (ACD) plasma containing a high titer of HB Ag (CF titer, 1:320 to 1:1,280; discontinuous CEP titer, 1:64 to 1:256) is obtained from an anicteric volunteer blood donor. The plasma is converted to serum by adding 1.5 to 2.0 ml of 1.0 M $CaCl_2$ per 100 ml, incubating the sample in a water bath at 37 C for 1 to 2 h to facilitate clot formation, then recovering the serum after centrifugation at 3,000 × *g* for 20 min. This preliminary step reduces the size and gelatinous quality of subsequent pellets without decreasing the concentration of HB Ag.

The serum is distributed into 25-ml portions and pelleted at 100,000 × *g* for 15 to 18 h at 4 C. The pellets are resuspended in 2.5 ml of 0.15 M NaCl and are disrupted by sonic treatment at peak output for 45 s at 4 to 10 C with a model W185 Sonifier Cell Disruptor (Heat Systems, Inc.) with a water-jacketed cup horn attachment. The samples are pooled, the volume is reconstituted to 25 ml with 0.15 M NaCl, and the material is repelleted for 5 h at 200,000 × *g* and 4 C. The pellet is reconstituted to 4 ml with 0.05 M potassium phthalate buffer, pH 2.4, and sonically disrupted as described above. The pH is readjusted to 2.4 and the sample is incubated at room temperature for 1 h.

The acid-treated sample is clarified at 12,000 × *g* for 10 min. Then 2-ml portions are layered over a 10 to 40% (wt/wt) CsCl gradient (ρ = 1.08 to 1.42 g/ml) prepared in 0.15 M saline containing 0.01 M total phosphates (1.096 g of anhydrous Na_2HPO_4 and 0.315 g of $NaH_2PO_4 \cdot H_2O$ per liter; PBS), pH 7.2, in SW41 cellulose nitrate centrifuge tubes (Beckman, no. 331370). After isopycnic centrifugation in a Spinco SW41 rotor at 286,000 × *g* (41,000 rpm) for 18 h at 4 C, two major bands are usually observed. The upper band, approximately one-third to one-half the distance from the top of the gradient, contains HB Ag at a density between 1.20 and 1.24 g/ml; the band in the lower one-third of the tube contains serum proteins at a density of 1.28 to 1.30 g/ml. Because the lower band often contains particulate material, collection of the upper band is best accomplished by side puncture or by collection from the top. Samples containing the HB Ag are combined, made up to 6.0 ml in PBS, and dialyzed against PBS at room temperature for at least 1 h to lower the density below 1.08 g/ml. A second equilibrium centrifugation in CsCl is performed as described above and the HB Ag-containing band is removed. Samples are dialyzed overnight at 4 C against two 100-volume changes of PBS. Final purification of this PBS-dialyzed HB Ag-rich fraction is accomplished by rate zonal centrifugation in an SW41 rotor at 41,000 rpm for 4 h at 4 C by layering the sample over a preformed linear 5 to 30% (wt/wt) CsCl gradient (ρ = 1.04 to 1.29 g/ml) prepared in PBS, pH 7.2. Fractions of 0.8 ml are collected by bottom puncture, HB Ag is determined by CF, and those fractions with peak antigenic activity are pooled. Most of the CF activity is found near the middle of the tube. Recovery of purified HB Ag from 100 ml of high-titered plasma by this method approaches 4 to 6 mg of protein (extinction coefficient for a 0.1% solution at an optical density of 280 nm is 3.726).

As with many highly purified preparations, aggregation of particles and loss of antigen by sticking to glassware must be prevented. All glassware is siliconized. Aggregation can be diminished by storing the antigen without removing the CsCl, then dialyzing it against saline or PBS when needed. Preparations are sterilized by filtration through a 0.22-μm membrane filter (Millipore Corp.) prior to storage. To avoid losing HB Ag during filtration, the filter is pretreated with 0.5 ml of 1% Tween 80 and then flushed with 100 ml of saline. A 10% stock solution of sterile polyethylene oxide in saline (PolyOx, WSRN-10, Union Carbide) is added to the filtrate to give a final concentration of 0.1%. PolyOx is a nonionic, water-soluble resin of 100,000 molecular weight which retards aggregation and prevents additional protein loss on glassware.

Production of hepatitis B antibody (6)

Satisfactory HB Ab for screening sera for HB Ag has been prepared in a variety of animals, including horses, goats, guinea pigs, rabbits, mice, rhesus monkeys, baboons, and chimpanzees. Antisera from multiply transfused individuals or other persons have also provided investigators with a rich source of HB Ab of moderate titer. The major advantage of human serum (or chimpanzee) is its freedom from anti-NHS contaminants.

Antibody with excellent antigen-precipitating capacity can be prepared in goats (6). It is not a good CF reagent because it fixes guinea pig complement poorly. In general, the antiserum is unsatisfactory for subtyping studies because of the large quantity of group-specific anti-*a* which invariably develops unless specimens are obtained early in the course of immunization. Conversely, this broad antigenic quality makes it an excellent screening reagent for all subtypes of HB Ag as used in the AGD, CEP, RIA, or RCA tests. Goats are inoculated intramuscularly in both flanks and both shoulders (1.0 ml/site) on days 0, 14, and 28, and are bled on day 42. The initial inoculum contains equal vlumes of purified HB Ag (50 μg/goat) and complete Freund's adjuvant diluted 1:5 in incomplete Freund's adjuvant. Subsequent inocula contain 35 μg of HB Ag per goat equally mixed with a 1:20 dilution of complete Freund's adjuvant. Goats reinjected on days 77 and 89 and bled on day 105 have shown an anamnestic response to HB Ag with decreased to absent levels of antibodies to NHS components. Titers range between 1:256 and 1:1,024 by discontinuous CEP, 1:32 to 1:128 by AGD, and over 1:10,000,000 by RIA and PHA.

Antiserum prepared in guinea pigs is an excellent reagent for the CF test, for subtyping, and as a screening reagent for AGD, CEP, and RIA procedures. Specificity of antisera produced against subtype *ay* is better than that produced against subtype *ad*, which suggests that the *a* subspecificity in the *ad* preparation may be more immunogenic, resulting in a more broadly reacting antiserum. Guinea pigs are inoculated initially in both hind footpads (0.25 ml/site) on day 0, reinoculated in the front footpads between days 14 and 18, and bled on day 42. The inocula contain equal volumes of purified HB Ag (5 to 10 μg/guinea pig) and complete Freund's adjuvant diluted 1:10 in incomplete Freund's adjuvant. Booster injections contain 5 to 10 μg of Ag/guinea pig in a 1:10 dilution of complete Freund's adjuvant. Titers range from 1:640 to 1:2,560 by CF, from 1:8

to 1:32 by AGD, and from 1:1,000,000 to 1:10,000,000 by RIA or PHA.

AGAR GEL DIFFUSION

AGD is the least sensitive method available for detecting HB Ag, but permits direct comparisons to be made between specimens regarding their identity, partial relatedness, or nonidentity. Correspondingly, AGD can be used to confirm positive reactions obtained by CEP.

A two-dimensional micro-Ouchterlony immunodiffusion test (19) is performed on microscope slides (1 by 3 inch [2.5 by 7.6 cm]) layered with 2.5 ml of 0.8% agarose in PBS, pH 7.2, containing 1:10,000 azide or thimerosal. A seven-well template is used (six peripheral wells surrounding a center well). The wells are 3 mm in diameter and 5 mm equidistant from each other. Reinforcement of weak precipitin lines is accomplished by placing reference HB Ag-positive specimens in peripheral wells 2, 4, and 6, and the unknown specimens in wells 1, 3, and 5. Thus, each test serum is adjacent to a positive serum. Because HB Ag is a large molecule and diffuses slowly compared with IgG antibody, preincubation of the slides for 2 h at room temperature in a humidified chamber prior to the addition of HB Ab in the center well permits precipitin lines to develop more distal to the peripheral well. The slides are observed for the development of precipitin lines at 24 and 48 h. Sensitivity can be improved by concentrating specimens with Lyphogel.

For subtyping antigens, the same reinforcement pattern can be used. Reference HB Ag subtype *ay* or *ad* is placed in peripheral wells 2, 4, and 6, and homologous subtype-specific HB Ab is added to the center well. Monospecific HB Ab containing anti-*d* or anti-*y* antibody only (see Red Cell Agglutination section) can be substituted for the reference antiserum to enhance specificity. Slides are observed for lines of identity or for the formation of a "spur" signifying different antigen reactants.

DISCONTINUOUS COUNTERIMMUNOELECTROPHORESIS

CEP has been the most widely applied method for detecting HB Ag on a large scale. The basic principle of the technique is that HB Ag, with an isoelectric pH between 4.4 and 5.2, migrates in an electrophoretic field toward the anode and, because of electroendosmosis, the gamma globulin (HB Ab) migrates toward the cathode. A precipitin line forms when optimal concentrations of the antigen and antibody meet. By reducing the ionic strength of the agarose buffer, as compared to the buffer used in the electrophoresis chambers, a discontinuous buffer system can be prepared which enhances the movement of acidic proteins toward the anode and globulins toward the cathode. This results in increased sensitivity and speed of reaction and in sharper, more easily read precipitin lines (24). Plates must be examined carefully for weak precipitin lines; a magnifying lens, a darkened room, and a good oblique viewing light are helpful. Artifacts may be encountered in this system which must not be confused with a true-positive reaction. These include a halo of precipitation around the well and movement of lipid over the surface of the agarose adjacent to the sample well. The latter artifact can easily be distinguished from a true precipitin reaction within the gel by wiping the area gently with a cotton swab.

Both specificity and sensitivity depend on the use of a potent precipitating antibody from which anti-NHS has been adsorbed. False-positive results are uncommon. However, precipitating antigen-antibody reactions unrelated to hepatitis B may sometimes occur, and this possibility should always be kept in mind. An imbalance between reactants, either excess HB Ag or HB Ab, can lead to the establishment of a prozone and a false-negative result. The prozone phenomenon which occurs in the region of HB Ag excess can be minimized by diluting the reagent antibody in normal homologous whole serum or its globulin fraction (7). Two-dimensional box titrations are essential to determine the optimal concentration of reagent antibody needed in subsequent tests.

Kodak lantern slides, 8.3 by 10.2 cm, are precoated with 5 ml of 1.0% agarose in distilled water and allowed to dry at room temperature overnight or at 110 C in an oven for 2 h. These coated slides can be stored indefinitely in a dust- and lint-free environment. Stock Veronal buffer (pH 8.6; ionic strength, 0.075 μ) is prepared with the use of 1.84 g of diethylbarbituric acid, 10.3 g of sodium diethylbarbiturate, and distilled water to make 1 liter. Sodium azide or thimerosal can be added as a preservative at a final concentration of 1:5,000. To perform the assay, 15 ml of 0.85% agarose is prepared in low ionic strength Veronal buffer (0.015 μ or a 1:5 dilution of the stock buffer) and layered over precoated slides placed on a leveling table. Wells cut into the agarose with a no. 1 cork borer or similar instrument are 4 mm in diameter and are separated by a distance of 9 mm between the centers of the wells. A satisfactory template which fits over the lantern slides can be prepared from a Linbro lucite plate, no.

IS-MRC-96, by drilling through the bottom of each well. Stock Veronal buffer (0.075 μ) is added to each chamber, and the chambers are bridged to the slides with filter-paper wicks. The chamber volume and the buffer-carrying capacity of the wick influence the endosmotic flux and temperatures of the gel and therefore the distortion which might occur. Each laboratory should standardize the system with its own equipment. Electrophoresis is conducted at room temperature. A constant current of about 3 mA/cm (25 mA/lantern slide) is applied across the narrow dimension of the slide which, under the conditions described, gives a starting voltage potential of approximately 275 V which falls to about 200 V by the end of the run. Slides are removed and read at 45 min. Weak precipitin reactions may not be visible immediately, and slides should be re-read at 2 h and after standing in a humidified chamber overnight. Staining has not enhanced detection of positive reactions. Commercial kits are available which utilize a discontinuous buffer system.

By employing a three-well configuration in which the unknown sample is placed in the center well, HB Ab is placed in the well on the anodal side, and HB Ag is placed in the cathodal well, simultaneous testing for antibody and antigen in the unknown can be accomplished. Low levels of HB Ab may be missed if the HB Ag reagent is in excess. In general, the CEP method is a relatively insensitive method for detecting HB Ab in human sera.

COMPLEMENT FIXATION

HB Ag titers obtained by the CF test are two- to fourfold greater than those obtained by CEP (Table 2). However, detection of HB Ag in sera from patients is equivalent since undiluted sera are examined by CEP compared with a starting dilution of 1:4 or 1:8 in the CF test. Equivalent sensitivity is observed when testing for HB Ab. Anticomplementary (AC) activity may be observed in some patients with hepatitis B but is also seen in hepatitis A, suggesting the presence of antigen-antibody complexes. Other causes of AC activity include the presence of aggregated gamma globulin due to repeated freezing and thawing, prolonged storage, or bacterial contamination. Prozones are occasionally observed with sera containing high titers of HB Ag, so several dilutions should be tested. Most prozones are <1:40. HB Ab which has a high precipitating efficiency may not bind complement effectively, illustrating the differences in quality as well as quantity among antibodies. It is important to use NHS-adsorbed antisera for the CF test to avoid false-positive results at high dilutions of human serum (6) or where testing protein-deficient specimens, e.g., urine. The procedure for the CF test is described in detail in chapter 71.

RADIOIMMUNOASSAY

The RIA technique is the most sensitive and specific method available today for detecting HB Ag. Its major disadvantages include time to complete the test, expense involved, and the need for radioisotopes with their associated hazards. Four basic RIA methods have been described for detecting HB Ag: a double antibody technique (1, 10, 14), a solid phase method (10), a chromatoelectrophoresis method (25), and a direct solid phase "sandwich" procedure (15). They differ primarily in the method used to isolate or detect the antigen-antibody complex and in the placement of the radioactive label, e.g., whether it is on purified HB Ab or purified HB Ag. The purity of the labeled preparation is an essential component to the specificity of the test. The methods most commonly used include the solid phase "sandwich" RIA technique and the double antibody RIA (RIA-DA) procedure.

Direct solid phase or "sandwich" method

The solid phase "sandwich" method (15) is comparable in sensitivity to the RIA-DA method, is less cumbersome, and is available in kit form (Ausria-I^{125} Abbott Laboratories, North Chicago, Ill.). Its present limitations are its specificity and reproducibility at the lower range of sensitivity.

HB Ab is fixed to the solid polystyrene or polypropylene surface of test tubes. A 0.1-ml sample of each specimen, tested in duplicate, is evenly distributed over the bottom of the HB Ab-coated test tube. The tubes are covered with an adhesive-coated paper and incubated for 16 to 18 h at room temperature. During this incubation period, HB Ag, if present, becomes fixed to the solid phase HB Ab at the liquid-surface interface. The contents are aspirated and the tubes are washed five times with 2 ml of 0.005 M tris(hydroxymethyl)aminomethane buffer, pH 7.1. For aspirating, a 1-ml disposable tip (Biotip, Schwarz-Mann, no. 0010-30) can be connected with rubber tubing to a vacuum system. The Biotip is pierced with an 18-gauge needle near the top to prevent the tip from touching the bottom of the tube. Rinse solution is added with a 2-ml Cornwall continuous pipetting outfit (Becton-Dickinson, no. 1251) and aspirated five times without removing the disposable tip. This prevents cross-contamination and removes any residual HB Ag or labeled

HB Ab. To the bottom of each washed tube is added 0.1 ml of purified ^{125}I-labeled HB Ab. To avoid diluting the labeled HB Ab, it is imperative that no residual rinse solution remain after the initial washing step. The tubes should be tapped gently to distribute the labeled antibody evenly. Care must be taken to avoid applying any labeled HB Ab to the sides of the tube as this can cause a false-positive result. The tubes are covered and incubated for 90 min at room temperature, during which time the labeled antibody becomes fixed to the previously bound antigen, resulting in an antibody-antigen-antibody "sandwich." The residual labeled antibody is aspirated, and the tubes are rinsed and aspirated five times as previously described. The radioactive counts retained in the tube are roughly proportional to the antigen concentration of the sample. To obtain reproducible results, it is essential that all tubes be incubated for 90 min in the presence of labeled HB Ab. Some variations in background between the first and last tube in a test will occur if incubation times are too dissimilar. The tubes are counted in a well-type gamma scintillation counter.

Each test should include one positive and six or seven negative control samples. From the negative controls, a mean counting rate (counts per minute) can be determined after subtracting the machine background from all samples. By dividing the counts per minute of the unknown sample by the control mean value, a ratio is obtained. Repeatable values $\geq$2.1 times the control mean are presumed to be positive, but their specificity must be confirmed by an inhibition or blocking test before informing the donor that he is an HB Ag carrier. To perform such a test, 0.1-ml samples of specimens are incubated with 0.01 to 0.02 ml of high-titering HB Ab, with normal guinea pig serum, or with NHS for 2 h at 37 C, and retested. Inhibition of a positive result by HB Ab but not by the guinea pig serum or normal human serum establishes the HB Ag specificity of an Ausria positive specimen.

Previous limitations of the Ausria test have concerned its reproducibility and the occurrence of false-positive results which were presumably due to the presence of cross-reacting antibodies in the unknown sample which reacted with the globulin fraction of the HB Ab (9, 21). Reproducibility and specificity were especially poor among equivocal or low-titered specimens. These methodological problems are currently under investigation and presumably can be resolved. The addition of excess guinea pig serum to the labeled HB Ab or the use of HB Ab produced in heterologous species for coating the tubes and for labeling has resulted in some improvement in specificity. More recently, the Bureau of Biologics has approved a reduction in the incubation time for Ausria-I^{125} from 16 h to 2 h for the initial incubation, and from 1.5 h to 1 h for the second incubation, provided that the incubation is carried out in a water bath at 45 C. This change in the test procedure has apparently improved both the sensitivity and the specificity of the procedure. Because plasma may clot and trap radioactive material at the elevated temperature, only serum or recalcified plasma should be used.

Double antibody radioimmunoassay procedure

The RIA-DA test is a useful research tool which measures the primary interaction between antigen and antibody and can be used for studying the kinetics of this reaction. It is highly sensitive, specific, and reproducible. The test is based on competition between HB Ag in the test sample with labeled purified HB Ag for a limited amount of HB Ab (first antibody). The antigen-antibody complexes which form are precipitated by heterologous anti-IgG (second, or immunoprecipitating, antibody) directed against the species of immunoglobulin-containing HB Ab. Decreased binding of labeled HB Ag to HB Ab, as illustrated by a reduced number of counts in the co-precipitate, is evidence for a positive reaction. The reduction is proportional to the concentration of HB Ag present in the unknown sample.

Purified HB Ag is labeled with ^{125}I by a modified chloramine-T method. To a siliconized 1-ml Kontes Microflex "V" reaction tube with Teflon cap is added 50 μliters of each of the following: 0.5 M phosphate buffer, pH 7.4, 2 mCi of carrier-free ^{125}I (high specific activity), and 5 to 10 μg of purified HB Ag. Next, 500 μg of freshly prepared chloramine-T in 100 μliters of 0.05 M phosphate buffer, pH 7.4, is added, and the mixture is incubated at room temperature for 3 min with constant mixing by inversion. The reaction is terminated by the addition of 1,000 μg of sodium metabisulfite in 100 μliters of 0.05 M phosphate buffer, pH 7.4, followed by 1,000 μg of KI in 100 μliters of the same buffer. An additional 100 ml of KI is subsequently used to rinse out the reaction tube. The sample is layered on a G-200 Sephadex column (1 by 30 cm) which has been pretreated with 200 mg of human serum albumin to prevent nonspecific binding of HB Ag to the Sephadex or to increase adsorption of damaged labeled antigen. The sample is eluted with PBS, pH 7.2, containing 1:10,000 sodium azide. Fractions of 1 ml are collected in 12 by 75 mm tubes containing 10 mg of human serum albumin in 0.1 ml to prevent nonspecific adsorption to the glass, and total radioactivity is determined in a well-type gamma counting system. HB Ag, with a molecular weight between 3.5×10^6 and 6.0×10^6 daltons, appears in the void volume, substantially removed from the free ^{125}I. Between 95 and 98% of the peak void volume (HB Ag) fractions contain protein as determined after precipitation with 10% trichloroacetic acid. These fractions are pooled, diluted in PBS with 0.5% human serum albumin to contain 3×10^6 counts per min per 0.3 ml, and stored in unsiliconized glass ampoules at −70 or −196 C. A typical iodination with the concentrations specified above should yield a preparation containing approximately 200×10^6 to 300×10^6 counts/min and a specific activity of 10 to 20 μCi/μg. This represents a labeling efficiency of 7 to 10%.

HB Ag is labeled routinely every 6 to 8 weeks. Previous studies in this laboratory showed that the sensitivity of the RIA-DA test was not significantly altered when tracer was varied over a 10-fold range. Thus, storage of ^{125}I-HB Ag for 8 weeks is not associated with any apparent changes in sensitivity. Each new lot of ^{125}I-HB Ag is evaluated for its immunoreactivity with HB Ab. Excess HB Ab binds from 85 to 95% of the label. A preliminary assay with controls and a standard curve is also performed, and the results are compared with previous lots of ^{125}I-HB Ag.

The procedure and reagents needed to perform the RIA-DA test for the detection of HB Ag are illustrated in Table 3. Specimens are tested in duplicate with the use of disposable unsiliconized glass culture tubes (12 by 75 mm). Six to 10 NHS, free from HB Ag or HB Ab, are used as negative controls. The standard curve samples represent 3 to 4 dilutions of purified HB Ag of known concentration diluted in NHS. The standard buffer consists of nonimmune serum of the same species as the HB Ab, diluted 1:400 in a buffer containing 0.05 M tetrasodium ethylenediaminetetraacetate (EDTA), 0.01 M sodium phosphate (1.096 g of anhydrous Na_2HPO_4 and 0.315 g of $NaH_2PO_4 \cdot H_2O$ per liter), 0.15 M NaCl, and 1:4,000 sodium azide, adjusted to pH 7.2 with 10 N HCl. The 1:400 dilution of nonimmune serum provides sufficient protein to prevent loss of HB Ab due to nonspecific adsorption to glass at the high dilutions used in the test (approximately 1:200,000 for guinea pig HB Ab and 1:640,000 for goat HB Ab). By titering the second antibody against this constant concentration of nonimmune globulin in the presence of HB Ab and ^{125}I-HB Ag, an optimal dilution within the zone of equivalence can be established (18). Thus, any homologous species HB Ab diluted above 1:400 in this standard buffer can be used without re-examining the conditions for equivalence. In addition, the 1:400 dilution of nonimmune globulin provides reasonable antigenic bulk to the final precipitate which permits decantation of the supernatant fluid without losing any precipitate. HB Ab (0.4 ml) is stored in siliconized vials at −70 C at a dilution of 1:50 in PBS, pH 7.2. Radioactivity is measured in a well-type gamma counting system.

In testing for HB Ag, 50 μliters of the appropriate sample is added to each tube (see Table 3) followed by 200 μliters of the standard buffer which contains a dilution of HB Ab that binds 30 to 50% of the ^{125}I-HB Ag. Standard buffer without HB Ab is added to the background control tubes. Since minor deviations in the amount of HB Ab or labeled HB Ag added to each tube can adversely affect the precision of the assay and lead to significant errors, use of an automatic micropipettor, e.g., Micromedic Systems, Inc., is recommended for these steps. The reactants are incubated for 36 to 48 h at 4 C before adding the labeled HB Ag. This initial preincubation step allows noncompetitive interaction of unlabeled HB Ag with HB Ab and significantly enhances the sensitivity of a nonequilibrium RIA-DA system.

The addition of 100 μliters of ^{125}I-HB Ag to each tube completes the second step in the RIA-DA procedure. Prior to use, the ^{125}I-HB Ag is thawed and refractionated on a G-75 Sephadex column. These columns are prepared in Corning disposable 10-ml pipettes (no. 3709C) and are pretreated with 100 mg of HSA. A small quantity of glass wool placed in the bottom of the pipette prevents the Sephadex from escaping. These inexpensive columns can be prepared in advance and stored at 4 C for at least 2 months if the PBS eluate contains 1:5,000 sodium azide. The refractionation process, which takes less than 45 min to perform, removes any residual free ^{125}I or damaged HB Ag which may be present. The label is collected in human serum albumin (final concentration, 0.5 to 1.0%), diluted in PBS, pH 7.2, containing 0.5% human serum albumin, and placed in a siliconized bottle to prevent adsorption of label to glassware. Approximately 10,000 counts/min of chilled label (4 to 8 C), containing 0.3 to 0.6 ng of HB Ag, is added to each sample with an automatic micropipettor. After a 24-h incubation period at 4 C, 100 μliters of the immunoprecipitating antibody, appropriately diluted in chilled PBS, is added to each tube. The co-precipitates are recovered 24 h later by adding 4.5 ml of cold (4 to 8 C) saline to each tube with a 5-ml Cornwall continuous pipetting outfit, centrifuging the specimens at 1,500 × *g* for 15 min at 4 C, and decanting the supernatant fluids into a radioactive waste container. Residual fluid is removed by touching the inverted lip of the tube to paper towels. Special precautions for decanting material containing HB Ag include the use of disposable gloves and thorough cleaning of the area with 0.5% sodium hypochlorite when finished. The tubes with their co-precipitates are placed into 16 by 125 mm polyethylene tubes which are then counted for 4 min or 10,000 total counts.

A positive reaction, indicating the presence of HB Ag, is determined by comparing the mean counts per minute of the unknown sample with the grand mean value of the normal reference sera from which a standard deviation has been obtained. An inhibition ≥5 SD from the HB Ag negative controls, which represents a reduction in counts per minute of 20% or more, has been shown to be unequivocally positive for HB Ag in this laboratory. False-positive results due to cross-reacting antibodies similar to those encountered in the direct solid phase RIA system have not been observed in the RIA-DA test. However, false-positive reactions can occur when testing human sera which contain HB Ab of high avidity. Such endogenously produced HB Ab can compete effectively with first antibody for ^{125}I-HB Ag. Since the endogenous HB Ab-tracer complex would not be precipitated by the immunoprecipitating antiserum which is directed against the gamma globulin of the first antibody, a decreased percentage of radioactivity would be recovered in the precipitate and result in a false-positive reaction. An appreciation of this problem is important since it can be nullified by utilizing a highly avid first antibody. Correspondingly, anti-human gamma globulin can be added to a duplicate set of specimens as the immunoprecipitating antibody to detect those which contain HB Ab (see below).

To evaluate the reliability of an RIA test, several parameters should be monitored from which the inter-assay and intra-assay error can be compared (18). Such quality-control data provide meaningful information on ways to improve the precision or reproducibility of the test (20). Parameters evaluated include a label control, background control, NHS control, and a standard curve (Table 3). Assessment of the stability and similarity of intra-assay experimental conditions (reproducibility) can be analyzed by including controls at the beginning, at the end, and sometimes in the middle of a test if it is a large one. Precision of the micropipetting system is evaluated by measuring the mean counts per minute and standard deviation of eight tubes containing label only. Counts should not deviate more than 1%. The background counts per minute should not exceed 3 to 5% of the label added to the test. The NHS

TABLE 3. *Flow diagram for detecting hepatitis B antigen (HB Ag) by the double antibody radioimmunoassay procedure*

Procedure	Volume (μliters)				
	Controls			Standard curve	Test (unknown)
	Label	Background	NHS[a]		
First reaction					
Step 1 (36–48 h, 4 C)					
Sample					
NHS[a]		50	50		
Standard curve				50	
Unknown					50
+					
Standard buffer					
with HB Ab			200	200	200
without HB Ab		200			
Step 2 (24 h, 4 C)					
^{125}I-HB Ag	100	100	100	100	100
Second reaction (24 h, 4 C)					
Immunoprecipitating antibody		100	100	100	100

[a] Normal human serum.

control indicates whether sufficient first antibody was added to bind 30 to 50% of the label. Two additional tubes receive a low dilution of antibody (1:1,000) to determine whether the immunogenicity of the ^{125}I-HB Ag has been altered on storage. From the standard curve, a slope is plotted on a logit scale—a convenient transformation resulting in a straight line for statistical analysis (20). Conversion of positive results to micrograms or nanograms of HB Ag per milliliter is not routinely done but could be determined from the standard curve if necessary.

Despite the long incubation period, the actual technician time needed to perform a test of 150 samples with controls (360 to 420 tubes) is approximately 8 h. Thus, one technician can test 500 specimens per week. The RIA-DA test can be shortened to 1 day or less by altering the incubation conditions, but at a loss of sensitivity and specificity. A 2-day test (step 1, 2 h at 37 C; step 2, 22 h at 4 C; second reaction, 24 h at 4 C) has a sensitivity only slightly less than that of the 4-day test. Recent tests have also demonstrated that the RIA-DA test can be conducted at 25 C with minimal loss of sensitivity or specificity if the various reagent concentrations and incubation parameters are properly evaluated.

To detect HB Ab with the RIA-DA method, 200 μliters of standard buffer without HB Ab is added to 50 μliters of a 1:15 dilution of the unknown specimen, followed by the addition of 100 μliters of ^{125}I-HB Ag. The reactants are incubated for 2 days at room temperature or for 4 days at 4 C. Anti-human gamma globulin (100 μliters) is added to each tube at a dilution experimentally found to be at equivalence with the gamma globulin in a 1:15 dilution of NHS. Incubation is continued for an additional 24 to 48 h at the respective temperatures, and the tubes are processed as previously described. A specimen is considered to contain HB Ab if the observed counts per minute are $\geq$1.5 times the mean of the negative control samples.

Modification of the RIA-DA test for subtyping can be accomplished by preincubating the unknown samples with broadly reacting unadsorbed HB Ab which contains anti-*d* and anti-*y* antibody (2). Purified HB Ag subtype *ad*, labeled with ^{131}I, and HB Ag subtype *ay*, labeled with ^{125}I, are simultaneously added to each tube and the test is continued as previously described. Radioactivity is determined in a dual-channel gamma counter, and the degree of inhibition of each labeled HB Ag is compared. Homologous inhibition is greather than heterologous, permitting discrimination of subtypes *ad* and *ay*. By substituting adsorbed mono-specific antisera (see Red Cell Agglutination section for preparation), subtyping specificity can be enhanced.

RED CELL AGGLUTINATION

The RCA method (11) is similar in sensitivity to the RIA procedure. Its most important advantage is that it utilizes the microtiter system which is familiar to most diagnostic virologists. The RCA microtiter method is easy to perform, uses relatively inexpensive equipment, can be completed in 3 h, lacks a radiation hazard, and can be adapted to commercially available automated microtiter systems. The method described for detecting HB Ag was developed in this laboratory (11) and can be modified for subtyping.

Human type O, Rh-negative erythrocytes are collected in EDTA or Alsever's solution, washed five times in 0.1 M phosphate buffer, pH 7.2, and resuspended as an 8% suspension. Stabilized cells are prepared according to the method of Hirata and Brandriss (8). One volume of 3% methyl glyoxal (pyruvaldehyde) diluted in 0.1 M phosphate buffer is added to one volume of an 8% suspension of washed erythrocytes, the pH is readjusted to pH 7.2 with NaOH, and the mixture is incubated for 18 h at 25 C. The cells are washed five times with 0.1 M phosphate buffer, filtered through four layers of surgical gauze, and resuspended to 8% (vol/vol). To 1 volume of this suspension is added an equal volume of 3% formaldehyde in 0.1 M phosphate buffer and the pH is readjusted to pH 7.2 with NaOH. This mixture is incubated for 18 h at 25 C with constant mixing. The suspension is filtered through gauze, washed five times with 0.1 M phosphate buffer, reconstituted to 10%, and stored at 4 C. No differences in coating efficiency have been observed when stabilized cells stored for at least 8 weeks are used.

High-titered HB Ab in goats or guinea pigs is prepared as previously described. Low concentrations of contaminating antibody to NHS proteins can be removed by adsorption to a water-insoluble preparation of pooled NHS cross-linked with glutaraldehyde according to the method of Avraemeas (4). The glutaraldehyde should be of E.M. grade (Polysciences, Inc.) to avoid variability in the preparation of these immunoadsorbents. Globulins are precipitated at 4 C by addition of an equal volume of neutral saturated ammonium sulfate. The precipitate is redissolved in 0.01 M phosphate buffer, pH 8.0, and dialyzed overnight against this buffer. Purified IgG containing HB Ab is obtained by eluting the equilibrated sample from a 2.5 by 30 cm column of diethylaminoethyl (DEAE) cellulose with 0.01 M phosphate buffer, pH 8.0.

The Formalin-treated pyruvaldehyde-stabilized human erythrocytes (FPHE) are washed once with 0.1 M acetate buffer, pH 4.0, and resuspended to 10%. A 1-ml amount of FPHE is added to a siliconized tube containing an equal volume of IgG/HB Ab diluted in the same acetate buffer. The volume is adjusted to 10 ml with the 0.1 M acetate buffer, pH 4.0, and the reactants are incubated for 60 min at 25 C with constant shaking. The cell suspension is washed five times in 0.15 M phosphate buffer, pH 7.2, and resuspended to 1%. To determine the optimal concentration of IgG needed to coat the red cells, various concentrations of the HB Ab/IgG preparation are used, and that dilution is selected which yields optimal titers against HB Ag-positive sera. In this laboratory, a range of 0.25 to 0.5 mg/ml has worked well.

The coated cells can be stored at 4 C for at least 1 month or at −70 or −196 C (10% suspension) for at least 4 months. To store cells in liquid nitrogen (−196 C), the 10% FPHE suspension is placed in a 5-ml syringe fitted with a 21-gauge needle and added dropwise to a receptacle containing liquid nitrogen. Each drop forms a sphere on contacting the liquid nitrogen, floats at the surface, and falls to the bottom as a pellet when frozen. Thawing of the FPHE pellets is done in saline at 37 C in a water bath, but temperature is not critical for these stabilized cells. They are washed once or twice in the RCA diluent which consists of 0.15 M phosphate buffer, pH 7.2, containing 0.4% gelatin and are resuspended as a 0.15% cell suspension. Reproducibility of results is enhanced by using a spectrophotometer to determine the correct cell suspension. A wavelength of 540 was selected and an OD reading of 1.500 was obtained for a 0.15% suspension (Gilford 240 spectrophotometer). Subsequent cell suspensions were compared with this value and appropriate dilutions were made to achieve the correct cell suspension; e.g., final OD_{540} of unknown divided by target OD_{540} of 1.500 times the original volume of cell suspension equals final volume.

Beginning at a 1:5 dilution, sera are diluted twofold (25 μliters) in the RCA diluent in Linbro Microtiter "V" plates (IS-MVC-96, processed, Linbro Chemical Co., New Haven, Conn.). To each well is added 25 μliters of the 0.15% coated FPHE with constant shaking. Control wells include dilutions of sera tested against FPHE coated with nonimmune IgG, and HB Ag positive and negative reference sera tested against HB Ab-coated FPHE. Plates are sealed with adhesive tape and incubated at room temperature for 3 h; the RCA patterns are then read. Hemagglutination is observed in the presence of HB Ag. Depending on the concentration of HB Ab present in the IgG preparation used to coat the cells, a prozone may occur with high-titered HB Ag positive sera. Therefore, several dilutions may be necessary to avoid a false-negative result. Sterility of the RCA diluent is important since bacterial contamination can result in nonspecific agglutination.

For subtyping, monospecific IgG containing anti-*d* or anti-*y* is obtained by adsorbing antisera with the heterologous HB Ag subtype which has been cross-linked with glutaraldehyde to form an insoluble immunoadsorbent (4). HB Ag used for cross-linking is concentrated from plasma by precipitation at pH 4.6 with polyethylene glycol 6000 at a final concentration of 8 g/100 ml. The pellet is redissolved in distilled water to its original volume, and is then repelleted at 176,000 × *g* for 5 h at 4 C. Anti-*a* can be recovered from the immunoadsorbent with 0.1 M glycine-HCl, pH 2.8, at 4 C for 30 min followed by dialysis against a 0.1 M phosphate buffer, pH 7.2. If necessary, the monospecific antibody can be concentrated by Amicon diafiltration with a PM-30 filter. These preparations are used to coat the red cells and can specifically detect their respective subtypes (11).

PASSIVE HEMAGGLUTINATION

The PHA technique is an excellent and rapid method for detecting HB Ab, rivaling the RIA for sensitivity (10, 22, 23). Human type O, Rh-negative erythrocytes are collected in Alsever's solution or EDTA and allowed to "age" at 4 C for 1 to 2 days prior to use. The plasma is separated from the cells and saved for later use, and the buffy coat is then removed. The cells are washed four times in 0.15 M NaCl by centrifugation at 1,500 × *g* for 15 min at 4 C. A 40% suspension is prepared in 0.15 M NaCl. Erythrocytes are sensitized by rapidly mixing (within 1 to 2 min) equal volumes (25 μliters) of the 40% cell suspension and purified HB Ag with varying dilutions of a freshly prepared and filtered 1% stock solution of chromic chloride ($CrCl_3 \cdot 6H_2O$) dissolved in water. All reactants used for sensitization must be diluted in 0.15 M NaCl since the presence of any buffer will result in the removal of chromium ions by the production of insoluble chromic hydroxide above pH 5.5 and a failure to sensitize the cells. The chromic chloride stock solution is approximately pH 2.8. It is important to establish optimal sensitization of the erythrocytes in a preliminary two-dimensional microtiter test by using various concentrations of purified HB Ag against several dilutions of $CrCl_3$ between 1:10 and 1:30. Appropriate saline controls are also included (10). In my experience, excellent sensitization occurs when HB Ag is used at concentrations from 50 to 400 μg/ml with a $CrCl_3$ dilution of 1:18 or 1:22. The cells are shaken at room temperature for 8 min, washed four times in saline, and then resuspended as a 0.2% suspension in the TPB-PBS test diluent (PBS, pH 7.2, containing 0.0025% polyvinylpyrrolidone K-90, 0.005% Tween 80, and 0.5% bovine albumin). An HB Ab and NHS titration is performed against each set of variables. Those conditions resulting in optimal sensitization without loss of specificity are used to prepare a larger batch of sensitized cells during which mixing time should be extended to 12 min.

Coated cells are prepared for storage at −196 C by use of a modification of the method originally described by Huntsman et al. (12). Equal volumes of a 50% suspension of coated cells in saline, autologous undiluted plasma, and 40% sucrose are mixed gently for 5 min, cooled to 4 C, and added dropwise with a 5-ml syringe and a 21-gauge needle to liquid nitrogen as previously described in the RCA test. Each pellet contains enough cells for one Microtiter plate. Unlike the stabilized red cells used in the RCA test, the temperature at which the $CrCl_3$-sensitized cells are thawed becomes critical if hemolysis is to be avoided. Pellets removed from the liquid nitrogen are added immediately to prewarmed (42 C) saline. These cells are then washed three times in saline, and a 0.2% suspension is prepared in TPB-PBS by use of the spectrophotometric method described in the RCA test. The target OD_{540} in this laboratory is 1.000 (Gilford 240 spectrophotometer).

Sera are diluted 1:4 in TPB-PBS diluent and heat-inactivated at 56 C for 20 min. Twofold dilutions (25 μliters) are prepared in Microtiter "V" plates (no. 220-25, Cooke) with the TPB-PBS diluent. The 0.2% sensitized cells (25 μliters) are added to each well and mixed by shaking. Control wells include serum dilutions with unsensitized erythrocytes (washed and stored in liquid nitrogen as described above) and positive and negative reference sera. The Microtiter plates are sealed with adhesive tape and incubated at room temperature (25 C) for 30 min, then at 4 C for 2 h. After this incubation period, the plates are placed in Microtiter centrifuge carriers (no. 200-18, Cooke) and centrifuged at 300 × *g* for 1 min at 4 C in an International PR-6 centrifuge with a no. 276 head. They are then placed at a 60° angle at 25 C for 60 min before being read. A positive result is represented by agglutinated cells which form a discrete button and which do not slide down the side of the wells. This pattern of agglutination is relatively stable. Although cells have been prepared with HB Ag subtype *ad* which have broad reactivity, some HB Ab directed against subtype *ay* may be missed. The use of cells sensitized with a mixture of *ad* and *ay* subtypes may alleviate this problem, or both subtypes may be used individually.

INTERPRETATION, EVALUATION, AND REPORTING OF RESULTS

Successful detection of HB Ag or HB Ab depends not only on the relative sensitivity of the test procedure but also on the availability of experienced personnel who comprehend the procedure and its idiosyncrasies, and who are meticulous in their performance of the test. Under these conditions, the final evaluation and interpretation of any positive test result will be determined by the specificity of the reagents used. It is essential for the diagnostic virologist to appreciate the difficulties encountered in preparing purified HB Ag which is completely free from NHS proteins. Purified antigen preparations almost invariably result in the production of low concentrations of antibodies to NHS during immunization. If this possibility remains unrecognized, a positive result may be falsely attributed to an HB Ag-HB Ab reaction rather than to a reaction between NHS proteins and their respective antibodies. The AGD, CEP, and CF tests are particularly predisposed to this kind of nonspecificity, whereas the RIA-DA and RCA tests are apparently unaffected. In general, such false-positive results do not occur with undiluted sera since the test is conducted in extreme antigen (NHS) excess. However, the testing of serum specimens at high dilutions, gradient fractions, or specimens containing low concentrations of human proteins, e.g., urine, stool, or saliva, can result in a false-positive reaction. This problem can be eliminated by preliminary adsorption of the antisera with an insoluble immunoadsorbent prepared from NHS. In other instances, the specificity of a test can be verified by a blocking or inhibition test in which 10 to 25 μliters of a high-titered human or experimental animal HB antiserum is mixed with 100 μliters of the sample. The reactants are incubated for 2 h at 37 C and then 18 h at 4 C, and the results are compared with those obtained with the same specimen incubated with NHS and with PBS.

It should be emphasized that the comparative sensitivity of a test is only one reason for choosing a specific assay system. The marked increase in sensitivity of the RIA or RCA tests when compared to the discontinuous CEP test should not imply that an equivalent increase in the number of HB Ag positive persons will be detected. Experience indicates that this is an unlikely possibility since low concentrations (below that detected by CEP) of HB Ag in the population are uncommon. This is especially true for the majority of clinical specimens sent to the laboratory.

The presence of HB Ag in the serum of a patient or blood donor indicates infection with type B hepatitis of unknown duration. The "carrier" designation should be limited to those individuals who continue to circulate HB Ag for a period of 3 months or longer. In a typical infection with HBV, HB Ag will be detected by the RIA test 2 to 4 weeks before the transaminase level becomes abnormally elevated and 4 to 6 weeks before the patient becomes jaundiced or develops other symptoms. HB Ab may develop shortly after jaundice appears, associated with a precipitous fall in the HB Ag titer, or antibody may not be detected until 1 or 2 months later. It is conceivable that a specimen might be obtained during a phase in which equivalent or near-equivalent proportions of HB Ag and HB Ab are present. Since this would result in a negative test reaction, a second specimen should be requested 4 weeks later if definitive diagnosis is important. Passive transfer of HB Ab is observed in approximately 40% of patients receiving HB Ab positive blood transfusions, and should not be confused with seroconversion due to exposure to HB Ag or infection with HBV. Passively transferred HB Ab is detected immediately after transfusion and gradually disappears over the next 2 months. HB Ab levels, once developed as a response to HB Ag, are remarkably stable over several years.

HB Ag results are currently reported as "positive" or "negative" without stipulating a titer. In most cases, no additional benefit is derived from titering the specimen, although in certain instances this may be requested. The RCA and CF tests are practical and rapid methods for obtaining the HB Ag titer.

Subtyping of specimens by the clinical laboratory provides additional information to the clinician or hospital epidemiologist, since the mutually exclusive *d* and *y* subdeterminants are virus-specific and not host-determined. This can be helpful in determining the source of infection or can provide epidemiological evidence for the relatedness among cases.

LITERATURE CITED

1. Aach, R. D., J. W. Grisham, and C. W. Parker. 1971. Detection of Australia antigen by radioimmunoassay. Proc. Nat. Acad. Sci. U.S.A. **68:**1056–1060.
2. Aach, R. D., E. J. Hacker, and C. W. Parker. 1973. Recognition of hepatitis B antigen determinants by a double label radioimmunoassay: a sensitive means of subtyping hepatitis B antigen. J. Immunol. **111:**381–388.
3. Almeida, J. D., D. Rubenstein, and E. J. Stott. 1971. New antigen-antibody system in Australia-antigen-positive hepatitis. Lancet **2:**1225–1227.
4. Avraemeas, S., and T. Ternynck. 1969. The cross-linking of proteins with glutaraldehyde and its use for the preparation of immunoadsorbents. Immunochemistry **6:**53–66.
5. Blumberg, B. S., A. I. Sutnick, W. T. London, and I. Millman. 1971. The discovery of Australia antigen and its relation to viral hepatitis. Perspect. Virol. **7:**223–240.
6. Dreesman, G. R., F. B. Hollinger, R. M. McCombs, and J. L. Melnick. 1972. Production of potent anti-Australia antigen sera of high specificity and sensitivity in goats. Infect. Immunity **5:**213–221.
7. Dreesman, G. R., F. B. Hollinger, and J. L. Melnick. 1972. Detection of hepatitis B antigen by counterimmunoelectrophoresis: enhancing role of homologous serum diluents. Appl. Microbiol. **24:**1001–1002.
8. Hirata, A. A., and M. W. Brandriss. 1968. Passive hemagglutination procedures for protein and polysaccharide antigens using erythrocytes stabilized by aldehydes. J. Immunol. **100:**641–646.
9. Hollinger, F. B. 1972. Radioimmunoassay for detection of hepatitis-associated antigen (HB Ag), p. 167–170. *In* G. N. Vyas, H. A. Perkins, and R. Schmid (ed.), Hepatitis and blood transfusion. Grune & Stratton, Inc., New York.
10. Hollinger, F. B., V. Vorndam, and G. R. Dreesman. 1971. Assay of Australia antigen and antibody employing double-antibody and solid-phase radioimmunoassay techniques and comparison with the passive hemagglutination methods. J. Immunol. **107:**1099–1111.
11. Hollinger, F. B., C. Wasi, G. R. Dreesman, and J. L. Melnick. 1973. Subtyping hepatitis B antigen using monospecific antibody-coated cells. J. Infec. Dis. **128:**753–760.
12. Huntsman, R. G., B. A. L. Hurn, E. W. Ikin, H. Lehmann, and J. Liddell. 1962. Blood groups and enzymes of human red cells after a year's storage in liquid nitrogen. Brit. Med. J. **2:**1508–1514.
13. Krugman, S., and J. P. Giles. 1970. Viral hepatitis. New light on an old disease. J. Amer. Med. Ass. **212:**1019–1029.
14. Lander, J. J., H. J. Alter, and R. H. Purcell. 1971. Frequency of antibody to hepatitis-associated antigen as measured by a new radioimmunoassay technique. J. Immunol. **106:**1166–1171.
15. Ling, C. M., and L. R. Overby. 1972. Prevalence of hepatitis B virus antigen as revealed by direct radioimmune assay with ^{125}I-antibody. J. Immunol. **109:**834–841.
16. London, W. T., H. J. Alter, J. Lander, and R. H. Purcell. 1972. Serial transmission in rhesus monkeys of an agent

related to hepatitis-associated antigen. J. Infec. Dis. **125**:382–389.
17. Melnick, J. L., and F. B. Hollinger. 1972. Hepatitis virology, p. 345–365. *In* H. Popper and F. Schaffner (ed.), Progress in liver diseases, vol. 4. Grune & Stratton, Inc., New York.
18. Midgley, A. R., Jr., G. D. Niswander, and R. W. Rebar. 1969. Principles for the assessment of the reliability of radioimmunoassay methods (precision, accuracy, sensitivity, specificity). Acta Endocrinol. (Copenhagen) **63**(Suppl. 142):163–180; 247–254.
19. Ouchterlony, Ö. 1958. Diffusion-in-gel methods for immunological analysis. Progr. Allergy **5**:1–78.
20. Rodbard, D., P. L. Rayford, J. A. Cooper, and G. T. Ross. 1968. Statistical quality control of radioimmunoassays. J. Clin. Endocrinol. **28**:1412–1418.
21. Sgouris, J. T. 1973. Limitations of the radioimmunoassay for hepatitis B antigen. N. Engl. J. Med. **288**:160–161.
22. Vyas, G. N., M. A. Mason, and E. W. Williams. 1972. Detection of hepatitis B antigen and antibodies by hemagglutination assay, p. 137–145. *In* G. N. Vyas, H. A. Perkins, and R. Schmid (ed.), Hepatitis and blood transfusion. Grune & Stratton, Inc., New York.
23. Vyas, G. N., and N. R. Shulman. 1970. Hemagglutination assay for antigen and antibody associated with viral hepatitis. Science **170**:131–132.
24. Wallis, C., and J. L. Melnick. 1971. Enhanced detection of Australia antigen in serum hepatitis patients by discontinuous counter-immunoelectrophoresis. Appl. Microbiol. **21**:867–869.
25. Walsh, J. H., R. Yalow, and S. A. Berson. 1970. Detection of Australia antigen and antibody by means of radioimmunoassay techniques. J. Infec. Dis. **121**:550–554.
26. Ward, R., and S. Krugman. 1962. Etiology, epidemiology and prevention of viral hepatitis. Progr. Med. Virol. **4**:87–118.
27. World Health Organization Consultation on Viral Hepatitis. 1970. Viral hepatitis and tests for the Australia (hepatitis-associated) antigen and antibody. Bull. World Health Organ. **42**:957–992.
28. World Health Organization Scientific Group. 1973. Viral hepatitis. World Health Organ. Tech. Rep. Ser. 512.
29. Zuckerman, A. J. 1972. Hepatitis-associated antigen and viruses, p. 187–201. American Elsevier Publishing Co., New York.

Chapter 90A
Classification of Viruses

JOSEPH L. MELNICK

Viruses are separated into groups on the basis of the type and form of the nucleic acid genome and the size, shape, substructure, and mode of replication of the virus particle. Within each group, subgroupings are usually based on antigenicity.

A significant development in classification and nomenclature of viruses was the first report of the International Committee on Nomenclature of Viruses (ICNV), published in 1971. The report deals with viruses of man, lower animals, insects, plants, and bacteria, and includes summaries of the properties of 43 groups of viruses for which current knowledge permits at least tentative classification. Two of the groups have been officially designated as virus families, *Papovaviridae* and *Picornaviridae*, and subgroups have been designated as genera. For other groups, the tentative status of a genus has been given, but official designation of family status for at least five of these (*Adenoviridae*, *Herpesviridae*, *Poxviridae*, *Togaviridae*, and *Reoviridae*) seems certain. For more detailed discussion of virus classification, nomenclature, and ultrastructure, the reader is referred to references 1–4.

In Tables 1 and 2, properties of the major groups of deoxyribonucleic acid (DNA)-containing and ribonucleic acid (RNA)-containing animal viruses are summarized. Since most of these groups are discussed more fully in the other chapters of this volume, the brief text which follows is confined to commentary on the tables, with some further discussion of certain virus groups whose members, although not currently considered major pathogens of man, may have future interest for clinical virology.

In Tables 1 and 2, the type of nucleic acid is indicated, but not its form. All of the virus groups listed in Table 1 have a genome of double-stranded DNA except the *parvovirus* (*picodnavirus*) group, whose DNA is single-stranded within the virion. This group includes viruses of rodents and swine, but also has some members, adeno-satellite serotypes, which are indigenous to man, although without known association with human disease. As indicated in Table 1, these very small viruses are about 20 nm in diameter, have cubic symmetry, naked virions, and are ether resistant. Some members also are resistant to high temperatures (60 C, 30 min). Replication and capsid assembly take place in the nucleus of the infected cell. The 32 capsomeres are each 2 to 4 nm in diameter. The molecular weight of the nucleic acid in the virion is relatively very small, 1.4×10^6, as compared, for example, with 160×10^6 for poxvirus DNA. It has been estimated that the number of genes making up the small parvovirus genome is approximately seven. *Subgenus A* of the parvovirus group includes the autonomously replicating parvoviruses: hamster osteolytic H viruses, latent rat viruses (Kilham rat virus, X14 virus), minute mouse virus, and a parvovirus of swine. The DNA of these nondefective, autonomously replicating members of the group appears to be single stranded both before and after extraction, indicating that strands of similar polarity are present in all virions. As will be seen below, this is in contrast to the nonautonomous, defective viruses of the other subgroup. *Subgenus B* consists of the adeno-associated satellite viruses, which are defective and cannot multiply in the absence of a replicating adenovirus which serves as a "helper virus." Herpesvirus can act as a partial helper; in cells co-infected with herpesvirus, infectious satellite DNA and capsid proteins are made, but they are not assembled into satellite virions. The single-stranded DNA genome has been shown to be present within the satellite virion as either plus or minus complementary strands in separate particles. Upon extraction, the minus and plus DNA strands unite to form a double-stranded helix.

Members of the *papovavirus* group (see Table 1) have DNA in double-stranded circular form. The human representatives are the papilloma or wart virus and an SV40-like virus isolated from patients with progressive multifocal leukoencephalopathy. Other members include papillomaviruses of rabbits and cattle, polyoma and K viruses of mice, and vacuolating viruses of monkeys (simian virus 40 [SV40]) and of rabbits. These viruses have relatively slow growth cycles characterized by replication within the nucleus. Papovaviruses produce latent and chronic infections in their natural hosts. All are tumorigenic in at least some animal host species. For this virus family, *Papovaviridae*, two genera have been designated: *Subgroup A* includes the agents producing papillomata in man and a variety of animals and *Subgroup B* includes mouse polyoma, monkey SV40, and the newly recognized human members mentioned above. When SV40 and adenoviruses replicate together, they may interact to form "hybrid" virus particles, in which a defective SV40 genome is covalently linked to adenovirus DNA and is carried within an adenovirus capsid.

Among the viruses with an RNA genome (Table 2), the *reovirus* group (family *Reoviridae*) is unique in having double-stranded RNA, in contrast to the single-stranded form characteristic of the other RNA-containing viruses. This property and other important characteristics are shared not only by the human and animal reoviruses but also by a number of other viruses, including the agents of Colorado tick fever, bluetongue, African horse-

TABLE 1. *Current classification of animal DNA viruses*[a]

Nucleic acid core				DNA	
Capsid symmetry			Cubic		Complex
Virion: naked or enveloped		Naked		Enveloped	Complex coats
Site of capsid assembly[b]		Nucleus		Nucleus	Cytoplasm
Site of nucleocapsid envelopment				Nuclear membrane	
Reaction to ether treatment		Resistant		Sensitive	Resistant
Number of capsomeres	32	72	252	162	
Diameter of virion (nm)[c]	18–22	43–53	70–90	100[d]	230 × 300
Molecular weight of nucleic acid in virion (× 10^6)	1.4	3–5	23	54–92	160
Virus group	Parvo- (Picodna-) virus	PAPOVA-VIRUS[e]	ADENO-VIRUS	HERPES-VIRUS	POXVIRUS
Typical member[f]	Adeno-associated satellite virus	SV40	Adenovirus	Herpes simplex virus	Vaccinia virus

[a] From reference 3, vol. 16, 1973.

[b] For the DNA viruses whose capsid assembly takes place in the nucleus, a phase of replication occurs in the cytoplasm, as evidenced by the detection of viral messenger RNA associated with polyribosomes.

[c] Diameter, or diameter × length.

[d] The naked virus is 100 nm in diameter; however, the enveloped virions range up to 150 nm.

[e] Where the group name is shown in capital letters, viruses have been given a family designation.

[f] The agents shown are among the most generally familiar members of the group, and are not in every instance the officially designated type species.

TABLE 2. *Current classification of animal RNA viruses*[a]

Nucleic acid core	RNA										
Capsid symmetry	Cubic					Helical			Unknown		
Virion: naked or enveloped	Naked			Enveloped		Enveloped			Enveloped		
Site of capsid assembly	Cytoplasm			Cytoplasm		Cytoplasm			Cytoplasm		
Site of nucleocapsid envelopment				Surface membrane	Intracytoplasmic membranes	Surface membrane			Surface membrane		Intracytoplasmic membranes
Reaction to ether treatment	Resistant			Sensitive	Sensitive	Sensitive			Sensitive		Sensitive
Number of capsomeres / Diameter of helix (nm)	32	32	92	32	?	6–9	18	18			
Diameter of virion[b]	20–30	60–80	75–80	40–70	40–50	90–120	150–300	70 × 175	About 100	50–150	70–120
Molecular weight of nucleic acid in virion ($\times 10^6$)	2–2.8	15	15	3	3	2–4	4–8	3–4	10–13	3.2	?
Virus group	PICORNA-VIRUS[c] Entero- Rhino- Calici- virus	Orbivirus (REOVIRUS)	Reovirus (REOVIRUS)	Alphavirus (TOGAVIRUS)	Flavivirus (TOGAVIRUS)	Orthomyxovirus[d]	Paramyxovirus[d]	Rhabdovirus	Oncornavirus	Arenavirus	Coronavirus
Typical member[e]	Poliovirus	Bluetongue virus	Reovirus	Sindbis virus	Yellow fever virus	Influenza virus	Newcastle disease virus	Vesicular stomatitis virus	Rous sarcoma virus	Lymphocytic choriomeningitis virus	Avian infectious bronchitis virus

[a] From reference 3, vol. 16, 1973.
[b] Diameter, or diameter × length.
[c] Where the group name is shown in capital letters, viruses have been given a family designation.
[d] Pneumonia virus of mice is intermediate between the orthomyxoviruses and paramyxoviruses, in that the diameter of its helix is 12 to 15 nm. Respiratory syncytial virus

sickness, and epizootic hemorrhagic disease of deer (EHD). For these latter viruses, a separate subgroup (genus) has been proposed, and the genus name *Orbivirus* (Latin *orbis*, ring) has been suggested, to represent the unusually large doughnut-shaped capsomeres, 10 to 15 nm wide, which they exhibit in negative contrast preparations.

Members of the *oncornavirus* (RNA tumor virus) group are of particular interest as animal models of oncogenic viruses, and also because of recent findings, in certain human leukemias, lymphomas and sarcomas, of particles containing high-molecular-weight (70*S*) RNA and reverse transcriptase characteristic of oncornaviruses. Established members of the oncornavirus group include the leukemia and sarcoma viruses of mice, cats, fowl, and monkeys. A relationship between the above-mentioned human particles and murine leukemia virus exists, in that the DNA product of the reverse transcriptase of the murine oncornavirus hybridizes with RNA of polysomes of human sarcoma cells. Reciprocally, the DNA synthesized by the human particles containing the 70*S* RNA and reverse transcriptase hybridizes with the RNA of the murine oncornavirus.

In addition, oncornaviruses are known to be the etiologic agents of mammary tumors of mice (MTV), and a similar virus has been isolated from a monkey mammary tumor. Particles resembling the murine mammary tumor virus (B type particles) have been recently detected in human mammary cancer and in the milk of women with a family history of mammary cancer. The infectious nature of these particles is unknown, but they also contain the high-molecular-weight 70*S* RNA and reverse transcriptase enzyme activity characteristic of oncornaviruses. Preliminary data indicate a relationship between these human particles and MTV, in that DNA derived from the RNA-DNA hybrid obtained in vitro by the MTV enzyme from MTV substrate has been shown to hybridize not only with messenger RNA derived from mouse mammary tumors but also with messenger RNA obtained from human mammary tumors.

Those members of the *coronavirus* group which cause respiratory illnesses in man are extremely fastidious in their growth requirements, making routine isolation difficult. However, serological evidence indicates that these agents may be a major cause of respiratory illness in adults during winter months when the prevalence of colds is high but the isolation of rhinoviruses or other respiratory viruses is low. The complement fixation test is a more sensitive index of human coronavirus infection than is virus isolation with the tissue culture or organ culture systems in use at present. Members of this group are enveloped, 70 to 120 nm in size, and the nucleocapsid is thought to be helical, 7 to 9 nm in diameter. They thus morphologically resemble the orthomyxoviruses, except that the surface projections of coronaviruses are petal shaped; this fringe of projections, resembling the solar corona, suggested the group name. The coronaviruses of man ("infectious bronchitis virus-like viruses") have been isolated from patients primarily through the use of human embryonic tracheal and nasal organ cultures. Coronaviruses of lower animals include avian infectious bronchitis virus, mouse hepatitis virus, transmissible gastroenteritis virus of swine, and probably rat pneumonotropic virus.

There are some human viral pathogens for which insufficient biochemical and biophysical data are available to permit their classification in any of the groups described in the tables. These include viruses which cause infectious and serum hepatitis (hepatitis A and B, respectively), and viruses responsible for certain immune complex diseases and neurological disorders characterized by a long latent period ("slow" virus diseases). In addition, a number of arboviruses remain unclassified except for their classic ecological and serological groupings; however, the rapidly growing body of information on their physical and chemical characteristics has made it possible to place many of these agents in the classification scheme described here, notably the arthropod-borne members of the togavirus family; other arboviruses belong to the rhabdovirus, reovirus, and arenavirus groups. Members of the large Bunyamwera supergroup are likely candidates for the next major entry of arboviruses into a classification based on properties of the virus particle.

LITERATURE CITED

1. Andrewes, C., and H. G. Pereira. 1972. Viruses of vertebrates, 3rd ed. The Williams & Wilkins Co., Baltimore.
2. Lwoff, A., and P. Tournier. 1971. Remarks on the classification of viruses, p. 1–42. *In* K. Maramorosch and E. Kurstak ed., Comparative virology. Academic Press Inc., New York.
3. Melnick, J. L. 1966–1974. Summaries on viral classification and nomenclature. Published annually in Progress in Medical Virology. Karger, Basel.
4. Wildy, P. 1971. Classification and nomenclature of viruses: first report of the International Committee on Nomenclature of Viruses. Monographs in Virology, vol. 5, Karger, Basel.

Section X

INFECTION PREVENTION—QUALITY CONTROL

Chapter 91

Control of Hospital-Associated Infections

A. Infection Surveillance and Control

RAYMOND C. BARTLETT

INTRODUCTION

About 2 million of the 30 million patients admitted to the nation's hospitals each year develop hospital-associated infections. This represents an attack rate of at least 5% and constitutes a waste of patient days of treatment representing an economic loss of at least $500,000,000 per year. This significant morbidity and mortality has resulted in a number of publications (2, 4, 5, 8–10), national and international conferences (6, 7), the National Nosocomial Infection Survey conducted by the Center for Disease Control (CDC), Atlanta, Ga., and a greatly expanded definition of the responsibility of hospital Infection Control Committees by the Joint Commission on Accreditation of Hospitals (JCAH; 1).

The majority of patients who develop these infections are afflicted without any clear evidence of cross-infection or contact with an identifiable environmental source. It is well established that substantial numbers are caused by bacteria which are brought into the hospital by the patient himself. These organisms become invasive only because normal body defense mechanisms become deranged by simultaneous occurrence of disease and exposure to drugs and mechanical irritants. These factors which predispose the host to infection, combined with the health and practices of personnel and the condition of the institutional environment, contribute in varying proportions to the risk of hospital-associated infection.

OBSTACLES TO CONTROL EFFORTS

Workers in individual hospitals have encountered numerous obstacles in attempting to develop effective measures for control of these infections. Superficial and inadequate systems for surveillance of incidence which depend upon reporting by physicians or nurses often result in a false impression of inconsequential numbers of cases. Few or no funds are allocated for materials and personnel to conduct a satisfactory surveillance and educational activity under the supervision of an Infection Control Committee. Physician members of Infection Control Committees usually have little time to participate directly in surveillance and control activities or to conduct special education programs for allied health personnel. Frequently these committees place the burden on the microbiologist by establishing environmental sampling as a substitute for a more comprehensive and effective program of infection surveillance, education, and control. To make matters worse, laboratory workers often are coerced into performance of sampling techniques for which no interpretative standards exist. Many physicians and administrators do not realize that the prevalence of microbial species in the hospital environment must be studied quantitatively and the results must be statistically analyzed with reference to well-established published standards if significant and useful epidemiological information is to be produced. The published recommendations of the JCAH have clearly stated the responsibility of the Infection Control Committee to be broad surveillance of the incidence of nosocomial infection as well as surveillance and control of predisposing factors among patients, personnel, and the environment (1). Microbiological sampling of the environment never has been a specific JCAH recommendation or requirement.

ORGANIZATION OF CONTROL EFFORTS

An Infection Control Committee requires adequate input to assess the frequency of nosocomial infection and factors predisposing to it. This will consist of efficient surveillance of all patients to provide rapid detection of such infections and evidence of routes of cross-infection. Selective monitoring of personnel and the hospital environment may be required from time to time to investigate specific problems. These activities require the time of a trained individual capable of interpreting medical records and of conducting studies of predisposing factors involving the patient, personnel, and the environment. This information must be analyzed by the committee which then may develop recommendations to control predisposing factors through improvements in institutional practices.

EDUCATION AND TRAINING OF PERSONNEL

Changes in personnel practices and institutional policies may be accomplished through written regulations and memorandums, but these must be supplemented by an outreaching educational program which will convince personnel that the recommendations are important and are based on supporting evidence. A physician member of the committee, usually the chairman, should meet periodically with members of the medical staff to review observations and recommendations of the committee. Effective infection control measures are practiced by hospital personnel only because they are convinced of their value and not because they have been legislated by a committee. This requires repeated contact with small numbers of personnel by a highly skilled and informed representative of the Infection Control Committee. Such an individual must have the ability to establish good rapport with all types of hospital workers, from staff physicians to building maintenance and housekeeping workers. Most hospitals have employed nurses for this task. Their broad clinical training and experience in direct patient care provide them with maximal insight into the complex human relationships which exist among doctors, nurses, and their patients, and the difficulty of maintaining a high priority for day to day practice of essential control measures. Medical technologists, microbiologists, and sanitarians have been delegated these responsibilities in some institutions. There is a natural tendency for all but the nurse to become excessively engaged in surveillance and control of environmental factors because of their greater knowledge and ease of operation in that setting, in contrast to the more human and subjective milieu of doctors, nurses, and patients, in which the most useful surveillance and control will be accomplished.

Many hospitals have allocated insufficient paid manpower to the functions of the Infection Control Committee. This has often restricted activity to collection of incidence data, leaving insufficient time for education of personnel. The committee and its epidemiologist, or other infection control officer, will "control" very little if there is insufficient time to do any more than collect information. One nurse epidemiologist or other worker assigned to this task should be provided for each 300 to 500 hospital beds.

Training programs for nurse epidemiologists are available at the CDC and at some hospitals with recognized infection control programs.

RECOGNITION AND CONTROL OF PREDISPOSING FACTORS

Although control measures should be related to observation of recognized predisposing factors through surveillance, every Infection Control Committee should review periodically control of commonly recognized predisposing factors. The following items are listed to draw attention to the diverse activities which may require evaluation and modification.

1. *Personnel factors:* (i) handwashing; (ii) standards and practices for isolation and selected precautions in accord with CDC recommendations (8); (iii) aseptic procedures for wound dressing changes, irrigation and soaks, percutaneous instrumentation, catheterization and instrumentation of veins and urinary bladders, suction and maintenance of respiratory tract, tracheostomy and use of inhalation therapy equipment, minor and major surgery, scrub and clothing practices in surgery, and nursery practices; (iv) traffic in intensive care, surgery, and nurseries; (v) infections in personnel (provide excused time at hospital expense); (vi) treatment of personnel exposed to communicable disease (only by employee health service); (vii) reporting of communicable disease (preferably by nurse epidemiologist).

2. *Environmental factors:* (i) housekeeping standards, procedures, materials, and actual practices in general patient care areas, in isolation units, and in the operating room; (ii) laundry standards—procedures, materials, and actual practices for contaminated linens, temperatures of washing and drying, and used mopheads; (iii) ventilation (air changes per minute, recirculation, humidification, filtration), repair of defects in floors, solid and liquid waste disposal, design and renovation of intensive care units, isolation units, and operating rooms, and maintenance and monitoring of autoclaves; (iv) standards and practices for cleaning, sterilizing, and storage of equipment in central service and operating rooms; (v) disinfection and antisepsis in nursing units and operating rooms; (vi) maintenance of inhalation therapy and anesthesia equipment; (vii) handling of contaminated drainage and suction systems; (viii) contamination of soaps, antiseptics, lotions, medications, ice machines, and water carafes; (ix) excessive storage and clutter in intensive care units and operating rooms; (x) dietary sources of pathogens, inadequate washing of tableware; (xi) contamination of intravenous fluid systems; (xii) hepatitis hazards (dis-

posal of needles, laboratory exposure); (xiii) control of sterility of irrigation water in cystoscopy; (xiv) skin preparation, maintenance of clippers, disposable razors; (xv) maintenance of bottle warmers in nurseries.

3. *Host factors:* (i) antibiotic usage; (ii) unnecessarily prolonged use of intravenous and urinary catheters, inhalation therapy, intubation, etc.; (iii) existence of diseases and physiological conditions predisposing to infection; (iv) protracted period of hospitalization before surgery; (v) risk of colonization with potential pathogens; (vi) immunosuppression.

The ability to evaluate and modify these activities depends on a basic knowledge of "nursing arts." Nurses should supplement this background with intensive training courses, reading, and several years of clinical experience. Others, including physicians and microbiologists, will have to acquire all of it from postgraduate programs and on-the-job experience. Considerable assistance will be required from medical specialists, pharmacists, sanitarians, engineers, and other professionals with unique training and experience. State health departments and the Bureau of Epidemiology of the CDC represent a valuable resource.

ROLE OF THE MICROBIOLOGIST

As a member of the Infection Control Committee

The JCAH recommends that someone, preferably the pathologist or microbiologist, represent the clinical laboratory on the Infection Control Committee (1). It should be obvious that an effective infection control program will depend upon a well-supervised and directed microbiology laboratory. This resource must be effectively and efficiently used by the Infection Control Committee. The microbiologist must be cognizant of the limitations of methods which may be used for evaluation of environmental contamination and the efficacy of disinfectants and antiseptics. No decision to culture personnel or the inanimate environment, or to evaluate disinfectants and antiseptics microbiologically, should be made by the committee without a complete discussion of the problem and potential courses of action.

Can microbiological evaluation contribute to definition of the problem? Can it support a decision to recommend action? Do members of the committee, especially representatives of the medical staff and administration, agree in advance to support any recommendations that might ensue? Too often, large numbers of cultures are taken, and after the data are examined it becomes apparent that no accepted values for interpretation exist. When interpretative standards are applicable and support recommendation for action, economic and administrative obstacles that could have been anticipated often preclude any change in institutional practice. These pitfalls must be avoided if the microbiologist is to prevent wasteful dissipation of time and resources.

Cost and technology

Current methods, criteria for microbial identification, and internal quality control of the precision and accuracy of performance of clinical microbiology in the hospital's laboratory provide essential support for an effective infection control program. Costly and time-consuming refinements often are proposed in laboratory procedures because they contribute to the collection of epidemiological data. The microbiologist should provide the hospital's administrative representative to the committee with an accounting of the cost of any existing or proposed work which is not a convenient byproduct of procedures used for diagnosis and treatment. If the committee agrees that the benefits appear to justify the cost, the procedure may be introduced, but the added cost should be allocated to infection control, not subsidized by the laboratory.

Recently, a few microbiologists have expressed the opinion publicly that routine anaerobic culture of all specimens and complete speciation of all isolates is essential for infection control. Such a recommendation is without scientific justification and fails to acknowledge increasing public reaction to rising health care costs. Similarly, serotyping of *Klebsiella pneumoniae* isolates has limited diagnostic and therapeutic significance. If this is to be conducted, the cost would be allocated to infection control. Reference laboratories may provide serotyping, phage typing, bacteriocin typing, etc., when this is of epidemiological value.

It has been recommended that all *Enterobacter* isolates be completely speciated because of the association of *E. agglomerans* with contaminated intravenous fluids. Although this observation is primarily of epidemiological interest, the opportunistic nature of this species compared with other *Enterobacter* species renders such a differentiation clinically useful. In this case, the added cost should be borne by the laboratory. Similarly, rapid reporting of presumptive isolation of enteric pathogens to physicians and nurse epidemiologists is important. Prompt reports should be rendered on Gram stains and preliminary culture results if there is any possibility that the information could result in isolation of a hazardous infection or a significant change in therapy. It should be appreciated that a positive culture does not establish an infection and a negative culture does not rule one out. Repeated cultures may be required to isolate enteric pathogens, especially in carriers.

Most laboratory workers, but too few physicians, appreciate the fact that specimens which are contaminated with fecal, oral, or cutaneous flora often require laboratory workers to expend needless effort in speciation and antimicrobial susceptibility testing. Reports from such cultures often are misleading and result in indiscriminate antimicrobial therapy of questionable infections. This contributes to predisposition of patients to other infections by alteration of normal flora and colonization with nosocomial strains. Laboratories should request repeat collection from wounds, lower respiratory tract, female genital tract, and urine when multiple species of gram-negative rods are isolated. This is especially desirable when Gram stains of exudate show evidence of cutaneous, oropharyngeal, or intestinal contamination and an absence of leukocytes. The microbiologist should establish firm policies, which can be agreed upon by the Infection Control Committee and clinicians primarily responsible for treatment of infectious disease, to confine identification and reporting to isolates which have a high probability of properly influencing diagnosis and treatment (3).

Increasing numbers of infections are being caused by microorganisms ordinarily considered of low virulence for humans. Differentiation of these from more commonly recognized and pathogenic related species was discussed previously. A former practice of ignoring the isolation of species assumed to be contaminants from such sources as blood or spinal fluid is no longer permissible.

Use of antimicrobial susceptibility data

Differences in antimicrobial susceptibility patterns are useful in identifying epidemiologically unique strains of bacteria. This information often is available earlier than data obtained by phage typing or serotyping. Indeed, many isolates are unavailable for such typing by the time a potential outbreak is recognized. Computer analysis is helpful but input data must be refined. For example, numerous isolates of the same species from one patient on one ward may create the impression that an outbreak has occurred if each report is entered. In addition, such data are often contaminated by entry of all cases without distinguishing between hospital-associated infection, infections present on admission, and contamination or colonization without evidence of infection. Profiles of antimicrobial susceptibility for commonly isolated species are useful to guide optimal therapy and allow recognition of unusual patterns which may assist recognition of cross-infection. Detection of methicillin-resistant *Staphylococcus aureus* through incubation at 35 C or less is essential.

Antimicrobial agents effective only for the treatment of urinary tract infections should not be tested against isolates from other sources, unless this is being done to provide markers for epidemiological purposes. The microbiologist should confer with the Infection Control Committee regarding choice of drugs for susceptibility testing. A requirement for consultation between the patient's physician and a member of the committee prior to testing certain drugs may reduce potential exposure to toxic antimicrobials and those which predispose to colonization and subsequent hospital-associated infection. This has eliminated routine testing of drugs such as chloramphenicol, kanamycin, gentamicin, and carbenicillin in a number of hospitals. There is general agreement that laboratory personnel, not the clinician, should decide which isolates are to be tested for antimicrobial susceptibility. The more liberal the approach to susceptibility testing of normal flora, colonizing bacteria, and contaminating bacteria, the greater will be the tendency toward indiscriminate antibiotic therapy.

Omission of culture in evaluation of infections

Improper or insufficient use of diagnostic microbiological services will undermine an infection control program. It will be helpful to include in surveillance a tabulation of cases which lack sufficient microbiological data to evaluate the existence and etiology of infection.

LITERATURE CITED

1. Accreditation Manual for Hospitals. 1973. Joint Commission on Accreditation of Hospitals. Chicago.
2. Bartlett, R. C. 1972. Control of hospital-associated infection. Progr. Clin. Pathol. **4**(7):259–282.
3. Bartlett, R. C. 1974. Medical microbiology, quality, cost and clinical relevance. Wiley Interscience, New York.
4. Infection Control in the Hospital (rev. ed.). 1970. American Hospital Association, Chicago.
5. LeRiche, W. H., C. E. Balcom, and G. Van Velle. 1966. The control of infections in hospitals. Univ. of Toronto Press, Toronto.
6. Proceedings of the International Conference on Nonsocomial Infection. 1971. American Hospital Association, Chicago.
7. University of Michigan, School of Public Health. 1966. Control of infections in hospitals. Continuing Educa-

tion Series No. 138, Continuing Education Services, Ann Arbor.

8. U.S. Department of Health, Education, and Welfare. 1973. Isolation techniques for use in hospitals. Public Health Service Publication No. 2054. U.S. Government Printing Office, Washington, D.C.

9. Williams, R. A., and R. A. Shooter. 1963. Infection in hospitals. F. A. Davis Co., Philadelphia.

10. Williams, R. E., R. Blowers, L. P. Garrod, and R. A. Shooter. 1966. Hospital infection. Lloyd-Luke, Ltd., London.

B. Microbiological Surveillance

RAYMOND C. BARTLETT, DIETER H. M. GRÖSCHEL, DONALD C. MACKEL, GEORGE F. MALLISON, AND EARLE H. SPAULDING

SURVEILLANCE OF PATIENTS

Microbiological surveillance of patients is rarely conducted except as a part of research projects to establish colonization rates. A number of reports have assessed the relation of colonization to subsequent infection (2, 12, 14, 16). Although an increased risk of infection has been associated with colonization by *Staphylococcus aureus* and various *Enterobacteriaceae*, the benefits of routine monitoring has not justified the added cost. An exception may be patients who are highly predisposed to infection by immunosuppression, in whom periodic blood, urine, and sputum cultures may help to anticipate acute life-threatening infections. *S. aureus* colonization rates of newborns do not appear to correlate sufficiently with infection to warrant monitoring. Instead, effort should be concentrated on signs of infection prior to discharge and prompt reporting by physicians of infections after discharge.

SURVEILLANCE OF PERSONNEL

The microbiologist should not accept cultures of personnel which are submitted to him without prior arrangement with the Infection Control Committee. The physician in charge of employee health services should be included in planning such an investigation. Routine cultures of personnel are not justified unless one is investigating a potential outbreak. A possible exception is routine stool culture of applicants for employment in dietary services. Although some hospitals culture applicants for nursing positions to determine carriage of *S. aureus*, there is no real justification for this practice. It is widely acknowledged that at least 30% of hospital employees are carriers of *S. aureus*. The culturing of nurses and other personnel for the carriage of *Salmonella* or enteropathogenic *Escherichia coli* is similarly unjustifiable in the absence of a suspected outbreak. Some authorities have recommended culturing of personnel as an adjunct to education. Culturing of personnel, especially students, in critical areas such as operating rooms or nurseries may provide visible evidence of bacterial contamination, augmenting an informal discussion of infection control measures.

If there is evidence that cross-infection has occurred, the chairman of the Infection Control Committee should be notified immediately. Investigation should be launched objectively through discussion with persons directly involved. These should include the nurse epidemiologist, the director of the department, individual physicians, nurses and their supervisors, and the microbiologist. It must be clearly understood by the medical staff that independent investigations, and the impulsive directives which frequently ensue, create confusion and obstruct an orderly investigation.

If the members of the committee and their consultants agree that cross-infection may have occurred, appropriate specimens from involved patients and personnel should be collected for culture. Personnel with any evidence of infection with the index agent should be treated and sent home without loss of pay. Carriers of intestinal pathogens should be treated. Physicians with minor infections, or those who prove to be carriers of nosocomial strains associated with an outbreak, must desist from operating or exposing themselves to predisposed patients in critical areas. This action will require strong staff support.

S. aureus carriers may be transferred to other areas of the hospital until the outbreak has been brought under control. Many of these carriers may have no relation to an outbreak. Antimicrobial susceptibility patterns or phage typing can pinpoint those which may be epidemiologically related. Staphylococci are most easily and frequently isolated from anterior nares, but carriers usually will demonstrate colonization of the skin of the hands and other portions of the body. The question of establishing whether a staphylococcal carrier is a "shedder" sometimes arises. No standard definition of a shedder has been established, and methods for collecting material are cumbersome. Carriers with exfoliative dermatitis or respiratory infection usually disseminate larger numbers of staphylococci, and this should be taken into consideration. *S. aureus* carriers who must continue to work in a critical area where cross-infection has been suspected or established should be placed on an intensive program of body hygiene involving regular use of antiseptic detergents and frequent bathing and changing of clothes. These measures, plus the use of a topical antimicrobial nasal ointment, may eliminate the carrier state temporarily. Systemic therapy may be used, but the individual is likely to be recolonized with the same or another strain of *S. aureus* a few weeks after the end of the treatment. Bacterial interference has been used to try to control colonization with epidemic strains of *S. aureus* but has not enjoyed general use (7).

Intestinal pathogens should be sought by obtaining at least three specimens. Rectal swabs should be taken if necessary. Streptococcal carriers may be identified by throat culture. Recently, an outbreak of streptococcal infection was associated with anal carriers; hence, this site should not be overlooked (15).

SURVEILLANCE OF THE ENVIRONMENT

The importance of coordinating environmental microbiological sampling with the broader objectives of the overall infection control program was described in part A of this chapter. A well-defined reason for collecting such samples along with standard methods and an organized protocol is essential. The procedure should be capable of producing information which can be used to provide convincing evidence that policies and methods for control of environmental contamination should be changed. Such sampling must be conducted proficiently, not in a haphazard manner.

Minimal program

It is recommended that the following portions of the environmental surveillance program be carried out routinely and be considered the minimal acceptable level.

Sterilizers. Physical, chemical, and biological indicators, as well as product sampling, have been used to monitor the autoclave sterilization process. Physical indicators such as thermometers and pressure gauges attached to the sterilizer, or melting point ampoules, will not monitor all parameters of a steam autoclave. All autoclaves should be equipped with time-temperature recorders to provide additional assurance of adequate exposure. Evidence that a sterilizing temperature was achieved for an adequate time does not assure sterilization, since this may require a longer time when the load is dense or large volumes of fluid are present. Residual air or superheat may cause false readings. Chemical monitors such as test tapes or other heat-sensitive color indicators are unsatisfactory, for they indicate only that the required temperature has been reached. Although product sampling may be the most reliable monitoring process for assuring sterility, it is impractical as a routine procedure for the hospital. Biological monitoring has generally been accepted as the most effective method of determining a successful sterilization process.

The microorganisms used as biological indicators are more resistant to the sterilization process than most naturally occurring contaminants, and to provide a margin of safety they are used in relatively high concentrations. Commercial biological monitors usually are filter paper strips impregnated with bacterial spores; for steam sterilizers, the thermophile *B. stearothermophilus* is used, and for dry heat and ethylene oxide, a *B. subtilis* strain (*globigii* or var. *niger*) is used. Because the spores of *B. stearothermophilus* are not very resistant to dry heat and ethylene oxide, nor those of *B. subtilis* to steam, the choice of the proper spore strip depends on the type of sterilization process to be monitored.

Steam and hot air sterilizers should be checked once a week, but every load of items subjected to ethylene oxide prior to use in deep tissues or in the vascular system should be checked because the types of apparatus used in hospitals provide a narrower margin of safety than does the autoclave, and malfunctions are not rare. Goods should not be released until it is known that the corresponding test cultures are negative. Commercially available spore strips should be placed in the largest package within the largest load and never on an open shelf in the autoclave. Either the center of the load or the bottom front near the exhaust valve is the location least likely to be exposed to sterilizing temperatures for an adequate length of time.

Spore strips are not valid indicators of sterilization of fluids. Instead, place an ampoule containing a spore suspension in the largest vessel. Alternatively, inoculate the fluid with a test culture: after autoclaving, subculture a generous inoculum to a tryptic digest casein soy (TS), or brain heart infusion (BHI) broth. Do not use spore suspensions to check the sterilization of culture media which have to be autoclaved at lower than usual temperatures and for shorter times to avoid overheating thermolabile constituents (13). It is advisable that a microbiologist be responsible for the selection, storage, and assay of the monitors.

After the sterilization cycle, the spore strips have to be handled carefully to prevent secondary contamination. All necessary data about the sterilization cycle should be recorded. In assaying the spore strips or ampoules, all recommendations of the manufacturer must be followed; *B. subtilis* will not grow at 56 C. *B. stearothermophilus* may not grow at 37 C. Thioglycolate broth is inhibitory and should not be used; TS broth is recommended. Sterile forceps and scissors are needed for the transfer. Alcohol flame technique should be avoided because alcohol may contain viable spores which may not be killed during the flaming process. Nonsterilized controls from the spore lot should be tested in parallel to assure the viability of the monitors. All positive test cultures and the controls must be subcultured to prevent misinterpretation due to secondary contamination during handling.

If a sterilizer is found to perform inadequately, it should be retested immediately under close scrutiny of thermometer and pressure gauge readings, type and size of load, etc. If it again fails to sterilize the monitors, the institution's maintenance engineer and/or an expert on autoclave technique should be consulted.

Sterilized objects. Routine sampling of items which have been properly packaged, autoclaved, and stored is not recommended. Although rare instances of contamination of presterilized commercial items have been observed, the frequency is insufficient to justify routine sampling. Instances of contamination of commercially prepared materials which have resulted in clinical infections are rare and are more economically detected through surveillance of infections in patients than by routine microbiological sampling.

Milk formulas. Several bottles of hospital-prepared infant formulas selected at random from each lot produced should be tested once a week. No more than 25 colonies of sporeformers per ml should be present (4). Sampling of commercially prepared formulas is less important but may be required by state health codes.

Instruments and equipment. Articles which are to be in direct contact with deep tissues must be sterile. Some of them are reused with different patients but are thermolabile and would be damaged by heat sterilization. Therefore, they must be subjected to a high-level chemical disinfection procedure capable of producing sterility. Examples of these critical items (see part C) are transfer forceps, instruments inserted into deep tissues or internal body cavities, thermolabile components or heart-lung oxygenators, and blood vessel catheters.

Some instruments and pieces of equipment are semicritical with respect to the risk of contributing to infection associated with their use. These make direct contact with skin and the mucous membranes of body orifices but not with deeper tissues. Parts of anaesthesia and inhalation therapy equipment, cystoscopes, and bronchoscopes are in this category. Here the criterion for satisfactory disinfection is the absence of recognized pathogens and opportunists known to be important causes of nosocomial infections. Thus, such articles do not have to be sterile when used, but they should be subjected to intermediate-level disinfection (see part C).

Sampling of articles after high-level disinfection should be conducted intermittently, whereas the frequency after intermediate-level will depend upon the nature of current sampling results, as well as the incidence of nosocomial disease in that institution. Isolates need to be identified to the extent of determining whether or not they are recognized causes of nosocomial infections, or are identical with clinical isolates from an institutional outbreak.

A point not sufficiently appreciated is the importance of thorough drying of inhalation therapy and similar equipment after cleansing and disinfection. "Water" bacteria and the other opportunists often involved in infections from this source can not grow in the absence of moisture.

Other indications for sampling

Many materials and objects become contaminated by direct contact with patients and personnel, and become potential avenues of cross-infection. These include water, ice, soap and soap dispensers, weak antiseptics, bedpans, thermometers, tubes of lubricant, multiple use and topical medications, and hydrotherapy equipment. *Routine* sampling of these items is not generally recommended. Such tests should be conducted only when surveillance of infections in patients implicates them as potential sources. Standard methods do not exist for sampling any of them; therefore, considerable expense is sometimes incurred in producing information that is not only worthless but also misleading.

Environmental sampling may have educational value despite the lack of standardized tests and an inability to draw valid epidemiological conclusions from the results. Culturing of the inner aspects of surgical masks and scrub suits after several hours of wear by student nurses and operating room technicians, for example, provides a useful demonstration of microbial buildup. This teaches students the need for frequent changes of masks and gowns despite the absence of recognized hazardous levels of microbial accumulation on these items. Even though no indication for routine environmental sampling exists, it may be desirable to do this periodically to obtain background levels of contamination, to maintain familiarity with sampling procedures, or as a check on the personnel who conduct sanitation procedures. Sampling of floors can be done, for example, as a part of quality control of housekeeping. Although the hazardous level of floor contamination has not been established, the numbers of microorganisms to be expected with standard cleansing methods are known (5, 11). Thus, a comparison of levels of contamination in one part of the hospital with those in another part may not produce epidemiologically significant information but it can detect neglected areas.

Sampling methods

Sampling of objects, hollow containers, and large surfaces is performed to detect the presence of recognized or potential pathogens and to obtain microbial counts (quantitation).

For quantitation, one may apply a moistened swab to a measured area, collect a rinse sample, or employ Rodac plates. Swab specimens can be immersed and wrung out in BHI broth supplemented with 0.5% beef extract in a screw-cap tube. After removal of the swab, the contents of the tube can be cultured for a rough quantitation and for pathogens in the manner described below.

The same broth may be used to sample objects which are more conveniently tested by rinsing. Samples are obtained from the inside of tubing by carefully introducing an appropriate volume (40 to 50 ml) of rinse broth while holding the tubing at both ends and alternately raising and lowering the ends 50 times. The broth is then allowed to flow into a sterile tube or flask.

Bottles and containers such as nebulizer reservoirs are sampled by adding 10 to 50 ml of rinse broth, inserting a sterile stopper if needed, shaking vigorously for about 30 s, and decanting or pipetting the broth into sterile 125-ml screw-capped flasks.

Plate counts are made as follows. Prepare a series of 10-fold dilutions in tubes of TS broth starting with 1 ml of the test sample. The number of dilutions to make depends upon the amount of contamination expected. From each dilution tube to be cultured, pipette 0.5 ml onto the surface of TS agar (TSA) plates supplemented with 5% sheep or rabbit blood. Rock the plates until the inoculum is thoroughly distributed and allow to dry at 35 to 37 C before inverting them (Fig. 1). Make colony counts after 24 h if colonies appear to be coalescing or spreading; otherwise make only 48-h colony counts.

For detection and identification of pathogens, we recommend that both a 4- and a 24-h enrichment procedure be carried out. The BHI

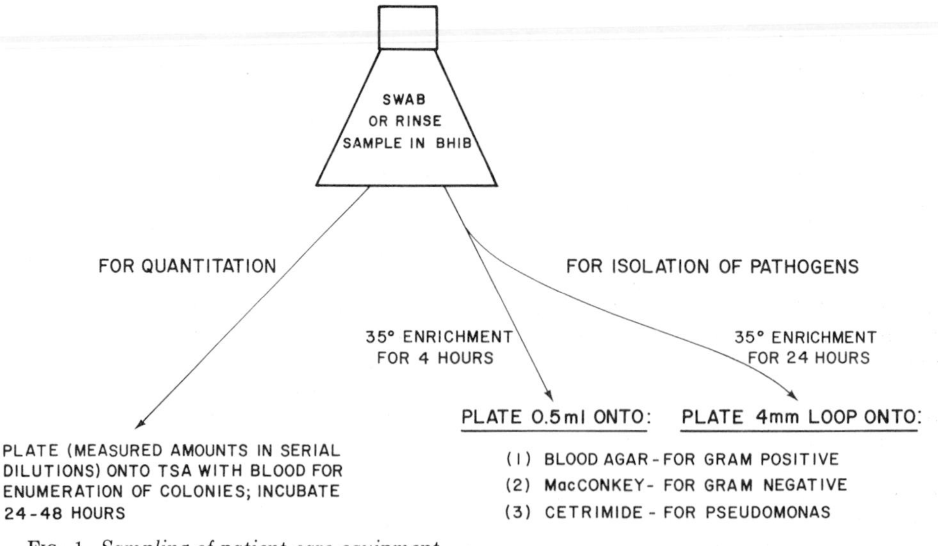

FIG. 1. *Sampling of patient-care equipment.*

broth rinse sample, minus the 1 ml used for a dilution count, is incubated for 4 h at 35 C. A 0.5-ml volume is pipetted onto the surfaces of TS blood agar, MacConkey agar, and Cetrimide agar plates. These are handled in the same manner as described for the quantitation step. The 24-h enrichment step is the continued incubation of the BHI broth rinse sample for a total of about 24 h with subcultures to the same three types of agar plates. The volume of inoculum may be different, however, in the case of the 24-h enrichment. If there is turbidity in the flask or tube, use only a film or biconvex loopful to streak the entire surface of the plate.

After incubation, examine the plate cultures for typical colonies. TS blood agar is a satisfactory general purpose medium and is particularly suitable for gram-positive varieties. MacConkey agar is useful for coliforms and other *Enterobacteriaceae*; Cetrimide agar for *Pseudomonas*. It is recommended that two colonies of each morphological (gross appearance) type be picked for presumptive identification. Identify each colony type by using standard microbiological criteria to determine the presence or absence of recognized or potential pathogens. Speciation should be carried out during epidemic situations.

Small objects which cannot be conveniently rinsed with broth may be completely immersed in flasks or tubes of BHI broth and shaken vigorously for 1 min. Plate counts and subcultures may be conducted as outlined above.

Although the broth rinse method produces quantitative results, these may bear no relationship to the actual risk of infection produced by use of the contaminated article. In the absence of such criteria, the results can help to detect and reduce the frequency and extent of contamination that is associated with various disinfection procedures.

Large surfaces such as floors which cannot be rinsed conveniently may be sampled either by the swab template method or by Rodac plates. The swab template method uses a sheet of heavy paper from which a square hole 5 cm by 5 cm has been cut out of the center. Several sheets can be enclosed together in a manila envelope or folded brown paper, sealed, and autoclaved. To perform this test, use a swab moistened with TS broth. Lay the paper template on the surface to be sampled. Slowly rub the swab, at the same time rotating it slightly, in close parallel streaks across the exposed area. Then repeat this step with the same swab but perpendicular to the first streaks. Place the swab in a tube of TS broth and, while doing so, break off the portion of the stick which was handled by pressing the swab against the side of the tube. Shake the tube 50 times. Make plate counts and identification of isolates as described earlier.

Rodac plates must be completely filled for sampling floors and other nonporous surfaces. This requires 16.5 ml of TS agar, preferably containing 0.07% lecithin and 0.5% polysorbate 80 as neutralizers of disinfectant (8). The number of plates to use will depend upon the size of the surface area to be sampled, the amount and heterogeneity of the contamination likely to be on that surface, and the level of statistical significance desired. At least 15 plates are needed to sample the floor of an average hospital room (5). Plates are touched to dry surfaces without producing a rotary or sliding motion. The colonies are counted after incubation for 48 h at 35 C.

Standards for acceptable levels of contamination of floors and overbed tables sampled by the above Rodac method have been suggested by a committee of the American Public Health Association (5): 25 or fewer colonies per plate is considered good; 26 to 50 colonies is considered fair; more than 50 colonies is considered poor. These figures are based on samplings taken about 0.5 h after cleansing and do not take into account the progressive accumulation of contamination which may occur between that time and the next cleansing. Counts below five colonies per Rodac plate are achievable in such critical areas as operating rooms but, to repeat, there is no evidence that these levels *must* be maintained in order to prevent infections or that any particular level of contamination in such areas is directly correlated with an increased risk of infection.

Sampling blood and intravenous fluids

Random units of blood from the Blood Bank should be cultured to assure sterility. The American Association of Blood Banks has recommended culturing 5-ml samples both aerobically and anaerobically at 30 to 32 C, or at both 20 to 22 C and 35 to 37 C (17). Bottles should be subcultured after 48 h of incubation, and again at the end of 7 days, to TS chocolate agar; the use of different media is optional.

If contamination is suspected in association with blood transfusion, the administration unit should be immediately disconnected from the patient with placement of sterile shields over the exposed ends of needles or tubing to prevent subsequent contamination. Samples of blood are withdrawn aseptically in the laboratory and subjected to the blood culture technique just described. In addition, at least two blood cultures should be collected by venipuncture from the patient.

Other ways contaminating microorganisms are introduced parenterally are by intravenous fluid administration, parenteral alimentation, or the development of contamination in indwelling intravenous catheters such as central venous pressure catheters and shunts used for dialysis. When there is a possibility that a contaminated fluid has been introduced, the system should be carefully disconnected to avoid extrinsic contamination of cannulae or needles. Two separate blood cultures should be collected from the patient using different venipuncture sites. The nature of the fluid and its lot number should be recorded on the patient's chart and in all subsequent laboratory records. The bottle and administration set should remain connected and be placed in a plastic bag to minimize contamination during delivery to the laboratory.

In the laboratory, withdraw aseptically 20 ml of fluid from the administration tubing. Use 1 ml to prepare a BHI-beef extract pour agar plate, and add the remainder to a blood culture bottle. Both cultures should be incubated aerobically overnight at 35 C and examined for turbidity each day for 7 days. If the fluid bottle or bag is more than half full, aseptically drain it to a level no more than one-half full and carefully add to the bottle an equal volume of double-strength BHI-beef extract broth. Incubate and examine as above. If bacteria are isolated, the state health department and a representative of the Food and Drug Administration should be contacted immediately.

Spurious contamination while handling these materials in the laboratory can be greatly minimized by conducting tests in a laminar flow cabinet. Any laboratory which does microbiological sampling of fluids and devices should be equipped with such a cabinet.

Parenteral introduction of microorganisms may also result from contamination of portions of the administration set or from a septic thrombophlebitis at the site of needle or catheter insertion. This can be minimized by good daily maintenance of venipuncture sites and by limiting the use of an indwelling catheter to a period of no longer than 48 h at any one site (10). If infection is suspected, remove needles and catheters and protect them with sterile shields, or place them in sterile containers and take them directly to the laboratory. The recommended procedure is to cut and culture separately the previously subcutaneous portion of catheters, free from that portion of the system previously exposed to skin and other superficial contamination; otherwise the "subcutaneous" portion of the device is likely to become contaminated before it reaches the laboratory. To do this, needles can be broken free from the contaminated hub portion by using a sterile clamp. The "subcutaneous" portion of the needle or catheter is cultured by the broth rinse technique described above; those portions of tubing which had been exposed to external contamination are cultured by carefully rinsing the interior as described earlier, provided the tubing is long enough.

Water and ice

Distilled or deionized water, or tap water which meets U.S. Public Health Service drinking water standards, frequently contains 10^2 to 10^6 or more microorganisms per ml, some of which may be opportunistic pathogens. Determination of microbial contamination of water (or ice, sampled after aseptic melting) may be carried out by use of a membrane filter procedure (Millipore Corp.) or by plate counts of undiluted and serial dilution inocula for quantitation. The 24-h enrichment method with BHI broth may be used if a comprehensive search is being made for a specific pathogen other than salmonellae. Substantial numbers of bacteria not generally associated with human infection may be isolated; there is no evidence that this situation is hazardous. On the other hand, the finding of a most probable number of 2.2 or more colonies of coliforms by the tube test, or four or more colonies per 100 ml by the membrane filter test per 100 ml suggests fecal pollution (3). The presence of staphylococci may indicate contamination from the hands of personnel. Also, *Pseudomonas aeruginosa* and other oxidative bacteria may be found in substantial numbers; again, there is no colony count figure generally recognized as hazardous. However, potential environmental sources of *P. aeruginosa* should be controlled by daily changes of stagnant water in flower vases and other containers.

Air sampling

Air sampling is not an essential activity for any infection control program. In major institutions conducting adequately staffed programs, the personnel and trainees should become familiar with the use of environmental surveillance methods and equipment as well as with the interpretation of results, because of the educational value and the potential usefulness of these methods in dealing effectively with important, and sometimes complex, epidemiological problems.

The occasional use of settling plates may produce results differing greatly from those obtained with simultaneous volumetric air samplers (9). Yet, low-count settling plates may serve a useful purpose by allaying the fears of physicians who may think that operating room air is excessively contaminated. It is also worth mentioning that no direct correlation has been established between levels of microbial contamination in hospital rooms and the infection rate in that hospital. A contamination level of 30 to 50 particles per ft^3 (0.028 m^3) with volumetric air sampling is acceptable and not uncommon in general patient care areas. Proper maintenance and ventilation in operating rooms should maintain levels at fewer than 5 particles per ft^3. Appropriate devices and detailed instructions for their use appear elsewhere (19).

Inhalation therapy equipment

Some inhalation therapy devices are composed of plastic and mechanical parts that cannot be steam-sterilized for one reason or another. Ethylene oxide gas or a high level liquid germicide is also used for disinfection. Regardless of the method of sterilization or disinfection, the mask and tubing should be changed daily and should never be used on more than one patient without being cleansed and either disinfected or sterilized. In addition to enforcing this rule, a program of intermittent sampling should be conducted, with the use of the broth rinse method. This program should also include sampling of the reservoirs of medication nebulizers and humidifiers. Cultures from masks and tubing will usually reveal mixed upper respiratory bacterial flora after they have been used by a patient for a short period of time; such sampling is of little value.

Some authorities have recommended sampling the aerosols produced by these devices since they may reach the terminal alveoli of patients. This may be accomplished with a mechanical air sampler or with the simplified technique described by Edmondson et al. (6) in which the aerosol that condenses on the wall of the tube is rinsed off with nutrient broth. Melted agar is added and the tube is slanted. The recovery of more than six colonies suggests an undesirable level of contamination emanating from the reservoir or nebulizer jet but not necessarily from other parts of the breathing circuit.

LITERATURE CITED

1. Bartlett, R. C. 1972. Control of hospital-associated infection. Progr. Clin. Pathol. **4**(7):259–282.
2. Bartlett, R. C. 1974. Medical microbiology, quality, cost and clinical relevance. Wiley Interscience, New York.
3. Committee of American Public Health Association, American Water Works Association, and Water Pollution Control Federation. 1971. Standard methods for the examination of water and waste water, 13th ed. American Public Health Association. Inc., New York.
4. Committee on Fetus and Newborn, American Academy of Pediatrics. 1971. Standards and recommendations for hospital care of newborn infants, 5th ed.
5. Committee on Microbial Contamination of Surfaces of Laboratory Section, American Public Health Association. 1970. A comparative microbiological evaluation of floor-cleaning procedures in hospital patient rooms. Health Lab. Sci. **7**:3–11.
6. Edmondson, E. B., and J. P. Sanford. 1966. Simple methods of bacteriological sampling of nebulization equipment. Amer. Rev. Resp. Dis. **81**:450–453.
7. Eichenwald, H. F., H. R. Shinefield, M. Boris, and J. C. Ribble. 1965. Bacterial interference and staphylococcal colonization in infants and adults. Ann. N.Y. Acad. Sci. **128**:365–380.
8. Fincher, E. L. 1966. Surface sampling—applications, methods and recommendations. Proc. Institute on Control of Infections in Hospitals, p. 189–199 (available from Center for Disease Control, Atlanta, Ga. 30333).
9. Fincher, E. L., and G. F. Mallison. 1972. Intramural sampling of airborne microorganisms, p. E1–E6. *In* Air sampling instruments, 4th ed. American Conference of Government Industrial Hygienists.
10. Fuchs, P. C. 1971. Indwelling intravenous polyethylene catheters: factors influencing the risk of microbial colonization and sepsis. J. Amer. Med. Ass. **216**:1447–1450.
11. Infection Control in the Hospital (rev. ed.). 1970. American Hospital Association, Chicago.
12. Johansen, W. G., A. K. Pierce, and J. P. Sanford. 1969. Changing pharyngeal flora of hospitalized patients. N. Engl. J. Med. **281**:1137–1140.
13. Perkins, J. J. 1969. Principles and methods of sterilization in health sciences. Charles C Thomas, Publisher, Springfield, Ill.
14. Redman, L. R., and E. Lockey. 1967. Colonization of the upper respiratory tract with Gram negative bacilli after operation, endotracheal intubation and prophylactic antibiotic therapy. Anesthesia **22**:220–227.
15. Schaffner, W., L. B. Lefkowitz, J. S. Goodman, and M. G. Koenig. 1969. Hospital outbreak of infections with Group A streptococci traced to an asymptomatic anal carrier. N. Engl. J. Med. **280**:1224.
16. Schlemker, J. D., and C. A. Hubay. 1973. Colonization of the respiratory tract and post operative pulmonary infections. Arch. Surg. **107**:313–318.
17. Standards for Blood Banks and Transfusion Services, 1970, 5th ed. American Association of Blood Banks, Chicago, Ill.

C. Hospital Disinfectants and Antiseptics

EARLE H. SPAULDING AND DIETER H. M. GRÖSCHEL

INTRODUCTION

Disinfection and sterilization constitute the principal means of preventing hospital-acquired infections. Both physical and chemical agents are used. Physical agents play the major role in sterilization, whereas chemical germicides in the form of disinfectants and antiseptics are the primary tools in disinfection procedures.

Many different kinds of disinfectants and antiseptics are used in American hospitals. A 1973 survey of 16 hospitals in various parts of the United States, with a combined bed capacity of more than 9,000, showed that the average number of different formulations per hospital was 14.5 with a range from 8 to 22 (4). The total for all 16 hospitals was 224, and 125 of them were proprietary products.

Thus, the hospital personnel responsible for the selection and use of chemical germicides are confronted with an extensive array of both nonproprietary formulations and commercial products, the latter supported by promotional claims which especially need to be evaluated. The purpose of this section of chapter 91 is to present information which can help to evaluate these agents correctly, to make appropriate selections for specific applications, and to use them properly.

STERILIZATION VERSUS DISINFECTION

Whereas sterilization achieves the destruction of all microbial life (at least within the limit of our present procedures), disinfection does not necessarily produce sterility as the end result. Whether a particular disinfection procedure does or does not result in sterilization in a particular situation depends upon a number of factors, each of which may have a significant effect upon the end result. Among these factors are the nature and number of contaminating microorganisms, and especially the presence of bacterial spores, the concentration of disinfectants, the length of time of application, the amount of organic "soil" present, the type and condition of the material to be disinfected, and the temperature. These factors influence both the rapidity and the level of the antimicrobial action. Thus, disinfection is a procedure which reduces the risk of infection, but there is a broad range of end results which extends from sterility at one extreme to a minimal reduction in the number of contaminating microorganisms at the other. Therefore, the distinction between sterilization and disinfection is important to remember if one is to select and use disinfectants properly.

Although both physical and chemical agents are used in disinfection, this discussion is limited to chemicals. Chemical disinfection is generally practiced with liquids, but gases are also used. Disinfection with a gas is often referred to in the vernacular as "gas sterilization," just as disinfection with chemical solutions becomes "chemical sterilization." Neither term is appropriate unless it has been established that the procedure in question will actually produce sterility when a substantial number, at least 10^5, of dried bacterial spores is present. The nature of the germicide per se does not determine this, for the manner of application is equally important. For example, glutaraldehyde, formaldehyde, and ethylene oxide are sometimes referred to as sterilizing agents. Such statements can be misleading. Even though these high-level germicides may be sterilants, they are often employed in hospitals in such a way that sterilization, though presumed, may not be achieved.

LEVELS OF GERMICIDAL ACTION

The greatest obstacle to the rapid sterilization of instruments with chemicals is the unique resistance of bacterial spores. Only a few strong germicides can kill large numbers of dried spores, and they require contact for several hours to destroy populations of the order of 10^5. Most disinfectants cannot achieve this level of antimicrobial activity.

Nonsporicidal germicides vary significantly in their levels of antimicrobial activity. Some of them are cidal within a few minutes for the ordinary vegetative forms of bacteria (i.e., staphylococci), fungi, lipid-containing viruses, tubercle bacilli, and nonlipid viruses. These germicides are intermediate in antimicrobial action between sporicides and a third group whose effective cidal range is limited to the ordinary vegetative forms of bacteria, most fungal forms, and the lipid-containing viruses. Thus, there are three levels of germicidal action: high, intermediate, and low (Table 1). A tacit but important part of these definitions (and of sterilization, too) is that the cidal effect must occur within a practicable period of time. What is practicable in any given situation is a decision for the operator to make.

TABLE 1. *Levels of germicidal action*

Level	Bacteria			Fungi[b]	Viruses[c]	
	Vegetative[a]	Tubercle bacillus	Spores		Lipid and medium size	Nonlipid and small
High	+[d]	+	+	+	+	+
Intermediate	+	+	−	+	+	+
Low	+	−	−	+	+	−

[a] Common forms of bacterial cells, e.g., staphylococcus.

[b] Includes usual asexual "spores" but not necessarily dried chlamydospores or sexual spores.

[c] Exclusive of the human hepatitis viruses.

[d] Plus signs indicate that a cidal effect can be expected when the usual use-concentrations of available disinfectants are properly employed.

High-level disinfection

Because certain critical items (see below, Nature of the Problem) are thermolabile and must be disinfected by chemicals, a question of great practical importance is whether high-level disinfectants can be depended upon to sterilize medical and surgical materials. In the absence of spores, they certainly can, and do so promptly. But the presence of spores cannot usually be predicted with certainty. Although the number will generally be small (12), the sporicidal capacity is, nevertheless, an essential property of high-level disinfectants.

Three high-level disinfectants are 8% formaldehyde solution, 2% glutaraldehyde in alkalinized solution, and gaseous ethylene oxide. All three of these can kill large numbers of resistant spores under severe test conditions, but they may require as long as 24 h to do so (8). On the other hand, sterilization may occur in 2 h or less if only a small number of spores is present (13).

As indicated earlier, whether or not the use of a high-level disinfectant results in sterilization depends upon its use. To illustrate, the sterilizing capacity of ethylene oxide varies widely with different procedures. The use in hospitals of the large autoclave type of ethylene oxide apparatus, with evacuation of the chamber and the potentiating action of additional humidification and heat, can be considered a sterilization method when sufficient exposure time is allowed. We must point out that exposure times as long as 12 h are sometimes needed for consistent sterilization of test objects heavily contaminated with thoroughly dry spores; prehumidification may reduce the time required for this (2). On the other hand, smaller bench-type apparatus providing ethylene oxide concentrations below 450 mg/liter and lacking one or more of the potentiating features just mentioned is less capable of producing sterility, despite the fact that some of the marketed pieces of equipment in the latter category are labeled with the word "sterilizer."

Intermediate-level disinfection

The tubercle bacillus is significantly more resistant to aqueous germicides than the ordinary vegetative bacteria. Although a tuberculocidal effect can be obtained with iodophors by increasing the concentration above that employed for general disinfection purposes (75 to 450 ppm), this higher level of cidal activity appears to be beyond the useful capability of quaternary ammonium compounds at any concentration (14).

The chemical resistance of viruses is also variable. Klein and Deforest reported that the small nonlipid viruses they tested were significantly more resistant than medium-sized viruses with lipid in their protein coats (6). Some of the most widely used liquid germicides failed to destroy picornaviruses, among which are the enterovirus group (poliomyelitis, echo, and coxsackie) and the rhinoviruses of the common cold. It might be anticipated that germicides with good tuberculocidal activity would also destroy the small nonlipid viruses, but this is apparently not the case. They found that isopropanol, a good tuberculocide, lacked this level of virucidal activity, whereas 70 to 95% ethanol rapidly killed both tubercle bacilli and picornaviruses.

Low-level disinfection

Some of the germicides in common use today can not be relied upon to destroy within a practicable period of time either tubercle bacilli or small nonlipid viruses. These low-level germicides are, nevertheless, useful in actual practice because they can rapidy kill the vegetative forms of bacteria and fungi, as well as the medium-sized and lipid-containing viruses (Table 1).

MICROBIAL RESISTANCE

Because bacteria exhibit a wide range of resistance to chemicals, the kinds of contaminating microorganisms known or most likely to be present determine the level of disinfection needed. The four major classes of microorganisms are bacteria, viruses, fungi, and animal parasites. For hospital disinfection, the last class can be disregarded; thus, the problem is how to destroy bacteria, fungi, and viruses.

The resistance of bacterial spores to germicides is enormously greater than that of the corresponding vegetative forms. The tetanus bacillus in its vegetative form, for example, has about the same resistance as the staphylococcus, but its spores can survive exposure to a use concentration of a widely used germicide, e.g., 1:750 aqueous "quat," for at least 3 weeks (14). Consequently, the statement that a certain germicide "kills sporeformers" is meaningless.

The differences in chemical resistance exhibited by various kinds of vegetative bacteria are relatively minor, except for tubercle bacilli, which, presumably because of their hydrophobic cell surfaces, are comparatively resistant to aqueous quaternaries, mercurials, and hexachlorophene. Among the ordinary vegetative bacteria, staphylococci and enterococci are slightly more resistant than most other gram-positive organisms. However, antibiotic-resistant "hospital" strains of staphylococcus are not discernibly more resistant to germicides than are susceptible strains. A number of gram-negative bacilli, such as *Pseudomonas*, *Klebsiella*, *Enterobacter*, *Serratia*, and "water bacteria", may show somewhat greater resistance to disinfectants and antiseptics. This fact is noteworthy because these species are among the emerging pathogens responsible for outbreaks of hospital infection, for example, as contaminants of inhalation therapy equipment (9, 11). However minor these differences in resistance are, they become significant in practice when low-level germicides are used, particularly at marginal concentrations. These slight differences may disappear when more concentrated solutions are substituted.

The differences in germicidal resistance among viruses have already been mentioned. Because pathogenic viruses can often be recovered from human mucous membranes, we have to assume that they may also be present on many surfaces in the hospital environment and should be destroyed. In that case, an intermediate germicide is needed.

Human hepatitis viruses constitute a formidable problem for chemical disinfection. Because the human is the only susceptible species, it has not been possible to carry out the definitive tests needed to determine the germicidal resistance of these viruses. Although it is unlikely that their resistance approaches that of bacterial spores, the serious nature of viral hepatitis makes it mandatory that a sterilization procedure be employed whenever the presence of these viruses is a possibility, especially with used needles and syringes. Steam autoclaving is preferable to ethylene oxide sterilization, but either is preferable to sterilization with a liquid disinfectant. When liquids *must* be used, it is advisable to allow exposure for at least 10 h to 8% aqueous or alcoholic formaldehyde or 2% activated (alkalinized) glutaraldehyde.

Apart from hepatitis, if disinfection of cannulas, tubings, syringes, etc. is attempted with liquid germicides, including high-level ones, be sure to dislodge by a thorough flushing any air bubbles which may be in the lumen.

NATURE OF THE PROBLEM

Hospital disinfection can be understood better and practiced more effectively if it is divided into three categories based upon the degree of risk of infection involved with the use of the disinfected materials. The first category covers the *critical* items, so called because they are introduced beneath the surface of the body or attached to other objects so used, e.g., transfer forceps, scalpel blades, cardiac catheters, plastic components of the heart-lung oxygenator, laparoscopes, and culdoscopes. Consequently, all contaminating microorganisms must be destroyed; the requirement is sterility.

The risk involved in using chemically disinfected endotracheal and aspirator tubes, bronchoscopes, thermometers, cystoscopes, and respiratory therapy equipment is considerably less, so that these can be classified as *semi-critical*. Although such objects come in contact with intact mucous membrane, they do not ordinarily penetrate body surfaces. Sterilization is desirable but not essential. A reasonable objective, therefore, is to employ a procedure which can be expected to destroy ordinary vegetative bacteria, most fungal spores, tubercle bacilli and the small nonlipid viruses.

Non-critical materials consist of a wide variety of objects, e.g., face masks, carafes, EKG electrodes, and X-ray machines, as well as surfaces which do not ordinarily come in contact with mucous membranes. Thus, their use carries relatively little risk of transmitting infection. Many individuals rely upon hot water or cleansing with detergent and water, but chemical disinfection is also widely practiced with low-level disinfectants, either alone or in addition to the cleansing.

CLASSES OF HOSPITAL GERMICIDES

Liquid versus gases

Most germicides are used as aqueous solutions. Water is the vehicle which brings the chemical in contact with the microorganisms, and without it the disinfection process ceases. A few germicidal chemicals have vapor pressures low enough to be gases at room temperature, and these compounds can be used as gaseous disinfectants or sterilizing agents. Table 2 contains the use-concentrations and activity levels of the major classes of germicides.

TESTING METHODS

Disinfectants are evaluated by in vitro laboratory tests and by in-use tests. In the United States, there is a set of "official" laboratory tests known as the A.O.A.C. tests (1). The A.O.A.C. Use-Dilution Method is the standard procedure for determining minimal acceptable low-level germicidal action and is the one most widely used. There are other A.O.A.C. tests designed specifically to determine whether proprietary germicides meet the minimal standards established for a sporicidal claim, tuberculocidal claim, fungicidal claim, etc.

The validity of in vitro laboratory tests for evaluating a disinfectant depends upon the intended application, the chemical nature of the product, and the level of antimicrobial activity needed. The A.O.A.C. Use-Dilution Method provides a standard rigorous enough to eliminate products of doubtful value, and insures that germicides which meet these standards are capable of achieving an acceptable level of antimicrobial activity if they are used as directed. One of the A.O.A.C. tests is very rigorous indeed. The Sporicidal Test uses a test carrier which may show counts as high as 10^7 (14). Since it takes longer to sterilize an object with that many spores than it does with only 10^5 or 10^3 spores (14), one may be justified in considering the Sporicidal Test a test for chemical sterilization.

TABLE 2. *Activity levels of selected classes of germicides*

Class	Use concentration	Activity level
GAS		
Ethylene oxide	450–800 mg/liter[a]	High
LIQUID		
Glutaraldehyde, alkaline, aqueous	2%	High
Formaldehyde + alcohol	8% + 70%	High
Formaldehyde, aqueous	3 to 8%	Intermediate to high
Iodine + alcohol	0.5% + 70%	Intermediate
Alcohols[b]	70 to 90%	Intermediate
Chlorine compounds	500 to 5000 ppm[c]	Intermediate
Phenolic compounds	1 to 3%[d]	Intermediate
Iodine, aqueous	1%	Intermediate
Iodophors	75 to 150 ppm[e]	Low to intermediate
Quaternary ammonium compounds	1:750 to 1:500	Low
Hexachlorophene	1 to 3%	Low
Mercurial compounds	1:1,000 to 1:500	Low

[a] In autoclave-type equipment at 55 to 60 C.
[b] Isopropanol not lethal for picornaviruses.
[c] Available chlorine.
[d] Dilution of concentrate containing 5 to 10% phenolics.
[e] Available iodine.

In-use tests

The A.O.A.C. test methods are laboratory, and not in-use, procedures. They provide a preliminary evaluation, but most of them do not approximate actual use conditions. In-use tests performed in the hospital environment would seem to be the ideal way to evaluate hospital disinfectants. This can be done with such items as thermometers under carefully controlled conditions so as to yield reliable, reproducible results. Similarly, it is possible to carry out meaningful in-use evaluation of chemical disinfection of hospital surfaces (3. 7). An in-use test to evaluate disinfection of inhalation therapy equipment (9) was described by Pierce et al. Often, however, reproducible results are difficult or impossible to achieve in practice.

Actually, laboratory tests can be controlled much more readily than most in-use tests, and so the best approach sometimes is to devise a laboratory test system which simulates the actual conditions under which the disinfection is to be used. When such tests are carefully designed, the results may be more meaningful than those obtained by in vitro methods or actual in-use testing in the hospital. The Use-Dilution Method, for example, can readily be modified in ways appropriate for various applications. It is important that the number of microorganisms to be destroyed in these tests be determined (not assumed), because this factor has a pronounced effect upon the time required to kill all of the microbial population. Such tests should also be adequately controlled for bacteriostasis.

Antiseptics must be tested by in vivo in-use methods. Most of them measure "degerming" action on human skin. The Price method (10), for example, evaluates surgical scrub antiseptics by washing (or scrubbing) the hands and arms in a series of 14 basins containing soap or detergent and water. Because this is time-consuming and arduous, simpler methods for evaluating degerming agents are favored. Some of the more popular ones are (i) rubbing the hands before and after application of antiseptic with swabs which are then inoculated to culture plates; (ii) placing finger tips before and after the use of the antiseptic on the surface of agar plates, (iii) determining the number of viable bacteria in the "juice" of surgical gloves which have been worn for 1 to 3 h, and (iv) skin stripping with pieces of sticky tape and placing the tape on culture plates (15). Unfortunately, these methods are not standardized and variations are often introduced by investigators which neglect adequate neutralization so that it is impossible to distinguish between killing and bacteriostasis.

SELECTION OF GERMICIDES

Even though the reader may have good working knowledge of the nature of microbial contamination, the principles of disinfection and the comparative value of available germicides, the following suggestions may be helpful in selecting the best one for a particular purposes.

1. Decide first upon the level of disinfection required. If it calls for disinfection of a critical item, select a high-level germicide, liquid or gaseous. When there is a chance of contamination with tubercle bacilli and/or viruses but not spores, a good tuberculocide (intermediate level) is indicated, except for hepatitis viruses. Consider the type of article to be disinfected.

2. Several hundred proprietary germicides are being sold in the United States on the basis

TABLE 3. *Disinfectants and antiseptics*[a]

Class	Disinfectant	Antiseptic	Other properties
GAS			
Ethylene oxide	+2 to +4[b]	0	Toxic; good penetration; requires relative humidity of 30% or more; bactericidal activity varies with apparatus used; absorbed by porous materials. Dry spores highly resistant; moisture must be present and presoaking is desirable.
LIQUID			
Glutaraldehyde, aqueous	+3	0	Sporicidal; active solution unstable; toxic.
Formaldehyde + alcohol	+2	0	Sporicidal; noxious fumes; toxic; volatile.
Formaldehyde, aqueous	+1 to +2	0	Sporicidal; noxious fumes; toxic;
Phenolic compounds	+3	±	Stable; corrosive; little inactivation by organic matter; irritates skin.
Chlorine compounds	+1	±	Flash action; much inactivation by organic matter; corrosive; irritates skin.
Alcohol	+2	+3	Rapidly cidal; volatile; flammable; dries and irritates skin.
Iodine + alcohol	0	+4	Corrosive; very rapidly cidal; causes staining; irritates skin; flammable.
Iodophors	+1	+3	Somewhat unstable; relatively bland; staining temporary; corrosive.
Iodine, aqueous	0	+2	Rapidly cidal; corrosive; stains fabrics; stains and irritates skin.
Quaternary ammonium compounds	+1	+2	Bland; inactivated by soap and anionics; absorbed by fabrics.
Hexachlorophene	0	+2	Bland; insoluble in water, soluble in alcohol; not inactivated by soap; weakly cidal.
Mercurial compounds	0	+1	Bland; much inactivated by organic matter; weakly cidal.

[a] *Comment.* More detailed information must be obtained from descriptive brochures, journal articles, and books. Selection of the most appropriate germicide for a particular situation should be made by the responsible personnel in each hospital and based upon: (i) whether it is to be used as a disinfectant or an antiseptic; (ii) estimation of the level of antimicrobial action needed; the hospital's scope of services, physical facilities, and personnel.

Instruments, apparatus and other objects should be cleansed to remove gross organic soil prior to the use of chemical disinfectants which coagulate protein so as to get good penetration of crevices and porous material. Instruments, as well as rubber and plastic tubing, must be rinsed or flushed with sterile water before coming into contact with skin and especially mucous membrane to avoid irritation. For the same reason, aeration is necessary after exposure to ethylene oxide.

Some of the above material was suggested, modified, or contributed by G. F. Mallison, U.S. Public Health Service, Center for Disease Control.

[b] Maximal usefulness is denoted by +4.

of the manufacturers' claims. There are so many that some have not yet been tested by the federal regulatory agency. Select those which are shipped in interstate commerce because they come under federal jurisdiction and may already have been tested in the laboratories of the Environmental Protection Agency. Ask for that information.

3. When considering an unknown disinfectant, ask for data comparing it with a well known germicide of the same class, for example, Zephiran if it is a "quat," Wescodyne if it is an iodophor, etc.

4. Before deciding whether a germicide will be useful for your purposes, consider the following questions. Is it compatible with the materials to be disinfected? Is it stable? How broad is its cidal action?

5. Ask for the manufacturer's report on local and systemic toxicity and allergenicity, especially if the preparation is to be used as an antiseptic. Certain phenolics have caused depigmentation of skin (5).

6. Consult Table 3.

LITERATURE CITED

1. Association of Official Analytical Chemists. 1970. Official methods of analysis, 10th ed. Association of Official Analytical Chemists, Washington, D.C.
2. Ernst, R. R., and J. J. Shull. 1962. Ethylene oxide gaseous sterilization. II. Influence of method of humidification. Appl. Microbiol. **10:**342–344.
3. Favero, M. S., J. J. McDade, J. A. Robertson, R. K. Hoffman, and R. W. Edwards. 1968. Microbiological sampling of surfaces. J. Appl. Bacteriol. **31:**336–343.
4. Greene, V. W., and T. Hortis. 1973. Germicide utilization survey. American Society for Microbiology *ad hoc* Committee on Microbiological Standards of Disinfection in Hospitals.
5. Kahn, G. 1970. Depigmentation caused by phenolic detergent germicides. Arch. Dermatol. **102:**177–187.
6. Klein, M., and A. Deforest. 1963. Antiviral action of germicides. Soap Chem. Spec. **39:**70–72, 95–97.
7. Kundsin, R. B., and C. W. Walter. 1961. In-use testing of bactericidal agents in hospitals. Appl. Microbiol. **9:**167–171.
8. Ortenzio, L. F. 1966. Collaborative study of improved sporicidal test. J. Ass. Offic. Anal. Chem. **49:**721–726.
9. Pierce, A. K., J. P. Sanford, G. D. Thomas, and J. S. Leonard. 1970. Long-term evaluation of decontamination of inhalation-therapy equipment and the occurrence of necrotizing pneumonia. N. Engl. J. Med. **282:**528–531.
10. Price, P. R. 1938. The bacteriology of normal skin: a new quantitative test applied to a study of the bacterial flora and the disinfectant action of mechanical cleansing. J. Infec. Dis. **63:**301–318.
11. Rhoades, E. R., R. Ringrose, J. A. Mohr, L. Brooks, B. A. McKown, and F. Felton. 1971. Contamination of ultrasonic nebulization equipment with gram-negative bacteria. Arch. Intern. Med. **127:**228–232.
12. Spaulding, E. H. 1939. Chemical sterilization of surgical instruments. Surg. Gynecol. Obstet. **69:**738–744.
13. Spaulding, E. H. 1971. Role of chemical disinfection in the prevention of nosocomial infections. Proceedings of the International Conference on Nosocomial Infections, p. 247–254. American Hospital Association, Chicago, Ill.
14. Spaulding, E. H. 1968. Chemical disinfection of medical and surgical materials, p. 517–531. *In* C. A. Lawrence and S. S. Block (ed.), Disinfection, sterilization and preservation. Lea & Febiger, Philadelphia.
15. Ulrich, J. 1964. Technics for skin sampling for microbial contaminants. Health Lab. Sci. **1:**133–136.

Chapter 92

Bacterial Food Poisoning

E. M. FOSTER, R. H. DEIBEL, CHARLES L. DUNCAN, J. M. GOEPFERT, AND H. SUGIYAMA

BACTERIAL FOOD POISONING

Humans may become ill after consuming food that is (i) naturally poisonous (e.g., toxic mushrooms), (ii) contaminated with toxic chemicals, or (iii) contaminated with pathogenic microorganisms or their toxic products. An outbreak of food poisoning usually is recognized by epidemiological and clinical signs, but the laboratory may be called upon to identify the responsible food and the causal agent. This chapter deals with the more common bacterial food poisonings that occur in the United States for which laboratory procedures applicable to the usual microbiological laboratory are available: salmonellosis, staphylococcal poisoning, botulism, and perfringens poisoning.

The etiology of these diseases is well established. There is, however, growing evidence to incriminate certain viruses in food-borne disease. Shigellae, members of the *Arizona* group of the *Enterobacteriaceae*, and enteropathogenic strains of *Escherichia coli* may be transmitted by foods. Illness may even result from eating large numbers of cells of *Bacillus* species (e.g., *B. cereus*). Several other organisms and even certain mycotoxins have been suspected of causing illness when consumed with food.

STAPHYLOCOCCAL POISONING

The active agent is one of several antigenically different enterotoxins produced by some strains of *Staphylococcus aureus* when they grow in a food prior to consumption. A test for enterotoxin has been described, but the necessary serological reagents are not yet generally available. Therefore, laboratory procedures are limited to the demonstration of potentially enterotoxigenic (coagulase-positive) staphylococci in a suspect food.

There is no simple way to determine whether a *Staphylococcus* culture can produce enterotoxin, but there is a relationship between enterotoxin production and formation of the enzyme coagulase. Enterotoxin-producing strains of *S. aureus* are coagulase-positive, but many coagulase-positive strains do not form enterotoxin. Foods suspected of involvement in a food-poisoning outbreak customarily are examined for a coagulase-positive *S. aureus* strain. Large numbers of these organisms (e.g., hundreds of thousands or more per gram) give presumptive evidence that the food may be involved. Small numbers, however, do not necessarily exonerate the product. *S. aureus* may grow and produce enterotoxin, and then die off; or heating the food may destroy the organism but not the relatively heat-stable enterotoxin. Thus, interpretation of *S. aureus* counts depends upon the nature of the food and its past treatment.

To quantitate *S. aureus* in a food product, prepare pour plates of egg yolk-pyruvate-tellurite-glycine agar (EYA). To dry the surface, place the inverted bottom of the plate over the rim of the cover and incubate at 35 or 45 C until visible moisture has disappeared.

Blend 10 g of the food sample with 90 ml of sterile water (or multiples of these quantities) for 3 min in a mechanical blendor *to make a 1:10 dilution.* Alternatively, add 10 g of sample to a 90-ml water blank containing glass beads or small pieces of broken glass and shake vigorously.

Prepare serial decimal dilutions and dispense 0.1-ml quantities of at least three successive dilutions onto the surface of EYA plates. Beginning with the highest dilution, spread the inoculum over the entire surface of each plate with a flame-sterilized glass rod bent in the shape of a hockey stick. Proceed rapidly to the next lower dilution, until all have been spread; it is not necessary to resterilize the glass rod between plates. Invert plates and incubate for 24 to 30 h at 35 C.

Typical *S. aureus* colonies are black and surrounded by a clear area showing proteolysis. On longer incubation (48 h), the area surrounding the colony will become opaque as a result of lipase activity (fats are hydrolyzed, yielding insoluble fatty acids).

Count the plate containing 30 to 300 colonies; then pick about 10 typical *S. aureus* colonies and inoculate into either brain heart infusion or Trypticase soy broth. Incubate overnight at 35 C and perform a coagulase test on each isolate.

Calculate the *S. aureus* count per gram by multiplying the number of colonies on the plate by the dilution and then by the percentage of isolates confirmed by the coagulase test. The following formula may be used:

$$\text{dilution on plate counted} \times 0.1 = \text{dilution factor}$$

$$\frac{1}{\text{dilution factor}} \times \text{no. of colonies counted} \times \frac{\text{no. of coagulase-positive isolates}}{\text{total colonies tested for coagulase}} = S.\ aureus \text{ count per gram}$$

Mannitol-salt-agar (MSA) or Staphylococcus Medium No. 110 (SM 110) may be used separately or in conjunction with EYA plates. If either MSA or SM 110 is used, the traditional pour-plating method can be employed. Incubate for 48 h at 35 C. Count total colonies, and test randomly selected colonies for coagulase as described above. MSA and SM 110 are less selective for *S. aureus* than is EYA.

SALMONELLOSIS

Demonstration of living salmonellae in a food product is sufficient evidence to show a potential hazard to health. The procedures employed are basically similar to those used for clinical specimens (see chapter 18). However, because of the diverse composition and the large quantities tested, special steps are necessary in examining food for salmonellae. Quantitation procedures (e.g., determination of most probable numbers) are laborious and usually are not attempted.

Pre-enrichment

Various food-manufacturing procedures (e.g., drying, curing, freezing, heating) may damage or debilitate the salmonellae so that the organism cannot tolerate the mild toxicity of the selective enrichment media. To alleviate this problem, add 100 g of food sample to 1 liter of nutrient broth or lactose broth. Adjust the pH of the inoculated medium to neutrality and incubate at 35 C for 20 to 24 h. Some foods (e.g., certain gums, spices, dyestuffs, and coffee) contain inhibitors and cannot be tested at the 100-g level. For such materials, reduce the sample size but not the quantity of medium. With foods that contain considerable lipid, add Tergitol 7 to a final concentration of 0.6% in the pre-enrichment culture, and shake to disperse the fat.

Enrichment

Transfer 1.0 ml of the pre-enrichment culture to 9.0 ml of selenite-cystine broth; transfer a like amount to 9.0 ml of tetrathionate broth. Incubate for 24 h at 35 C. Both enrichment media are used because some salmonellae will not grow in one or the other. If Tergitol 7 was used in the pre-enrichment step, there is sufficient carry-over in the transfer so that further addition of this compound is unnecessary. When adding iodine to complete the tetrathionate broth, be sure to follow the manufacturer's directions and shake well to insure reaction of all of the iodine before inoculation.

Foods (e.g., raw meat and poultry) that are not subjected to rigorous processing treatments and materials that have been thawed or rehydrated prior to arrival at the laboratory may be inoculated directly into the enrichment media at a level not exceeding 50 g per liter of broth. Do not use a higher ratio of sample to medium, as it may disrupt the finely balanced selective system. If the food has high lipid content, use Tergitol 7 as described under Pre-enrichment.

Selective plating

Streak a loopful of each enrichment culture on plates of Brilliant Green-agar or Brilliant Green-sulfa-agar, Salmonella-Shigella agar or deoxycholate-citrate-lactose-sucrose-agar, and bismuth sulfite-agar. Incubate at 35 C for 24 h. It is imperative that isolated colonies be obtained. Preferably, use all three selective media; if this is not possible, select the order listed.

Typical reactions of the salmonellae on these media are as follows:

1. Brilliant Green- and Brilliant Green-sulfa-agar—colorless, pink, or gray colonies; area surrounding colonies shows no change, pink or deep red color.
2. Salmonella-Shigella and deoxycholate-citrate-lactose-sucrose-agar—translucent to opaque colonies, with or without black centers; agar around colonies unchanged or yellow.
3. Bismuth sulfite-agar—glistening colonies of black, dark brown, or dark green color; may or may not have a metallic sheen; agar around colonies may or may not be black.

Suspicious colonies are isolated and identified by biochemical and serological procedures.

BOTULISM

Examination for botulinal toxin

Demonstration in a suspect food of one of the types of neurotoxin produced by *Clostridium botulinum* is used to confirm a clinical diagnosis of botulism. Avoid unnecessary destruction of the thermolabile toxin by keeping the sample refrigerated until tested. Handle specimens aseptically.

Use liquid portion of the food directly. If only the food container is available, rinse with 5 to 10 ml of sterile saline. Use all of the solid sample if the amount can be handled conveniently; otherwise, take representative portions.

To prepare an extract of solid food, add an equal volume (wt/vol) of gelatin-phosphate buffer. Homogenize in a mechanical blendor at low speed to avoid overheating. Alternatively, grind with a pestle in a prechilled mortar containing sterile sand. When results are needed as soon as possible, centrifuge homogenate or sample fluid immediately at high speed (e.g., 10,000 × *g*) for 30 min (preferably in a refrigerated centrifuge). Otherwise, refrigerate overnight to achieve better extraction of toxin. Collect supernatant fluid, avoiding particles and fat.

Inject 0.5 ml of sample (with and without trypsinization) into mice to determine the presence of botulinal toxin and its type (see chapter 39). Save unused portions in a refrigerator until tests are completed.

Food extracts may contain nonbotulinal factors which are lethal for mice. If this is indicated by the death of all mice, inject a 1:10 dilution made with gelatin-phosphate buffer. Freeze the extract (−6 to −20 C) overnight before animal injections if nonspecific factors still interfere with the test.

Mice may develop the botulism syndrome but the typing results may be inconclusive. In such cases, inject a 1:10 dilution to see if a high botulinal toxicity is exceeding the protective limits of the antitoxin. A rare alternative is the presence of more than one type of botulinal toxin.

Examination for C. botulinum

Finding the organism does not necessarily incriminate the food as the responsible vehicle; the existence of viable organisms does not always mean that toxin has been formed. Nevertheless, it may be desirable to know whether *C. botulinum* is present. Demonstration of botulinal toxin in enrichment cultures inoculated with the food is acceptable evidence for the presence of the organism. Use of replicate cultures in different media increases the chances of positive findings. A minimum of nine cultures are recommended when the type of *C. botulinum* being sought is not known.

Add 1 to 2 g of food homogenate or other available sample to the bottom of each tube of cooked-meat medium. If the medium is not prepared on the day of use, place tubes in a boiling-water bath for 5 min and cool in tap water before inoculating. Divide the inoculated tubes into three equal sets. Heat one set in a water bath at 60 C for 15 min, heat a second at 80 C for 30 min, and leave the third set unheated. Incubate one culture from each set at 35, 30, and 25 C; special precaution to maintain anaerobic condition is not needed. These various cultural procedures are used because of differences in heat resistance of spores and the optimal temperature of growth among *C. botulinum* strains. If possible, prepare a second series of cultures in Trypticase-peptone-glucose medium.

Test the culture supernatant fluids for toxin by injection into mice when gas production and turbidity indicate vigorous growth. This usually occurs within 2 to 4 days, but cultures are held 10 days before being considered negative.

Isolation

Streak plates of egg yolk agar with the enrichment cultures at the time they are tested for toxin. Incubate plates for 48 h at 30 C under anaerobic conditions. Colonies of *C. botulinum* (and a few other species) have a pearly iridescence which extends from the colony and over the zone of heavy precipitate in the agar. Pick several of these colonies into cooked meat medium, incubate 2 to 4 days, and test for toxin.

Chances of successful isolation are increased by an additional procedure. After RCM has been streaked, mix the enrichment culture, let the heavy particles settle, and transfer 2 ml of supernatant fluid to a sterile tube. Add an equal volume of absolute ethyl alcohol, mix, and hold for 1 h at room temperature with occasional agitation. Streak plates as described above.

PERFRINGENS POISONING

Demonstration of large numbers (usually hundreds of thousands or more per gram) of *Clostridium perfringens* cells in a suspect food supports a diagnosis of perfringens poisoning based on clinical and epidemiological evidence. Further support is provided if the same serotype of organism is recovered from the food and the stools of patients. Cooked meat and poultry dishes are the foods most commonly involved.

Quantitation in foods

Refrigerate food specimens as soon as they are received, but do not freeze them. Promptly Gram stain a direct smear of the sample and look for thick, gram-positive rods which are 1.0 to 1.5 by 4.0 to 8.0 μm in size. The cells may or may not contain endospores.

Add 10 g of food to 90 ml of sterile 0.1% peptone-water and blend for 2 min at slow speed with a mechanical mixer to obtain a 1:10

dilution. Prepare serial decimal dilutions (through 10^{-7}) with peptone-water. Make duplicate surface platings of each dilution, using 0.1-ml amounts, on tryptose-sulfite-cycloserine (TSC) agar (chapter 95). After the agar has dried, overlay the surface with an additional 4 to 5 ml of TSC agar from which the egg yolk emulsion has been omitted. Alternatively, make duplicate pour plates of each dilution with either sulfite-polymyxin-sulfadiazine (SPS) agar (chapter 95) or tryptone-sulfite-neomycin (TSN) agar (chapter 95), using 1 ml of dilution to about 15 ml of agar. After the pour plates solidify, cover with an additional 4 to 5 ml of the agar. Invert the plates and incubate them anaerobically for 24 h at 37 C.

SPS and TSN agar may be inhibitory to some strains of *C. perfringens* and therefore less useful than TSC agar, which reportedly allows virtually complete recovery of most *C. perfringens* strains.

Select plates containing 30 to 300 black colonies, which may be surrounded by a zone of precipitate on the TSC agar (as a result of lecithinase production) but not on SPS or TSN agar. Using a Quebec colony counter with a piece of white tissue paper on the glass to provide a white background, count all black colonies and calculate the average number of colonies in the duplicate plates.

Select at least 10 representative black colonies and determine the ratio of *C. perfringens* among these colonies. Inoculate each colony into a tube of fluid thioglycolate medium (FTG). Incubate for 4 h in a water bath at 46 C, or overnight at 35 C. Rapid growth with profuse gassing occurs at 46 C if *C. perfringens* is present. After incubation, examine for the presence of gram-positive rods with blunt ends; endospores usually are not produced in this medium.

Stab-inoculate each FTG culture containing these cells into two tubes of motility-nitrate medium (chapter 95) and incubate at 35 C. After 24 h, read for motility and test one culture of each pair for reduction of nitrate to nitrite. If nitrate has not been reduced, incubate the second tube for an additional 24 h and repeat the test.

Cultures which are nonmotile and reduce nitrate are confirmed as *C. perfringens*. Calculate the number of viable *C. perfringens* per gram of food sample by multiplying the number of colonies by the dilution plated and then by the percentage of colonies confirmed as *C. perfringens*. In the case of TSC agar in which only 0.1 ml of the dilution was surface plated, 0.1 should be multiplied times the dilution plated to obtain the proper dilution factor. The following formula may be used:

$$\text{average count of colonies} \times \frac{1}{\text{dilution in plates counted}} \times \frac{\text{colonies confirmed as } C.\ perfringens}{\text{total colonies tested}} = C.\ perfringens \text{ per gram}$$

Isolation from feces

Inoculate two tubes containing 25 ml of FTG with about 1 g of feces, or 5 ml if the fecal sample is liquid. Heat one tube for 20 min in a water bath at 75 C; then cool in tap water. Incubate both tubes for 4 h at 46 C or for 18 to 24 h at 35 C. After incubation, streak from the cultures onto the dry surface of McClung-Toabe egg yolk agar (chapter 95) to obtain isolated colonies. Incubate the plates in an anaerobic jar.

Examine the plates for circular, slightly raised colonies which are surrounded by a zone of precipitate (indicating lecithinase production). Pick representative lecithinase-positive colonies to FTG, and proceed as before to confirm isolates as *C. perfringens* by motility and nitrate reduction tests.

Save for serotyping at least two *C. perfringens* isolates from the incriminated food and three or more from the feces of each patient. In large outbreaks, save cultures from each of 10 different patients. Since antisera for typing are not generally available to the usual laboratory, arrangements for serotype identification must be made with a laboratory equipped for this work.

Chapter 93

Quality Control in the Microbiology Laboratory

RUTH L. RUSSELL

In the past 50 years, clinical laboratory science has developed from a simple and relatively unimportant branch of medicine into a highly complex science that provides physicians with information vital to the diagnosis and treatment of many diseases. Since the first description of the use of control charts for recording quality control data in the clinical laboratory by Levey and Jennings in 1950 (26), there has been increasing concern that control measures to assure reliability and reproducibility of laboratory results have not kept pace with the tremendous expansion and automation in laboratory medicine, the complexity of modern laboratory tests, and the increasing importance of test results in the practice of medicine. Since the latter part of the 1960's, this concern for quality control has led to Federal legislation establishing the Clinical Laboratories Improvement Act of 1967 and to the laboratory standards included in the Medicare Act. Private accreditation agencies, such as the College of American Pathologists and the Joint Commission on the Accreditation of Hospitals, have imposed more stringent standards for quality control. In addition, a number of state and local public health agencies have developed regional standards and regulations for quality control in clinical laboratories within their jurisdictions. An increasing number of clinical laboratories in the United States are under the quality control standards of one or more of these agencies. Numerous publications are related to the philosophy and implementation of quality control regulations in clinical laboratories (1, 2, 4, 5, 13–15, 17, 19, 20, 22).

The more quantitative disciplines in clinical laboratory medicine, such as clinical chemistry, have practiced quality control for some years and, in general, the necessity for quality control techniques has been accepted by technologists in the quantitative disciplines. However, clinical microbiology is one of the least quantitative and most subjective of the laboratory disciplines, and there has been some reluctance to accept the mandatory intrusion of quality control techniques into clinical microbiology laboratories. Some consider it unnecessary, and others believe that, although quality control techniques may be desirable, the techniques available to microbiologists are too indirect, too esoteric, or too expensive, especially for the small laboratory. Although there is some truth in the above allegations, sources of error in the clinical microbiology laboratory and the need for quality assurance has been well documented (1–8, 13, 17, 25, 29, 32).

A well-designed quality control program for microbiology includes many simple and direct methods for monitoring, as well as other techniques, and should be viewed as an asset, not a liability, to the laboratory. However, personnel faced with the immediate necessity of establishing a quality control program might overlook some of the positive factors provided by a well-designed program; for example, (i) monitoring of media and reagents before use on clinical specimens eliminates the potential errors inherent if inadequate materials were employed for the isolation and subsequent identification of clinically significant microorganisms, (ii) routine monitoring and maintenance of equipment helps to prevent serious and costly breakdowns, (iii) it will permit more expedient and accurate laboratory reports by preventing the use of inadequate media, equipment, and techniques, (iv) it is a learning technique to help identify subtle problems that otherwise might be overlooked or might result in major problems, (v) it is a good administrative tool to assist a busy supervisor in detecting current or potential deficiencies by periodic review of quality control data, and (vi) it bolsters the morale of laboratory personnel to know that all practicable measures have been taken to assure the quality of materials and techniques and therefore to enhance the reliability of test results emanating from their laboratory. A feeling of quality assurance among laboratory personnel is a very valuable asset.

There are many viewpoints as to the scope of a quality control program and manual. Some interpret quality control in a broad sense encompassing all aspects of "quality" in the laboratory, and their manuals may include such items as the philosophy and goals of a quality control program, safety precautions including immunization schedules for laboratory personnel, and addresses of suppliers of laboratory reagents and equipment. Two very valuable compendia for guidelines for the development of quality control programs are *Quality Control in Clinical Microbiology* by Bartlett et al. (5) and the *Manual of Quality Control Procedures for Microbiological Laboratories* currently in the working draft stage of development at the Center for Disease Control (12). A quality control manual, as well as all other laboratory workbooks, should be reviewed and revised at periodic intervals not exceeding 1 year.

A very important facet of any quality control program is the log sheets utilized for recording and reviewing quality control data generated by the program. Two features are essential in the design of these logs: (i) the amount of writing or other notations needed to describe the quality control data should be minimal, and (ii) the log charts should be organized so that data can be quickly reviewed and easily interpreted by persons involved in quality control. Since several persons may be involved in the recording and/or reviewing of quality control data, vague terms such as "OK" should be avoided and more precise terms or abbreviations should be utilized. The space allowed for recording of quality control data should take into consideration the terms or abbreviations necessary to describe adequately the information needed. For example, if a laboratory wished to record certain physical characteristics of specimens it received, more space on log sheets would be needed for entering such data than would be needed for recording the temperatures of incubators. There are two major formats for log sheets used for recording temperatures of equipment in the laboratory. In laboratories with only a few pieces of equipment, it may be desirable to have a separate sheet for each piece of equipment and attach the sheet to the equipment. When a number of pieces are to be monitored, it may be more expedient to attach a sheet or sheets listing the various pieces of equipment to a clipboard to be carried by the person monitoring the equipment. Although there are certain basic elements in all quality control programs, there are many variations in their implementation that can be tailored to fit the needs of individual laboratories. Examples of the diversity of quality control programs and log sheets designed by different laboratories are provided by references 5, 7, 12, 15, 16, 21, 29, 31, and 33.

The quality control program described below is a modification of the program developed by the Microbiology Section of the Memorial Hospital Medical Center of Long Beach, a large, modern, teaching hospital with primary service obligations. The program was implemented in 1968 and the cooperation of the staff in the initiation and performance of the program has been excellent. One technologist is designated the responsibility for directing the program, but the entire staff and the medical technology trainees are involved in its implementation.

QUALITY CONTROL PROGRAM FOR MICROBIOLOGY

The quality control program is organized into the sections outlined below. Detailed procedural instructions, including microorganisms to be utilized in monitoring procedures, are presented in each section followed by logs for the recording and reviewing of quality control data. Failures in quality control are recorded in the appropriate section in which they occur and also in the Failures in Quality Control Log.

I. Mechanical equipment
II. Media
III. Reagents
   A. Chemical
   B. Disk
   C. Antisera
   D. Water
IV. Specimens
V. Personnel and procedures
   A. Written protocols
   B. Internal unknowns
   C. External unknowns (proficiency tests)
   D. Departmental conferences
   E. Education of personnel in quality control procedures
   F. Continuing in-service education
VI. Failures in quality control log
Appendix I. Maintenance of stock cultures
Appendix II. Log of selected clinical isolates
Appendix III. References in quality control

I. Mechanical equipment (an abstract of an Equipment Control Log is presented in Fig. 1)
   A. Temperatures are checked at the start of each day on incubators, water baths, hot blocks, refrigerators, and freezers. Hi-Lo thermometers are employed in most equipment, and recording thermometers are employed in walk-in refrigerators and incubators and on autoclaves.
   B. "Kilit tests" are performed weekly on all steam autoclaves.
   C. The gaseous environment for anaerobic and carbon dioxide incubation is checked both chemically and biologically each day. A methylene blue indicator is used for chemical testing of anaerobic conditions and a Fyrite

Carbon Dioxide testing device is used for chemically measuring the CO_2 content of capneic incubators. Biological testing is performed by the monitor culture technique. *Clostridium hemolyticum* inoculated onto blood-agar plates is employed in anaerobic jars and incubators, and a CO_2-dependent strain of *Neisseria gonorrhoeae* inoculated on chocolate-agar is employed in capneic incubators.

D. The cold catalyst utilized in GasPak jars is reactivated each time it is used by heating a hot air oven at 350 F (177 C) for 1 h.

E. Mechanical rotators are checked weekly for correct oscillation speed and orbit.

F. The face velocity of biological hoods is checked at monthly intervals for the desired rate of 50 ft/min (15.2 meters/min) and filter pads are replaced at 6-month intervals.

G. All mechanical equipment is closely observed for defects; if defects are suspected, the equipment is checked by qualified personnel.

II. Media

A. Source

1. Most media utilized in the laboratory are prepared from dehydrated media and media supplements purchased from reputable manufacturers. A record is kept in the Media Source Log (Fig. 2) on each bottle, giving the name of the manufacturer, control number, date of receipt, and date bottle was opened. The dehydrated media are stored at room temperature and the media supplements are kept in a refrigerator.
2. Prepared media are purchased from reliable sources and are dated and logged upon receipt in the laboratory.

B. Preparation, sterility testing, and storage

1. All dehydrated media are reconstituted with deionized water, and the directions supplied by the manufacturer are explicitly followed.
2. All agar media that are dispensed after autoclaving are maintained in a water bath at 50 C for not longer than 1 h before dispensing.
3. Ten percent of all noninhibitory media that are dispensed after autoclaving are sterility-checked by overnight incubation at 35 C.
4. Those inhibitory media that do not require sterilization are sterility-checked by overnight incubation at 35 C of 10% of the plates or tubes; the incubated media are observed and discarded. If contamination is present in the incubated media, the remainder of that batch of medium is discarded.
5. A record is kept in the Media Performance Log (Fig. 3) of the date of media preparation and receipt of prepared media in the laboratory; all batches of media are dated.
6. Thiol and thio are stored at room temperature in the dark; all other media are stored in a refrigerator.

C. Performance testing

1. The quality of each batch of medium is tested before use on clinical specimens by inoculation of appropriate organisms to produce positive and negative results.

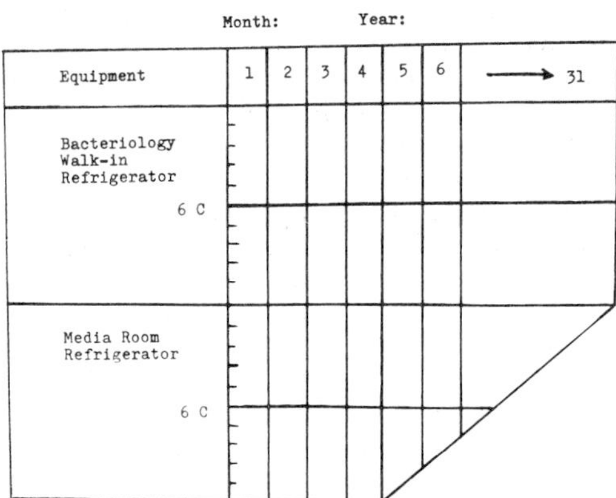

Month: Year:

Equipment	1	2	3	4	5	6	→ 31
Bacteriology Walk-in Refrigerator							
6 C							
Media Room Refrigerator							
6 C							

FIG. 1. *Abstract of an equipment control log.*

Month: Year:

Media	Source	Control Number	Date Rec'd	Date Bot' Opened	Source →
Media: Plates					
Blood Azide					
Chlamydospore					
Hektoen-Enteric					
MacConkey's					
Mannitol Salt					
Mueller-Hinton					

FIG. 2. *Abstract of a media source log.*

Month: Year:

Date	1	2	3	4	5	6	7	→ 31
Media: Plates								
Blood Azide								
Chlamydospore								
Hektoen-Enteric								
MacConkey's								
Mannitol-Salt								
Mueller-Hinton								

FIG. 3. *Abstract of a media performance log.*

Methods used include the inoculation of separate tubes of fermentation medium with fermentative and nonfermentative organisms and the inoculation of selective media with organisms that should grow and others that should be inhibited. Isolation media are lightly inoculated with diluted suspensions of organisms that should grow in an attempt to simulate the small quantity of potential pathogens that may be present in clinical specimens.

2. Those few media that are kept more than 1 month are retested at monthly intervals.
3. A record is kept in the Media Performance Log.

III. Reagents

A. Chemical

1. Source
The chemicals purchased are of approved quality and all bottles are dated upon receipt, recorded in the Chemical Reagent Log, and stored in tightly closed containers. Chemicals are purchased in small quantities to help assure freshness and stability.

2. Preparation and storage of reagents
The reagents are carefully prepared, and labels include the data and the name of the technologist who prepared them. A record is kept in the Chemical Reagent Log of the date of preparation and the lot or control number of the chemicals used in preparation of the reagents. Most reagents are stored in opaque, tightly closed bottles at room temperature; however, some reagents such as H_2O_2 and coagulase plasma must be stored in a refrigerator.

3. Performance testing
All reagents are tested for correct reactions with known positive and negative controls before they are used on clinical specimens, and most reagents are retested at monthly intervals. Tests on the Gram and acid-fast stains are performed weekly, and controls are used each time the niacin and other infrequently performed tests are run on clinical specimens. The results of performance testing are recorded in the Chemical Reagent Log.

B. Disk

1. Source and storage
All disks are obtained from reputable manufacturers and are stored with the desiccant supplied by the manufacturer. Antimicrobial disks are stored at −20 C until placed in dispensers; other disks, e.g., "A" and "N," are stored in a refrigerator. A record is kept in the Disk Reagent Control Log of the date of receipt, manufacturer, lot or control number, and the expiration date.

2. Performance testing
The disks are tested on a lot or control number basis before they are used on clinical specimens. Three randomly selected disks are tested on appropriate organisms and the results are recorded in the Disk Reagent Control Log. The antimicrobial disks are tested by the Bauer-Kirby technique (7) on the Seattle strains of *Escherichia coli* (ATCC 25922) and *Staphylococcus aureus* (ATCC 25923) and are retested at weekly intervals.

C. Antisera

1. Source and storage
All antisera are purchased from reputable manufacturers and a record is kept in the Antisera Reagent Log of the date of receipt, manufacturer, lot or control number, date of rehydration, and expiration date. The directions supplied by the manufacturer for the rehydration and storage of sera are rigidly followed.

2. Performance testing
The antisera are tested for correct reactions with appropriate cultures before use on clinical specimens and are retested at monthly intervals. The results of performance testing are recorded in the Antisera Reagent Log.

D. Water
The deionized water is tested daily for chemical purity by a conductance bridge, and plate counts are performed weekly on Plate Count Agar. The results of testing are recorded in the Water Reagent Log.

IV. Specimens
Personnel who collect specimens are instructed in the methods and importance of proper collection and handling of specimens. Concise written instructions and appropriate containers and transport media are provided in convenient locations throughout the hospital. Specimens are logged, labeled with prenumbered pressure tapes, and processed within 1 h after receipt in the laboratory.

V. Personnel and procedures

A. Written protocols
A complete workbook of all laboratory procedures and pertinent Public Health regulations is present in the laboratory. In addition, specific procedural instructions are provided in work areas in the laboratory.

B. Internal unknowns

1. The supervisor introduces especially inoculated unknown specimens into the regular flow of clinical microbiology specimens accompanied by routine laboratory slips.
2. When the results are obtained, the supervisor notifies the technologists that it was an internal unknown and discusses the techniques and results with them.
3. A minimum of two unknowns are introduced each month, and their content is rotated so that all of the specialties within the department are checked periodically.

C. External unknowns (proficiency tests)

1. Four sets of specimens a year are received from the Survey Program of the College of American Pathologists and four sets a year

are received from the Check Sample Program of the Commission on Continuing Education of the American Society for Clinical Pathologists.

2. The specimens are processed in a routine manner, and the procedures and results obtained are compared and evaluated by the pathologist and supervisor with the critiques and computer print-outs supplied by the associations. The pathologist and supervisor discuss the results with the technologists, and the results are reported to the Department of Pathology's weekly administrative meeting.

D. Departmental conferences
A weekly departmental conference is held to discuss problems, potential changes, and other matters of concern to the microbiology department.

E. Education of personnel in quality control procedures
1. The supervisor presents an orientation to the philosophy and techniques of quality control to all new personnel.
2. Technologists and student technologists are assigned to read the quality control manual and to participate in all aspects of quality control as the procedures are performed in the laboratory.
3. Technicians are required to read those sections of the quality control manual pertinent to their duties and to participate in those procedures performed by technicians.
4. An evaluation of the employees' performance in quality control procedures is incorporated in the periodic evaluation report of all personnel.

F. Continuing in-service education
1. All technologists and student technologists are required periodically to review Kodachromes and microscope slides of microorganisms which are of medical importance but are not commonly encountered in clinical specimens.
2. Technologists are encouraged to attend workshops and seminars and to read journal articles in the field of clinical microbiology.
3. Periodic review sessions are held for personnel assigned to the afternoon and evening shifts to evaluate, and if necessary to refresh, their capabilities in basic microbiological procedures.

VI. Failures in quality control log
All failures detected by quality control monitoring are listed in this section. They are accompanied by notes on the corrective measures taken to prevent recurrences and with the signature of the supervisor.

During the first year of implementation, the quality control program revealed a number of subtle problems with media, antimicrobial disks, procedures, and equipment that might have remained undetected without a surveillance system. In addition, several gross media deficiencies were detected that would have resulted in a number of erroneous or delayed laboratory reports if there had not been a monitor system for performance testing of media before use on clinical specimens. The detection of problems has permitted corrective measures to be taken that have markedly reduced the number of problems and has resulted in more accurate and expedient laboratory reports.

A very important consideration in a quality control program is the selection of an appropriate battery of microorganisms for the sensitive monitoring of media, reagents, and gaseous conditions of incubators and for the preparation of internal unknowns. A few criteria to be considered in the selection of quality control monitor organisms may be of assistance in the development of a quality control program. For ease of maintenance, as small a number of cultures should be chosen as will provide for adequate surveillance. Organisms that are strongly positive or negative in their reactions, in general, do not provide for adequate detection of subtle problems. For example, weakly gram-positive and gram-negative bacteria such as *Bacillus subtilis* and *Neisseria catarrhalis* would be more sensitive indicators of deficiencies in Gram stain reagents and techniques than would more strongly gram-positive and gram-negative bacteria such as *Staphylococcus aureus* and *Escherichia coli*. In the selection of a positive control for enteric selective and enrichment media, a relatively delicate enteric pathogen such as *Shigella flexneri* would be more sensitive than the more hardy *Shigella sonnei* or the even hardier *Salmonella* species. Since the most common deficiency in chocolate-agar is inactivation of the heat-labile "V" factor, a microorganism that requires the "V" factor, such as *Haemophilus influenzae*, would be an appropriate positive control in checking for nutritional adequacy of that medium.

Performance testing of media is one of the most time-consuming aspects of a microbiological quality control program. This is primarily due to the necessity of having available a relatively large battery of control organisms in the correct physiological state for media monitoring. During the past few years, laboratories with media monitoring programs have learned that there is a greater percentage of deficiencies in media that contain inhibitory substances than in media that do not, and that the pH of Mueller-Hinton medium influences the zone diameter of many antimicrobial agents tested by the Bauer-Kirby technique. As more information of this type becomes available, it will permit the establishment of priorities for media performance testing. Nagel and Kunz (28) suggested that the commercial manufacturers of prepared media be given the responsibility for quality assurance of media and relieve the consumer of that time-consuming obligation. This is an excellent suggestion and, since most of the larger and many of the smaller manufacturers currently have good quality control programs, placing the responsibility for preparation of good media on the manufacturer would not be a major problem for reliable companies. Currently, the major problem is to provide adequate environmental conditions to maintain the quality of media during shipment, particularly during extreme weather conditions and to laboratories at locations inconvenient to shipment. It was suggested in 1969 that one of the alternatives to performance testing of prepared media in the consumer laboratory was to depend upon the quality control of reliable manufacturers (29). Obviously, shipping conditions as well as the preparation of good media by the manufacturer must be taken into consideration.

MAINTENANCE OF MICROBIAL CULTURES

Many quality control procedures in clinical microbiology are dependent in part on viable cultures possessing physiological and morphological characteristics that are typical and reproducible. Cultures should be selected with care to insure that they are typical for the desired characteristics and they should be maintained in a manner to minimize mutations. Mutations can be minimized by permitting only minimal amounts of growth of the microorganisms and by providing optimal environmental conditions. Minimal growth includes both minimal periods for growth of cultures, e.g., 6 to 10 h for staphylococci and enteric organisms, and limited numbers of subcultures.

For convenience, maintenance of cultures will be separated into three major catagories: stock cultures, semistock cultures, and working cultures.

Stock cultures

Stock cultures are those cultures held in reserve in a culture "bank" from which working or semistock cultures are made. Stock cultures are maintained in a manner as close as possible to animated suspension to minimize physiological and genetic activity and therefore potential mutation. The two major methods for preservation of stock cultures are lyophilization (freeze-drying) and ultrafreezing. Grow cultures on suitable agar plates or slants, suspend in a medium high in protein or glycerol, dispense in 0.25- to 0.5-ml portions, and quick-freeze. For maximal viability, bacterial cultures should be young but past the logarithmic growth phase, and fungus cultures should be young but well sporulated. There are many formulations for suspending media, but, in general, skim milk or serum is employed for lyophilization and blood or a rich buffered broth, e.g., Brucella Broth, with 15% reagent-grade glycerol is employed for ultrafreezing.

Lyophilization. Make a heavy suspension of young culture in sterile skim milk (or substitute), dispense into thin-walled tubes with constrictions, shell-freeze by rotating in a bath of dry ice-ethanol or dry ice-ethylene glycol, attach to a lyophile apparatus, dry by vacuum, cut tubes off with a torch while still under vacuum, and store in the dark at room temperature or preferably in a refrigerator. Cultures preserved in this manner will remain viable nearly indefinitely. Details of lyophilization are described in references 5, 9, 18, 23, and 24.

The lyophile apparatus may vary in complexity from simply a heavy-duty vacuum pump with appropriate tubing to a sophisticated machine specifically designed for the purpose. There are two major safety precautions to be followed, particularly with pathogens. (i) During lyophilization do not permit the culture to be carried by vacuum from the tube into the lyophile apparatus. This can be prevented by having a small cotton plug pushed about 1 cm down from the top of the lyophile tube. (ii) Do not permit the formation of aerosols when opening lyophile tubes for culture. Any measure that will prevent a rapid influx of air into the lyophile tube will minimize aerosol formation. A simple precaution is to place cellophane tape around the tube after etching but before breaking the tube. Although lyophilization is the most time-consuming method of maintenance of stock cultures, it has the advantages of ease of storage and shipment of cultures and maximal storage life of delicate microorganisms.

Ultra freezing in a dry-ice chest or in an electric ultrafreezer. Make a heavy suspension of young culture in Brucella Broth containing 15% reagent-grade glycerol (or substitute), dispense in 0.25- to 0.5-ml portions into small test tubes or screw-capped vials, seal cap with Parafilm Self-Sealing Tape, and either shell-freeze or place directly into a deep freeze. With freezers that attain −45 C or lower, cultures will keep for an extended period of time. With this basic method, it is necessary to thaw the suspension to obtain cells for culture, and, except with very hardy organisms, the remaining suspension should not be refrozen with the anticipation of obtaining viable cells for culture at a later time. There have been a number of modifications of this basic technique that employ a variety of glass beads or alundum to serve as inert carriers to be coated with the suspension of organisms. Cultures can be made repeatedly from such frozen stocks, if care is taken not to thaw the culture, by removing a bead or a few grains of alundum with sterile forceps. In one technique that employs alundum and defibrinated blood, a well is made in the center of the alundum with the pipette used to dispense the suspension into the vial containing the alundum (27). The well permits faster freezing and greater ease of removal of particles. With all freezing methods utilizing beads or alundum, it is essential to have only a minimal coating of suspension on the carriers so that the carriers can be easily removed while the rest of the culture remains frozen. Details of various techniques for ultrafreezing of cultures are described in references 9, 12, 23, 24, 27, and 30.

Ultrafreezing by storage in liquid nitrogen. Make a heavy suspension of a young culture in Brucella Broth containing 15% reagent-grade glycerol (or substitute), dispense in 0.25- to 0.5-ml portions in special ampoules, seal ampoules by torch, and place in a special apparatus specifically designed for storage of materials in liquid nitrogen. This method preserves cultures for extended periods of time, and the apparatus is nearly maintenance free. Details of this procedure, including the necessary safety precautions, are available in brochures describing commercially available liquid nitrogen apparatus and in references 5, 9, 12, 23, and 24.

Semistock cultures

The term semistock refers to maintenance of cultures for periods intermediate between the relative permanence of stock cultures and the relative impermanence of working cultures. There is a very wide temporal range of viability among various microorganisms when maintained by these relatively simple techniques that require only minimal time and apparatus. Of the five techniques listed, only the freezing technique is suitable for anaerobes (11). Some laboratories utilize semistock cultures in place of stock cultures, and other laboratories use them to reduce the frequency of starting new working cultures from stock cultures.

Freezing in a conventional freezer. Conventional freezers attain temperatures from −10 to −25 C. Prepare cultures in the same manner as for ultrafreezing. Hardy organisms will survive several years and less hardy ones from 6 to 12 months. The lower the temperature, the longer the survival period will be. This method is used primarily for bacteria and yeasts.

CTA stab cultures. Inoculate a screw-capped tube of cystine Trypticase Soy agar by stabbing about 2 cm below the surface, incubate until moderate growth appears, tighten the cap, and store in the dark at room temperature or preferably in a refrigerator. This method is suitable for yeasts and all but anaerobic and very fastidious bacteria. Hardy organisms will survive for about 1 year and relatively delicate organisms for several weeks.

Drying in gelatin disks. Cut circles of waxed paper to fit into glass petri dishes, place in petri dishes, and sterilize by autoclaving at 15 psi for 15 min. Prepare suspending fluid consisting of nutrient broth with 10% (wt/vol) gelatin powder and 0.25% (wt/vol) ascorbic acid, dispense into tubes, and autoclave at 15 psi for 15 min. If the tubes are not to be used immediately, omit the ascorbic acid and add it from a concentrated stock solution just before use. Heat the gelatin suspending medium to 30 C, make a relatively heavy suspension of young culture in the suspending medium, place individual drops of the suspension on the waxed paper in the petri dish with a capillary pipette, and transfer the dish to a vacuum desiccator containing phosphorus pentoxide. Evacuate the desiccator with a vacuum pump. When the disks have dried, aseptically place them in sterile screw-capped bottles or tubes, and store in a refrigerator. To make a culture from the disks, aseptically remove a disk and place in a suitable broth medium. This method is known as Stamp's method in honor of its originator and is suitable for most aerobic, nonfastidious bacteria of medical importance.

Mineral oil overlay of slant cultures. This method is used primarily for fungi but may be used for relatively hardy bacteria. To young but well-sporulated cultures, add sufficient sterile, medicinal-grade mineral oil to cover the slant of the culture completely, tighten the cap of the container, and store in the dark, preferably in a refrigerator. Cultures will remain viable from 6 months to several years by this method. To assure the sterility of mineral oil, it should be autoclaved at 15 psi for 45 min.

Storage in sterile soil. This method is used primarily for fungi and spore-bearing bacteria. Sterilize soil in test tubes or vials by autoclaving at 15 psi for 1 h. Make a heavy suspension of young but well-sporulated culture, allow to dry at room temperature, and store in a refrigerator.

Working cultures

Working cultures are in a convenient form ready to be utilized for quality control and other purposes in the laboratory. For those procedures requiring 24-h cultures, e.g., the Gram stain, it will be necessary to subculture from the working stocks if the working stocks are more than 24 h old.

Relatively hardy bacteria. Working cultures are prepared by plating out from stock or semistock cultures, transferring young colonies to Trypticase Soy agar slants (or substitute), incubating slants for a minimal time for good growth to occur, and storing in a refrigerator. The working slants are transferred to new working slants at monthly intervals for 6 months and then new working cultures are prepared from stock or semistock cultures.

Delicate bacteria. Working cultures of delicate bacteria, e.g., *Neisseria meningitidis* and *Streptococcus pyogenes*, are prepared by plating out from stock or semistock cultures and are maintained on suitable plates or slants. They are transferred at weekly intervals, incubated for 24 h, and stored in a refrigerator. After a series of six consecutive transfers to new plates, new working cultures are prepared from stock or semistock cultures.

Very delicate bacteria. Working cultures of very delicate bacteria, e.g., gonococci and pneumococci, are prepared by plating out from stock or semistock cultures and incubating for 24 to 48 h. After a series of six consecutive transfers to new plates, new working cultures are prepared from stock or semistock cultures.

Anaerobic bacteria. Working cultures of most anaerobes can be maintained in chopped-meat medium or in thioglycolate broth with 0.5% sodium carbonate added before autoclaving. Working cultures are incubated for 24 to 48 h and are stored at room temperature. Working cultures of relatively hardy organisms are transferred at monthly intervals and relatively delicate organisms are transferred at 2-week intervals. After a series of six consecutive transfers, new working cultures are prepared from stock or semistock cultures.

Fungi. Working cultures of most fungi can be maintained on Sabouraud agar (or substitute); however, a few relatively delicate fungi should be maintained on Sabouraud agar containing blood (or substitute). Cultures should be incubated at room temperature until good growth and sporulation appear and then stored in a refrigerator. Working cultures should be transferred at 2-month intervals, and new working cultures should be prepared from stock or semistock cultures after six consecutive transfers of working cultures.

Commercially available working cultures. There are currently available two sets of bacterial semistock cultures prepared by commercial companies in the form of water-soluble disks impregnated with a standardized number of bacteria. They are stored in a refrigerator and are stable for 1 year. The number of organisms presently available is too limited to serve all of the needs of a comprehensive quality control program; however, the sets will serve many of the procedures and include the Seattle strains of *Escherichia coli* and *Staphylococcus aureus*. Bact-Chek (Roche Diagnostics, Division of Hoffmann-La Roche, Inc., Nutley, N.J.) has been available for several years and has been found satisfactory (10). Bactrol Disks (Difco) have become available very recently. It is hoped that commercial companies will increase the number of types of cultures available in a convenient form for use in medical laboratories.

Sources of cultures

There are a number of sources of cultures for the establishment of a culture collection. (i) Cultures isolated and completely identified in a medical laboratory may be saved and placed in a culture collection. Ideally, identification should be confirmed by another laboratory. (ii) Cultures received as proficiency test specimens serve as excellent sources for a culture collection. (iii) Cultures may be purchased from a reputable organization such as the American Type Culture Collection.

LITERATURE CITED

1. Anonymous. 1970. Total quality control for the medical laboratory. Amer. J. Clin. Pathol. **54**(No. 3, Part II):435–530.
2. Anonymous. 1973. Bacterial surveillance. Laboratory Management **11**:32–33.
3. Barry, A. L., and G. D. Fay. 1972. A review of some common sources of error in the preparation of agar media. Amer. J. Med. Technol. **38**:241–245.
4. Barry, A. L., and K. L. Feeney. 1968. The role of quality control in the clinical bacteriology laboratory. Amer. J. Med. Technol. **34**:195–201.
5. Bartlett, R. C., G. O. Carrington, and C. Mielert. 1968. Quality control in clinical microbiology. American Society of Clinical Pathologists Commission on Continuing Education, Chicago.
6. Bauer, A. W., W. M. M. Kirby, J. C. Sherris, and M. Turck. 1966. Antibiotic susceptibility testing by a standardized single disc method. Amer. J. Clin. Pathol. **45**:493–496.
7. Blazevic, D. J., M. H. Koepcke, and J. M. Matsen. 1972. Quality control testing with the disk antibiotic susceptibility test of Bauer-Kirby-Sherris-Turck. Amer. J. Clin. Pathol. **57**:592–597.
8. Branson, D. 1966. Problems and errors in the clinical microbiology laboratory. Amer. J. Med. Technol. **32**:349–357.
9. Clark, W. A. 1970. The American Type Culture Collection: experiences in freezing and freeze-drying microorganisms, viruses, and cell-lines, p. 309–318. *In* H. Iizuka and T. Hasegawa (ed.), Culture collections of microorganisms. University Park Press, Baltimore.

10. Douglas, G. W., A. Balows, D. Rhoden, K. Tomfohrde, and P. B. Smith. 1973. In-use evaluation of a commercially available set of quality control cultures. Appl. Microbiol. **25:**230–234.
11. Dowell, V. R., Jr., and T. M. Hawkins. 1973. Laboratory methods in anaerobic bacteriology. CDC Laboratory Manual, Center for Disease Control, Atlanta, Ga.
12. Ellis, R. J. 1973. Manual of quality control procedures for microbiological laboratories, working draft copy. Center for Disease Control, Atlanta, Ga.
13. Fodor, A. R. 1968. Microbiological reagents in search of precision. Health Lab. Sci. **5:**5–11.
14. Forney, J. E. 1973. Who should regulate whom? Health Lab. Sci. **10:**277–279.
15. Glasser, L., G. S. Bosley, and J. R. Boring. 1971. A systematic program of quality control in clinical microbiology. Amer. J. Clin. Pathol. **56:**379–383.
16. Halstead, E. G., R. A. Quevedo, and W. H. Gengerich. 1971. A quality control program for the bacteriology laboratory. Amer. J. Med. Technol. **37:**15–20.
17. Harding, H. B. 1965. Quality control in microbiology. I and II. Hospital topics. **43:**77–80; 81–85.
18. Heckley, R. J. 1961. Preservation of bacteria by lyophilization. Advan. Appl. Microbiol. **3:**1–76.
19. Hicks, H. A. 1973. Philosophy of laboratory control. Health Lab. Sci. **10:**268–270.
20. Isenberg, H. D. 1973. License to practice laboratory medicine. Health Lab. Sci. **10:**271–276.
21. Jennings, E. R., J. W. Reynolds, R. L. Russell, and G. A. Schmidt. 1970. Quality control program for microbiology. Memorial Hospital Medical Center, Long Beach, Calif.
22. Kaufmann, W. 1973. Quality control of physician office laboratories. Health Lab. Sci. **10:**284–286.
23. Lapage, S. P., J. E. Shelton, and T. G. Mitchell. 1970. Media for the preservation of bacteria, p. 1–134. *In* J. R. Norris and D. W. Ribbons (ed.), Methods in microbiology, vol. 3A. Academic Press Inc., New York.
24. Lapage, S. P., J. E. Shelton, T. G. Mitchell, and A. R. Mackenzie. 1970. Culture collections and preservation of bacteria, p. 134–228. *In* J. R. Norris and D. W. Ribbons (ed.), Methods in microbiology, vol. 3A. Academic Press Inc., New York.
25. Laskaris, T., and A. L. Chaney. 1969. Reliability of biologic autoclave sterilization indicators. Amer. J. Clin. Pathol. **52:**495–500.
26. Levey, S., and E. R. Jennings. 1950. The use of control charts in the clinical laboratory. Amer. J. Clin. Pathol. **20:**1059–1066.
27. Microbial Diseases Laboratory. 1973. Instructions for freezing cultures. State of California-Health and Welfare Agency, Department of Health, Berkeley.
28. Nagel, J. G., and L. J. Kunz. 1973. Needless retesting of quality-assured, commercially prepared culture media. Appl. Microbiol. **26:**31–37.
29. Russell, R. L., R. S. Yoshimori, T. F. Rhodes, J. W. Reynolds, and E. R. Jennings. 1969. A quality control program for clinical microbiology. Tech. Bulletin **39:**195–201.
30. Raper, K. B. 1963. General methods for preserving cultures, p. 81–93. *In* S. M. Martin (ed.), Culture collections: perspectives and problems. University of Toronto Press, Toronto.
31. Smith, J. P., and C. Sandlin. 1969. Quality control in bacteriology. Amer. J. Med. Technol. **35:**531–539.
32. Vera, H. D. 1971. Quality control in diagnostic microbiology. Health Lab. Sci. **8:**176–189.
33. Woods, D., and J. F. Byers. 1973. Quality control recording methods in microbiology. Amer. J. Med. Technol. **39:**79–85.

Chapter 94

Biological Safety in the Clinical Laboratory

ROBERT H. HUFFAKER

In every clinical laboratory, *biological safety is the responsibility of management.* This responsibility can be delegated, reassigned, abandoned, or ignored but, when an accident occurs, it ultimately returns, unforgivingly, to the supervisor who allowed the causative situation to develop. Collecting and processing clinical specimens are accompanied by a varying degree of risk of infection to hospital and laboratory personnel. This chapter contains suggestions on how to minimize these risks. Detailed information on specific safety items such as laboratory design, methods of sterilization and decontamination, or special pieces of laboratory safety equipment will be found in other publications, some of which are cited here.

ASSESSMENT OF RISK

It is difficult to quantitate the risk of acquiring an infection when handling etiological agents in a laboratory. With the majority of them, the degree of hazard depends as much on the quantity of agent present as on its inherent virulence and on its form (colonies on agar, in broth, or freeze dried, for example), the manipulations used (aerosolization, animal inoculation, sonic treatment, etc.), the presence of vectors (*Aedes aegypti* in conjunction with yellow fever virus), and other factors. Some agents, such as *Francisella tularensis*, are so virulent that any procedure involving them may cause laboratory infections. The safety factors described below are applicable to all procedures involving etiological agents; in many cases, however, more stringent precautions may be required.

LABORATORY DESIGN

Whenever possible, operations involving etiological agents should be done in special rooms which are set aside for this purpose, are not used for other work, and have at least 10 air changes per hour. Air exhausted from these areas should not be recirculated unless it is first freed from infectious material by filtering through High Efficiency Particulate Air (HEPA) filters. Air balance must be maintained to ensure air flow from the areas of lesser risk to areas of greater risk, i.e., from clean halls and corridors into suites of rooms where etiological agents are processed, and within the suites from areas of lesser potential contamination to these of greater potential contamination.

RESTRICTED ACCESS

Areas of high risk, such as tuberculosis laboratories, should be marked by appropriate signs, stating, for example, "Caution, do not enter without permission of (name of supervisor)" and displaying the standard biohazard symbol (Fig. 1). Access to infectious disease laboratory areas should be restricted to persons who need to be there; no casual visitors or children under 12 years of age should be allowed to enter.

VACCINATION

Everyone working with etiological agents should be immunized in advance against all of those for which Bureau of Biologics approved vaccines are available. Only vaccinated personnel should be allowed to enter work areas where the staff is so protected.

Determination of antibody titers after immunization or prior to beginning work with an agent provides valuable information concerning the immune status of the worker and assists in selecting the optimal medical management of individuals in whom a subsequent accidental exposure to an agent occurs. This is done by taking an annual sample of at least 5 ml of blood serum from each employee, storing it at −20 C in a serum bank, and pairing it with serum samples taken after an illness or suspected illness for comparison of antibody levels. In many instances, increases in antibody titers indicate exposure to an infectious agent.

Live virus vaccine should not be administered to a pregnant employee, nor should she be exposed to any viral agents to which she is not known to be immune. This includes Australian antigen, as there is evidence that transplacental infection may occur. Women of childbearing age should never be subjected to exposure to known teratogenic agents.

FIG. 1. *Standard biohazard symbol.*

Personnel records of each employee should contain complete records of immunizations, of serum stored in the serum bank, of accidental exposures to etiological agents, and of job-related and other significant illnesses.

MEANS OF LABORATORY INFECTION

The most frequently recognized causes of laboratory infections are accidental oral aspiration of infectious material through a pipette, accidental inoculation with syringe needles, sprays from loose needles on syringes, centrifuge accidents, and animal bites. To prevent oral aspiration of etiological agents, mouth pipetting must be forbidden and replaced by the use of safety pipetting devices. When inoculating etiological agents, only syringes to which the needle is firmly fixed by threads (Luer Lok or equal) should be used. Screw-capped safety cups should be used when centrifuging etiological agents in an open laboratory area. Small, tabletop model centrifuges without safety cups can be used to process etiological agents if the centrifuge is operated in a closed box, if the box is under negative air pressure, and if exhausted air is filtered or incinerated. Neither smoking nor the consumption of food and drink shall be permitted in areas in which etiological agents are handled.

ANIMAL CARE

Animals infected with etiological agents which may be transmitted to humans via urine, feces, or other body discharges are more safely housed in cages with solid bottoms and sides than in wire cages. Such animals should be housed in cages with filter tops or in isolator cages through which all exhaust air is filtered. All cages or rooms holding animals inoculated with etiological agents should be labeled accordingly. Necropsy of animals inoculated with highly hazardous etiological agents must be carried out in ventilated safety cabinets or, when this is impracticable, by requiring personnel to wear appropriate safety equipment (i.e., gloves, gowns, face shields, etc.). Carcasses of animals infected with etiological agents must be placed in leak-proof containers such as plastic bags and incinerated.

STERILIZATION

All etiological agents and equipment or apparatus contaminated with them must be sterilized by autocalving or by other equally effective means before being washed or discarded. Stock solutions of disinfectants known to be effective against the etiological agents used must be maintained in each laboratory and used in routine cleaning of tables and work surfaces after use. Past experience has taught that manufacturers' and salesmen's claims for disinfectant effectiveness are no substitute for a use-test performed against etiological agents that are processed in the laboratory.

EMERGENCY PLAN

Every laboratory working with etiological agents must have an emergency plan, including a clean-up procedure, to follow if an accident contaminates personnel or environment. The supervisor must ensure that everyone in the laboratory is familiar both with the hazards associated with the work and with the emergency plan. He should be notified of an accident as soon as possible. When an accident likely to produce a large aerosol occurs, staff should leave the area at once before any action is taken to contain the hazard. Thereafter, no one should enter the room, except to save life, until the extent of the hazard has been determined. Wait and consider the best method to be used before beginning clean-up operations. In most cases, the risk decreases as time passes and aerosols settle. Protective clothing, including a respirator equipped with a particulate filter, should be worn during cleanup if infectious aerosols are likely to be present.

OCCUPATIONAL SAFETY AND HEALTH ACT

The Occupational Safety and Health Act (OSHA) of 1970 (Public Law 91-596) establishes minimal safety standards for many work situations. These standards are not specific for a particular work area, such as diagnostic laboratories. They do define standards for particular hazards such as: storing compressed gases and flammable solvents, allowable airborne amounts of various pollutants, wearing of safety equipment, and many other things. The Center for Disease Control (CDC) is attempting to identify those OSHA standards that will apply to laboratories and, when requested (Office of

Table 1. *Index to operational requirements*[a]

OID	Agent	PC
	BACTERIA	
1	*Actinobacillus*—all species (except *A. mallei*)	D
2	*Actinobacillus mallei*	BB
3	*Antinomyces*—all species	D
4	*Aeromonas salmonicida*	D
5	*Arizona arizonae*—all serotypes	D
6	*Bacillus anthracis**	AA
7	*Bartonella*—all species	N
8	*Bordetella*—all species	D
9	*Brucella*—all species	BB
10	*Clostridium botulinum**	AA
11	*Clostridium tetani**	G
12	Clostridia—other species	D
13	*Corynebacterium diphtheriae**	G
14	Corynebacteria—other species	A
15	*Erysipelothrix insidiosa*	D
16	*Haemophilus ducreyi, H. gallinarum, H. influenzae*	D
17	*Herellea vaginicola*	A
18	*Klebsiella*—all species	A
19	*Leptospira*—all species	D
20	*Listeria*—all species	D
21	*Mima polymorpha*	A
22	*Mycobacterium avium, M. bovis, M. johnei, M. tuberculosis*	CC
23	Mycobacteria—all other species	D
24	Mycoplasma—all species	D
25	*Neisseria gonorrhoeae* and *N. meningitidis*	D
26	*Pasteurella pestis,* P. tularensis,* P. multocida* (type B)	AA
27	*Pasteurella*—all other species	D
28	*Pseudomonas pseudomallei*	BB
29	*Salmonella typhi**	G
30	*Salmonella*—all other species	D
31	*Shigella*—all species	D
32	*Sphaerophorus necrophorus*	D
33	*Staphylococcus aureus*	D
34	*Streptobacillus moniliformis*	D
35	*Streptococcus pneumoniae*	D
36	*Streptococcus agalactiae, S. equi, S. equisimilis, S. pyogenes* of Lancefield's groups A, B, C, G	D
37	*Treponema pallidum, T. pertenue, T. carateum*	D
38	*Vibrio comma**	K
39	*Vibrio fetus*	D
40	*Yersinia enterocolitica*	D
	PARASITES	
41	*Echinococcus granulosus*	C
42	*Echinococcus multilocularis*	C
43	*Leishmania braziliensis*	N
44	*Leishmania donovanii*	N
45	*Leishmania mexicana*	N
46	*Leishmania tropica*	N
	PARASITES	
47	*Naegleria gruberi*	L
48	*Plasmodium falciparum*	F
49	*Plasmodium malariae*	F
50	*Plasmodium ovale*	F
51	*Plasmodium vivax*	F
52	*Pneumocystis carinii*	T
53	*Schistosoma haematobium*	H
54	*Schistosoma japonicum*	H
55	*Schistosoma mansoni*	H
56	*Taenia solium*	B
57	*Toxoplasma gondii*	T
58	*Trypanosoma cruzi*	N
59	*Trypanosoma gambiense*	D
60	*Trypanosoma rangeli*	B
61	*Trypanosoma rhodesiense*	D
	VIRUSES, RICKETTSIA, BEDSONIA	
62	Adenoviruses—all types	I
63	Arboviruses—general	Y
64	B virus	CC
65	Coxsackie A and B—all types	J
66	Cytomegalovirus	I
67	Echoviruses—all types	I
68	Encephalomyocarditis virus	L
69	Hepatitis—infectious and serum	I
70	Herpesviruses except B	L
71	Infectious bronchitis-like virus	L
72	Influenza virus—all types*	I
73	K virus	P
74	Langat	R
75	Lassa virus	EE
76	Marburg virus	EE
77	Measles virus*	K
78	Murine viruses, including ectromelia, LCM, murine hepatitis, etc.	E
79	Mumps virus*	K
80	Newcastle disease virus	I
81	Polioviruses*	M
82	Psittacosis, LGV	U
83	Q fever,* *R. prowazeki**, and all other rickettsia except *R. rickettsii*	Z
84	Rabies—fixed and attenuated	I
85	Rabies—Street virus*	S
86	Reoviruses	I
87	Respiratory syncytial virus	J
88	Rhinovirus	I
89	*Rickettsia rickettsii**	DD
90	Rubella*	K
91	Simian viruses (except B virus and Marburg)	J
92	Smallpox virus, major and minor*	DD
93	Tacaribe group viruses except Tamiami	EE
94	Tamiami virus	L

[a] OID = organism identification number; PC = precaution category. Vaccines are available for agents marked with an asterisk. (Adapted from *Lab Safety at the Center for Disease Control.*)

TABLE 1—*Continued*

OID	Agent	PC	OID	Agent	PC
	VIRUSES, RICKETTSIA, BEDSONIA			FUNGI	
95	Tick-borne viral encephalitis (Russian-Spring-Summer-Encephalitis* and all other viruses of complex except Langat)	X	102	*Blastomyces dermatitidis*	O
96	Vaccinia*	P	103	*Cryptococcus neoformans*	O
97	Varicella	J	104	Paracoccidioides	O
98	Venezuelan encephalitis virus—exotic strains	Y	105	*Histoplasma capsulatum*	Q
99	VEE-domestic and vaccine strains	W	106	*Coccidioides immitis*	Q
100	Vesicular stomatis and other rhab-doviruses	V	107	*Sporothrix schenckii*	O
101	Yellow fever*	X			

Biosafety, CDC, Atlanta, Ga. 30333), will provide these citations.

REFERENCES

The following safety guides prepared for use at the CDC are available from the Office of Biosafety upon request. Each is a short issuance on a single subject and most concepts are applicable in any laboratory.

- Standards for Handling Nonhuman Primates
- CDC Hazard Warning Signs
- Standards for Handling Compressed Gases in Cylinders
- Ultraviolet Lights—Use and Maintenance
- Laboratory Exposure to Dangerous Chemicals or Infectious Agents
- Control of Air Flow in Laboratory Areas
- Use of Laminar Air Flow Equipment
- Laboratory Accident Investigation Board
- Storage of Flammable Solvents in CDC Laboratories
- Exposure to Teratogenic Agents in Laboratories
- Use of Hazardous Biological Agents
- Use of Vacuum Equipment
- Labeling of Equipment Sent in for Maintenance/Repair
- Please Keep Your Laboratory Doors Closed!
- Visitors in Laboratory Areas
- Eye Wash Bottles
- Caustic Chemicals and Eye Protection

The CDC has also published two larger books dealing with infectious agents and with laboratory safety: *Classification of Etiologic Agents on the Basis of Hazard* and *Lab Safety at the Center for Disease Control*. Other useful references are listed in the Literature Cited (1–11).

The following is taken from the introduction to *Lab Safety at the Center for Disease Control* (Department of Health, Education, and Welfare Publication No. [HSM] 72-8118).

This section presents certain safety requirements for handling specific hazardous microorganisms. These requirements derive from judgment based on present knowledge; as further knowledge accumulates and additional vaccines are developed, the requirements for some agents will change. The operational requirements are also based, in part, on the existing facilities and resources at CDC. Similar precautions may not be feasible in many other institutions.

In the following tables on operational requirements for safety in the laboratory, no attempt was made to cover all microbiologic agents. All known microorganisms that are not listed, however, can be handled safely in the laboratory without special equipment, techniques, or immunization of personnel.

Precautions are indicated only when they are clearly required for the safety of laboratory workers or others. Optional or debatable items have been excluded; only those items deemed absolutely necessary for safety are presented. Thus, the following table of operational requirements presents only minimal safety criteria. For example, it is highly desirable that all laboratories be under negative air pressure; however, the absence of negative air pressure in laboratories working with certain agents may not be associated with an infection hazard.

Several additional operational principles and habits might be routine in laboratories even though they may not be required for safety with all microorganisms. As a general principle, doors to laboratories should be kept closed except for necessary entrances and exits, and visits by extraneous persons should be discouraged. Eating, drinking, or smoking in the laboratory is undesirable. Handwashing by laboratory personnel should be encouraged, and bulb pipetting, a good laboratory procedure, can be generally recommended. Disinfection of work surfaces after working with a disease agent is strongly recommended as a routine measure. All of these general recommendations are desirable, even if they are not specifically needed for the safe handling of certain agents.

Table 1 lists hazardous microorganisms within the basic categories of Bacteria, Parasites, Viruses (including Rickettsia and Bedsonia), and Fungi. Each agent has been given a number and an alphabetic

TABLE 2. *Operational requirements for safe laboratory handling of hazardous microorganisms*[a]

Precaution category	Geographic isolation	Controlled access	Negative air pressure	Hoods and cabinets	Disinfection			Bulb pipetting required	Special protective equipment			Special precautions with work involving		Special aerosol precautions (centrifuge, blendor, etc)	Immunization available and required	Organisms requiring these precautions
					Work surfaces	Entire work area	Material before leaving work area		Gloves	Masks	Other special clothing or guards	Insects	Animals			
A					+											14, 17, 18, 21
B								+								56, 60
C													+			41, 42
D					+			+								1, 3, 4, 5, 8, 12, 15, 16, 19, 20, 23, 24, 25, 27, 30, 31, 32, 33, 34, 35, 36, 37, 39, 40, 59, 61
E							+	+								78
F												+	+			48, 49, 50, 51
G					+			+							+	11, 13, 29
H					+			+	+				+			53, 54, 55
I					+		+	+								62, 66, 67, 69, 72, 80, 84, 86, 88
J				+	+		+	+								65, 87, 91, 97
K					+		+	+							+	38, 77, 79, 90
L				+	+		+	+						+		47, 68, 70, 71, 94
M				+	+		+	+							+	81
N				+	+			+				+	+			7, 43, 44, 45, 46, 58
O		+		+	+		+	+						+		102, 103, 104, 107
P				+	+		+	+						+	+	73, 96
Q		+	+	+	+		+	+						+		105, 106
R				+	+		+	+				+	+	+		74
S					+		+	+	+				+		+	85

TABLE 2—*Continued*

Precaution category	Geographic isolation	Controlled access	Negative air pressure	Hoods and cabinets	Disinfection			Bulb pipetting required	Special protective equipment			Special precautions with work involving		Special aerosol precautions (centrifuge, blendor, etc)	Immunization available and required	Organisms requiring these precautions
					Work surfaces	Entire work area	Material before leaving work area		Gloves	Masks	Other special clothing or guards	Insects	Animals			
T	+	+		+	+			+	+				+	+		52, 57
U	+	+	+	+	+		+	+						+		82
V	+			+	+		+	+				+	+	+		100
W			+	+	+		+	+				+	+	+		99
X	+	+	+	+	+	+	+	+				+	+	+	+	95, 101
Y	+	+	+	+	+	+	+	+	+			+	+	+	+	63, 98
Z	+	+	+	+	+	+	+	+		+	+	+	+	+	+	83
AA	+	+	+	+	+	+	+	+	+	+		+	+	+	+	6, 10, 26
BB	+	+	+	+	+	+	+	+	+	+		+	+	+		2, 9, 28
CC	+	+	+	+	+	+	+	+	+	+	+		+	+		22, 64
DD	+	+	+	+	+	+	+	+	+	+	+	+	+	+	+	89, 92
EE	+	+	+	+	+	+	+	+	+	+	+	+	+	+		Newly discovered agents and 75,76, 93

[a] An explanation of column headings is given in the text. The numbers used in the last column are the organism identification numbers listed in Table 1. (From *Lab Safety at the Center for Disease Control.*)

letter that identifies its "precaution category" (PC). Table 2, the operational requirements table, contains precaution categories in alphabetic order; the specific requirements for handling a particular agent are indicated by "+" entries under the various columns. Microorganisms that require the same set of precautions are grouped within the same precaution category and, to conserve space, are identified by their code numbers. Comments on each column heading in Table 2 follow.

Explanation of column headings in Table 2

Precaution category: The explanation is given above.

Geographic isolation: The action of isolating in a separate room or building in which no other work is concurrently conducted. A ventilating system to the room that prevents recirculation of air is implied. Exhaust air may be passed through High Efficiency Particulate Air (HEPA) filters or incinerated. For extremely hazardous agents, an air lock should also be used.

Controlled access: The exclusion of extraneous persons from areas where certain agents are being handled. Such control decreases the probability of distractions resulting in accidents and limits the number of exposed individuals should an accident occur.

Negative air pressure: Ideally, the air pressure in all laboratories should be negative in relation to the pressure in surrounding corridors, thus helping to prevent agents from leaving the work area. When negative pressure is required, as shown in Table 2, it is essential for safety. Even when cultures are manipulated under hoods, negative pressure in the general laboratory area in relation to that in surrounding corridors is still highly desirable. In addition, doors to all laboratories should be closed except for necessary entrances and exits.

Hoods and cabinets: These include protected work areas such as the CDC Bio-Safety Cabinet, glove boxes, laminar flow safety cabinets, and gastight isolators.

Disinfection: Standard methods suitable for disinfection of work surfaces, entire work area, and material before leaving work area have not been presented. Disinfection should routinely take place when work with agents is completed, and each laboratory should be cleaned, work surfaces decontaminated, and all contaminated material either covered in discard pans or autoclaved at the end of the work day.

Bulb pipetting required: This heading is self-explanatory.

Protective equipment: Gloves, including gloves on cabinet or hood ports, should be worn whenever one is handling organisms which call for this precaution. Gloves prevent the direct invasion of microorganisms through intact skin and greatly reduce the hazards of indirect spread. Masks should be worn to protect against the aerosol spread of certain organisms. Such masks should be worn except when (i) the work is done in a sealed cabinet in rooms with isolated ventilation systems with exhaust control, or (ii) effective immunizing agents have been given to all who might be exposed. High efficiency, disposable surgical masks are recommended; they are capable of reducing by 2 logs the number of airborne microorganisms that are inhaled. Special respirators or supplied air equipment may have essentially complete respiratory protection. Other special clothing or guards, such as face masks or shields, caps, safety gloves, booties, or even complete changes of clothing, may be indicated for aerosol work with certain very hazardous agents. No attempt has been made to specify which special equipment may be needed for which special agents.

Special precautions with work involving insects and animals: These precautions have been stipulated for hazardous agents that might be capable of spread to humans through insects and animal vectors. Containment facilities should be secure before work is begun. The excretions and secretions of infected animals and insects may be infectious to humans, and personnel who must come in contact with them should routinely use special protective equipment. In some instances, discharges are capable of establishing disease in nature. These wastes must be decontaminated before they are released from the facility.

Special aerosol precautions: Centrifuges, blendors, and other equipment capable of creating aerosols should be operated in separate "isolation" rooms or hoods. Special care should be taken in loading centrifuges to avoid accidental breakage during operation. Safety equipment to prevent the formation of aerosols is available and should be used.

Immunization available and required: Immunization is generally recommended for all diseases against which effective, safe, and licensed vaccines have been developed. However, there are no vaccines against many highly virulent organisms, and some vaccines for such agents are investigational and without clear documentation of efficacy in humans. Nonetheless, in certain circumstances, the seriousness of the disease and the absence of other effective therapy may dictate their use.

LITERATURE CITED

1. Benarde, M. (ed.). 1970. Disinfection. Marcel Dekker, Inc., New York.
2. Bodily, H. L. 1970. General administration of the laboratory, p. 1–28. *In* H. L. Bodily, E. L. Updyke, and J. O. Mason (ed.), Diagnostic procedures for bacterial, mycotic, and parasitic infections, 5th ed. American Public Health Association, Inc., New York.
3. Braker, W., and A. L. Mossman. 1971. Matheson gas data book. Matheson Gas Products, East Rutherford, N.J.
4. Chatigny, M. A. 1961. Protection against infection in the microbiology laboratory—devices and procedures. Advan. Appl. Microbiol. **3:**131–192.
5. Darlow, H. M. 1969. Safety in the microbiological laboratory, p. 169–204. In J. R. Norris and D. W. Ribbons (ed.), Methods in microbiology. Academic Press Inc., New York.
6. Lawrence, C. A., and S. S. Block (ed.). 1971. Disinfection, sterilization and preservation. Lea and Febiger, Philadelphia.
7. Proceedings. 1970. Seminar on clinical laboratory planning and design. State of Washington Department of Health, Olympia.
8. Runkle, R. S., and G. B. Phillips (ed.). 1969. Microbial

contamination control facilities. Van Nostrand Reinhold Environmental Engineering Series. Van Nostrand Reinhold Co., New York.

9. Shapton, D. A., and R. G. Board (ed.). 1972. Safety in microbiology. Academic Press Inc., New York.
10. Steere, N. V. (ed.). 1971. Handbook of laboratory safety, 2nd ed. The Chemical Rubber Co., Cleveland.
11. Sulkin, S. E., and R. M. Pike. 1969. Prevention of laboratory infections, p. 66–78. *In* E. H. Lennette and N. J. Schmidt (ed.), Diagnostic procedures for viral and rickettsial infections, 4th ed. American Public Health Association, Inc., New York.

Section XI

MEDIA, REAGENTS, AND STAINS

Chapter 95
Culture Media

HARRIETTE D. VERA AND MORRIS DUMOFF

INTRODUCTION

All media are described in the last part of this chapter, in alphabetical order. These culture media are devised and used for cultivation of microorganisms. The cultivation may be for many different purposes, e.g., isolation and identification of organisms, sterility testing, food and water analysis, environmental control, production of biological products (toxoids, vaccines, etc.), antibiotic and vitamin assays, and industrial testing.

As living cells, microorganisms require sources of nitrogen, carbon, and many other elements. The autotrophic bacteria can utilize free nitrogen, and some organisms can use simple compounds such as ammonia or nitrate, so that media for such organisms can be chemically very simple. On the other hand, heterotrophic organisms, with limited synthetic ability, require more complex nitrogen compounds. For the latter organisms, media containing crude natural protein sources may be used. However, since cells cannot always obtain their nitrogen requirements directly from protein, they may require protein hydrolysates which provide nitrogenous compounds in a more available form. Such hydrolysates, generally known as peptones, are water-soluble materials derived from proteins by means of acid, alkali, or added or intrinsic enzymes.

COMPOSITION

Peptones

The characteristics of a peptone depend upon the purity and quality of the proteinaceous material employed and the method of hydrolysis (75, 129). Acid and alkaline hydrolysis tend to destroy the vitamin content of the protein, and part of the amino acid content may also be lost. Enzymatic hydrolysis tends to preserve the vitamins and to keep the amino acid content intact. For example, pure casein contains no carbohydrates and has a high tryptophan and vitamin content. A casein peptone made by tryptic digestion should, therefore, contain no sugar and should be useful for fermentation and indole tests (USP). A casein peptone made by acid hydrolysis has no tryptophan and no carbohydrate, and it can be used as an ingredient in media for assaying vitamin content of serum or of pharmaceutical preparations (47, 56).

A peptone made from gelatin by enzymatic hydrolysis should contain neither tryptophan nor carbohydrate, because neither is present in pure gelatin. By contrast, peptones made from milk, meat, or yeast cells contain the respective carbohydrates present in the original materials. Consequently, such peptones should not be present in media used for fermentation tests (128; USP). For sterility testing, two media are required, and they must be made with defined peptones. A number of other media will be included in the 19th edition of the U.S. Pharmacopeia, for determining the microbiological attributes of drugs.

Most microbiological yeast extracts are really yeast peptones, the digestion of the yeast cells being due to their own autolytic enzymes. The principle employed in manufacture is, thus, the same phenomenon commonly seen in a pneumococcus broth culture—the broth becomes cloudy as growth takes place and then gradually clears as incubation is continued.

Infusions and extracts

Infusions and extracts of meat and other tissues were in use before peptones were developed and are, to a lesser extent, still in use today. Strictly speaking, they are poorly defined water-soluble materials, including sugars, derived from proteinaceous materials without the use of enzymes, the proteins themselves usually being heatcoagulated. However, the methods used, and especially the time involved often permit some microbial enzymatic action, without which the nutritional quality and consequent replicability and reliability are likely to be poor.

Examination of peptones, infusions, and extracts for microbial content. Excessive microbial contamination of peptones, infusions, and extracts or other ingredients makes them unreliable for scientific purposes, although they usually support growth of other organisms. If any of these materials are prepared in a laboratory, contamination tests should always be made prior to use (1). This is easily done by the modified Breed test, which is performed as follows. Dissolve 1 g of the material to be examined in 10.0 ml of purified water. Spread 0.01 ml over a 1-cm^2 area of a glass slide, air-dry, and stain by the Gram method. Examine 10 fields with an oil immersion lens. There should be no more than 50 microorganisms, or clumps, visible in 10 fields (129; USP). If the materials have been contaminated, either during the preparation, or afterward by exposure to moist air, rodents, etc., the visible organisms are usually too numerous to count.

Solidifying agents

Gelatin, agar, silica, and polyacrylic gels have been used as solidifying agents. Gelatin is now rarely used for this purpose, and silica gel is used mostly in soil microbiology. Agar derived from certain red sea weeds, the *Rhodophyceae*, which is suitable for microbiological use, should be clean and free from debris, should melt at 80 C, and should gel at no more than 30 C. A 2% aqueous solution should be clear, or nearly so. Certain polyacrylic gels appear to be nontoxic to microorganisms and fully functional in agar plates. Agarose is a neutral polysaccharide which, along with agaropectin, is a dissociation product from agar. It is used in immunoelectrophoretic diffusion tests where clarity is especially important.

Other components: indicators, selective agents, and reducing agents

Colorimetric indicators. Colorimetric indicators may be included in media. The pH indicators most used today are phenol red, bromothymol blue, bromocresol purple, and neutral red. They have largely replaced the more crude and variable litmus and Andrade indicators. These indicators are used mainly to demonstrate the production of acid from a carbohydrate contained in the medium. As many organisms do not lower the pH sufficiently for the change to be detected by bromocresol purple, phenol red, which is more sensitive in this pH range, is more generally useful than other pure chemical indicators. Bromocresol purple and neutral red are used mostly with media for enteric bacilli. Bromothymol blue tends to fade more than phenol red.

Methylene blue and resazurin are the most popular E_h indicators at present. Some lots of pH and E_h indicators may be toxic to some organisms and should be tested prior to use.

Selective agents. Selective agents which permit growth of some organisms and inhibit growth of others may be incorporated into media. They are *very* useful for detecting the presence of specific pathogens in a mixed flora, and for identification. Many selective agents have been tried, and some are very valuable and widely used. Dyes were probably the first selective agents employed. Examples of these are crystal violet and brilliant green, which are used to inhibit gram-positive organisms. Sodium chloride in high concentrations will inhibit growth of most bacteria, but is well tolerated by staphylococci. Sodium azide, sodium citrate and tellurite, sodium lauryl sulfate, sodium selenite, iodine, and phenylethanol are used to provide selectivity. Crude bile preparations are still used, but pure bile salts, especially sodium deoxycholate, are now in use also.

A medium may also be made selective by adjusting the reaction to a very high or very low pH in order to permit growth of some organisms and to inhibit others. A well-known example is the use of pH 5.6 for Sabouraud medium for growth of yeast and molds. Another example is the use of media adjusted to a reaction of pH 8.0 to 9.0 for the isolation of *Vibrio cholerae*.

The newest group of materials now incorporated into culture media to make them selective are antimicrobial agents developed for therapeutic purposes. For reliable use in culture media, heat-stable agents are preferable because they can be put into the medium before autoclaving. At present, chloramphenicol, cycloheximide, and the sulfonamides are popular. Neomycin, colistin, trimethoprim, vancomycin, and nalidixic acid are relatively stable agents. Pencillin G and streptomycin have been used, but they require aseptic manipulation and they deteriorate in solution. Both penicillin G and streptomycin plus nystatin or amphotericin are often used in tissue culture media to inhibit growth of bacterial contaminants, but these formulas usually are sterilized by filtration. Kanamycin is used to inhibit growth of *Mycoplasma* and also to facilitate isolation of anaerobes.

Reducing agents. Reducing agents may be incorporated to promote anaerobiosis. One or more compounds, such as the following, may be used: ascorbic acid, sodium thioglycolate, sodium formaldehyde sulfoxalate, thiomalic acid, sodium hydrosulfite, and cysteine. Addition of 0.5 to 1.0 g of agar per liter of an appropriate broth may limit convection currents and thus provide suitable conditions for growth of some organisms, if the broth is used at once or is boiled and cooled without agitation just prior to use. Many media which do not contain reducing agents and are normally used for cultivation of aerobes can be employed for cultivation of organisms having special requirements, by incubation in propane, hydrogen, methane, or other gases.

Special types of media

In addition to formulas made for cultivation and identification, and solid media for selective isolation of bacteria and fungi, there are other formulations which deserve some comment.

Enrichment media. Enrichment media are generally broths designed to promote growth of microorganisms present, especially possible pathogens. They may or may not contain selective agents, such as sodium selenite, brilliant green, and others noted above. A good example of a general enrichment medium suitable for many kinds of specimens is thioglycolate medium without indicator, which has a defined casein soy peptone nutrient base. Enrichment media should not be confused with transport media, which are designed to transport or "hold" specimens, and in which little or no growth should occur.

Maintenance media. Satisfactory maintenance media may be quite different from the media which yield the heaviest and most rapid growth of an organism. Best growth may be obtained in a medium which also gives the fastest death. For example, *Clostridium botulinum*, pneumococci, and *Neisseria* grow very well in media with dextrose. However, sufficient acid may be produced from the dextrose to destroy the vegetative cells and to prevent sporulation. Maintenance in the same medium may be possible when calcium carbonate is added prior to sterilization, or maintenace is possible in suitable media that do not contain dextrose (127). Occasional cultures may, of course, require dextrose or other sugars to grow; in such cases, the sugar must be included, and incorporation of calcium carbonate may be necessary (126). Incorporation of selective agents in maintenance media should normally be avoided to prevent changes in cultures. In the presence of selective agents, the culture may not be able to develop typically, as in the case of certain fungi.

Media for assays. Media for assays of vitamin and amino acid content of serum or other materials are usually very complex. They may or may not be synthetic, but they are generally made up from a large number of salts, vitamins, and amino acids, with at least one vitamin or amino acid absent. Varying amounts of the test materials are added to the media, and the growth responses in these tubes are compared with that in the control tubes which contain various amounts of the specific vitamin or amino acid. The test organism cannot grow in the absence of the vitamin or amino acid and will show a growth response to small increments. The test organisms include special strains of various streptococci, lactobacilli, *Ochromonas*, *Euglena*, and *Tetrahymena* (56). Extreme care—such as washing and rinsing, as well as baking, all glassware—must be taken with such media, because they can easily become chemically contaminated.

Tissue and organ culture media. Media for culture of tissues and organs are often very nearly as complex as assay media. Many have a mixture of amino acids, vitamins, dextrose, and salts, plus enrichment with serum or plasma. Phenol red is commonly included and, as noted above, antibiotics may be added to inhibit growth of bacterial contaminants. Doubtless many formulas could be greatly simplified, as has occurred in bacterial culture work.

Protozoa and other small animals are grown on media similar to, or even the same as, media for bacteria. Hirsch charcoal agar was devised for cultivation of *Mycobacterium tuberculosis*, and it is also used, with a Locke solution overlay, for growth of *Entamoeba histolytica* (82). Other media for *E. histolytica* utilize USP pancreatic digest of casein plus serum and inoculation with *Trypanosoma cruzi* (18, 97). Or streptobacilli are used in thioglycolate or thiomalic broths (99, 102).

Trichomonas species are readily grown in serum broths containing pancreatic digest of casein and cysteine. For diagnostic work, chloramphenicol is added to inhibit bacterial growth, and nystatin may be added if *Candida* inhibition is desirable. For assaying activity of drugs on *Trichomonas* and for maintaining cultures, no antibiotic is added (69).

Crithidia, *Tetrahymena*, and *Ochromonas* have been grown on peptone agar or broth, with blood added for the *Crithidia* (56). Cultivation of exoerythrocytic stages of malaria parasites has been carried out with tissue cultures in several tissue culture media (51). Flukes have been grown on a yeast extract, salt, serum, and egg albumin medium, as well as other media (132).

SELECTION

Selection of media is important and may be something of a problem. Available commercially are literally hundreds of formulations in dehydrated or complete form. Historically, culture media were natural materials, or infusions thereof, used for human nutrition—milk, eggs, potatoes, meat, etc. These materials are still in use today, but most modern media formulations frequently contain more defined components, such as the peptones described in the U.S. Pharmacopeia and pure chemicals. The trend has been toward the use of better defined or even entirely synthetic media.

Still in use, because of demand, are media which were used 25 to 50 years ago. Many of them should not now be used because ingredients of better quality made specifically for culture work are available, and the resultant newer formulas are often more efficient. All too frequently, people continue to use formulas *only* because those formulas were used in their schools or in training courses. However, new media may or may not be better than the older formulations and should be carefully tested and evaluated before being accepted. A laboratory may elect to purchase a large variety of prepared and pretested media, ready to use in tubes, bottles, or plates, or may elect to prepare its own media from numerous ingredients, including certain groceries, such as hamburger, peas, eggs, etc.

The most efficient laboratory is not necessarily the one with the greatest variety of media. The microbiologist will likely have relatively few media, carefully chosen and stored for most efficient performance and results. Some general criteria or guidelines for selection are as follows:

1. Select prepared media if the laboratory lacks efficient facilities or personnel for preparation and testing of ingredients and media.

2. Choose defined, rather than undefined, media. They will be more replicable and reliable. Preferably, for scientific work, they should not contain unidentified peptones, infusions, or extracts.

3. Choose media with the most potentialities as being more economical of space and time. Why have two or six media to do one job? Select one highly nutritive medium which will grow the greatest variety of organisms rapidly, and which can also serve as a base for hemolytic reactions of both aerobes and anaerobes. Because of improved growth, sensitivity test zones of enteric cultures will be smaller than on the "poor medium," but adequate growth of fastidious organisms will make more sensitivity tests possible and readable earlier.

4. In situations where a selective medium is desirable, choose another that is not selective. For example, if a medium selective for streptococci is employed, use a blood plate or a thioglycolate broth, or both, in addition. The patient may have another infection, instead of, or in addition to, the streptococcal infection.

5. For most miscellaneous specimens, include a broad-spectrum enrichment medium.

6. If there is a new, improved form of a medium, try the improved one. Triple sugar iron (TSI) agar is, for example, considerably more informative than the ancestral Russell medium. New media that, in published comparative studies, appear to be better than those currently in use should be tried in parallel with—not instead of—those in routine use.

7. When two or more selective media are employed, select formulas with *different* levels of selectivity to obtain organisms of different types. For example, use brilliant green bile agar with xylose lysine deoxycholate (XLD) agar, rather than with bismuth sulfite agar.

PREPARATION

Preparation of finished media from dehydrated materials should be in accordance with directions (7, 20, 96). Only chemically clean equipment and glassware should be used. Distilled or demineralized water should be used routinely unless otherwise specified. Accurate weighing of dry materials and correct measurement of water are essential. Heat should be direct or in a boiling-water bath or steam-jacketed container with agitation. Heating to effect solution of ingredients and sterilization of the completed medium should normally be done in the shortest possible time. Excessive heating at any time during the preparation should be avoided. Homogeneity is essential also, especially for media containing gelation agents.

When media are rehydrated from dry materials, they should have the correct appearance and pH. Microorganisms have requirements for acidity and alkalinity within a range beyond which growth will not take place. Most bacteria, yeasts, and molds encountered in clinical specimens grow best at a pH near neutrality. The laboratory should regularly check the pH of the final medium after autoclaving. This is particularly important for dehydrated media which have been previously opened, as they may undergo changes which may be detected by determination of the pH.

Sterilization is accomplished in various ways, usually by autoclaving or filtration. Most media are sterilized at 121 C for 15 min for volumes up to 500 ml. For larger volumes, the time should be extended to 20 to 30 min or more, as needed.

Media containing heat-stable carbohydrates are probably best autoclaved at a temperature not exceeding 116 to 118 C. However, heat-labile carbohydrates should preferably be sterilized by filtration and added aseptically to the cooled, autoclaved base medium. With the addition of certain carbohydrates, the reaction of the medium should be readjusted before sterilization to obtain the correct pH. Another efficient method of adding carbohydrates is by means of impregnated paper disks.

Filtration of carbohydrates or other materials may be accomplished with various filters, including asbestos Seitz filters, very small Swinney filters, and membrane filters, some of which can be used to process very large quantities. All collection equipment must be sterile and aseptically manipulated.

When enrichments, such as blood, are added, precautions must be taken that the base medium is as cool as possible. Admixture should be aseptic and also gentle to achieve homogeneity without froth or bubbles. Media containing such enrichments should *not* normally be incubated. To check sterility, representative plates or tubes should be incubated at 20 to 25 C or 30 to 35 C for several days, or for 1 week. The majority of the lot should be put into a refrigerator for storage, as soon as it is cool, to minimize drying and discoloration. The incubated samples should be discarded as soon as the results have been recorded; they should not be employed in clinical test procedures. The productivity of blood-agar media, for example, can be markedly impaired by incubation prior to use.

Enrichment with blood or serum, for nutrition or for determination of hemolysis, should be done with care. The blood or serum should be from animals fed on diets free from antimicrobial agents. Blood from different animal species, including human blood, is used to demonstrate bacterial hemolysins, and their performance is not necessarily identical.

1. Defibrinated sheep blood is probably the most efficient for routine work because (i) hemolytic reactions of streptococci are "correct" and (ii) growth of *Haemophilus hemolyticus*, a "non-pathogen," is inhibited. Colonies of this organism may be mistaken for hemolytic streptococci.

2. Defibrinated rabbit blood is the second choice because hemolytic reactions are "correct." Unfortunately, *H. hemolyticus* will grow, but *H. influenzae* will also grow on suitable media prepared with unheated rabbit blood.

3. Defibrinated horse blood may give "incorrect" hemolytic reactions. Some streptococci, e.g., group D, give hemolytic reactions on horse blood, but not on sheep blood, and may be mistakenly called group A if definitive tests are not performed.

4. Blood bank blood is often used because of availability. It has the disadvantages of containing citrate and dextrose. The citrates may be inhibitory to the organisms under test, and the dextrose may cause hemolytic streptococci to show greening rather than true hemolysis. The presence of antibodies and antimicrobial agents must also be considered.

A sterility test should be performed on added filtered solutions, bloods, etc. prior to use. The test should be in accordance with the requirements of the U.S. Pharmacopeia for the appropriate direct or membrane-filter methods for solutions.

In addition to performance of sterility tests, it is strongly recommended that all dispensing of sterile media and/or addition of sterile enrichments and other solutions should be carried out in a laminar-flow hood with sterile precautions, including the use of masks and gloves.

QUALITY CONTROL

In principle, control testing in the laboratory should be similar for all sizes and kinds of laboratories (129). Storage, equipment and environmental controls are the same. The specific media and procedures which are performed in the laboratory determine how much and exactly what kind of physical and cultural control are needed. Small laboratories or those receiving limited types of specimens obviously need fewer control cultures. This is particularly true of those laboratories which mainly do isolation, susceptibility testing, and generic identification, but refer isolates elsewhere for more definitive ancillary identification or epidemiological studies.

Some of the following recommendations apply to all culture media, while others apply only to those prepared by the using laboratory (7, 20, 96; C. W. Griffith and H. D. Vera, Amer. Pub. Health Ass. Meet., Philadelphia, 1969).

Water

USP Purified Water is recommended for general use. Purified water is water obtained by distillation or by ion-exchange treatment. The quality of the water employed should be checked both chemically and bacteriologically, at intervals, to determine whether it is of suitable quality. Impurities in the water may cause media to be cloudy and may very likely cause errors in other laboratory procedures as well.

Equipment

1. Recording thermometers on incubators and refrigerators are highly desirable; if these items

are not so equipped, manual recordings can be done in the morning before, or when the doors are first opened. Most incubators should be set at 35 C so that they will be unlikely to go above 37 C at any time. General information as to temperature requirements of most organisms indicates that temperatures below 37 C are optimal. Some *Neisseria* strains may be killed by temperatures very little above 37 C, but grow well at 35 C. Incubators for a temperature of 20 to 25 C, as for sterility testing or for growth of fungi, *Leptospira*, and *Listeria*, may require cooling devices, or a closed cupboard in a well air-conditioned room may suffice.

2. Autoclaves, ovens, and other sterilizers should be checked for performance, and temperatures should be recorded. Inclusion of spore controls is recommended to test efficiency.

3. Meters for measuring pH should be checked once or twice daily and preferably cross-checked with two standards, e.g., 4.0 and 7.0. Buffer tablets and solutions should be dated and should be used only while in good condition and without evidence of water loss or contamination.

4. Glassware (pipettes, syringes, etc.) should be discarded if etched or chipped. Rinsing should be thorough enough to remove all traces of chemical contaminants. Glassware which has been sterilized should be tested for freedom from microbial contamination. Accuracy of delivery should be retested before reuse.

5. Disposable plastic items should be checked for sterility and possible inhibitory properties.

Dehydrated media

1. Date containers on receipt and rotate so that the oldest is used first. The stock should be inspected regularly and records should be kept to insure that the supply is adequate and in good condition.

2. Make sure that the size of the container fits the rate of use.

3. Store media in a cool, dry place, away from hot ducts or pipes, preferably at a temperature below 30 C. Assay and other sensitive media should be stored in a freezer or refrigerator, as directed on the label.

4. Check performance of finished media, especially when made from previously opened containers, and discard the containers if the results are unsatisfactory. Such materials may undergo deterioration, even though they show no visible signs of change such as caking or browning.

5. Check the pH of the cool, finished medium or medium base each time a lot is made. The pH should be ±0.2 of the desired figure.

Media performance

1. The clinical laboratory should ordinarily maintain a set of stock cultures for minimal testing. The number of cultures need not be large, but the cultures must be well chosen for many kinds of check tests, should represent both common and uncommon organisms, and should be typical, highly stable, and homogeneous. If the cultures are selected from routine work, they should be from single colonies, unlikely to vary, and repeatedly tested. Such cultures should serve for: (i) check tests on media, (ii) teaching new technologists, (iii) keeping familiarized with relatively unusual, important pathogens, (iv) control tests on specimens, and (v) control tests on reactions.

2. The actual testing of culture media should be in accordance with the end use. For broad-spectrum media, testing should be mainly qualitative and should make use of a variety of fastidious genera or species. Some quantitative testing should also be done with serial dilutions of selected cultures, portions of which may be added to tubed media or to sterilized and cooled fluid agar media for plate counts.

3. Selective media can be tested more simply. The control cultures should be chosen for typical characteristics or to test for the presence of specific selective agents (especially those that are not visible in uninoculated media), or for both purposes. Cultures should represent groups that should grow well and those that should be partially or mostly inhibited. It is not wise to use strains with unusual characteristics, because a medium sufficiently selective to inhibit 100% of the undesirables would also be likely to inhibit some cultures that should grow and be detected. Most *Proteus* species are, for example, highly sensitive to chloramphenicol, but an occasional strain may grow well in its presence. Thus, selection of the unusually resistant *Proteus* for a test of chloramphenicol activity in selective media for fungi would be impractical.

4. Identification media should also be tested with cultures possessing *typical* characteristics. The cultures should include those causing both positive and negative reactions for each specific test for all reactions which the medium under test may give. Uninoculated controls should be included for comparison in test procedures, and are often helpful when included in the diagnostic procedures on unknown specimens or cultures. Some examples are listed in Table 1.

5. Prepared media should normally be stored in a refrigerator. Certain media, such as thioglycolate broths and cystine-tryptophan-peptone-agar (CTA) medium, should be refriger-

TABLE 1. *Some biochemical reactions in common use*

Reaction	Species suitable for demonstration		Medium
	Positive	Negative	
Bile solubility	*D. pneumoniae*	*S. pyogenes*	Typticase soy broth and deoxycholate reagent
Catalase	*B. subtilis*	*L. casei*	Eugonagar or L agar
Chromogenesis	*S. aureus*	*G. tetragena*	Eugonagar
	P. aeruginosa	*P. vulgaris*	Trypticase soy broth
Fermentation			
Monosaccharide			
Dextrose	*C. botulinum*	*C. tetani*	Trypticase dextrose agar
	S. aureus	*P. aeruginosa*	
Disaccharide			
Maltose	*N. meningitidis*	*N. catarrhalis*	CTA medium
Sucrose	*C. perfringens*	*C. septicum*	Trypticase sucrose agar
	P. vulgaris	*E. coli*	
Hemolysis	*C. perfringens*	*C. multifermentans*	Anaerobic agar without dextrose or Trypticase soy agar
	S. pyogenes	*S. lactis*	Trypticase soy agar
Hydrogen sulfide	*S. typhi*	*S. flexneri*	TSI agar or Trypticase lactose iron agar
IMViC reactions			
Indole	*E. coli*	*E. aerogenes*	Indole-nitrite medium
Methyl red	*E. coli*	*E. aerogenes*	MR-VP medium
Voges-Proskauer	*E. aerogenes*	*E. coli*	MR-VP medium
Citrate	*E. aerogenes*	*E. coli*	Koser citrate medium or Simmons citrate agar
Nitrate reduction	*C. perfringens*	*C. butyricum*	Indole-nitrite medium
	E. aerogenes	*G. tetragena*	Indole-nitrite medium or nitrate agar
Oxidase	*N. meningitidis*	*S. aureus*	Eugonagar
Proteolysis			
Gelatin	*C. sporogenes*	*C. spheroides*	Thiogel medium
	P. aeruginosa	*E. aerogenes*	
Serum	*C. sporogenes*	*C. butyricum*	Thioglycolate medium with Loeffler medium
Tartrate utilization	*S. enteritidis*	*S. schottmuelleri*	Phenol red tartrate agar

ated, if in sealed containers; if the containers are *not* sealed, these media should be stored at room temperature and used within a relatively short period. Quantity, age, and condition should be monitored. Media should be discarded that show signs of water loss or drying of the surface, discoloration, or microbial contamination. Stock should be dated on receipt and rotated. Less culture control work is necessary than for media prepared from raw or dehydrated materials. Tests should usually be similar, but less extensive. If necessary, check tests with control cultures and clinical specimens can be run concurrently. Actually, such direct comparisons can be helpful.

FORMULAS AND INSTRUCTION FOR PREPARATION AND USE OF CULTURE MEDIA

The formulas submitted by the contributing authors are reproduced essentially as received, except for changes made in the interest of uniform presentation.

To save space, the following general instructions are not repeated for each medium. For *media containing agar*, suspend the specified amount of ingredients in purified water, USP, unless tap water is specified. Heat with agitation and boil for 1 min. *Heating should be minimal.* Do not allow a mixture to stand in a steamer for more than 10 min. For *fluid media*, weigh out the dry material and suspend it in water unless otherwise specified. Heat with agitation until solution is obtained. Usually broths may also be heated to boiling, if desired, to insure homogeneity and to minimize the period of autoclaving.

The pH, unless otherwise specified, is that of the finished medium when it is ready for inoculation. It is determined at room temperature. If a medium or base is sterilized by heat, the pH prior to sterilization is usually *not* the same as it is afterward. In research work, to properly make adjustments, it is necessary to sterilize, or otherwise process, several small samples (e.g., 100-ml amounts) to which have been added known increments of selected reagents, in order to determine exactly how much acid or alkali should be added to convert (e.g., 1 liter of) the bulk volume into correct finished medium. Hot samples can, of course, be cooled rapidly in cold or cool water. Nonsterile solutions should not be held more than an hour or so, because of the possibilities of water loss and of microbial growth. Moreover, nonsterile solutions should not be held at high temperatures, because of the likelihood of damage by heat over prolonged periods. If the medium contains phosphates or other active buffers, the kind of buffer salt should be adjusted to obtain the proper pH, rather than, for example, using an alkaline salt and adding acid, thus changing the salt into its acid form. In general, precautions should be taken, when adjusting pH, to minimize any increase in concentrations of any salts, and thus changing of the formulation.

To determine the pH of the finished medium, remove the agar or broth to the cup or beaker used with the meter. If preferred, tubes of agar or egg media can be broken and the contents can be transferred to the meter container. Macerate solid media if necessary, but do not add water; if there is sufficient moisture for culture growth, there is sufficient for meter readings. Surface electrodes are convenient for testing plated media.

Wherever possible, the generic names for peptones are given, and in some cases trade names are also noted. Many of the media listed by the individual authors are available from commercial sources under different terminologies and spellings (e.g., thioglycolate is sometimes spelled thioglycollate). This information can frequently be obtained from the manufacturers. Note that media or components designated by an asterisk (*) are available commercially in dehydrated or prepared form. The composition of the commercial preparation may be either identical or comparable to the formula submitted by the author, and this may be determined by comparing the formulas.

Water of hydration is included when submitted by the author. The form used here, while not traditional or chemically correct, was selected for the sake of convenience and simplicity. Where commercial media are used, preparation should be in accordance with the manufacturer's directions. Media for viruses are listed in Tables 2–4.

A medium of King* (66)
Pseudomonas agar for detection of pyocyanin USP*
Tech agar* Pseudomonas agar P*

*Throughout chapter 95, asterisks (*) designate compounds or media which are available commercially.

TABLE 2. *Composition of Hanks and Earle balanced salt solutions (BSS)*

Components	Hanks BSS	Earle BSS
Sodium chloride	8.00 g	6.80 g
Potassium chloride	0.40 g	0.40 g
Calcium chloride	0.14 g	0.20 g
Magnesium sulfate · $7H_2O$	0.20 g	0.20 g
Disodium phosphate · $12H_2O$	0.12 g	—
Monosodium phosphate	—	0.125
Monopotassium phosphate	0.06 g	—
Sodium bicarbonate	0.35 g[a]	2.20 g[b]
Dextrose	1.00 g	1.00 g
Phenol red, 1% aqueous	1.60 ml[c]	1.60 ml
Purified water USP	1.00 liter	1.00 liter

[a] Prepared as a 2.8% stock solution and added at the time of use.
[b] Prepared as an 8.8% stock solution and added at the time of use.
[c] If a somewhat deeper red color is preferred, 2.0 ml may be used.

Bacto peptone or Gelysate pancreatic digest of gelatin	20.0 g
Magnesium chloride, anhydrous	1.4 g
Potassium sulfate, anhydrous	10.0 g
Agar (dried)	(13.6 g
or not dried	15.0 g
Glycerol, chemically pure	10.0 ml
Distilled water	1.0 liter
Final pH 7.2	

Dispense in tubes for slants with deep butts and autoclave at 118 to 121 C for 15 min.

Acetate agar* (123)

Sodium acetate	2.00 g
Sodium chloride	5.00 g
Magnesium sulfate	0.20 g
Monoammonium phosphate	1.00 g
Dipotassium phosphate	1.00 g
Bromothymol blue	0.08 g
Agar (dried)	(17.00 g)
or not dried	20 g
Distilled water	1.00 liter
Final pH 6.7 ± 0.2	

Dissolve and dispense into tubes for 2.5-cm butts and 3.8-cm slants. Autoclave at 121 C for 15 min.

Inoculate and incubate in the same manner as Simmons citrate agar.

Actinomyces agar
Actinomyces broth* plus agar

Potassium phosphate	15.00 g
Ammonium sulfate	1.00 g
Magnesium sulfate	0.20 g
Calcium chloride	0.01 g
Infusion broth	25.00 g
Dextrose	5.00 g
Cysteine	1.00 g
Pancreatic digest of casein USP	4.00 g

TABLE 3. *Composition of three synthetic media employed in diagnostic virology*

Component	Medium 199	Eagle minimum essential medium	Leibovitz medium 15 (L-15)
	mg	*mg*	*mg*
Amino acids			
L-Alanine	50.00[a]		450[a]
L-Arginine	70.00	105	500[b]
L-Asparagine			250
L-Aspartic acid	60.00[a]		
L-Cysteine	0.10		120[b]
L-Cystine	20.00	24	
L-Glutamic acid	150.00[a]		
L-Glutamine	100.00	292	292
Glycine	50.00		200
L-Histidine	20.00	31	250[b]
Hydroxy-L-proline	10.00		
L-Isoleucine	40.00[a]	52	250[a]
L-Leucine	120.00[a]	52	125
L-Lysine	70.00	58	75
L-Methionine	30.00[a]	15	150[a]
L-Phenylalanine	40.00	32	250[a]
L-Proline	40.00		
L-Serine	50.00		200
L-Threonine	60.00[a]	48	300
L-Tryptophan	20.00[a]	10	20
L-Tyrosine	40.00	36	320
L-Valine	50.00[a]	46	200[a]
Vitamins			
p-Aminobenzoic acid	0.050		
Biotin	0.010		
Calcium pantothenate	0.010	1.0	1.0
Choline chloride	0.500	1.0	1.0
Folic acid	0.010	1.0	1.0
i-Inositol	0.050	2.0	2.0
Niacin	0.025		
Niacinamide	0.025	1.0	1.0
Pyridoxal HCl	0.025	1.0	1.0
Pyridoxine HCl	0.025		
Riboflavine	0.010	0.1	0.1
Thiamine HCl	0.010	1.0	1.0
Vitamin A	0.100		
Ascorbic acid	0.050		
α-Tocopherol phosphate	0.010		
Calciferol	0.100		
Menadione	0.010		
Nucleic acid derivatives			
Adenine	10.0		
Guanine · HCl	0.3		
Hypoxanthine	0.3		
Thymine	0.3		
Uracil	0.3		
Xanthine	0.3		
Adenylic acid	0.2		
Carbohydrates			
2-Deoxy-D-ribose	0.5		
D-Ribose	0.5		
Dextrose	1,000.0	1,000.0	
Galactose			900.0

TABLE 3.—*Continued*

Component	Medium 199	Eagle minimum essential medium	Leibovitz medium 15 (L-15)
	mg	*mg*	*mg*
Miscellaneous			
Sodium acetate	50.00		
Sodium pyruvate			550.0
Polysorbate (Tween) 80	5.00		
Cholesterol	0.20		
Glutathione	0.05		
Adenosine triphosphate	10.00		
Phenol red	20.00	20.0	10–20
Salts			
Sodium chloride	6,800	6,800	8,000
Potassium chloride	400	400	400
Calcium chloride	200	200	140
Magnesium chloride · $6H_2O$		200	200
Magnesium sulfate · $7H_2O$	200		200
Monosodium phosphate · H_2O	140	140	
Disodium phosphate · H_2O			70
Potassium phosphate			60
Ferric nitrate · $9H_2O$	0.1		
Sodium bicarbonate	2,200	2,200	
Purified water USP	1.0 liter	1.0 liter	1.0 liter

[a] Amount of DL form of amino acid rather than L form.
[b] Free base form.

Yeast extract	5.00 g
Soluble starch	1.00 g
Agar	20.00 g
Distilled water	1.00 liter
Final pH 6.9	

Heat with agitation to obtain solution. Dispense and autoclave at 118 to 121 C for 10 min. May also be used as a semisolid (7 g of agar) medium.

Agar deep slants

See Brucella agar.

Albizo-Surgalla serum agar

1. Dilute filtered *Pasteurella pestis* antiserum with 0.85% NaCl solution.
2. Warm to 37 C in a water bath.
3. Admix gently with sterile double-strength (8%) blood agar base, sterilized and cooled to 55 C.
4. Pour rapidly into disposable petri plates, 8 to 10 ml per plate.
5. Tilt plates immediately to distribute the medium evenly.

TABLE 4. *Composition of two media employed for the cultivation and maintenance of primary cell cultures*

Component	Melnick medium A[a]	Melnick medium B[b]
Sodium chloride	8.00 g	6.80 g
Potassium chloride	0.40 g	0.40 g
Magnesium sulfate · $7H_2O$	0.20 g	0.20 g
Monopotassium phosphate	0.60 g	—
Disodium phosphate · $7H_2O$	0.09 g	—
Monosodium phosphate · H_2O	—	0.14 g
Calcium chloride, anhydrous	0.14 g	0.20 g
Sodium bicarbonate	0.35 g	2.20 g
Dextrose	1.00 g	1.00 g
Phenol red	0.02 g	0.01 g
Lactalbumin hydrolysate	5.00 g	5.00 g
Calf serum	20.00 ml	20.00 ml
Purified water USP	1.00 liter	1.00 liter

[a] Recommended for the initial culture of monkey kidney epithelium and other primary cells.
[b] Recommended for the continued growth and maintenance of cells. Before cells are used for culture of viruses, the medium should be changed to one which has the same ingredients but without calf serum.

6. Place in plastic bags immediately after the medium is solidified and store at 4 C.

Incubate at 37 C for 40 h, after which time *P. pestis* colonies are 0.5 to 1 mm in diameter. Expose plates to chloroform vapors for 1 min by inverting them over a glass petri dish cover containing 2 ml of chloroform on a gauze sponge (5 × 5 cm, 12 ply). Remove plates and leave inverted (agar surface down) in a tilted position for 10 min to eliminate chloroform vapor. Incubate at 37 C and examine after 2, 4, 6, and 24 h for precipitation ring formation. Observe with a dissecting microscope and oblique transmitted light.

Albumin fatty acid broth, Ellinghausen and McCullough, Modified* (59)

Leptospira medium and enrichment EMJH*

Basal medium

Disodium phosphate	1.0 g
Monopotassium phosphate	0.3 g
Sodium chloride	1.0 g
Ammonium chloride, 25% aqueous	1.0 ml
Thiamine, 0.5% aqueous	1.0 ml
Glycerol, 10% aqueous	1.0 ml
Distilled water	997.0 ml

Mix and adjust to pH 7.4. Autoclave at 121 C for 20 min.

Albumin-fatty acid supplement

Bovine Albumin Fraction V*	20.0 g
Calcium chloride-$2H_2O$ and magnesium chloride · $6H_2O$, aqueous solutions, 1% each salt	2.0 ml
Zinc sulfate · $7H_2O$, 0.4% aqueous	2.0 ml
Copper sulfate · $5H_2O$, 0.3% aqueous	0.2 ml
Ferrous sulfate · $7H_2O$, 0.5% aqueous	20.0 ml
Vitamin B_{12}, 0.02% aqueous	2.0 ml
Polysorbate (Tween) 80, 10% aqueous	25.0 ml
Distilled water to	200.0 ml

1. Add the bovine albumin slowly with careful stirring (to avoid foaming) to 100 ml of water.
2. Add remaining ingredients (prepared as stock solutions) slowly to the albumin solution with constant stirring.
3. Adjust the pH to 7.4 and add water to 200 ml final volume.
4. Sterilize by filtration through a membrane or Seitz filter (porosity, 0.2 to 0.3 μm).
5. Store at 4 C or −20 C.

Aseptically combine one part of supplement with nine parts of basal medium and dispense in sterile containers.

Note. If deionized water is used, preheat it to 56 C for 30 min to destroy naturally occurring water leptospires, which are not retained by membrane and asbestos filters (0.2 μm).

Alginate medium (19)

As for Acetate agar, except with 2.5 g of sodium alginate instead of 2.0 g of sodium citrate.

Inoculate and incubate in the same manner as Simmons citrate agar.

Alkaline peptone water*

Alkaline peptone broth

Peptone *or* Gelysate *or* pancreatic digest of casein USP	10 g
Sodium chloride	5 g
Distilled water	1 liter

1. Dissolve and adjust pH to about 8.4 or 8.5 with 1 N NaOH.
2. Dispense in 10-ml amounts in test tubes.
3. Alternatively, dispense in 0.5- to 1-ml amounts for transportation of rectal swab specimens.
4. Autoclave at 121 C for 15 min.

Amies transport medium* (3)

Sodium chloride	8.0 g
Potassium chloride	0.2 g
Calcium chloride	0.1 g
Magnesium chloride	0.1 g
Monopotassium phosphate	0.2 g
Disodium phosphate	1.5 g
Sodium thioglycolate	1.0 g
Charcoal, finely powdered	10.0 g
Agar	3.6 g
Distilled water	1.0 liter

1. Mix and heat gently to dissolve soluble ingredients.
2. Dispense in small screw-capped vials filled within 5 mm of the top.
3. Tighten caps and sterilize at 121 C for 15 min.
4. Invert vials just before gelation to suspend the charcoal evenly. Retighten caps if necessary.

5. Use sterile nontoxic swabs or boil swabs in Sorensen phosphate buffer 0.067 M, pH 7.4, and dry before use.

6. After a swab has been dipped into a specimen, insert it deep into the medium of a vial. Cut off the stick and replace the cap tightly.

Ammonium nitrate agar
Trichophyton agars 6 and 7*

Ammonium nitrate	1.5 g
Dextrose	40.0 g
Magnesium sulfate	0.1 g
Monopotassium phosphate	1.8 g
Agar	20.0 g
Distilled water	1.0 liter

Adjust pH to 6.8 and dispense in 100-ml amounts into flasks.

For *Histidine ammonium nitrate agar*, add 2 ml of histidine solution, 150 mg/100 ml of water. Tube, sterilize at 121 C for 15 min, and slant.

Andrade carbohydrate broths
A. *For Erysipelothrix, chapter 14*

Beef extract	3 g
Bacto peptone or Gelysate or proteose pancreatic digest of gelatin	10 g
Sodium chloride	5 g
Andrade indicator (see below)	10 ml
Distilled water	900 ml

1. Make up broth in excess of 900 ml. Adjust the pH to 7.2 with 4% NaOH and autoclave for 15 min at 121 C.
2. To each 900 ml of broth, add 10 ml of Andrade's indicator.
3. Prepare 10% solutions of carbohydrates in distilled water which has been previously autoclaved for 30 min. Arabinose and xylose must be sterilized by filtration; the others may be autoclaved for 12 min.
4. Aseptically add 100 ml of 10% carbohydrate solution.

Andrade indicator

Acid fuchsin	0.5 g
Distilled water	100.0 ml
Sodium hydroxide, 1 N	16.0 ml

Allow to decolorize before use. Add an additional 1 or 2 ml of alkali, if necessary. Autoclave at 121 C for 20 min.

B. *For Enterobacteriaceae, chapter 18*

Prepare 1,000 ml of basal medium. Prepare and add carbohydrates as follows, and tube with inverted insert tubes.

1. Add 1.0% dextrose, lactose, sucrose, and mannitol (20).
2. Add 0.5% dulcitol, salicin, and other carbohydrates.
3. Add dextrose, mannitol, dulcitol, salicin, adonitol, and inositol prior to sterilization.
4. Sterilize disaccharides, such as lactose and sucrose, in 10% concentration.
5. Sterilize arabinose and xylose separately.

C. *For Dermatophilus, chapter 17*

Prepare 1,000 ml of medium in demineralized water, omitting beef extract. Adjust pH to 7.4 to 7.5 and add 10% filter-sterilized carbohydrate solutions in a 1% final concentration.

Antibiotic medium 5 FDA*

See Streptomycin assay agar with yeast extract.*

Antibiotic medium 20 FDA*
Yeast beef broth*

Yeast extract	6.50 g
Beef extract	1.50 g
Peptone *or* Gelysate pancreatic digest of casein	5.00 g
Pancreatic digest of casein	10.00 g
Dextrose	11.00 g
Sodium chloride	3.50 g
Dipotassium phosphate	3.68 g
Monopotassium phosphate	1.32 g
Purified water	1.00 liter
Final pH 6.6	

1. Heat to boiling to dissolve.
2. Dispense and autoclave at 121 C for 15 min.

Auxanographic agar media

For carbohydrate assimilation tests

1. Prepare 10× concentration of yeast nitrogen base* (YNB) but omit asparagine and dextrose. Sterilize by filtration.
2. Autoclave a 2% aqueous solution of washed agar. Autoclave at 121 C for 15 min and cool to 50 C.
3. Pipette 2.0 ml of the YNB into each petri plate. Mix 20 ml of sterile agar; allow medium to solidify.
4. Use a sterile swab to streak an actively growing yeast culture from a Sabouraud slant for confluent growth. Allow surface to dry.
5. Place carbohydrate disks near the periphery of each plate. Use dextrose, maltose, sucrose, lactose, galactose, cellobiose, melibiose, xylose, raffinose, inositol, trehalose, and dulcitol.
6. Incubate at 25 C and examine for growth around disks.

For nitrate assimilation tests

1. Use 10× yeast carbon base (YCB) and proceed as above.
2. Add disks containing potassium nitrate or peptone (or amino acids).

B medium of King, Ward, and Raney* (66)
Pseudomonas agar for detection of fluorescin USP*
Flo agar,* Pseudomonas agar F*

Pancreatic digest of casein USP	10.0 g
Peptic digest of animal tissues USP	10.0 g
Dipotassium phosphate anhydrous	1.5 g
Magnesium sulfate $\cdot 7H_2O$	1.5 g
Agar (dried)	(14.0 g)
or not dried	15 g
Distilled water	1.0 liter
Final pH 7.2	

Dissolve and add 10 ml of glycerol. Dispense in 7-ml amounts in 15 by 125 mm tubes for slants with deep butts.

Baird-Parker agar USP*
Egg yolk pyruvate tellurite glycine agar

Pancreatic digest of casein USP	10 g
Beef extract	5 g
Yeast extract	1 g
Sodium pyruvate	10 g
Glycine	12 g
Lithium chloride	5 g
Agar (dried)	(17 g)
or not dried	20 g
Distilled water	1 liter
pH 6.8	

1. Autoclave at 121 C for 15 min.
2. Cool to about 50 C, and add 50 ml of egg yolk emulsion* and 10 ml of sterile 1% (or 3 ml of 3.5%) potassium tellurite solution.*
3. Mix well and pour into plates.

Balamuth egg infusion medium (5)

Liver extract solution

Powdered liver extract	5 g
Distilled water	100 ml

Boil, filter through paper, and autoclave at 121 C for 20 min.

0.067 M Buffer solution

1. Dipotassium phosphate	87.09 g
Distilled water	500.00 ml
2. Monopotassium phosphate	13.61 g
Distilled water	100.00 ml

Mix 4.3 parts of stock solution 1 with 0.7 parts of solution 2 and dilute 1:14 with distilled water.

1. Mix well yolks of four hard-boiled eggs with 125 ml of 0.85% NaCl, preferably in a blender.
2. Heat in covered double boiler for 20 min at 80 C. Add 20 ml of distilled water to make up for evaporation.
3. Filter through several layers of no. 2 paper in Büchner funnel under reduced pressure.
4. Autoclave filtrate for 20 min at 121 C. Cool below 10 C and filter again.
5. Into the filtrate, admix an equal amount of 0.067 M buffer solution.
6. Add one part of liver extract solution to the buffered yolk infusion. Autoclave at 121 C for 20 min, and tube in 7- to 10-ml quantities.
7. Just prior to use, add to each tube approximately 30 mg of sterile rice powder, previously heated for 2.5 h at 150 C dry heat.

Balamuth's egg infusion medium is an all-liquid egg infusion medium to which liver has been added. It is good for isolating most intestinal protozoa, and, as an additional advantage, it may be stored for several months without marked deterioration. The techniques for inoculation and examination are similar to those described for Boeck and Drbohlav's medium (8).

Beef heart charcoal agar (60, 85)

Soluble starch	10.0 g
Yeast extract	3.5 g
Agar	20.0 g
Heart infusion broth (infusion broth)	25.0 g
Distilled water	1.0 liter

1. Dissolve by heating and add 4.0 g of charcoal (Norit FQP).
2. Autoclave at 121 C for 15 min.
3. Cool and add 30 units of penicillin per 100 ml of medium just before dispensing.

Beef heart infusion agar* with blood*

Beef heart, infusion from	450 g
Peptone	10 g
Sodium chloride	5 g
Agar	15 g
Demineralized water	1 liter
Final pH 7.2.	

1. Infuse meat in 500 ml of water overnight at 4 to 6 C. Remove fat.
2. Add peptone, heat slowly to boiling, and boil for 30 min. Strain through colander.
3. Filter through paper, make up weight, and adjust to pH 7.6 to 8.0.
4. Boil 10 min and make up weight.
5. Dissolve agar and sodium chloride in remaining water by autoclaving.
6. Combine the agar with the broth and mix thoroughly. Adjust to pH 7.4.
7. Filter through glass wool and dispense in 900-ml amounts in 2-liter flasks.
8. Autoclave at 121 C for 30 min. Cool to 45 C and add 50 ml of defibrinated sterile horse blood per 900 ml of base.
9. Dispense as required. Store at 2 to 8 C.

Beef infusion agar*

Ground defatted beef, infusion from	453.6 g
Peptone	10.0 g
Sodium chloride	5.0 g
Agar	20.0 g
Distilled water	1.0 liter

1. Allow meat to infuse in water overnight at 4 to 5 C. Cook for 1 h at 80 to 90 C. Allow to stand for 2 h and filter through muslin.
2. Add peptone and salt, and adjust to pH 7.6 with 4% NaOH. Filter.
3. Add agar and autoclave. Filter through cotton or several layers of milk filter disks. Autoclave again.

Beef infusion broth*
As above, but omit the agar.

Beef infusion-peptone broth

Beef, infusion from	450.0 g
Proteose *or* Thiotone peptic digest of animal tissue USP	20.0 g
Sodium chloride	5.0 g
Dextrose	0.5–1.5 g
Demineralized water	1.0 liter

1. Infuse the meat overnight in 1,000 ml of demineralized water at 4 to 6 C. Remove fat and sample for sugar test (quantitative Benedict's).

2. Add peptone and salt, heat to boiling, and boil for 30 min. Strain through cheese cloth.

3. Add needed glucose, weigh, and adjust pH to 8.2+.

4. Autoclave for 30 min. Weigh and adjust reaction up to 7.8 to 8.0, if necessary.

5. Boil for 5 to 10 min. Filter, dispense, and autoclave at 115 to 118 C for 30 min. The final reaction should be pH 7.4 to 7.6.

Bennett agar

Pancreatic digest of casein USP	2 g
Yeast extract	1 g
Beef extract	1 g
Dextrose	10 g
Agar	15 g
Demineralized water	1 liter
Final pH 7.3.	

Heat with agitation to dissolve. Dispense and autoclave.

Recommended for production of aerial hyphae and spores by *Nocardia* and *Streptomyces*.

Bile esculin agar*

Beef extract	3.0 g
Peptone	5.0 g
Agar	15.0 g
Oxgall	40.0 g
Ferric citrate	0.5 g
Water	1 liter

1. Dissolve first three ingredients in 400 ml of water. Dissolve oxgall in 400 ml of water. Dissolve the ferric citrate in 100 ml of water.

2. Combine the solutions and mix well. Heat to 100 C for 10 min.

3. Autoclave at 121 C for 15 min. Cool to 50 C.

4. Aseptically add 100 ml of water containing 1 g of esculin previously heated gently to obtain solution and filter-sterilized.

5. Dispense in sterile screw-capped tubes. Tighten caps and cool in the slanted position.

6. Alternatively, use dehydrated medium of this formula and prepare according to directions.

7. Optional: add 50 ml of horse serum to the sterile cool base.

Bile test broth, for anaerobes

For the bile test, thioglycolate medium "without added dextrose" is used with the addition of 0.5% dextrose and 20% concentration of either crude ox bile (must be green) or reconstituted oxgall. Before using the bile (fresh or reconstituted) in the medium, add sodium deoxycholate in a concentration of 1.0% (final concentration in the medium is 0.1%). Dispense in 9-ml portions in 16 by 125 mm screw-capped tubes. Also prepare a control medium as above, but omit bile.

Bird seed agar

See Staib agar.

Bismuth sulfite agar, modified* (133–135)
Wilson-Blair Base*

Base

Beef extract	5 g
Peptone: Thiotone *or* Thiopeptone *or* Polypeptone	10 g
Dextrose	5 g
Sodium chloride	5 g
Agar	25 g
Distilled water	1 liter

Autoclave at 121 C for 15 min. Cool to about 50 C and add 70 ml of the following:

Bismuth sulfite solution

1. Dissolve 200 g of anhydrous sodium sulfite in 1 liter of distilled water.

2. Dissolve 50 g of bismuth ammonium citrate in 500 ml of distilled water. Add 1 ml of concentrated ammonium hydroxide. Allow to stand until clear. Add several more milliliters of ammonium hydroxide if necessary. Add to 1.

3. To the mixture of 1 and 2, admix 100 g of anhydrous dibasic sodium phosphate.

4. Dissolve 10 g of ferric ammonium sulfate in 100 ml of distilled water. Add to mixture 3.

5. Heat the combined solution at 100 C for 2 or 3 min. Stopper the container and store in the dark at room temperature. Do not refrigerate and do not autoclave.

Shake the mixture of base and bismuth sulfite solution thoroughly. Add 4 ml of 1% aqueous solution of brilliant green (43, 44). Cool to 40 to 50 C and pour into plates.

Blood agar base*
Heart infusion agar

Beef heart muscle, infusion from	375 g
Tryptose *or* thiotone peptic digest of animal tissue USP	10 g
Sodium chloride	5 g
Agar	15 g
Distilled or demineralized water	1 liter
pH 7.3 or pH 6.8.	

Autoclave at 121 C for 15 min. Cool to 50 C and add 5% sterile defibrinated rabbit blood, if desired.

For aerobic actinomycetes, chapter 17, add defibrinated horse blood, 50 ml/900 ml of base.

Blood agar media for anaerobes

See Brain heart infusion agar and Brucella agar.

Blood agar, diphasic, for trypanosomes and leishmania, NIH method (55)

Lean beef, desiccated	25.0 g
Neopeptone* or other	10.0 g
Agar	10.0 g
Sodium chloride	2.5 g
Distilled water	500.0 ml

1. Infuse the beef and distilled water in a water bath for 1 h. Heat for 5 min at 80 C.
2. Filter through filter paper.
3. Add the rest of the above ingredients and adjust the pH to 7.0 to 7.4 with NaOH.
4. Autoclave at 120 C for 20 min.
5. Cool to 45 C and aseptically add 10% defibrinated rabbit blood.
6. Dispense 5-ml quantities in sterile tubes. Slant and cool.
7. Just prior to inoculation, overlay with 2 ml of sterile Locke solution.

Locke solution

Sodium chloride	8.0 g
Potassium chloride	0.2 g
Calcium chloride	0.2 g
Monopotassium phosphate	0.3 g
Dextrose	2.5 g
Distilled water	1.0 liter

Editors' note. The author recommends Difco ingredients.

Blood-free medium (124)

Tryptose broth with thiamine *or* Biosate broth	26.00 g
Dextrose	10.00 g
L-Cysteine hydrochloride	1.20 g
Ferrous sulfate	0.05 g
L-Histidine hydrochloride	1.00 g
Hydroxymethyl aminomethane	3.00 g
Potassium chloride	0.20 g
Distilled water	1.00 liter

1. Dissolve and adjust pH to 7.0 with concentrated HCl.
2. Add 15 g of agar, dissolve, and autoclave at 121 C for 20 min.
3. Cool to 48 C and add aseptically, from stock solutions containing 100,000 units/ml each: penicillin G, 1 ml; polymyxin B, 3 ml; nystatin, 1 ml.
4. Dispense aseptically.

Boeck and Drbohlav medium, modified* (8, 98)

*Locke solution, modified**

Sodium chloride	8.00 g
Calcium chloride·$2H_2O$	0.20 g
Potassium chloride	0.20 g
Magnesium chloride·$6H_2O$	0.01 g
Disodium phosphate, anhydrous	2.00 g
Sodium bicarbonate	0.40 g
Monopotassium phosphate, anhydrous	0.30 g
Distilled water	1.00 liter

Boil for 10 min. Cool to room temperature and filter through paper to remove precipitate. Dispense and autoclave at 121 C for 15 min.

1. Wash and break four fresh eggs into a sterile 1-liter flask containing a few glass beads (or into a blender).
2. Add 50 ml of sterile Locke solution and emulsify by shaking.
3. Filter through gauze and dispense into sterile 16 by 125 mm test tubes for 4- to 5-cm slants with short butts.
4. Inspissate in an autoclave: (i) allow the jacket to reach 15 lb of pressure; (ii) place tubes in chamber in desired slanted position; (iii) close door and all exhaust valves to entrap air; (iv) allow steam to enter chamber as fast as possible until pressure is 15 lb; (v) hold for 15 min and turn off steam; (vi) allow pressure to drop gradually with door and valves closed.
5. Allow slants to cool and cover with Locke solution to a depth of 5 to 6 cm.
6. Sterilize at 121 C for 15 min. Allow pressure to drop gradually.
7. Incubate at 37 C for 24 h and check for sterility.
8. If overlay is clear, refrigerate for use within 1 month.
9. Just prior to use, add sterile rice powder. *See* Balamuth medium.
10. Also add to one of each pair of tubes penicillin and streptomycin to a final concentration of 200 to 250 units (penicillin) or μg (streptomycin) per ml of overlay (95, 112).

Inoculate fecal specimen into two tubes of warmed medium, one containing antibiotics. If specimen is liquid or semisolid, add about 0.5 ml to each tube with a large-bore pipette. Mix carefully with overlay to add as little air as possible. If specimen is formed, use portion the size of a small pea and mix carefully with overlay by rubbing against side of the tube. Choose portions from any mucus, blood, or abnormally appearing areas. Incubate at 37 C for 24 h and examine microscopically. Remove a few drops of sediment, with a sterile large-bore pipette, to a slide and cover with a cover slip.

The amoebae grow at the bottom of the culture or on the surface of the slant near the bottom. If the culture shows no trophozoites or an insufficient number for identification, transfer about half of the sediment to media without antibiotics and incubate the original cultures and the subcultures for 48 h. The sediment of cultures revealing organisms or questionable objects should be mixed in vials with polyvinyl alcohol fixative. Prepare permanently stained films and examine under oil immersion objective (94).

Bordet Gengou agar, modified*
Without Peptone

Potatoes, washed, peeled, sliced	125.0 g
Glycerol	10.0 ml
Sodium chloride	5.6 g
Agar	22.5 g
Distilled water	1.0 liter

1. Place potatoes in loose gauze bag. Submerge in mixture of glycerol and half of the water. Boil until potatoes are soft. Strain through gauze and allow fluid to stand in tall cylinders until relatively clear supernatant fluid can be decanted.
2. Restore to volume with water.
3. Add salt and stir to dissolve. Heat.
4. Add agar and stir vigorously. Heat to boiling to dissolve agar. Check volume and add water if necessary.
5. Dispense in 250-ml amounts in 16-oz screw-capped bottles.

6. Autoclave at 121 C for 15 min and cool to 45 C.
7. Aseptically add 50 ml of defibrinated sheep blood to each 250 ml of agar base and mix carefully to avoid bubbles.
8. Dispense into sterile plates. Incubate at 35 ± 1 C to check sterility.

Note. For diagnostic medium, also add 125 units of penicillin to each 250 ml of base prior to dispensing.

Brain heart infusion agar*

Calf brains, infusion from	200.0 g
Beef heart, infusion from	250.0 g
Proteose *or* Gelysate pancreatic digest of gelatin	10.0 g
Dextrose	2.0 g
Sodium chloride	5.0 g
Disodium phosphate	2.5 g
Agar	15.0 g
Distilled or demineralized water	1.0 liter
Final pH 7.4	

Dispense and autoclave at 121 C for 15 min.

For Actinomyces, the use of freshly poured plates is recommended.

Brain heart infusion broth*

As above, but without agar

Additives

A. For yeasts: Add Neopeptone, 5 g/liter.
B. For fungi: Add Neopeptone, 5 g, and dextrose, 20 g/liter.
C. For sheep blood medium (131):
   1. Heat 1 liter of broth to boiling.
   2. Add 10% defibrinated sheep blood while hot; shake for 5 min.
   3. Filter through Schleicher and Schuell filter paper.
   4. Dispense the filtrate in 10-ml quantities in 12.5-cm screw-capped tubes.
   5. Autoclave at 120 C for 15 min.

Brain heart infusion* supplemented* (BHIS) broth (49)

Brain heart infusion broth	100.0 ml
Yeast extract	5.0 g
Distilled water	900.0 ml
Resazurin solution, 0.025% (*see* Cary and Blair, modified)	4.0 g
Cysteine hydrochloride	0.5 g

1. Mix and heat to obtain solution.
2. Tube in 10-ml volumes and autoclave at 121 C for 15 min.
3. Aseptically add to each tube 0.1 ml of vitamin K-heme solution (55), prepared as follows:
   a. Dissolve 10 mg of vitamin K_1 (menadione) in 20 ml of 95% ethanol, and filter sterilize.
   b. Dissolve 50 mg of hemin in 1 ml of 1 N sodium hydroxide or in 10 ml of commercial ammonia water. Dilute to 100 ml with water. Autoclave at 121 C for 15 min.
   c. Add 1 ml of vitamin K_1 solution to 100 ml of hemin solution. Use 1 ml of mixture per 100 ml of medium.

Brain heart infusion supplemented (BHIS) with agar

As above with 1.5% agar incorporated. If desired, after sterilization and cooling to 50 C, add 50 ml of sterile defibrinated sheep blood. Omit hemin and add 1 ml of vitamin K_1 solution only. *See* Brucella agar, additives for anaerobes.

Brilliant green agar* (62, 63, 68)

Proteose No. 3 *or* Polypeptone	10.0 g
pancreatic digest of casein USP	(5.00 g)
peptic digest of animal tissue USP	(5.00 g)
Yeast extract	3.00 g
Sodium chloride	5.00 g
Lactose	10.00 g
Sucrose	10.00 g
Agar	20.00 g
Phenol red (4 ml per liter of 2% phenol red prepared by dissolving 1 g in 40 ml 0.1 N NaOH and made up to 500 ml with distilled water)	0.08 g
Brilliant green (2 ml per liter of 0.5% brilliant green)	12.50 mg
Distilled water	1.00 liter
Final pH 6.9 ± 0.2.	

Autoclave at 121 C for 15 min. Cool and pour 25 to 30 ml per plate. Store in dark.

Brilliant green sulfa agar*

As above, with incorporated sodium sulfapyridine, 1 g/liter, or sodium sulfadiazine, 8 to 16 mg per 100 ml (36).

Bromocresol purple milk*
B C P milk

Purple milk	100 g
Demineralized water	1 liter

Mix to obtain a homogeneous uspension and dispense 2- to 2.5-ml amounts in 11 by 75 mm tubes. Autoclave at 115 to 118 C for 15 min.

This medium is recommended for determining proteolytic properties of the aerobic actinomycetes. Observe for peptonization. *Nocardia asteroides* does not peptonize but usually turns this medium alkaline. Incubate an uninoculated control with every set of tests.

Bromothymol blue "teepol" agar* (71)

For Vibrio, chapter 21

Yeast extract	3 g
Peptone or Gelysate	10 g
Sucrose	20 g
Sodium chloride	40 g
Bromothymol blue	0.04 g
Thymol blue	0.04 g
Agar	15 g
Gardinol-type detergent "teepol" (Shell Oil Co., 110 W. 51st St., New York, N.Y. 10020)	2 ml
Distilled water	1 liter
Final pH 7.8 ±	

1. Heat with agitation to obtain solution.
2. Dispense and autoclave at 121 C for 15 min.

Brucella agar*

Pancreatic digest of casein USP	10.0 g
Peptic digest of animal tissues USP	10.0 g
Dextrose	1.0 g
Yeast autolysate	2.0 g
Sodium chloride	5.0 g
Sodium bisulfite	0.1 g
Agar	15.0 g
Distilled water	1.0 liter
Final pH 7.0 ± 0.2	

Heat with agitation until dissolved. Dispense and autoclave at 121 C for 15 min. Cool to 50 C.

Additives for anaerobes (119)

For nonselective media

1. 50 ml of sterile defibrinated sheep, rabbit, or horse blood and 1 ml of vitamin K_1 solution per liter. *See* BHIS media and Note below.
2. 50 ml of laked blood and 1 ml of vitamin K_1 per liter.

Note. Prepare and use vitamin K_1 (119) solution as follows:

a. Weigh 0.2 g on previously flamed aluminum foil square.
b. Aseptically place 20 ml of absolute alcohol in a sterile tube.
c. Add foil with sterile forceps.
d. When solution has occurred, remove foil. Concentration is 0.01 g/ml.
e. Use 1 ml/liter in agar media (concentration, 10 μg/ml).
f. For fluid media, dilute stock solution 1:100 in sterile water. Use 0.01 ml/liter (concentration, 0.1 μg/ml).

For selective media

1. For *Bacteroides* (119; *see* chapter 38). Kanamycin, 100 μg/ml, to either Brucella agar or BHIS agar before autoclaving. Cool and add blood and vitamin K_1 solution. Also add filter (0.45 μm)-sterilized aqueous vancomycin to a concentration of 7.5 μg/ml.
2. For *B. melaninogenicus*. Add as for 1 but first lyse the blood by freezing and thawing.
3. For certain *Fusobacterium*, *Eubacterium* and *Clostridium* species. Rifampin, 50 μg/ml, and blood just prior to pouring plates.
4. *For Fusobacterium* and *Veillonella*. Neomycin, 100 μg/ml, before autoclaving; add blood, vitamin K_1, and 7.5 μg vancomycin/ml just prior to pouring plates.
5. For *Clostridium* and anaerobic cocci. Neomycin, 100 μg/ml, before autoclaving. Add blood and vitamin K_1 just prior to pouring plates.

Brucella broth*

As above, but without agar.

For Campylobacter (4, 130)

Use Brucella broth with 0.16% agar added prior to dissolving, dispensing, and sterilization. Tube about 7.6 cm deep in 16 by 150 mm screw-capped tubes.

To this base the following materials may be added prior to sterilization to prepare:

A. Glycine medium. Add 1% glycine.
B. Catalase medium. Add 1% dextrose.
C. Hydrogen sulfide medium. Add 0.02% cysteine hydrochloride. Use lead acetate test paper above medium for 6 days.
D. Dextrose medium. Add 8%.
E. Sodium chloride. Add 3.5%.

Buffered gelatin

Gelatin	2 g
Disodium phosphate, anhydrous	4 g
Distilled water	1 liter

Adjust pH to 7.0 and autoclave at 121 C for 20 min.

Buffered glycerol saline solution* (100, 122)
Buffered glycine saline base for transportation

Sodium chloride	4.200 g
Dipotassium phosphate, anhydrous	3.100 g
Monopotassium phosphate, anhydrous	1.000 g
Phenol red	0.003 g
Distilled water	700.000 ml
Glycerol	300.000 ml
Final pH 7.2	

Dispense and autoclave at 121 C for 10 or 15 min.

Calymmatobacterium granulomatis defined medium (42)

Lactalbumin hydrolysate *or* papaic digest of soy meal USP	20.0 g
Sodium chloride	2.5 g
Dipotassium phosphate	1.5 g
Sodium thioglycolate	0.6 g
L-Cystine	0.4 g
Distilled water	1.0 liter

1. Dissolve with heat, cool, and adjust to pH 7.2.
2. Dispense in 20- to 22-ml amounts in screw-capped tubes.
3. Autoclave at 121 C for 15 min and tighten caps to maintain reduced conditions.

Campylobacter media

See Brucella broth.

Carbohydrate media

See Andrade broth, C T A medium, Elrod-Braun solution, Fermentation basal medium, Fermentation broths for anaerobes, Phenol red broths.

Carlquist ninhydrin broth* (10)

Pancreatic digest of casein USP	15 g
Potassium phosphate	2 g
Dextrose	1 g
Distilled water	1 liter

1. Dissolve and dispense in 5-ml amounts in screw-capped tubes.
2. Autoclave at 121 C for 15 min.
3. Close tubes during storage and after addition of alkali and chloroform to cultures.

This procedure has its greatest value in the study of pseudomonads as a confirmatory rather than essential test for the recognition of *P. maltophilia*.

Cary and Blair transport (holding) medium* (11)

Sodium thioglycolate .... 1.5 g
Disodium phosphate .... 1.1 g
Sodium chloride .... 5.0 g
Agar .... 5.0 g
Distilled or demineralized water ...... 991.0 ml

1. Prepare in chemically clean glassware rinsed with Sorensen's 0.067 M buffer (pH 8.1).
2. Heat with agitation until the solution just becomes clear.
3. Cool to 50 C, add 9 ml of freshly prepared aqueous 1% $CaCl_2$, and adjust the pH to about 8.4.
4. Dispense 7 ml into previously rinsed and sterilized 9-ml screw-capped vials.
5. Steam vials for 15 min, cool, and tighten caps.

Cary and Blair transport medium, modified (PRAS)

Sodium thioglycolate .... 1.5 g
Calcium chloride .... 0.1 g
Disodium phosphate .... 0.1 g
Sodium chloride .... 5.0 g
Sodium bisulfite .... 0.1 g
Agar .... 5.0 g
Resazurin solution .... 4.0 ml
Distilled water .... 1 liter

1. Mix and boil ingredients to dissolve.
2. Gas out with carbon dioxide.
3. Add 0.5 g of L-cysteine hydrochloride.
4. Adjust so that final pH is 8.4.
5. Tube in roll tubes gassed out with nitrogen.
6. Stopper with butyl stoppers.
7. Steam for 15 min on three successive days.

Note. Prepare resazurin solution (119) by dissolving 0.05 g of resazurin in 20 ml of 95% ethanol and adding 180 ml of distilled water or dissolve one 11-mg tablet* (12) in 44 ml of water.

Casein agar
Trichophyton agars 1–5*

A. *With casein peptone for fungi*

Casein, 10% acid-hydrolyzed, vitamin-free *or* .... 25.0 ml
Acid hydrolysate of casein .... 2.5 g
Dextrose .... 40.0 g
Magnesium sulfate .... 0.1 g
Monopotassium phosphate .... 1.8 g
Agar .... 20.0 g
Distilled water, to .... 1.0 liter

1. Adjust pH to 6.8.
2. Dissolve by heating, distribute 100-ml quantities in flasks, and autoclave at 121 C for 15 min.
3. Contents of several flasks may be distributed into test tubes and slanted for use as vitamin-free controls.
4. To 100 ml of sterile, melted casein agar, add autoclaved vitamin solutions as follows: thiamine, 2 ml of a stock solution containing 10 mg/liter of water; inositol, 2 ml of a stock solution containing 250 mg/100 ml of water; thiamine-inositol, 2 ml of each of above stock solutions; nicotinic acid, 2 ml of a stock solution containing 10 mg/100 ml of water.
5. Tube and slant.

B. *With skim milk for aerobic actinomycetes, chapter 17.*

Skim milk .... 75 g
Agar .... 20 g
Demineralized water .... 1 liter

1. Add the milk to 500 ml of water, a little at a time, stirring constantly; do not leave lumps.
2. Autoclave at 113 to 115 C for 20 min.
3. Dissolve the agar in 500 ml of water and autoclave.
4. Cool the solutions to 60 to 65 C and pour the agar solution into the skim milk suspension.
5. Mix gently and pour 20 ml per plate while hot.

Recommended for differentiation of species of aerobic actinomycetes. Streak a pure culture heavily on duplicate plates and incubate at room temperature or 37 C for up to 2 weeks. Observe for growth and clearing of medium.

Casein soy peptone agar

See Soybean-casein digest agar* USP.

Cetrimide agarR USP (9, 65)
Pseudosel agar*

Gelysate pancreatic digest of gelatin .. 20.0 g
Magnesium chloride .... 1.4 g
Potassium sulfate .... 10.0 g
Agar (dried) .... 13.6 g
Cetrimide* .... 0.3 g
Distilled water .... 1 liter
Final pH 7.2±

Suspend ingredients in the water and add 10 ml of glycerol. Heat with frequent agitation and boil for 1 min. Dispense and autoclave at 118 to 121 C for 15 min.

Cetrimide agar, non-USP (65)

A. *For miscellaneous gram-negative bacteria, chapter 24*

Heart infusion agar .... 40.0 g
Cetrimide (hexadecyltrimethyl-ammonium bromide) .... 0.9 g
Distilled water .... 1 liter
Final pH 7.2

Heat to dissolve. Dispense in 5-ml amounts in 15 by 125 mm test tubes, shaking flask to insure even distribution of sediment.

Note. Lots of cetrimide vary and amount needed must be determined with known cultures.

B. *For enterics, chapters 18 and 21* (E. O. King, personal communication)

Prepare as above, but with 0.5% cetrimide. Incubate inoculated slants at 37 C for 7 days. Growth of the organism is considered a positive test.

Chocolate agars

Use one of the following as preferred, or as required to obtain satisfactory growth:

Beef infusion agar*
Blood agar base*

Casein peptone agar*
Eugonic agar*
Mueller-Hinton agar*

In addition, G C Agar Base* or G C Medium Base* may be employed.

Pancreatic digest of casein USP	7.5 g
Peptic digest of animal tissue USP	7.5 g
or other peptone	(15.0 g)
Corn starch	1.0 g
Dipotassium phosphate	4.0 g
Monopotassium phosphate	1.0 g
Sodium chloride	5.0 g
Agar	10.0 g
Distilled water	1.0 liter

Prepare sterile base. Add sterile 5 to 10% defibrinated blood and heat at about 80 C for 15 min or until the color is chocolate-brown.

Variations

1. Add chemical supplement. *See* Thayer-Martin agar.
2. Add yeast supplements.
3. Prepare double-strength medium and add an equal volume of sterile 2% hemoglobin. Also add chemical supplement, especially for *Neisseria* and *Haemophilus*.

See also Fildes enrichment agar and Levinthal agar.

Chopped meat

See Cooked meat medium.

Citrate agar, Christensen* (15)
Christensen citrate sulfide agar

Sodium citrate	3.000 g
Dextrose	0.200 g
Yeast extract	0.500 g
Cysteine hydrochloride	0.100 g
Ferric ammonium citrate	0.400 g
Monopotassium phosphate	1.000 g
Sodium chloride	5.000 g
Sodium thiosulfate	0.080 g
Phenol red	0.012 g
Agar	15.000 g
Distilled water	1.000 liter

Final pH 6.7

1. Dissolve, tube, and sterilize at 121 C for 15 min.
2. Cool in the slanted position for 2.5-cm butt and 3.8-cm slant.
3. The ferric ammonium citrate and sodium thiosulfate may be omitted, if desired.

Inoculate over the entire surface of the slant. Incubate at 37 C for 7 days. Positive reactions are indicated by development of a red color, particularly on the slant.

Citrate agar* (106)
Simmons citrate agar

Sodium citrate	2.00 g
Sodium chloride	5.00 g
Magnesium sulfate	0.20 g
Monoammonium phosphate	1.00 g
Dipotassium phosphate	1.00 g
Agar (dried)	(15.00 g)
or not dried	20.00 g
Bromothymol blue	0.08 g
Distilled water	1.00 liter

Final pH 6.9

Dispense in tubes, autoclave at 121 C for 15 min, and cool in the slanted position for 2.5-cm butt and 3.8-cm slant.

Inoculate the slant with a straight wire from a saline suspension of a young agar culture. Incubate at 37 C for 4 days. If equivocal results are obtained as sometimes happens with members of the *Providencia* genus, for example, the test should be repeated and incubated at room temperature for 7 days.

Clostridial agar, reinforced

See Reinforced clostridial agar.

Cooked meat medium*
Chopped meat medium

A. *For C. botulinum, chapter 92*

Ground beef, lean (connective tissue trimmed off before putting meat through grinder)	500 g
Distilled water	1 liter
Sodium hydroxide, 1 N	25 ml

1. Mix, heat to boiling, and simmer for 20 min with frequent stirring.
2. Cool and check pH, which should be about 7.4.
3. Filter through several layers of gauze; squeeze out excess liquid.
4. Spread particles to dry. When dried, place in test tubes to depth of 2.5 cm.
5. Prepare broth as follows:

Beef extract	10 g
Peptone, pancreatic digest of gelatin	10 g
Sodium chloride	5 g
Yeast extract	5 g
Soluble starch	2 g
Dextrose	3 g
Distilled water	1 liter

Dissolve and adjust pH to 7.5.

6. Add broth to tubes of meat and fill tubes half full.
7. Autoclave at 121 C for 20 min.

When dried meat particles are not available, add 10 ml of an aqueous solution containing 0.2% soluble starch and 0.5% glucose to tubes (16 by 150 mm) containing 1.25 g of commercially available dehydrated cooked meat medium. Mix thoroughly and allow particles to become thoroughly wetted. Autoclave at 121 C for 15 min.

B. *For Anaerobes, chapter 38*

1. Prepare meat particles as for *C. botulinum*, but do not dry.
2. Separate meat particles by filtering through several layers of cheesecloth. Dispense meat in tubes 1.3 cm deep.

3. Filter fluid through three coarse filter papers and one fine filter paper.

4. Adjust volume of fluid to 1 liter and to each 500 ml of fluid add the following:

Pancreatic digest of casein USP	15.00 g
Yeast extract USP	2.50 g
Dipotassium phosphate	2.50 g
Cysteine	0.25 g
Resazurin, 25 mg/100 ml of water	2.00 ml

5. Adjust pH to 7.8. Dispense in meat tubes, about 6 ml per tube.

6. Autoclave at 121 C for 20 min.

7. If desired, add 0.5% dextrose for enrichment.

Note. Chopped meat glucose (CMG) broth*: complete formula not provided.

Cornmeal Polysorbate 80 agar*

Cornmeal	40 g
Polysorbate (Tween) 80	3 ml
Water	1 liter
Agar (not dried)	20 g

1. Simmer the cornmeal and water for 1 h.

2. Filter through gauze. Restore filtrate to 1 liter.

3. Add agar. Mix and heat to melt the agar. Filter again if necessary.

4. Add polysorbate 80. Add glycerol, 20 to 30 ml, if desired.

5. Autoclave at 121 C for 15 min.

6. Cool to 45 to 50 C and dispense into sterile petri dishes.

Corn oil medium

See Lipase medium with corn oil.

CTA medium* (127)
Cystine tryptophan agar medium

Cystine	0.500 g
Pancreatic digest of casein USP	20.000 g
Agar	2.500 g
Sodium chloride	5.000 g
Sodium sulfite	0.500 g
Phenol red	0.017 g
Distilled water	1.000 liter

Final pH 7.3.

Mix and heat with agitation until solution occurs. Dispense and autoclave at 115 to 118 C for 15 min.

Cycloheximide chloramphenicol agar* (39)
Myocosel agar, Mycobiotic agar, etc.

Sabouraud dextrose agar	1.00 liter
Agar	5.00 g
Cycloheximide, in 10 ml of acetone	0.50 g
Chloramphenicol, in 10 ml of 95% alcohol	0.05 g

Heat to dissolve the agar and the Sabouraud dextrose agar. Dispense in tubes and autoclave at 121 C for 10 min. Cool in a slanted position.

Recommended for the routine isolation of most pathogenic fungi. For species sensitive to cycloheximide, the medium can be prepared without it.

Cysteine gelatin medium, modified (48)

Bacto peptone or Gelysate	5 g
Beef extract	3 g
Gelatin	125 g
Bromothymol blue, 0.2%	40 ml
Distilled water	1 liter

1. Dissolve 1.5 g of cysteine HCl in 25 ml of hot distilled water and add slowly to basic broth.

2. Adjust pH to 7.0 by addition of NaOH. Tube in 4-ml amounts in 13 by 100 mm screw-capped tubes.

3. Autoclave at 121 C for 20 min.

Inoculate with a loopful of growth from a 24-h agar slant, incubate at 37 C for 7 days, and read daily. Acid production and a marked precipitate that appears first in the upper part of the medium are evidence of a positive test.

Cystine heart agar* plus blood and antibiotics

Beef heart, infusion from	500 g
Proteose or Polypeptone	10 g
Dextrose	10 g
Sodium chloride	5 g
L-Cystine	1 g
Agar	15 g
Water	1 liter

Final pH 6.8

1. Mix and heat to obtain complete solution.

2. Autoclave at 121 C for 15 min. Cool to 45 to 48 C.

3. Aseptically add 25 ml of packed human blood cells or add 50 ml of defibrinated rabbit blood.

4. Aseptically add antibiotics—1 ml each of solutions containing: penicillin, 100,000 units/ml; polymyxin B sulfate, 100,000 units/ml; and cycloheximide, 0.1 mg/ml.

Cystine tellurite blood agar

Heart infusion agar	500 ml
Agar	2.5 g

1. Adjust pH to 7.4 and autoclave at 121 C for 15 min.

2. Cool to 56 C and add 25 ml of defibrinated rabbit or sheep blood, 75 ml of sterile 0.3% potassium tellurite, and 22 mg of L-cystine.

3. Stir while pouring plates to keep cystine suspended.

4. Store plates at 5 C and use within 1 month.

Czapek agar*
Czapek Dox solution agar

Sucrose	30.00 g
Sodium nitrate	2.00 g
Dipotassium phosphate	1.00 g
Magnesium sulfate	0.50 g
Potassium chloride	0.50 g
Ferrous sulfate	0.01 g
Agar	15.00 g

Demineralized water	1.00 liter
Final pH 7.3	

1. Mix and heat to boiling to dissolve completely. Dispense and autoclave at 121 C for 15 min.

2. Recommended for colonial appearance, pigment, and sporulation of *Nocardia* and *Streptomyces.*

Decarboxylase broths, Falkow (33)

Bacto peptone *or* Gelysate pancreatic digest of gelatin	5 g
Yeast extract	3 g
Dextrose	1 g
Bromocresol purple, 1.6%	1 ml
Distilled water	1 liter

1. Adjust to pH 6.7 to 6.8, if necessary.
2. Divide into four parts; tube one as a control, and add 0.5% L-arginine monohydrochloride, L-lysine dihydrochloride, and L-ornithine dihydrochloride to the remaining portions. Alternatively, add 1% DL-amino acids.
3. Readjust pH of ornithine portion.
4. Tube in 3- to 4-ml amounts in 13 by 100 mm screw-capped tubes and autoclave at 121 C for 10 min.
5. A small amount of floccular precipitate in the ornithine does not interfere with its use.

Inoculate test and control portions lightly from a young agar slant culture. Cover with a 4- to 5-mm layer of sterile mineral (paraffin) oil. Incubate at 37 C and examine daily for 4 days. Positive reactions are indicated by alkaline (purple) reaction. The media turn yellow first due to acid production from dextrose. Comparative studies have shown that this medium can be used successfully in most areas of the *Enterobacteriaceae*, but it is not recommended for *Klebsiella* and *Enterobacter*. Most positive reactions occur in 1 or 2 days.

Decarboxylase broths, Moeller* (87)

Peptic digest of animal tissue USP	5.000 g
Beef extract	5.000 g
Bromocresol purple	0.010 g
Cresol red	0.005 g
Dextrose	0.500 g
Pyridoxal	0.005 g
Distilled water	1.000 liter
Final pH 6.0.	

Prepare as for Falkow medium except that 1% L-amino acids or 2% DL-amino acids are used.

See Falkow's medium for use and interpretation, except that Moeller's medium may be used for all families of the *Enterobacteriaceae*.

Deoxycholate agar* (73)

Bacto peptone *or* Polypeptone Pancreatic digest of casein USP	5.000 g
Peptic digest of animal tissue USP	5.000 g
Lactose	10.000 g
Sodium chloride	5.000 g
Dipotassium phosphate	2.000 g
Ferric citrate	1.000 g
(*or* Ferric ammonium citrate)	(2.000 g)
Sodium citrate	1.000 g
Sodium deoxycholate	1.000 g
Neutral red	0.033 g
Agar	16.000 g
Distilled water	1.000 liter
Final pH 7.3.	

Heat with agitation and boil for 1 min. Cool and pour into plates. Alternatively, the medium may be heated in flowing steam for 20 to 30 min.

Deoxycholate citrate agar, modified* (73)

Meat, infusion from	330 *or* 375.00 g
Peptic digest of animal tissue USP	10.00 g
Lactose	10.00 g
Sodium citrate	20.00 g
Ferric citrate	1.00 g
(*or* Ferric ammonium citrate)	(2.00 g)
Sodium deoxycholate	5.00 g
Neutral red	0.02 g
Agar (dried)	(17.00 g)
or not dried	20 g
Distilled water	1.00 liter
Final pH 7.3	

Heat with agitation until the medium boils for 1 min. Do not autoclave. Cool and pour into plates.

Deoxycholate citrate lactose sucrose agar*
DCLS agar

Sodium deoxycholate	2.50 g
Sodium citrate	10.50 g
Lactose	5.00 g
Sucrose	5.00 g
Polypeptone	
Pancreatic digest of casein USP	3.50 g
Peptic digest of animal tissues USP	3.50 g
Meat extract *or* beef extract	3.00 g
Sodium thiosulfate	5.00 g
Neutral red	0.03 g
Agar	12.00 g
Distilled water	1.00 liter
Final pH 7.2	

Heat to boiling to dissolve completely. Do not autoclave. Cool and pour into plates.

Diphasic blood agar for trypanosomes and leishmania (NIH method)

See Blood agar, diphasic.

Deoxyribonuclease test agar* (84)
DNase test agar*

Deoxyribonucleic acid	2 g
Pancreatic digest of casein USP	15 g
Papaic digest of soy meal USP	5 g
Sodium chloride	5 g
Agar	15 g
Distilled water	1 liter
Final pH 7.3	

Inoculate culture heavily over a 1 cm^2 area of the plate. Several cultures may be tested on the same plate. Incubate for 18 to 24 h and flood with 1 N HCl. A zone of clearing around the colony indicates a positive deoxyribonuclease test.

Dubos broth*

Pancreatic digest of casein USP	0.50 g
Asparagine	2.00 g
Monopotassium phosphate	1.00 g
Disodium phosphate	2.50 g
Ferric ammonium citrate	0.50 g
Magnesium sulfate	0.01 g
Polysorbate 80	0.20 g
Calcium chloride	0.50 mg
Zinc sulfate	0.10 mg
Copper sulfate	0.10 mg
Glycerol (optional)	50.00 ml
Water	1.00 liter

1. Dissolve the other ingredients in 180 ml of water or in 170 ml of water plus 10 ml of glycerol.
2. Autoclave at 121 C for 15 min.
3. Enrich as desired, e.g., by aseptic addition of 20 ml of sterile serum or of 5% fraction V albumin in saline.

Dubos oleic acid agar*

Pancreatic digest of casein	0.50 g
Asparagine	1.00 g
Monopotassium phosphate	1.00 g
Disodium phosphate	2.50 g
Ferric ammonium citrate	0.05 g
Magnesium sulfate	0.01 g
Agar	15.00 g
Calcium chloride	0.50 mg
Zinc sulfate	0.10 mg
Copper sulfate	0.10 mg
Water	1.00 liter

1. Heat with agitation and boil for 1 min.
2. If desired, add 0.5 or 1.0% polysorbate 80 or glycerol.
3. Autoclave at 121 C for 15 min.
4. Cool to 50 C and add enrichments, such as Oleic acid albumin complex* made as follows:
   a. Dissolve 0.12 ml of oleic acid in 10 ml of 0.05 N NaOH.
   b. Dissolve 4 g of bovine albumin fraction V in 100 ml of 0.85% saline.
   c. Add 5 ml of solution a to 95 ml of solution b. Warm at 55 C for 30 min.
   d. Sterilize by filtration.
   e. Add 20 ml to 180 ml of agar base.

Dulaney slants (23)

Aseptically remove yolks from 5- to 8-day hen egg embryos and place in an equal volume of sterile Locke solution containing glass beads. Homogenize. Dispense the homogenate in slanted tubes and coagulate with steam at 80 C for 15 min.

Prepare Locke Solution as follows:

Sodium chloride	0.900 g
Calcium chloride	0.024 g
Potassium chloride	0.042 g
Sodium carbonate	0.020 g
Dextrose	0.250 g
Distilled water	100.000 ml

Egg yolk agars

A. *Blood agar base*

B. *Brain heart infusion agar*

C. *Soy bean-casein digest agar USP or other*

Alternatively use commercial suspension as directed.

D. *McClung and Toabe agar*

For *B. anthracis*, chapter 15

Pancreatic digest of casein USP	40.0 g
Disodium phosphate	5.0 g
Monopotassium phosphate	1.0 g
Sodium chloride	2.0 g
Magnesium sulfate	0.1 g
Dextrose	2.0 g
Agar	25.0 g
Distilled water	1.0 liter

1. Dissolve and adjust the pH to 7.6.
2. Autoclave at 121 C for 15 min.
3. Cool to 50 to 55 C.
4. Meanwhile, scrub, then soak, an antibiotic-free hen's egg in 95% ethanol for 1 h. Aseptically aspirate or separate egg yolk.
5. Add one egg yolk to 500 ml of agar base and stir to smooth suspension with a sterile pipette. Alternatively, add commercial egg yolk emulsion* as directed.

E. *McClung and Toabe agar, modified* (79)

For lecithinase and lipase tests

Proteose #2 peptone* or Polypeptone*	40.0 g
Disodium phosphate	5.0 g
Monopotassium phosphate	1.0 g
Sodium chloride	2.0 g
Magnesium sulfate	0.1 g
Dextrose	2.0 g
Hemin solution, 5 mg/ml	1.0 ml
Agar	20.0 g
Water	1.0 liter

1. Suspend ingredients and adjust pH to 7.6.
2. Mix and boil to dissolve.
3. Dispense and autoclave at 118 C for 15 min.
4. Cool to 50 C and add 10 ml of egg yolk emulsion* to each 90 ml of medium. Use an emulsion of equal volumes of egg yolk in sterile saline. *See* D above.

For Clostridium (119)

1. Add neomycin, 100 μg/ml, medium base prior to autoclaving.
2. Cool and add egg yolk emulsion.

For C. botulinum

Yeast extract	5.0 g
Pancreatic digest of casein	5.0 g
Proteose #2 peptone* or Polypeptone*	20.0 g
Sodium chloride	5.0 g
Sodium thioglycolate	1.0 g
Agar	20.0 g
Distilled water	1.0 liter

1. Sterilize and cool the medium base to 45 to 50 C.
2. Add 80 ml of sterile egg yolk suspension.
3. Mix and pour plates immediately.
4. Dry plates and store in a refrigerator.

Egg yolk pyruvate tellurite glycine agar

See Baird Parker agar.

Ellinghausen and McCullough albumin fatty acid broth, modified

See Albumin fatty acid broth

Elrod-Braun solution (modified)

Magnesium sulfate	0.2 g
Calcium chloride	0.1 g
Sodium chloride	0.2 g
Dipotassium phosphate	0.2 g
Bromothymol blue, 0.2% aqueous	20.0 ml
Distilled water	880.0 ml

1. Sterilize by filtration.
2. Sterilize 10% carbohydrate solutions by filtration.
3. Aseptically mix 1 ml of carbohydrate with 9 ml of salts solution.
4. Tube aseptically in 0.5-ml volumes.

Emerson agar

Beef extract	4.0 g
Gelysate pancreatic digest of gelatin	4.0 g
Sodium chloride	2.5 g
Yeast extract	1.0 g
Dextrose	10.0 g
Agar	20.0 g
Final pH 7.0 ±	

1. Heat with frequent agitation and boil for 1 min to insure solution.
2. Add cycloheximide,* 0.05 g per liter, if desired.
3. Dispense and sterilize at 118 to 121 C for 15 min.

Emerson broth

As above, but with meat peptone substituted for meat extract and agar omitted.

Enriched heart infusion agar for Streptobacillus

1. Prepare 1 liter of beef heart infusion agar, but adjust to pH 7.6 with 5 N NaOH prior to sterilization. Dispense in 85-ml volumes in screw-capped tubes.
2. To sterile fluid medium at 50 C, add 10 ml of sterile horse serum (previously heated for 30 min at 56 to 60 C) and 5 ml of 10% sterile yeast extract solution (previously adjusted to pH 7.0 and filtered through 0.01-μm Seitz or 0.45-μm membrane filter). Mix and pour into plates, e.g., 15 by 60 mm size.

Enriched heart infusion basal medium for Streptobacillus

As above, but using only 750 ml of water.

Enriched heart infusion broth for Streptobacillus

As for the enriched agar, but omit the agar.

Eosin methylene blue agar, modified* (50)

Bacto peptone, or Gelysate pancreatic digest of gelatin	10.000 g
Lactose	5.000 g
Sucrose	5.000 g
Dipotassium phosphate	2.000 g
Agar (dried)	13.500 g
Eosin Y	0.400 g
Methylene blue	0.065 g
Distilled water	1.000 liter
Final pH 7.2.	

Heat with agitation until the medium boils. Autoclave at 121 C for 15 min. Mix frequently while pouring plates.

Erysipelothrix selective broth

Disodium phosphate	12.02 g
Monopotassium phosphate	2.09 g
Beef extract	3.00 g
Peptone: Tryptose or Biosate Pancreatic digest of casein USP and Yeast extract USP	15.00 g
Sodium chloride	5.00 g
Distilled water	1.00 liter

1. Filter through cotton or filter paper and autoclave.
2. Cool and add aseptically: serum, horse, bovine or other, 50 ml; kanamycin, 400 mg; neomycin, 50 mg; vancomycin, 25 mg.
3. Dispense aseptically. Store at 4 to 5 C but not longer than 2 weeks.

Esculin agar, modified (110)

Esculin	1.0 g
Ferric citrate	0.5 g
Heart infusion agar* (blood agar base)	40.0 g
Distilled water	1.0 liter

Heat to dissolve. Cool to 55 C; adjust *p*H to 7.0. Dispense in 5-ml amounts in 16 by 125 mm cotton-plugged tubes. Autoclave at 121 C for 15 min. Cool in a slanted position.

Esculin broth (125)

A. *For enteric organisms*

Peptone or Gelysate	5.0 g
Dipotassium phosphate	1.0 g
Andrade indicator (*see* Andrade carbohydrate broths)	10.0 ml

Esculin	0.3 g
Ferric citrate	0.5 g
Distilled water	1.0 liter

Heat to dissolve. Tube and sterilize at 121 C for 10 min.

Inoculate and incubate as with any carbohydrate media. Observe for black precipitate.

B. *For anaerobes* (21)

Heart infusion broth	1 liter
Esculin	1 g
Agar	1 g

1. Dissolve ingredients by boiling. Cool and adjust pH to 7.0.
2. Dispense and autoclave at 121 C for 15 min.

Eugonagar,* modified for Bifidobacterium (119)

Trypticase peptone	15.0 g
Phytone peptone	5.0 g
Sodium chloride	4.0 g
Sodium sulfite	0.2 g
L-Cystine	0.7 g
Dextrose	5.5 g
Maltose	10.0 g
Yeast extract	5.0 g
Hemin solution, 5 mg/ml	1.0 ml
Agar	15.0 g
Water	1.0 liter

1. Mix thouroughly and boil to dissolve.
2. Dispense and sterilize at 118 C for 15 min. Eugonagar* to which maltose, yeast extract, and hemin are added may be used.

Feinberg medium (34)

Proteolyzed liver, Panmede (Harrisons and Crossfield Inc., P.O. Box 39, Bronxville, N.Y. 10708)	12.5 g
Sodium chloride	3.3 g
Dextrose	2.5 g
Horse serum (inactivated at 57 C for 25 min)	40.0 ml
Distilled water	500.0 ml
Penicillin	500,000 units
Streptomycin	250,000 units

Combine and adjust pH to 6.5 with sodium hydroxide. Filter through a Seitz filter. Dispense aseptically into 100 by 13 mm screw-capped tubes, filling them half full. Store at 4 C.

Fermentation basal medium (109)

Diammonium phosphate	1.0 g
Potassium chloride	0.2 g
Magnesium sulfate	0.2 g
Yeast extract	0.2 g
Agar	15.0 g
Distilled water	1.0 liter
Bromocresol purple, 0.04%	20.0 ml

Tube and sterilize. Filter-sterilize the appropriate sugar and add 10 to 15% after the basal medium has cooled.

Fermentation broths, for anaerobes

Thioglycolate medium without dextrose or indicator*

Pancreatic digest of casein	20.00 g
Sodium chloride	2.50 g
Sodium thioglycolate	0.50 g
L-Cystine	0.50 g
Agar	0.75 g
Final pH 7.2	

1. Heat with agitation until solution occurs. Add stable carbohydrates, and hemin, if desired. Do not add yeast extract because of high carbohydrate content.
2. Dispense in screw-capped tubes and autoclave at 118 to 121 C for 15 min. Close caps while hot.
3. Boil, cool, and add sterile heat-labile carbohydrates or carbohydrate disks when ready to use.
4. To prepare urea medium, add 1 ml of urea broth concentrate to 9 ml of the fermentation base.

Fildes enrichment agar (35)

Fildes enrichment*

Sodium chloride, 0.85%	150 ml
Hydrochloric acid	6 ml
Defibrinated sheep blood	50 ml
Pepsin, granular	1 g

1. Mix in a glass-stoppered bottle. Shake thoroughly.
2. Place in a water bath at 55 C for 4 h. Shake occasionally.
3. Add about 6 ml of 5 N sodium hydroxide to obtain a pH of 7.0 or slightly less.
4. Add 0.25 ml chloroform and shake thoroughly. Store at 4 C.
5. Before use, gently heat in water bath to remove chloroform.
6. Add 4 to 10 ml of enrichment to 200 ml of sterile nutrient agar melted and cooled to 56 C. Pour into plates.

Flagella broth (76)

Tryptose or Biosate	10..0 g
Dipotassium phosphate	1.0 g
Sodium chloride	2.5 g
Distilled water	1.0 liter

1. Dissolve ingredients and adjust the pH to 7.0.
2. Dispense in 5-ml volumes in 15 by 125 mm test tubes.
3. Autoclave at 121 C for 15 min.

Fletcher semisolid medium*

Pancreatic digest of casein USP *or* pancreatic digest of gelatin	0.3 g
Beef extract	0.2 g
Sodium chloride	0.5 g
Agar	1.5 g
Water	920.0 ml
Final pH 7.4 to 8.0	

1. Suspend ingredients in cold water and heat to boiling to dissolve. Autoclave at 121 C for 15 min.

2. Cool to 56 C and add filter-sterilized rabbit serum.
3. Dispense in screw-capped tubes in 5- to 7-ml amounts.
4. Inactivate the medium by placing the tubes in a water bath at 56 C for 1 h on two successive days.

Fluid thioglycolate medium USP*

Pancreatic digest of casein USP	15.000 g
L-Cystine	0.500 g
Dextrose anhydrous	5.000 g
Yeast extract USP	5.000 g
Sodium chloride	2.500 g
Sodium thioglycolate	0.500 g
Agar	0.750 g
Resazurin	0.001 g
Purified water	1.000 liter
Final pH 7.1	

Heat to dissolve. Dispense in test tubes, filling them at least half full. Sterilize at 118 to 121 C for 15 min. Just before use, heat to boiling, or expose in flowing steam for 10 min to remove dissolved oxygen. Cool rapidly in tap water.

Note. The reazurin may be omitted, but its presence is legally required in sterility testing. *See* the USP.

Fluorouracil leptospira medium

1. Dissolve 1.0 g of 5-fluorouracil in approximately 50 ml of distilled water; add 1.0 to 2.0 ml of 2 N NaOH and heat gently (less than 56 C) for 1 to 2 h or until soluble. Adjust the pH to 7.4 to 7.6 with 1 N HCl and bring volume to 100 ml with distilled water.
2. Sterilize by filtration and store in a refrigerator.
3. Add aseptically just before use 0.1 ml of 5-fluorouracil solution (Roche Laboratories, Nutley, N.J.) for each 5 ml of Albumin fatty acid broth or Fletcher medium or Stuart leptospiral broth.

FM medium, modified* (93)

Peptone	20.0 g
Papaic digest of soy meal USP	1.5 g
Peptonized whale serum	6.75 g
Liver extract powder	0.6 g
Meat extract of whale powder	5.0 g
Beef extract powder	1.15 g
Yeast extract powder	0.10 g
Hemin	0.003 g
Dextrose	3.0 g
Monosodium phosphate	2.5 g
Sodium chloride	3.0 g
Soluble starch	5.0 g
L-Cysteine hydrochloride	0.3 g
Sodium thioglycolate	0.3 g
Neomycin	0.2 g
Crystal violet	0.01 g
Agar	14.70 g
Water	1.0 liter

Heat with agitation and boil for 1 min. Pour into petri dishes and use on the day of preparation.

Gastric mucin virulence medium

Gastric mucin, granular	5 g
Distilled water	95 ml

Suspend and mix in blender for 5 min. Autoclave. Cool and adjust to pH 7.3 with sterile NaOH. Test for sterility and store under refrigeration for not more than a few months.

G C medium base

See Chocolate agars

Gelatin phosphate buffer

1. Dissolve 2 g of gelatin in 500 ml of distilled water with heat.
2. Mix 200 ml of 0.2 M disodium phosphate with 300 ml of 0.2 M monopotassium phosphate and adjust pH to 6.4, if necessary.
3. Autoclave solutions separately at 121 C for 15 min.
4. Aseptically mix equal volumes of gelatin and phosphate buffer.

Gelatin liquefaction

See Nutrient gelatin and Heart infusion broth.

Gelatin medium, for anaerobes

Thioglycollate medium without indicator* plus hemin	1 liter
Gelatin	50 g

1. Mix and heat with agitation to dissolve.
2. Dispense in screw-capped tubes filled at least half full and autoclave at 118 C for 15 min.

Note. Alternatively, use dehydrated thioglycollate gelatin (Thiogel)* medium plus hemin.

Glucose cysteine agar with thiamine* (22)

Pancreatic digest of heart muscle	3.00 g
Papaic digest of soyameal	10.00 g
Sodium chloride	5.00 g
Cysteine hydrochloride	1.00 g
Dextrose	25.00 g
Agar	14.00 g
Thiamine	0.05 mg
Purified water	1.00 liter
Final pH 6.8	

1. Heat with agitation and boil for 1 min.
2. Autoclave at 118 to 121 C for 20 min.
3. Cool to 45 to 48 C.
4. Aseptically add 25 ml of packed, human blood cells or 50 ml of defibrinated rabbit blood.
5. Add antibiotics: 1 ml each of penicillin, 100,000 units/ml; polymyxin B sulfate, 100,000 units/ml; cycloheximide, 0.1 mg/ml.
6. Mix thoroughly and pour into plates.

10% glucose and lactose agars (13)

Phenol red agar base* plus carbohydrates

Pancreatic digest of casein USP	10.000 g
Sodium chloride	5.000 g

Agar	15.000 g
Phenol red	0.018 g
Carbohydrate	100.000 g
Distilled water	1.000 liter

Dissolve with heat, cool, and adjust the glucose-agar to pH 7.7. (Not necessary to adjust the lactose agar.) Dispense 5 ml in 15 by 125 mm tubes and autoclave at 118 C for 15 min. Cool in a slanted position.

Glycerol fuchsin broth (116)

Meat extract *or* beef extract	1 g
Peptone *or* Gelysate	2 g
Tap water	100 ml

1. Adjust *p*H to 8 and add the following:

Basic fuchsin, 10% in alcohol	0.20 ml
Sodium sulfite, 10% in water (anhydrous, fresh)	1.66 ml
Glycerol	1.00 ml

2. Tube and autoclave at 121 C for 12 min.

Inoculate from an agar slant and incubate at 37 C. Observe daily for 8 days, noting the development of a deep-red color as compared with an uninoculated control tube incubated simultaneously.

G N broth*

Gram-negative enrichment broth

Pancreatic digest of casein	10.0 g
Peptic digest of animal tissue	10.0 g
Dextrose	1.0 g
D-Mannitol	2.0 g
Sodium citrate	5.0 g
Sodium deoxycholate	0.5 g
Dipotassium phosphate	4.0 g
Monopotassium phosphate	1.5 g
Sodium chloride	5.0 g
Distilled water	1.0 liter
Final pH 7.0.	

Dissolve, dispense, and sterilize by autoclaving at 116 C for 15 min. Alternatively, steam for 30 min at 100 C.

Gohar preservative solution (40, 41)

Peptone or Gelysate pancreatic digest of gelatin USP	1 g
Purified water	100 ml

1. Adjust pH to 7.8 to 8.0.
2. Autoclave at 121 C for 15 min. Cool.
3. Add 0.2 ml of sterile 1% aqueous potassium tellurite.* Dispense as for Monsur preservative or Alkaline peptone water.

H antigen broth for salmonella*

H broth*

Use any good broth. A mixture of equal parts of casein soy broth and tryptose or Biosate broth may be used. Tube in 10-ml amounts in 18-mm tubes and autoclave at 121 C for 15 min.

Incubate for 18 to 20 h at 35 to 37 C or in a water bath at 37 C (use heavy inoculum) for 4 to 6 h. Add an equal volume of formalinized saline solution (0.5 or 0.85% sodium chloride plus 0.6% formalin). Mix thoroughly and allow to stand for *1 h* before use.

Heart infusion agar

Same as Blood agar base, but no blood added.

A. *With tyrosine*

For miscellaneous gram-negative bacteria, chapter 24

1. Add 1 g of tyrosine to heart infusion agar prior to sterilization.
2. Dispense in 7-ml volumes in test tubes. Plug with cotton.
3. Autoclave at 121 C for 15 min and cool in a slanted position.

B. *Additives for isolation of fungi*

1. Penicillin, 20 units/ml, and streptomycin, 40 units/ml.
2. Chloramphenicol, 0.05 mg/ml, and cycloheximide, 0.5 mg/ml.
3. Gentamicin, 100 μg/ml, and chlortetracycline, 100 μg/ml.

Heart infusion agar enriched for Streptobacillus moniliformis

See Enriched heart infusion agar

Heart infusion broth

Infusion broth

Same as Blood agar base or Heart infusion agar.

A. *With gelatin*

Gelatin may be added, 120 g/liter. Adjust pH to 7.4. Dispense 5 ml per tube in 16 by 25 mm screw-capped tubes. Sterilize at 121 C for 15 min.

B. *With sodium hippurate*

For Streptococci, chapter 8

Add 10 g per liter. Dispense in screw-capped tubes and autoclave at 121 C for 15 min. Tighten caps to prevent evaporation. (Omit blood.)

C. *For salt tolerance test of streptococci*

For Streptococci, chapter 8

Heart infusion broth	1 liter
Sodium chloride	60 g
Dextrose	1 g
Bromocresol purple, 1.6% in ethanol	1 ml

1. Dissolve and dispense in screw-capped tubes.
2. Autoclave at 121 C for 15 min.

Hektoen enteric agar*

Hektoen agar

Peptone, e.g., Peptic digest of animal tissue USP	12.0 g
Yeast extract	3.0 g
Bile salts	9.0 g
Lactose	12.0 g
Sucrose	12.0 g

Salicin	2.0	g
Sodium chloride	5.0	g
Sodium thiosulfate	5.0	g
Ferric ammonium sulfate	1.5	g
Bromothymol blue	0.064	g
Acid fuchsin	0.10	g
Agar (dried)	13.5	g
Water	1	liter

Final pH 7.6

1. Heat with agitation until solution occurs; *do not autoclave.*
2. Cool to 45 to 50 C and pour into plates.

Hemolysis culture broth (52)

Pancreatic digest of casein USP	10.0 g
Sodium chloride	8.5 g
Purified water	1.0 liter

1. Dispense in tubes and autoclave at 121 C for 15 min.
2. For the test add 1 ml of 18-h culture in this broth to 1 ml of a 5% suspension of washed sheep erythrocytes in saline. Incubate for 2 h and then refrigerate at 4 to 6 C for 24 h. Observe for clearing (lysis) of the suspended erythrocytes.

Hickey and Tresner agar

Dextrin	10 g
Pancreatic digest of casein USP	2 g
Beef extract	1 g
Yeast extract	1 g
Agar	20 g
Cobalt chloride $\cdot 6H_2O$	20 mg
Demineralized water	1 liter

Dissolve and dispense for agar deeps. Autoclave at 121 C for 30 min. For pour slides, melt in a water bath and pipette 0.5 to 1.0 ml per slide.

Recommended for production of aerial hyphae, arthrospores, and pigment by *Nocardia* and *Streptomyces*. For best results, allow surface to dry well before inoculation.

Indole nitrite medium*

Pancreatic digest of casein USP	20 g
Disodium phosphate	2 g
Dextrose	1 g
Agar	1 g
Potassium nitrate	1 g
Distilled water	1 liter

Final pH 7.2

Add 2 g of agar if for use in motility tests. Heat with agitation until the medium boils. Dispense in tubes filled at least half full. Autoclave at 118 to 121 C for 15 min.

Indole test broth or tryptophan broth* (53)

A. *For Enterobacteriaceae, Pseudomonas, and other bacteria*

Peptone, e.g., pancreatic digest of casein USP	10, 15, *or* 20 g
Sodium chloride	5 g
Distilled water	1 liter

Final pH 7.1.

Do not adjust reaction. Dispense and autoclave at 121 C for 15 min.

B. *For miscellaneous gram-negative bacteria*

Prepare a 2% solution of peptone. Adjust to pH 7.3 ± 0.1 and dispense 4 ml per 16 by 125 mm tube. Autoclave at 121 C for 15 min.

Note. Any peptone with a high tryptophan content, as required by the USP for Pancreatic Digest of Casein, may be used.

Kelley Borrelia medium A

Disodium phosphate $\cdot 7H_2O$	26.52 g
Monosodium phosphate $\cdot H_2O$	1.03 g
Sodium chloride	1.20 g
Potassium chloride	0.85 g
Magnesium chloride $\cdot 6H_2O$	0.68 g
Dextrose	12.75 g
Peptone: Proteose No. 2 or Polypeptone	5.95 g
Pancreatic digest of casein USP	2.55 g
Sodium pyruvate	1.06 g
Sodium citrate $\cdot 2H_2O$	0.47 g
N-acetylglucosamine	0.53 g
Distilled water	1.00 liter

1. Dissolve and store at −20 C.
2. Prepare a 10% aqueous solution of bovine albumin fraction V. Adjust pH to 7.8 with NaOH.
3. Dissolve 4.5 g of sodium bicarbonate in 100 ml of water. Use fresh.
4. Prepare a 7% aqueous solution of gelatin autoclaved at 115 C for 15 min. Store at 4 C.
5. Prepare an aqueous 0.5% solution of phenol red and refrigerate.
6. Combine 80 ml of solution 1, 34 ml of 2, 4 ml of 3, 0.7 ml of 5, and 1.3 ml of water. Sterilize by filtration under pressure through an 0.22 μm membrane filter.
7. Dispense aseptically in 6-ml portions into 13 by 100 mm, sterile, borosilicate screw-capped tubes with Teflon liners.
8. To each tube aseptically add 2 ml of the gelatin solution (4) liquefied by immersion in warm water.
9. Aseptically add 0.5 ml of pooled sterile rabbit serum to each tube. Mix by inversion.
10. Store at room temperature. Use within 30 days.

2-Ketogluconate broth (90)

Monopotassium phosphate	5.4 g
Potassium nitrate	2.0 g
Potassium gluconate	20.0 g
Distilled water	1.0 liter

Final pH 6.5.

Sterilize by filtration. Dispense aseptically, 1 ml per sterile 13 by 100 mm tube.

3-Ketolactonate medium (6)

Yeast extract	1.0 g
Agar	2.0 g
Distilled water	100.0 ml

1. Mix and heat to obtain solution.
2. Dispense in 20 by 150 mm test tubes, using 20 ml per tube.
3. Autoclave at 121 C for 15 min.
4. While agar is still melted, aseptically admix 2.0 ml of 10% filtered aqueous lactose per tube.

King's medium for pyocyanin production

See A medium of King.

King's medium for fluorescein production

See B medium of King

Kliger iron agar*

Peptone	20.0	g
Meat extract (optional)	3.0	g
Yeast extract (optional)	3.0	g
Lactose	10.0	g
Dextrose	1.0	g
Sodium chloride	5.0	g
Ferric ammonium citrate	0.5	g
Sodium thiosulfate	0.5	g
Agar	12 to 15.0	g
Phenol red	0.025	g
Water	1	liter

Final pH 7.4 ±

1. Mix and heat with agitation until solution occurs.
2. Dispense for deep slants and autoclave at 121 C for 15 min.

KSCN broth

See Potassium thiocyanate broth.

Lactose broth USP*

Beef extract	3 g
Peptone *or* Gelysate pancreatic digest of gelatin	5 g
Lactose	5 g
Distilled water	1 liter

Final pH 6.9.

Autoclave at 121 C for 15 min.

Levinthal agar and broth

Brain heart infusion broth* ....100 ml
1. Heat to boiling, and add:
Defibrinated horse blood .... 10 ml
2. Filter through Whatman filter paper no. 12, then through a Seitz filter to sterilize.
3. Dissolve:

Peptone phosphate agar* *or* Proteose no. 3 agar	45 g
Agar	15 g
Distilled water	1 liter

4. Dispense the agar base in 100-ml amounts and autoclave. Cool.
5. Mix equal parts of sterile, fluid agar base and the horse blood broth. Pour into plates.

Lipase medium with corn oil* (19)
Spirit blue agar* without oil

Peptone component	10 g
Yeast extract	3 g
Sodium chloride	5 g
Agar	20 g
Victoria blue, 1:500	100 ml
Distilled water	900 ml
Corn oil	50 ml

Final pH 7.8.

Mix thoroughly, using a magnetic stirrer or a blender or sonic oscillator. Dispense in tubes. Autoclave at 115 C for 30 min. Solidify in a slanted position with long slants.

Litmus milk*

Litmus milk	105 g
Distilled water	1 liter

Mix to obtain a homogeneous suspension. Dispense 6 ml per tube (16 by 125 mm). Autoclave at 121 C for 10 min.

Littman oxgall agar*

Oxgall	15.00 g
Peptone	10.00 g
Dextrose	10.00 g
Agar, undried	20.00 g
or (dried)	(16.00 g)
Crystal violet	0.01 g
Water	1.00 liter

Final pH 7.0 ±

1. Mix and heat with agitation and boil for 1 min.
2. Autoclave at 121 C for 15 min.
3. Cool to 45 to 50 C and add 3 ml of 1% aqueous solution of streptomycin.
4. Mix and dispense aseptically into sterile tubes or plates.

Littman oxgall agar* with birdseed extract

Prepare as above but use only 800 ml of water and 200 ml of birdseed extract in the basic medium.
Birdseed extract is prepared as follows:
1. Grind 70 g of *Guizottia abyssinica* seeds in a blender.
2. Add 300 ml of water.
3. Autoclave at 115 C for 10 min.
4. Filter through gauze.

Loeffler medium*

A. *For gram-negative bacteria, chapter 24, and Dermatophilus, chapter 17*

Beef extract	3 g
Peptone	10 g
Sodium chloride	5 g
Dextrose	10 g
Demineralized water	1 liter

1. Combine and dissolve with heat. Cool to 55 C.
2. Admix 3,000 ml of horse serum and filter the mixture through infusorial earth in a Büchner funnel.

3. Sterilize by filtration and dispense aseptically, 2 to 3 ml in 16 by 100 mm screw-capped tubes.
4. Do not flame tubes and avoid formation of bubbles.
5. Slant and inspissate at 95 to 98 C for 50 min.
6. Cool and then tighten caps.
7. Incubate for 24 h at 35 to 37 C and for 48 h at 20 C.
8. Store at 4 to 6 C.

B. *For corynebacteria, chapter 12*

Mammalian serum, nonhuman	750.0 ml
Infusion broth	250.0 ml
Dextrose	2.5 g

1. Mix well, but carefully to avoid bubbles.
2. Dispense and slant in an autoclave with a manually operated air-escape valve. Close the door and air-escape valve, to avoid foaming, and raise the pressure immediately to 15 lb. After 10 min, open the valve *very slightly* so that steam enters and air escapes slowly, maintaining 15 lb of pressure.
3. When the temperature reaches 121 C, close the valve and hold for 15 min.
4. Turn off the steam, but do not open the autoclave until the pressure slowly falls to zero and the autoclave is cool.
5. Admit air *slowly* to the cooled autoclave.

Lowenstein-Jensen medium*

Monopotassium phosphate, anhydrous	2.40 g
Magnesium sulfate·$7H_2O$	0.24 g
Magnesium citrate	0.60 g
Asparagine	3.60 g
Potato flour	30.00 g
Glycerol	12.00 ml
Distilled water	600.00 ml
Homogenized whole eggs	1,000.00 ml
Malachite green, 2% aqueous	200.00 ml

1. Dissolve the salts and asparagine in the water.
2. Admix the glycerol and potato flour, autoclave at 121 C for 30 min, and cool to room temperature.
3. Scrub eggs, not more than 1 week old, in 5% soap solution. Allow to stand for 30 min in soap solution: then rinse thoroughly in cold running water.
4. Immerse in 70% ethyl alcohol for 15 min.
5. Break eggs into a sterile flask. Homogenize by hand shaking and filter through four layers of gauze.
6. Add 1 liter of homogenized eggs to the potato-salt mixture.
7. Prepare the malachite green and admix thoroughly.
8. Dispense 6 to 8 ml in 20 by 150 screw-capped tubes.
9. Slant and inspissate at 85 C for 50 min.
10. Incubate for 48 h at 37 C to check sterility and store at 4 to 6 C with caps tightly closed.

Lysine iron agar* (27, 58)

Bacto peptone *or* Gelysate pancreatic digest of gelatin	5.00 g
Yeast extract	3.00 g
Dextrose	1.00 g
L-Lysine	10.00 g
Ferric ammonium citrate	0.50 g
Sodium thiosulfate	0.04 g
Bromocresol purple	0.02 g
Agar	15.00 g
Distilled water	1.00 liter

Final pH 6.7.

Dispense in 4-ml amounts and autoclave at 121 C for 12 min. Cool in slanted position to form slants with deep butts.

Inoculate with a straight wire by stabbing to the base of the butt and by streaking the slant. Incubate at 37 C for 18 to 24 h. The medium was designed originally for the examination of backened colonies on bismuth sulfite agar plates.

MacConkey agar* (45, 57, 80, 81)

Bacto peptone *or* Gelysate	17.000 g
Peptone: Proteose *or* Polypeptone	3.000 g
Lactose	10.000 g
Bile salts	1.500 g
Sodium chloride	5.000 g
Agar	13.500 g
Neutral red	0.030 g
Crystal violet	0.001 g
Distilled water	1.000 liter

Final pH 7.1.

Sucrose may be added to give a final concentration of 1% (54). Autoclave at 121 C for 15 min. Use in plates or as slants.

Malonate broth, modified* (72)

Yeast extract	1.000 g
Ammonium sulfate	2.000 g
Dipotassium phosphate	0.600 g
Monopotassium phosphate	0.400 g
Sodium chloride	2.000 g
Sodium malonate	3.000 g
Dextrose	0.250 g
Bromothymol blue	0.025 g
Distilled water	1.000 liter

Final pH 6.7.

Autoclave at 121 C for 15 min.

Inoculate from a young agar slant or preferably with a 3-mm loopful of a broth culture. Incubate at 37 C and observe after 24 and 48 h. Positive results are indicated by a change in the color of the indicator from green to Prussian blue.

Mannitol salt agar USP*

Beef extract	1.000 g
Peptone *or* Polypeptone	10.000 g
Sodium chloride	75.000 g
Mannitol	10.000 g
Agar	15.000 g
Phenol red	0.025 g
Distilled water	1.000 liter

Final pH 7.4.

Heat to dissolve and autoclave at 121 C for 15 min.

McBride listeria medium*

Peptone: Tryptose *or* Biosate	10.0 g
Beef extract	3.0 g
Sodium chloride	5.0 g
Glycine anhydride	10.0 g
Lithium chloride	0.5 g
Phenylethanol	2.5 g
Agar	15.0 g
Distilled water	1.0 liter

Final pH without blood, 7.3.

Autoclave at 121 C for 15 min. Cool to 45 to 50 C and add sterile defibrinated sheep blood to a final concentration of 5%.

Meat extract agar
Nutrient agar modified

For Vibrio cholerae, chapter 21

Beef extract	3 g
Peptone or Gelysate pancreatic digest of gelatin	10 g
Sodium chloride	5 g
Agar (not dried)	20 g
Distilled water	1 liter

1. Adjust pH to 7.6 with 1 N sodium hydroxide.
2. Autoclave at 121 C for 15 min.
3. Cool to 45 to 50 C and dispense in petri dishes.

Middlebrook 7H9 broth*

Monopotassium phosphate	1.000 g
Disodium phosphate	2.500 g
L-Glutamic acid	0.500 g
Sodium citrate	0.100 g
Ammonium sulfate	0.500 g
Pyridoxine	0.001 g
Ferric ammonium citrate	0.040 g
Magnesium sulfate	0.050 g
Zinc sulfate	0.001 g
Copper sulfate	0.001 g
Biotin	0.50 mg
Calcium chloride	0.50 mg
Water	900 ml

1. Dissolve and add 0.5 ml of polysorbate 80 *or* 2 ml of glycerol, but not both. Add 2 g of dextrose if desired.
2. Dispense and autoclave at 121 C for 15 min.
3. Cool and to each 180 ml add 20 ml of Oleic acid albumin complex.* *See* Dubos oleic acid agar.

Middlebrook and Cohn 7H10 agar*
7H10 agar

Stock solutions

Solution 1. Store at room temperature

Monopotassium phosphate	15 g
Disodium phosphate	15 g
Distilled water	250 ml

Solution 2. Store at 4 to 10 C.

Ammonium sulfate	5.0 g
Monosodium glutamate	5.0 g
Sodium citrate·$2H_2O$ USP	4.0 g
Ferric ammonium citrate	0.4 g
Magnesium sulfate ($7H_2O$) ACS	0.5 g
Biotin, in 2 ml of 10% NH_4OH	5.0 mg
Distilled water to	250.0 ml

Solution 3. Store at 4 to 10 C.

Calcium chloride·$2H_2O$ ACS	50 mg
Zinc sulfate·$7H_2O$ ACS	100 mg
Copper sulfate·$5H_2O$ ACS	100 mg
Pyridoxine hydrochloride	100 mg
Distilled water to	100 ml

Solution 4. Glycerol, reagent.
Solution 5. Malachite green, 0.01% aqueous.

1 To 975 ml of distilled water, add:

Solution 1	25 ml
Solution 2	25 ml
Solution 3	1 ml
Solution 4	5 ml

2. Adjust pH to 6.6 by adding approximately 0.5 ml of 6 N HCl.
3. Add 2.5 ml of solution 5 and 15 g of agar.
4. Autoclave at 121 C for 15 min. Cool to 56 C and add 100 ml of O A D C Enrichment*:

Bovine albumin fraction V	50 g
Sterile saline, 0.85%	900 ml

Dissolve and add 30 ml of the following:

Oleic acid	0.6 ml
Distilled water to	30.0 ml
Sodium hydroxide, 6 M	0.6 ml

Warm to 56 C: swirl until solution occurs.

5. Adjust reaction to pH 7.0, measured electrometrically.
6. Add 40 ml of sterile 50% aqueous dextrose. Sterilize by filtration.
7. Heat at 56 C for 1 h, incubate overnight, and heat again at 56 C; again incubate overnight at 37 C for sterility.
8. Add 100 ml of this solution to the agar base.
9. Add also 2 ml of freshly prepared, membrane filter-sterilized, catalase solution containing 1,000 μg/ml.
10. Dispense the complete medium completely into petri plates or tubes.
11. Store at 4 to 8 C; unsealed and unprotected containers should be used for no longer than 1 week.
12. During preparation and storage, protect from light.

Monsur agar (88)

Pancreatic digest of casein USP	10 g
Sodium chloride	10 g
Sodium taurocholate	5 g
Sodium carbonate	1 g
Gelatin	30 g
Agar	15 g
Distilled water	1 liter

Autoclave at 121 C for 15 min. Cool to 45 to 50 C. Add sterile potassium tellurite solution to a final concentration of 1:200,000. Pour into plates.

Monsur preservative solution (88, 89)

1. As for Monsur agar, but omit agar and gelatin. Sterilize and cool. Add 0.002% potassium tellurite for a final concentration of 1:200,000.
2. Dispense in 25-ml amounts in 80-ml screw-capped bottles or in 0.5- to 1-ml amounts in tubes.

Morris selective medium for Pasteurella (91)

Tryptose *or* Biosate agar	4g
Distilled water	950 ml

Autoclave at 121 C for 15 min. Cool to 50 C and admix aseptically:

Peptic digest of sheep blood	50 ml
Novobiocin	10 mg
Potassium tellurite	5 mg
Erythromycin	5 mg
Cycloheximide	100 mg

Distribute in 20-ml amounts into petri dishes. When solidified, incubate for 2 h at 37 C to eliminate excess moisture. Store at 40 C for not more than 7 days.

Motility indole ornithine medium* (24)

MIO medium*

Pancreatic digest of casein USP	14.00 g
Pancreatic digest of gelatin, or equal	5.00 g
Yeast extract	3.00 g
Dextrose	1.50 g
L-Ornithine monohydrochloride	5.00 g
Bromocresol purple	0.02 g
Agar	2.00 g
Purified water	1.00 liter
Final pH 6.6 ± 0.2	

1. Heat with agitation until solution occurs.
2. Dispense in tubes, about 5 ml per tube.
3. Autoclave at 118 to 121 C for 15 min.

Motility nitrate medium (M-N)

Beef extract	3.0 g
Peptone *or* Gelysate	5.0 g
Potassium nitrate	1.0 g
Agar	3.0 g
Distilled water	1.0 liter
Final pH 7.0	

Dispense 10 ml per 150 by 16 mm screw-capped tube. Autoclave at 121 C for 15 min.

Motility test medium*

A. *For Enterobacteriaceae, chapter 18*

Beef extract	3 g
Peptone *or* Gelystate	10 g
Sodium chloride	5 g
Agar	4 g
Distilled water	1 liter
Final pH 7.4	

Dispense about 8 ml per tube. Autoclave at 121 C for 15 min.

B. *For Pseudomonas, chapter 23*

Pancreatic digest of casein USP	10 g
Yeast extract	3 g
Sodium chloride	5 g
Agar	3 g
Distilled water	1 liter
Final pH 7.2.	

Dispense 3.5 ml per 13 by 100 mm tube. Autoclave at 121 C for 15 min.

See chapter 96 for discussion of motility testing.

C. *For miscellaneous gram-negative bacteria, chapter 24*

Tryptose or Biosate	8 g
Sodium chloride	5 g
Agar	4 g
Nutrient broth	500 ml
Distilled water	500 ml

1. Mix and heat to dissolve ingredients.
2. Dispense in test tubes and autoclave at 121 C for 15 min.

MR-VP broth

Dipotassium phosphate	5 g
Polypeptone *or* buffered peptone	7 g
Dextrose	5 g
Distilled water	1 liter
Final pH 6.9	

Tube and autoclave at 118 to 121 C for 15 min. *See* chapter 96 for procedure.

Mueller-Hinton agar*

Beef, infusion from	300.0 g
Acid hydrolysate of casein	17.5 g
Starch	1.5 g
Agar	17.0 g
Distilled water	1.0 liter
Final pH 7.4.	

Dispense and autoclave at 116 to 121 C for 15 min. Cool to 45 to 50 C and add blood, if desired.

Mueller-Hinton broth*

As above, but with omission of agar.

Mycobacteria 7H11 agar*

Seven H11 agar

Middlebrook and Cohn 7H10 agar	1 liter
Pancreatic digest of casein USP	1.0 g

Mycobactosel agar*

Mycobactosel 7H11 agar

Mycobacteria 7H11 agar	1 liter
Cycloheximide	0.360 mg
Lincomycin	0.002 mg
Nalidixic acid	0.020 g

Mycobactosel L-J medium*

Lowenstein-Jensen medium	1,600 ml
Cycloheximide	0.64 g

Lincomycin	3.2 mg
Nalidixic acid	0.056 g

Myocoplasma media (103, 104)

E agar

Papaic digest of soy meal USP	20 g
Sodium chloride	5 g
Purified water	1 liter
Agar	10 g

1. Heat with agitation to obtain solution.
2. Cool and adjust pH to 7.4 with 1 N sodium hydroxide.
3. Dispense and autoclave at 121 C for 15 min. Cool to 50 C.
4. To 65 ml of solution add 10 ml of yeast dialysate, 25 ml of horse serum, 2 ml of penicillin (10,000 units/ml), and 1 ml of 3.3% aqueous thallium acetate.
5. Dispense in 5-ml amounts in 10 by 35 mm petri dishes and incubate overnight at room temperature.

Note. Prepare yeast dialysate as follows: Suspend 450 g of active dried yeast (e.g., Fleischman) in 1,250 ml of water at 40 C. Heat in an autoclave at 121 C for 5 min.

Place in dialysis casing and dialyze against 1 liter of water at 4 C for 2 days. Discard casing and contents.

Autoclave dialysate at 121 C for 15 min. Store frozen.

E broth

Papaic digest of soy meal USP	20 g
Sodium chloride	5 g
Dextrose	10 g
Purified water	1 liter
Phenol red, 2% aqueous	2 ml

1. Dissolve and adjust pH to 7.6.
2. Dispense and autoclave at 121 C for 15 min. Cool.
3. To 65 ml of broth aseptically add same solutions as for E agar (step 4).

Diphasic E medium

Dispense E agar in 3-ml amounts in 16 by 125 mm screw-capped tubes, allow to solidify, and overlay with 3 ml of E broth. Store at room temperature. Tubes must have good closures to avoid excessive elevation of pH upon loss of CO_2 from some lots of horse serum.

Dialysate broth base

1. Dissolve 300 g of papaic digest of soy meal USP in 2 liters of water and place in dialysis casing.
2. Autoclave 250 g of active dried yeast (e.g., Fleischman) in 2 liters of water for 5 min. Place in dialysis casing.
3. Dialyze both casings in 10 liters of water at 4 C for 2 days. Discard casing and contents.
4. Add 0.5% sodium chloride and 0.04% phenol red to dialysate. Adjust pH to 7.3 with 1 N sodium hydroxide.
5. Autoclave at 121 C for 15 min.

Medium for production of complement-fixing antigen for M. pneumoniae

Dialysate broth base	87 ml
Agamma horse serum	10 ml
Penicillin, 10,000 units/ml	2 ml
Thallium acetate, 3.3%	1 ml

1. Combine and dispense aseptically.
2. Inoculate with 1 to 5% actively growing cultures.
3. Agitate or stir with spin bars. Incubate for 5 to 8 days until haze is observed and pH begins to drop.
4. Harvest by centrifugation at 8,000 × *g* and wash three times with saline.
5. Resuspend in a volume 1/100 to 1/1,000 of the original culture.

Mes agar

Papaic digest of soy meal USP	20.00 g
Sodium chloride	5.00 g
2-(*N*-morpholino) ethane sulfonic acid (Mes* Calbiochem)	4.25 g
Water	1.00 liter
Agarose	10.00 g

1. Dissolve, adjust pH to 6.0 at 37 C, autoclave at 121 C for 15 min and cool to 50 C.
2. To 65 ml of solution add 10 ml of yeast dialysate, 25 ml of horse serum, and 2 ml of penicillin (10,000 units/ml).
3. Dispense in plates as for E agar.

Urea broth

Dialysate broth base	75 ml
Urea, 1% aqueous, filter-sterilized	4 ml
Horse serum	20 ml
Penicillin (10,000 units/ml)	2 ml

Combine aseptically and dispense in 3-ml amounts in sterile 16-mm test tubes.

Urea test reagent (104)

Urea	1.0 g
Manganous chloride	0.8 g
Water	100.0 ml

Place several drops on a plate with visible colonies and not over 48 h old. T colonies will be surrounded by a brown color. *M. hominis* colonies do not react.

Neopeptone meat infusion broth

For pneumococci, chapter 9

Chopped meat	450 g
Neopeptone or equivalent	10 g
Sodium chloride	5 g
Tap water	1+ liter

1. Add 1 liter of tap water to 450 g of finely chopped fresh beef heart previously freed from fat and fascia.
2. Heat slowly while stirring to 85 C and maintain at 85 C for 45 min.
3. Filter through paper and drain thoroughly.
4. Add water to restore volume, peptone, and sodium chloride.
5. Heat to boiling and adjust to pH 7.8 to 8.0 while hot, using approximately 14 ml of 1 N NaOH.
6. Boil vigorously for 1 min.
7. Filter through paper, dispense, and autoclave at 121 C for 20 min.

Neopeptone meat infusion with agar

For pneumococci, chapter 9

1–4. Prepare infusion as above.
5. Add 17 g of agar and boil.
6. Adjust pH to 7.6 while hot and boil vigorously for 1 min.
7. Filter through cotton. Do not press.
8. Dispense and autoclave.

Nitrate broth

Chapter 24

Bacto peptone *or* Gelysate pancreatic digest of gelatin	1 liter
Potassium nitrate	2 g
Final *p*H 7.0	

Dispense 4 ml in 16 by 125 mm tubes containing Durham vials. Autoclave at 121 C for 15 min.

Nitrate broth enriched

Chapter 24

Heart infusion broth* *or* infusion (heart) broth	25 g
Potassium nitrate	2 g
Distilled water	1 liter

Dispense 4 ml per tube with inverted insert tubes. Autoclave at 121 C for 15 min.

Nitrate reduction test medium

Chapter 18

Pancreatic digest of casein	5.0 g
Neopeptone *or* other peptone, e.g., peptic digest of animal tissue USP	5.0 g
Agar	2.5 g
Distilled water	1.0 liter

Boil, adjust pH to 7.3 to 7.4, and add:

Potassium nitrate (nitrite-free)	1.0 g
Dextrose	0.1 g

Autoclave at 121 C for 15 min.

Nitrate reduction broth

Chapter 23

Pancreatic digest of casein	10 g
Yeast extract	3 g
Potassium nitrate	2 g
Distilled water	1 liter
Final pH 7.1	

Dispense in 4-ml amounts in 13 by 100 mm test tubes containing Durham vials. Autoclave at 121 C for 15 min.

Nitrite reduction broth

For miscellaneous gram-negative bacteria, chapter 24

Heart infusion broth	1 liter
Potassium nitrite, c.p.	1 g
Adjust to pH 7.0	

Dispense 4-ml amounts in 15 by 125 mm tubes containing Durham vials. Autoclave at 121 C for 15 min.

Nutrient agar*

Beef extract	3 g
Peptone *or* Gelysate pancreatic digest of gelatin	5 g
Agar	15 g
Distilled water	1 liter
Final pH 6.8	

Autoclave at 121 C for 15 min.

Nutrient agar modified

See Meat extract agar.

Nutrient broth*

As for Nutrient agar, but without agar.

Nutrient gelatin*

A. *For Enterobacteriaceae, chapter 18*

Nutrient broth	1 liter
Gelatin	120 g

Autoclave at 121 C for 12 min.

Inoculate by stabbing with a wire and incubate at 20 C for 30 days. Nutrient gelatin is recommended as the "standard" method in taxonomic work, since the rate of gelatin liquefaction is important in the characterization of members of certain groups and subgroups within the family *Enterobacteriaceae*. Some of the rapid methods are excellent for diagnostic work in which one is not interested in rate of liquefaction. In those areas where the rate of liquefaction is of differential value (e.g., within the tribe *Klebsielleae*), positive tests obtained by the rapid methods should be repeated using the conventional methods. If the above-mentioned limitations are borne in mind, certain rapid methods can be recommended.

Gelatin liquefaction demonstration by rapid methods (67, 70)

Prepare Nutrient gelatin, using 15 g/100 ml of distilled water. Add 3 to 5 g of powdered charcoal, mix thoroughly, cool, and pour into petri dishes or other flat containers to a depth of 3 mm. (Apply a thin film of Vaseline to containers first.) After medium has set, remove the sheet of gelatin and place in 10% formalin for 24 h. Cut the sheet into pieces 1 cm by 5 to 8 mm. Wrap in gauze and wash in running tap water for 24 h. Place in wide-mouth, screw-capped jars or bottles and cover with distilled water. Sterilize by exposure to flowing steam for 30 min on 3 successive days. After sterilization, the water may be decanted. Check sterility by placing pieces in tubes of Nutrient broth.

Suspend the growth from an 18- to 24-h agar plate culture in 3 ml of 0.85% sodium chloride solution containing 0.01 M calcium chloride in a small test tube (e.g., 13 by 100 mm). The suspension should be very dense, since the rapidity of the reaction appears to be a function of density and temperature of incubation. The agar plates should be thick; i.e., they should contain 35 to 40 ml of infusion agar medium. Three or four drops of a broth culture should be spread over the entire surface so as to obtain maximal confluent growth.

With aseptic precautions, add a piece of denatured charcoal to each dense suspension prepared as above. Add 0.1 ml of toluene to each suspension and shake the tube. Toluene appears to have an activating effect upon the reactions of strains that ordinarily are slow liquefiers of gelatin. Incubate at 37 C, and examine after 5 or 6 h and daily for 14 days. Positive reactions are indicated by the release of charcoal particles which collect in the bottom of the tube.

Advantage may be taken of the bactericidal effect of toluene: distribute 3-ml amounts of saline solution containing 0.01 M calcium chloride in small tubes and autoclave at 121 C for 15 min. Place a piece of charcoal-gelatin and 0.1 ml of toluene in each tube, and stopper with corks that have been soaked in hot paraffin. Store until needed.

B. *For aerobic actinomycetes, chapter 17*

Prepare as for Medium A, but with demineralized water.

Inoculate just below the surface of the solidified medium. Incubate at room temperature or 37 C, together with an uninoculated control. When growth is sufficient, place tests and control in refrigerator until control solidifies; then observe tests for liquefaction.

C. *For Erysipelothrix, chapter 14*

Medium A is recommended.

D. *For miscellaneous gram-negative bacteria, chapter 24*

Heart infusion broth* *or* infusion (heart) broth	25 g
Gelatin	120 g
Distilled water	1 liter

Heat to boiling to dissolve. Cool to 55 C and adjust to *p*H 7.4. Dispense 5 ml per screw-capped 16 by 125 mm tube and autoclave at 121 C for 15 min.

Organic acid media (29, 64)

Bacto peptone *or* Gelysate pancreatic digest of gelatin	10 g
Bromothymol blue, 0.2%	12 ml
Distilled water	1 liter

1. Divide the basal medium into three equal portions and add, respectively, 1% sodium potassium tartrate, sodium citrate, and mucic acid.

2. After addition of the tartrate and the citrate, adjust the pH to 7.4 with 5 or 10 N NaOH and tube 3-ml amounts in 13 by 100 mm tubes. Autoclave at 121 C for 15 min.

3. The portion to which mucic acid is to be added is sterilized in bulk. Weigh the mucic acid aseptically and add to the hot basal medium. Add sufficient NaOH (5 or 10 N) slowly to bring the mucic acid into solution as sodium mucate and to adjust the final pH to 7.4. Tube, aseptically, in 3- or 4-ml amounts and incubate for sterility. If care is taken to make certain the mucic acid is in solution, it may be added prior to autoclaving.

Inoculate each medium with a 3-mm loopful from an overnight Nutrient broth culture. Incubate at 37 C and observe daily for 14 days, beginning at 20 h. Development of an acid reaction indicates utilization of D-tartrate, citrate, or mucate. In addition, 0.5 ml of a 50% neutral lead acetate solution is added to the tubes of D-tartrate and citrate media, as well as to uninoculated control tubes, after 14 days of incubation. Multiple tubes of each medium may be inoculated, and lead acetate solution may be added at different intervals of incubation. Utilization of these substances is indicated by a diminution in the volume of precipitate formed in comparison with that in the control tubes.

Oxidation-fermentation test medium (54)

OF basal medium*

A. *For Corynebacterium, chapter 12, Enterobacteriaceae, chapter 18, Aeromonas, chapter 20, and Pseudomonas, chapter 23*

Peptone, e.g., pancreatic digest of casein	2.00 g
Sodium chloride	5.00 g
Dipotassium phosphate	0.30 g
Bromothymol blue	0.03 g
Agar	3.00 g
Distilled water	1.00 liter
Final *p*H 7.1	

1. Dispense 3 or 4 ml per 13 by 100 mm test tube. Autoclave at 121 C for 15 min.

2. Cool and add 10% dextrose solution in distilled water for a final concentration of 1% dextrose. Other carbohydrates may be substituted for dextrose, if desired.

3. Dispense aseptically.

This medium aids in the differentiation of organisms that utilize carbohydrates oxidatively rather than fermentatively and, therefore, is helpful, in the identification of pseudomonads and members of the tribe *Mimeae*. It also aids in the identification of organisms that do not utilize dextrose in either way (e.g., *Alcaligenes*). Inoculate (stab) lightly two tubes of medium from a young agar slant culture. Cover one of the tubes with a layer (about 5 mm) of sterile melted petrolatum or sterile paraffin oil. Incubate at 37 C and observe daily for 3 or 4 days. Acid formation in the open tube only indicates oxidative utilization of dextrose. Acid formation in both the open and sealed tubes is indicative of a fermentative reaction. Lack of acid production in either tube indicates that the organism does not utilize dextrose by either method.

B. *For miscellaneous gram-negative bacilli, chapter 24*

Pancreatic digest of casein	0.2 g
Phenol red, 1.5% aqueous	0.2 ml
Distilled water	100.0 ml

1. Warm to dissolve the peptone and adjust to pH 7.3.

2. Dissolve 0.3 g of agar by heating.

3. Dispense 6 ml per 16 by 125 mm tube. Autoclave at 121 C for 15 min.

4. While basal agar is melted, add Seitz-filtered carbohydrate (dextrose, D-xylose, D-mannitol, lactose, sucrose, or maltose) aseptically to a final 1% concentration.

"Pablum" cereal agar

Pablum precooked cereal	100 g
Agar	18 g
Chloramphenicol	50 mg

Distilled water	1 liter

Mix and autoclave at 121 C for 15 min.

Packer agar*

Tryptose *or* Biosate	15 g
Beef extract	3 g
Sodium chloride	5 g
Agar	18 g
Distilled water	1 liter

1. Heat to dissolve and filter through cotton or several layers of milk filter disks. Autoclave at 121 C for 15 min. Cool to 50 C and add aseptically the following sterile fluids: crystal violet, 0.25% aqueous, autoclaved, 4 ml; sodium azide, 4% aqueous, autoclaved, 25 ml; equine serum or blood, 50 ml.

2. Mix thoroughly and dispense into sterile plates or into tubes for slants.

Pai medium*

A. *For stock cultures of S. typhi*

Whole egg	2 parts
Sodium chloride solution, 0.85%	1 part

Mix well, dispense in tubes, and sterilize by inspissation or a method suitable for egg medium.

B. *For corynebacteria, chapter 12*

Whole eggs	1,000.0 ml
Distilled water	500.0 ml
Glycerol	120.0 ml
Dextrose (optional)	5.0 g

Beat eggs and water; filter through two layers of gauze, add glycerol, and mix well. Dispense, slant, and sterilize as for Loeffler medium B.

Pectate medium (115)

Yeast extract	0.50 g
Sodium hydroxide, 1 N	0.90 ml
Calcium chloride $\cdot 2H_2O$, 10%	0.60 ml
Bromothymol blue, 0.2%	1.25 ml
Sodium Polypectate No. 24 (Sunkist Growers, Inc., Ontario, Calif.)	3.00 g
Distilled water	100.00 ml

1. Mix in a beaker. Add sodium pectate last and slowly.

2. Dissolve pectate with constant stirring while warming in a boiling-water bath. Color should be blue-green (ca. pH 7.3). Further adjustments of pH cannot be made.

3. Dispense 3 to 4 ml in small tubes. Autoclave at 121 C for 15 min. Resulting color should be yellowish-green (ca. pH 6.4).

4. Allow tubes to cool in an upright position. The medium cannot be reheated.

Certain bacteria, presently classified as *Erwinia* and now referred to as *Pectobacterium*, occasionally may be seen, and their differentiation from *Enterobacteriaceae* may be somewhat difficult. However, these bacteria produce pectinases and *Enterobacteriaceae* are not known to possess them. Hence, a medium containing pectin is of value in the differentiation of these bacteria.

Inoculate from a young agar slant culture by stabbing deep into the column of medium. Incubate at 37 C for 7 days. Observe for evidence of liquefaction as with nutrient gelatin medium. (Changes in the color of the medium may occur during growth of *Enterobacteriaceae*. This apparently is of no importance as far as *Enterobacteriaceae* are concerned.)

Peptone iron agar

Peptone or Gelysate	15.00 g
Proteose or Thiotone	5.00 g
Ferric ammonium citrate	0.50 g
Dipotassium phosphate	1.00 g
Sodium thiosulfate	0.08 g
Agar	15.00 g
Distilled water	1.00 liter

Final pH 6.7

Dissolve, dispense in tubes, and autoclave at 121 C for 15 min. Allow to cool in an upright position.

Inoculate by the stab method, incubate at 37 C, and observe for 7 days for blackening caused by hydrogen sulfide production.

Peptone yeast glucose maltose broth
PYGM Broth

Peptone	5.00 g
Yeast extract	2.50 g
Dextrose	1.25 g
Maltose	2.50 g
Distilled water	250.00 ml
Resazurin, 0.025%	1.00 ml
Combined salt solution (A and B) containing	10.00 ml
A. Dipotassium phosphate	1 g
Monopotassium phosphate	1 g
Sodium bicarbonate	10 g
Sodium chloride	2 g
Cobalt chloride $\cdot 6H_2O$	Trace
Sodium molybdate $\cdot 2H_2O$	Trace
Distilled water combined with	1 liter
B. Calcium chloride $\cdot 2H_2O$ and	0.25 g
Magnesium sulfate	0.20 g
Distilled water, boiling less than	5.00 ml

Mix thoroughly. Boil until bubbles are large and color becomes yellowish. Cool in ice water (preferably under bubbling oxygen-free CO_2) until the outside of the flask is cold. Add 0.125 g of cysteine and adjust pH to 7.0. Tube, preferably under bubbling oxygen-free N_2. Autoclave at 121 C for 15 min.

Phenol red broth*

Beef extract (optional)	1.000 g
Peptone, e.g., Proteose *or* trypticase pancreatic digest of casein USP	10.000 g
Sodium chloride	5.000 g
Phenol red	0.018 g
Distilled water	1.000 liter

Final pH 7.4

Autoclave at 118 to 121 C for 15 min.

Phenol red lactose agar*

Pancreatic digest of casein	10.0	g
Sodium chloride	5.0	g
Agar	15.0	g
Phenol red	0.018	g
Lactose	10.0	g
Water	1.	liter

Final pH 7.4

1. Heat with agitation and boil for 1 min.
2. Dispense and autoclave at 121 C for 15 min.

Phenylalanine agar* (32)

Yeast extract	3 g
DL-Phenylalanine	2 g
(*or* L-phenylalanine)	(1 g)
Disodium phosphate	1 g
Sodium chloride	5 g
Agar	12 g
Distilled water	1 liter

Final pH 7.3

Tube and autoclave at 121 C for 10 min. Solidify in a slanted position with a long slant.

This medium is used to test for deamination of phenylalanine to phenylpyruvic acid. Inoculate with a fairly heavy inoculum from an agar slant culture. Incubate at 37 C for 4 h or 18 to 24 h, if desired. Allow 4 or 5 drops of a 10% (wt/vol) ferric chloride solution to run down over the growth on the slant. If phenylpyruvic acid has been formed, a green color develops in the syneresis fluid and in the slant.

Phenylethyl alcohol agar*
Phenylethanol agar*

Pancreatic digest of casein USP	15	g
Papaic digest of soya meal USP	5	g
Sodium chloride	5	g
Phenylethyl alcohol	2.5	g
Agar	15.0	g
Distilled water	1.0	liter

Final pH 7.3

Dissolve with heat, autoclave at 118 C for 15 min, cool, and pour into plates. Add 5% defibrinated sheep blood if desired.

Polysorbate dextrose agar
Tween dextrose agar

Nutrient agar*	100.0 ml
Polysorbate (Tween) 40	0.5 ml

Autoclave at 121 C for 15 min and cool to 60 C. To each 95 ml, add 5 ml of filtered 20% aqueous dextrose solution. Dispense in tubes or plates.

Potassium cyanide medium (26, 28, 86)
Moeller KCN broth base*

Peptic digest of animal tissue USP	10.000 g
Sodium chloride	5.000 g
Monopotassium phosphate	0.225 g
Disodium phosphate	5.640 g
Distilled water	1.000 liter

1. Adjust to pH 7.6 and autoclave at 121 C for 15 min.
2. Refrigerate until thoroughly chilled. To the *cold* medium add 15 ml of a 0.5% KCN solution prepared in *cold* sterile distilled water.
3. Dispense about 1 ml per small sterile tube. Stopper *quickly* with corks sterilized in heated paraffin.
4. May be stored at 4 C for 2 weeks.

Inoculate with one loopful (3-mm loop) of a 24-h broth culture grown at 37 C. Incubate at 37 C and observe daily for 2 days. Positive results are indicated by growth in the presence of KCN.

Potassium thiocyanate broth
KSCN broth

Potassium thiocyanate	37.5 g
Tryptose *or* Biosate	20.0 g
Dextrose	2.0 g
Sodium chloride	5.0 g
Disodium phosphate	2.5 g
Distilled water	1.0 liter

Autoclave at 121 C for 15 min.

Potato dextrose agar* (107)
Recommended to induce sporulation in all fungi.

Potatoes (white, not new), diced	200 g
Dextrose	10 g
Agar	18 g

1. Simmer the potatoes in water for 1 h. Filter through coarse paper.
2. Add the dextrose and agar, dissolve by heat, and filter through cotton and gauze. Restore volume to 1 liter.
3. Tube and autoclave at 121 C for 10 min.

Pseudomonas agar for detection of fluorescein USP

See B medium of King et al.

Pseudomonas agar for detection of pyocyanin USP

See A medium of King

Purple broth base*

Peptone: Proteose *or* peptic digest of animal tissue USP	10.000 g
Beef extract	1.000 g
Sodium chloride	5.000 g
Bromocresol purple	0.015 g
Distilled water	1.000 liter

Final pH 6.8

Autoclave at 121 C for not more than 15 min. Add sugars, alcohols to 1% weight by volume.

Reinforced clostridial agar*
RCM agar

Yeast extract	3.0 g
Beef extract	10.0 g
Peptone, e.g. pancreatic digest of casein USP	10.0 g
Dextrose	5.0 g
Soluble starch	1.0 g
Sodium chloride	5.0 g
Sodium acetate	3.0 g
Cysteine hydrochloride	0.5 g
Agar	60.0 g
(*or* dried)	(13.5 g)
Distilled water	1.0 liter
Final pH 6.8	

1. Add additional agar to 60 g/liter, if desired, to reduce spreading.
2. Heat with frequent agitation until dissolved. Cool to 50 to 60 C.
3. Autoclave at 115 C for 15 to 20 min. Pour about 20 ml per plate.
4. Dry agar surface thoroughly before using.

Rice grain medium

White rice (not enriched)	8 g
Distilled water	25 ml

Place in 125-ml Erlenmeyer flask and autoclave at 121 C for 15 min.

This medium is recommended for the differentiation of *Microsporum* spp. *M. canis* and *M. gypseum*, as well as other dermatophytes, grow and sporulate well on this medium. *M. audouini* produces only negligible growth.

Sabhi agar, modified

Brain heart infusion broth	18.60 g
Calf brains, infusion from	50.00 g
Beef heart, infusion from	62.50 g
Proteose or Gelysate pancreatic digest of gelatin	2.50 g
Dextrose	20.50 g
Sodium chloride	1.25 g
Neopeptone	5.00 g
Disodium phosphate	0.625 g
Agar	7.50 g
Distilled water	1.00 liter

Dissolve and autoclave at 121 C for 15 min.

Sabouraud dextrose agar*

Dextrose	40 g
Neopeptone *or* Polypeptone	10 g
Pancreatic digest of casein USP	(5 g)
Peptic digest of animal tissue USP	(5 g)
Agar	20 or 15 g
Demineralized water	1 liter
Final pH 5.6	

Heat to dissolve completely. Dispense in tubes (18 to 25 mm diameter) and autoclave at 121 C for 10 min.

Sabouraud dextrose agar Emmons* (30)
Sabouraud agar Emmons

Dextrose	20 g
Bacto peptone *or* Polypeptone	10 g
Pancreatic digest of casein USP	(5 g)
Peptic digest of animal tissue USP	(5 g)
Agar, not dried	20 g
(or dried)	(17 g)
Distilled water	1 liter
Final pH 6.9	

Dispense and autoclave at 118 to 121 C for 10 min.

Salmonella flagellar H antigen broth

See H antigen broth.

Salmonella-Shigella agar* (20, 105)
SS agar

Beef extract	5.000 g
Proteose *or* Polypeptone	5.000 g
Lactose	10.000 g
Bile salts	8.500 g
Sodium citrate	8.500 g
Sodium thiosulfate	8.500 g
Ferric citrate	1.000 g
Agar	13.500 g
Neutral red	0.025 g
Brilliant green	0.330 mg
Distilled water	1.000 liter
Final pH 7.0	

Heat to boiling. Do not autoclave. Cool to 42 to 45 C, and pour into plates. For slants, prepare the medium in a sterile flask, using sterile water. Dispense aseptically, 5 ml per sterile 16 by 125 mm tube.

Salt tolerance of streptococci

See Heart infusion broth.

Schaedler broth*

Trypticase soy broth (Soybean-casein digest broth USP)	1 liter
Polypeptone or equivalent	5.0 g
Dextrose	5.0 g
Yeast extract	5.0 g
Tris(hydroxymethyl)aminomethane	3.0 g
Hemin	0.01 g
L-Cystine	0.40 g
Agar (dried)	13.50 g
Final pH 7.6	

1. Heat with frequent agitation and boil for 1 min.
2. Dispense and sterilize at 121 C for 15 min.
3. Cool to 50 C and add 5% sheep blood if desired.

Selenite broth* (74)
Selenite-F broth

Peptone: Polypeptone *or* tryptone	5 g
Lactose	4 g
Disodium phosphate	10 g
Sodium acid selenite	4 g
Distilled water	1 liter
Final pH 7.0	

Dispense in sterile tubes to a depth of at least 5 cm. Sterilization is not necessary if medium is used immediately. If not to be used immediately, expose tubes to flowing steam for 30 min. Do not autoclave.

Selenite cystine broth USP*

Peptone: Polypeptone *or* tryptone	5.00 g
Lactose	4.00 g
Disodium phosphate	10.00 g
Sodium acid selenite	4.00 g
L-Cystine	0.01 g
Distilled water	1.00 liter

Final pH 7.0

Dispense in bottles or flasks. Do *not* autoclave. Heat in flowing steam for 20 min.

Semisolid agar media

A. *Semisolid medium for isolation of phases (flagellar)*, chapter 18 (semisolid agar of Edwards and Bruner*)

Bacto peptone *or* Thiotone peptic digest of animal tissue USP	10 g
Gelatin	80 g
Meat or beef extract	3 g
Agar	4 g
Sodium chloride	5 g
Distilled water	1 liter

Dissolve the gelatin in 600 ml of water and the remaining ingredients in 400 ml of water. Mix, leave reaction unadjusted, tube, and autoclave at 121 C for 15 min.

B. *For Listeria, chapter 13*, use any of the following:

1. Casein soy peptone broth* plus 0.4% agar.
2. Tryptose or Biosate phosphate broth plus 0.4% agar.
3. Motility test medium.

Semisynthetic medium for Calymmatobacterium granulomatis

See Calymmatobacterium granulomatis defined medium.

Serum dextrose agar

Stock serum dextrose solution

Horse or ox serum	5 ml
Dextrose	1 g

The serum should be proved free from brucella agglutinins and inactivated at 56 C for 30 min.

Pass through Seitz filter, test for sterility, and store in refrigerator or freezer until used.

Complete medium

Nutrient agar	95 ml
Serum-dextrose stock	5 ml

1. Autoclave the nutrient agar at 121 C for 15 min.
2. Cool to 50 C and add the serum-dextrose stock solution.
3. Dispense in tubes or plates.

Sodium bicarbonate agar

Trypticase soy agar* or brain heart infusion agar* sterile fluid at 45 to 50 C	90 ml
Sodium bicarbonate, 7%, aqueous, filter-sterilized	10 ml

Sodium hippurite broth

See Heart infusion broth.

Soybean-casein digest agar* USP

Trypticase soy agar, tryptic soy agar, tryptone soya agar, casein soy peptone agar, etc.

Pancreatic digest of casein USP	15 g
Papaic digest of soy meal USP	5 g
Sodium chloride	5 g
Agar	15 g
Distilled water	1 liter

Final pH 7.3

Heat with agitation until the medium boils. Dispense and autoclave at 118 to 121 C for 15 min.

Soybean-casein digest broth* USP

Trypticase soy broth, tryptic soy broth, tryptone soya broth, casein soy peptone broth, etc.

Pancreatic digest of casein USP	17.0 g
Papaic digest of soy meal USP	3.0 g
Sodium chloride	5.0 g
Dipotassium phosphate	2.5 g
Dextrose	2.5 g
Distilled water	1.0 liter

Final pH 7.3

Dissolve, dispense, and autoclave at 118 to 121 C for 15 min.

SPS agar*

Sulfite polymyxin sulfadiazine agar

Pancreatic digest of casein USP	15.0 g
Yeast extract USP	10.0 g
Iron citrate	0.5 g
Agar (dried)	(13.9 g)
not dried	15.0 g
Distilled water	1.0 liter

Final pH 7.0

Autoclave at 121 C for 15 min. Add aseptically the following filter-sterilized solutions to each liter of sterile medium:

Sodium sulfite·$7H_2O$ (freshly prepared, 10%)	5.0 ml
Polymyxin B sulfate, 0.1%	10.0 ml
Sodium sulfadiazine, 12 mg/ml	10.0 ml

Staib agar, modified (113)

Birdseed agar

Guizottia abyssinica seeds (niger or thistle seeds)	70.00 g
Creatinine	0.78 g
Dextrose	10.00 g
Chloramphenicol (one 50-mg capsule)	0.05 g
Agar	20.00 g
Distilled water	1.00 liter
Diphenyl	100.00 mg

1. Grind seed powder in blender. Add 300 ml of water and autoclave at 115 C for 10 min.
2. Filter through gauze and bring volume to 1 liter.

3. Add other ingredients except diphenyl and autoclave at 121 C for 15 min.
4. Cool to 50 C.
5. Add diphenyl to 10 ml of 95% ethyl alcohol and add aseptically to medium.
6. Stir and pour into plates.

Standard mineral base (SMB)

A. *SMB with β-hydroxybutyrate* (114)

Disodium phosphate and monopotassium phosphate buffer, 1 M, pH 6.8	40.00 ml
Vitamin-free mineral solution (*see below*)	20.00 ml
Ammonium sulfate	0.20 g
DL-β-Hydroxybutyrate	5.00 g
Distilled water to	1.00 liter

Dispense 4-ml amounts in 13 by 100 mm tubes. Autoclave at 121 C for 15 min. The precipitate dissolves at room temperature.

Inoculate with a needle. Prepare smears from turbid cultures which develop in 1 to 3 days and stain with Sudan Black (*see* chapter 96).

Vitamin-free mineral solution (17)

Nitrilotriacetic acid	10.000 g
Magnesium sulfate	14.450 g
Calcium chloride $\cdot 2H_2O$	3.335 g
Ferrous sulfate $\cdot 7H_2O$	0.099 g
Ammonium molybdate $\cdot 4H_2O$	9.300 mg

Dissolve and neutralize the nitrilotriacetic acid with KOH, about 7.3 g. Add the salts and 50 ml of concentrated metals solution (*see below*), adjust to pH 6.8, and add distilled water to make 1 liter.

Concentrated metals solution (17)

Ethylenediaminetetraacetic acid	2.500 g
Zinc sulfate $\cdot 7H_2O$	10.950 g
Ferrous sulfate $\cdot 7H_2O$	5.000 g
Manganese sulfate $\cdot H_2O$	1.540 g
Copper sulfate $\cdot 5H_2O$	0.392 g
Cobalt nitrate $\cdot 6H_2O$	0.248 g
Sodium borate $\cdot 10H_2O$	0.177 g
Sulfuric acid	Few drops
Distilled water to	1.000 liter

B. *SMB with p-hydroxybenzoate* (114)

Buffer, as for A	40 ml
Vitamin-free mineral solution	20 ml
Ammonium sulfate	1 g
Agar, e.g., Ionagar 2	10 g
p-Hydroxybenzoate	5 g
Distilled water to	1 liter

Autoclave at 121 C for 15 min. Cool to 45 C and pour into plates.

To demonstrate cleavage of protocatechuate, harvest the growth from SMB with *p*-hydroxybenzoate, and suspend in 2 ml of Tris buffer, prepared by dissolving 2.24 g of tris(hydroxymethyl)aminomethane in 1 liter of distilled water, final pH 8.0. Add 4 drops of toluene and 0.1 ml of 3% protocatechuate solution. Mix the suspension. If *meta* cleavage occurs, the suspension turns bright yellow within a few minutes. Cultures giving negative tests are incubated at 30 C for 1 h and tested for the presence of β-keto groups of β-ketoadipate. Keto groups are detected by the nitroprusside test (Rothera reaction). Add 0.5 to 1 g of ammonium sulfate to each tube followed by 2 drops of concentrated ammonium hydroxide and 2 drops of 5% sodium nitroprusside solution. Mix the suspension. A positive *ortho* cleavage becomes purple. Each test must be controlled by inoculating the above medium without parahydroxybenzoate.

C. *SMB with testosterone*

Prepare as for B, but omit *p*-hydroxybenzoate. Boil to dissolve and autoclave at 121 C for 15 min. Suspend 2 g of testosterone in 50 ml of distilled water by 9-kc 50-W sonic oscillation for 30 min (83). Add the suspension to the hot SMB. Cool to 45 C and pour into plates.

Organisms which use testosterone as the sole source of carbon and energy clear the agar medium of suspended testosterone around the colonies. Each test must be controlled by inoculating the above medium without testosterone.

Stanier nitrate medium (17, 114)

Disodium phosphate and monopotassium phosphate, 1 M, pH 6.8	40.0 ml
Vitamin-free mineral solution, Hutner's (18)	20.0 ml
See Standard mineral base	
Ammonium sulfate	1.0 g
Glycerol	10.0 g
Potassium nitrate	10.0 g
Yeast extract	5.0 g
Distilled water q.s.	800.0 ml

1. Combine above and heat slightly in a double water bath to effect solution.
2. Filter-sterilize.
3. Dissolve 1 g of Ionagar 2 or equal in 200 ml of water, and autoclave at 121 C for 15 min.
4. Combine 2 and 3 aseptically and dispense in 5-ml volumes in sterile 16 by 125-mm screw-capped tubes.

Staphylococcus medium 110*

Yeast extract	2.5 g
Pancreatic digest of casein USP	10.0 g
Gelatin	30.0 g
Lactose	2.0 g
Mannitol	10.0 g
Sodium chloride	75.0 g
Dipotassium phosphate	5.0 g
Agar	13.0 g
Distilled water	1.0 liter
Final pH 7.0	

Autoclave at 121 C for 15 min.

Starch agar

Nutrient agar*	23 g
Potato starch	10 g
Demineralized water	1 liter

Dissolve Nutrient agar medium in 500 ml of water. Dissolve starch in 250 ml of water by boiling. Combine and make up to 1 liter volume. Adjust pH and autoclave at 121 C for 30 min.

This medium is useful for differentiation of species of aerobic actinomycetes. Inoculate as for Casein agar. When good growth is obtained, test for hydrolysis by flooding a small portion of the plate with Gram's or Lugol's iodine; this does not contaminate the plate, which may subsequently be retested if necessary. In a negative test, the agar immediately around the growth becomes (temporarily) dark blue; if it becomes red or remains unstained, partial or complete hydrolysis is shown.

Stock culture medium

Beef infusion agar or (heart) infusion agar* without added carbohydrate. Dispense in 13 by 100 mm tubes for short slants with deep butts. Autoclave at 121 C for 15 min.

Inoculate by stabbing the butt once or twice and streaking the slant. Seal with cork stoppers (no. 3) that have been soaked in hot paraffin. *Stock cultures should be kept at room temperature in the dark.*

Alternatively, use a medium prepared by mixing equal parts of meat extract agar and nutrient broth. Do not slant and inoculate by stabbing. Seal and store as above.

Streptomycin assay agar with yeast extract*
Antibiotic medium 5 FDA

Peptone or Gelysate	6.0 g
Yeast extract	3.0 g
Beef extract	1.5 g
Agar	15.0 g
Purified water	1.0 liter
Final pH 7.9 ± 0.2	

1. Mix until a uniform suspension is obtained.
2. Heat with agitation and boil for 1 min.
3. Dispense and sterilize at 121 C for 15 min.

Stuart Leptospira broth, modified*

Modified by the Department of Veterinary Medicine, Walter Reed Army Institute of Research, Washington, D.C.

Glycerol asparagine salt solution

Sodium chloride	1.930 g
Ammonium chloride	0.340 g
Magnesium chloride·$6H_2O$	0.190 g
D-Asparagine	0.130 g
Disodium phosphate	0.666 g
Monopotassium phosphate	0.087 g
Glycerol, optional	5.000 ml
Distilled water	995.000 ml
Final pH 7.5	

Dissolve each ingredient separately in 100-ml portions of water. Mix and make up to 1 liter with water. Autoclave at 121 C for 15 min. Cool and add 100 ml of filter-sterilized rabbit serum, previously inactivated in a 56 C water bath for 30 min. Dispense.

Stuart transport medium, modified (2)
Transport medium,* Cary and Blair transport medium*

Agar	4.00 g
Distilled water	1.00 liter
Heat until dissolved and add while hot:	
Sodium chloride	3.00 g
Potassium chloride	0.20 g
Disodium phosphate, anhydrous	1.15 g
or disodium phosphate·$12H_2O$	(2.90 g)
Monopotassium phosphate	0.20 g
Sodium thioglycolate	1.00 g
Calcium chloride, 1% aqueous, freshly prepared	10.00 ml
Magnesium chloride·$6H_2O$, 1% aqueous	10.00 ml

Final pH 7.3

1. Stir until dissolved. Add 10 g of pharmaceutical neutral charcoal.
2. Dispense 5 to 6 ml per 13 by 100 mm screw-capped tube, stirring to keep the charcoal evenly suspended (avoid cooling or gelling).
3. Autoclave at 121 C for 20 min. Invert tubes prior to solidification in order to distribute the charcoal uniformly. Store in refrigerator.

Note. Avoid prolonged heating at any time.

Sucrose agar for Neisseria

Heart infusion broth	25.00 g
Yeast extract	3.00 g
Ionager 2 *or* washed agar	10.00 g
Sucrose	50.00 g
Calcium chloride, 1.0 M	0.50 ml
Distilled water	1.00 liter

1. Dissolve the sucrose in 250 ml of water.
2. Dissolve the broth, yeast extract, and agar in 750 ml of water.
3. Dissolve 0.735 g of $CaCl_2$ in 10 ml of water.
4. Autoclave all solutions separately and cool to 50 C. Combine aseptically and pour into plates.

Sulfite-polymyxin-sulfadiazine agar

See SPS agar.

Tartrate agar* (61)
Phenol red tartrate agar

Bacto peptone *or* Trypticase	10.000 g
Sodium potassium tartrate	10.000 g
Sodium chloride	5.000 g
Agar	15.000 g
Phenol red	0.024 g
Distilled water	1.000 liter
Final pH 7.6	

Dispense about 10 ml per tube. Autoclave at 121 C for 10 min. Allow tubes to cool in the upright position.

Inoculate by stabbing deep into the medium with a straight wire and incubate at 37 C for 24 h.

Taurocholate gelatin agar (108)

Pancreatic digest of casein USP	10 g
Gelatin	30 g
Sodium taurocholate	5 g
Sodium chloride	10 g
Yeast extract	1 g
Agar	15 g
Distilled water	1 liter

1. Mix and heat with agitation.
2. Autoclave at 121 C for 15 min. Cool and dispense in petri dishes.

Note: May be used without sodium taurocholate.

TCBS agar*
Thiosulfate citrate bile salts sucrose agar

Sodium thiosulfate	10.00 g
Sodium citrate	10.00 g
Oxgall	5.00 g
Sodium cholate	3.00 g
Sucrose	20.00 g
Pancreatic digest of casein USP	5.00 g
Peptic digest of animal tissue USP	5.00 g
Yeast extract	5.00 g
Sodium chloride	10.00 g
Iron citrate	1.00 g
Thymol blue	0.04 g
Bromothymol blue	0.04 g
Agar (dried)	14.00 g
Distilled water	1.00 liter
Final pH 8.6	

Heat with agitation and boil for 1 min. Cool to 45 to 50 C and pour into plates. Do not autoclave.

Tellurite taurocholate gelatin agar

See Monsur agar.

Tellurite taurocholate peptone water

See Monsur preservative solution.

Tetrathionate broth base* (62, 92)

Polypeptone *or* Proteose	5 g
Bile salts	1 g
Calcium carbonate	10 g
Sodium thiosulfate	30 g
Distilled water	1 liter

1. Heat to boiling. Cool to less than 45 C.
2. To each 100 ml of basal medium, add 2 ml of iodine solution:

Iodine	6 g
Potassium iodide	5 g
Distilled water	20 ml

3. Do not heat after the addition of the iodine solution.
4. One ml of 1:1,000 solution of brilliant green may also be added to 100 ml of the base medium (62, 63). Sulfathiazol (0.125 mg per 100 ml of medium) may be added to prevent excessive growth of *Proteus* (37).

TGY agar* (46)
Tryptone (Tryptophan peptone) glucose yeast agar

Pancreatic digest of casein USP	5 g
Dextrose	1 g
Yeast extract	5 g
Dipotassium phosphate	1 g
Agar	15 g
Distilled water	1 liter

Combine all ingredients except agar and warm to dissolve. Adjust to pH 6.8 to 7.0. Add agar and heat to boiling. Dispense 5 ml per 16 by 125 mm tube and autoclave at 121 C for 15 min.

Thayer-Martin agar*

Combine sterile solutions, with the agar base cooled to 50 C.

GC agar base* sterile, double-strength, 100 ml (*see* Chocolate agars).

Hemoglobin,* 2% aqueous, 100 ml, *or* Chocolated defibrinated blood, 5%.

Antibiotic inhibitors* to give final concentrations per 100 ml of medium of: vancomycin, 300 μg; colistin, 750 μg; and nystatin, 1,250 units.

Chemical enrichment, e.g., 1% IsoVitalex*

Vitamin B_{12}	0.010 g
L-Glutamine	10.000 g
Adenine	1.000 g
Guanine hydrochloride	0.030 g
p-Aminobenzoic acid	0.013 g
L-Cystine	1.100 g
Dextrose	100.000 g
Diphosphophyridine nucleotide oxidized (coenzyme 1)	0.250 g
Cocarboxylase	0.100 g
Ferric nitrate	0.020 g
Thiamine hydrochloride	0.003 g
Cysteine hydrochloride	25.900 g
Distilled water	1.000 liter

Other supplements, e.g., Supplement "B,"* may be used instead of the defined chemical enrichment.

Also see Transgrow agar.

Thioglycolate medium without indicator,* plus hemin

Pancreatic digest of casein USP	17.00 g
Papaic digest of soy meal USP	3.00 g
Dextrose	6.00 g
Sodium chloride	2.50 g
Sodium thioglycolate	0.50 g
Agar	0.70 g
L-Cystine	0.25 g
Sodium sulfite	0.10 g
Purified water	1.00 liter
Hemin	5.00 mg

1. Mix and heat with agitation to obtain solution. Omit hemin, if desired.
2. Dispense in tubes with calcium carbonate chips or powder, approximately 0.1 g per tube, to promote

viability, spore formation, and maintenance of cultures.

3. Boil (or steam for 10 min) and cool to room temperature just prior to use.

4. Add filter-sterilized sodium bicarbonate to a concentration of 1 mg/ml and vitamin K_1 to a concentration of 0.1 g/ml.

5. Other supplements may be added, if desired, by introducing a pipette to the bottom of the tube and withdrawing the pipette as the supplement is added, e.g., 5% Fildes enrichment *or* 10% sterile animal serum. Do not shake or invert tubes.

Thioglycollate medium with gelatin*
Thiogel medium

As above, but with gelatin, 50 g.

Threonine deamination test broth
Buffered peptone yeast glucose medium plus threonine

Pancreatic digest of casein USP	0.50 g
Yeast extract	0.50 g
Dipotassium phosphate	0.20 g
Dextrose	0.05 g
DL-Threonine	0.30 g
Distilled water	100.00 ml
Resazurin (25 mg/100 ml of water)	0.40 ml
Salts solution (*see* PYGM broth)	4.00 ml

Boil until colorless. Cool, preferably under bubbling oxygen-free CO_2. Add 0.05 g of L-cysteine HCl. Adjust pH to 7.0 with 2 N NaOH and dispense in tubes, preferably under oxygen-free N_2. Autoclave at 121 C for 15 min. The control medium is identical except that threonine is omitted.

Tinsdale agar, Moore and Parsons, modified*

Proteose No. 3 *or* Thiotone peptic digest of animal tissue USP	20.00 g
L-Cysteine	0.24 g
Sodium chloride	5.00 g
Sodium thiosulfate	0.43 g
Agar (dried)	(14.00 g)
or not dried	20 g
Distilled water	1.00 liter
Final pH 7.4.	

1. Heat with agitation and boil for 1 min. Dispense.

2. Autoclave at 121 C for 15 min. Cool to 56 C and, to each 100 ml of base, add:

Sterile serum, e.g., bovine	10 ml
Potassium tellurite, 1% aqueous	3 ml

3. Alternatively, the thiosulfate may be dissolved in 1.7 ml of water and added separately. It must be prepared fresh each time the medium is prepared. The cystine may be dissolved in 6 ml of 0.1 N HCl and added separately, in which case it may be necessary to add 6 ml of 0.1 N NaOH to make sure that the final pH is correct.

Todd-Hewitt broth*

Beef heart, infusion from	500.0 g
Peptone component	20.0 g
Dextrose	2.0 g
Sodium chloride	2.0 g
Disodium phosphate	0.4 g
Sodium carbonate	2.5 g
Distilled water	1.0 liter
Final pH 7.8	

Dissolve, dispense, and autoclave at 121 C for 15 min.

Toxigenicity test agar, Elek

Proteose *or* Thiotone peptic digest of animal tissue USP	20.0 g
Maltose	3.0 g
Lactic acid	0.7 g
Sodium chloride	5.0 g
Agar	15.0 g
Sodium hydroxide, 40% aqueous	1.5 ml
Distilled water	1.0 liter

1. Add with agitation, to 500 ml of water, the peptone, maltose, lactic acid, and sodium hydroxide.

2. Heat to boiling and filter through Whatman no. 2 filter paper.

3. Adjust the reaction of the filtrate to pH 7.8, using 1 N HCl.

4. Add the agar and salt dissolved in 500 ml of water.

5. Mix and dispense 10-ml quantities in screw-capped tubes.

6. Autoclave at 115 C for 10 min. Store at room temperature with caps closed.

Transgrow agar*

1. Prepare as for Thayer-Martin agar, except with added dextrose, 0.15%, and the agar increased to 2% in the GC agar base.

2. Gas bottles with 20% CO_2 in air and tighten caps securely.

3. Trimethoprim lactate, 5 mg/liter, may be added to either Thayer-Martin or Transgrow agars, if desired, especially for examination of rectal specimens.

Transport media for anaerobes (PRAS)

A. *Without peptones*

Ionagar 2 or equivalent	2.00 g
Resazurin solution	0.40 ml
See Cary and Blair transport medium, modified (PRAS)	
L-Cysteine hydrochloride	0.05 g
Distilled water	100.00 ml

1. In a flask, boil above ingredients except cysteine.

2. When dissolved, gas with carbon dioxide.

3. Add cysteine. When dissolved, adjust pH to 6.8 with 20% sodium hydroxide.

4. Cap the flask with a rubber stopper, pass into an anaerobic chamber, and dispense aseptically into tubes.

B. *PYG medium*

Peptone or Gelysate, pancreatic digest of gelatin	1.00 g
Yeast extract	1.00 g
Dextrose	1.00 g
Resazurin solution	0.40 ml
Distilled water	100.00 ml
L-Cysteine hydrochloride	0.05 g
Salts solution	4.00 ml

1. Boil ingredients except cysteine until colorless.
2. Cool to 45 C while gassing with carbon dioxide.
3. Add cysteine. When dissolved, adjust pH to 6.8 with 20% sodium hydroxide.
4. Cap the flask with a rubber stopper, pass into an anaerobic chamber and dispense aseptically into tubes.

Note. Salts solution formula:

Calcium chloride	0.2 g
Magnesium sulfate	0.2 g
Dipotassium phosphate	1.0 g
Monopotassium phosphate	1.0 g
Sodium bicarbonate	10.0 g
Distilled water	1.0 liter

C. *See Cary and Blair media*

Triple sugar iron agar*
TSI agar

Pancreatic digest of casein USP	10.00 g
Peptic digest of animal tissue USP	10.00 g
or	
Beef extract	(3.00 g)
Yeast extract	(3.00 g)
Peptone components	(20.00 g)
Dextrose	1.000 g
Lactose	10.000 g
Sucrose	10.000 g
Ferrous sulfate *or* ferrous ammonium sulfate	0.200 g
Sodium chloride	5.000 g
Sodium thiosulfate	0.300 g
Agar	12.000 g
or	13.000 g
Phenol red	0.024 g
Distilled water	1.000 liter

Dispense for 2.5-cm butts and 3.8-cm slants. Autoclave at 121 C for 15 min.

This medium is recommended for the detection of hydrogen sulfide production by the *Enterobacteriaceae* (*see also* Peptone iron agar). Inoculate by stabbing into the butt and streaking the slant. Incubate at 37 C and observe daily for 7 days for blackening. Changes in pH in the butt and on the slant are recorded after 18 to 24 h only.

Tryptic soy agar

See Soybean casein digest agar USP.

Tryptic soy broth

See Soybean casein digest broth USP.

Trypticase peptone glucose (TPG) broth
Tryptophan peptone glucose broth

Pancreatic digest of casein USP	50 g
Peptone: e.g., Gelysate pancreatic digest of gelatin	5 g
Dextrose	4 g
Sodium thioglycolate	2 g
Distilled water	1 liter

Dissolve and adjust to pH 7.0. Fill test tubes half full and autoclave at 121 C for 15 min. If not to be used immediately, omit the thioglycolate and add aseptically, just before use, a 10% sterile thioglycolate solution to give a 0.2% final concentration.

Trypticase soy agar

See Soybean casein digest agar USP.

Trypticase soy broth

See Soybean casein digest broth USP.

Tryptone broth

See Indole test broth.

Tryptone glucose yeast agar slants

See TGY agar.

Tryptone-sulfite-neomycin agar

See TSN agar.

Tryptone yeast glucose medium, buffered

See Threonine deamination test broth.

Tryptose or Biosate agar*

A. *Brucella, chapter 25*

Tryptose	20.000 g
and Thiamine hydrochloride	0.005 g
or Biosate (high in thiamine)	20.000 g
Sodium chloride	5.000 g
Dextrose	1.000 g
Agar	15.000 g
Water	1.000 liter
Final pH 7.2	

Dissolve, dispense, and autoclave at 121 C for 15 min.

B. *Erysipelothrix, chapter 14*

As above, with 5% whole blood or serum added aseptically to the sterile, fluid agar medium at 50 C before dispensing.

C. *Listeria, chapter 13*

Peptone, Tryptose *or* Biosate	20.0 g
Dextrose	2.0 g
Sodium chloride	5.0 g
Disodium phosphate	2.5 g
Agar	20.0 g
Distilled water	1.0 liter
Final pH 7.3	

Autoclave at 121 C for 15 min.

Tryptose or Biosate broth*

A. *Brucella, chapter 25*

As for the solid medium A, but without agar.*

B. *Listeria, chapter 13*

As for the solid medium C, but without agar.*

Tryptose or Biosate extract agar*

Erysipelothrix, chapter 14

Beef extract	3 g
Peptone: Tryptose *or* Biosate	15 g
Sodium chloride	5 g
Agar	18 g
Distilled water	1 liter
Final pH 7.6	

Heat to dissolve and filter through cotton or several layers of milk filter disks. Autoclave at 121 C for 15 min and dispense; 5% whole blood or serum may be added aseptically before dispensing, if desired.

Tryptose or Biosate extract broth

As above, but without agar.

TSC agar

Tryptose or Biosate	15.00 g
Papaic digest of soya meal	5.00 g
Yeast extract	5.00 g
Sodium metabisulfite	1.00 g
Ferric ammonium citrate	1.00 g
Agar	20.00 g
Distilled water	1.00 liter

1. Adjust pH to 7.6.
2. Autoclave at 121 C for 10 min.
3. Cool to 50 C and add 40 ml of 1% filter-sterilized cycloserine.
4. Add 80 ml of sterile 50% egg yolk emulsion, if medium is not used for overlaying plates.
5. Dispense in petri dishes and air-dry for 24 h prior to use.

TSN agar*

Tryptophan peptone sulfite neomycin agar

Pancreatic digest of casein USP	15.00 g
Sodium sulfite	1.00 g
Neomycin sulfate	0.02 g
Polymyxin sulfate	0.05 g
Yeast extract	10.00 g
Ferric citrate	0.50 g
Agar (dried)	13.50 g
Purified water USP	1.00 liter
Final pH 7.2 ±	

1. Heat with agitation and boil to dissolve.
2. Dispense in screw-capped containers and autoclave, with caps loose, at 118 C for 12 min. Close caps while the medium is very hot. Store in a refrigerator.
3. When remelting the medium, remelt only once with minimal heat exposure and not in the autoclave.

Tween-dextrose agar

See Polysorbate dextrose agar.

Tyrosine or xanthine agar

Nutrient agar*	23 g
Tyrosine *or*	5 g
Xanthine	4 g
Demineralized water	1 liter

1. Dissolve the nutrient agar in 500 ml of water.
2. Add tyrosine or xanthine and mix to distribute the crystals evenly.
3. Adjust to pH 7.0 and autoclave at 121 C for 15 min.
4. Dispense in plates, 20 ml per plate, with the crystals evenly distributed.

Recommended for differentiation of species of aerobic actinomycetes. Use as for Casein agar.

Urease test agar* (14)

Urea agar base, Christensen

A. *For Enterobacteriaceae, chapter 18*

Urea concentrate

Peptone or Gelysate	1.000 g
Pancreatic digest of gelatin	
Sodium chloride	5.000 g
Dextrose	1.000 g
Monopotassium phosphate	2.000 g
Phenol red	0.012 g
Urea	20.000 g
Distilled water	100.000 ml

Adjust to pH 6.8 and sterilize by filtration. Dissolve 15 g of agar in 900 ml of water and autoclave at 121 C for 15 min. Cool to 50 to 55 C in a water bath and add 100 ml of sterile urea concentrate. Cool in a slanted position to form slants with deep butts.

Inoculate heavily over the entire surface of the slant and incubate at 37 C. Examine at 2 h, 4 h, and after overnight incubation. Negative tubes should be observed daily for 4 days in order to detect delayed reactions given by members of certain groups other than *Proteus*. Urease-positive cultures produce an alkaline reaction evidenced by a red color.

B. *For aerobic actinomycetes, chapter 17*

Prepare agar base by dissolving 20 g of agar in 500 ml of demineralized water; dissolve the salts, peptone, and glucose in the remaining 500 ml of water. Combine and adjust to pH 6.9. To 1 liter of base cooled to 50 C, add 100 ml of 20% filter-sterilized urea solution. Dispense, slant, and inoculate as above.

Urease test broth* (117)

Urea solution

Yeast extract	0.100 g
Monopotassium phosphate	0.091 g
Disodium phosphate	0.095 g
Urea	20.000 g
Phenol red	0.010 g
Distilled water	1.000 liter

Sterilize by passing through Seitz filter and dispense 3-ml amounts in tubes. Alternatively, prepare basal medium in 900 ml of distilled water and autoclave at 121 C for 15 min. After cooling, 100 ml of

20% filter-sterilized urea solution is added and the medium is dispensed in sterile tubes.

Inoculate with three loopfuls (2-mm loop) from an agar slant culture, and shake to suspend the bacteria. Incubate in a water bath at 37 C and read after 10 min, 60 min, and 2 h.

USAMU medium (38)

L-Cysteine hydrochloride (should be from pretested lots)	5.0 g
Sodium thioglycolate	2.0 g
Tryptose broth with thiamine *or* Biosate broth	26.0 g
Dextrose	9.0 g
Agar	15.0 g
Distilled water	1.0 liter

1. Place the L-cysteine hydrochloride and sodium thioglycolate in a dry flask and add the water. Dissolve by mixing, but do not heat.
2. Add Tryptose broth with thiamine or Biosate broth and the dextrose, and mix with magnetic stirrer. Adjust to *p*H 7.2 with 0.1 N NaOH.
3. Add agar and autoclave at 121 C for 20 min.
4. Cool and add 50 ml of defibrinated rabbit or sheep blood (should be from pretested lots).
5. Add antibiotics as in Glucose cysteine blood agar.

Virology media

See Tables 2–4.

Voges-Proskauer broth (16)

See also MR-VP broth.

For Bacillus anthracis, chapter 15

Peptone component	5 g
Dextrose	5 g
Sodium chloride	5 g
Distilled water	1 liter

Dispense in 5-ml amounts in 18-mm tubes and autoclave.

Wagatsuma agar* (101)

For Vibrio, chapter 21

Yeast extract	3 g
Peptone	10 g
Sodium chloride	70 g
Dipotassium phosphate	5 g
Mannitol	10 g
Crystal violet	0.01 g
Agar	15 g
Distilled water	1 liter

1. Heat in flowing steam or boiling water until agar is melted. The pH should be about 8.0.
2. Do not autoclave.
3. Cool to 50 C in a water bath and add 5% thrice-washed (in saline) rabbit or human erythrocytes.
4. Mix and pour into petri plates.

Editors' note. The author states that Bacto peptone must be used.

Weed agar

Fresh meat extract broth	1 liter
Agar	15 g
Peptone *or* Gelysate	10 g
Sodium chloride	5 g

Adjust to *p*H 7.2. Dispense in 100-ml portions and autoclave at 121 C for 15 min. Store base at 4 C. Melt one 100-ml portion, cool to 55 C, and aseptically add:

Sheep blood	5 ml
Bacitracin	2,500 units
Polymyxin	590 units
Cycloheximide	10 mg

Pour into six plates.

Wickerham broths

A. *For carbohydrate assimilation tests*

1. Use 100 ml of Yeast Nitrogen Base (YNB),* 10×, without asparagine and dextrose.
2. Add 10 g of carbohydrate, except 20 g of raffinose. *See* Auxanographic media.
3. Filter-sterilize.
4. Add 0.5 ml of this concentrate to tubes containing 4.5 ml of sterile distilled water.

B. *For nitrate assimilation tests*

1. Use 100 ml of YCB,* 10×.
2. Add 0.78 g of potassium nitrate or of peptone.
3. Sterilize by filtration and follow the procedure for carbohydrate assimilation tests with Wickerham media.

Note. Inoculation for both tests should be with a suspension of starved yeast which gives at least 95% T at 530 nm in a spectrophotometer. Incubate at 25 to 30 C with shaking. Examine tubes for growth as indicated by turbidity.

Wickerham media, modified

Bromocresol purple, 1.6%	1.0 ml
Deionized water	450.0 ml
Sodium hydroxide, 0.1 N	5.0 ml
Washed agar	10.0 g

Mix and heat to dissolve. Cool to 45 to 50 C.

A. *For carbohydrate assimilation*

1. To 50 ml of YNB, 10×, without asparagine and dextrose, add 5.0 g of carbohydrate.
2. Admix to the melted basal medium.
3. Dispense in 5-ml amounts in sterile screw-capped tubes.
4. Autoclave at 115 C for 10 min. Cool in the slanted position.
5. Test each lot with standard control cultures of *Candida krusei, C. guillermondii, C. tropicalis,* and *Cryptococcus neoformans.*

B. *For nitrate assimilation*

1. To 50 ml of YCB, 10×, add 0.5 g of peptone or potassium nitrate and filter-sterilize.
2. Admix to the melted basal medium.
3. Proceed as above for 3, 4, and 5.

Wolin-Bevis agar (136)

Polysorbate (Tween) 80	3.00 ml
Dextrose	0.25 g
L-Histidine hydrochloride	6.25 g
Ammonium sulfate	1.00 g
Monopotassium phosphate	1.00 g
Agar	20.00 g
Distilled water	1.00 liter

Dissolve and autoclave at 121 C for 15 min.

Worfel-Ferguson agar*

Sodium chloride	2.00 g
Potassium sulfate	1.00 g
Magnesium sulfate	0.25 g
Sucrose	20.00 g
Yeast extract	2.00 g
Agar	15.00 g
Distilled water	1.00 liter

Do not adjust pH. Autoclave at 121 C for 15 min.

This medium is recommended for the enhancement of capsule production in *Klebsiella* cultures. The agar may be omitted, as in the original formula of Worfel and Ferguson, and the mixture is then employed as a liquid medium.

Xanthine agar

See Tyrosine agar.

Xylose lysine deoxycholate agar USP* (121)
X L D agar,* X L agar base*

Xylose	3.50 g
L-Lysine	5.00 g
Lactose	7.50 g
Sucrose	7.50 g
Sodium chloride	5.00 g
Yeast extract	3.00 g
Phenol red	0.08 g
Agar (dried)	13.50 g
Sodium deoxycholate	2.50 g
Sodium thiosulfate	6.80 g
Ferric ammonium citrate	0.80 g
Distilled water	1.00 liter

Final pH 7.4.

Heat with agitation just until the medium boils. Transfer *at once* to 45 to 50 C water bath. Pour into plates *as soon as* the medium has cooled.

Alternatively, prepare the base (as above except last three ingredients). Autoclave, cool, and admix: (i) 20 ml of aqueous solution containing 34% sodium thiosulfate and 4% ferric ammonium citrate; (ii) 25 ml of 10% aqueous sodium deoxycholate.

Yeast ascospore agar (78)

Potassium acetate	10.0 g
Yeast extract	2.5 g
Dextrose	1.0 g
Agar	30.0 g
Distilled water	1.0 liter

Dissolve, tube, and autoclave at 121 C for 15 min.

Ascospores are obtained in 2 to 6 days at room temperature (23 to 25 C).

Yeast beef broth*

See Antibiotic medium 20.

Yeast carbon base* (YCB), 10×
Wickerham carbon base broth

Boric acid	0.500 mg
Copper sulfate	0.040 mg
Potassium iodide	0.100 mg
Ferric chloride	0.200 mg
Manganese sulfate	0.400 mg
Sodium molybdate	0.200 mg
Zinc sulfate	0.400 mg
Biotin	0.002 mg
Calcium pantothenate	0.400 mg
Folic acid	0.002 mg
Inositol	2.000 mg
Niacin	0.400 mg
p-Aminobenzoic acid	0.200 mg
Pyridoxine	0.400 mg
Riboflavine	0.200 mg
Thiamine hydrochloride	0.400 mg
L-Histidine hydrochloride	0.001 g
DL-Methionine	0.002 g
DL-Tryptophan	0.002 g
Potassium phosphate	1.000 g
Magnesium sulfate	0.500 g
Sodium chloride	0.100 g
Calcium chloride	0.100 g
Dextrose	10.000 g
Water	1.000 liter

Final pH of the base 4.5 ±

Dissolve and sterilize by filtration.
Dispense aseptically.

Yeast nitrogen base,* 10×, supplemented with asparagine and dextrose
For susceptibility tests

Boric acid	500.0 μg
Copper sulfate	40.0 μg
Potassium iodide	100.0 μg
Ferric chloride	200.0 μg
Manganese sulfate	400.0 μg
Sodium molybdate	200.0 μg
Zinc sulfate	400.0 μg
Biotin	2.0 μg
Calcium pantothenate	400.0 μg
Folic acid	2.0 μg
Inositol	2000.0 μg
Niacin	400.0 μg
p-Aminobenzoic acid	200.0 μg
Pyridoxine hydrochloride	400.0 μg
Riboflavine	200.0 μg
Thiamine hydrochloride	400.0 μg
L-Histidine monohydrochloride	10.0 mg
DL-Methionine	20.0 mg
DL-Tryptophan	20.0 mg
Magnesium sulfate	500.0 mg
Sodium chloride	100.0 mg
Calcium chloride	100.0 mg
Ammonium sulfate	5.0 g
Monopotassium phosphate	1.0 g
L-Asparagine	1.5 g

Dextrose	10.0 g
Purified water	100.0 ml

Dissolve, sterilize by filtration, and dispense aseptically.

LITERATURE CITED

1. American Public Health Association. 1967. Standard methods for the examination of dairy products, 12th ed., p. 236. American Public Health Association, Inc., New York.
2. Amies, C. R. 1967. A modified formula for the preparation of Stuart's transport medium. Can. J. Pub. Health **58**:296–300.
3. Amies, C. R., and J. I. Douglas. 1965. Some defects in bacteriological transport media. Can J. Pub. Health **56**:27.
4. Anaerobe Laboratory. 1972. Outline of clinical methods in anaerobic bacteriology. Anaerobe Laboratory, Virginia Polytechnic Institute, Blacksburg.
5. Balamuth, W. 1946. Improved egg yolk infusion for cultivation of *Entamoeba histolytica* and other intestinal protozoa. Amer. J. Clin. Pathol. **16**:380.
6. Bernaerts, M. J., and J. DeLey. 1963. A biochemical test for crown gall bacteria. Nature (London) **197**:406–407.
7. Bioquest. 1968. BBL manual of products and laboratory procedures, 5th ed., p. 88. Bioquest, Division of Becton, Dickinson and Co., Cockeysville, Md.
8. Boeck, W. C., and J. Drbolav. 1925. The cultivation of *Endamoeba histolytica*. Amer. J. Hyg. **5**:371–407.
9. Brown, V. I., and E. J. Lowbury. 1965. Use of an improved cetrimide agar medium and other culture methods for *Pseudomonas aeruginosa*. J. Clin. Pathol. **18**:752–756.
10. Carlquist, P. R. 1956. A biochemical test for separating paracolon groups. J. Bacteriol. **71**:339–341.
11. Cary, S. G., and E. B. Blair. 1964. New transport medium for shpment of clinical specimens. I. Fecal specimens. J. Bacteriol. **88**:96–98.
12. Cato, E. P., et al. 1970. Outline of clinical methods in anaerobic bacteriology, p. 100. Anaerobe Laboratory, Virginia Polytechnic Institute & State Univ. Blacksburg, Va.
13. Chilton, M. L., and M. Fulton. 1946. A presumptive medium for differentiating paracolon from *Salmonella* cultures. J. Lab. Clin. Med. **31**:824–827.
14. Christensen, W. B. 1946. Urea decomposition as a means of differentiating Proteus and paracolon cultures from each other and from Salmonella and Shigella types. J. Bacteriol. **52**:461–466.
15. Christensen, W. B. 1949. Hydrogen sulfide production and citrate utilization in the differentiation of enteric pathogens and coliform bacteria. Research Bulletin No. 1, p. 3. Weld County Health Department, Greeley, Colo.
16. Coblentz, L. M. 1943. Rapid detection of the production of acetyl-methyl-carbinol. Amer. J. Public Health **33**:815–817.
17. Cohen-Bazire, G., W. R. Sistrom, and R. Y. Stanier. 1957. Kinetic studies of pigment synthesis by non-sulfur purple bacteria. J. Cell. Comp. Physiol. **49**:25–68.
18. Committee on Cultures, Society of Protozoologists. 1958. A catalogue of laboratory strains of free-living and parasitic protozoa. J. Protozool. **5**:1–3.
19. Davis, B. R., and W. H. Ewing. 1964. Lipolytic, pectolytic, and alginolytic activities of Enterobacteriaceae. J. Bacteriol. **88**:16–19.
20. Difco. 1953. Manual of dehydrated culture media and reagents, 9th ed., p. 16–22 and 134. Difco Laboratories, Detroit, Mich.
21. Dowell, V. R., Jr., and T. M. Hawkins. 1973. Laboratory methods in anaerobic bacteriology. CDC Laboratory Manual, Department of Health, Education, and Welfare Publ. No. 73-8222.
22. Downs, C. M., L. L. Coriell, S. S. Chapman, and A. Klauber. 1947. The cultivation of Bacterium tularense in embryonated eggs. J. Bacteriol. **53**:89–100.
23. Dulaney, A. D., K. Guo, and H. Packer. 1948. *Donovania granulomatis:* Cultivation, antigen preparation and immunological tests. J. Immunol. **59**:335–340.
24. Ederer, G. M. and M. Clar. 1970. Motility-indole-ornithine medium. Appl. Microbiol. **2**:849–850.
25. Edwards, P. R., and W. H. Ewing. 1962. Identification of Enterobacteriaceae, 2nd ed. Burgess Publishing Co., Minneapolis, Minn.
26. Edwards, P. R., and M. A. Fife. 1956. Cyanide media in the differentiation of enteric bacteria. Appl. Microbiol. **4**:46–48.
27. Edwards, P. R., and M. A. Fife. 1961. Lysine-iron agar in the detection of *Arizona* cultures. Appl. Microbiol. **9**:478–480.
28. Edwards, P. R., M. A. Fife, and W. H. Ewing. 1956. Newer biochemical methods in the recognition of shigellae and salmonellae. Amer. J. Med. Technol. **22**:28.
29. Ellis, R. J., P. R. Edwards, and M. A. Fife. 1957. The differentiation of the *Salmonella* and *Arizona* groups by utilization of organic acids. Pub. Health Lab. **15**:89.
30. Emmons, C. W., C. H. Binford, and J. P. Utz. 1963. Medical mycology. Lea and Febiger, Philadelphia.
31. Ewing, W. H. 1960. *Enterobacteriaceae:* biochemical methods for group differentiation. Pub. Health Serv. Publ. 734.
32. Ewing, W. H., B. R. Davis, and R. W. Reaves. 1957. Phenylalanine and malonate media and their use in enteric bacteriology. Pub. Health Lab. **15**:153.
33. Falkow, S. 1958. Activity of lysine decarboxylase as an aid in the identification of salmonellae and shigellae. Amer. J. Clin. Pathol. **29**:598.
34. Feinberg, J. G., and M. J. Whittington. 1957. A culture medium for *Trichomonas vaginalis* Donne and species of Candida. J. Clin. Pathol. **10**:327–329.
35. Fildes, P. 1920. A new medium for the growth of *B. influenzae*. Brit. J. Exp. Pathol. **1**:129–130.
36. Galton, M. M., W. D. Lowery, and A. V. Hardy. 1954. *Salmonella* in fresh and smoked pork sausage. J. Infec. Dis. **95**:232.
37. Galton, M. M., J. E. Scatterday, and A. V. Hardy. 1952. Salmonellosis in dogs. I. Bacteriological, epidemiological and clinical considerations. J. Infec. Dis. **91**:1–5.
38. Gaspar, A. J., H. B. Tresselt, and M. K. Ward. 1961. New solid medium for enhanced growth of *Pasteurella tularensis*. J. Bacteriol. **82**:564–569.
39. Georg, L. K., L. Ajello, and C. Papegeorge. 1954. Use of cycloheximide in the selective isolation of fungi pathogenic to man. J. Lab. Clin. Med. **44**:422–428.
40. Gohar, M. A., and M. Makkawi. 1948. Cholera in Egypt, laboratory diagnosis and protective inoculation. J. Trop. Med. Hyg. **51**:95–99.
41. Gohar, M. A., and M. Makkawi. 1948. Isolation of the cholera vibrio. J. Roy. Egypt. Med. Ass. **31**:462.
42. Goldberg, J. 1959. Studies on granuloma inguinale. IV. Growth requirements of *Donovania granulomatis* and its relationship to the natural habitat of the organism. Brit. J. Vener. Dis. **35**:266–268.
43. Hajna, A. A. 1951. Preparation and application of Wilson and Blair's bismuth sulfite agar medium. Pub. Health Lab. **9**:48–50.
44. Hajna, A. A., and S. R. Damon. 1956. New enrichment

and plating media for the isolation of *Salmonella* and *Shigella* organisms. Appl. Microbiol. **4**:341-345.
45. Harvey, R. W. W. 1956. Choice of a selective medium for the routine isolation of members of the *Salmonella* group. Mon. Bull. Min. Health Public Health Lab. Serv. **15**:118-124.
46. Haynes, W. C. 1951. *Pseudomonas aeruginosa*—its characterization and identification. J. Gen. Microbiol. **5**:939-950.
47. Herbert, V. 1956. Aseptic addition method for *L. casei* assay of folate activity in human serum. J. Clin. Pathol. **19**:12-16.
48. Hinshaw, W. R. 1941. Cysteine and related compounds for differentiating members of the genus *Salmonella*. Hilgardia **13**:583-621.
49. Holdeman, L. V., and W. E. C. Moore. 1972. Anaerobe laboratory manual. Anaerobe Laboratory, Virginia Polytechnic Institute & State Univ., Blacksburg, Va.
50. Holt-Harris, J. E., and O. Teague. 1916. A new culture medium for the isolation of *Bacillus typhosus* from stools. J. Infec. Dis. **18**:596-600.
51. Huff, C. G. 1964. Cultivation of the exoerythrocytic stages of malarial parasites. Amer. J. Trop. Med. Hyg. **13**:171-177.
52. Hugh, R. 1965. A comparison of the proposed neotype strain and 258 isolates of *Vibrio cholerae* Pacini. Int. Bull. Bacteriol. Nomen. Taxon. **15**:13-24.
53. Hugh, R. 1966. A comparison of the neotype strain and 119 isolates of *Vibrio eltor* Pribram 1933. Indian J. Med. Res. **54**:839-848.
54. Hugh, R., and E. Leifson. 1953. The taxonomic significance of fermentative *versus* oxidative metabolism of carbohydrates by various gram-negative bacteria. J. Bacteriol. **66**:24-26.
55. Hunter, G. W., III, W. W. Frye, and J. C. Swartzwelder. 1966. A manual of tropical medicine, 4th ed. W. B. Saunders Co., Philadelphia.
56. Hutner, S. H., A Cury, and H. Baker. 1958. Microbiological assays. Anal. Chem. **30**:849-867.
57. Jameson, J. E., and N. W. Emberley. 1956. A substitute for bile salts in culture media. J. Gen. Microbiol. **15**:198-204.
58. Johnson, J. G., L. J. Kunz, W. Barron, and W. H. Ewing. 1966. Biochemical differentiation of the *Enterobacteriaceae* with the aid of lysine-iron-agar. Appl. Microbiol. **14**:212-217.
59. Johnson, R. C., and V. G. Harris. 1967. Differentiation of pathogenic and saprophytic leptospires. I. Growth at low temperatures. J. Bacteriol. **94**:27-31.
60. Jones, G. L., and P. L. Kendrick. 1969. Study of a blood-free medium for transport and growth of *Bordetella pertussis*. Health Lab. Sci. **6**:40-45.
61. Jordan, E. O., and P. H. Harmon. 1928. New differential medium for paratyphoid group. J. Infec. Dis. **42**:238-241.
62. Kauffman, F. 1935. Weitere erfahrungen mit den kombinierten Anreicherungs verfahren fur Salmonellabacillen. Z. Hyg. Infectionskr. **117**:26-32.
63. Kauffman, F. 1954. *Enterobacteriaceae*, 2nd ed. Einar Munksgaard, Copenhagen.
64. Kauffman, F., and A. Peterson. 1956. The biochemical group and type differentiation of *Enterobacteriaceae* by organic acids. Acta. Pathol. Microbiol. Scand. **38**:481-491.
65. King, E. O. 1960. The identification of unusual pathogenic gram negative bacteria. Communicable Disease Center, Atlanta, Ga.
66. King, E. O., M. K. Ward, and D. E. Raney. 1954. Two simple media for the demonstration of pyocyanin and fluorescein. J. Lab. Clin. Med. **44**:301-307.
67. Kohn, J. 1953. A preliminary report of a new gelatin liquefaction method. J. Clin. Pathol. **6**:249.
68. Kristensen, M., V. Lester, and A. Juergens. 1925. Use of trypsinized casein, brom-thymol-blue, brom-cresol-purple, phenol-red and brilliant green for bacteriological nutrient media. Brit. J. Exp. Pathol. **6**:291-299.
69. Kupferberg, A. B., G. Johnson, and H. Sprince. 1948. Nutritional requirements of *T. vaginalis*. Proc. Soc. Exp. Biol. Med. **67**:304-308.
70. Lautrop, H. 1956. A modified Kohn's test for the demonstration of bacterial gelatin liquefaction. Acta Pathol. Microbiol. Scand. **39**:357.
71. LeClair, R. A., H. Zen-Hoji, and S. Sakai. 1970. Isolation and identification of *Vibrio parahaemolyticus* from clinical specimens. J. Conf. Pub. Hlth. Lab. Dir. **28**:82-92.
72. Leifson, E. 1933. The fermentation of sodium malonate as a means of differentiating Aerobacter and Escherichia. J. Bacteriol. **26**:329-330.
73. Leifson, E. 1935. New culture media based on sodium desoxycholate for the isolation of intestinal pathogens and for the enumeration of colon bacilli in milk and water. J. Pathol. Bacteriol. **40**:581-599.
74. Leifson, E. 1936. New selenite enrichment media for the isolation of typhoid and paratyphoid (*Salmonella*) bacilli. Amer. J. Hyg. **24**:423-432.
75. Leifson, E. 1943. Preparation and properties of bacteriological peptones. Bull. Johns Hopkins Hosp. **72**:179-199.
76. Leifson, E. 1960. Atlas of bacterial flagellation. Academic Press Inc., New York.
77. Levine, M., and H. W. Schoenlein. 1930. A compilation of culture media for the cultivation of microorganisms. Society of American Bacteriologists, Monographs on Systematic Bacteriology, vol. 2. The Williams & Wilkins Co., Baltimore.
78. McClary, D. O., W. L. Nulty, and G. R. Miller. 1959. Effect of potassium versus sodium in the sporulation of Saccharomyces. J. Bacteriol. **78**:362-368.
79. McClung, L. S., and R. Toabe. 1947. The egg yolk plate reaction for the presumptive diagnosis of *Clostridium sporogenes* and certain species of the gangrene and botulinum groups. J. Bacteriol. **53**:139-147.
80. MacConkey, A. T. 1905. Lactose-fermenting bacteria in faeces. J. Hyg. **5**:333-379.
81. MacConkey, A. T. 1908. Bile salt media and their advantages in some bacteriological examinations. J. Hyg. **8**:322-344.
82. McQuay, R. M. 1956. Charcoal medium for the growth and maintenance of large and small races of *E. histolytica in vitro*. Amer. J. Clin. Pathol. **26**:1137-1141.
83. Marcus, P. I., and P. Talalay. 1956. Induction and purification of alpha- and beta-hydroxysteroid dehydrogenases. J. Biol. Chem. **218**:661-674.
84. Martin, W. J., and W. H. Ewing. 1967. The desoxyribonuclease test as applied to certain gram negative bacteria. Can. J. Microbiol. **13**:616-618.
85. Mishulow, L., L. S. Sharpe, and L. L. Cohen. 1953. Beef-heart charcoal agar for the preparation of pertussis vaccine. Amer. J. Pub. Health **43**:1466-1472.
86. Moeller, V. 1954. Diagnostic use of the Braun KCN test within the *Enterobacteriaceae*. Acta Pathol. Microbiol. Scand. **34**:115-126.
87. Moeller, V. 1955. Simplified tests for some amino acid decarboxylases and for the arginine dihydrolase system. Acta Pathol. Microbiol. Scand. **36**:158-172.
88. Monsur, K. A. 1961. A highly selective gelatin-taurocholate-tellurite medium for the isolation of *Vibrio cholerae*. Trans. Roy. Soc. Trop. Med. Hyg. **55**:440-442.

89. Monsur, K. A. 1963. Bacteriological diagnosis of cholera under field conditions. Bull. World Health Organ. **28**:387–389.
90. Moore, H. B., and M. J. Pickett. 1960. *The Pseudomonas-Achromobacter* group. Can. J. Microbiol. **6**:35–42.
91. Morris, E. J. 1958. Selective media for some *Pasteurella* species. J. Gen. Microbiol. **19**:305–311.
92. Mueller, L. 1923. Un nouveau milieu d'enrichissement pour le recherche du bacille typhique et des parathyphiques. C. R. Soc. Biol. **89**:434–437.
93. Ninomiya, K., F. Ohtani, S. Koosaka, H. Kamiya, K. Ueno, S. Suzuki, and T. Inoue. 1972. Simple and expedient methods of differentiation among Bacteroids, Sphaerophorus and Fusobacterium. Jap. J. Med. Sci. Biol. **25**:63–73.
94. Norman, L., and M. M. Brooke. 1955. The effectiveness of the PVA-fixative technique in revealing intestinal amebae in diagnostic cultures. Amer. J. Trop. Med. Hyg. **4**:479–482.
95. Norman, L., and M. M. Brooke. 1955. The use of penicillin and streptomycin in the routine cultivation of amebae from fecal specimens. Amer. J. Trop. Med. Hyg. **4**:472–478.
96. Oxoid. 1965. The Oxoid manual, 3rd ed., p. 13–18. Oxoid Laboratories, London.
97. Phillips, B. P. 1951. Comparative effects of certain species of *Trypanosomidae* on the growth of *E. histolytica*. Amer. J. Trop. Med. **31**:290–294.
98. Reardon, L. V., and C. W. Rees. 1939. The cultivation of *Endamoeba histolytica* without serum. J. Parasitol. **25**(Suppl.):13–14.
99. Reeves, R. E., H. E. Meleney, and W. W. Frye. 1957. A modified Shaffer-Frye technique for the cultivation of *E. histolytica*. Amer. J. Hyg. **66**:56–62.
100. Sachs, A. 1939. Difficult association with bacteriological diagnosis of bacillary dysentery. J. Roy. Army Med. Cor. **73**:235–239.
101. Sakazaki, R., K. Tamura, T. Kato, Y. Obara, S. Yamai, and K. Hobo. 1968. Studies on the enteropathogenic faculatively halophilic bacteria, *Vibrio parahaemolyticu*. Jap. J. Med. Sci. Biol. **21**:325–331.
102. Shaffer, J. G., and V. Iralu. 1963. Studies on the growth requirements of *E. histolytica*. Amer. J. Trop. Med. **12**:19–21.
103. Shepard, M. C. 1967. Cultivation and properties of T-strains of Myocoplasma associated with nongonococcal urethritis. Ann. N.Y. Acad. Sci. **143**:505–514.
104. Shepard, M. C. 1973. Differential methods for identification of T-mycoplasmas on demonstration of urease. J. Infec. Dis **127**:S22–S25.
105. Shipolini, R., G. Konstantinow, A. A. Triponawa, and S. Atanassowa. 1959. Apocholat-Citrat-agar zur Isolierung von Shigella und Salmonella-Bakterien. Zentralbl. Bakteriol. Parasitenk. Infektionskr. Hyg. Abt. I Orig. **174**:75–80.
106. Simmons, J. S. 1926. A culture medium for differentiating organisms of typhoid-colon aerogenes group and for isolation of certain fungi. J. Infec. Dis. **39**:201–214.
107. Skinner, C. E., C. W. Emmons, and H. M. Tsuchiya, 1963. Henrici's molds, yeasts, and actinomycetes, 2nd ed. John Wiley & Sons, Inc., New York.
108. Smith, H. L., R. Freter, and F. J. Sweeney. 1961. Enumeration of cholera vibrios in fecal samples. J. Infec. Dis. **109**:31–34.
109. Smith, M. R., R. E. Gordon, and F. E. Clark. 1952. Aerobic sporeforming bacteria. U.S. Dep. Agr. Monograph No. 16.
110. Sneath, P. H. A. 1956. Cultural and biochemical characteristics of the genus *Chromobacterium*. J. Gen. Microbiol. **15**:70–98.
111. Society of American Bacteriologists. 1957. Manual of microbiological methods. McGraw-Hill Book Co., Inc., New York.
112. Spingarn, C. L., and M. H. Edelman. 1952. Further observations on the use of streptomycin and penicillin the cultivation of *Endamoeba histolytica* from stools. Amer. J. Trop. Med. **1**:412–416.
113. Staib, F. 1962. Zur Kreatinin-Kreatin-Assimilation in der Hefepilz-diagnostik. Zentralbl. Bakteriol. Parasitenk. Infektionskr. Hyg. Abt. I Orig. **191**:429–432.
114. Stanier, R. Y., N. J. Palleroni, and M. Doudoroff. 1966. The aerobic pseudomonads: a taxonomic study. J. Gen. Microbiol. **43**:159–271.
115. Starr, M. P. 1947. Causal agent of bacterial root and stem disease of guayule. Phytopathology **37**:291.
116. Stern, W. 1916. Studien zur differenzierung der Bakterien der Coli Typhus Gruppe mittele gefarbter, flussiger Nahrboden. Bietrage zur Biologie der Bakteriengruppe Paratyphosus B-Enteritidis. Zentralbl. Bakteriol. Parasitenk. Infektionskr. Hyg. Abt. I **78**:481–492.
117. Stuart, C. A., E. van Stratum, and R. Rustigian. 1945. Further studies on urease production by Proteus and related organisms. J. Bacteriol. **49**:437–444.
118. Stuart, R. D. 1959. Transport medium for specimens in public health bacteriology. Publ. Health Rep. **74**:431–438.
119. Sutter, V. L., H. R. Attebery, J. E. Rosenblatt, K. S. Bricknell and S. M. Finegold. 1972. Anaerobic bacteriology manual. Extension Division, Univ. of California, Los Angeles.
120. Sykes, G. (ed.). 1956. Constituents of bacteriological culture media. Soc. Gen. Microbiol. Special Report. Cambridge Univ. Press, Cambridge.
121. Taylor, W. I. 1965. Isolation of shigellae. I. Xylose lysine agars; new media for isolation of enteric pathogens. Amer. J. Clin. Pathol. **44**:471–475.
122. Teague, O., and A. W. Clurman. 1916. A method for preserving typhoid stools for delayed examination and a comparative study of the efficacy of eosin brilliant-green agar, eosin methylene-blue agar, and Endo agar for the isolation of typhoid bacilli from stools. J. Infec. Dis. **18**:653–671.
123. Trabulsi, L. R., and W. H. Ewing. 1962. Sodium acetate medium for differentiation of *Shigella* and *Escherichia* cultures. Pub. Health Lab. **20**:137–140.
124. Tresselt, H. B., and M. K. Ward. 1964. Blood-free medium for the rapid growth of *Pasteurella tularensis*. Appl. Microbiol. **12**:504–507.
125. Vaughn, R. H., and M. Levine. 1942. Differentiation of the "intermediate" coli-like bacteria. J. Bacteriol. **44**:487–505.
126. Vera, H. D. 1944. A comparative study of materials suitable for the cultivation of clostridia. J. Bacteriol. **47**:59–69.
127. Vera, H. D. 1948. A simple medium for identification and maintenance of the gonococcus and other bacteria. J. Bacteriol. **55**:531–536.
128. Vera, H. D. 1950. Relation of peptones and other culture media ingredients to the accuracy of fermentation tests. Amer. J. Pub. Health **40**:1267–1272.
129. Vera, H. D. 1971. Quality control in diagnostic microbiology. Health Lab. Sci. **8**:176–189.
130. Veron, M., and R. Chatelain. 1973. Taxonomic study of the genus *Campylobacter* Sebald and Veron and designation of the Neotype strain for the type species, *Campylobacter fetus* (Smith and Taylor) Sebald and Veron. Int. J. Syst. Bacteriol. **23**:122–134.
131. Warren, L. G. 1960. Metabolism of *Schizotrypanum cruzi* Chagas. J. Parasitol. **46**:529–540.
132. Williams, M. O., C. A. Hopkins, and M. R. Wyllie. 1961. The *in vitro* cultivation of strigeid trematodes. Exp. Parasitol. **11**:121–127.

133. Wilson, W. J., and E. M. McV. Blair. 1926. Combination of bismuth and sodium sulfite affording enrichment and selective medium for typhoid and paratyphoid groups of bacteria. J. Pathol. Bacteriol. **29:**310.
134. Wilson, W. J., and E. M. McV. Blair. 1927. Use of a glucose bismuth sulfite iron medium for the isolation of *Bacillus typhosus* and *Bacillus proteus*. J. Hyg. **26:**374–391.
135. Wilson, W. J., and E. M. McV. Blair. 1931. Further experience of the bismuth sulfite media in the isolation of *Bacillus typhosus* and *Bacillus paratyphosus* from faeces, sewage, and water. J. Hyg. **31:**138–161.
136. Wolin, H. L., M. L. Bevis, and N. Laurora. 1962. An improved synthetic medium for the rapid production of chlamydospores by *Candida albicans*. Sabouraudia **2:**96–99.

Chapter 96

Reagents, Stains, and Miscellaneous Test Procedures

GEORGE PAIK AND MORRIS T. SUGGS

REAGENTS AND TEST PROCEDURES

All-glass impinger collecting fluid (30)

Buffered gelatin

Gelatin . . . . .2 g
Disodium phosphate anhydrous . . . .4 g
Distilled water .1 liter

Adjust reaction to pH 7.0 and autoclave at 121 C for 20 min.

Aspirates from liver abscesses—examination for amoebae

Liver abscesses suspected of being caused by *Entamoeba histolytica* are often drained, and the aspirate is examined in an attempt to determine the etiological agent. Demonstrating amoebae in the thick pus removed from the abscesses is frequently difficult. Several factors contribute to this difficulty: (i) most of the organisms are in the peripheral area of the abscess and often relatively few are free in the abscess contents; (ii) the organisms may be partially immobilized by coagulum; (iii) since the fluid is sterile, amoebae will not grow in culture when the material is inoculated in the manner routinely used for the stool cultures.

The Amoebiasis Research Unit, Durban, South Africa, has reported great success in freeing the amoebae from aspirates of liver abscesses. The following procedure incorporates the Unit's recommendations (9) and personal communication from Elsdon-Dew (1960).

1. During aspiration, a minimum of two portions of exudate are removed. These are kept separate. The first portion withdrawn, usually yellowish-white in color, seldom contains amoebae and is not examined routinely. Later portions, which are reddish in color, are likely to include organisms. The final portion containing most of the material from near the wall is most likely to be positive. (Collapse of the abscess and inflowing blood is believed to release amoebae from the tissue.) Portions obtained on later aspirations, performed after appropriate rest periods, have a greater chance of revealing organisms.

2. Ten units of the enzyme streptodornase are added to each 1 ml of thick pus, and the mixture is incubated for 30 min at 37 C with repeated shaking. This process frees the amoebae from coagulum.

3. Centrifuge the mixture at 1,000 rpm for 5 min. The sediments may be microscopically examined in wet mounts or used to inoculate culture media.

4. In culturing the material, the egg slant medium overlaid with Locke's solution is conditioned by inoculation with *Clostridium perfringens*. This can be done at the time of the inoculation with the amoebic pus, though it is preferable, if possible, to precondition the medium for 24 h at 37 C. Sterile rice powder is added at the time of inoculation of the pus. Overlay with a mixture of paraffin and petrolatum (1:1). The cultures are incubated at 37 C and examined for amoebae after 24 and 48 h.

Bacitracin grouping for group A streptococci

See chapter 8.

Bile solubility test

Reagent

Sodium deoxycholate . . . . .1 g
Distilled water, sterile . . . . .9 ml

Test procedure. To test for bile solubility, prepare two tubes, each containing a sample of fresh culture (a light suspension of the organism in buffered broth, pH 7.4). To one tube, add a few drops of a 10% solution of sodium deoxycholate. A comparable volume of sterile physiological salt solution may be added to the second tube. If the cells are "bile soluble," the tube containing the bile salt should lose its turbidity in 5 to 15 min and show an increase in viscosity concomitant with clearing.

Buffered saline

Sodium chloride, 0.85% buffered to pH 7.2 with 0.067 M potassium phosphate mixtures.

Catalase test

The organism should be grown on an agar slant heavily inoculated from a colony of the organism to be tested. The slant is usually incubated for 18 to 24 h at optimal temperature. To test for catalase, set the slant in an inclined position and pour 1 ml of a 3% solution of hydrogen peroxide over the growth. The appearance of gas bubbles indicates a positive test.

An alternative to conducting the test with a slant culture is to emulsify a colony in one drop of 30% hydrogen peroxide (superoxol) on a glass slide. Immediate bubbling is indicative of a positive catalase test. Extreme care must be exercised if a colony is taken from a blood-agar plate. The enzyme catalase is present in red blood cells, and the carry-over of blood cells with the colony can give a false-positive reaction.

Coagulase test

Tube test

To 0.5 ml of undiluted or 1:4 diluted rabbit plasma, add one loopful of growth from an 18- to 24-h-old agar culture, 0.1 ml of broth culture or a single colony from a blood-agar plate. Incubate in a water bath at 37 C and examine for clotting at intervals of 30 min for 4 h; if no clot is observed at the end of this period, examine the tubes again at 6 and 24 h. A known coagulase-positive, a coagulase-negative, and, if possible, a weak coagulase producer must be set up as controls with each test.

A positive coagulase test is represented by any degree of clotting—from a loose clot suspended in plasma to a solid clot. The majority of coagulase-positive strains will produce a clot within the first 4 h, many within 1 h. False-positive tests may occur with mixed cultures or with pure cultures of some gram-negative rods, e.g., *Pseudomonas*, but the mechanism of clotting is different. Organisms which utilize the citrate, which is used as the anticoagulant in the plasma, will produce a clot. Therefore, the organism to be tested must first be determined to possess characteristics consistent with the genus *Staphylococcus*.

Slide test

1. Emulsify a colony in a drop of water on a glass slide to produce a dense, uniform suspension. If any evidence of autoagglutination is noted before the plasma is added, the culture is not suitable for the slide test.
2. Add one loopful or drop of fresh plasma to the suspension and mix by a continuous circular motion for 5 s.
3. A positive reaction is indicated by easily visible, white clumps which usually appear immediately or within 5 s.
4. Known coagulase-positive and -negative strains must always be set up in parallel.
5. All negative tests must be confirmed by the tube test.

Darkfield examination

See chapters 3, 4, and 36.

Formalin-ether concentration technique for stool examination (24)

This concentration procedure is efficient in recovering protozoan cysts and helminth eggs and larvae, including operculated and schistosome eggs. Less distortion of cysts occurs with this technique than with the zinc sulfate method, and it is more effective in concentrating formalin-treated specimens.

If permanently stained slides are to be made, the smears should be prepared before the specimen is used for concentration. If a portion of the specimen is to be preserved in polyvinyl alcohol (PVA) fixative, this should be done before proceeding with the concentration procedure.

Procedure with fresh specimens

1. Comminute a portion of the stool specimen in sufficient saline so that upon centrifugation 10 ml of emulsion will yield about 2 ml of sediment. A portion about the size of a walnut is usually enough. The suspension can be prepared in the carton in which it is submitted or in a beaker or flat-bottom paper cup.
2. Using a small glass funnel, strain about 10 ml of the emulsion through one or two layers of wet gauze into a 15-ml pointed centrifuge tube. With wide-mesh gauze, use two layers; with narrow-mesh material, use one layer. To conserve glassware, a cone-shaped paper cup with the point cut off can be substituted for the funnel.
3. Centrifuge at 2,000 to 2,500 rpm for 1 min. Decant supernatant fluid.
4. Resuspend the sediment in fresh saline, centrifuge, and decant as before. This step may be repeated if a cleaner sediment is desired.
5. Add about 10 ml of 10% formalin to the sediment, mix thoroughly, and allow to stand for 5 min.
6. Add 3 ml of ether, stopper the tube, and shake vigorously in an inverted position for a full 30 s. Remove the stopper with care.

7. Centrifuge at 1,500 rpm for about 1 min. Four layers should result as follows: (i) ether at top, (ii) plug of debris, (iii) formalin solution, and (iv) sediment.

8. Free the plug of debris from the sides of the tube by ringing with an applicator stick, and carefully decant the top three layers. Use a cotton swab to remove any debris adhering to the sides of the tube.

9. Mix the remaining sediment with the small amount of fluid that drains back from the sides of the tube (or, if necessary, add a small amount of formalin or saline), and prepare iodine and unstained mounts in the usual manner for microscopic examination.

Procedure with formalin-preserved specimens

1. Thoroughly stir the formalin-treated specimen.

2. Depending on the size and density of the specimen, strain a sufficient quantity through gauze into a 15-ml pointed centrifuge tube to give the desired amount of sediment indicated below.

3. Add tap water, mix thoroughly, and centrifuge at 2,000 to 2,500 rpm for 1 min. The resulting sediment should be about 1 ml.

4. Decant supernatant fluid and, if desired, wash again with tap water.

5. Add about 10 ml of 10% formalin to the sediment and mix thoroughly.

6. Complete as for fresh specimens, beginning with step 6.

Gluconate oxidation to 2-ketogluconate (21)

Chapter 23

Inoculate a loopful of 24-h broth culture into a tube of 2-ketogluconate medium and incubate for 18 to 24 h. Add 0.3 ml of double-strength Benedict's solution to each tube. Place the tubes in a boiling-water bath for 10 min. Oxidation of gluconate to 2-ketogluconate is indicated by the presence of red-brown copper precipitate.

Hemolysis (13)

For Vibrio, chapter 21

Cultures to be tested are cultivated for 18 h in a medium prepared by adding 1.0% Casitone to isotonic sodium chloride (0.85%) solution. This medium is dispensed in tubes and sterilized at 121 C for 15 min. A 1-ml amount of each culture is added to 1 ml of a 5% suspension of washed sheep erythrocytes in physiological saline solution. These mixtures are incubated at 37 C for 2 h and then placed in a refrigerator at 4 to 6 C for 24 h. Hemolysin production is indicated by clearing (lysis) of the erythrocyte suspension.

Indole test

A. *For Enterobacteriaceae, chapter 18*

Kovacs' reagent (11)

Amyl or isoamyl alcohol	150 ml
p-Dimethylaminobenzaldehyde	10 g
Hydrochloric acid, concentrated	50 ml

Dissolve aldehyde in alcohol and then slowly add acid. The dry aldehyde should be light in color. Alcohols that result in indole reagents which become deep brown in color should not be used. The above-mentioned reagent is stable at room temperature and has a light color. Some authors recommend preparation of only small quantities, which are stored in a refrigerator when not in use.

Test procedure. Add about 0.5 ml of Kovacs' reagent to a 40- to 48-h peptone-water culture incubated at 37 C and shake the tube gently. A deep-red color develops in the presence of indole. Tests for indole may be made after 24 h of incubation, but, if this is to be done, 1 or 2 ml of culture should be removed aseptically for testing. If the test is negative, the remaining portion of the culture should be reincubated for an additional 24 h.

B. *For miscellaneous gram-negative bacteria, chapter 24*

Ehrlich's reagent

Ethyl alcohol, 95%	95 ml
p-Dimethylaminobenzaldehyde	1 g
Hydrochloric acid, concentrated	20 ml

Dissolve aldehyde in alcohol and then slowly add acid. The dry aldehyde should be light straw in color. Ehrlich's reagent should be prepared in small quantities and stored in a refrigerator when not in use.

Test procedure. Add 1 ml of xylene to a 48-h 2% tryptone broth culture incubated at 35 to 37 C. Shake vigorously to extract the indole. Allow to stand 1 to 2 min for the xylene extract to layer on top. Add 0.5 ml of Ehrlich's reagent down the side of the tube so that it forms a layer between the broth and the xylene. Do not shake the tube after the reagents are added. If indole is present, a red ring will develop just below the xylene layer.

Indophenol (cytochrome) oxidase test (7, 10)

Solution A

α-Naphthol	1 g
Ethyl alcohol, 95 to 96%	100 ml

Solution B

p-Aminodimethylaniline hydrochloride .... 1 g
Distilled water .... 100 ml

(Reagent B should be prepared frequently and should be stored in a refrigerator when not in use.)

Test procedure. The test is performed on nutrient agar slant cultures incubated at 37 C or at a lower temperature if required. Add 2 or 3 drops of each reagent and tilt the tube so that the reagents are mixed and flow over the growth on the slant. Positive reactions are indicated by the development of a blue color in the growth within 2 min.

The majority of positive cultures produce a strong reaction within 30 s. Any weak or doubtful reaction that occurs after 2 min should be ignored. Plate cultures may be tested by allowing an equal-parts mixture of the reagents to flow over isolated colonies.

Lancefield grouping procedures for streptococci

See chapter 8.

McFarland nephelometer barium sulfate standards

1. Prepare 1% aqueous barium chloride and 1% aqueous sulfuric acid solutions.
2. Add the amounts indicated in Table 1 to clean, dry ampoules. Ampoules should have the same diameter as the test tube to be used in subsequent density determinations.
3. Seal the ampoules and label them.

TABLE 1. *Preparation of McFarland nephelometer barium sulfate standards*

Tube	Barium chloride 1% (ml)	Sulfuric acid, 1% (ml)	Corresponding approx density of bacteria (million/ml)
1	0.1	9.9	300
2	0.2	9.8	600
3	0.3	9.7	900
4	0.4	9.6	1,200
5	0.5	9.5	1,500
6	0.6	9.4	1,800
7	0.7	9.3	2,100
8	0.8	9.2	2,400
9	0.9	9.1	2,700
10	1.0	9.0	3,000

Mercuric iodide solution (2)

Stock solution

Mercuric iodide .... 1 g
Potassium iodide .... 4 g
Distilled water .... 100 ml

Working solution

Stock solution .... 10.00 ml
Sodium chloride, 0.5 or 0.85% .. 90.00 ml
Formalin .... 0.05 ml

Both of these solutions keep indefinitely.

Methyl red test

Methyl red indicator

Methyl red .... 0.1 g
Ethyl alcohol, 95% .... 300.0 ml

Dissolve dye in alcohol and add sufficient distilled water to make 500 ml.

Test procedure. Inoculate buffered glucose-peptone broth lightly from a young agar slant culture. Incubation at 37 C for 48 h is sufficient for the majority of cultures. Tests should not be made with cultures incubated less than 48 h. If the results are equivocal, repeat the test with cultures that have been incubated for 4 or 5 days. In such instances, duplicate tests should be incubated at 25 C.

Add 5 or 6 drops of reagent for each 5 ml of culture. Reactions are read immediately. Positive tests are bright red. Weakly positive tests are red-orange, and negative tests are yellow.

Motility tests

A. For the *Enterobacteriaceae*, chapter 18, a medium containing 0.4% agar is recommended. Inoculate by stabbing into the top of the column of medium to a depth of about 5 mm. Incubate at 35 C for 1 or 2 days. If negative, follow with further incubation at 21 to 25 C for 5 days. For special purposes, such as enhancement of the motility and flagellar development in poorly motile cultures, it is often advisable to passage cultures first through a semisolid medium containing 0.2% agar tubed in Craigie tubes or in U tubes. Subsequent passages may be made in the 0.4% agar medium.

B. The following discussion on motility testing was submitted for *Aeromonas* and *Pseudomonas*, chapters 20 and 23. Motility media containing concentrations higher than 0.3% produce gels through which many motile organisms cannot spread. Spreading in a semisolid medium is judged by macroscopic examination of the medium for a diffuse zone of growth emanating from the line of inoculation. Many aerobic pseudomonads fail to grow deep in semisolid medium in a test tube. Organisms possessing "paralyzed" flagella are nonmotile and cannot spread in the medium. Some filamentous organisms spread in or on semisolid medium but are nonmotile and nonflagellated. Although cultures may grow at 37 C or higher temperatures, the flagellar proteins of some organisms are not synthesized optimally at this temperature; hence, motility medium should be incubated at temperatures near 18 to 20 C. These observations require judicious interpretation of motility, and limit, to some extent, the reliability of using spreading in semisolid agar as the sole taxonomic criterion to delineate related species.

A deep layer of motility medium, 18 to 20 ml, in a 100-mm diameter petri dish, is useful for selecting motile strains from a predominantly nonmotile stock. The plate is inoculated in the center, and motile descendants are "fished" from the periphery of the giant colony after organisms have spread through the semisolid agar.

Nitrate reduction

Solution A

Sulfanilic acid	8 g
Acetic acid, 5 N	1 liter

Solution B

N,*N*-dimethyl-1-naphthylamine	6 ml
Acetic acid, 5 N	1 liter

(The 5 N acetic acid consists of 1 part glacial acetic acid to 2.5 parts distilled water.)

Although *N*,*N*-dimethyl-1-naphthylamine has not been listed as a carcinogen, as has α-naphthylamine, by the Occupational Safety and Health Administration (OSHA), Department of Labor (*Federal Register*, Vol. 39, No. 20, Tuesday, January 29, 1974), its structural similarity to α-naphthylamine would indicate that such safety precautions as avoidance of aerosols, mouth pipetting, and contact with the skin should be followed.

Test procedure for Enterobacteriaceae, chapter 18. Inoculate semisolid medium or fluid medium tubed with inverted Durham tubes and incubate at 37 C for 24 h. Immediately before testing, mix equal parts of solutions A and B, and add 0.1 ml of the mixture to the culture. Positive tests for reduction of nitrate are indicated by the development of a red color within a few minutes. The occasional culture that gives apparently equivocal results should be retested after 1, 2, 3, and 4 days of incubation. Negative tests for nitrite should always be confirmed by adding a minute amount of zinc dust to the tube. The development of a red color indicates the presence of unreduced nitrate. Almost all strains of *Enterobacteriaceae* except *Enterobacter agglomerans* (approximately 18% nitrate negative) are nitrate positive.

Test procedure for Pseudomonas, chapter 23, and miscellaneous gram-negative bacteria, chapter 24. Inoculate a fluid medium tubed with inverted Durham tubes, incubate at 30 C (or 35 C), and examine after 24 and 48 h for reduction of nitrate to nitrogen gas, which accumulates in the Durham tube. After 48 h, test for nitrite by the addition of 0.5 ml of each of reagents A and B. A red color indicates a positive test, provided the uninoculated control medium is negative. Negative tests should be confirmed by the addition of zinc dust to convert unreduced nitrate to nitrite.

Nitrite reduction—test for miscellaneous gram-negative bacteria, chapter 24

Inoculate nitrite reduction broth containing inverted Durham tubes, incubate at 35 C, and examine after 24 and 48 h for reduction of nitrite to nitrogen gas which accumulates in the Durham tubes. After 48 h, test for nitrite by the addition of 0.5 ml of each of reagents A and B. The test is positive if there is no color change, provided a red color develops in the uninoculated control.

ONPG test—test for β-D-galactosidase (19)

Buffer, 1 M monosodium phosphate, pH 7.0

Monosodium phosphate·H_2O	6.9 g
Sodium hydroxide, 30% (wt/vol)	ca. 3.0 ml
Distilled water to	50.0 ml

Dissolve the monosodium phosphate in approximately 45 ml of distilled water. Add the sodium hydroxide and adjust to pH 7.0. Bring volume to 50 ml with distilled water and store in refrigerator (about 4 C).

Test reagent (0.75 M ONPG reagent)

O-nitrophenyl-β-D-galactopyranoside	80 mg
Distilled water	15 ml
Monosodium phosphate, 1 M, pH 7.0	5 ml

Dissolve the ONPG in the distilled water at 37 C and add the monosodium phosphate solution. The solution should be colorless and should be stored in a refrigerator. Warm to 37 C before use.

Test procedure. The test is performed on cultures grown for 18 h on triple sugar iron agar slants. Emulsify a loopful of growth in 0.25 ml of physiological saline to make a heavy suspension.

Add one drop of toluene and shake well (to liberate the enzyme). Allow the tubes to stand for about 5 min at 37 C. Add 0.25 ml of buffered 0.75 M ONPG reagent and incubate in a water bath at 37 C. Tubes are examined at intervals, and incubation is continued for 18 to 24 h. A positive test is indicated by the development of a yellow color due to the liberation of *o*-nitrophenol.

Optochin test

See chapter 9.

Oxidase test

A. For Neisseria, chapters 10 and 11

The preferred reagent is a 1% solution of tetramethyl-*p*-phenylenediamine dihydrochloride prepared fresh daily or refrigerated for not longer than 1 week. Kovacs' method as described by Steel (27) is a recommended procedure. Remove a portion of a colony with a sterile platinum loop (iron-containing wire gives a false-positive reaction) and rub on a strip of filter paper impregnated with the oxidase reagent. The moist paper were the bacteria are deposited turns dark purple within 10 s. A delayed positive reaction (color development in 10 to 60 s) is not typical of *Neisseria;* a strain showing this reaction should be reexamined, with a young culture used for the second test. A delayed reaction may also be encountered if the bacteria are taken from an acid environment (medium containing a utilizable carbohydrate); the test should be repeated using an 18-h culture on blood agar.

Alternatively, the test may be done with a 1% solution of dimethyl-*p*-phenylenediamine hydrochloride. This reagent is dropped on the culture plate. Oxidase-positive colonies develop a pink color which successively becomes maroon, dark red, and finally black. This reagent is less sensitive and more toxic than tetramethyl-*p*-phenylenediamine dihydrochloride. The bacteria may be dead by the time they are black. Also, viscid colonies may appear oxidase negative because of poor penetration of the reagent.

B. For miscellaneous gram-negative bacteria, see chapter 24

PVA fixative technique for stool examination

Trophozoites of intestinal amoebae disintegrate rapidly; consequently, obtaining laboratory confirmation of suspected cases of amoebic dysentery or amebiasis is often difficult. The polyvinyl alcohol (PVA) fixative technique (3) furnishes a means of preserving these fragile organisms for later examination and therefore is applicable particularly to central diagnostic or public health laboratories which receive specimens through the mails. Fresh specimens, feces, or other materials suspected of containing trophozoites are mixed with PVA fixative—a mixture of fixative and water-soluble resin. Immediately, or months later, permanently stained films can be prepared from the preserved material. Trophozoites and cysts, if originally present, can be demonstrated by microscopic examination with oil immersion objectives.

PVA powder, produced by E. I. Dupont de Nemours & Co., is designated as Elvanol. In addition to the original grade, Elvanol 90-25, other grades of high hydrolysis medium-viscosity PVA (71-24, 71-30) have proved satisfactory. PVA powder and PVA fixative solution may be purchased from Delkote, Inc. (Wilmington, Del.). When ordering PVA powder, specify the pretested powder for use in PVA fixative. Lot RM 132 is most satisfactory.

PVA powder is also produced by Shawinigan Resins Corp. (Springfield, Mass.) and designated as Gelvatol Resin. The grade 3-60 has been found satisfactory for use in preparing PVA fixative.

Preparation of the PVA fixative

1. Add 5 g of PVA powder to 100 ml of Schaudinn's fixative at room temperature, stirring constantly.

Modified Schaudinn's fixative

Glacial acetic acid	5.0 ml
Glycerol	1.5 ml
Schaudinn's fixative	93.5 ml

(Schaudinn's fixative contains 2 parts saturated aqueous solution of mercuric chloride and 1 part 95% ethyl alcohol.)

2. Heat to about 75 C or higher until powder dissolves and suspension clears.

3. When cooled to room temperature, the solution should be clear and free from lumps. Solutions prepared with some lots of PVA may remain turbid and may exhibit some precipitate upon cooling. Unless these conditions are excessive, they will not interfere with satisfactory use of the solution. PVA fixative remains satisfactory for several months and can be used either at room temperature or heated to 50 C.

Preservation of specimens and preparation of PVA films

To obtain the full advantage of PVA fixative as a preservative, specimens should be thoroughly mixed with the solution immediately after their passage from the patient and before the organisms lose their characteristic morphology.

On microscope slides. A drop of dysenteric stool or other material is placed on a microscope slide and mixed with 3 drops of PVA fixative. With an applicator stick, the mixture is then spread (*not* smeared like a blood film) over approximately one-third of the glass surface, with care to extend the smear to the sides of the slides to reduce later peeling, and is allowed to dry *thoroughly* (preferably overnight at 37 C). Dried films remain satisfactory for staining for several weeks.

In vials. A quantity of specimen is thoroughly mixed in a vial containing 3 or more parts of PVA fixative. Films for staining can be prepared immediately or weeks later by spreading 2 or 3 drops of the mixture over the surface of the microscope slide. The smear should cover about one-third of the slide surface and, to reduce peeling during staining, should extend to the edge of the side of the slide. Not having the films too thick and allowing them to dry thoroughly is very important. If the specimen in the vial jells, it can be liquefied by heating in a water bath before making the films.

Staining of PVA films. PVA films are permeable to all commonly employed staining reagents. The films are, therefore, handled in the same way as smears fixed in the conventional manner with Schaudinn's fixative.

A variety of staining techniques can be used, but the long Heidenhain iron-hematoxylin procedure gives best results. The Wheatley trichrome method (29) is a more rapid procedure that gives satisfactory results for diagnostic purposes.

Regardless of the staining procedure to be used, dried films are first placed in 70% alcohol containing iodine for approximately 20 min to remove mercuric chloride crystals. After staining, the film is mounted with a cover slip and examined with an oil immersion objective.

A distinct advantage of PVA fixative is that it makes possible successful staining of organisms occurring in fluid specimens such as diarrheic specimens and the sediments of cultures (23). The solution serves as an adhesive as well as a preservative and prevents loss of organisms during the staining procedure.

Two-vial method of shipping specimens

PVA fixative was developed primarily to preserve trophozoites of intestinal amoebae. The method is not recommended for the diagnosis of larvae and helminth eggs. Therefore, to make possible the recovery of all stages and types of organisms occurring in stools, a two-vial method for shipping specimens is recommended (3). A portion of *freshly* passed feces is introduced into one empty vial (or one containing 5 to 10% formalin) and into one containing PVA fixative. The samples are thoroughly mixed with the preservatives in the ratio of 3 parts fixative to 1 part feces. Permanently stained films can be prepared from the PVA-fixed portion and examined for trophozoites and cysts. Concentration procedures can be performed on the other portion and examined for protozoan cysts and helminth eggs and larvae.

Slide culture technique

In the study of fungi, it is often necessary to observe the undisturbed relationship between reproductive structures and mycelium. This may be accomplished by growing the fungi on glass slides in a moist chamber. The operator should be aware of the infectious hazards of this procedure. This technique should *never* be used for the systemic pathogenic molds *Coccidioides immitis*, *Histoplasma capsulatum*, *Blastomyces dermatitidis*, and *Paracoccidioides braziliensis*.

1. Place a slide on a bent-glass rod in the bottom of a petri dish, add a cover slip, cover, and sterilize.
2. Prepare Sabouraud dextrose agar plates with about 15 ml of agar per plate. Allow to solidify and dry. Cut agar blocks about 1 cm square.
3. Place a block of agar, using sterile technique, on the slide in a petri dish.
4. Inoculate the central portion of the four sides of the block with a small fragment of the fungus being studied.
5. Cover inoculated block with a sterile cover slip.
6. Add 8.0 ml of sterile water to bottom of petri dish.
7. Incubate at 25 C until sporulation occurs. The slide preparation may be checked periodically under the low power of a microscope.
8. When sporulation is complete, carefully lift off cover slip and lay aside with fungus growth up.
9. Lift agar block from slide and discard.
10. Place a drop of lactophenol cotton blue in

the center of growth on the slide and cover with a fresh cover slip. Place another drop in the center of growth on the cover slip and drop into place on another clean slide.

11. Blot away excess mounting fluid from the two preparations, and allow to dry. Seal edges with nail polish or preferably with a synthetic resin (Harleco).

Stoll egg-counting technique, modified

Since the special equipment necessary to perform this technique is not readily available, a modification is recommended.

1. Fill a graduated 15-ml centrifuge tube to the 14-ml mark with 0.1 N sodium hydroxide.
2. Using two applicators, add sufficient feces to raise the fluid level to the 15-ml mark.
3. If the feces is hard, allow the preparation to stand for a while.
4. Shake vigorously for 1 min to secure a *homogenous suspension.*
5. The eggs and debris will begin to settle immediately after the shaking is stopped. Quickly pipette 0.15 ml from the middle area of the sample.
6. Expel the entire contents onto a 3 by 1.5 inch (7.6 by 3.8 cm) slide, and cover with a 22 by 40 mm no. 2 cover slip.
7. Examine under low power (10×). Using a mechanical stage, count all hookworm eggs present both under and at the sides of the cover slip.
8. Multiply the number obtained by 100. This will yield the number of eggs per milliliter of formed feces.

A clinical classification used in hookworm surveys is shown in Table 2.

"String" test (H. L. Smith, personal communication, 1962)

This test is performed by emulsifying a small amount of growth from an agar slant culture (20 to 24 h) or a gelatin agar plate in a drop of an aqueous solution of sodium deoxycholate (0.5%) on a slide. This is examined for a mucous-like "string" extending from the drop to a loop as the loop is lifted away from the slide. Three distinct patterns may occur:

1. ++ A string occurs soon after emulsifying growth and can still be obtained 45 to 60 s later. All *Vibrio cholerae* and most biotype El Tor cultures gave this type of reaction, with the delayed string being even stronger than the initial. Most ++ *Vibrio* species and the few ++ aeromonads give a weaker delayed reaction than that occurring initially.
2. +− A string occurs initially but is absent 45 to 60 s later. Most *Vibrio* species give this pattern.
3. − No string occurs either initially or delayed.

TABLE 2. *Clinical classification based on number of hookworms in feces*

Intensity grouping (eggs/ml of feces)	Clinical classification
100–699	Very light
700–2,599	Light
2,600–12,599	Moderate
12,600–25,099	Heavy
25,100 and over	Very heavy

Urease test reagent (25)

For mycoplasmas, chapter 32

Urea	1.0 g
Manganous chloride	0.8 g
Water	100 ml

Test procedure. Place several drops on an agar plate with visible colonies. A brown color surrounding T strain colonies, but not *M. hominis*, immediately results. Colonies should not be more than 48 h old.

Voges-Proskauer test

Method 1

Reagent O'Meara, modified

Potassium hydroxide	40.0 g
Creatine	0.3 g
Distilled water	100.0 ml

Dissolve the alkali in the water and add creatine. The reagent should be prepared frequently and should be refrigerated when not in use (17, 26). The reagent may be used for 2 to 3 weeks but deteriorates rapidly thereafter.

Test procedure. The test is performed on the culture grown in buffered peptone glucose broth incubated at 37 C for 48 h. Add 1 ml of reagent to 1 ml of culture and place at 37 C or at room temperature, after shaking to aerate. A positive test is indicated by the development of a pink color. The test depends on the formation of acetylmethylcarbinol which is oxidized in alkaline medium, in the presence of air, to form diacetyl. Diacetyl reacts with creatine to form the pink compound. Final readings are made after 4 h. If equivocal results are obtained, repeat the test with cultures incubated at 25 C.

Method 2, Barritt

Solution A

α-Naphthol	5 g
Ethyl alcohol, absolute	100 ml

Solution B

Potassium hydroxide	40 g
Distilled water	100 ml

Test procedure. Add 0.6 ml of solution A and 0.2 ml of solution B to 1 ml of culture. Shake well after the addition of each reagent. Positive reactions occur at once or within 5 min and are indicated by the production of a red color. The development of a copper color in some tests should be disregarded.

Method 3, Coblentz (5)

MR-VP medium	1.7 g
Distilled water	100.0 ml

Dispense in 2.0 ml volumes in 18 by 150 mm cotton-plugged tubes. Autoclave at 121 C for no longer than 10 min to prevent caramelization of the glucose.

Test procedure. Inoculate the medium with a massive inoculum consisting of a loopful (2 to 3 mm) of an 18-h agar slant culture. Incubate at 30 C for 6 to 7 h and add 0.6 ml of α-naphthol (5.0 g of α-naphthol in 100.0 ml of 95% ethyl alcohol) followed by 0.2 ml of 40% KOH containing 0.3% creatine. The tubes are then shaken vigorously for 30 s to 1 min.

Zinc sulfate concentration technique for stool examination, modified

The zinc sulfate flotation procedure was the first concentration technique developed for the recovery of both helminth eggs and larvae *and* protozoan cysts. Operculated eggs and those of schistosomes are not recovered, however.

The original method, developed by Faust et al. (8), included two steps which are omitted in the modified procedure described below. These were (i) preparation of a fecal-water suspension, and (ii) straining a portion of the suspension through gauze into a small tube. In addition, the number of washings by centrifugation is reduced to one, unless the specimen is very oily. The method is further simplified by superimposing a cover slip on the meniscus to remove the concentrate.

Preparation of zinc sulfate solution

1. Add 331 g of $ZnSO_4$ (USP) to 1 liter of warm tap water. A technical-grade $ZnSO_4$ can also be used if the insoluble salts are removed from the solution by filtering.

2. After it is thoroughly dissolved, *check the specific gravity with a hydrometer*. It should read 1.18. If the reading is not correct, adjust the specific gravity by adding water or zinc sulfate as needed.

3. Some workers prefer a specific gravity of 1.20, which is prepared by using a slightly larger amount of zinc sulfate and by similarly checking with a hydrometer. This solution of higher specific gravity should always be used when a Formalin-preserved fecal specimen is to be examined.

Technique

1. Using two applicators, comminute a fecal sample about the size of a small pea in a Wasserman tube (13 by 100 mm) half filled with tap water. Make certain that all obvious particles are broken up and that an even suspension is formed.

2. Add additional tap water until the tube is two-thirds full.

3. Centrifuge this preparation for 1 min at approximately 2,500 rpm.

4. Pour off the supernatant fluid into a container holding a disinfectant, for example, cresol.

5. Repeat this washing only if the stool is extremely oily.

6. Add enough zinc sulfate solution to fill the tube half full.

7. Using an applicator, break up the packed sediment very thoroughly.

8. Add additional zinc sulfate solution to fill the tube to within 1.3 cm of the top.

9. Centrifuge this suspension for 1 min at 2,500 rpm.

10. Without shaking or spilling the solution, carefully place the tube in a rack.

11. Slowly fill the tube brimful with zinc sulfate *without allowing any runover*.

12. Place a clean, grease-free no. 1 cover slip (22 by 22 mm) on top of the tube so that the under surface touches the meniscus. Leave undisturbed for about 10 min.

13. Deftly remove the cover slip with a straight, upward motion. A drop containing eggs and cysts will adhere to the underside of the cover slip.

14. Lower this onto a drop of iodine stain placed on a clean slide (7.6 by 5 cm). Seal the preparation.

15. Examine under a microscope for eggs and cysts.

ıoroughly in mortar. Add 1 g of mixture ml of distilled water.

› stain (Hiss method)

ı loopful of physiological saline suspen-rowth with a drop of normal serum on a ide. Allow the smear to air-dry and . Flood the smear with crystal violet (1% s solution). Steam the preparation or 1 min, and rinse with copper sulfate queous solution). Capsules appear as ue halos around dark blue to purple

zol Black E staining technique for tinal protozoa in feces and in tissue

also chapter 65 for discussion of this ıre.

azol Black E staining technique (14) is a procedure in which fixation and stain-e place in a single solution. No destain-ıecessary. The modified stain technique y be used for staining protozoa in fecal or in tissues.

procedure gives good results with fresh mears but is less satisfactory for PVA-ıaterial. (PVA-fixed specimens are better by iron-hematoxylin or trichrome This technique would be of value in spital or clinic laboratories where fresh ens are usually obtained, since the steps d are fewer than in other available pro-s and require less attention.

optimal staining dilution and time for iter of stain prepared must be deter-. The stock stain may be kept indefinitely ain dilutions may be used repeatedly. er, repeated use "wears out" the stain n, and when slides appear visibly red than greenish-black at the end of the g period the dilution should be discarded. ximately 20 slides can be satisfactorily d in a 50-ml Coplin jar of diluted stain be-eterioration makes change necessary. De-tion of the stain is dependent on use stained) and not on time, since satisfac-ains may be obtained with stain dilutions 30 days old if the number of slides stained ıt been excessive. Slides that appear red restained in fresh stain.

ration of solutions

sic solution

alcohol, 90%	170 ml
yl alcohol	160 ml
c acid, glacial	20 ml
ıl, liquid	20 ml
ıhotungstic acid, 1%	12 ml
led water	618 ml

Add alcohols and acids to distilled water and mix thoroughly. (Prepare 1% phosphotungstic acid by dissolving 1 g of phosphotungstic acid crystals in 100 ml of distilled water.)

B. *Stock stain solution*

Chlorazol Black E dye	5 g
Basic solution	1 liter

Weigh out dye, put in mortar, and grind for at least 3 min. Add a small amount of basic solution and grind until a smooth paste is obtained. Add more solution and grind for 5 min. Allow particulate matter to settle for a few minutes, and pour off the liquid into a separate dry, clean container. Add more basic solution and continue the grinding, mixing process until all of the dye appears to be in solution. Add any remaining basic solution, bottle the stain, and put aside for 4 to 6 weeks to ripen. A black sediment settles out within a few days, leaving black-cherry colored liquid which is the fixa-tive-stain. Filter the stain through Whatman no. 12 filter paper before use. Keep the filtered stain in a stoppered bottle protected from moisture, dust, and dirt.

C. *Carbol-xylol*

Liquefy phenol crystals by placing jar in a waterbath. (Do *not* heat over direct flame.)

Phenol, liquid	1 part
Xylol	2 parts

Preparation of fecal smears

The smears should be prepared in the usual fashion by spreading a thin, even layer over approximately one-third of the slide. Care should be taken not to make the smear too thick. The smear should be placed immediately in the fixative-stain dilution. It should not dry to any degree between preparation and staining, because the organism will be distorted.

Procedure for staining

Determination of optimal dilution and staining time. The optimal dilution and staining time must be determined for each liter of fixative-stain. The following series of dilutions and staining periods are recommended for this purpose.

Fixative-stain	*Basic solution*	*Time (h)*
Undilute	—	2–3
1	1	2–4-overnight
2	1	2–4
1	2	2-overnight
1	3	4-overnight

STAINING PROCEDURES

Buffered methylene blue solutions for wet mount preparations

For staining intestinal protozoa in wet mount preparations, Nair (22) determined that the pH of the solution is the deciding factor in bringing out the morphological details of the nucleus. As a result of this finding, a satisfactory stain for wet mounts can be made by simply dissolving biological dyes in an appropriately buffered solution. For staining trophozoites of *Entamoeba histolytica*, the exact pH is not critical, and the optimal range may vary with the buffer system and dyes employed. Directions for prepared acetate buffers with the pH range of 3.6 to 4.8 are given below. (If desired, commercially available buffer tablets can be used. Coleman Buffer tablets [Coleman Instruments, Inc., Maywood, Ill.] composed of potassium acid phthalate and sodium phosphate will give a pH range of 3.8 to 6.0.)

Preparation of acetate buffer solution

Stock solution A: 0.2 M solution of acetic acid (11.55 ml in 1,000 ml).

Stock solution B: 0.2 M solution of sodium acetate (16.4 g of $C_2H_3O_2Na$ or 27.2 g of $C_2H_3O_2Na \cdot 3H_2O$ in 1,000 ml).

Proportions of A and B for specific pH. Mix amounts of A and B indicated in Table 3, and dilute with distilled water to a total of 100 ml.

Temporary stain

Biological dyes like methylene blue and pyronine may be used. The quantity of dye that should be dissolved in the buffer solutions can be determined by a little experience. The quantity will depend upon the solubility of the dye in the buffer at different pH levels. In practice, a small quantity of methylene blue (0.06%) in acetate buffer at pH 3.6 has given satisfactory results.

Technique. A small amount of feces is picked up with an applicator sti
mixed with a large drop of t
ene blue solution. The mixtu
cover slip and sealed. After
the trophozoite nuclei are s
lighter blue cytoplasm. The
lar to that described for
resembles a permanent
preparation. Inclusions in
also stained. After a time
become over-stained and n
The preparation should b
approximately 30 min. Fl
do not stain well.

TABLE 3. *Proportions of solutions A and B for specific pH*

pH	A (ml)	B (ml)
3.6	46.3	3.7
3.8	44.0	6.0
4.0	41.0	9.0
4.2	36.8	13.2
4.4	30.5	19.5
4.6	25.5	24.5
4.8	20.0	30.0

Buffers for malarial stai

Stock solutions

(*Note.* These solutions
refrigerator in Pyrex glass

Solution A: 0.067 M dis

Disodium phosphate
(Na_2HPO_4) ....
Distilled water to .....

Place the phosphate sa
metric flask; add a smal
water to dissolve, and di
distilled water.

Solution B: 0.067 M m

Monosodium phosphat
($NaH_2PO_4 \cdot 2H_20$) ..
Distilled water to ....

Place the phosphate s
metric flask; dilute to t
water.

Working solutions

Buffered water, pH 7.
Solution A ....
Solution B ....
Distilled water ....

Buffered water, pH 7.
Solution A ....
Solution B ....
Distilled water ....

Buffered water, pH 6
Solution A ....
Solution B ....
Distilled water ...

Buffered water for thick films (6:5 pho

Disodium phosphate
Monopotassium pho

A solution producing good overnight staining does not appear to over-stain when left for periods of several days.

Trial smears should be stained with each dilution according to the technique given below, and the optimal dilution and time should be selected for routine staining with the "batch" of stain concerned. More than one dilution-time combination may be satisfactory, and the choice of which to use will depend on the laboratory schedule and the urgency of diagnosis. The range most commonly found satisfactory is a 1:2 dilution for 2 h or a 1:3 dilution for 4 h or overnight. However, for best results, the exact combination should be determined.

Technique of staining

1. Fixative-stain dilution (for routine use, use dilution and time predetermined) 2 h-overnight
2. Ethyl alcohol, 95% .... 10–15 s
3. Carbol-xylol .... 5 min

   or

   Ethyl alcohol, 100% ...... 5 min
4. Xylol .... 5 min
5. Mount in Permount or other suitable media

Staining of protozoa in tissue

Preparation of tissue section slides. Tissue slides are prepared following the usual histological procedures for fixing, embedding, sectioning, and preparing slides. The sections are treated in xylol and alcohol as usual to remove the paraffin and prepare them for staining. Good stains have been obtained on sections of 5 to 7 μm thickness.

Preparation of stain. For staining protozoa in tissue, use the optimal stain dilution as determined for protozoa in feces, but substitute distilled water for basic solution as the diluent.

Fixative-stain	*Distilled Water*	*Time (h)*
Undilute	—	4–6
1	1	4–8-overnight
2	1	4–8
1	2	4-overnight
1	3	8-overnight

Note that the staining time is twice as long for tissue as for fecal smears. The most common satisfactory time is about 6 to 7 h with the optimal dilution.

Technique

1. Fixative-stain (as determined) ....4 h-overnight
2. Alcohol, 95% ....10–15 s
3. Carbol-xylol .... 5–10 min
4. Xylol .... 5–10 min
5. Mount in Permount or other suitable media

Stain reactions. Protozoa in fresh fecal specimens stain green to gray-green; in older stools, organisms are gray to black. Nuclei, chromatoid bodies, karyosomes, and cell membranes stain dark green to black. Ingested red cells may vary from pink to black. *Entamoeba coli* cysts may stain pink or green, and, rarely, *E. histolytica* cysts stain faintly pink. Trophozoites in tissue have the same appearance as those in feces.

Flagellar stain (16)

Chapter 23

Leifson flagellar stain

Pararosaniline acetate	3 parts
Pararosaniline hydrochloride	1 part
95% ethyl alcohol	

Reagents should be certified for flagellar staining.

Tannic acid	3.0 g
Distilled water	100.0 ml
NaCl	1.5 g
Distilled water	100.0 ml

Prepare the stain by making three separate solutions: (i) 1.5% NaCl in distilled water, (ii) 3.0% tannic acid in distilled water, and (iii) 1.2% of a dye mixture (3 parts pararosaniline acetate and 1 part pararosaniline hydrochloride) in 95% ethyl alcohol. Allow the alcoholic dye solution to stand overnight at room temperature to assure complete solution. Mix equal volumes of the three solutions, shake and let stand for 2 h. Store in a tightly stoppered bottle in a refrigerator. The precipitate which settles to the bottom of the bottle on storage should not be disturbed. If stored at room temperature, the solution stains flagella satisfactorily for only a few days. It can be used for about 2 months if stored in a refrigerator and will keep indefinitely at freezer temperatures. Frozen stain solution must be thoroughly mixed after thawing since the water separates from the alcohol. After mixing, the precipitate should be allowed to settle to the bottom.

Test procedure. Cultures to be stained are grown in brain heart infusion broth, or other suitable peptone broth, at room temperature for 18 to 20 h. Formalin (0.25 ml) is added to 4 ml of the overnight broth culture which is allowed to stand for 15 min after mixing. The tube is filled with fresh distilled water, mixed, and centrifuged. Remove the supernatant fluid carefully by decanting. Add distilled water, mix, and recentrifuge. Remove the supernatant fluid, resuspend the organisms in 1 to 2 ml of distilled water, and then dilute until the suspension is barely turbid.

A clean glass slide (1 by 3 inches) is heated in the blue portion of a burner flame. While the slide is hot, make a heavy line with a wax pencil across the slide one-third of the distance from one end and around the margin of two-thirds of the slide. The smear is made on the ringed portion of the slide. Place a large loopful of the bacterial suspension at the end of the cooled slide and tilt the slide to cause the liquid to flow lengthwise to the opposite waxed pencil line. Allow the film to dry at room temperature and do not fix with heat.

A 1-ml amount of clear, supernatant, stain solution, warmed to room temperature, is applied to the smear on the glass slide. As the alcohol evaporates from the solution on the slide, a precipitate forms in the solution within 5 to 15 min. Freshly prepared solution will stain flagella more quickly than will old stain solution. As soon as precipitate forms over the entire smear, the staining is completed and the stain is carefully washed off of the slide by flooding with water. Air-dry.

Giemsa stain for demonstrating Dermatophilus in smears

Giemsa's blood stain (stock solution), Matheson, Coleman and Bell, 257	1 ml
Distilled water	49 ml

Staining procedure. Fix the film with methyl alcohol for 30 s. Apply dilute stain for 45 min. Rinse with distilled water and air-dry.

Giemsa stain for demonstrating Dermatophilus in paraffin sections

Stock solution

Giemsa powder	4 g
Methyl alcohol	264 ml
Glycerol	264 ml

Working solution

Stock solution	1.25 ml
Methyl alcohol	1.50 ml
Distilled water	50.00 ml

Staining procedure. Pass slide through xylol, absolute alcohol, and 95% alcohol. If section was fixed in Zenker's solution, remove the mercury precipitates by placing in iodine for 5 min and then in 5% sodium thiosulfate until clear. Wash in water and rinse in distilled water. Flood with working Giesma solution and steam gently for 10 min. Wash in tap water. Differentiate in rosin alcohol (95% alcohol and a few drops of 10% rosin) to a macroscopic purplish-pink color; usually three swishes are sufficient. Pass through two changes each of absolute alcohol and xylol, and mount.

Giemsa stain for malaria

Use certified liquid or prepare as below.

Giemsa stain, powdered (certified)	0.75 g
Methyl alcohol, pure	65.00 ml
Glycerol, pure	35.00 ml

Shake well in bottle with glass beads. Keep tightly stoppered at all times. Filter if necessary. *See* chapter 67 for procedure.

Gram stain (1)

A. *Modified Hucker's crystal violet*

Solution A

Crystal violet (certified)	2 g
Ethyl alcohol, 95%	20 ml

Solution B

Ammonium oxalate	0.8 g
Distilled water	80.0 ml

Mix solutions A and B. Store fore 24 h before use. Filter through paper into staining bottle.

B. *Gram's iodine*

Iodine	1 g
Potassium iodide	2 g
Distilled water	300 ml

Grind the dry iodine and potassium iodide in a mortar. Add water, a few milliliters at a time, and grind thoroughly after each addition until solution is achieved. Rinse the solution into an amber glass bottle with the remainder of the distilled water.

C. *Decolorizers*

1. Ethyl alcohol, 95%: slowest agent
2. Acetone: fastest agent
3. Acetone-alcohol: intermediate (95% ethyl alcohol, 100 ml; acetone, 100 ml).

With experience, any one of the three decolorizing agents will yield good results.

D. *Counterstain*

Stock solution

Safranine O (certified)	2.5 g
Ethyl alcohol, 95%	100.0 ml

Working solution

Stock solution	10 ml
Distilled water	90 ml

Staining procedure. Flood smear with crystal violet solution and let stand for 1 min. Wash smear briefly with tap water and drain off excess water. Flood smear with iodine solution and let stand for 1 min. Wash with tap water and decolorize until the solvent flows colorlessly from the slide. Wash briefly with tap water. Counterstain with safranine for 10 s. Wash briefly with tap water, blot dry, and examine. Gram-positive organisms are blue; gram-negative, red.

Gram stain for actinomycetes and other bacteria

Aniline crystal violet solution

Aniline	40 ml
Water	1 liter
Crystal violet, saturated alcohol solution	114 ml

Shake aniline and water in a closed container until mixed. Filter through four sheets of paper moistened with water. Add crystal violet solution to filtrate.

Gram's iodine solution

Iodine	1 g
Potassium iodide	2 g
Water	300 ml

Grind iodine and potassium iodide in mortar until well blended. Add water slowly to dissolve.

Safranine

Safranine, saturated alcohol solution (about 2.5 g/100 ml of 95% alcohol)	10 ml
Water	90 ml

Staining procedure. Stain with crystal violet for 2 min, wash, and dry. Apply Gram's iodine for 1 min, wash, and dry. Decolorize with 95% alcohol for 30 s and wash in running tap water. Counterstain with safranine for 30 s, wash, and blot dry.

Gram-Weigert stain for actinomycetes in tissues (18)

Lithium carmine solution

Carmine	4 g
Lithium carbonate, saturated aqueous	100 ml
Thymol	1 g

Dissolve the carmine in the lithium carbonate solution and boil for 10 to 15 min. When cool, add thymol. Filter before use.

Crystal violet solution

Solution A

Absolute alcohol	33 ml
Aniline oil	9 ml
Crystal violet to saturate (4.5 g/100 ml of water)	in excess

Solution B

Crystal violet	2 g
Distilled water	100 ml

Working solution

Solution A	3 ml
Solution B	27 ml

Stock solutions keep well. Working solution will keep about 1 week.

Gram's iodine solution

Iodine	1 g
Potassium iodide	2 g
Distilled water	300 ml

Staining procedure. The tissue should be fixed in absolute alcohol, Carnoy's, or alcohol-formalin. Process in paraffin and cut sections at 6 mm. Pass slide through xylene, absolute alcohol, 95% alcohol, and distilled water. Stain nuclei for 2 to 5 min with lithium carmine stain. Transfer directly to acid alcohol for a few seconds (will not hold red without this step). Wash thoroughly in water. Stain for 8 min in working solution of crystal violet. (Use slide rack; pour solutions on slides.) Drain and blot with filter paper. Pour Gram's iodine over the sections. Allow to stand for 5 to 10 min. Drain, and blot with filter paper. Differentiate in a mixture of equal parts of aniline oil and xylene from a dropping bottle. Blot, and pour on fresh aniline-xylene serveral times until the section is well differentiated and no more purple washes out. Be sure to check slides so differentiation will not be carried too far. Blot; rinse in several changes of xylene to remove aniline. Mount in Permount or balsam.

Results. Fibrin: blue to blue-black. Gram-positive bacteria: blue to blue-black. Nuclei: red. Russell bodies: blue.

Grocott-Gomori methenamine silver nitrate stain for actinomycetes and fungi in tissue sections

Solution A

Borax, 5%	8 ml
Distilled water	100 ml

Solution B

Silver nitrate, 10%	7 ml
Methenamine, 3%	100 ml

Add equal parts of solutions A and B to make working methenamine silver nitrate solution. These solutions should be made up fresh.

Stock light green solution

Light green S. F. (yellow)	0.2 g
Distilled water	100.0 ml
Glacial acetic acid	0.2 ml

Staining procedure. Deparaffinize and bring to distilled water. Oxidize in 5% chromic acid for 1 h. Wash in running tap water for a few seconds. Rinse in 1% sodium bisulfite for 1 min to remove residual chromic acid. Wash in tap water for 5 to 10 min. Wash in three or four changes of distilled water. Place in working methenamine silver nitrate solution in oven (58 to 60 C) for 30 to 60 min. When section turns yellowish-brown, use paraffin-coated forceps to remove slide from silver nitrate solution. Dip slide in distilled water and check with microscope for adequate silver impregnation. Fungi should be dark brown in color at this stage. Rinse in six changes of distilled water. Tone in 0.1% gold chloride for 2 to 5 min. Rinse in distilled water. Remove unreduced silver with 2% sodium thiosulfate for 2 to 5 min. Wash in tap water. Counterstain for 1 min with fresh 1:5 dilution in distilled water of stock light green solution. Dehydrate, clear, and mount.

Hematoxylin and eosin stain for mycetoma granules and Dermatophilus in paraffin sections

Cut sections at 5 mm.

1. Two changes of xylol, 2 min each.
2. Two changes of absolute alcohol, 1 min each.
3. One change of 95% alcohol, 1 min.
4. One change of 90% alcohol, 0.5 min.
5. One change of 80% alcohol, 0.5 min.
6. One change of 60% alcohol, 0.5 min.
7. Two changes of distilled water or until slides have cleared.
8. Harris' hematoxylin with glacial acetic acid (5 ml of acetic acid/100 ml of hematoxylin), 1 to 2 min.
9. Rinse in distilled water.
10. Place in tap water to which 20 to 40 drops of ammonium hydroxide have been added for about 3 s (section will turn blue immediately).
11. Rinse in two changes of tap water to remove the ammonia.
12. Counterstain in picro-eosin solution for about 30 s.
13. Two changes of 95% alcohol, 1 min each.
14. Two changes of absolute alcohol, 1 min in first, 2 min in last.
15. Two changes of xylol, 1 min each.
16. Mount in neutral xylol damar.

Note. Zenker-fixed tissue at step 5 is placed in Lugol's iodine for 5 min; washed in tap water for 0.5 min; placed in 5% sodium thiosulfate solution (hypo) about 0.5 min or until color is removed; (i) wash in tap water, 1 min; (ii) rinse in distilled water; (iii) triple the staining time in hematoxylin; (iv) then stain the same as for other fixatives.

Harris' alum hematoxylin

Hematoxylin crystals (National Aniline Division, Allied Chemical Corp.)	5.0 g
Absolute alcohol	50.0 ml
Ammonium or potassium alum	100.0 g
Distilled water	1.0 liter
Mercuric oxide (red)	2.5 g

Dissolve hematoxylin in alcohol; dissolve alum in water with the aid of heat. Remove from heat and mix the two solutions. Bring to a boil as rapidly as possible. Remove from heat and add the mercuric oxide slowly. Reheat until solution is dark purple, remove from flame immediately, and plunge vessel into a basin of cold water until cool. The stain is ready for use as soon as it cools. Filter before use.

Picro-eosin solution

Eosin Y, water-soluble (National Aniline Division, Allied Chemical Corp.)	10 g
Potassium dichromate	5 g
Picric acid, saturated, aqueous ...	100 ml
Absolute alcohol	100 ml
Distilled water	800 ml

Neutral xylol damar

1. Place approximately 10 oz (283.5 g) of damar (Singapore gum damar, A. D. Mackay Inc., New York, N.Y.) in beaker and cover with xylol.
2. Heat on a closed electric hot plate until damar has dissolved.
3. Filter through coarse filter into 1-liter graduate.
4. Add approximately 2 g of calcium carbonate and let settle to bottom of graduate.
5. Pour off small amount of damar into evaporating dish.
6. Heat on a closed electric hot plate to desired thickness (remember that it thickens on cooling).
7. Store in bottles for use.

India ink mount for Cryptococcus neoformans capsules

1. Mix the specimen (pus, exudate, tissue, sputum or sediment of centrifuged spinal fluid) with a small drop of India ink on a clean slide. Cover with a 22 by 40 mm no. 2 cover slip. The mount should be thin. Gentle pressure may have to be applied on the cover slip for pus, exudate, tissue, or sputum to obtain a thin mount. Pelikan Drawing Ink, 17 Black, Gunther Wagner, Germany, is recommended.

2. Scan under low power using reduced lighting. Switch to high power to examine for presence of encapsulated cells. The mucoid capsules appear as a clear halo that surrounds the yeast cell or lies between the cell wall and the surrounding black mass of India ink particles. Capsules may be broad or narrow. The yeast cells may be round, oval, or elongate; buds may be absent, single, or rarely multiple. The buds may be detached from the mother cell but enclosed in a common capsule attached.

Iodine solutions for wet mount preparations

Iodine solutions are used to stain protozoan cysts in wet mounts. A weak rather than a strong iodine solution is best. The strong iodine tends to coagulate the fecal particles and to destory the refractile nature of the organism.

Several iodine solutions can be used satisfactorily. The two described below have been widely used and are simply prepared. The one recommended by Dobell and O'Connor (6) is a weak iodine that should be prepared fresh about every 10 days for best results. Lugol's iodine *must be diluted* about five times with distilled water, since the full strength solution is too strong. Lugol's iodine should be prepared fresh about every 3 weeks. Gram's iodine used for bacteriological work is not satisfactory for staining protozoan cysts.

Dobell and O'Connor's iodine solution (6)

Iodine (powdered crystals)	1 g
Potassium iodine	2 g
Distilled water	100 ml

The KI is dissolved in the distilled water, and the iodine crystals are added slowly and shaken thoroughly. Filter or decant.

Lugol's iodine solution

Iodine (powdered crystals)	5 g
Potassium iodide	10 g
Distilled water	100 ml

The KI is dissolved in the distilled water, and the iodine crystals are added slowly and shaken until dissolved. Filter and place in tightly stoppered bottle. Dilute 1:5 with distilled water for use in staining protozoan cysts.

Technique. A small portion of feces is comminuted in a drop of the iodine solution, mounted with a cover slip, and sealed with a heated paraffin-Vaseline mixture.

In a correctly stained cyst, the glycogen appears reddish-brown, the cytoplasm appears yellow, and the nuclei stand out as lighter refractile bodies. The location of the karyosomes may be more easily determined, but the chromatoid bodies are less visible than in saline solution. Since glycogen is a reserve food, it will not usually appear in older cysts.

Kinyoun acid-fast stain

Kinyoun carbol-fuchsin

Basic fuchsin	4 g
Alcohol, 95%	20 ml
Phenol crystals	8 g
Distilled water	100 ml

Acid alcohol

Hydrochloric acid, concentrated	3 ml
Ethyl alcohol, 95%	97 ml

Methylene blue counterstain

Methylene blue	0.3 g
Distilled water	100.0 ml

Staining procedure. Flood fixed smear with Kinyoun carbol-fuchsin and let stain for 2 min (no heat necessary). Wash with tap water and decolorize by dropping acid alcohol over the smear until the alcohol flows colorless from the slide. Wash with tap water and counterstain for 20 to 30 s. Wash, blot dry, and examine. Acid-fast organisms stain red; the background and other organisms stain blue.

Kinyoun acid-fast stain, modified for actinomycetes

Staining procedure. The solutions are the same as those described above except that 2.5% methylene blue in 95% ethyl alcohol is used as the counterstain. Stain with Kinyoun carbol fuchsin for 3 min without heat. Wash. Decolorize for 5 to 10 s with acid alcohol. Wash. Counterstain for 30 s. Wash in water and blot dry.

KOH solution

Potassium hydroxide	10 or 20 g
Distilled water	100 ml

1. Mix specimen (pus, exudate, tissue) with a

drop of 10 or 20% solution on a clean slide, cover with no. 2, 22 by 40 mm cover slip, and press gently to make a thin mount. Gentle warming may aid in clearing the mount. Viscid specimens may require overnight storage in a moist chamber. (Place slide on applicator stick supports over moist filter paper in a petri dish, or place in a screw-capped Coplin jar laid on its side.)

2. Scan under low power with reduced lighting. Switch to high power to check presence of suspected fungus elements.

Koster's stain, modified for Brucella

Staining procedure. Stain for 1 min with a freshly prepared mixture of two parts saturated aqueous safranine solution and five parts 1 N potassium hydroxide. Wash in tap water. Decolorize twice with 0.1% sulfuric acid within 10 to 20 s. Wash in tap water. Counterstain with 1% carbol methylene blue. Brucellae stain orange-red against blue background. The direct staining method can be utilized in enzootic abortion field studies.

Lactophenol cotton blue mounting solution

Phenol crystals	20 g
Lactic acid	20 ml
Glycerol	40 ml
Distilled water	20 ml

Dissolve the ingredients by heating the container in a hot water bath. Add 0.05 g of cotton blue (Poirrier's blue).

Methylene blue phosphate stain for malaria

Methylene blue, medicinal	1 g
Disodium phosphate, anhydrous	3 g
Monopotassium phosphate, anhydrous	1 g

All of these are thoroughly mixed in a dry mortar, and 1-g quantities are placed in well-stoppered vials. For use, 1 g is dissolved in 250 to 350 ml of distilled water. Filter if necessary.

Spore stain (Wirtz-Conklin)

Flood the entire slide with 5% aqueous malachite green. Steam for 3 to 6 min, and rinse under running tap water. Counterstain with 0.5% aqueous safranine for 30 s. Spores are seen as green spherules in red-stained rods or with red-stained debris.

Sudan black B fat stain (4)

Sudan black B	0.3 g
Ethyl alcohol, 70%	100.0 ml

Shake the solution thoroughly at intervals during the day and allow it to stand overnight before use.

Staining procedure. Dry and fix the smear with heat. Stain the slide with Sudan black for 10 min, drain, and blot dry. Wash and clear the smear with xylol. Counterstain with 0.5% aqueous solution of safranine for 10 to 15 s. Wash in tap water; blot dry. The cells stain red; the highly refractile poly-β-hydroxybutyrate granules are blue-black.

Trichrome technique for staining intestinal protozoa

In many instances, permanently stained preparations of the fecal specimen must be made for the diagnosis of protozoan infections. Such preparations facilitate detection and identification of cysts and trophozoites and afford a permanent record of the organism encountered. Small organisms which are missed by other examinations may be found on stained films. The trichrome technique of Wheatley (29) is a rapid and simple procedure of staining intestinal protozoa for routine diagnostic work. It is not necessary to mordant before staining. The stain solution is stable and may be used repeatedly, the lost volume being replaced by adding stock solution. Staining over 15 smears daily (in 50 ml of stain), however, tends to weaken the stain. If the stain is allowed to stand and evaporate in open air for 3 to 8 h, its strength will return.

The staining of fresh and PVA-fixed material differs chiefly in that the latter requires increased time, and, since the material in the PVA solution is already fixed, the fixative step is omitted.

Preparation of solutions

1. *Fixative (Schaudinn's solution)*

Ethyl alcohol, 95%	1 part
Mercuric chloride, saturated aqueous (approx. 14 g/100 ml of water)	2 parts

Before use, add 5 ml of glacial acetic acid to 100 ml of solution.

2. *Iodine alcohol*

Prepare a stock solution by adding enough iodine crystals to 70% alcohol to make a dark, concentrated solution. For use, dilute some of the stock with 70% alcohol until a port-wine-colored solution is obtained. The exact concentration of this solution is not important.

3. *Trichrome stain*

Chromotrope 2R	0.60 g
Light green SF	0.15 g
Fast green FCF	0.15 g
Phosphotungstic acid	0.70 g
Acetic acid, glacial	1.00 ml
Distilled water	100.00 ml

Good stain is purple in color and is obtained by adding 1 ml of glacial acetic acid to dry components of stain. This mixture is allowed to stand ripening for 15 to 30 min; then 100 ml of distilled water is added.

4. *Destaining solution*

Acid alcohol

Acetic acid	0.45 ml
Ethyl alcohol, 90%	99.55 ml

5. *Carbol-xylene*

Add 1 volume of carbolic acid (phenol) to 3 volumes of xylene. Phenol crystals can be liquefied in a water bath.

Preparation of the smear for staining

From fresh specimens. Using an applicator stick, make a thin smear of the fecal sample on a clean 7.6 by 2.5 cm slide. If necessary, dilute feces with physiological saline. Immerse slide immediately into Schaudinn's fixative (solution 1). The smear must not be permitted to dry from the time it is made until it is mounted. *This is very important.* If the staining schedule must be interrupted, slides may be stored for long periods in the last 70% alcohol (step before staining).

From specimens preserved in PVA fixative. With an applicator stick, 2 or 3 drops of the preserved specimen are spread (not smeared) over approximately one-third of the surface of a microscope slide. The films are allowed to dry thoroughly, either overnight in a 37 C incubator or at room temperature. It is important that the films dry thoroughly to prevent the material from washing off the slide during staining.

Staining procedure with fresh specimens

1. Schaudinn's fixative (solution 1): 5 min at 50 C, 1 h at room temperature.
2. Alcohol (70%) plus iodine (solution 2): 3 min.
3. Alcohol 70% (1): 3 min.
4. Alcohol 70% (2): 3 min.
5. Stain, trichrome (solution 3): 2 to 8 min.
6. Alcohol, 90%, acidified (1 drop of glacial acetic acid in 10 ml of alcohol; solution 4): 10 to 20 s or until stain barely runs from smear. Prolonged destaining in 90% alcohol (over 20 s) may differentiate organisms poorly, although larger trophozoites, particularly those of *E. coli*, may require slightly longer periods of decolorization.
7. Alcohol, 95 or 100%: rinse twice.
8. Alcohol, 100%, or carbol-xylene (solution 5): 3 min.
9. Xylene: 3 min or until refraction at smear-xylene interface ends.
10. Mount with cover slip using Permount, balsam, or other mounting media.

Staining procedure with PVA films

1. Alcohol, 70%, plus iodine (solution 2): 10 to 20 min.
2. Alcohol, 70% (1): 3 to 5 min.
3. Alcohol, 70% (2): 3 to 5 min.
4. Stain, trichrome (solution 3): 6 to 8 min.
5. Alcohol, 90%, acidified (1 drop of glacial acetic acid in 10 ml of alcohol; solution 4): 10 to 20 s or until stain barely runs from smear.
6. Alcohol, 95% (1): rinse.
7. Alcohol, 95% (2): 5 min.
8. Carbol-xylene (solution 5): 5 to 10 min.
9. Xylene: 10 min.
10. Mount with cover slip using Permount, balsam, or other mounting media.

Stain reactions (trichrome)

The cytoplasm of thoroughly fixed and well-stained cysts and trophozoites is blue-green tinged with purple. Occasionally, *E. coli* cysts may stain slightly more purplish than cysts of other species. The nuclear chromatin, chromatoid bodies, and ingested red cells and bacteria stain red or purplish red. Other ingested particles, such as yeasts or molds, usually stain green, but variations frequently occur in the color reaction of ingested particles. Background material usually stains green, and a color contrast with the protozoa results. In contrast with hematoxylin-stained preparations, trichrome smears have a transparency which makes it possible to identify embedded protozoa, even in thicker smears. Protozoa and eggs are less subject to distortion, however, in thinner smears. Eggs and larvae usually stain red and contrast strongly with green background. Thin-shelled eggs often collapse when placed in mounting medium, although if the smear is examined immediately, they may retain some diagnostic features.

Nonstaining cysts and those staining predominantly red are most frequently associated with incomplete fixation. Obtaining unsatisfactorily stained organisms from specimens submitted in PVA fixative usually indicates incomplete fixation associated with poor emulsification. Thorough emulsification of preferably *soft* stools will yield critically stained cysts and trophozoites. Degenerate forms stain pale green. Organisms may also appear green if understained or overdestained.

Mononuclear and polymorphonuclear leukocytes as well as *Blastocystis* present the same diagnostic problems with this technique as with the technique using hematoxylin. The cytoplasm of pus and tissue cells, however, does stain more greenish than that of the protozoa.

Smears should be examined with an oil immersion lens. Occasionally, large protozoa may be detected with the lower power (10×) objective, and smaller forms, with high dry lenses. Details are more distinct, however, with oil immersion. A 43× or 44× oil immersion objective is useful in examining the smears.

Truant's Auramine-Rhodamine stain for mycobacteria (28)

Solutions

A. *Fluorescent dyes*

Auramine O Cl 41000	1.50 g
Rhodamine B Cl 749	0.75 g
Glycerol	75.00 ml
Phenol	10.00 ml
Distilled water	50.00 ml

Combine dyes with phenol and 25 ml of water and mix well. Add the remainder of the water and the glycerol, and mix well with a magnetic stirrer, if desired. Clarify by filtration through glass wool. The solution may be stored for several months at 4 C or at room temperature.

B. *Decolorizer*

Acid alcohol, 0.5% HCl in 70% ethyl alcohol.

C. "*Counterstain*"

Potassium permanganate, 0.5% aqueous solution.

Staining procedure

1. Prepare smears and fix with heat.
2. Stain for 15 min at room temperature or at 37 C.
3. Rinse off with distilled water.
4. Decolorize for 2 to 3 min; then rinse thoroughly with distilled water.
5. Flood smear with counterstain for *2 to 4 min*. Longer exposure results in loss of brilliance. The precise function of the "counterstain" is not completely understood but it renders tissue and its debris nonfluorescent, thus reducing the possiblity of artifacts.
6. Rinse, dry, and examine.

Wayson's stain

Solution A

Basic fuchsin (90% dye content)	0.20 g
Methylene blue (90% dye content)	0.75 g
Ethyl alcohol, 95%	20.00 ml

Solution B

Phenol, 5%	200.00 ml

Pour solution A slowly into solution B, and filter.

Staining procedure. Stain smears for 10 to 20 sec. Wash with water and blot dry. The stain is especially useful for demonstrating polar staining.

Wright's stain for malaria

Use certified liquid or prepare as below.

Wright's stain, powdered	0.30 g
Glycerol, neutral, chemically pure	3.00 ml
Methyl alcohol, absolute, acetone-free	97.00 ml

Grind powder in a mortar. Add glycerol and grind thoroughly. Add methyl alcohol and mix. Let stand overnight in tightly stoppered container. Filter. Age for a few days before use. Store in a dark colored bottle. *See* chapter 67 for procedure.

Ziehl-Neelsen acid-fast stain for actinomycetes in tissues (20)

Carbol-fuchsin solution

Phenol crystals, melted	2.5 ml
Alcohol, 95%	5.0 ml
Basic fuchsin	0.5 g
Distilled water	50.0 ml

Dissolve fuchsin in alcohol, add phenol and water, and let stand overnight. Filter through paper and then through filter candle to remove any acid-fast bacilli. Store at room temperature, and filter before use.

Acid alcohol, 3%

Hydrochloric acid, concentrated	3.0 ml
Alcohol, 70%	99.0 ml

Working methylene blue solution

Methylene blue chloride	0.5 g
Glacial acetic acid	0.5 ml
Distilled water	100.0 ml

Shake and filter twice.

Staining procedure. Any well-fixed tissue may be used. Cut sections at 4 to 6 μm. Deparaffinize sections through two changes of xylene and run through absolute and 95% alcohols to distilled water as usual. Remove mercury precipitates through iodine and hypo solutions, if necessary. Stain with freshly filtered carbol fuchsin for 10 min. Rinse well in tap water. Decolorize with 3% acid alcohol until sections are pale pink. Wash thoroughly with running tap water for 8 min. Counterstain by dipping one slide at a time in working methylene blue solution for 15 to 30 s. Sections should be pale blue. Overstaining will mask bacilli. Wash with tap water and distilled water. Dehydrate with two changes of 95% alcohol and absolute alcohol; clear with two or three changes of xylene and mount in Permount. Acid-fast actinomycetes are bright red; erythrocytes are yellowish orange, and other tissue elements are pale blue.

Ziehl-Neelsen stain modified, for staining brucella

Stock carbol fuchsin

Basic fuchsin	1 g
Methyl alcohol, absolute	10 ml
add to	
Phenol, 5%	90 ml

Staining procedure. Stain for 10 min with a 1:10 dilution of stock carbol fuchsin. Wash in tap water. Decolorize with 0.5% acetic acid for 20 to 30 s. Wash thoroughly. Counterstain with 1% methylene blue. Wash and blot dry. *Brucella* stain red against a blue background.

Ziehl-Neelsen stain for mycobacteria

Carbol fuchsin stain

Basic fuchsin	0.3 g
Ethyl alcohol, 95%	10.0 ml
Phenol, melted crystals	5.0 ml
Distilled water	95.0 ml

Dissolve the basic fuchsin in the alcohol; the phenol in the water. Mix the two solutions. Let stand for several days before use.

Acid alcohol

Ethyl alcohol, 95%	97 ml
Hydrochloric acid, concentrated	3 ml

Methylene blue counterstain

Methylene blue	0.3 g
Distilled water	100.0 ml

Staining procedure. Flood entire slide with carbol-fuchsin and heat slowly to steaming point. Use low or intermittent heat to maintain steaming for 3 to 5 min. Cool. Wash briefly with tap water and decolorize until no more stain comes off. Wash with tap water and counterstain for 20 to 30 s. Wash, dry, and examine. Acid-fast organisms are red; the background and non-acid-fast organisms are blue.

LITERATURE CITED

1. Bartholomew, J. W. 1962. Variables influencing results, and the precise definition of steps in gram staining as a means of standardizing the results obtained. Stain Technol. **37**:139–155.
2. Bridges, R. F. 1951. The dysentery reference laboratory. Brit. Med. Bull. **7**:200–203.
3. Brooke, M. M., and M. Goldman. 1949. Polyvinyl alcohol-fixative as a preservative and adhesive for protozoa in dysenteric stools and other liquid materials. J. Lab. Clin. Med. **34**:1554–1560.
4. Burdon, K. L. 1946. Fatty material in bacteria and fungi revealed by staining dried, fixed slide preparations. J. Bacteriol. **52**:665–678.
5. Coblentz, L. M. 1943. Rapid detection of the production of acetyl-methyl-carbinol. Amer. J. Pub. Health. **33**:815–817.
6. Dobell, C., and F. W. O'Connor. 1921. Intestinal protozoa of man. William Wood, New York.
7. Ewing, W. H., and J. G. Johnson. 1960. The differentiation of *Aeromonas* and C27 cultures from *Enterobacteriaceae*. Int. Bull. Bacteriol. Nomencl. Taxon. **10**:223.
8. Faust, E. C., J. S. D'Antoni, V. Odum, M. J. Miller, C. Peres, W. Sawitz, L. F. Thomen, J. E. Tobie, and J. H. Walker. 1938. A critical study of clinical laboratory technics for the diagnosis of protozoan cysts and helminth eggs in feces. Amer. J. Trop. Med. **18**:169–183.
9. Freedman, L., S. E. Maddison, and R. Elsdon-Dew. 1958. Moxenic cultures of *Entamoeba histolytica* derived from human liver abscesses. S. Afr. J. Med. Sci. **23**:9–12.
10. Gaby, W. L., and C. Hadley. 1957. Practical laboratory test for the identification of *Pseudomonas aeruginosa*. J. Bacteriol. **74**:356–358.
11. Gadebusch, H. H., and S. Gabriel. 1956. Modified stable Kovac's reagent for the detection of indole. Amer. J. Clin. Pathol. **26**:1373–1375.
12. Gleason, N. N., and G. R. Healy. 1965. Modification and evaluation of Kohn's one-step staining technique for intestinal protozoa in feces or tissue. Amer. J. Clin. Pathol. **43**:494–496.
13. Hugh, R. 1965. A comparison of the proposed neotype strain and 258 isolates of *Vibrio cholerae* Pacini. Int. Bull. Bacteriol. Nomencl. Taxon. **15**:13–24.
14. Kohn, J. 1960. A one stage permanent staining method for fecal protozoa. Dapim. Rafuiim Med. Quart. Israel **19**:160–161.
15. Leifson, E. 1951. Staining, shape, and arrangement of bacterial flagella. J. Bacteriol. **62**:377–389.
16. Leifson, E. 1960. Atlas of bacterial flagellation. Academic Press Inc., New York.
17. Levine, M., S. S. Epstein, and R. H. Vaughn. 1934. Differential reactions in the colon group of bacteria. Amer. J. Pub. Health **24**:505.

18. Lillie, R. D. 1954. Histopathologic technic and practical histochemistry. The Blakiston Co., Inc., New York.
19. Lubin, A. H., and W. H. Ewing. 1964. Studies on beta-D-galactosidase activities of *Enterobacteriaceae*. Pub. Health Lab. **22**:84–97.
20. Mallory, F. B. 1942. Pathological technique, p. 75. W. B. Saunders Co., Philadelphia.
21. Moore, H. B., and M. J. Pickett. 1960. The *Pseudomonas-Achromobacter* group. Can. J. Microbiol. **6**:35–42.
22. Nair, C. P. 1953. Rapid staining of intestinal amoebae on wet mounts. Nature (London) **172**:1051.
23. Norman, L., and M. M. Brooke. 1955. The effectiveness of the PVA-fixative technique in revealing intestinal amebae in diagnostic cultures. Amer. J. Trop. Med. Hyg. **4**:479–482.
24. Ritchie, L. S. 1948. An ether sedimentation technique for routine stool examinations. Bull. U.S. Army Med. Dep. **8**:326.
25. Shepard, M. C. 1973. Differential methods for identification of T-mycoplasmas based on demonstration of urease. J. Infect. Dis. **127**:S22–S25.
26. Smith, M. R., R. E. Gordon, and F. E. Clark. 1952. Aerobic sporeforming bacteria. U.S. Dep. Agr. Monograph No. 16.
27. Steel, K. J. 1961. The oxidase reaction as a taxonomic tool. J. Gen. Microbiol. **25**:297–306.
28. Truant, J. P., W. A. Brett, and W. Thomas, Jr. 1962. Fluorescence microscopy of tubercle bacilli stained with auramine and rhodamine. Henry Ford Hosp. Med. Bull. **10**:287–296.
29. Wheatley, W. B. 1951. A rapid staining procedure of intestinal amoebae and flagellates. Amer. J. Clin. Pathol. **21**:990–991.
30. Wolf, H. W., L. B. Hall, P. Skaliy, M. M. Harris, H. M. Decker, C. M. Dahlgren, and L. M. Buchanan. 1959. Sampling microbiological aerosols. Pub. Health Serv. Monograph 60.

AUTHOR INDEX

SUBJECT INDEX